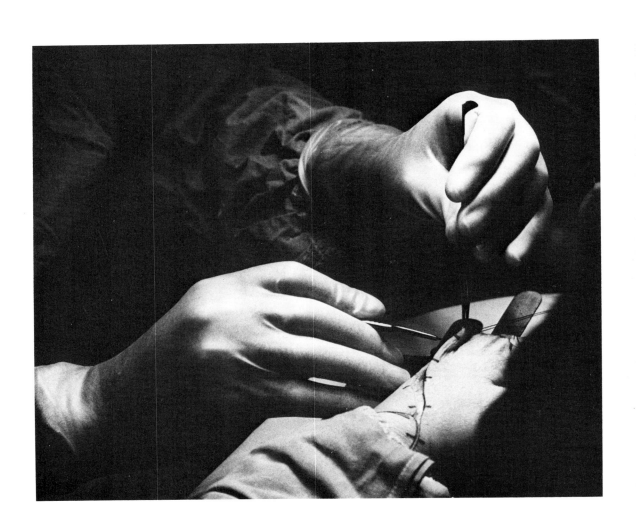

The HAND

Volume III

Edited by

RAOUL TUBIANA, M.D.

Director of the Hand Institute (Paris)
Associate Professor of the Cochin Faculty of Medicine
Attending Surgeon of the American Hospital of Paris
Former President of the International Federation of
  Societies for Surgery of the Hand

1988

W. B. SAUNDERS COMPANY
Harcourt Brace Jovanovich, Inc.

Philadelphia•London•Toronto•Montreal•Sydney•Tokyo

W. B. SAUNDERS COMPANY
Harcourt Brace Jovanovich, Inc.

The Curtis Center
Independence Square West
Philadelphia, PA 19106

Library of Congress Cataloging in Publication Data

(Revised for Volume 3)
Main entry under title:

The Hand.

Includes bibliographical references and index.
1. Hand—Surgery. 2. Hand. I. Tubiana, Raoul.
   [DNLM: 1. Hand.   WE 830 H2306 1981]

RD559.H357   617'.575059   80-27141

ISBN 0–7216–8907–8 (v. 1)
ISBN 0–7216–8908–6 (v. 2)
ISBN 0–7216–8909–4 (v. 3)

Editor: Albert E. Meier
Designer: Karen O'Keefe
Production Manager: Frank Polizzano
Manuscript Editor: Kate Mason
Illustration Coordinator: Peg Shaw
Indexer: W. B. Saunders Staff

Front cover illustration: Rembrandt's *The Anatomy Lesson* (detail). Courtesy Mauritshuis Museum, The Hague, Netherlands.

The Hand

ISBN 0–7216–8909–4

Last digit is the print number: 9   8   7   6   5   4   3   2   1

CONTRIBUTORS

WALTER MANNA ALBERTONI, M.D.

Professor, Paulista School of Medicine, São Paulo

YVES ALLIEU, M.D.

Professor of Orthopaedic Surgery, University of Montpellier, Chief of Orthopaedic and Hand Surgery Services, University Hospital Center, Montpellier.

JEAN-YVES ALNOT, M.D.

Professor of Orthopedic Surgery, Hand Surgery Unit, Bichat Hospital, Paris.

PHILIPPE AMEND, M.D.

Resident in Surgery, University Hospital Center, Nancy.

GÉRARD ASENCIO, M.D.

Assistant Orthopaedic Surgeon, Saint Charles Hospital, Montpellier.

PIERRE BALDET, M.D.

Assistant Professor of Anatomy, Faculty of Medicine, Montpellier; Biologist, Anatomic Pathology Service, Guy de Chauliac Hospital Center, Montpellier.

JACQUES BAUDET, M.D.

Professor of Surgery, Hand Plastic and Reconstructive Surgery Service, Saint Andre Hospital, Bordeaux.

SERGE BAUX, M.D.

Professor of Orthopedic and Reconstructive Surgery, Rothschild Hospital, Paris.

CORINNE BECKER, M.D.

Brussels.

HILTON BECKER, M.D., F.R.C.S.

Consultant Plastic Surgeon, Good Samaritan Hospital, West Palm Beach; West Boca Medical Center, Boca Raton.

PAOLO BEDESCHI, M.D.

Professor of Orthopaedic Surgery, University of Modena.

JACQUES BERES, M.D.

Surgeon, University of Paris Hospitals.

ALFRED BERGER, M.D.

Professor and Director of the Clinic for Plastic and Reconstructive Surgery of the Hand, Eastern City Hospital, Hannover.

CONRADO C. BONDOC, M.D.

Assistant Professor of Surgery, Harvard Medical School, Associate Visiting Surgeon, Massachusetts General Hospital and Shriners Burn Institute, Boston.

FRANÇOIS BONNEL, M.D.

Professor of Anatomy, Department of Orthopedics and Traumatology, University of Montpellier.

JOHN A. BOSWICK, JR., M.D.

Attending Surgeon, St. Joseph's Hospital, Rose Medical Center, and Veterans Administration Hospital, Denver.

F. M. BRAUN, M.D.

Nancy.

DONAL M. BROOKS, M.A., F.R.C.S.

Lately Consultant in Charge, Peripheral Nerve Injury Unit, Royal National Orthopaedic Hospital, Consultant Orthopaedic Surgeon, King Edward VII Hospital For Officers, London.

GIORGIO BRUNELLI, M.D.

Professor of Orthopedic Surgery, University of Brescia.

UELI BÜCHLER, M.D.

Chief of Hand Surgery, Inselspital, Berne.

DIETER BUCK-GRAMCKO, M.D.

Professor of Hand Surgery and Plastic Surgery, University of Hamburg, Chief of Hand Surgery and Plastic Surgery, Accident Hospital, Consultant Hand Surgeon, Children's Hospital, Hamburg.

HARRY J. BUNCKE, M.D.

Clinical Professor of Plastic Surgery, University of California School of Medicine, San Francisco; Assistant Clinical Professor of Surgery, Stanford University Medical Center, Palo Alto; Chief, Replantation-Transplantation Service, Ralph K. Davies Medical Center, San Francisco.

JOHN F. BURKE, M.D.

Helen Andrus Benedict Professor of Surgery, Harvard Medical School, Chief, Trauma Services, and Visiting Surgeon, Massachusetts General Hospital, Boston.

TI-SHENG CHANG, M.D.

Professor of Plastic and Reconstructive Surgery, Shanghai Second Medical University, Advisor of Ninth People's Hospital of Shanghai Second Medical University.

JEAN-JACQUES COMTET, M.D.

Professor of Surgery, Claude Bernard University, Chief, Emergency Orthopaedic Service, Edouard Herriot Hospital, Lyon.

RICHARD T. D'ALONZO, M.D.

Assistant Clinical Professor, Thomas Jefferson University, Philadelphia; Senior Attending, Wilmington Medical Center and St. Francis Hospital, Wilmington.

WILSON DE MOURA, M.D.

Hand Institute, Balneario, Brazil.

CLAUDE DUFOURMENTEL, M.D.

Professor of Surgery, University of Paris, Honorary Surgeon, University of Paris Hospitals.

JERRY L. ELLSTEIN, M.D.

Assistant Professor of Clinical Orthopaedics, Division of Hand Surgery, State University of New York at Stony Brook; Attending Hand and Orthopaedic Surgeon, Huntington Hospital; Attending Hand Surgeon, Northport Veterans Administration Hospital, Northport.

JOEL ENGEL, M.D.

Professor of Orthopedic Surgery, Sackler School of Medicine, Tel-Aviv University; Director of Hand Surgery Service, Chaim Sheba Medical Center, Tel-Hashomer.

P. ESTEVE, M.D.

Paris.

MARIUS FAHRER, M.D., F.R.A.C.S.

Director (Senior Specialist in Charge), Central Development Unit—Prostheses Orthoses, Department of Veterans' Affairs, Melbourne.

GUY FOUCHER, M.D.

Director of the Emergency Hand Service, Clinique de l'Orangerie, Strasbourg.

C. FRANCHESCHI, M.D.

Radiology Service, Saint Joseph Hospital, Paris.

ABRAHAM GANEL, M.D.

Senior Lecturer, Orthopedic Surgery, Sackler School of Medicine, Tel-Aviv University; Staff, Department of Orthopedic Surgery, Chaim Sheba Medical Center, Tel-Hashomer.

ALAIN GILBERT, M.D.

Surgeon, Hand Institute, Paris.

TIMOTHY GILL, M.D.

Clinical Assistant Professor of Orthopedic Surgery, University of South Dakota, Chief of Orthopedics, Rapid City Regional Hospital, Rapid City, South Dakota.

JULIEN GLICENSTEIN, M.D.

Surgeon, The American Hospital, Paris.

STANLEY GORDON, M.D.

Professor of Orthopedic Surgery and Chief of Division of Orthopedic Surgery, State University of New York, Downstate Medical Center, Brooklyn.

JOHN A. I. GROSSMAN, M.D.

Assistant Professor of Surgery (Plastic Surgery), Brown University Program in Medicine, Attending Plastic Surgeon, Rhode Island Hospital, Chief, Plastic Surgery, Veterans Administration Medical Center, Providence.

ROBERT W. HARRIS, M.Sc., F.R.C.S.(C)

Cornwall, Ontario.

JOHN A. E. HOBBY, F.R.C.S.

Consultant Plastic Surgeon, Wessex Centre for Reconstructive and Maxillofacial Surgery, Odstock Hospital, Salisbury.

JOHN T. HUESTON, M.D., M.S., F.R.A.C.S., F.R.C.S. (E)

Consultant Plastic Surgeon, Royal Melbourne Hospital, Victoria.

JAMES M. HUNTER, M.D.

Professor of Orthopaedic Surgery, Jefferson Medical College of Thomas Jefferson University, Chief, Hand Surgery Service, Department of Orthopaedic Surgery, Thomas Jefferson University Hospital, Philadelphia.

SCOTT H. JAEGER, M.D.

Clinical Instructor, Department of Orthopaedic Surgery, Jefferson Medical College of Thomas Jefferson University, Philadelphia.

JESSE B. JUPITER, M.D.

Assistant Professor of Orthopedic Surgery, Harvard Medical School, Assistant Orthopedic Surgeon, Massachusetts General Hospital, Boston.

ADALBERT I. KAPANDJI, M.D.

Orthopedic Surgeon, Yvette Clinic, Longjumeau.

HAROLD E. KLEINERT, M.D.

Clinical Professor of Surgery, University of Louisville School of Medicine and Indiana University–Purdue University School of Medicine.

†JAMES ELLSWORTH LAING, F.R.C.S.

Late Senior Consultant Plastic Surgeon, Wessex Centre for Plastic and Reconstructive Surgery, Odstock Hospital, Salisbury.

CAROLINE LECLERCQ, M.D.

Surgeon, Hand Institute, Paris.

LARRY G. LEONARD, M.D., F.A.C.S.

Associate Professor (Clinical), Division of Plastic Surgery, University of Utah School of Medicine, Active Staff, Latter Day Saints Hospital, Holy Cross Hospital, Primary Children's Hospital, St. Mark's Hospital, Salt Lake City.

CLAUDE LE QUANG, M.D.

Surgeon, Saint Joseph Hospital, Paris.

DOMINIQUE LE VIET, M.D.

Attending Surgeon, Boucicaut Hospital, Paris.

W. LITTLER, M.D.

Professor of Clinical Surgery, College of Physicians and Surgeons of Columbia University, Attending Surgeon, Roosevelt Hospital, New York.

†Deceased.

GÖRAN LUNDBORG, M.D.

Hand Surgical Unit, Department of Orthopaedic Surgery I, Sahlgren Hospital, Göteborg.

EVELYN J. MACKIN, L.P.T.

Director of Hand Therapy, Hand Rehabilitation Center, Ltd., Philadelphia.

MICHINOBU MAEDA, M.D.

Instructor of Orthopaedic Surgery, Shinshu University School of Medicine, Surgeon, Shinshu University Hospital, Matsumoto.

ALAIN MASQUELET, M.D.

Surgeon, Hand Institute, Paris.

TAKESHI MATSUI, M.D.

Associate Professor of Orthopaedic Surgery, Shinshu University School of Medicine, Associate Director, Department of Orthopedic Surgery, Shinshu University Hospital, Matsumoto.

PHILLIP MATTHEWS, F.R.C.S., F.R.C.S. (E)

Senior Lecturer, Welsh National School of Medicine, Consultant Orthopaedic Surgeon, West Glamorgan Health Authority, Consultant in Hand Surgery, Neath General and Port Talbot Hospitals.

P. MAURER, M.D.

Professor of Orthopedic Surgery, Cochin Hospital, Paris.

PETER MCMENIMAN, M.D.

Brisbane.

JEAN-PIERRE MELKI, M.D.

Radiologist, Neuroradiology and Therapeutic Angiography Service, Lariboisière Hospital, Paris.

JEAN-JACQUES MERLAND, M.D.

Associate Professor of Radiology, Neuroradiology and Therapeutic Angiography Service, Lariboisière Hospital, Paris.

MICHEL MERLE, M.D.

Associate Professor of Surgery, Nancy Faculty of Medicine, Surgeon, University Hospital Center, Nancy.

VIKTOR E. MEYER, M.D.

Attending Surgeon, Reconstructive Surgery Service, University Hospital, Zürich.

JACQUES MICHON, M.D.

Professor of Orthopaedic Surgery, Nancy Faculty of Medicine, Chief of Plastic and Reconstructive Surgery of the Hand, University Hospital Center, Nancy.

LEE W. MILFORD, JR., M.D.

Professor of Orthopedic Surgery, University of Tennessee, Medical Staff Director, Baptist Memorial Hospital, Chief of Staff, Campbell Clinic, Memphis.

HANNO MILLESI, M.D.

Head, Department of Plastic and Reconstructive Surgery, Director, First Surgical Clinic, University of Vienna Medical School.

JEAN-CLAUDE MIRA, D.SC.

Senior Lecturer, René Descartes University, Paris.

VLADIMIR MITZ, M.D.

Attending Surgeon, Boucicaut Hospital, Paris.

EZIO MORELLI, M.D.

First Department of Plastic Surgery of the Hand, Legnano City Hospital, Milano.

WAYNE A. MORRISON, M.B., F.R.A.C.S.

Associate, Department of Surgery, University of Melbourne, Assistant Plastic Surgeon and Deputy Director, Microsurgery Research Unit, St. Vincent's Hospital, Melbourne.

ALGIMANTAS O. NARAKAS, M.D.

Associate Professor of Surgery, University of Lausanne, Surgeon, University Hospital Center, Lausanne.

GEORGE E. OMER, JR., M.D., M.S., F.A.C.S.

Professor of Orthopaedic Surgery and Chairman, Department of Orthopaedics and Rehabilitation, School of Medicine, University of New Mexico, Chief of Staff, University of New Mexico Hospital, Acting Medical Director, Carrie Tingley Hospital for Crippled Children, Albuquerque.

E. PANEVA-HOLEVICH, M.D.

Professor of Orthopaedics and Traumatology, Academy of Medicine, Sofia.

RODGER D. POWELL, M.D.

Gainesville, Florida.

SARAH PRI-CHEN, M.SC.

Director, Microsurgery Laboratory, Chaim Sheba Medical Center, Tel-Hashomer.

†ROBERT GUY PULVERTAFT, M.D., M.CHIR., F.R.C.S.

WILLIAM C. QUINBY, JR., M.D.

Associate Clinical Professor, Surgery, Emeritus, Harvard Medical School, Associate Visiting Surgeon, Massachusetts General Hospital, Boston.

PIER LUIGI RAIMONDI, M.D.

Staff, Legnano City Hospital, Milano.

JEAN-PIERRE RAZEMON, M.D.

Associate Professor of Surgery, University of Lille, Surgeon, Haubourdin Hospital, Lille.

DANIEL REIZINE, M.D.

Resident in Radiology, Neuroradiology and Therapeutic Angiography Service, Lariboisière Hospital, Paris.

---

†Deceased.

MARIE-CLAIRE RICHE, M.D.

Neuroradiology and Therapeutic Angiography Service, Lariboisière Hospital, Paris.

SARAH RIMON, PH.D.

Head, Department of Biochemistry, and Senior Lecturer in Biochemistry, G. S. Weiss Faculty of Life Sciences, Tel-Aviv University.

JACQUES ROULLET, M.D.

Consultant Surgeon, Lyon.

MAURICE ROUSSO, M.D.

Senior Lecturer in Orthopedics, Hebrew University, Chief of the Hand Surgery Unit, Department of Orthopedics, Hadassah Mount Scopus University Hospital, Jerusalem.

JEAN-CLAUDE ROUZAUD

Physical Therapist, Saint Charles Hospital, Montpellier.

P. SAFFAR, M.D.

Surgeon, Hand Institute, Paris.

RICARDO SALAZAR LOPEZ, M.D.

Hand Institute, Bogota, Colombia.

BRUCE SCHLAFLY, M.D.

St. Louis.

LAURENT SEDEL, M.D.

Associate Professor of Surgery, University of Paris VII, Surgeon, Department of Orthopedics and Traumatology, Saint Louis Hospital, Paris.

YEHESKELL SHEMESH, M.D.

Instructor in Physical Medicine and Rehabilitation, Sackler School of Medicine, Tel-Aviv University; Staff, Department of Neurologic Rehabilitation, Chaim Sheba Medical Center, Tel-Hashomer.

JOHN SIEBERT, M.D.

Plastic Surgery Resident, New York University Hospital.

DANIEL I. SINGER, M.D.

Assistant Professor of Orthopedic Surgery, Jefferson Medical College, Attending Surgeon, Hand Surgery Service, Department of Orthopedic Surgery, Thomas Jefferson University Hospital, Philadelphia.

CLIFFORD C. SNYDER, B.S., M.D., F.A.C.S.

Professor and Chairman Emeritus, Division of Plastic Surgery, University of Utah School of Medicine, Attending Staff, University of Utah Medical Center, Chief, Plastic Surgery, Shriners Hospital for Crippled Children, Salt Lake City.

JAMES B. STEICHEN, M.D.

Clinical Associate Professor of Orthopaedic Surgery, Indiana University School of Medicine, Indianapolis.

JAMES W. STRICKLAND, M.D.

Clinical Professor of Orthopedic Surgery, Indiana University School of Medicine, Chief, Hand Surgery Section, St. Vincent Hospital and Health Care Center, Indianapolis.

SYDNEY SUNDERLAND, M.D., B.S., D.Sc., F.R.A.C.P., F.R.A.C.S.(Hon.)

Professor Emeritus of Experimental Neurology, University of Melbourne, Consultant, Royal Melbourne, Alfred and Prince Henry's Hospitals, Melbourne.

JULIA K. TERZIS, M.D., PH.D.

Director, Microsurgical Research Center, and Associate Professor, Department of Plastic Surgery, Eastern Virginia Medical School, Norfolk.

GUY TRENGOVE-JONES, M.D., F.R.C.S., F.R.C.S.(E)

Assistant Professor of Orthopedic Surgery, Eastern Virginia Medical School, Norfolk.

MAURICE TUBIANA, M.D.

Director, Gustave Roussy Institute, Villejuif.

RAOUL TUBIANA, M.D.

Director, Hand Institute, Associate Professor, Cochin Faculty of Medicine, Attending Surgeon, The American Hospital of Paris.

FREDERICK A. VALAURI, M.D.

Clinical Instructor, Department of Plastic and Reconstructive Surgery, New York University–Bellevue Medical Center, Attending Surgeon, Department of Plastic Surgery, Hand Surgery Service and Microsurgery Service, Bellevue Hospital, New York.

CLAUDE E. VERDAN, M.D.

Professor of Surgery, University of Lausanne, Chief of Surgical Service, University Hospital Center, Lausanne.

L. VIDAL, M.D.

Bayonne.

EDWARD R. WEBER, M.D.

Associate Professor of Orthopedic Surgery and Head, Section of Hand Surgery, University of Arkansas College of Medicine, Little Rock.

MENACHEM RON WEXLER, M.D.

Associate Professor of Plastic Surgery, Hebrew University Medical School, Head, Department of Plastic Surgery, Hadassah University Hospital, Jerusalem.

C. B. WYNN PARRY, M.B.E., D.M., F.R.C.S.

Director of Rehabilitation and Consultant Rheumatologist, Royal National Orthopaedic Hospital, Stanmore.

BATIA YAFFE, M.D.

Lecturer in Hand Surgery, Sackler School of Medicine, Tel-Aviv University; Director of Microsurgery Service, Chaim Sheba Medical Center, Tel-Hashomer.

PREFACE

The third volume of *The Hand* addresses several subjects of considerable practical interest, such as traumatic lesions of tendons, nerves, and blood vessels and burns and mutilations. Each of these subjects is analyzed from different perspectives by several authors, thus providing the reader with a more complete view of the subject.

Some of these chapters are synthesized to bring about a more general understanding.

The first section is on extensor and flexor tendon repairs of the hand, which have benefited in the last decade from considerable progress in surgical techniques. This progress is related to a better understanding of physiology and the biologic process of tendon repair as well as to improvements in surgical methods and postoperative follow-up.

Peripheral nerve repair poses problems of great complexity. Research with practical applications has been done in the last few years in three major directions, including measures to improve coaptation and orientation of divided nerves, measures to limit proliferation of injury, and measures to bridge the gap between injured nerves of the extremities. Epineural, perineural, interfascicular, and mixed suture repairs have individual indications that have become progressively more accurate according to the nerve and the lesion levels. Although the use of thin interfascicular nerve grafts has made incontestable progress over that of thick truncal nerve grafts, the actual tendency is for primary immediate microscopic nerve suture repair for management of vascular lesions.

The occurrence of brachial plexus lesions has multiplied with the increased number of two-wheel vehicle accidents. The essential clinical problem of these lesions depends on the lesion level, their distribution, and the nature of the nerve injury. It is a difficult diagnosis to make clinically and often requires surgical exploration, which permits early nerve repair. The results of primary suturing, grafts, neurolysis, and nerve transfers are analyzed by the surgeons with the greatest experience in these fields.

To this section on nerves is added a chapter on clinical examination of the paralyzed limb, including the testing protocols for all the muscles of the upper limb.

Burns of the hand can be treated in diverse ways according to (1) the extent of the area of the burn, (2) the age of the patient, and (3) the center of treatment, e.g., a specialized burn institution.

In cases of war catastrophes, a large number of burn victims demand simple and economic methods of treatment that are adapted to mass treatment and also to the conditions of developing countries.

Last, the section on mutilation describes the multiple varieties from fingertip to limb amputations. Emergency reimplantation and late reconstruction are both discussed, and the respective indications for numerous techniques are elaborated. A procedure must not be used because it is technically possible but because it is best adapted to the patient's particular need. The use of microsurgery, which has been a great advance in the treatment of mutilations, does not exclude conventional techniques of reconstructive surgery. The desirable association of traditional and modern techniques often increases the efficacy of both. Numerous examples of hand reconstruction demonstrate this point.

RAOUL TUBIANA

CONTENTS

PART THREE—SURGERY OF VESSELS

PART FOUR—SPECIAL INJURIES

Section 1 Burns

Part One

SURGERY OF TENDONS

INTRODUCTION

Raoul Tubiana

Tendon injuries in the hand are extremely frequent, and in an organ whose main attribute is its mobility they are an important cause of functional incapacity. Tendon repairs, regarded for so long as minor surgical procedures, are in fact complex procedures with many problems that have not been resolved.

This part of the book is divided into two sections. The first deals with methods of repair and the second with the applications of these repairs to specific injuries.

The first portion includes the history of treatment of tendon injuries in the hand and anatomical, pathological, and biological considerations complimentary to those discussed by Peacock in Volume I. The general principles of treatment are also discussed.

The second section includes discussions of traumatic injuries of extensor and flexor tendons. Tendon transfers in cases of paralysis are considered with nerve lesions, and the tendon lesions commonly seen in rheumatoid arthritis are discussed in the section on that disease in Volume IV.

SURGICAL TECHNIQUES

Chapter 1

HISTORICAL SURVEY OF THE TREATMENT OF TENDON LESIONS IN THE HAND

Raoul Tubiana

Lesions of the tendons in the hand have long been considered together with tendon lesions elsewhere in the body. Only in the early part of this century was it realized that because of their greater excursion repair of the flexor tendons of the hand required special reconstructive techniques in order to preserve their gliding function. A better understanding of the mechanism of extension of the fingers, which has led to more physiological methods of repair, is also a relatively recent advance.

Although surgery of the tendons is not new, the repair of tendon lesions in the hand has not yet been precisely defined. The results are still unpredictable in many cases. The frequency of tendon lesions and the difficulty in their repair explain the interest they provoke, and the advances in their treatment have largely paralleled the development of hand surgery.

As early as the tenth century, Avicenna (980–1037) of Boukhara, in Persia, advocated surgical suturing of tendons, but this practice did not reach the West until much later. This delay was due primarily to Galen (130–201), who, having mistaken the tendons for nerves, stated that interfering with these structures could only result in pain and convulsions. Owing to medical conformism, this erroneous teaching was passed on through the centuries until the eighteenth century when Galen's dogma was officially refuted at the Sorbonne. However, adventurous surgeons such as Guy de Chauliac in France, Roger in Parma, Italy, and others had performed tenorrhaphies as early as the thirteenth century; this subject was mentioned by Ambroise Paré (1510–1590).

In the seventeenth century Bienaise in Paris, and later Dionis, performed numerous tendon repairs in the hand. In his *Surgical Lecture* (of which there is a contemporary English translation [1710]) Dionis gave a detailed description of three suturing techniques and reported Bienaise's experimental tendon sutures in the dog. In 1770 Missia, another French surgeon, transplanted an extensor tendon of the index finger to repair an extensor of the middle finger. According to Waterman (1902), this was the original attempt at tendon transfer. Tenotomies were performed mainly to correct deformities of the feet by Lorenz (1789), Sartorius (1806), and Strohmeyer (1831) in Germany and by Delpech (1816) in Montpellier.

3

The mechanism and treatment of clubfoot by means of tenotomies were fashionable surgical topics in Paris in the early nineteenth century. Among the best known publications are those by Velpeau (1839), Malgaigne (1841), and Bouvier (1838). Later Nicoladoni (1880) in Germany applied tendon transfers to the treatment of paralysis.

The progress of tendon surgery was hampered by the risks of infection and adhesions and the lack of basic knowledge about the repair of tendons. The works of Albrecht von Haller (1752) in Germany on the sensibility and irritability of various tissues demonstrated the insensibility of tendons and finally led to the discrediting of Galen's theories.

Duchenne de Boulogne in France (1867) was the first to give an accurate account of the action of each muscle, particularly those in the hand, but his work was long ignored by surgeons. Codovilla (1889) in Bologna studied the prevention of adhesion formations following tendon transfers and described the role of tendon sheaths in making possible the gliding of transferred tendons.

The introduction of tendon grafts represented a huge step forward in tendon surgery. The exact date of the first attempt is not known for certain but probably lies near the end of the nineteenth century. The exact dating has been made more difficult by the confusion surrounding the term transplant, which should be used only to describe a graft, although it is frequently and inaccurately used (even today) to signify a transfer.

In 1882 Heuck, a German surgeon, removed a segment of the extensor pollicis longus while attempting its repair; the segment of tendon was replaced as a free graft. In 1886, at the Surgical Society of Paris, Peyrot reported a case of "transplantation in man of the tendon of a dog" to replace the flexor tendons of a middle finger "which had been destroyed"; this resulted in "good healing with partial functional recovery." One year later (1887) Monod reported at a meeting of the same society a case in which a 5 cm. tendon graft taken from the Achilles tendon of a rabbit was successfully used to repair the extensor pollicis longus. Robson (1888) took a tendon from an injured digit to fashion an extensor graft on the same hand.

The beginning of the twentieth century saw extensive clinical and experimental work being done, especially in Germany, by Lange (1900), Kirschner (1909), Rehn (1910), and more particularly by Biesalski (1910) of Berlin. The latter reconsidered the problem of adhesions and the action of tension on sutures, and his work had a profound influence on his contemporaries. In 1912 Lexer, of Iena, published the results in the first series of 10 autografts of flexor tendons. However, it was in the United States that tendon surgery saw the greatest advance.

In 1911 Lewis and Davis made an experimental study of direct tendon and fascial transplant. Leo Mayer, who had worked in Lange's department in Munich, in 1912 published a number of works, including three articles (1916) on "The Physiological Method of Tendon Transplantation." In these he described the anatomy and physiology of the peritendinous structures and mentioned the necessity for a precise surgical technique, which he called the "physiological method." He also stressed the importance of insuring the correct tension in the transfer and the necessity for preserving the gliding planes, and he recommended that the surgeon himself supervise the postoperative care and resumption of movements.

While the clinical applications of Mayer's work were directed more toward the foot and the ankle joint, Bunnell in San Francisco turned his interest increasingly toward surgery of the hand. Between the time of his first article on tendon repair in the fingers, published in 1918, and his masterly book, *Surgery of the Hand*, whose first edition was in 1944, he formulated the principles that now form the basis of tendon surgery. Such surgery respects the mechanisms of tendon gliding and the pulley system and attempts to prevent the scar fibrosis and stiffness that may follow infection and surgical trauma. It was he who emphasized the importance of atraumatic surgical technique, the use of nonreactive suture material, its removal by means of a pullout wire, and the position for immobilization of joints.

With the work of Bunnell and his school, surgical technique took a giant leap forward. Yet this was still inadequate to solve the major surgical problem in flexor tendon repair, namely, primary healing with subsequent recovery of an adequate range of movement.

Atraumatic techniques represent a vital

step toward obtaining good results in tendon surgery, but they are in fact a "negative" step in that they consist mainly in the elimination of iatrogenic lesions. It becomes evident that "biological" methods must succeed the simply "anatomical or mechanical" ones in order to bring about a significant advance in this form of surgery. This is why in the section of research in Volume I we have allowed ample space for Peacock's work on tendon healing.

In this volume, which deals mainly with treatment, we frequently refer to Peacock's chapters, and we advise the reader to become familiar with these concepts before studying this section. Recent works on the nutrition of tendons having repercussions on techniques for repair will be discussed here.

Chapter 2

GENERAL ORGANIZATION OF THE TENDON (INTRATENDINOUS STRUCTURE)

FRANÇOIS BONNEL
AND PIERRE BALDET

Lying as it does between muscle and bone, a tendon acts primarily as mechanical transmitter, but it also serves to regulate muscular contraction. Accordingly the tendon is structurally programmed to fulfill these functions, which are especially delicate in such a multifunctional and precise organ as the hand.

The tendon is incompressible, can glide, and is inextensible, flexible, and mechanically resistant, a set of properties making it particularly well adapted to its function as a transmitter. In addition, its diversified internal structure provides a degree of elasticity and resistance intermediate between those of bone and muscle.

Unlike many other structures that are fixed, the tendon must move silently and efficiently in spite of friction. For this purpose it is fitted with a synovial sheath in the flexion zones. Because of its precarious blood supply, it is highly vulnerable to trauma. Through its rich and complex nerve supply it helps to regulate the force of a movement.

The tendinous continuation of a muscle is the essential element in the relationship. Tendons are classified into two main groups—the uniarticular tendon, which crosses a single joint, and a biarticular or multiarticular tendon, which crosses two or more joints.

Uniarticular muscles are sufficiently long and extensible to enable a joint to extend and flex fully. Multiarticular muscles, by contrast, are not perfectly adapted to all the combined movements possible at the joints. Thus, if the wrist is in full palmar flexion, full flexion of the fingers is painful. We are left wondering therefore why two types of muscles are necessary and why one of them is ill adapted.

The fingers have a wide range of mobility. If only uniarticular muscles were used, the extensor digitorum and flexor digitorum would lie very close to their phalangeal insertions. Such distal positioning of the muscles would significantly increase the weight of the hand and the mechanical work needed, which would be incompatible with good function. For these reasons the muscle masses are situated higher up the limb and are connected to the extremities by lengthy tendons.

THE BODY OF THE TENDON

Tendons are cylindrical or flattened fibrous cords connecting the muscles to the skeleton. In man, tendons are of the composite type, i.e., made up by the association of several tendinous fibers, or fascicles, separated by connective tissue septa of the first and second orders. The whole organ is enclosed within a connective tissue envelope or paratenon.

Microscopic examination of a fascicle reveals thick collagen fibers that run parallel to the lines of force of the tendon. These bundles have a uniform caliber that varies from muscle to muscle. They are separated by flat longitudinal cells with a dense, sometimes linear, nucleus. These cells, which tend to form regular alignments, are reminiscent of specialized fibroblasts. Orcein staining also shows the presence of a few elastic fibers scattered among the collagen fibers and running parallel to them.

Ultrastructural examination of the tendon cells shows an intracellular organization identical to that of fibroblasts. The nucleus is round or oval and has a large nucleolus. The cytoplasm contains an abundant endoplasmic reticulum, which is sometimes dilated, and a well developed Golgi apparatus. Also visible are numerous microfilaments arranged in bundles. The plasma membrane is irregular, is raised by microvacuoles, and is in close contact with the collagen fibrils of the extracellular environment. Like all connective tissue cells, the tendinocyte can manufacture the four great families of macromolecules found in the intercellular matrix—proteoglycans, structural glycoproteins, elastin, and especially collagen.

Proteoglycans are complexes of proteins and long chains of acid mucopolysaccharides. In the tendon, the most common are dermatan sulfates and the 4- and 6-chondroitin sulfates. After impregnation with phosphotungstic acid or ruthenium red, proteoglycans appear as a scanty, osmiophilic, granular material that bathes the collagen fibers.

Structural glycoproteins form microfibrillary aggregates, which are clearly visible with electron microscopy. They are present in tendons, especially in elastin structures, but in small amounts in relation to other connective tissues.

Elastin is manufactured from subunits, known as tropoelastin, synthesized by fibroblasts. By a process of reticulation (aggregation and lateral bridging) elastin forms elastic sheets and fibers. This process is carried out in close collaboration with the microfibrils of structural glycoproteins, which act as guides to elastogenesis. Human tendon contains relatively few elastic fibers. These have a characteristic infrastructure: they are made up of a homogeneous amorphous substance that can be electron dense or transparent according to the degree of maturation of the fiber. The elastin fraction is crossed by microfibrils, which also form denser central areas and a peripheral network and consist of structural glycoproteins.

Collagen remains the basic component of tendons. This fibrous protein is made up of three peptide chains, called alpha chains, which are coiled into a triple helix. Collagen synthesis starts in the fibroblast with a nuclear phase where the structural genes are translated into mRNA (Fig. 2–1).

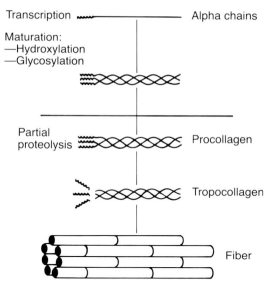

Figure 2–1. Collagen synthesis.

The transcription of mRNA onto the polysomes of the endoplasmic reticulum results in the separate synthesis of the polypeptide chains, which differ with regard to the nature of the amino acids and their sequence in the molecule. There are four $\alpha 1$-chains (known as $\alpha 1^I$, $\alpha 1^{II}$, $\alpha 1^{III}$, and $\alpha 1^{IV}$) and one $\alpha 2$-chain. Recently, two new chains, known as αA and αB, have been isolated in the collagen of the basal membranes.

These chains undergo a series of so-called post-transcriptional maturation reactions and recombine to form the triple helices of procollagen, which in turn form into different genotypes depending on the mode of combination (Table 2–1). Tendon collagen, which belongs to genotype 1, results from the combination of two 1-chains and one 2-chain.

After partial proteolysis, procollagen appears in the extracellular spaces in the form of elementary units of tropocollagen. By a process of end to end and lateral bridging, the latter gives rise to microfibrils and then to fibers, which on electron microscopy show a characteristic longitudinal periodicity of 640 to 650 Å. Tendon collagen of type I consists of thick fibers of a more variable diameter than type III collagen, which is more homogeneous and occurs in the walls of the larger vessels and in dermal collagen.

Histological examination of a tendon under 125 per cent tension shows elongated cells and gently undulating fibers. A tension of 150 per cent straightens the collagen fibers

Table 2–1. STRUCTURE AND DISTRIBUTION OF THE VARIOUS TYPES OF COLLAGEN

Type	Composition of the Triple Helix		Organ
I	$(\alpha 1^I)2$	$\alpha 2$	Tendon, skin, bone
II	$(\alpha 1^{II})3$		Embryonic cartilage
III	$(\alpha 1^{III})3$		Aorta, skin
IV	$(\alpha 1^{IV})3$		
V	$(\alpha A(\alpha B))2$		Basal membranes

and brings them into close contact with the elastin fibers (Fig. 2–2).

STRUCTURAL VARIATIONS

During the aging process the secretion of macromolecules of the intercellular matrix undergoes various qualitative and quantitative changes that in turn lead to structural modifications. This phenomenon, about which little is known as yet, is of considerable surgical importance because it determines the possibilities of repair.

Working on the rabbit, Ippolito et al. studied the histological and biochemical changes that occur during maturation and aging of the tendon. In the newborn animal the tendon cells are relatively numerous and arranged in chains. On transverse sections they seem to be interconnected by fine cytoplasmic projections, which outline collagen bundles of the first order. They show all the signs of synthetic activity with, in particular, a well developed endoplasmic reticulum. The intercellular substance is made up of loose fine collagen fibers that are constant in size that are no larger than 550 Å. The elastic fibers are slender and always lie close to the tendinocytes. Finally, as in all growing tissue, there is a rich capillary network.

As early as the age of two months, structural changes are discernible. The cell to matrix ratio tends to diminish, suggesting cellular regression and increased synthesis of intercellular material. The capillaries thus seem less abundant. The tendinocytes are larger, often with a distended endoplasmic reticulum and longer cytoplasmic expansions. The collagen fibers condense, and their diameter becomes more variable, some becoming much bulkier (in the newborn reaching a size of 1660 Å). The elastic fibers are more numerous and their structure is more clearly defined. This development is accompanied by an increase in collagenic material. By contrast, the polysaccharide content is reduced, and this reduction becomes more marked with age.

In the four year old rabbit the cellular depletion becomes more obvious and areas of necrosis start to develop. The tendinocytes may appear to be retracted and their nuclei almost fill the cytoplasm, suggesting that intracellular synthetic activity is on the ebb. Extracellular collagen increases further and some fibers now have a diameter of up to 200 Å. There is a progressive laying down of an insoluble, highly polymerized collagen, a characteristic feature of aging in connective tissue. There is a simultaneous reduction in the elastic network, which may disappear altogether. Indeed elastic fibers are not renewed after the stage of young adulthood, and in the older animal the elastic tissue content decreases progressively with a markedly reduced repair potential. Finally biochemical studies confirm the presence of water and mucopolysaccharides observed in the younger animal.

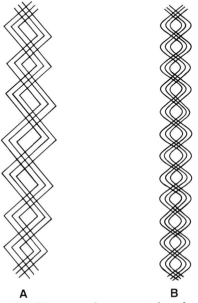

A   **B**

Figure 2–2. Diagrammatic representation of a tendon at rest (*A*) and under tension (*B*).

These changes explain the clinical observation that with advancing age the tendons become less supple and more fragile and heal more slowly. The local conditions then favor metaplastic changes—calcification and bony and cartilaginous metaplasia.

JUNCTIONAL ZONES

At one extremity the tendon is continuous with the muscle; at the other it is inserted onto a bone or cartilage. At the muscular insertion the tendon fibers splay out and become continuous with the aponeurotic sheath and the fibrous intramuscular septa. At a cartilaginous insertion the fibers of the tendon enter the perichondrium, from which they become inseparable, and disappear into the basic substance. This produces an intermediate fibrocartilaginous zone.

Most tendons, however, are inserted onto a bone. The peripheral fibers mingle with the fibers of the periosteum, which disappears around the tendon insertion. The central (Sharpey's) fibers penetrate the cortex and become lost within the bone.

Microscopic studies of these junctions have thrown some light on the ultrastructure of these junctions. Continuous with the tendon proper is a strip of fibrocartilage within which the collagen fibers continue their course. The tendon cells undergo changes at this level: they become spherical, form into groups of two or three cells, and become surrounded with an extracellular matrix that keeps them separate from the collagen fibers, an arrangement commonly found in cartilage. The cells have a well developed endoplasmic reticulum, a Golgi apparatus, and a lysozomal system. The plasma membrane sends out fine extracellular expansions, and dense vesicles appear in the cytoplasm. The overall picture is that of active chondrocytes.

The deep portion of the fibrocartilage, which lies close to the bone, becomes calcified. This zone, which is 100 to 300 microns thick, is clearly demarcated from the nonmineralized part by a basophilic horizontal blue line, also known as the tide mark or cement line.

The collagen fibers continue their course, and the cellular pattern is the same as for the nonmineralized zone. Some of the fibers, however, show signs of nuclear and cytoplasmic degeneration. Within the intercellular substance can be seen needle shaped crystals of hydroxyapatite, which lie neatly between the collagen fibers. These calcific deposits are particularly abundant in the deeper part of the calcified zone, concealing the connective tissue fibers. Beyond the calcified fibrocartilage can be seen the first lamellae of cortical bone, tendon collagen mingling with the collagen of the matrix.

The "progression" of the different histological layers results in a more harmonious transmission of the forces between the muscle, with its low Young modulus, and bone, which has an elastic modulus of 1800.

THE TENOSYNOVIAL SHEATH

For most of its course the tendon runs within a synovial sheath, which facilitates its gliding. The sheath is made up of two sheets—an internal one, which is applied to the tendon itself, and an external one, which is continuous with the surrounding connective tissue. The two synovial layers become continuous at each extremity, forming a cavity whose blind ends fold and unfold during flexion and extension.

At certain points along its course, the sheath is not completely wrapped around the tendon, which thus retains direct connections with the adjacent connective tissue (mesotenon) through a fibrous tract, or mesotenon. The latter is inserted on the body of the tendon along a longitudinal line, or hilum, from which fibers are given off that splay out on the surface of the tendon to form the epitenon. Some fibers of the mesotenon penetrate the tendon itself and mingle with the primary and secondary internal septa. The mesotenon forms a pathway for the blood vessels, lymphatics, and nerves supplying the tendon. It also limits the mobility of the tendon within its sheath.

Histologically the tendon sheaths are very similar to the synovial sheaths. The inner aspect of each sheet is lined by one layer of cubical or endothelioform mesenchymal cells. These are similar to the synoviocytes and lie on a very vascular connective tissue of variable density.

In some parts of the tendon, and especially under the joint capsules, small cushions of fatty tissue can be seen between the two sheets (Jaffe).

The space between the two synovial layers contains a small amount of substance identical to synovial fluid and secreted by the cells lining the space. At the blind ends the layer gives off fringes or tufts, which appear to increase the surface area for the production or absorption of tenosynovial fluid.

NERVE SUPPLY

The tendon, with its rich supply of nerve endings, can be regarded as a tensiometer involved in the regulation of muscle contraction. It was Golgi who in 1880 first described in detail the "terminal musculotendinous nerve organs."

In the lumbrical muscles the neurotendinous organs lie at the musculotendinous junction. They vary widely in size: according to Rabischong (1961), their length ranges from 840 to 2892 microns and their width from 34 to 164 microns. The muscle spindles are made up of several encapsulated tendon fascicles, the unit being some 10 to 25 microns wide. Its nerve supply comes from a Ib sensory nerve, which gives off four ramifications: type I, large myelinated fibers from the Ib afferent nerve; type II, unmyelinated fibers lined by Schwann cells and by a basal membrane; type III, unmyelinated fibers lined by either a single layer of Schwann cells or a basal membrane; and type IV, simple bare unmyelinated fibers coming into direct contact with the spindle fibers.

On the surface and in the body of the tendon can be found Golgi-Mazzoni corpuscles, 200 to 540 microns long and 20 to 58 microns wide. These respond to lateral pressure.

The distribution of nerve endings is different from flexor and for extensor tendons. In the flexors the nerve fibers are more numerous at the joints, the most common endings being the Vater-Pacini corpuscles (Becton, 1966). The flexor tendons, both superficial and deep, receive their nerve supply through the vincula, and the nerve endings are located close to them.

REFERENCE

Rabischong, P.: Recherches sur la morphologie et la distribution des organes neuro-tendineux et des récepteurs encapsulés intra-musculaire et épitendineux des muscles lombricaux humains. C. R. Ass. Arch. Anat., 44:327–349, 1961.

Chapter 3

TENDON LESIONS: ANATOMICAL, PATHOLOGICAL, AND BIOLOGICAL CONSIDERATIONS

RAOUL TUBIANA

The treatment of tendon lesions in the hand requires a knowledge of anatomy, biomechanics, physiology, and biology. The basic facts have been discussed in the first volume of this work, but for the sake of clarity, we believe it appropriate at this stage to reconsider some of these facts, which are essential for a full understanding of the evolution of tendon surgery.

ANATOMICAL AND PATHOLOGICAL CONSIDERATIONS

A tendon transmits to the skeletal segment to which it is attached the movement produced by contraction of the muscle of which it is a continuation.

The tendon has an organized connective tissue structure. It consists of bundles of parallel collagen fibers separated by the connecting septa of the endotenon. The septa, which penetrate all the interstices of the tendon, carry the vessels and nerves. The tendon is surrounded by a thin connective envelope—the epitenon (or peritenon). Adult tendons, with their paucity of cellular elements, have low metabolic requirements, but healing after trauma considerably increases their needs.

The anatomy of the tendons of the fingers is illustrated schematically in Figures 3–1 and 3–2.

THE GLIDING APPARATUS

The straight segments of a tendon are surrounded by the paratenon, a thin layer of loose cellular tissue containing long elastic fibers, which lengthen during tendon movements. Thus the tendon does not glide through the paratenon; it only increases the tension within its elastic structures.

At the points where the course of a tendon deviates, the tendon is held down by a fibrous band or pulley (e.g., flexor and extensor retinacula and fibrous pulleys of the digits). Between the fibrous sheath and the tendon proper there is a synovial sheath that provides the true gliding surface. It is made up of a parietal and a visceral layer between which the delicate mesotenon transmits the vessels. The synovial sheaths are poorly developed on the extensor side, but on the flexor tendons five individual digital sheaths and three carpal sheaths (lateral, middle, and medial) are recognized. The lateral carpal sheath usually communicates with that of the thumb and the medial sheath with that of the little finger, thus forming the lateral and medial digitocarpal sheaths.*

TENDON LESIONS

In the hand, traumatic lesions are most common, although "dystrophic" lesions also form an important group. Neoplastic lesions are rare.

Although displacement or nodular thickening of the tendon poses specific problems,†

---

*The arrangement of the synovial sheaths is considered in detail in the section on anatomy in Volume I.

†See chapter on rheumatoid arthritis in Volume IV.

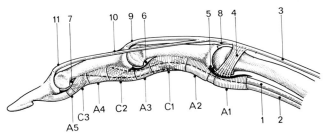

Figure 3–1. The extrinsic tendons of the fingers. In each finger, the superficial (1) and deep (2) tendons surrounded by their synovial sheath are closely applied to the phalanges by their fibrous sheath. These include five annular pulleys (A1, A2, A3, A4, A5) and three cruciform portions (C1, C2, C3) offering no resistance to joint flexion.

The extensor digitorum communis has five terminal insertions: the most proximal is made up by the sagittal bands (4), which insert to the volar plate (5) on each side of the metacarpophalangeal joint. The insertion at the base of the proximal phalanx is not constant. The insertion of the central (or middle) extensor tendon to the base of the middle phalanx (9) is the most important. Finally, the two lateral extensor tendons insert to the base of the distal phalanx.

1 = Flexor digitorum profundus; 2 = flexor digitorum superficialis; 3 = extensor digitorum communis; 4 = sagittal band inserting to the volar plate of the metacarpophalangeal joint; 5 = volar plate of the metacarpophalangeal joint; 6 = volar plate of the proximal interphalangeal joint; 7 = volar plate of the distal interphalangeal joint; 8 = insertion of the extensor digitorum communis to the base of the proximal phalanx (inconstant); 9 = insertion of the middle extensor tendon to the base of the distal phalanx; 10 = lateral extensor tendon; 11 = terminal extensor tendon inserting to the base of the distal phalanx; A1, A2, A3, A4, A5 = annular fibers of the fibrous sheath of the flexor tendons forming five pulleys; C1, C2, C3 = cruciform portions of the sheath of the flexor tendons.

lacerations, ruptures, and obstructive adhesions constitute the major part of tendon surgery for trauma surgeons.

Open Wounds

It is important to distinguish a clean division from a contused wound with a frayed tendon in which functional recovery is likely to be less complete. A tendon may be completely or partially severed, and a partial section may later become complete. These injuries demand special treatment.*

Because of muscle tone and the action of antagonists, the cut edges tend to pull apart but to different degrees. If the tendon is free, as is the case with intrasynovial tendons, retraction of the proximal segment may be considerable; this may be reduced by the

*See Chapter 38 on therapeutic indications.

presence of intertendinous anastomoses or resistant mesotenons. In the flexor tendons, the greater the flexion when the tendon is divided, the greater the retraction will be.

When a tendon is sectioned within a sheath, there is little tendency for it to regenerate. The retracted proximal segment becomes rounded and remains relatively free. Local trauma is responsible for the fibrous reaction around the tendon: the adhesions arise not from the extremity of the tendon but from the adjacent connective tissue.

In some cases the tendon becomes a dull yellow color and the extremities may even undergo lysis. This type of lesion occurs earlier in the proximal segment. Histological examination shows the loss of the parallel arrangement of the tendon fibers, with sparse, widely scattered nuclei, the whole tendon becoming a mass of scar tissue.

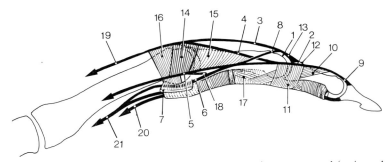

Figure 3–2. Diagrammatic view of the profile of a finger showing the insertions of the intrinsic and extrinsic muscles and the retinacular ligaments. There is a symmetry between the fibrous formations at the level of the metacarpophalangeal joint and the proximal interphalangeal joint. 1 = central or middle extensor tendon, 2 = lateral extensor tendon, 3 = central band of the long extensor, 4 = lateral band of the long extensor, 5 = interosseous tendon, 6 = lumbrical tendon, 7 = deep transverse intermetacarpal (or interglenoid) ligament, 8 = central band of the interosseous muscle, 9 = terminal extensor tendon, 10 = oblique retinacular ligament, 11 = transverse retinacular ligament, 12 = triangular ligament, 13 = insertion of the extensor digitorum into the second phalanx, 14 = transverse fibers of the interosseous hoods, 15 = oblique fibers of the interosseous hoods, 16 = sagittal bands, 17 = fibrous sheath of the flexor tendons, 18 = insertion of the interosseous muscle on the base of the proximal phalanx, 19 = tendon of the extensor digitorum, 20 = superficial flexor tendon, 21 = deep flexor tendon.

The peritendinous gliding structures undergo the same type of degeneration. They become disorganized and form undifferentiated connective tissue which adheres to the tendon. That ischemia is an important factor in this degenerative process is suggested by the early advent of the lesions, their variability, and the fact that the bony and muscular insertions are partially or totally spared.

Infection of the divided tendon may occur unless correct treatment is begun as early as possible. If the infection is mild, the tendon becomes covered with granulation tissue, which forms adhesions by growing into the adjacent structures. If the infection persists, the tendon undergoes partial or total necrosis as the vascular structures are destroyed by the infection. Because of the poor blood supply, elimination of the necrosed segment is slow. The tissue debris, which behaves like a foreign body and encourages suppuration, must be removed.

It appears therefore that the tendon is a specialized yet fragile connective tissue that degenerates under trauma and undergoes scarring fibrosis. Surgical trauma may induce the same type of reaction; a clumsy initial repair may aggravate the original lesion and jeopardize later attempts at repair.

Apart from the tendinous injury proper, two factors affect the prognosis and treatment: the site of the tendon lesion and the nature of concomitant lesions. These considerations will be amplified subsequently.

Rupture

The term rupture implies a break in the continuity of the tendon in the absence of skin injury.

Ruptures in the hand are common. They tend to occur immediately after sudden, often violent trauma in young subjects, especially during ball games. Ruptures also occur in the aged as a result of minor trauma, e.g., while making the bed. Frequently the injury is quite old or untraceable and the rupture is then recorded as "spontaneous." We must mention here "occupational" ruptures such as those of the extensor pollicis longus following repetitive minor traumas in drummers, as well as those that occur after fractures of the wrist. In all such cases mechanical wear and the degenerative processes of ischemic origin must be kept in mind as potential contributing factors.

Pathological rupture remains a complex subject; thus tendon ruptures in rheumatoid arthritis have been attributed to ischemia, to synovial involvement (Vainio), and to erosion by bony spicules (Vaughan Jackson). Ruptures, unlike open injuries, have the advantage of asepsis, but the presence of a pathological or dystrophic process means that healing is likely to be slow and unpredictable.

HEALING IN TENDONS

To say that a good repair should be based on a sound knowledge of tendon healing might seem like a statement of the obvious, and yet until only a few years ago our knowledge of this subject was fragmentary and inaccurate.

Experimental work had indeed been done but mostly on extrasynovial animal tendons, so that the results could hardly be applied to the tendons of the human hand. In this context, Iselin appropriately quoted the remark of Lecenne: "Experimental study too often consists of extrapolating from the healthy animal to the diseased human."

Thus the long digital flexors with their excursion of up to 7 cm. have no laboratory animal equivalent. Also experimental conditions do not exactly reproduce the normal situation.

Surgical repair of such tendons should aim at producing a solid scar while reconstructing a good gliding plane, two apparently incompatible objectives. Connective tissue proliferation, which is the usual healing process in most wounds, tends to tether the mobile structures.

The two main questions asked are: How does a tendon heal, and how is the scar remodeled and gliding restored?

It is interesting to consider that with the progress made by increasingly sophisticated experimentation, claims and counterclaims for and against have been made in regard to the importance of the endotendinous cells in the healing process, the influence of the synovial sheath on nutrition, and the role of tension and immobilization on the solidity of repair.

We shall consider the constitution of the scar and the re-establishment of free gliding.

SCAR FORMATION

Healing in a tendon requires a nutritional supply that will support the connective tissue scar. This nutrition is supplied by blood vessels and lymphatics, and also in intrasynovial tendons by synovial fluid.*

Vascularization

A study of the blood supply of tendons, which had long been neglected, proved indispensable for understanding degeneration and healing in this tissue. Until the work of Kolliker (1850) and Sappey (1888), tendons had been regarded as avascular structures that derived their nutrition by imbibition of synovial fluid. Only very recently have surgeons been prepared to recognize the importance of vascularization in tendon repair, and that following the work of Mayer (1916), Edwards (1946), Braithwaite (1951), Skoog and Persson (1954), Brockis and Brockis (1953), Peacock (1959), Gambier et al. (1962), Smith (1965), Colville et al. (1969), Caplan et al. (1975), Lundborg (1975), and Matsui (1979).

Although the tendon in normal circumstances has a low metabolic rate, the reparative process considerably augments its nutritional needs. It can survive for some time by diffusion of gas and liquid, as shown by Peacock (1959), but its ultimate survival depends on the re-establishment of vascular connections with the surrounding tissues. A tendon deprived of vascularization degenerates and dies (Skoog and Persson, 1954).

The importance of the blood supply in tendon repair is now widely accepted. It has also been proved that vascularization of tendons is both intrinsic and extrinsic, from the muscular origin and bony insertion and from the paratenon and mesotenon. Smith and Conway (1966), using microdissection techniques, have shown that throughout the extent of the tendon, and not only at the level of the synovial sheaths, there exists a thin membrane, the mesotenon, which provides the tendon with arterial arcades similar in arrangement to those found in the intestinal mesentery.† In the digits the mesotenon condenses into vincula.

The distribution and importance of the vascularization vary with the anatomical site and the age of the subject (see the following chapters by Matsui and by Maeda). The vascularization of the cut ends of the tendon

is threatened not only by the initial trauma but also by the retraction of the proximal end, which tears the mesotenon. Surgical treatment produces supplementary vascular damage. In a following chapter we shall discuss the measures that must be taken to limit this damage.

The lymphatic circulation of tendons has been neglected for an even longer period than its vascularization, although it is relatively more abundant. It is described by Verdan and Setti in the first volume of this work.

The Role of Synovial Fluid

It was believed that the purpose of the fluid contained in the synovial sheaths was essentially to help the tendons to glide. It also plays a role in nutrition, insuring diffusion of metabolites (Potenza, 1964).

Eiken et al. (1975) and Lundborg and Rank (1978) observed healing of a cut rabbit tendon that had been placed within the synovial cavity of the knee joint.

The experimental work of Matthews and Richards (1974, 1976) led them to recommend suturing of the synovial sheath during primary repair of flexor tendons to provide better tendon nutrition and to prevent the formation of adhesions. Experimental work on animals implies a primary role for synovial nutrition, the blood supply being of relatively less importance (Manske et al., 1978).

Weber* noted the presence of intratendinous canaliculi through which the synovial fluid circulates. Movements of the flexor tendons in their tight digital sheath act as a pump mechanism to aid the diffusion of synovial fluid.

Since synovial fluid diffusion is believed to be the predominant source of nutrients (Lundborg, 1980; Manske, 1983) to the flexor tendons in zone II, closure of the digital sheath has been performed with increasing frequency after tendon repair. However, Katsumi et al. (1981) have shown that not only synovial fluid but also extracellular tissue fluid is capable of nourishing flexor tendons. In a recent study, Peterson, Manske, and Lesker (1986) confirmed this view. The nutrient pathways to the flexor tendons in zone II do not appear to be affected by varying degrees of sheath integrity. Although closure of the sheath after primary flexor tendon

---

*See Chapter 4, "The Nutrition of Flexor Tendons," by G. Lundborg.

†Smith reports the results of his studies on this topic in the first volume of this work.

---

*See Chapter 5.

repair does not appear to be necessary for tendon nutrition, "it is possible that sheath closure may affect tendon gliding. Additional studies to examine the effect of sheath integrity on tendon gliding should be carried out" (Peterson et al., 1986).

Tendon Healing

Experimental studies of tendon healing have given rise to different interpretations of the role of endotendinous and extratendinous cells in the process of healing. On the basis of his experimental studies, Schwarz (1922) concluded that intrinsic tendon cells do not play an active role in healing and stated that repair takes place from the peripheral tissues.

Mason and Shearon (1932) suggested that peripheral connective tissue proliferation was followed by proliferation of the tendon cells themselves: "The tendon itself takes an important part in healing, but because of its scanty blood supply and the very nature of its tissue, it begins its proliferation late. . . . This tardiness of tendon response is compensated, however, by the early response of the sheath."

Thus Lindsay and Thomson (1960) believed that all the tissues present in a tendon, and especially the least differentiated connective tissue cells of the endotenon and peritenon, take part in the healing process. Others, such as Iselin and Lafaury (1950), and Skoog and Persson (1954), believed that healing originated in the paratenon.

The work of Potenza, which started in 1962, appeared for a time to have received approval from most workers in the field. His results suggested that the tendon plays no part in the healing process and that the most important single factor is invasion by fibroblasts from outside the tendon.

Iselin and Lafaury (1950) had observed that no healing occurred at the site of a tendon suture where the sutured segment was wrapped in a polyethylene sheath. The same experiments were repeated by Gonzalez (1959) and Ashley et al. (1959, 1962) with a variety of materials. Potenza (1963) showed that when contact between a tendon and its sheath is prevented by means of an interposed impermeable membrane or by a millipore tube, tendon healing is delayed until granulation tissue has grown around the end of the tube and has reached the tendinous breach by creeping along the surface of the

tendon. Mittelmeier (1963) performed similar experiments using polyethylene tubes, which he slit to create a mesotenon.

It should be remembered that the wounds of the skin, subcutaneous tissue, tendons, and tendon sheaths are continuous and are subject to the same scarring process. This is the "one wound scar" concept, which Peacock has described. The scarring process in the tendon wound edges cannot be isolated from that which occurs in adjacent tissues. Wound repair is achieved by proliferation of fibrous tissue, of which collagen is the main constituent. Tissue differentiation occurs later. Collagen synthesis is a highly specialized process, which is accomplished by fibroblasts derived from parent cells that are normally found in the loose connective tissue lining the smaller blood vessels. Peacock believes that adult tendons and synovial sheaths are virtually free of fibroblasts. When a tendon is divided within an intact sheath, the retracted end does not hypertrophy. On the contrary, it atrophies, and the fibroblasts are mobilized from the loose connective tissue of adjacent structures, fibrous sheath, aponeurosis, ligaments, and periosteum when these have been injured. Every structure makes its contribution to the cicatrization in response to the insult it has itself sustained, either at the time of the tendon injury or following the superimposed surgical trauma. It then becomes connected to the tendon through adhesions, which carry the blood supply as well as the cells responsible for initiating the scarring process. This concept of tendon cicatrization has been summarized by Potenza (1975): "Flexor tendons are not healed by an intrinsic tenoblastic response of their own to injury but rather by the proliferative fibroblastic vascular reaction of surrounding tissues whose own integrity has been violated either by accidental injury or surgery."

When conditions are favorable, these adhesions may be remodeled and become sufficiently loose to allow tendon mobility.

Thus it was generally agreed that adhesions were inevitable during healing and that their formation provided "useful" nutritional and physiological pathways (Lindsay and Birch, 1964). This concept has been recently discussed by Matthews and Richards (1976). For them the absence of repair activity in the connective tissue cells of the tendon is difficult to accept. They believe that this observation reflects unfavorable conditions created by the experiment or by surgical repair. Their experiments show that when conditions are ideal (partial section of a rabbit's tendon without synovial excision, without suturing, and without immobilization), the tendon is capable, like any tissue, of repairing itself by the activity of its own connective tissue cells without the creation of adhesions. Surgical suturing is the principal factor in adhesion formation, but excision of the sheath and immobilization also contribute. The gap in the excised sheath is filled by undifferentiated scar tissue. Immobilization prevents the pump action of the flexor tendons in their enclosed sheaths, which impairs venous and lymphatic drainage. The circulatory stasis enhances edema and ischemia.

When the surgical trauma of repair is associated with sheath excision and immobilization, adhesions with neighboring structures predominate and intrinsic tendon activities tend to disappear. McDowell and Snyder (1977) have confirmed the studies of Matthews and Richards.

Surgical Trauma and Adhesions

Experience has shown that the results of surgical tendon repairs depend on surgical technique, and Potenza (1962) has shown quite convincingly that surgical trauma does induce the formation of adhesions.

In one series of experiments in which the tendons were either pricked with a needle or crushed with artery forceps, the number and extent of the adhesions were directly proportional to the severity of the trauma inflicted. An attempt was then made to determine the effect of surgical trauma to adjacent structures on the formation of adhesions.

In one group of dogs the tendon sheath around a scarred flexor profundus tendon was excised; the result was the same as in a series of equivalent cases when the sheath around the sutured tendon had been sutured. This suggested that the adhesions surrounding the tendon suture were gradually absorbed and that a new synovial sheath was formed that allowed the tendon to glide.

The author then studied the effect of removal of the flexor superficialis tendon on the healing of the flexor profundus. In one group of dogs the two bands of flexor superficialis were completely excised, while in a second group flexor superficialis was divided opposite the proximal phalanx, immediately

proximal to the vincula, thus preserving the blood supply to the tendon extremity. In the latter group, limited adhesions formed between the sheath and the tendon suture; none grew from the divided ends of the flexor superficialis tendon. But in the first group in which the flexor superficialis had been completely excised, extensive adhesions developed from the whole exposed surface of the bone, thus tethering the sutured flexor profundus.

Ischemia caused by tendon suture and excision of the synovial sheath create unfavorable nutritional conditions that are responsible for the absence of activity of tendon cells and the development of adhesions (Bergljung, 1968; Matthews and Richards, 1976).

It appears, therefore, that adhesion formation results not only from the initial injury but also secondarily from the surgical trauma, and that restoration of the gliding planes depends on the severity and nature of these adhesions.

Solidity of the Healing Scar

The experiments of Mason and Allen (1941) performed on the extensor carpi radialis longus and flexor carpi radialis in the dog showed that the resistance of a sutured tendon diminishes rapidly until the fifth day; this is the "lag time." After this time it increases slowly until the fifteenth day, when the resistance returns to what it was on the day of the suturing. The resistance of the healing scar then continues to increase progressively for six weeks. Studying the influence of mobilization on the formation of the scar, the authors noted that early mobilization may lead to rupture or induce gross hypertrophy. They concluded that a repaired tendon should be immobilized in a relaxed position for a minimum of 15 days and then mobilized with restriction over a period of three weeks.

The work of Lindsay, Thomson, and Walker (1960) on intrasynovial tendons (flexor tendons of chickens' legs) showed that a gap frequently persisted between the sutured tendon extremities, the diastasis resulting in scar hypertrophy, more numerous adhesions, disorientation of cellular architecture, and reduced gliding. Immobilization for only three weeks would appear to be insufficient and to result in most cases in diastasis at the suture site. This is due primarily to the traction exerted by the muscle proximally and can be prevented by sectioning, at a distance, of the tractor muscle or by a longer period of immobilization (more than four weeks).

These experiments refute the theory of the usefulness of traction on the arrangement of tendon architecture (Biesalski, 1910). However, Ketchum et al. (1977) stated that in the absence of tension or mobilization, the strength at the level of repair was weaker at the third week but increased rapidly thereafter.

All researchers admit the existence of a gap, which can reach a few millimeters between the two tendon ends during the first week following suturing. It seems obvious that the strength of repair would be stronger if the gap between the tendon ends were less significant and could be more quickly reduced. Many factors are responsible for this gap. Bergljung (1968) focused attention on the constricting effects of certain types of sutures on the microcirculation of the tendon ends, Ketchum (1977) stated that tension is probably the essential factor in disturbing the microcirculation.

Other factors also have an influence on the strength of the repaired tendon: suture technique, material used, and agents like β-amino proprionitrile (Peacock and Madden, 1969) or triamcinolone (Ketchum, 1971). It is probable that local conditions due to the trauma also have an influence, particularly the state of vascularization. Associated lesions of the neurovascular bundles definitely prejudice the quality of tendon repair. The state of the synovial sheath is also important.

RESTORATION OF GLIDING

The mobility of a repaired tendon requires the remodeling of newly formed scar tissue. Little is known concerning the factors that induce remodeling, and no explanation has yet been given as to why the scar between the tendon ends remains solid while the peritendinous scar tissue undergoes remodeling and allows movement of the tendon.

To understand these processes, we need a better knowledge of the mechanisms of synthesis, maturation, and breakdown of collagen. These questions have been the subject of numerous electron microscopic studies in the last decade, and we are just now reaching the stage of examining the factors that may influence this cycle. The ultimate aim is the local pharmacological control of collagen synthesis as well as the ability to influence its physical orientation and metabolism. This goal is not as idealistic as it may seem (Bora et al., 1972; Peacock and Madden, 1969).

Because adhesions are difficult to eliminate in the vicinity of sutures, it is important that the latter be placed away from bone and fibrous sheaths, which are fixed anatomical structures. This principle is in fact commonly applied by those who resect the sheath around the suture line, or again by using a tendon graft so that the optimal suture site can be chosen.

Resection of the Sheaths

This procedure is not without problems, both mechanical and biological. The mechanical function of the fibrous sheath is an important one, and we know that active flexion is significantly diminished if the pulleys are removed. Biomechanical studies by Caffinière (1972) and Brand (1975) have also shown that the rhythm and strength of flexion and lateral deviation of the fingers are grossly altered even by partial excision of the pulley.* Conservation and reconstruction of pulleys constitute an important operative step in tendon repair.†

From the biological point of view, the significance of excising the sheaths is still debated. Because the process of healing is initiated by peritendinous structures, some authors (e.g., Bloch and Bouvet, 1929) believed that the synovial sheath acts like a screen, which separates the tendon ends from the adjacent connective tissue. Because a repaired tendon increases in volume during the period of healing, it was thought advisable to perform a wide resection of the sheaths while preserving narrow pulleys.

On the other hand, experimental studies by Lindsay, Thomson, and Walker (1960) and by Potenza (1975) tend to show that the presence or partial removal of the synovial sheath (which "regrows" rapidly) makes little difference in the healing of a sutured tendon. In fact, a grossly damaged sheath does not behave like a true sheath, because it is soon

---

*See chapter on the physiology of finger flexion in Volume I.

†See Chapter 30, "Flexor Tendon Grafts in the Hand."

converted into a fibrous scar, which tends to promote local connective tissue reactions. If, however, trauma to the synovium is minimal, adhesion formation is limited because the intact sheath contains few, if any, cells capable of synthesizing collagen.*

Using tritiated thymidine as a radioactive label, Lindsay and Birch (1964) studied the origin and migration of fibroblasts during healing. They found that these cells travel along the adhesions that join the tendon to its synovial sheath, suggesting that the sheath does not take an active part in healing. It also confirms the view that adhesions between sheath and tendon result from the trauma, which allows granulation tissue to penetrate inside the synovial sheath.

When local conditions are favorable, some surgeons are tempted not to perform any resection of the sheath. Matthews and Richards (1976) advocated suture of the synovial sheath. Richards (1977) has published encouraging results in 275 cases of primary flexor tendon suturing in which this principle was applied.

Similarly, Eiken et al. (1980) reconstitute a synovial sheath before inserting a tendon graft. In a preliminary operation the scar tissue is excised, and the synovial sheath is reconstructed around a silicone rod by autografts of synovium taken from the great toe, the wrist, or occasionally the suprapatellar bursa. The tendon graft is inserted 10 to 12 weeks later. This separates the wound into two compartments, one containing the healing tendon graft and the other comprising the skin and subcutaneous tissues. The skin and surrounding tissue scar and the tendon scar are thus kept apart; the one-scar relationship is broken. The application of these principles has produced good results following tendon grafting—88 per cent good results in 48 grafts (Eiken et al., 1981).

Tendon Grafts

Tendon grafting is an ingenious attempt at solving the problems of tendon repair; it has been the subject of numerous publications which in turn have given rise to a variety of different methods.

We shall consider in turn the healing of autogenous grafts, the influence of the presence or absence of paratenon around the grafts, and the various sources of grafts.

Healing in Autogenous Grafts. The fate of the cells in the transplant is the subject of much controversy. According to some, the tendon cells die and the transplant is little more than a support along which regeneration occurs (Flynn and Graham, 1962; Iselin, 1955; Nageotte, 1926; Skoog and Persson, 1954). Others believe that the transplant survives (Mason and Allen, 1941; Peer, 1955). This view is supported by the work of Lindsay and McDougall (1961) and of Potenza (1964). But although the earlier authors talked of survival, healing, and regeneration in the transplant, Potenza noted that a flexor profundus graft showed little alteration when the sheaths and the flexor superficialis were intact. Adhesions were restricted to the immediate vicinity of the suture line. Poor results in flexor tendon grafts within the so-called "no man's land" may have been due largely to surgical trauma.

Effect of the Presence or Absence of Paratenon Around the Transplant. Some surgeons prefer a pad of adipose tissue around the transplant to facilitate gliding. But Potenza's studies (1964) on intrasynovial (flexor profundus tendon) and extrasynovial (with paratenon) transplants have shown that not only is paratenon not essential for survival of the transplant, but it even gives rise to more adhesions. This agrees with the observation of Peacock and van Winkle (1970) that the transplanted paratenon abounds in collagen synthesizing cells.

We may conclude therefore that the presence of paratenon around the graft is neither desirable nor necessary, the important factors being a healthy untraumatized transplant.

Allografts (Homologous Grafts) and Xenografts (Heterografts). As Cordrey, McCorkle, and Hilton (1963) have stated in their historical review, the possibility of using preserved grafting material has been considered for a long time. This would allow the creation of tendon banks and obviate the need for autogenous grafts. It is generally agreed, however, that the best results are obtained with autogenous grafts, and very few surgeons would use a nonautogenous transplant to replace a flexor tendon.

Other studies have concentrated on preservation methods such as freeze drying and chemical substances (Iselin et al., 1964), on the fate of allografts (Potenza, 1964), and on heterografts (Flynn and Graham, 1962).

---

*See Peacock's chapter on "Research in Tendon Healing" in Volume I (pp. 511–540).

For many years Iselin (1955) has advocated the use of acellular grafts preserved in a mercurial solution of Cialit, 1 in 5000 (1 gm. of Cialit powder in 5 liters of sterile water). These grafts are easy to handle and are immunologically less active than fresh grafts containing live cells. Seiffert and Schmidt (1971) have followed the life cycle of these grafts by radioactive labeling techniques (^{14}C proline) and have shown that the collagen is gradually replaced and that the allograft is repopulated in six to eight weeks.

In a series of experiments in dogs in which homologous freeze dried grafts were transplanted into the digital sheaths, Potenza showed that the graft is well tolerated and that its repopulation by the recipient's cells is not accompanied by adhesion formation in the sheath.

As Potenza has pointed out, the term "dead graft" is too often applied to allografts and heterografts, for although the cells themselves disappear, extracellular collagen remains. An important question is whether this collagen is denatured in the course of transplantation. If doubts persist concerning heterografts (Flynn and Graham, 1962), there is now ample evidence that tendon allografts are well tolerated.

Peacock has carried out a series of fascinating experiments on homologous transplantation of the whole flexor tendinous apparatus of the digits with a view to applying his methods to the human.* His basic premise is that adult tendons and their sheaths are devoid of cells capable of synthesizing collagen. If the tendon sheath could be taken intact with its contents, the scarring would proceed between the recipient's bed and the outside of the sheath and not between the inside of the sheath and the tendons. Animal experiments confirm this view and show that immunological reactions are of little significance.

This method has been used successfully in man by several surgeons (Hueston et al., 1967; Peacock and Madden, 1967). (Hueston describes this technique and its applications later in this section.) Although the taking of such grafts is a long and difficult procedure, which precludes their use for everyday practice, the possibility of preserving and banking freeze dried, composite homografts may well widen their application in selected cases.

Chacha (1974) has used composite autogenous grafts taken from the flexor apparatus of the toes (second toe), first in the monkey and then in man, with interesting functional results.

Reconstructing the Tendon Sheath

Another method for restoring gliding consists of creating a good quality permeable sheath. Attempts to use foreign material (glass or metal "sheaths") are not new (Mayer and Ransohoff, 1936), but for biological reasons they were doomed to failure because the presence of a foreign body excites collagen formation, which is the opposite of the function of a normal synovial sheath.

The introduction of substances that are almost inert, such as silicone, has induced some authors to reconsider the problem (Carroll and Basset, 1963; Hunter, 1965; Nicolle, 1969). A peculiar reaction follows the implantation of Silastic, a purified silicone for medical use. A smooth shiny membrane is formed, which remains mobile in relation to adjacent planes. When, two months later, the implant can be removed and replaced by a graft introduced through the extremity of the new sheath, the latter does form some loose adhesions with its new sheath, but a double gliding plane exists around the tendon and around the sheath itself. Hunter's study now comprises several hundred cases, and the results, which he discusses in Chapter 32, are encouraging. Seiffert and Schmidt (1971) have also transplanted an allograft to a bed prepared by a silicone implant.

REFERENCES

The references for this chapter can be found at the end of Chapter 8.

---

*See Chapter 52 on Research in Tendon Healing by Peacock in Volume I.

Chapter 4

THE NUTRITION OF FLEXOR TENDONS*

Göran Lundborg

The special problems associated with trauma to the flexor tendon structures within the synovial sheath regions of the hand are well known to every hand surgeon. Numerous methods for surgical repair of tendon injuries in this region have been suggested, but no matter what method is used, the results are still often unpredictable and disappointing. The reason for this may theoretically be based on cellular as well as nutritional factors:

1. The tenocytes—according to the classic concept—may lack the potential for repair. If so, we might face a biological problem without a solution, consitituted by a requirement for extrinsic cellular support to achieve tendon healing. Adhesions would then be essential and would make impossible the restoration of the delicate gliding mechanisms and the considerable amplitude in motion of tendons normally seen in this highly differentiated region. However, because an increasing number of reports during recent years have indicated that the tenocytes really do possess an intrinsic potential for repair (Furlow, 1976; Gelberman et al., 1984; Lindsay and Thomson, 1960; Lundborg, 1976, 1977; Lundborg et al., 1985; Manske and Lester, 1984; Manske et al., 1985; Matthews and Richards, 1974, 1976; McDowell and Snyder, 1977), this proposed explanation appears less attractive than the alternative.

2. The injury and the surgical intervention may deprive the tendon of its normal nutrition, leaving the tendon ends more or less devitalized. If so, one could not expect healing based upon tenocyte activity, because devitalized cells could not participate in the healing of a wound. Necrosis of the tendon ends is handled by the body according to general biological mechanisms, i.e., resorption of devitalized and necrotic tissue and ingrowth of cells and vessels from surrounding tissues—adhesion formation. The human flexor tendons within synovial sheaths have a well developed intrinsic vascular system, based upon the segmental vinculum system and the longitudinal vessels running inside the tendons (Bergljung, 1968; Brockis, 1953; Caplan et al., 1975; Edwards, 1946; Leffert et al., 1974; Lundborg, 1975; Lundborg and Myrhage, 1977; Lundborg et al., 1977; Peacock, 1959; Schatzker and Brånemark, 1969; Smith, 1965). This vascularization may easily be jeopardized by the injury as such or by a surgical procedure involving extensive dissection and the introduction of various types of suture material into the tendon substance.

During recent years evidence has been presented indicating that diffusion from the synovial fluid in the tendon sheath also constitutes an important nutritional mechanism for the tendon (Eiken et al., 1975; Furlow, 1976; Lundborg, 1976; Lundborg and Myrhage, 1977; Lundborg and Rank, 1978; Manske et al., 1978a,b,c, 1979, 1982; Mathews, 1976; Potenza, 1963). In this respect the tendon, in whole or in part, is believed to receive its nutrition in the same manner as does the cartilage of a joint. The synovial fluid is produced by the membranous synovial sheath, and thus the fate of the synovial sheath has proved to be a significant factor in hand surgery. Paradoxically this sheath used to be regarded as a structure to be resected to facilitate the nutrition of damaged

*Study supported by grants from the Swedish Medical Research Council (Projects 5188 and 2543), the Swedish Antirheumatoid League, Svenska Livförsäkringsbolagens nämnd för Medicinsk Forskning, the Swedish Work Environment Fund, and the Trygg-Hansas fond för personskadeforskning.

tendons or tendons grafts by ingrowth of vessels from surrounding tissues, i.e., formation of adhesions.

Current concepts regarding nutritional mechanisms of flexor tendons are reviewed in this chapter. The review is based primarily upon our own experiments on tendon vascularization and tendon nutrition via diffusional pathways from the synovial fluid.

GENERAL BACKGROUND

Our present knowledge regarding the nutritional and healing mechanisms of flexor tendons within the synovial sheath region is based mainly on experiments carried out on chickens, rabbits, and dogs as well as primates. In experiments carried out on chicken flexor tendons to elucidate the nutritional roles of vessels and synovial fluid, it was found that the vessels have essentially no nutritional role at all (Manske et al., 1978a,b). However, it should not be forgotten that the intratendinous vascular system of chicken flexor tendons differs fundamentally from that of human tendons (Lundborg and Myrhage, 1979). Histochemical studies have shown that chicken flexor tendons have very few vessels, which are located only in their most dorsal parts, whereas the greatest part of each tendon is devoid of vessels (Fig. 4–1). In more recent studies it has also been demonstrated that flexor tendons of primates are to a great extent nourished by diffusion from the synovial fluid (Manske et al., 1978c, 1982). Thus, there are reasons to believe that human tendons are also to some extent dependent on synovial fluid—an assumption that correlates with the microstructure of tendon tissue (see below).

THE VASCULARIZATION OF THE HUMAN FLEXOR TENDON SYSTEM

All the studies to be discussed were performed on human arms and hands that had been amputated because of malignant tumors. Shortly after amputation the main arteries were cannulated and perfused with India ink at a moderate pressure (Lundborg and Myrhage, 1977; Lundborg, et al., 1977). After adequate fixation each specimen was meticulously dissected, and the superficial vascular systems of tendons as well as tendon sheaths were studied by use of a dissecting

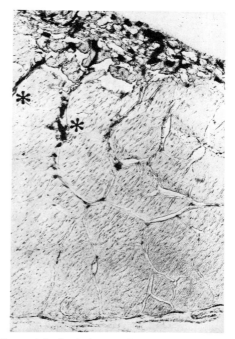

Figure 4–1. Intrinsic vascular pattern in a chicken flexor tendon as indicated by adenosine triphosphatase activity in endothelial cells (black). Asterisks indicate transverse vascular loop formations. All vessels are concentrated in the dorsal parts of the tendon (at the top of the picture), while the volar areas are avascular.

microscope. After clarification, the vessels in the deeper layers of the structure could be observed. Some specimens were analyzed by histochemical methods in which adenosine triphosphate activity indicated the endothelial cells. Thus, this method did not require perfusion of the vascular system with a contrast medium.

THE EXTRINSIC VASCULAR SUPPLY

Proximal to the tendon sheath region the flexor tendons have a well developed vascular system on their surfaces as well as in their interiors, where vessels are distributed in the endotenon between the collagen bundles. On the surface there is a vascular network of a "paratenon type," characterized by a main longitudinal system with numerous vessels anastomosing in all directions (Fig. 4–2). As the flexor tendons pass into the tendon sheath, their vascular characteristics change dramatically. Inside the sheath their intrinsic vascularization is based upon a longitudinal vascular system. Proximally this system represents a distal continuation of intratendinous

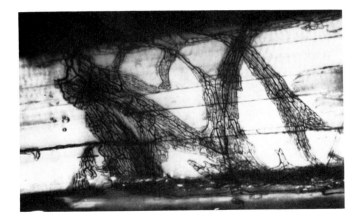

Figure 4–2. The vascular pattern on the surface of the flexor digitorum profundus tendon in the palm proximal to the entrance into the tendon sheath. The tendon here is embedded in paratenon, showing a well developed vascular net.

vessels from the palmar region, reinforced by vessels running in the accordion-like folds of the proximal synovial sheath reflection. Along the course of the tendons there is a segmental vascular supply based upon the vincula structures—the vinculum longum and the vinculum breve (Fig. 4–3). At the insertion of the tendons, vessels might also run into the tendons in the tendon-periosteum-bone attachments.

Bone vincula breve, situated close to the insertions of the deep and superficial flexor tendons, are well developed structures. The vinculum breve to the flexor digitorum superficialis originates in the groove just volar and proximal to the head of the proximal phalanx, inserting on the dorsal aspect of the chiasm formed by this tendon close to its insertion on the middle phalanx (Fig. 4–3). Volar to this chiasm, a vinculum longum, composed of a long slender slip, crosses the synovial space to reach the dorsal surface of the flexor digitorum profundus tendon. Thus, this vinculum longum has an intimate connection with the vinculum breve of the superficialis tendon and can be regarded as a continuation of this structure. In many specimens there are also several vincula longa or one, running from the dorsal part of the tunnel to the slips of the superficialis tendon where these slips fold dorsally over the profundus tendon. Occasionally there are also tiny bands connecting one slit of the superficialis tendon with the profundus tendon at

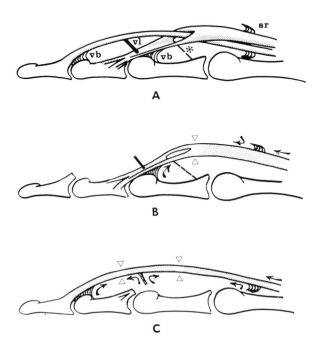

Figure 4–3. A, The anatomy and the general organization of the segmental vascular supply to both flexor tendons within the digital synovial sheath. vb = vinculum brevis; vl = vinculum longus; sr = synovial sheath reflection; the asterisk indicates a vinculum longus that is not always present. B, The flexor digitorum superficialis vascular system is demonstrated separately. The triangles indicate the critical poorly vascularized segments. There are two separate vascular systems. The proximal system originates from longitudinal vessels inside the tendon in continuity from the palm and from nutrient vessels in the reflection of the proximal synovial sheath. The distal vascular system originates from the vinculum brevis and the inconstant vinculum longus. C, The flexor digitorum profundus tendon. There are three vascular systems with different origins. A proximal system originates from nutrient vessels in the synovial reflection and longitudinal intratendinous vessels from the palm region. An intermediate system originates from the vinculum longus, while a distal segment originates from the vinculum brevis. (Reproduced from Lundborg, Myrhage, and Rydevik, 1977, with permission of the authors and publisher.)

this level. In the proximal reflection of the synovial tendon sheath, i.e., the "cul de sac," numerous vessels approach the tendons in the synovial folds.

INTRINSIC MICROVASCULAR SYSTEM

When the flexor tendons gain their entrance into the tendon sheath, their vascular pattern changes dramatically (Fig. 4–4). The surface of the most proximal centimeters of the flexor tendons inside the sheath shows a well developed vascular network, which, however, ends distally in numerous terminal vascular loops. Distal to these loops the volar surface, i.e., the friction surface of the tendons, appears to be more or less avascular with the exception of small loops piercing transversely from deeper layers of the tendon. In the profundus tendon the superficial vessels appear again on the volar side when the tendon approaches its insertion in the distal phalanx. On the dorsal, nonfriction side there is, however, a continuous longitudinal vascular pattern sending transverse vessels along the side of the tendon. However, these vessels end in terminal loop formations at a point about halfway along the side, very reminiscent of the terminal vascular loops seen in a joint in the border zone between synovial membrane and cartilage (Fig. 4–16).

The intrinsic vascular pattern of the profundus tendon changes dramatically at a level corresponding to the bifurcation of the superficialis tendon. Here many of the longitudinal vessels end in terminal loops, and a short segment of the tendon appears to be poorly vascularized (Fig. 4–3). However, distal to this level the intrinsic vascularization of the tendon is again well developed, the extrinsic vascular supply here being the vinculum longum at the level of the proximal interphalangeal joint. Within this segment of the tendon the intrinsic vessels show special characteristics: vertical vascular loops penetrate the tendon substance toward the volar surface, but about 1 mm. dorsal to the surface they very distinctly turn back in terminal loop formations, leaving the most volar part of the tendon avascular (Fig. 4–5). Histological sections from this part of the tendon show a differentiation of the tendon cells into cartilage-like cells—a cartilaginous differentiation (Fig. 4–6).

Figure 4–4. *A,* The superficial vascular pattern of the flexor tendons just distal to the entrance into the sheath. The synovial reflection is at the left. Proximally in the sheath, the tendons have a characteristic vascular plexus, which, however, ends after a few centimeters in numerous terminal loops. These superficial terminal loops anastomose with a deeper vascular system, continuing more distally. *B,* The area in *A* at higher magnification, showing the terminal capillary loops. Asterisk indicates loops penetrating toward the surface from deeper layers. (Reproduced from Lundborg, Myrhage, and Rydevik, 1977, with permission of the authors and publisher.)

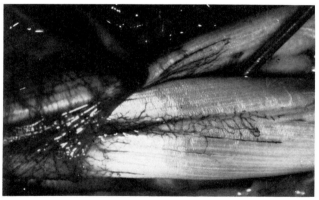

A

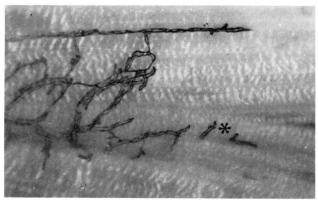

B

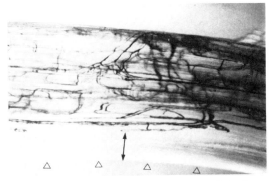

Figure 4–5. The intrinsic vascular system of the flexor digitorum profundus tendon (clarified) at the level of the proximal interphalangeal joint. Triangles indicate the volar friction surface. The volar part of the tendon (*arrow*) is devoid of vessels. (After Lundborg and Myrhage, 1977, with permission of the authors and publisher.)

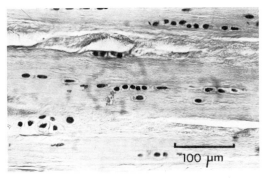

Figure 4–6. Histological section from the volar part of the profundus tendon at the level of the proximal interphalangeal joint. There is cellular diferentiation into chondrocyte-like cells within the whole area. Hematoxylin and eosin. (After Lundborg, Myrhage, and Rydevik, 1977, with permission of the authors and publisher.)

Just distal to the vinculum longum there is again a poorly vascularized part of the tendon, but as we approach the vinculum breve at the insertion the tendon substance again appears to be well vascularized (Fig. 4–3). In summary, the profundus tendon appears to be segmentally vascularized, showing three more or less separated systems along its course. Between these structures there are poorly vascularized parts: at the level of the superficialis bifurcation and just distal to the vinculum longum (Fig. 4–3).

The superficialis tendon also appears to be segmentally vascularized, the border zone between the two systems being situated at the bifurcation (Fig. 4–7). The proximal system is supplied by intrinsic longitudinal vessels in the tendon, whereas the distal system is supplied by the vinculum breve at the insertion and occasionally by a slender vinculum longum. Numerous vessels are seen on both slips of the tendon, but they end in terminal loops when the two slips meet, i.e., where the bifurcation starts. The "confluence," i.e., the dorsal part of the tunnel, situated in association with the bifurcation, is extremely well vascularized.

FLEXOR POLLICIS LONGUS

The flexor pollicis longus tendon differs in many respects from the other flexor tendons with regard to microanatomy and vascularization. This tendon runs inside a tendon sheath, starting at the level of the wrist joint and ending just distal to the interphalangeal joint of the thumb. There are three pulley structures: at the metacarpophalangeal and interphalangeal joints and in the proximal phalanx, where there is an oblique pulley structure.

Distally there is a well developed vinculum brevis, often extending proximally to the mid-

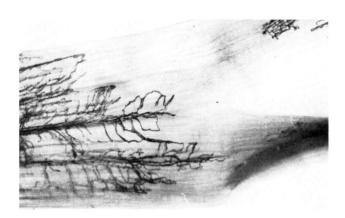

Figure 4–7. The flexor digitorum superficialis tendon (clarified) where it bifurcates into two slips in the base phalanx level. There is an avascular zone between the proximal and distal vascular segments. (Reproduced from Lundborg, Myrhage, and Rydevik, 1977, with permission of the authors and publisher.)

brevis, often extending proximally to the middle of the proximal phalanx. At the metacarpophalangeal joint level a tiny vinculum longum–like structure occasionally can be found. However, proximal to the metacarpophalangeal joint a "mesotenon" of variable shape and caliber is always found (Fig. 4–8). This structure usually has a length of 3 to 4 cm. and is often separated into several parts by one or more perforations. The most distal part of the mesotenon is sometimes condensed into a slender vinculum-like structure at the metacarpal neck region, already referred to (Fig. 4–9).

Along its course the flexor pollicis longus tendon describes an S form, with a volar concave shape distal to the metacarpophalangeal joint and a dorsal concave shape proximal to this level. Thus, proximal to the

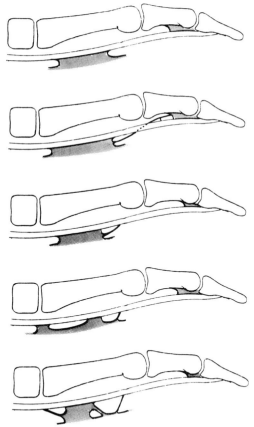

Figure 4–8. Variations in the appearance of the extrinsic vascular supply to the flexor pollicis longus tendon as observed in five dissection specimens. Distally a well developed vinculum brevis is consistently found. Proximally there is a mesotenon that varies in appearance, originating from the volar-ulnar (nonfriction) side of the tunnel. (After Lundborg, 1979, with permission of the publisher.)

level of the metacarpophalangeal joint the friction forces act on the dorsal parts of the tendon. This explains why the mesotenon at this level originates from the volar-ulnar part of the tunnel, approaching the tendon on the corresponding nonfriction side (Fig. 4–8).

The intratendinous vascular system of the flexor pollicis longus tendon presents a longitudinal pattern that remains uninterrupted along its entire length.

THE TENDON SHEATH

The tendons run in a tunnel, dorsally limited by the periosteum and the volar plates of the small joints. The volar part of this tunnel is usually referred to as the "tendon sheath." The tendon sheath comprises rigid fibrous components referred to as annular ligaments or "pulleys," as well as membranous synovial components. The macroanatomy and microanatomy of these structures have been outlined by Doyle and Blythe (1975) and Lundborg and Myrhage (1977).

Histologically the membranous parts of the sheath have the characteristics of a synovial membrane—a loose fibrovascular tissue covered by a layer of polyhedral cells. There is a well developed capillary network showing numerous characteristic loop formations (Figs. 4–10 and 4–11). In the region of the pulleys, however, no vessels can be seen. In fact, the friction surface of the pulleys appears to be completely avascular. In histological sections it can be seen that the vascular plexus of the synovial membrane is in continuity on the outside of the pulleys (Fig. 4–12A), so that the pulleys in this respect are situated on the inside of the synovial membrane. No distinct synovial cells can be found on the friction side of the pulleys; instead histological sections show metaplasia to cartilage-like cells (Fig. 4–12B). Also macroscopically the pulleys appear to be situated "inside" the synovial parts of the sheath, as indicated by deep pouch formations in the border zones between membranous and fibrous parts of the tunnel (Lundborg and Myrhage, 1977). Most noticeably a sharp border is formed by the distal opening of the second annular ligament, situated in the middle of the proximal phalanx (Fig. 4–15). This distinct anatomical structure may constitute a considerable hindrance to tendon motion, e.g., in cases of rheumatoid nodule formation inside the profundus tendon at the vinculum longum level.

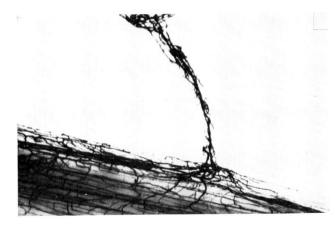

Figure 4–9. The appearance and distribution of vessels of a vinculum longus, here represented by the most distal condensed part of the mesotenon to the flexor pollicis longus tendon. The tendon is at the bottom of the picture. (After Lundborg, 1979, with permission of the publisher.)

In summary, the vascularization of the tendons as well as the tendon sheath follows a logical pattern based upon functional demands and is absent in areas of maximal friction and bending forces. Tissues subjected to pressure often show a differentiation into cartilage cells in connective tissue (Pauwels, 1960). This is beautifully illustrated by the volar parts of the tendons and the dorsal parts of the pulleys, i.e., the structures subjected to pressure in the flexor system. In these regions there are no vessels; a vessel cannot be expected to function under such mechanical stress. Instead these areas are probably adopted to nutrition via diffusional pathways.

THE ROLE OF THE SYNOVIAL FLUID

THE KNEE JOINT MODEL

Experiments designed to study the role of the synovial fluid have used as an experimental model segments of flexor tendons extirpated from the synovial sheath regions of rabbits, introduced into the knee joints of the same animals (Eiken et al., 1975; Lundborg, 1976; Lundborg and Rank, 1978). Each tendon segment was placed as a free body in a synovial pouch lateral to the femoral condyle. In one series of experiments the tendon was divided into two pieces, which were

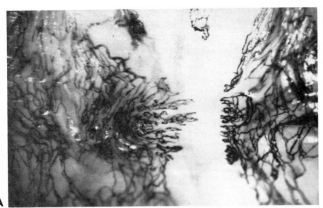
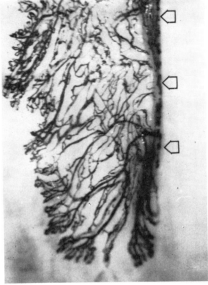

Figure 4–10. A, The capillary pattern of the membranous synovial sheath. Thin fibrous bands representing cruciform ligaments can be seen in some areas woven into the synovial membrane—here, such a band passes transversely over the picture. B, Typical vascular formation of the synovial tendon sheath, shown here in the membranous area between the first (AI) and second (AII) annular ligaments. The arrows indicate the very sharp border constituted by the AII ligament.

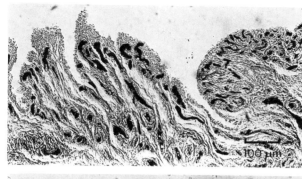

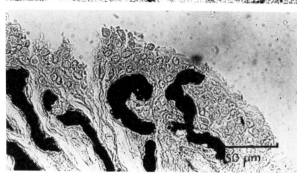

Figure 4–11. *A*, The histoangiographic appearance of the human synovial tendon sheath. The perfused capillaries (black) are evident superficially in the villus-like synovial formations. *B*, The same area at higher magnification. (After Lundborg and Myrhage, 1977, with permission of the authors and publisher.)

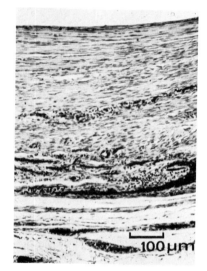

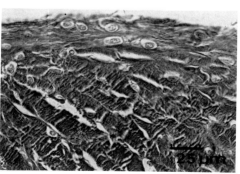

Figure 4–12. *A*, Transsection of the second annular ligament (AII), showing a concentration of vessels in the periphery of the pulley. The friction surface (at the top) is devoid of vessels. *B*, Friction surface of the same annular ligament at high magnification. There is a differentiation into chondrocyte-like cells. (Reproduced from Lundborg and Myrhage, 1977, with permission of the authors and publisher.)

sutured back together by two single stitches before the tendon was placed in the joint. After various periods, sometimes as long as three months, the tendon specimens were removed and subjected to analysis by histological and ultrastructural techniques (transmission and scanning electron microscopy).

The results indicated that tendons can survive for a long time in the synovial fluid environment. The tendons remained free bodies in the fluid, and adhesions did not form. On the contrary, the terminal ends rapidly became smooth and rounded owing to the formation of new tissue, and the superficial parts of the anastomosis site were bridged by smooth glistening tissue, which histologically was found to comprise proliferating fibroblasts and newly formed collagen (Fig. 4–13A, B). The gliding surface of the tendon remained white, glistening, and striated. Histologically the tendon as a whole was found to remain viable for at least three weeks. However, in the central parts of the tendon, an area of tissue necrosis developed after the third week, which continued to increase in size.

These experiments demonstrated a capacity of the synovial fluid to function as a nutritional medium for flexor tendons and a capacity of the tendon cells to proliferate and synthesize collagen without an "extrinsic cellular supply." Because the tendons were deprived of all their vascular supply, the synovial fluid was the only available nutrient medium in these experiments, and the cells of the tendons showed not only histological criteria of viability but also proliferation and collagen synthesis. These observations indicate that the synovial fluid may play a role as a nutrient medium normally as well as during repair. There may of course be limits to the diffusing capacity of tendons, and the necrotic picture in the centers of the tendons may thus reflect a critical diffusion distance. A cell seeding from the synovial fluid may play a role in restoring the gliding surface of the tendon but could not be a mechanism for cellular proliferation in the intermediate layers of the tendon.

In the experimental model described here raw tendon tissue with cut collagen bundles and exposed suture material was exposed to an intact membranous synovial membrane. The tendon was continuously surrounded by synovial fluid. Under these circumstances adhesions were not formed in the tendon or

synovial membrane, the tendon cells proliferated and synthesized collagen, and the gliding surface was rapidly restored over the suture site. These observations indicate that non-damaged synovium, producing synovial fluid, is a remarkable tissue, which certainly may have a central role in the basic biological mechanisms of flexor tendon healing.

SYNOVIAL NUTRITION VERSUS VASCULAR SUPPLY—THE DIFFUSION CAPACITY OF FLEXOR TENDONS

In an experimental study performed in dogs, the transport into the flexor tendons of intravenously infused [^{3}H] methyl glucose was studied under various experimental conditions (Lundborg and Holm, 1980). The aim was to study the relative importance of the intratendinous vascular system and the synovial fluid in the tendon sheath in providing nutrition of the tendon. For this purpose the following experimental conditions were created in three different series: (1) normal state—tendon and tendon sheath intact; (2) tendon sheath excised, metal foil wrapped around the intact tendon (intratendinous circulation noninterrupted); (3) tendon sheath intact but intratendinous vessels excluded (sheath carefully opened at two levels, tendon transversely cut at the corresponding levels, between which no vinculum was present; sheath then sutured). After 15 minutes the tendon was removed and cut into slices 200 μm. thick (the slicing pattern is shown in Fig. 4–14). The radioactivity of the slices was then determined and the counts at all levels of the transsection area of the tendon plotted in a diagram (Fig. 4–14). In this way the transport patterns of the tracer into the flexor tendon under the various experimental conditions could be evaluated.

It was found that within 15 minutes the tracer concentration in the synovial fluid of the tendon sheath corresponded exactly to the tracer concentration measured in the blood. The transport pattern into the tendon in cases in which the intratendinous vessels were excluded but the synovial sheath was preserved corresponded relatively closely to the normal state in which both vessels and tendons were preserved. By contrast, when the synovial fluid was excluded by excision of the sheath, the intratendinous vessels

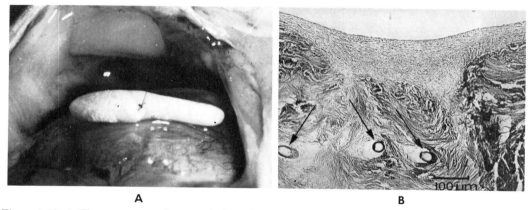

Figure 4–13. *A,* The appearance of a sutured piece of tendon, kept as a free body in the knee joint for two weeks. There are no adhesions. The surface of the tendon is white and glistening, showing normal striations. The suture region is covered by a smooth, newly formed tissue of intrinsic origin. (Reproduced from Lundborg, 1976, with permission of the publisher.) *B,* The histological appearance of the suture region after three weeks. The gap is bridged by proliferating cells and newly synthesized collagen. The surface is smooth. Arrows indicate suture material. (van Gieson stain.)

showed no (or only a minimal) capacity to supply the tendon tissue with tracer: counting showed an extremely low uptake of tracer.

These results indicate that in the dog, there is rapid transport of tracer from the blood to the synovial fluid, equilibrium being reached within 15 minutes after intravenous injection. A diffusional pathway from the synovial fluid plays the greater role in the transport of tracer into the tendon, while the intratendinous vessels apparently are of little importance in this context. The results attribute an important nutritional role to the synovial fluid

in this model. Similar results have been obtained in studies on flexor tendons in primates (Manske et al., 1978c, 1982).

THE HUMAN FLEXOR TENDON SYSTEM—A JOINT ANALOGY

The nutrition of human flexor tendons seems to result from the combined effects of vascularization and diffusion from the synovial fluid. The superficial avascular areas show a cellular differentiation toward carti-

Figure 4–14. Normalized tracer concentration profiles across the flexor tendon 15 minutes after intravenous injection of methyl-³H-glucose. Also included is a schematic diagram showing the transectional slicing pattern. Considering the short circulation time, the interest should be focused on the peripheral parts of the tendon. When the vessels are excluded, there is only a slight decrease in uptake of tracer. However, when the tendon sheath is excluded but the intratendinous vessels are still intact, there is a marked decrease in uptake. For further explanation see text. (Reproduced from Lundborg and Holm, 1979, with permission of the authors and publisher.)

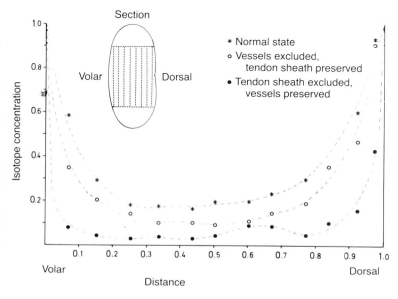

lage cells and are probably nourished by diffusion from the synovial fluid. The interior of the tendon has a well developed vascular system, concentrated in the dorsal parts of the tendon, sending down volar loops approaching the volar avascular areas from the inside (Fig. 4–15). Dorsally and on the sides of the tendon the vascular plexus sends loops toward the avascular parts, loops that, however, never go farther down than the midlateral line" of the tendon The arrangement is similar to that of the vascular loops seen in the interface between bone and cartilage in joints, i.e., the reflection of the synovial membrane (Fig. 4–16).

The avascular parts of the tendon (the volar gliding surface) glide against the pulleys of the tendon sheath, which has a glistening avascular surface with cellular differentiation toward cartilage. (cf. Fig. 4–12B). The production of synovial fluid is secured by the membranous parts of the tendon sheath, which are not subjected to any mechanical stress.

Thus, the avascular surfaces of the tendon and the pulleys are comparable to the cartilaginous surfaces of the components in a joint. Synovial fluid is a dialysate of blood plasma, and it has been proposed that the nutrition of cartilage is derived, totally or in part, from this synovial fluid (Ekholm, 1951; Hodge and Mackibbin, 1969; Honner and Thompson, 1971; Mankin, 1963; Maroudas et al., 1968). It is believed that in the joint cartilage the nutritive fluid reaches the chondrocytes by diffusion through the intercellular substance by joint movements (Ekholm, 1951; Salter and Field, 1960). The cartilage was described by McCutchen (1962) as acting like a sponge, soaking up the synovial fluid

after the fluid had been squeezed out during weight bearing. A similar mechanism may govern the nutrition of the avascular gliding surfaces of the flexor tendons and pulleys.

Thus, the flexor tendon system of the fingers in many respects could be looked upon as a specialized joint, sliding longitudinally and having an extremely wide range of motion between the components involved (cf. Fig. 4–15). The analogy is obvious when one considers the nature of rheumatoid lesions in the flexor tendon system, and the operative technique of tenosynovectomy in severe cases of rheumatoid arthritis. The rheumatoid lesion of the sheath as well as the tendon usually follows the localization of the vessels. Thus, in the tendon, the nodules are usually concentrated in the best-vascularized areas (cf. Fig. 4–3). In the sheath the membranous parts may be involved, but the insides of the pulleys are always unaffected, because there are no vessels. On the outsides of the pulleys, however, there may be many granulations. Synovectomy can be radically performed by extirpating the pathological membranous sheath, but the pulleys corresponding to the joint cartilage usually can be completely spared (Lundborg and Hagert, unpublished data). The philosophy of this procedure can best be understood if it is regarded as an intervention in a joint—an arthrosynovectomy—in which the cartilaginous surfaces are not to be touched.

CONCLUDING REMARKS

The vascular structure of the human flexor tendon indicates that the majority of the tendon is nourished from intratendinous vessels, although some areas, including the glid-

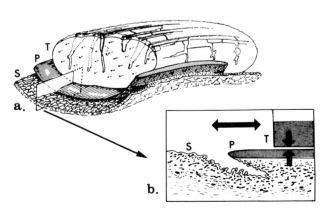

Figure 4–15. Schematic representation of the relationship between the flexor tendon (T), the pulley (P), and the synovial tendon sheath (S). *a*, This drawing is based upon our observations in the area at the distal border of the second annular ligament (AII). Close to the sharp edge of the pulley there is a deep pocket in the synovial sheath (see below). *b*, The "critical zone" around the sharp edge of the pulley. The shaded areas indicate the *avascular parts* of the tendon and the pulley, respectively, where cellular differentiation into chondrocyte-like cells can be observed (compare with Figs. 4–6 and 4–12B). The thick arrows indicate the traction and compression forces involved in active finger flexion. The vascular network of the synovial sheath is in continuity on the "outside" of the pulley. (Reproduced from Lundborg, G., and Myrhage, R.: The vascularization and structure of the human digital tendon sheath. Scand. J. Plast. Reconstr. Surg., *11*:195, 1977.)

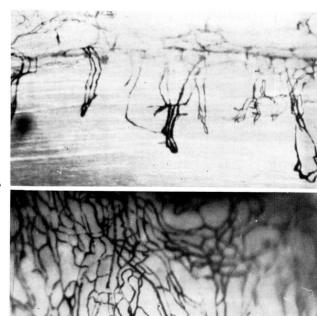

Figure 4–16. *A,* Capillary loop formations on the dorsolateral surface of the human flexor tendon at the proximal interphalangeal joint level. The volar-lateral surface (bottom of the picture) is avascular, and the cells in this area show differentiation toward cartilage. Compare with the vascular appearance shown in the schematic Figure 4–15. *B,* Capillary loop formations in the synovial reflection metacarpophalangeal joint. The cartilage is at the bottom of the picture. The appearance strongly corresponds to the transverse capillary formations in the mediolateral line on the surface of the flexor tendon (compare above), further illustrating the physiological similarities between joints and flexor tendons in the synovial sheath region.

ing surfaces, receive their nutrition via diffusional pathways from the synovial fluid. This appears to be the normal condition, but one should not exclude an increased role of synovial fluid nutrition when the blood flow in the tendon is jeopardized. Such situations may occur when a tendon is severed and its intrinsic longitudinal circulation is thereby interrupted, or when sutures in the tendon strangle the intratendinous vessels, as demonstrated experimentally by Bergljung (1968). Exclusion of the alternative nutritional source—the synovial fluid—also could be disastrous for the tendon in such cases. Thus, preservation of the membranous tendon sheath in such situations could be of critical importance for tendon survival.

The concept of preservation of the membranous tendon sheath in order to secure the nutrition of tendon tissue was applied clinically by Eiken et al. (1975), in association with flexor tendon grafting. These authors showed that the more membranous tendon sheath that could be preserved, the better were the clinical results.

The vessels in the tendon, and especially those in the vincula, may be jeopardized by an increase in pressure inside the closed ten-

don sheath. This is probably one contributory factor in the tendon necrosis sometimes seen after advanced septic tenovaginitis in the fingers. Decompression of the tendon by opening its sheath in these cases may be the essential procedure. A corresponding mechanism has been put forward as an explanation for the ruptures of the extensor pollicis longus tendon sometimes seen after distal nondisplaced fractures of the radius. In these cases the trauma is slight enough not to disrupt the sheath, but great enough to induce a critical increase in the pressure inside the nonruptured sheath (Engkvist and Lundborg, 1978).

In summary, experimental evidence indicates that intratendinous vessels as well as the synovial fluid produced by the membranous synovial sheath are significant in the provision of nutrition of flexor tendon. Thus, there are strong reasons to handle the flexor tendon as well as the membranous tendon sheath with utmost care. The main objectives in handling of flexor tendon injuries should therefore be to use tendon sutures that interfere as little as possible with the intratendinous microcirculation and to preserve the membranous tendon sheath as much as possible.

REFERENCES

Bergljung, L.: Vascular reactions after tendon suture and tendon transplantation. A stereo-microangiographic study of the calcaneal tendon of the rabbit. Scand. J. Plast. Reconstr. Surg., Suppl. 4, 1968.

Brockis, J. G.: The blood supply of the flexor and extensor tendons of the fingers in man. J. Bone Joint Surg., 35B:131, 1953.

Caplan, H. S., Hunter, J. M., and Merklin, R. J.: The intrinsic vascularisation of flexor tendons in the human. In: AAOS Symposium on Tendon Surgery. St. Louis, The C. V. Mosby Company, 1975, p. 48.

Doyle, J. R., and Blythe, W.: The finger flexor tendon sheath and pulleys: anatomy and reconstruction. In AAOS Symposium on Tendon Surgery. St. Louis, The C. V. Mosby Company, 1975, p. 81.

Edward, D. A. W.: The blood supply and lymphatic drainage of tendons. J. Anat., 80:147, 1946.

Eiken, O., Lundborg, G., and Rank, F.: The role of the digital synovial sheath in tendon grafting. An experimental and clinical study on autologous tendon grafting in the digit. Scand. J. Plast. Reconstr. Surg., 9:182, 1975.

Ekholm, R.: Articular cartilage nutrition. How radioactive gold reaches the cartilage in rabbit knee joints. Acta Anat., Suppl. 15, 1951.

Engkvist, O., and Lundborg, G.: Rupture of the extensor pollicis longus tendon after radius fracture—a clinical and experimental study. Hand, 11:28, 1979.

Furlow, L. T.: The role of tendon tissues in tendon healing. Plast. Reconstr. Surg., 57:39, 1976.

Gelberman, R. H., Manske, P. R., Vande Berg, J. S., Lesker, P. A., and Abeson, W. H.: Flexor tendon repair in vitro: A comparative histological study of the rabbit, chicken, dog and monkey. J. Orthop. Res., 2:39, 1984.

Hodge, L., and McKibbin, B.: The nutrition of mature and immature joint cartilage in rabbits. J. Bone Joint Surg., 51B:140, 1969.

Honner, R., and Thompson, R. C.: The nutritional pathways of articular cartilage. J. Bone Joint Surg., 53A:742, 1971.

Leffert, R. D., Weiss, C., and Athanasoulis, C. A.: The vincula. J. Bone Joint Surg., 56A:1191, 1974.

Lindsay, W. K., and Thomson, H. G.: Digital flexor tendons: experimental study. Part I. Br. J. Plast. Surg., 12:289, 1959-1960.

Lundborg, G.: The microcirculation in rabbit tendon. In vivo studies after mobilisation and transsection. Hand, 7:1, 1975.

Lundborg, G.: Experimental flexor tendon healing without adhesion formation—a new concept of tendon nutrition and intrinsic healing mechanisms. A preliminary report. Hand, 8:235, 1976.

Lundborg, G., and Hagert, C. G.: Unpublished data.

Lundborg, G., and Holm, S.: The role of the synovial fluid and tendon sheath for flexor tendon nutrition. J. Plast. Reconstr. Surg. 14:99, 1980.

Lundborg, G., and Myrhage, R.: The vascularization and structure of the human digital tendon sheath as related to flexor tendon function. Scand. J. Plast. Reconstr. Surg., 11:195, 1977.

Lundborg, G., and Myrhage, R.: Unpublished data.

Lundborg, G., Myrhage, R., and Rydevik, B.: The vascularization of human flexor tendons within the digital synovial sheath region—structural and functional aspects. J. Hand Surg., 2:417, 1977.

Lundborg, G., and Rank, F.: Experimental intrinsic healing of flexor tendons based upon synovial fluid nutrition. J. Hand Surg., 3:21, 1978.

Lundborg, G., Rank, F., and Heinan, B.: Intrinsic tendon healing: A new experimental model. Scand. J. Plast. Reconstr. Surg., 19:113, 1985.

Mankin, H. J.: Localization of tritiated thymidine in articular cartilage of rabbits. J. Bone Joint Surg., 45A:529, 1963.

Manske, P. R., and Lesker, P. A.: Nutrient pathways of flexor tendons in primates. J. Hand Surg., 7:436, 1982.

Manske, P. R., and Lesker, P. A.: Biochemical evidence of flexor tendon participation in the repair process: An in vitro study. J. Hand Surg., 9:117, 1984.

Manske, P. R., Whiteside, L. A., and Lesker, P. A.: Nutrient pathways to flexor tendons using hydrogen washout technique. J. Hand Surg., 3:32, 1978a.

Manske, P. R., Bridwell, K., and Lesker, P. A.: Nutrient pathways in flexor tendons of chicken using tritiated proline. J. Hand Surg., 3:352, 1978b.

Manske, P. R., Bridwell, K., Whiteside, L. A., and Lesker, P. A.: Nutrition of flexor tendon in monkeys. Clin. Orthopaed. Rel. Res., 36:294, 1978c.

Manske, P. R., Lesker, P. A., and Bridwell, K.: Experimental studies in chickens on the initial nutrition of tendon grafts. J. Hand Surg., 4:565, 1979.

Manske, P. R., Gelberman, R. H., Vande Berg, J., and Lesker, P. A.: Flexor tendon intrinsic repair: A morphological study in vitro. J. Bone Joint Surg., 67A:385, 1984.

Maroudas, A., Bullough, P., Swanson, S. A. V., and Freeman, M. A. R.: The permeability of articular cartilage. J. Bone Joint Surg., 50B:166, 1968.

Matthews, P.: The fate of isolated segments of flexor tendons within the digital sheath—a study in synovial nutrition. Br. J. Plast. Reconstr. Surg., 29:216, 1976.

Matthews, P., and Richards, H.: The repair potential of digital flexor tendons. J. Bone Joint. Surg., 56B:618, 1974.

Matthews, P., and Richards, H.: Factors in the adherence of flexor after repair. J. Bone Joint Surg., 58B:230, 1976.

McCutchen, C. E.: The frictional properties of animal joints. Wear, 5:1, 1962a.

McCutchen, C. E.: Animal joints and weeping lubrication. New Scientist, 15:412, 1962b.

McDowell, C. L., and Snyder, D. M.: Tendon healing: An experimental model in the dog. J. Hand Surg., 2:122, 1977.

Pauwels. F.: Eine neue Theorie über den Einfluss mechanischer Reize auf die Differenzierung der Stutzgeweve. Z. Anat. Entwicklungsgesch., 121:478, 1960.

Peacock, E. E., Jr.: A study of the circulation in normal tendons and healing grafts. Ann. Surg., 149:415, 1959.

Potenza, A. D.: Critical evaluation of flexor-tendon healing and adhesion formation within artificial digital sheaths. J. Bone Joint Surg., 45A:1217, 1963.

Salter, R. B., and Field, P.: The effects of continuous compression on living articular cartilage. An experimental investigation. J. Bone Joint Surg., 42A:31, 1960.

Schatzker, J., and Brånemark, P.-I.: Intravital observations on the microvascular anatomy and microcirculation of the tendon. Acta Orthop. Scand., Suppl. 126, 1969.

Smith, J. W.: Blood supply of tendons. Am. J. Surg., 109:272, 1965.

Chapter 5

OPTIMIZING TENDON REPAIRS WITHIN THE DIGITAL SHEATH

EDWARD R. WEBER

THE PROBLEM

The results of tendon surgery are unpredictable, especially in the area of the digital sheath. In the past 10 years new information regarding the nutrition of the flexor tendons in this region has provided the basis for repair techniques that have improved the results of tendon surgery. In this chapter we examine these advances and suggest methods of tendon surgery to optimize the utilization of these normal physiological processes.

THE BEGINNING

The modern basis for tendon surgery was provided by the work of Potenza (1962). His elegant experiments demonstrated that tendons heal by the proliferation of fibrous tissue nourished by new vascular growth in the form of granulation tissue. Because of these experiments, the tendon pulley system was viewed as an impediment to healing. Excision of the sheath, following repair, was the logical application of this experimental evidence.

NEW EVIDENCE

In 1979 Matthews sectioned a profundus tendon and placed it in the digital sheath. These free pieces of tendon healed on the surface but not in their central core. Matthews, working with Richards (1976), partially lacerated flexor tendons and allowed them to retract into the flexor tendon sheath. These tendons healed without evidence of granulation tissue. In fact Matthews believed that they healed by tenoblastic proliferation.

Lundborg (1976) placed a flexor tendon specimen in the synovial pouch of the knee and demonstrated healing of the tendon. He repeated this experiment, including a semipermeable membrane to exclude cellular seeding. Again healing of the tendon was demonstrated, although the central core did not heal. These findings were similar to those of Matthews' early work.

All these studies demonstrate that the flexor tendons can provide a tenoblastic response that can result in healing. They presented the possibility of tendon healing without adhesions. The process of tenoblastic proliferation appeared to be a primary or intrinsic response of the tendon to an injury. In practical terms of repair, however, this goal has been difficult to achieve. While working in our laboratory, Sterusky demonstrated that three conditions affected the amount of adhesion formation within the digital sheath—motion of the tendon, damage to the digital sheath, and the presence of suture material in the damaged tendon. If only one of these variables was changed, a primary healing response took place; if two variables were altered, moderate adhesion formation ensued. If all three variables were involved, dense adhesion formation resulted.

THE ROLE OF NUTRITION

In 1978 Manske carried out hydrogen washout studies indicating that the tenosynovial fluid was the major nutritional source for the flexor tendons. In later studies he demonstrated utilization of tritiated proline, from the tenosynovial fluid, in collagen production by the tendon. Finally, working with primates, he demonstrated that the nutritional source is not constant throughout the digital sheath. The vascular supply to the tendon offered a second system of nutrition by perfusion. The effect of this system was most evident in the distal tendon segment. Manske concluded that the process of nutrition by diffusion was predominant, supplying all areas of the tendon within the digital sheath.

These studies indicate that in the digital sheath tenosynovial fluid is the major source of nutrition for the flexor tendon. The nutrition provided by the tenosynovial fluid is sufficient to support tenoblastic activity and produce a healing response from the tendons themselves. Finally, they indicate that tendon healing within the digital sheath can take place without adhesion formation.

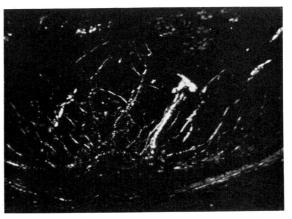

Figure 5–2. Transverse section of a profundus tendon, polarized light micrograph. The fibers are oriented at 90 degrees to the tendon tissue.

THE ROLE OF MOTION

In order to apply our knowledge of tenosynovial nutrition to tendon repair, a greater understanding of the means by which synovial fluid interfaces with the tenocytes was necessary. We examined the flexor tendons of chickens by scanning and transmission electron microscopy; additional information was supplied by polarized light microscopy (Figs. 5–1 to 5–3). These studies demonstrated the presence of a system of channels within the flexor tendon that are situated advantageously to allow the transportation of teno-

synovial fluid through the interstices of the tendon. These channels are associated with a system of nonparallel collagen fibers within the tendon. The channels transport an electron dense fluid to the tenocytes. We believe that this electron dense material is synovial fluid. In another experiment we injected fluorescein intravascularly and harvested specimens at time intervals of two to 20 minutes. These studies demonstrated that body fluid entered the flexor tendon from its nonvascular area, with a predilection for a diffusional pathway (Fig. 5–4). The addition of histologic information made it evident that a purposeful delivery system existed.

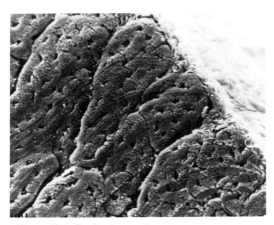

Figure 5–1. Profundus tendon of a chicken, scanning electron microscopic view. Note the series of channels approaching the tendon surface. A second smaller system of channels is located within the tendon bundles. (Magnification: 1 cm. = 40 μm.)

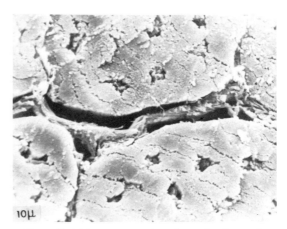

Figure 5–3. Transverse section of a profundus tendon, scanning electron microscopic view. Note the fibrous septum within the channel. The fibers of this septum are oriented at 90 degrees to the main bundles of the tendon. (Magnification: 1 cm. = 10 μm.)

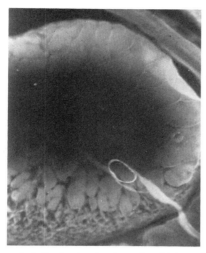

Figure 5–4. Profundus tendon of a chicken, fluorescent micrograph. This photograph, taken 15 minutes after injection of fluorescein dye, shows the ultraviolet luminescence demonstrating penetration of fluorescein-labeled synovial fluid from the nonvascular volar surface of the tendon.

The effect of motion on the delivery of fluorescein was then studied by awakening one of the subjects and allowing movement prior to sacrifice. Motion of the tendon obtained by this method doubled the rate of penetration of the tendon by the fluorescein tag.

THE MECHANISM (MOTION PUMP)

On the basis of these experiments, we postulate the following mechanism of tendon nutrition (Fig. 5–5). We view the system as a flow-through system, the tenosynovial fluid being pumped into the channels of the flexor tendon by the pressure difference created by the transitions between the heavy (pulleys) and thin (membranous) portions of the digital sheath. The pressures exerted on the palmar surface of the tendon tend to aid this process. The tenosynovial fluid is pumped through the channels where it interfaces with the tenocytes, providing nutrition. The excess fluid and waste products are then passed to the dorsal portion of the tendon where a looped vascular bed is present. We postulate that this bed absorbs the excess fluid and removes it from the tendon. Thus, the major role of tendon vascularity is played by the egress portion of the tendon circulation.

CONSISTENCY OF THE MOTION PUMP MECHANISM

This view of tendon nutrition is consistent with the previous work of other authors. The discrepancy of central necrosis and surface healing of isolated tendon segments within the fibro-osseous tunnel (Matthews) and in the knee cavity (Lundborg) is explained by the lack of a pumping mechanism. Their specimens were disconnected from their muscle source and therefore were not subjected to the pressures necessary to propel the tenosynovial fluid into the tendon in sufficient quantity to effect healing of the central core. The surface, however, could use the available tenosynovial fluid on a diffusional system alone. The three variables identified by Sterusky—i.e., integrity of the sheath, motion, and tendon suture—are also compatible with this mechanism. The intact sheath is necessary to provide the synovial fluid and the pumping surface. Motion is necessary to force the tenosynovial fluid into the tendon in sufficient quantity to provide nutrition for the healing response. The results obtained by

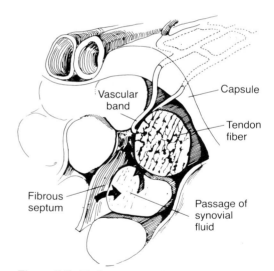

Figure 5–5. Motion pump. This drawing represents our concept of the way in which tenosynovial fluid passes through the flexor tendon. The fluid is pumped through the superficial tendon by the sliding motion of the tendon on its volar surface. The fluid is forced along the channels created by the nonparallel collagen fibers. The fluid then penetrates the individual tendon bundles where it provides nutrition to the tenocytes. The excess fluid is then returned to the intrabundle spaces where it comes into contact with a looped vascular bed in the dorsal portion of the tendon. This bed picks up the excess fluid and removes it from the tendon, making room for a fresh supply.

Potenza are also consistent with this model. If the sheath is discarded, healing by neovascularization must ensue. If the tendon repair is isolated from both the tenosynovial fluid and vascularity, as was the case when polyethylene tubes were placed around the tendons, no healing would be expected. Finally, the characterization of tenosynovial fluid as containing macromolecules in platelike configurations is that of a distillate. The small molecules are pumped through the tendon, and the larger molecules remain behind and are subjected to shearing forces, resulting in the platelike configurations.

USE OF THE FLOW-THROUGH CONCEPT IN TENDON REPAIR

The ideal tendon repair would allow full gliding and force transmission immediately, the digital sheath having been returned to its prelaceration condition. In this circumstance the majority of flexor tendon injuries would heal by a primary mechanism without any adhesions. Full function of the repaired tendon could be anticipated. Unfortunately such a suture technique is not yet available and the restoration of full function remains an idealized goal. However, several steps in the tendon repair process bring us closer to this ideal. These steps are categorization of the injury and improvements in suture technique, management of the tendon sheath, and aftercare.

CATEGORIZATION OF FLEXOR TENDON INJURIES

The purpose of categorizing flexor tendon injuries is to determine the mechanism by which they are likely to heal. An injury involving crushing of the tendon or loss of the tendon sheath has no chance of healing by a primary tenoblastic process. However, a partial laceration of a flexor tendon that occurred in flexion so that the fibro-osseous tunnel was not damaged has every possibility of undergoing primary tenoblastic repair. Most wounds fall between these two extreme examples. The question that must be posed prior to operative intervention is, can the wound be reconstructed so that a tenoblastic repair process is possible? If the answer to this question is yes, every effort to restore the patient to the preinjury state should be undertaken. If the answer is no, conditions favorable to the granulation repair process should be created.

In categorizing tendon injuries, the type of trauma, the nature of the wound, the environment in which the accident occurred, the nature of the loss of continuity, injury of surrounding tissue, age of the patient, and time are important. In general, all sharply lacerated tendon injuries repaired by surgical intervention within 24 hours after occurrence are candidates for a tenoblastic healing process if the proper circumstances can be created—restoration of the tenosynovial sheath, utilization of a suture technique that allows free motion of the tendon within the sheath, and an aftercare program that ensures safe gliding of the tendon during the healing process. In most injuries both healing systems are utilized. The degree to which adhesions form is proportional to the failure of the intrinsic healing system.

SUTURE TECHNIQUE

A suture technique avoiding tissue constriction while providing sufficient strength to allow early passive motion is essential. The technique discribed by Kessler (1973) is commonly used to this end. My preference for a transverse laceration of the flexor tendon is the modified Kessler repair. Other repairs that fulfill the requirements are the Verdan and Becker methods; the Becker method is preferred for long oblique lacerations. In order to achieve the second requirement of full motion, an epitendinous running suture is necessary; this prevents the edge of the cut tendon from snagging on the surrounding lacerated tissues.

RESTORATION OF THE FIBRO-OSSEOUS TUNNEL

Restoring the fibro-osseous tunnel is the next important step. Consideration should be given to the dorsal and palmar surfaces of the sheath system. Thus, the superficial flexor tendon should be repaired not only to provide full finger power but also because it is part of the important bed of the profundus system. The sheath itself should be restored. The goal of the sheath repair is to re-establish a

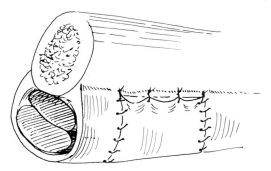

Figure 5–6. Fibro-osseous sheath repair. Repair of the tendon sheath is accomplished by placing two to four anchoring sutures in the thickened ridge of tissue next to the phalanx. The volar portion of the sheath is then opposed with a running suture of 6–0 or 7–0 Dacron.

SUMMARY

Experimental evidence of synovial fluid nutrition of flexor tendons within the digital sheath is presented. Concepts governing the repair of flexor tendon lacerations in this region are presented. The old concept of wound healing and tendon repair has been challenged. In its place a compartmental healing process is suggested, based on a physiologic nutrition system. In reality both intrinsic healing (synovial fluid supported tenoblastic healing) and extrinsic healing (granulation tissue supported fibroblastic healing) are operative. The system predominating can be altered by the surgeon at the time of surgery and during aftercare.

smooth surface for the flexor tendon to glide upon. Restoring the volar portion of the sheath is therefore the critical point in the repair. The sheath system thickens near its attachment with the phalanx. These ridges provide anchorage for sutures that provide the base for sheath repair. I usually place two to four figure-of-eight sutures of 5-0 Dacron in this area. Gaps in the repair are usually present, but these gaps are unimportant along the side of the tendon. The volar surface of the sheath is then repaired with fine running sutures of 6-0 or 7-0 Dacron (Fig. 5–6).

There are some injuries that are destined to heal exclusively by an extrinsic process. The lacerated sheath, in the area of the tendon suture, acts as a deterrent to successful repair. In these cases excision of the noncritical areas of the sheath is appropriate. This approach is usually reserved for untidy wounds in which the sheath has been damaged over a large area.

Rarely an untidy laceration of the sheath is associated with a tidy tendon laceration. In this instance a graft to the damaged sheath area is indicated. Appropriate graft material may be obtained from the extensor retinaculum on the dorsum of the wrist, as described by Lister (1979).

Finally, an aftercare program to allow safe sliding of the tendon is necessary for intrinsic healing. The programs outlined by Kleinert and by Duran and Houser succeed in this regard. In addition to aiding the movement of tenosynovial fluid into the tendon, these motion programs also may allow earlier remodeling of the scar produced by the extrinsic healing system.

REFERENCES

Becker, H., Orak, F., and Duponselle, E.: Early active motion following a beveled technique of flexor tendon repair. Report on fifty cases. J. Hand Surg., 4:454, 1979.

Duran, R. J., and Houser, R. G.: Controlled passive motion following flexor tendon repair in zones two and three. *In* AAOS Symposium on Tendon Surgery in the Hand. St. Louis, The C. V. Mosby Company, 1975, p. 165.

Kessler, I.: The grasping technique for tendon repair. Hand, 5:253, 1973.

Kleinert, H. E., and Bennett, J. B.: Digital pulley reconstruction employing the always present rim of the previous pulley. J. Hand Surg., 3:297, 1978.

Lister, G. D.: Reconstruction of pulleys employing extensor retinaculum. J. Hand Surg., 4:461, 1979.

Lister, G. D., Kleinert, H. E., Kutz, J. E., and Atasoy, E.: Primary flexor tendon repair followed by immediate controlled mobilization. J. Hand Surg., 2:441, 1977.

Lundborg, G.: Experimental flexor tendon healing without adhesion formation—a new concept of tendon nutrition and intrinsic healing mechanisms. A preliminary report. Hand, 8:235, 1976.

Lundborg, G., Myrhage, R., and Rydevik, B.: The vascularization of human flexor tendons within the digital synovial sheath region—structural and functional aspects. J. Hand Surg., 2:417, 1977.

Lundborg, G., and Rand, F.: Experimental intrinsic healing of flexor tendons based upon synovial fluid nutrition. J. Hand Surg., 3:21, 1978.

Manske, P. R., Birdwell, K., Lesker, P. A.: Nutrient pathways to flexor tendons of chickens using tritiated proline. J. Hand Surg., 3:52, 1978.

Manske, P. R., Lesker, P. A.: Nutrient pathways of flexor tendons in primates. J. Hand Surg., 7:436, 1982.

Manske, P. R., Whiteside, L. A., and Lesker, P. A.: Nutrient pathways to flexor tendons using hydrogen washout technique. J. Hand Surg., 3:32, 1978.

Matthews, P.: The pathology of flexor tendon repair. Hand, 11:233, 1979.

Matthews, P., and Richards, H. J.: The repair potential of digital flexor tendons. J. Bone Joint Surg., *56B*:618, 1974.

Matthews, P., and Richards, H. J.: Factors in the adherence of flexor tendons after repair. J. Bone Joint Surg., *58B*:230, 1976.

Ochiai, N., Matsue, T., Miyaji, N., Merklin, R. J., and Hunter, J. M.: Vascular system and blood supply of the profundus system in the digital sheath. J. Hand Surg., *4*:321, 1979.

Potenza, A. D.: Tendon healing within the flexor digital sheath in the dog. J. Bone Joint Surg., *44A*:49, 1962.

Potenza, A. D.: Concepts of tendon healing and repair. *In* AAOS Symposium on Tendon Surgery in the Hand. St. Louis, The C. V. Mosby Company, 1975, p. 88.

Potenza, A. D.: The healing process in wounds of the digital flexor tendons and tendon grafts. An experimental study. *In* Verdan, C. (Editor): Tendon Surgery of the Hand. Edinburgh, Churchill Livingstone, 1979, p. 40.

Sterusky, M.: Personal communication.

Verdan, C.: Reparative surgery of flexor tendons in the digits. *In* Verdan, C. (Editor): Tendon Surgery of the Hand. Edinburgh, Churchill Livingstone, 1979, p. 57.

Chapter 6

THE EFFECTS OF AGING AND VARIATIONS IN VINCULA ON FLEXOR TENDON VASCULARIZATION

TAKESHI MATSUI
AND JAMES M. HUNTER

Following Mayer's great achievements in studying the arrangement of blood vessels in tendons (Mayer, 1916), the profuse vascularization of the human digital flexor tendons has been described in detail utilizing recent advances in injection technique and methods of infusion. During this period there has been much disagreement about the arrangement and course of blood vessels in the tendons (Brockis, 1953; Caplan et al., 1975; Edwards, 1946; Lundborg et al., 1977; Manske and Lesker, 1982; Miyaji et al., 1978; Smith, 1965, Young and Weeks, 1971). Except for two publications (Matsui et al., 1979; Ochiai et al., 1979), no agreement has been reached because of lack of consideration of the changes that occur with age in blood vessel distribution in tendons and the variations in the vincula.

This discussion, which is intended to clarify the effects of aging on flexor tendon vascularization and the variations in patterns of the vincula, is based on the study of 38 hands.

MATERIALS AND METHODS

Thirty-eight fresh autopsy or amputation specimens were used. The age distribution of the patients is shown in Table 6–1.

Perfusion with saline was carried out through the subclavian artery in newborns and through both the ulnar and radial arteries of the forearm in other subjects. Infusion with diluted India ink–latex solution was con-tinued until the skin of the whole hand was stained black so that the capillary bed could be filled with the injection fluid. The specimen was next fixed in formalin and dissected under magnification. It was dehydrated with alcohol and cleared by using a mixture of tricresyl phosphate and tri-n-butyl phosphate. The clarified specimen was then photographed by the transillumination technique and observations recorded as described by Caplan et al. (1975), Miyaji et al. (1978), and Ochiai et al. (1979).

BASIC PATTERN OF TENDON VASCULARIZATION

The typical blood vessel distribution in the flexor digitorum profundus tendon is shown schematically in Figure 6–1. Two separate vascular systems are defined. The proximal

Table 6–1. AGE DISTRIBUTION OF SPECIMENS USED IN STUDY OF 38 HANDS (JEFFERSON MEDICAL COLLEGE AND SHINSHU UNIVERSITY SCHOOL OF MEDICINE)

Age	No. of Specimens
0–10	7
11–20	1
21–30	3
31–40	1
41–50	2
51–60	7
61–88	17

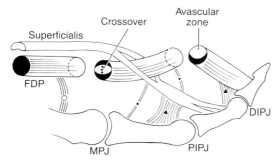

Figure 6–1. Schema of vascular distribution of flexor digitorum profundus tendon (FDP). MPJ = metacarpophalangeal joint, PIPJ = proximal interphalangeal joint, DIPJ = distal interphalangeal joint.

vascular system, supplied by palmar longitudinal channels and vessels of the synovial reflection, runs proximal to the base of the proximal phalanx. Distal to the base of the proximal phalanx one finds the vascular system, which is derived from long and short vincula. The distal vascular system is located mainly at the dorsal portion of the flexor profundus tendon; the proximal system is situated mainly at the volar-central portion of the tendon. There is a crossover of vessels between these longitudinal vascular systems at the base of the proximal phalanx. In the distal vascular system an avascular zone is recognized at the volar portion of the profundus tendon; most of the blood vessel channels course longitudinally on the dorsal side of the tendon.

EFFECTS OF AGING ON TENDON VASCULARIZATION

In newborns the flexor tendons have a rich vascularization (Fig. 6–2). In the profundus tendon, however, an avascular zone is recognized at the volar site in the distal vascular system. A crossover of longitudinal blood vessel channels is also found at the base of the proximal phalanx.

The specimens of older tendons show poor vascularity (Fig. 6–3), but a crossover of longitudinal blood vessels and an avascular

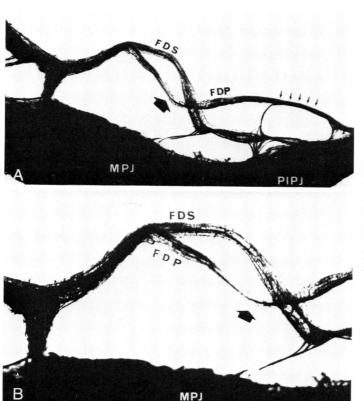

Figure 6–2. *A,* Middle finger, 10-hour-old newborn. *B,* Detail of *A* at the metacarpophalangeal joint. The large arrow points to a crossover of longitudinal blood vessels. The small arrows indicate an avascular zone of the profundus tendon. FDP = flexor digitorum profundus tendon, FDS = flexor digitorum superficialis tendon, MPJ = metacarpophalangeal joint, PIPJ = proximal interphalangeal joint.

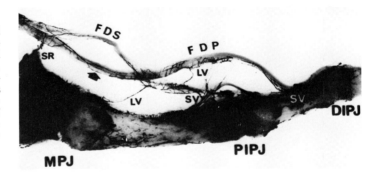

Figure 6–3. Ring finger, 52-year-old individual. The arrow points to a crossover of the intratendinous longitudinal blood vessels of the profundus tendon. FDS = flexor digitorum superficialis tendon, FDP = flexor digitorum profundus tendon, SR = synovial reflection, SV = short vincula, LV = long vincula, MPJ = metacarpophalangeal joint, PIPJ = proximal interphalangeal joint, DIPJ = distal interphalangeal joint.

zone at the volar site are observed in the profundus tendon. Thus the basic pattern in the tendon of the aged subject is similar to that in the newborn.

In the second and third decades the flexor tendons are well vascularized (Fig. 6–4). The blood vessel arrangement of the profundus tendon also has a crossover at the base of the proximal phalanx and an avascular zone at the volar site in the distal vascular system.

The vascularity of the flexor tendons becomes poor with age. Especially in subjects beyond the sixth decade, fewer blood vessels are found in the tendons, although the basic pattern of the vascular distribution remains unchanged. The characteristic features of the profundus tendon blood vessel distribution are a crossover of blood vessels at the base of the proximal phalanx and an avascular zone at the volar site in the distal vascular system.

VARIATIONS IN THE VINCULA

The short vincula of the flexor digitorum superficialis and the flexor digitorum profundus tendons are present in the proximal part

Figure 6–4. *A,* Middle finger, 26-year-old individual. *B,* Detail of the profundus and superficialis tendons in *A.* The small arrows indicate an avascular area of the profundus tendon. The large arrow points to a crossover of longitudinal blood vessels of the profundus tendon. FDS = flexor digitorum superficialis tendon; FDP = flexor digitorum profundus tendon, MPJ = metacarpophalangeal joint, PIPJ = proximal interphalangeal joint, DIPJ = distal interphalangeal joint.

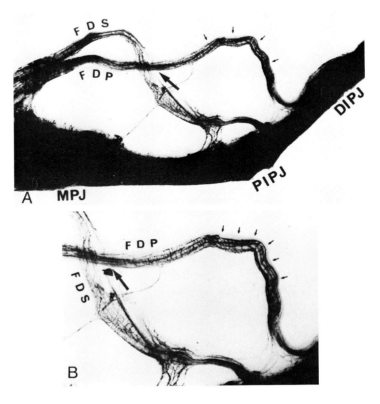

of the bony attachment and morphologically are almost constant. By contrast, the patterns of the long vincula of the tendons vary greatly.

Typically the long vincula of the flexor digitorum profundus tendon appear to receive blood vessels from the short vinculum of the flexor digitorum superficialis tendon by way of Camper's chiasm (Fig. 6–5A). In Figure 6–5B the long vinculum of the profundus tendon is shown to be supplied directly from the long vinculum of the flexor digitorum superficialis tendon. Occasionally the long vinculum arises from the synovial mem-

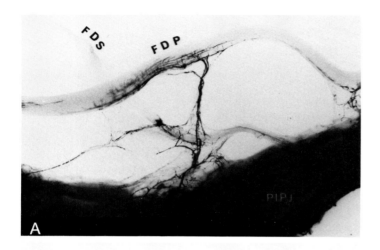

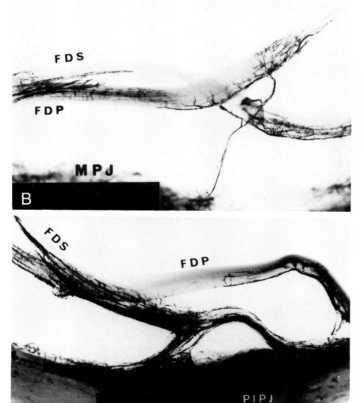

Figure 6–5. Variations in the long vinculum of the profundus tendon. A, Little finger, 52-year-old individual. B, Index finger, 52-year-old individual. C, Ring finger, 42-year-old individual. FDS = flexor digitorum superficialis tendon, FDP = flexor digitorum profundus tendon, MPJ = metacarpophalangeal joint.

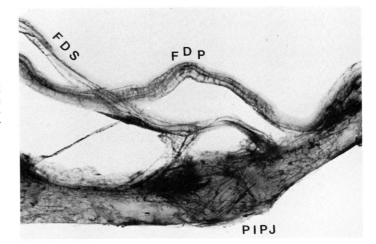

Figure 6–6. Ring finger, 26-year-old individual. There are no vincula of the profundus tendon. FDS = flexor digitorum superficialis tendon, FDP = flexor digitorum profundus tendon, PIPJ = proximal interphalangeal joint.

brane between the two tendinous slips proximal to Camper's chiasm of the flexor digitorum superficialis tendon (Fig. 6–5C). Rarely the long vincula may be absent (Fig. 6–6).

The long vincula of the flexor digitorum profundus tendon shown in Figure 6–7A consists of two slender vincula from Camper's chiasm and broad ones lying more proximally. The flexor digitorum superficialis ten-

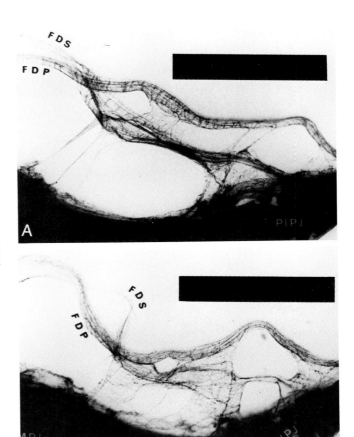

Figure 6–7. Mesotenon-like vincula. A, Index finger, 8-year-old child. B, Little finger, 8-year-old child. FDS = flexor digitorum superficialis tendon, FDP = flexor digitorum profundus tendon.

don shown in Figure 6–7*B* is hypoplastic, with membranous vincula extending from bones to the profundus tendon via the flexor digitorum superficialis tendon. These vincula can be described as mesotenon-like. The long vincula of the superficialis tendon also show variations. Although the long vincula patterns of the flexor tendons vary among the fingers, typical patterns exist in each finger. The details of variation in the vincula have been discussed by Ochiai et al. (1979).

CONCLUSIONS

1. Our study of the vascularization of the flexor digitorum profundus tendon within the human digital fibrous tendon sheath reveals that the tendon has two separate vascular systems—proximal and distal. A crossover of blood vessels is found at the base of the proximal phalanx. An avascular zone is present at the volar site of the distal blood vessel system.

2. The distribution of blood vessels varies with age; the vascularity of the flexor tendons is poorer in aged than in young and newborn subjects.

3. In investigating the distribution pattern of blood vessels in the tendons, the changes with age, as well as the variations in the vincula, should be taken into consideration.

REFERENCES

Brockis, J. G.: The blood supply of the flexor and extensor tendons of the fingers in man. J. Bone Joint Surg., *35B*:131–138, 1953.

Caplan, H. S., Hunter, J. M., and Merklin, R. J.: Intrinsic vascularization of flexor tendons. *In* Symposium on Tendon Surgery in the Hand. St. Louis, The C.V. Mosby Company, 1975, pp. 48–58.

Edwards, D. A. W.: The blood supply and lymphatic drainage of tendons. J. Anat., *80*:147–152, 1946.

Lundborg, G., Myrhage, R., and Rydevik, B.: The vascularization of human flexor tendons within the digital synovial sheath region—structural and functional aspects. J. Hand Surg., *2*:417–427,1977.

Manske, P. R., and Lesker, P. A.: Nutrient pathways of flexor tendons in primates. J. Hand Surg., *7*:436–444, 1982.

Matsui, T., Merklin, R. J., and Hunter, J. M.: A microvascular study of the human flexor tendons in the digital fibrous sheath—normal blood vessel arrangement of tendons and effects of injuries to tendons and vincula on distribution of tendon blood vessels. J. Jpn. Orthop. Assoc., *53*:307–320, 1979.

Mayer, L.: The physiological method of tendon transplantation. 1. Historical; anatomy and physiology of tendons. Surg. Gynecol. Obstet., *182*:182–197,1916.

Miyaji, N., Hunter, J. M., and Merklin, R. J.: A study of microvascularization of human finger flexors. J. Jpn. Orthop. Assoc., *52*:687–694, 1978.

Ochiai, N., Matsui, T., Miyaji, N., Merklin, R. J., and Hunter, J. M.: Vascular anatomy of flexor tendons. 1. Vincular system and blood supply of the profundus tendon in the digital sheath. J. Hand Surg., *4*:321–330, 1979.

Smith, J. W.: Blood supply of tendons. Am. J. Surg., *109*:272–276, 1965.

Young, L., and Weeks, P. M.: Profundus tendon blood supply within the digital sheath. Surg. Forum, *21*:504–506, 1971.

Chapter 7

THE DISTRIBUTION OF BLOOD VESSELS IN THE EXTENSOR APPARATUS OF THE HUMAN DIGIT

MICHINOBU MAEDA
AND TAKESHI MATSUI

The extensor tendon of the human digit differs from the flexor tendon in its characteristic anatomical structure and gliding mechanism. The only digital sheath present on the extensor surface of the hand is the synovial sheath; the fibrous sheath, which acts as a pulley in the flexor mechanism, is absent. In the region of the finger, the extensor apparatus forms a complex extensor mechanism. The extensor apparatus is wrapped only by the paratenon and fascia in this region. Although the extensor tendon has many unique features, the blood supply seems to play an important role as a nutrient pathway, just as in the flexor tendon. Because less interest is usually paid to extensor tendon injuries than those of the flexor tendon, there are very few detailed reports concerning extensor tendon circulation, which is a factor that is considered to exert a great influence in the healing process of injured tendons. We investigated the distribution of blood vessels of the extensor apparatus by means of microangiography.

MATERIALS AND METHOD

The arms of fresh cadavers were amputated at the level of the forearm and catheters were inserted and fixed into the radial and ulnar arteries. A mixture of India ink and latex was prepared with a volume ratio of 2:1 as the injection for angiography. This was then diluted approximately seven-fold using physiological saline. After perfusion with physiological saline, the injection was performed through both arteries by manual pressure. When back-flow of the injection from the stumps of the veins was observed, a tourniquet was applied immediately to prevent further leakage of the injected fluid, and injection was continued until the entire skin was stained black to an adequate level. After fixation in 10 per cent formalin for about one week, the desired tissue was dissected under magnification. The isolated tissue was then dehydrated in alcohol for two days and was observed following clarification in an 11:2 mixture of tricresyl phosphate and tri-n-butyl phosphate.

RESULTS AND DISCUSSION

The blood vessels of the flexor tendon and its digital sheath originate from the proper digital artery. Some branches from the transverse digital artery are distributed through the vincula to the intratendinous vessels of the flexor tendon. Consequently, the blood vessels on which angiography was performed were not observed macroscopically on the surface of the flexor tendon within the fibrous digital sheath. However, the distribution of the blood vessels to the extensor apparatus differs completely from that of the flexor tendon. Close to the interphalangeal joint, branches originating from the proper digital artery are distributed to both sides of the extensor apparatus surface (Fig. 7–1). In addition to the relatively wide vessels that run longitudinally on both sides of the extensor communis tendon in the dorsal region of the extensor apparatus, there are also numerous fine blood vessels that are interconnected with each other by microvascular anastomoses (Fig. 7–2A). The distribution of blood vessels on the dorsal surface appears to be slightly more abundant in the region of each interphalangeal joint than in other regions. Blood vessels were observed on the tendon surface at the metacarpus and proximal phalanx level on the volar surface, but in the region distal to the proximal interphalangeal joint they were greatly reduced (Fig. 7–2B). In particular, no blood vessels detectable by the microangiography method were observed in the region of contact with the proximal interphalangeal and distal interphalangeal joints. One of the cardinal functions of the extensor apparatus is its ability to slide and so this surface must be very smooth. The

evidence of rather poor vascularization in the sliding surface would be a natural adaptation to this function. However, smaller vessels that are not detected by the microangiography method may be present on the gliding surface. The blood vessels were observed extending along the entire length of the extensor apparatus in the cleared specimen (Fig. 7–3A). Fine blood vessels can be seen running through the extensor communis tendon and the lateral band in the extensor apparatus (Fig. 7–3B). Among these blood vessels, there are branches that interconnect with vessels of the interosseous and lumbrical muscles. The distal tip of the cleared specimen corresponds to the terminal tendon. In this region, the extensor apparatus is narrow and paper-thin, yet there is a dense distribution of fine blood vessels.

The anatomical structure of the extensor mechanism in the thumb differs from that in other digits (Fig. 7–4A), but it displays a similar irregular meshlike distribution of blood vessels extending along the entire length of the extensor apparatus (Fig. 7–4B).

When the fingers are flexed, the extensor apparatus stretches passively, causing displacement and increased pressure in the soft tissue. The meshwork of the blood vessels adapts to this displacement. When the vessels are not able to supply blood to an area of increased pressure, this meshwork is able to provide alternative collateral pathways.

We have already reported on the aging phenomenon occurring in the blood vessel distribution of the flexor tendon and its digital sheath, whereby a reduction in the number of blood vessels occurs with increasing age. The same phenomenon can also be found in the blood vessel distribution of the extensor apparatus. Figure 7–5 shows an extensor apparatus (Fig. 7–5A) and the cleared specimen of a 52-year-old male's left index finger (Fig. 7–5B). It is difficult to quantify the vascular distribution to make comparisons, but the number of blood vessels distributed in the extensor apparatus is apparently reduced compared with that of a young person.

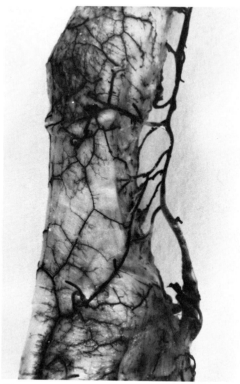

Figure 7–1: Oblique view from the dorsal side of the finger at the level of the proximal phalanx. Blood vessels branch from the proper digital artery and supply the surface of the extensor apparatus.

SUMMARY

1. The distribution of blood vessels in the extensor apparatus was investigated by means of microangiography.

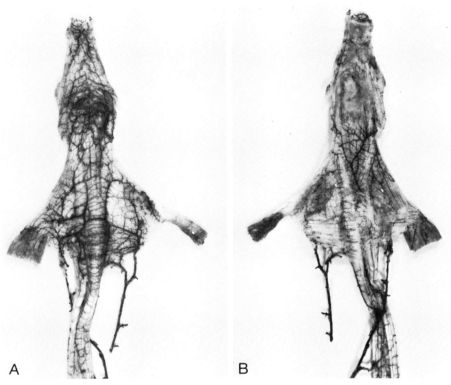

Figure 7–2. Index finger of a 6-year-old boy. *A,* Dorsal view of the extensor apparatus. *B,* Volar view. Many blood vessels are found on the dorsal side. However, the vascularity of the volar side is poor compared with that of the dorsal side.

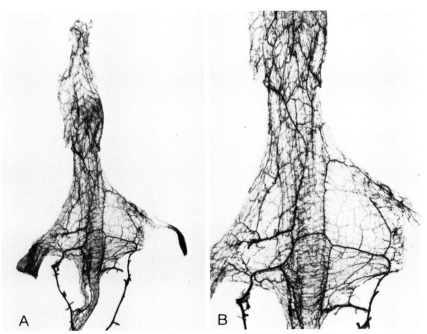

Figure 7–3. Many blood vessels are found along the full length of the extensor apparatus. *A,* Clarified specimen of the finger shown in Figure 7–2. *B,* Close-up view of the finger shown in Figure 7–2.

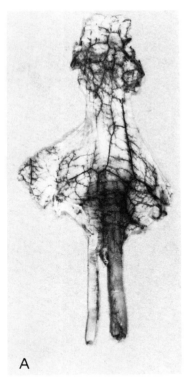
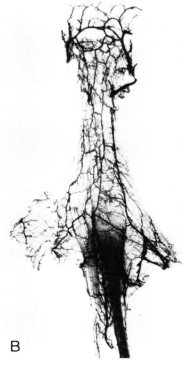

Figure 7–4. Extensor apparatus of the right thumb of a 6-year-old boy. *A,* Dorsal view. *B,* Clarified specimen.

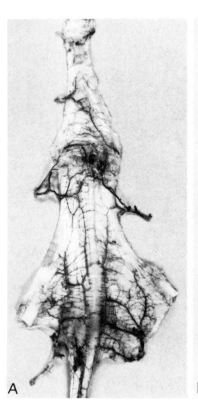
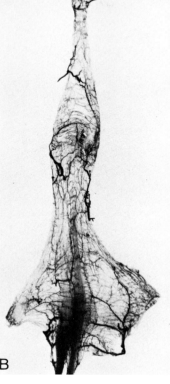

Figure 7–5. Left index finger of a 52-year-old man. *A,* Dorsal view. *B,* Clarified specimen. The vascularity of the extensor apparatus is poor compared with that of the specimen shown in Figures 7–2 and 7–3.

2. Many blood vessels that branched from the proper digital arteries were distributed on the surface of the extensor apparatus. They were found along the full length of the extensor apparatus in the cleared specimens, were connected with each other, and formed microvascular anastomoses.

3. A reduced vascular distribution was observed in the volar surface compared with that of the dorsal surface of the extensor apparatus.

4. The vascularity of the extensor apparatus is reduced with age.

REFERENCES

Caplan, H. S., Hunter, J. M., and Merklin, R. J.: *In* Symposium on Tendon Surgery in the Hand. St. Louis, The C. V. Mosby Company, 1975.

Gajisin, S., Zubrodowski, A., and Grodecki, J.: Vascularization of the extensor apparatus of the finger. J. Anat., *137*:315, 1983.

Maeda, M., Hunter, J. M., and Merklin, R. J.: An experimental study on the healing of injured flexor tendons. Part 3. A microvascular study of the human flexor tendon sheath. Orthop. Surg., *34*:1544, 1983.

Matsui, T., Merklin, R. J., and Hunter, J. M.: A microvascular study of the human flexor tendons in the digital fibrous sheath. J. Jpn. Orthop. Assoc., *53*:307, 1979.

Chapter 8

GENERAL PRINCIPLES OF TREATMENT OF TENDON LESIONS

Raoul Tubiana

Although repair of traumatic lesions of the tendons of the hand is one of the most common surgical problems, the results are all too often disappointing. Recent progress as a result of improved and less traumatic surgical techniques has reduced iatrogenic lesions to a minimum.

It is difficult to present a chapter on the subject of tendon lesions without again stressing the technical aspects of repair.

GENERAL PRINCIPLES OF TECHNIQUE

Surgeons who are concerned with tendon repairs in the hand must master a technique that is totally aseptic and "atraumatic," to use Bunnell's expression. One must reduce surgical trauma to a minimum in order to preserve vascularization and gliding planes.

MINIMIZING VASCULAR DAMAGE

Because retraction of the proximal end of the tendon tears the mesotenon, one must keep the hand in a relaxed position after the injury, with the wrist and fingers in flexion for injured flexor tendons or in extension for extensor damage.

In acute cases there may be an advantage in repairing the vessels to improve nutrition. In injuries to the volar aspect of the wrist associated with tendon and vessel divisions, it is essential to re-establish flow in at least one of the major vessels, e.g., the radial or ulnar artery. In the digits, when the two palmar bundles are severed, re-establishment

of one artery with the aid of microvascular surgery will improve the chances for tendon healing.*

When the proximal end of the tendon is retracted, it should be sought through the same wound using external maneuvers or massage. One should never make a proximal incision to exteriorize the cut tendon and then reintroduce it into its bed. Such a maneuver increases vascular damage and tears more mesotenon.

Merle, Foucher, and Michon (1977) proposed the introduction of a silicone rubber implant into the wound via the empty sheath in a retrograde fashion (Fig. 8–1). This allows the surgeon to locate the extremity of the cut tendon and the site for a small counterincision and permits the tendon end to be sutured to the Silastic prosthesis and advanced along the sheath.

Excessive tension at the site of tendon suture diminishes the intratendinous microcirculation (Ketchum, 1977).

The suture technique must avoid strangulation of the tendon and ensure the least possible damage to the intratendinous circulation. Because the longitudinal intratendinous vessels are on the dorsal aspect of the flexor tendon, it is better to place the suture more volarly.

In flexor tendons, the vinculum longus to the profundus tendon arises in common with the retinaculum brevis to the superficialis tendon at the level of the proximal interphalangeal joint. This explains why the vascularization of the profundus tendon is deprived by removal of the superficialis at this level.

---

*See the chapter on wounds of the hands by Michon in Volume II.

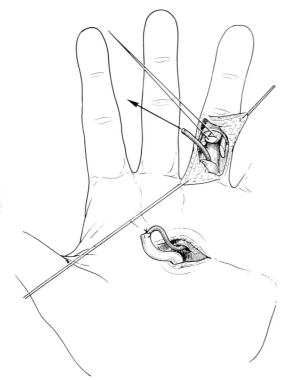

Figure 8–1. Extraction of the proximal end of the tendon with a flexible catheter. A silicone tube can also be used.

PRESERVING GLIDING PLANES

We will briefly review the most important rules for atraumatic surgery discussed in the chapter on surgical technique in Volume II.

1. The incision must not follow directly the course of the tendon (Fig. 8–2).
2. The instrumentation must be delicate and adapted to this special form of surgery.
3. Magnification facilitates dissection and suturing.
4. The neurovascular bundles are isolated with vessel loops.
5. The tendon ends and grafts are manipulated by traction sutures (Fig. 8–3).

The surgical technique has an undoubted influence on results. A technique based on gentleness, careful suturing, and careful hemostasis is vital in achieving optimal results.

METHODS OF TENDON REPAIR

There are two broad categories of tendon repair: Reconstructive methods aim to restore anatomical continuity by suturing, graft-

ing, or reinsertion. Palliative methods include transfer, tenodesis, and arthrodesis.

END TO END SUTURING

Studies of flexor tendon healing have shown that the extremities of the tendon must be held in apposition for at least three weeks if union is to occur, the suture material should be nonabsorbable and as nonirritating as possible, and the suturing technique should be "atraumatic."

Keeping the Tendon Ends Apposed

The methods used to keep the tendon ends apposed depend on the "physical" property of the suture and aim to produce an apposition strong enough to resist traction forces. The suturing techniques most commonly used are described later in this chapter. Experiments have shown that the sutured extremities of a tendon undergo some degeneration and that the resistance to traction offered by the suture diminishes over the first two weeks. To keep the ends apposed, therefore, it is essential to prevent their retraction. This can be achieved by using an appropriate

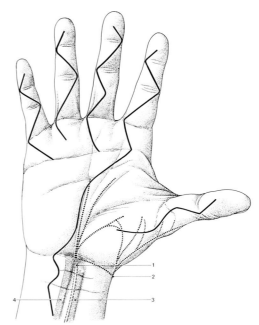

Figure 8–2. Zigzag incision for access to flexor tendons. 1 = palmar sensory branch of median nerve, 2 = sensory branches of radial nerve, 3 = flexor carpi radialis, 4 = palmaris longus.

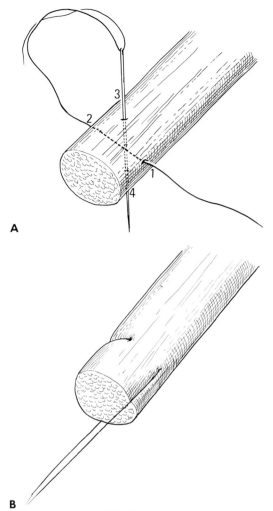

A

B

Figure 8–3. *A* and *B,* The extremities of the tendons are manipulated by traction sutures. These sutures are passed through twice at right angles.

The suture material should be as inert as possible. Any suture material acts as a foreign body and is a potential source of inflammatory reaction and adhesions. Catgut, linen, and silk have been held responsible for a number of failures. In the chapter on suture materials we have shown that stainless steel and synthetic fibers (polyester and silicone threads) are tolerated best of all. We use multifilament synthetic sutures, which are easier to handle than monofilament sutures and are covered by an impermeable coating that prevents fibroblastic infiltration and decreases local tissue reaction. Other authors prefer monofilament nylon or polypropylene.

The caliber of the suture used in tendon repair varies between 3-0 and 7-0. We avoid the use of metallic sutures adjacent to bony prominences. For example, in extensor tendons repaired with metal near the metacarpophalangeal joint, the suture tends to fragment when mobilized.

Because the suture is only necessary to maintain end to end contact for three or four weeks, Bunnell devised a removable suture by passing a pullout wire through a loop of

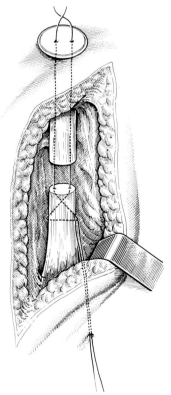

Figure 8–4. Bunnell removable suture with pullout wire.

suturing technique and immobilizing the joints in a relaxed position.

Reducing the Complications Due to the Suture

The suture should not traumatize the tendon or strangle it. Multiple loops, which result in extensive necrosis, should be avoided. Great care should be taken not to damage the epitenon.

Every suture material induces a local reaction and may give rise to peritendinous adhesions. As much of the suture as possible should be buried within the substance of the tendon.

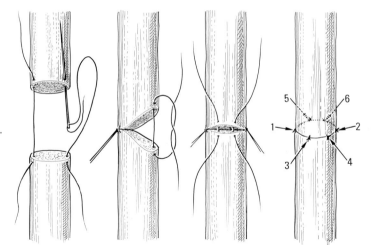

Figure 8–5. Peripheral suture.

the suture (Fig. 8–4). Other types of removable sutures have been introduced since, but the use of a pullout suture is not necessary if one uses fine, well tolerated material.

Suturing Procedures

The following procedures are best performed with the help of a magnifying device.

Peripheral Sutures. Sutures can be placed around the periphery of the tendon, in the epitenon, in an interrupted or continuous fashion (Fig. 8–5). This type of suture, comparable to a nerve suture, provides good contact but lacks strength. Interrupted mattress sutures, which are used when the tendon is flat (like the flexor superficialis near its insertion), are preferable to simple sutures (Fig. 8–6).

Crisscross Sutures. This method, although one of the most commonly used, is seldom performed correctly. It requires burying as much of the suture as possible and avoiding multiple loops, which are known to produce necrosis. A straight atraumatic needle, passed obliquely into one cut end, traces a crisscross pattern in one end and a symmetrical pattern in the other and emerges from the other cut end, the knot being buried between the two ends (Fig. 8–7). A few fine inverting sutures to appose the edges are inserted.

The Square Suture. This suture is passed at right angles to the axis of the tendon fibers to produce more resistant tethering. In certain cases, Bunnell inserts two square sutures about 5 mm. from the cut edge (Fig. 8–8). Because they cross the tendon at right angles

and diagonally, these sutures hold well and by their "basket" effect produce reasonable apposition.

The Grasping Suture. The use of grasping sutures was originated in Chicago by Koch, Mason, and Allen (1940). Two small sutures, which grasp the lateral tendon fibers, are placed about 1 cm. from the tendon ends. At this level they traverse the tendon to gain a firm hold and are then tied to their opposites in the other tendon end. This type of grasping suture was reintroduced by Kessler (1973) (Fig. 8–9): the transverse portion of the suture should be superficial with respect to the longitudinal one. Kessler placed a separate suture in each tendon end, with the knots buried between the cut tendon ends. Each knot produces a foreign body reaction which reduces the strength of the repair. A slight modification uses only one suture passed through both ends; one knot is then sufficient (Fig. 8–9C). Zechner et al. (1985) preferred to bury the knot inside the proximal end of the tendon (Fig. 8–9D). A grasping suture disturbs the intratendinous vascularization less than the crisscross suture.

Another suture technique done microscopically has been described by Tsuge et al. (1977): the looped nylon suture is placed within the longitudinal axis of the tendon

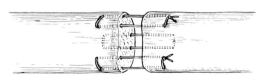

Figure 8–6. Interrupted mattress suture.

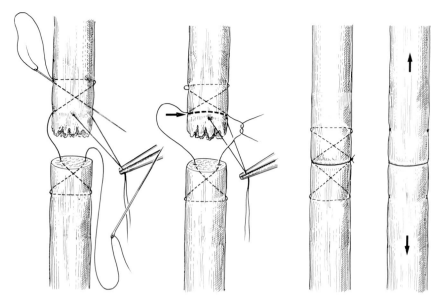

Figure 8–7. Crisscross suture.

(Fig. 8–10). Two additional small peripheral sutures are used to prevent twisting.

These grasping suturing procedures now tend to replace the others.

The Pullout Suture. Bunnell popularized this technique whereby a tension absorbing suture placed through the proximal end of the tendon resists muscle traction. When exposure is limited and little suturing area is available, as in the fingers, Bunnell places, in addition to the apposing stitch and proximal to it, a looped suture, which pulls against the muscle traction and is tethered to a button or a bolus of tulle gras on the skin. The whole suture complex can be removed after three weeks by means of pullout wire.

Duparc and Alnot (1973) suggested that the tether should emerge not in the hand but at the wrist where the risk of adhesions is reduced.

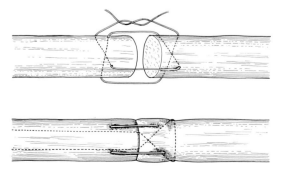

Figure 8–8. Square suture.

The tethering suture itself can be used by itself. With a double ended suture a loop is made with both arms emerging through the proximal cut end; these are then passed obliquely into the distal segment for a distance of about 2.5 cm. They are then brought out through the skin and fixed to a button, as already described.

Fixation on the proximal end of the tendon can be effected by a small harpoon mounted on a suture, that is, the "barbed wire" devised by Jenning and Yeager (1959). This technique has been used in extensor tendons on the dorsal aspect of the hand because it permits early mobilization. It is also useful for reinserting small avulsed fragments of bone with ligaments or tendons. It seems to be contraindicated for the flexor tendon, with the exception of an avulsion of the insertion.

The Blocked Suture. The aim in using blocked sutures again is to reduce the tension on the tendon suture by tethering both tendon extremities (Fig. 8–11). This procedure has been advocated in zones of great mobility, such as the fingers. The two tendon ends and the skin can be transfixed transversely by a pin (Montant, 1938) or by a needle (Fruchaud and Verdan, 1952, Fig. 8–12). Becker (1978) introduced the "bevel" technique for flexor tendon repair (Fig. 8–13). It provides enough strength to allow immediate postoperative mobilization while respecting the vascularity of the cut tendon ends (see Chapter 29).

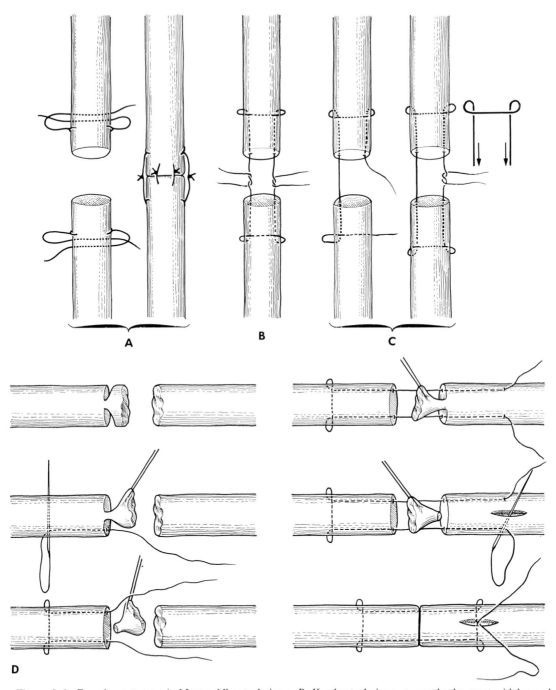

Figure 8–9. Grasping sutures. *A*, Mason Allen technique. *B*, Kessler technique, currently the most widely used. *C*, Technique of Kessler modified by Kleinert (1982) with only one knot between the tendon ends. It is important that the horizontal suture be superficial in relation to the longitudinal one. *D*, Zechner et al. (1985) bury the knot in the interior of the proximal end of the tendon to decrease the amount of reaction around the knot, a reaction that weakens the anastomosis.

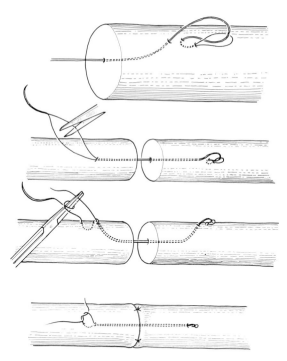

Figure 8–10. Looped nylon suture (Tsuge) using a needle mounted with both ends of the same suture material.

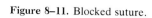

Figure 8–11. Blocked suture.

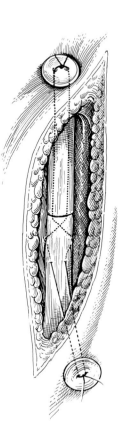

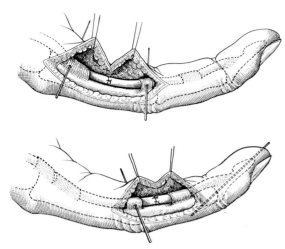

Figure 8–12. The two types of Verdan blocked suture.

The Surface Apposition Suture. The area of contact between the two tendon extremities is much more extensive than an end to end suture. Frontal splitting of the tendinous extremities permits broad surface contact of the ends. This technique is particularly useful in cases of tendon lengthening in the forearm.

The Transfixion Suture. One tendon end is transfixed by one or more passes of the other end (Fig. 8–14). This procedure is used to unite tendons of different calibers, the thinner tendon being threaded through the broader one. The extremity of the broader one may be opened like a "fish mouth" and molded around the thinner one (Pulvertaft, 1965; Fig. 8–15). At each transfixion a U suture is passed through both. Union is solid, but the junction is bulky.

The Buckling Suture. Buckling sutures are used when multiple anastomoses are needed. Thus, in forearm injuries a tendon may be used to transfix a number of severed tendons and then be sutured to itself.

Bone Insertion. Sometimes it is possible to insert the extremity of the tendon into the bone. These procedures are used to repair the long flexor of the thumb and the deep flexors of the fingers when the tendon has been sectioned near the insertion, or to fix the extremity of a tendon graft. The tech-

nique is described in Chapter 30 dealing with flexor tendon grafts (Fig. 8–16).

It is sometimes possible to lengthen the tendon in a favorable zone in order to diminish tension at the insertion, for instance, at the level of the musculotendinous junction in the forearm for the long flexor of the thumb (Rouhier, 1950).

Indications for Different Types of Sutures

The indications depend on the site of the suture, the power of the muscle whose tendon is to be repaired, and the projected date of mobilization.

Urbaniak et al. (1975) classified the sutures into three groups:

In the first group is the suture that is placed parallel to the collagen bundles, such as interrupted sutures placed circumferentially, or the Nicoladoni type of suture, which is the weakest type.

With the second group of sutures longitudinal tension is transformed into an oblique or transverse force on the extremities of the tendon; the resistance to rupture is greater. This group comprises loop sutures and figure of eight and grasping sutures. If one compares loop sutures (described by Bunnell) and grasping sutures (used by Kessler), their resistance is equivalent at the beginning, but at the fifth day the grasping suture is three times stronger. However, this difference disappears by the tenth day. A study by Greulich et al. (1977) has confirmed the better resistance afforded by grasping sutures. The gap resulting in various experiments was 2.5 mm. after placement of Kessler sutures, 6.7 mm. after the Bunnell sutures, and 9.8 mm. after the Lengeman sutures (interrupted peripheral sutures).

The third group of sutures comprising transfixion sutures, such as Pulvertaft's suture, yield the strongest anastomoses. Traction on the tendon exerts a compressive force applied from one tendon to the other, but the volume of the anastomosis prohibits use of such a suture in areas of confinement. In those areas (for example, in the finger) only end to end anastomoses are used.

Other elements affect the resistance of the suture. For instance, tying a knot weakens the material and alters its tensile strength but to different extents, depending on the material used (Urbaniak et al., 1975). The extent

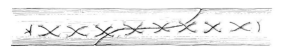

Figure 8–13. Becker's "bevel" technique.

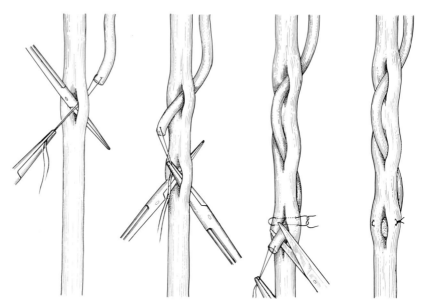

Figure 8–14. Transfixion suture.

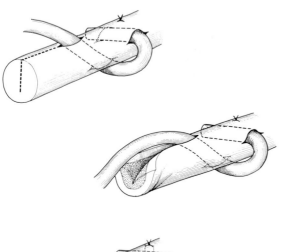

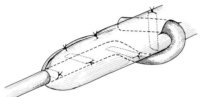

Figure 8–15. Pulvertaft "fish mouth" technique used to join two tendons of different caliber.

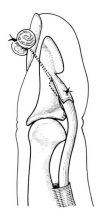 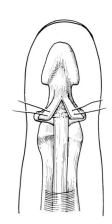

Figure 8–16. Bone insertion of the tendon extremity using a transosseous suture tethered on a button with a pullout wire.

of ischemia differs with the type of suture. Interrupted peripheral sutures are the least dangerous sutures, and peripheral grasping sutures (Kessler) are probably less dangerous to vascularization than loop sutures. Ketchum (1977) has shown that regardless of the type of suture, excessive tension produces the same effect of the microcirculation.

Immobilization Following Tendon Suturing

The length of the immobilization period following tendon repair is a complex and controversial subject and many factors are involved. One must strike a balance between the effect of mobilization and the effect of tension on the suture line. Mobilization of the tendons (in particular, the flexors, which are in confined sheaths) aids venous and lymphatic drainage. Stasis following immobilization is a factor in ischemia, edema, and adhesion formation. Prolonged immobilization of the finger can result in joint stiffness, which may persist for a long time if the joints are immobilized in unfavorable positions.

On the other hand, if one considers that adhesions are unavoidable in tendon repair because of the tendinous blood supply, it seems illogical to allow early excessive mobilization and incur the risk of rupturing the adhesions. Mobilization also increases tension at the suture line and accentuates the tendency for a gap to occur at the site of the suture.

Experiments done by Mason and Shearon (1932) have shown that early active mobili-

zation increases the inflammatory reaction of the tendon and risks disrupting the suture. They concluded that it would be difficult to trust the strength of the anastomosis, for the divided ends of the tendon undergo a degenerative process (perhaps due to the suturing technique), and recommended immobilization for at least three weeks.

Yet, there is now proof (Matthews and Richards, 1976; Celli et al., 1979; Gelberman, 1982) that early mobilization does not prevent the formation of adhesions, but affects their physical properties by limiting the formation of rigid adhesions between the tendon and the fibrous structures which surround it and by altering the orientation of the scar tissue and vessels; however, this also requires that this mobilization not be accompanied by tension on the repair.

Numerous surgeons have now adopted a method for early passive mobilization of the interphalangeal joints, provided by an elastic band traction (Young and Harmon, 1942). Since 1954 this technique has been used by Kleinert following flexor tendon repair (Fig. 8–17). The publication of his results has widened the use of this procedure. (This is described by its author in Chapter 28.)

Elastic traction causing flexion of the fingers, while the wrist and metacarpophalangeal joint are maintained in flexion, allows only limited passive mobilization. Merle, Foucher, and Michon (1976) established radiographically that the amplitude of movement in the area of the suture is only 3 to 4 mm. within the digital canal (Fig. 8–18). They also verified, as Lister did (1977), by electromyography the lack of activity in the flexors during passive mobilization just as during active finger extension (Fig. 8–19). This minimal movement, in the area of the suture, limits the formation of restricting adhesions. This is of much less magnitude than a total active finger mobilization where the amplitude of movement in the digital canal reaches 1 cm., with a much greater danger of rupture. Early passive mobilization is particularly indicated when both flexors are repaired in order to avoid the formation of dense adhesions between the two sutured tendons. Duran and Hauser (1975) described a method of mobilizing each of the repaired tendons by passive movements separately at the proximal interphalangeal and then the distal interphalangeal joints. Duran estimated that no traction should be exerted on the suture

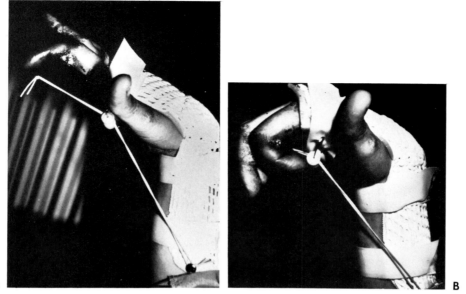

Figure 8–17. *A* and *B*, Splinting with rubber band traction used after suture of the flexor tendons of the index finger (after Kleinert and modified by Foucher and Merle, who insert a pulley overlying the proximal transverse palmar crease).

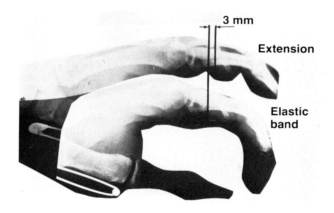

Figure 8–18. Displacement of tendon suture line of the flexor profundus in zone 2 mobilized by a rubber traction according to Kleinert technique (Merle, Foucher, and Michon).

Figure 8–19. Electromyogram of the flexor digitorum muscles during extension of a flexor tendon primary suture with repair and splinting by the Kleinert technique (Paquin, Merle, and Foucher).

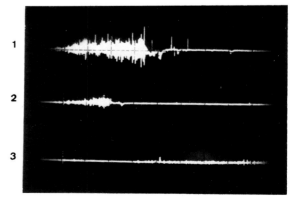

for about four and one-half weeks because he feels early mobilization weakens the repair. The strength of a tendon suture submitted to no tension is weaker during the first weeks following repair than a suture under moderate tension (Ketchum). This method of early passive mobilization is also applicable after repair of the extensor tendons.*

In a comparative study on the effect of immobilization or early passive mobilization on the results of primary flexor tendon repair in zone 2 (see Chapter 37), Strickland and Glogovac (1980) reported more secondary ruptures after immobilization than after early mobilization. Lister et al. (1977) as well as Duran and Hauser (1975) similarly report a low incidence of rupture following early mobilization.

Experience has shown that there is less need for tenolysis following early mobilization.

The evidence now available seems to indicate that, provided there is no tension at the suture line, early mobilization is one of the elements that have contributed to the improvement in results of primary flexor tendon repair. One cannot directly extrapolate these results to those obtained with tendon grafting, in which the physiological problems and nutritional needs are different. However, the need for a similar appraisal of technique is obvious.

EARLY ACTIVE MOBILIZATION

Rarely do surgeons trust the physical qualities of the suture and allow early active mobilization after flexor tendon repair (Kessler, 1969; Becker, 1977; Brunelli, 1980). Several strategies have been proposed for avoiding any tension in the area of the suture during mobilization: maintenance of the proximal joints with the repaired tendon in a relaxed position, the proximal anastomosis of the tendon sutured to the neighboring active flexor tendon (Furlow, 1976), and digital suture supported by a button (Mantero, 1974) (Fig. 8–20).

Early active mobilization of extensor tendons on the back of the hand and wrist has been applied by numerous surgeons (Allieu, 1971; Bertolotti, 1979).

---

*See Chapter 23, "Protected Passive Mobilization after Suturing of the Extensor Tendons of the Hand."

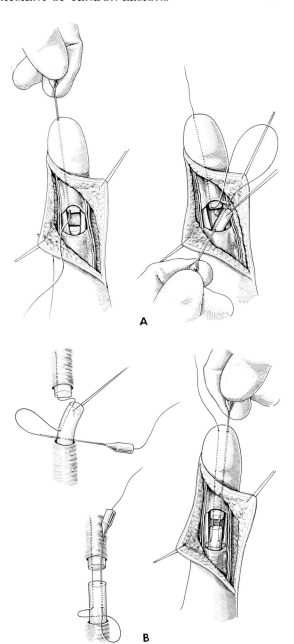

Figure 8–20. *A* and *B*, Mantero technique for suture of flexor tendons with distal fixation to a button, permitting early mobilization. A similar technique, using a double mounted needle, has been described by Brunelli.

TENDON GRAFTS

A tendon graft is used to compensate for a loss of substance. It offers the advantage that the sutures are tension-free and can be placed in an optimal position, away from the fibrous pulleys. The graft can be inserted between the two tendinous segments (bridge or segmental graft). More commonly a terminal graft is used, which is inserted directly into the bone.

Sources of Tendon Grafts

These transplants come from several sources. In practice most grafts are autogenous, but as we have seen in the previous chapter, allografts and xenografts have been used. Further experimentation with nonautogenous grafts will reveal more about their value in the hand and perhaps will lead to the setting up of tendon banks. Despite the availability of conserved tendons, few surgical centers are using them at this time (Iselin, 1975).

Some surgeons prefer a graft with a caliber analogous to that of the tendon being repaired for reasons of strength and ease of suturing. Thin grafts are reincorporated better and they slide more easily. Pulvertaft (1956) has described how to join two tendon extremities of unequal caliber in a congruous manner.

A wide range of autografts is available, and the choice depends on the length, caliber, and accessibility of each. The technique for taking these grafts is described in Chapter 30 on flexor tendon grafts.

The most common source for a transplant is the palmaris longus: it is long, slender, resistant, and readily accessible. Admittedly it is not a constant structure, but its absence is easily detected clinically. Although the muscle fibers sometimes have a low insertion, the tendon can usually be relied upon to provide a graft 11 cm. in length in an adult, i.e., sufficiently long to run from the distal phalanx of a digit to the proximal part of the palm.

The plantaris tendon can also be used with no loss of function, but it is too inconstant and its absence can only be detected surgically. It is sometimes too slender and may have multiple attachments to the soleus tendon, but on the whole it constitutes excellent transplant material. Its length is such that it can be used to graft two flexor tendons. Because of its slimness, it is the transplant of choice to replace the digital extensors and the flexor digiti minimi and to reconstruct the flexor profundus while preserving the flexor superficialis.

When there is more than one tendon to be replaced, it may be convenient to use the long extensor tendons of the toes, whose action (apart from that of the fifth toe) is supplemented by the extensor brevis tendons.

The tendons of the flexor digitorum superficialis, although bulkier and intrasynovial, can be used as grafts in multiple injuries of the hand. When a digit is amputated, both its flexor and extensor tendons can be used for the repair of other tendons in the hand.

Finally, one can use the extensor proprius or extensor communis of the fingers as a thin graft for a specific use (pulley reconstruction, bridge graft).

A tendon, part of a tendon, or a strip of tensor fascia lata can be used as a graft following sheath reconstruction using a Silastic implant.

Tendon Anastomoses and Transfers

The action of an injured tendon can be supplemented by a muscle in close proximity either by effecting a simple anastomosis to the distal extremity of the severed tendon or by the transfer of an adjacent tendon.

Transfers must follow certain basic rules for treatment of paralysis:*

1. The transferred muscle must be healthy.
2. The transferred tendon must pass through a bed that allows it to glide easily.
3. As far as possible, the tendon should have a straight line of pull, for angulation of the transfer could reduce its effective force.
4. The amplitude of movement of the tendon should be sufficient so that the desired movement can be performed.
5. The transfer of one tendon to supplement the action of two tendons of different amplitudes should be avoided.

The transfer is fixed either directly to the bone at the point of insertion of the destroyed tendon or on the distal extremity of the severed tendon.

Tenodesis and Arthrodesis

When restoration of a lost movement cannot be expected as a result of tendon repair or tendon transfer, one may have to employ tenodesis or arthrodesis to prevent deformities.

Tenodesis consists of tethering the proximal end of the injured tendon in such a way

---

*See chapter on treatment of paralysis in Volume IV.

as to restrict the mobility of the joint and prevent a fixed deformity. When the joint keeps its mobility through the action of an antagonist, the tenodesis is active and may serve a useful function.

Arthrodeses are performed following irreparable tendon injuries to correct a fixed deformity or to stabilize a mobile articulation that has lost its active motor muscles.

Artificial Tendons

A variety of materials have been tried for this purpose, but replacement of the tendons of the hand poses particularly difficult problems. Favorable short term results are often the subject of hurried publications, but figures from long term studies are rarely seen reported. Among these publications, we can mention those by Sarkin (1956), Grau (1958), Bader and Curtin (1971), and Hunter (1965 and 1986). Research is progressing in several centers with the use of more inert and more resistant materials or materials that guide the growth of connective tissue. Totally inert implants are not yet available, and living tissue is subject to wear and tear, not to mention the as yet unsolved problem of fixation. All these obstacles can only stimulate the imagination of the researcher.

REFERENCES

Adamson, J. E., and Wilson, J. N.: The history of flexor tendon grafting. J. Bone Joint Surg., 43A:709, 1961.

Allieu, Y., and Romieu, C.: L'utilisation du "Barb-Wire de Jenning" dans les sutures tendineuses: Absence d'immobilisation post-opératoire. Ann. Chir., 25:19–20, 987–994, 1971.

Allieu, Y.: L'utilisation du Barb-Wire de Jenning en chirurgie de la main. Ann. Chir., 31(4):359–361, 1977.

Ashley, F. L., et al.: Experimental and clinical studies on the application of monomolecular cellulose filter tubes to create artificial tendon sheaths in digits. Plast. Reconst. Surg., 23:526–534, 1959.

Ashley, F. L., Polak, R., Stone, R. S., and Marmor, L.: An evaluation of the healing process in avian and mammalian digital flexor tendons following the application of an artificial tendon sheath (silastic). In Proceedings of the American Society for Surgery of the Hand. J. Bone Joint Surg., 44A:1038, 1962.

Bader, K., and Curtin, J. W.: Clinical survey of silicone underlays and pulleys in tendon surgery in hands. Plast. Reconst. Surg., 47(6):576, 1971.

Becker, H.: Repair of flexor tendons in the hand. Hand, 10:37, 1978.

Bergljung, L.: Vascular reactions after tendon suture and tendon transplantation. A stereo-microangiographic study on the calcaneal tendon of the rabbit. Scand. J. Plast. Reconst. Surg., Suppl. 4, 1968.

Biesalski, K.: Ueber Sehnenscheidenauswechslung. Deutsche Med. Wochnschr., 36:1615–1618, 1910.

Bloch, J. C., and Bonnet, P.: Plaies des tendons de la main. Congrès Français de Chirurgie, 1929.

Bora, F. W., Lane, J. M., Heppenstall, R. B., and Prockop, D. J.: The alteration of scar by collagen inhibitors. Am. Soc. for Surg. of the Hand. Annual Meeting Washington, 1972.

Bouvier, H.: Mémoire sur la section du tendon d'Achille dans le traitement des pieds-bots. Mem. Acad. Med. (Paris), 7:411, 1838.

Boyes, J. H., and Stark, H. H.: Flexor tendon grafts in the fingers and thumb. A study of factors influencing results in 1,000 cases. J. Bone Joint Surg., 53A:1332, 1971.

Braithwaite, F., and Brockis, J.: Vascularisation of a tendon graft. Br. J. Plast. Surg., 4:130, 1951.

Brand, P. W.: Tendon grafting. J. Bone Joint Surg., 43B:444, 1961.

Brand, P. W., Cramer, K. C., and Ellis, J. C.: Tendon and pulleys at the M. P. Joint of the finger. J. Bone Joint Surg., 57A:779, 1975.

Brockis, J. G.: The blood supply of the flexor and extensor tendons of the fingers in man. J. Bone Joint Surg., 35B:131, 1953.

Brunelli, G., and Monini, L.: Technique personnelle de suture des tendons fléchisseurs des doigts avec mobilisation immédiate. Annales Chir. Main, 1:92–96, 1982.

Buck-Gramcko, D.: Verletzungen der Beugesehen. In Nigst, H., Buck-Gramcko, D., and Millesi, H. (Editors): Handchirurgie. Vol. II. Stuttgart, Thieme, 1983, Chap. 28.

Bunnell, S.: Repair of tendons in the fingers and description of two new instruments. Surg. Gynec. Obstet., 26:103, 1918.

Bunnell, S.: Surgery of the Hand. Philadelphia, Lippincott, 1944.

Caplan, H. S., Hunter, J. M., and Merklin, R. J.: The intrinsic vascularisation of flexor tendons in the human. In Proceedings, American Society of the Hand. J. Bone Joint Surg., 57A:726, 1975.

Carroll, R. E., and Bassett, A. L.: Formation of tendon sheath by silicone rod implants. J. Bone Joint Surg., 45A:884–885, 1963.

Chacha, P.: Free autologous composite tendon grafts for division of both flexor tendons within the digital theca of the hand. J. Bone Joint Surg., 56A:5, 1974.

Codivilla, A.: Sur trapianti tendinei nella practica ortopedica. Arch. Orthop., 16:225–250, 1889.

Colville, J., Callison, J. R., and White, W. L.: Role of the mesotendon in tendon blood supply. Plast. Reconst. Surg., 43:53, 1969.

Cordrey, L. S., McCorkle, H., and Hilton, E.: A comparative study of fresh autogenous and preserved homogenous tendon grafts in rabbits. J. Bone Joint Surg., 45B:182–195, 1963.

Dionis, P.: "Chief Chirurgeon to the late Dauphiness and to the present Duchess of Burgundy." A Course of Chirurgical Operations Demonstrated in the Royal Garden at Paris, Jacob Tonson, London, 392, 1710.

Duchenne, G. B.: Physiologie des mouvements. Paris, Baillières, 1867. Trans. Kaplan, E. Philadelphia, Lippincott, 1949.

Duparc, J., Alnot, J. Y., Nordin, J. Y., and Pidhorz, L.: Plaies récentes des tendons fléchisseurs au doigt. Ann. Chir., 27:(5):467–478, 1973.

Duran, R. J., and Hauser, R. G.: Controlled passive motion following flexor tendon repair in zones two and three. *In* AAOS Symposium on tendon surgery in the hand. St. Louis, The C. V. Mosby Co., 1975, p. 105.

Duran, R. J., Hauser, R. G., Coleman, C. R., et al.: A preliminary report in the use of controlled passive motion following flexor tendon repair in zones II and III. J. Hand Surg., *1*:79, 1976.

Edwards, D. A. W.: The blood supply and lymphatic drainage of tendons. J. Anat., *80*:147, 1946.

Eiken, O., Lundborg, G., and Rank, I.: The role of the digital synovial sheath in tendon grafting. An experimental and clinical study on autologous tendon grafting in the digit. Scand. J. Plast. Reconstr. Surg., *9*:182, 1975.

Eiken, O., Holmberg, J., and Ekerot, L.: Restoration of the digital tendon sheath. A new concept of tendon grafting. Scand. J. Plast. Reconstr. Surg., *14*:89–97, 1980.

Eiken, O., Hagberg, L., and Lundborg G.: Evolving biologic concepts as applied to tendon surgery. Clin. Plast. Surg., *8*:1–12, 1981.

Flynn, J. E., and Graham, J. H.: Healing following tendon suture and tendon transplants. Surg. Gynec. Obst.,*115*:467–472, 1962.

Foucher, G., Merle, M., and Michon, J.: Place de la microchirurgie dans la réparation de l'appareil fléchisseur de la main. Actual. Chirur., *3*:129–130, 1977.

Foucher, G., and Merle, M.: La suture des tendons fléchisseurs selon la technique de Kleinert. Ann. Chir. Main, *3*:170–172, 1984.

Fruchaud: Chirurgie de guerre, 1939.

Furlow, L. T.: The role of tendon tissues in tendon healing. Plast. Reconstr. Surg., *57*:39, 1976.

Galien (Galen): Œuvres Anatomiques, Physiologiques et Médicales, traduites par Ch. Daremberg. Baillière, Paris, 1854.

Gambier, R., Asvasadurian, A., and Venturini, G.: Recherches sur la vascularisation des tendons. Rev. Chir. Orthop.,*48*:225, 1962.

Gelberman, R. H., Woo, S. L., Lothringer, K. et al.: Effects of early intermittent passive mobilization on healing canine flexor tendons. J. Hand Surg., *7*:170–175, 1982.

Gonzalez, R. I.: Experimental use of teflon in tendon surgery. Plast. Reconstr. Surg., *23*:535–539, 1959.

Grau, H. P.: Le tendon artificiel:étude experimentale. Plast. Reconstr. Surg., *22*:564–566, 1958.

Greulich, M., Lanz, V., and Glockner, J.: Sennennaht im Bereich der Sehnenscheide. Experimentelle untersuchungen. Handchirurgie, *9*(3):113–118, 1977.

Von Haller, A.: Von den empfindlichen und reizbaren Teilen des menschlichen Korpens. Leipzig, 1752.

Heuck, G.: Ein Beitrag zur Sehnenplastik. Zentralbl. Chir., *9*:289–292, 1881.

Hueston, J. T., Hubble, B., and Rigg, B. R.: Homografts of the digital flexor tendon system. Aust. N. Zeal. J. Surg., *36*:269, 1967.

Hunter, J. M.: Artificial tendons. Early development and application. Am. J. Surg., *109*:325, 1965.

Iselin, F.: Preliminary observations on the use of chemically stored tendinous allografts in hand surgery. *In* AAOS Symposium on tendon surgery in the hand. St. Louis, The C. V. Mosby Co., 1975, p. 66.

Iselin, M.: Chirurgie de la Main. Masson édit., Paris, 1955.

Iselin, M., and LaFaury, G.: Pathologie du tendon fléchisseur sectionné chez l'homme. Mém. Ac. Chir., *76*:789, 1950.

Iselin, M., de La Plaza, R., and Flores, A.: Surgical use of homologous tendon grafts preserved in cialit. Plast. Reconstr. Surg., *32*:401, 413, 1963.

Jenning, E. R., and Yeager, G. H.: Suture tendineuse avec Barb-Wire. Arch. Surg., *70*(4):566–569, 1959.

Kessler, I.: The grasping technique for tendon repair. Hand, *5*:253–255, 1973.

Ketchum, L. D.: Effects of triamcinolone on tendon healing and function. Plast. Reconstr. Surg., *47*:471, 1971.

Ketchum, L. D.: Primary tendon healing: a review. J. Hand Surg., *2*(6):428–435, 1977.

Ketchum, L. D., Martin, N., and Kappel, D.: Factors affecting tendon gap and tendon strength at the site of tendon repair. Plast. Reconstr. Surg., *59*:1977.

Kirschner, M.: Ueber freie Sehnen und Fascientransplantation. Beitr. Klin. Chir., *65*:472–503, 1909.

Kleinert, H. E., Kutz, J. E., Atasoy, E., et al.: Primary repair of flexor tendons. Orthop. Clin. N. Am., *4*:865, 1973.

Kleinert, H. E., Kutz, J. E., and Cohen, M. J.: Primary repair of zone 2 flexor tendon lacerations. *In* AAOS Symposium on tendon surgery in the hand. St. Louis, The C. V. Mosby Co., 1975, p. 91.

Kleinert, H. E., and Smith, D. J.: Primary and secondary repairs of flexor and extensor tendon injuries. *In* Flynn, J. E. (Editor): Hand Surgery, 3rd ed. Baltimore, Williams and Wilkins, 1982.

Kolliker , von A.: Mikroskopische Anatomie oder Bewebelehre des Menschen (quoted by Mayer). Leipzig, Engelmann, 1850.

La Caffinière, J. Y. de: Chirurgie de la poulie proximale dans les plaies des tendons longs fléchisseurs des doigts. Ann. Chir. Plast. *19*:201–211, 1974.

Lane, M. J., Black, J., and Bora, F. W.: Gliding function following flexor tendon injury. J. Bone Joint Surg., *58A*(7):985–989, 1976.

Lange, F.: Ueber periostale Sehnenverpflanzungen bei Lahmungen. Münchener Med. Wochnschr., *47*:486–490, 1900.

Leffert, D. R., and Weiss, C.: The Vincula. J. Bone Joint Surg., *50A*:1191–1192, 1974.

Lewis, D., and Davis, C. B.: Experimental direct transplantation of tendon and fascia. J. Am. Med. Assn., *57*:540–546, 1911.

Lexer, E.: Die Verwertung der freien Sehnentransplantation. Langenbecks Arch. Klin. Chir., *98*:818–852, 1912.

Lindsay, W. K., and Thomson, H. G.: Digital flexor tendons: an experimental study. Part I. The significance of each component of the flexor mechanism in tendon healing. Br. J. Plast. Surg., *12*:289–316, 1960.

Lindsay, W. K., Thomson, H. G., and Walker, F. G.: Digital flexor tendons: an experimental study. Part II. The significance of a gap occurring at the line of suture. Br. J. Plast. Surg., *13*:1, 1960.

Lindsay, W. K., and McDougall, E. P.: Digital flexor tendons: an experimental study. Part III. The fate of autogenous digital flexor tendon grafts. Br. J. Plast. Surg., *13*:293–304, 1961.

Lindsay, W. K., and Birch, J. R.: The fibroblast in flexor tendon healing. Plast. Reconstr. Surg., *34*:223, 1964.

Lister, G. D., Kleinert, H. E., Kutz, J. E., and Atasoy, E.: Primary flexor tendon repair followed by immediate controlled mobilization. J. Hand. Surg., *2*(6):441–451, 1977.

Lister, G. D.: Incision and closure of the flexor sheath during primary tendon repair. Hand, *15*:123–135, 1983.

Lundborg, G.: The microcirculation in rabbit tendon. In vivo studies after mobilisation and transection. An experimental study. Hand, 7:1, 1975.

Lundborg, G., Myrhage, P. D., and Rydevik, B.: The vascularization of human flexor tendons within the digital synovial sheath region, structural and functional aspects. J. Hand Surg., 2(6):417–427, 1977.

Lundborg, G., and Rank, F.: Experimental studies on cellular mechanisms involved in healing of animal and human flexor tendons in synovial environment. Hand, 12:3–11, 1980.

Lundborg, G., and Rank, F.: Experimental intrinsic healing of flexor tendons based upon synovial fluid nutrition. J. Hand Surg., 3(1):21–31, 1978.

McMaster, P. E.: Tendon and muscle ruptures. Clinical and experimental studies on the causes and location of subcutaneous ruptures. J. Bone Joint Surg., 15:709, 1933.

Malgaigne, J. F.: Œuvres Complètes d'Ambroise Paré. Vol. III. Baillière, Paris, 1841, p. 42.

Manske, P. R., Whiteside, L. A., and Lesker, P. A.: Nutrient pathways to flexor tendons using hydrogen washout technique. J. Hand Surg., 3:(1):32–36, 1978.

Manske, P. R., and Lesker, P. A.: Nutrition pathways of flexor tendons in primates. J. Hand Surg., 7:436–444, 1982.

Mason, M. L.: Primary and secondary tendon suture. Surg. Gynec. Obstet., 70(2-A):392–402, 1940.

Mason, M. L., and Shearon, C. G.: Process of tendon repair. Arch. Surg., 25:615–692, 1932.

Mason, M. L., and Allen, H. S.: Rate of healing of tendons. Ann. Surg., 113:424–459, 1941.

Matthews, P., and Richards, H.: The repair potential of digital flexor tendons. J. Bone Joint Surg., 56B:618, 1974.

Matthews, P., and Richards, H.: Factors in the adherence of flexor tendons after repair. J. Bone Joint Surg., 58B:230, 1976.

Mayer, L.: The physiological method of tendon transplantations. I. Historical: anatomy and physiology of tendons. Surg. Gynec. Obstet. 22:182, 1916.

Mayer, L.: The physiological method of tendon transplantations. II. Operative technic. Surg. Gynec. Obstet. 22:198, 1916.

Mayer, L.: The physiological method of tendon transplantations. III. Experimental and clinical experiences. Surg. Gynec. Obstet. 22:472, 1916.

Mayer, L.: Reconstruction of digital tendon sheaths. J. Bone Joint Surg., 18:607–616, 1936.

Mayer, L., and Ransohoff, N.: reconstruction of the digital tendon sheath. A contribution to the physiological method of repair of damaged finger tendons. J. Bone Joint Surg., 18:607, 1936.

McDowell, L. C., and Snyder, M. D.: Tendon healing: an experimental model in dog. J. Hand Surg., 2(2):122–126, 1977.

Merle, M., Foucher, G., and Michon, J.: Extraction atraumatique du bout proximal du tendon fléchisseur. Ann. Chir., 31(4):357, 1977.

Michon, J., and Vilain, R.: Lésions traumatiques des tendons de la main. Masson édit., Paris, 1974.

Mittelmeier, H.: Experimentalle Untersuchungen zur Pathologie und Verhütung der post-traumatischen Sehnenverwachsung. Hefte Unfallheilk, 73:186, 1963.

Monod: Plaies des tendons: greffe tendineuse. Bull. Mem. Soc. Chir. Paris, 13:297–299, 1887.

Montant, R.: Section des tendons fléchisseurs des doigts. Technique réparatrice personnelle. Mem. Acad. Chir., 64:1344–1346, 1938.

Nageotte, J.: Résultats éloignés de la greffe morte employée pour réparer les pertes de substance des tendons chez l'homme. C.R. Soc. Biol., 95:1552, 1926.

Nicoladoni, C.: Ein Vorschlag zur Sehnennaht. Wien. Med. Wschr., 30:144, 1880.

Nicolle, F. V.: A silastic tendon prosthesis as an adjunct to flexor tendon grafting. An experimental and clinical evaluation. Br. J. Plast. Surg., 22:224, 1969.

Nigst, H.: Chirurgie des Beugesehnen. Basler Handchirurgische Arbeitstagung. Handchirurgie, 8:225, 1976.

Paneva-Holevich, E.: Two stage tenoplasty in injury of the flexor tendon of the hand. J. Bone Joint Surg., 51A:21–32, 1969.

Paneva-Holevich, E.: Résultats de traitement des lésions multiples des tendons fléchisseurs des doigts par greffe effectuée, en deux temps. Rev. Chir. Orthop., 58:481–489, 1972.

Paneva-Holevich, E.: Reconstructive Surgery of the Flexor Tendons of the Hand. Sofia, Medicina i Fizkultura, 1977.

Paré, A.: Les Œuvres de M. Ambroise Paré. Paris, Chez Gabriel Buon, 1575.

Peacock, E. E.: A study of the circulation in normal tendons and healing grafts. Ann. Surg., 149:415, 1959.

Peacock, E. E., and Van Winkle, W.: Surgery and Biology of Wound Repair. Philadelphia, W. B. Saunders Co., 1970.

Peacock, E. E., and Madden, J. W.: Human composite tissue tendon allografts. Ann. Chir., 166:624, 1967.

Peacock, E. E., and Madden, J. W.: Some studies on the effects of beta-aminopropionitrile in patients with injured flexor tendons. Surgery, 66:215, 1969.

Peer, L. A.: Transplantation of Tissues, Cartilage, Bone, Fascia, Tendon and Muscle. Baltimore. Williams & Wilkins Co., 1955, pp. 277–295.

Peterson, W. W., Manske, P. R., and Lesker, P. A.: The effect of flexor sheath integrity on nutrient uptake by primate flexor tendons. J. Hand Surg., 111:413–416, 1986.

Peyrot: Transplantation chez l'homme d'un tendon emprunté à un chien. Guérison avec rétablissement partiel de la fonction. Bull. Mem. Soc. Chir. Paris, 12:356–361, 1886.

Potenza, A. D.: Tendon healing within the flexor digital sheath in the dog. J. Bone Joint Surg., 44A:49–64, 1962.

Potenza, A. D.: Effect of associated trauma on healing of divided tendons. J. Trauma, 2:175–184, 1962.

Potenza, A. D.: Critical evaluation of flexor tendon healing and adhesion formation within artificial digital sheaths. J. Bone Joint Surg., 45A:1217–1233, 1963.

Potenza, A. D.: Prevention of adhesions to healing digital flexor tendons. J.A.M.A., 187:187–191, 1964.

Potenza, A. D.: The healing of autogenous tendon grafts within the flexor digital sheath in dogs. J. Bone Joint Surg., 46A:1462–1484, 1964.

Potenza, A. D.: Concepts of tendon healing and repair. In AAOS Symposium on Tendon Surgery in the Hand. St. Louis. The C. V. Mosby Co., 1975, p. 18.

Pulvertaft, R. G.: Tendon grafts for flexor tendon injury in the fingers and thumb. J. Bone Joint Surg., 38B:175, 1956.

Pulvertaft, R. G.: Suture materials and tendon junctures. Am. J. Surg., 109:346–352, 1965.

Rehn, E.: Die homoplastiche Sehnentransplantation in Tierexperiment. Beitr. Klin. Chir., 68:417–447, 1910.

Richards, H. J.: Digital flexor tendon repair and return of function. Ann. R. Coll. Surg., England, 59:25–32, 1977.

Robson, A. W. H.: A case of tendon grafting. Tr. Clin. Soc. London, 22:289, 1889.

Rouhier, F.: La restauration due tendon long fléchisseur du pouce, sans sacrifice du tendon primitif. J. Chir., 66:8–9, 1950.

Sappey, P. C.: Traité d'Anatomie. Paris, Delahaye et Lecrosnier Edit., 1888.

Sarkin, T. L.: Le remplacement plastique des tendons fléchisseurs des doigts traumatisés. Br. J. Surg., 44:232–240, 1956.

Schwarz, W.: Ueber die anatomischen Vorgänge bei der Sehnenregeneration und dem plastichen Ersatz von Sehnendefekten durch Sehne, Fascie und Bindegewebe. Deutsche Ztschr. Chir., 173:301, 1922.

Seiffert, K., and Schmidt, K. P.: Preserved tendon grafts in hand surgery. Trans. Fifth Internat. Congr. Plast. Surg., London, Butterworths, 1971.

Skoog, T., and Personn, B. H.: An experimental study of the early healing of tendons. Plast. Reconstr. Surg., 13:384–399, 1954.

Smith, J. W.: Blood supply of tendons. Am. J. Surg., 109:272, 1965.

Smith, J. W., and Conway, H.: La dynamique du glissement des tendons normaux et greffés. Rev. Chir. Orthop., 53:185, 1966.

Strickland, J. W., and Glogovac, S. V.: Digital function following flexor tendon repair in zone II: a comparison of immobilization and controlled passive motion techniques. J. Hand Surg., 5:535–543, 1980.

Tsuge, K., Ikuta, Y., and Matshuishi, Y.: Repair of flexor tendons by intratendinous tendon suture. J. Hand Surg., 2(6):436–440, 1977.

Tubiana, R.: Incisions and technics in tendon grafting. Am. J. Surg., 109(3):339–345, 1965.

Tubiana, R.: La réparation des tendons fléchisseurs. Etat actuel des recherches biologiques. Rev. Chir Orthop., 58(7):637–648, 1972.

Tubiana, R.: Les voies d'abord dans la chirurgie des tendons de la main. Ann. Chir. Plast., 2:99–109, 1960.

Tubiana, R.: La réparation des tendons fléchisseurs dans la zone 2. Ann. Chir., 32:619–626, 1978.

Urbaniak, J. R., Cahill, J. D., and Mortension, R. A.: Tendon suturing methods: analysis of tensile strengths. In AAOS Symposium on tendon surgery in the hand. St. Louis, The C. V. Mosby Co., 1975, p. 70.

Vainio, K.: Surgery of the rheumatoid hand. In Graham, W. D. (Editor): Orthopaedics. Vol. 5. London, Butterworths, 1967, Chap. 10, pp. 219–236.

Vaughan Jackson, O. J.: Rheumatoid hand deformities considered in the light of tendon imbalance. J. Bone Joint Surg., 44B:764, 1962.

Velpeau, A. A.: Nouveaux Éléments de Médecine Opératoire. Augmentée d'un Traité des Bandages de Petite Chirurgie. 2nd ed. Paris, J. B. Baillière, 1839.

Verdan, C.: Chirurgie Réparatrice et Fonctionnelle des Tendons de la Main. Paris, Expansion Scientifique Française, 1952.

Verdan, C., and Michon, J.: Le traitement des plaies des tendons fléchisseurs des doigts. Rev. Chir. Orthop., 47:287, 1961.

Verdan, C.: Half a century of flexor tendon surgery. J. Bone Joint Surg., 54A:472, 1972.

Verdan, C.: Chirurgie des Tendons de la Main. Monographie du G.E.M. Paris, Expansion Scientifique Française, 1976.

Waterman, J. H.: Tendon transplantation: its history, indications and technic. Med. News, 81:54, 1902.

Young, R. E. S., and Harmon, J. M.: Repair of tendon injuries of the hand. Am. Chir., 151(4):562–566, 1960.

Zechner, W., Buck-Gramcko, O., Lohmann, H., et al.: Ueberlegungen zur Verbesserung der Nahttechnik bei beugesehnenverletzungen. Klinische und experimentelle Studie. Handchirurgie, 17:8–13, 1985.

Chapter 9

TENOLYSIS

Claude E. Verdan

A frequent sequel to trauma or inflammation in the hand is the formation of tendinous adhesions, which markedly limit motion. In selected cases tenolysis serves to free the intact tendon from this adherent bed and thereby restore satisfactory function to the affected hand.

A traumatized tendon heals by the ingrowth of richly vascular fibroblastic connective tissue. Limited motion resulting from this adherent tissue is the inevitable result if the tendon is immobilized for a prolonged period in this environment. There are many causes of traumatized adherent tendons, including fractures, infections, foreign bodies, untidy wounds, and chemical or thermal burns. Adhesions are sometimes seen following tendon repair or grafting and other types of surgery, such as ganglion or tumor resection.

Tenolysis disrupts these adhesions, and with prompt early institution of motion, new adhesions are converted into a mobile and nutritive mesotenon that allows adequate tendon gliding. Thus, the fundamental conditions for successful tenolyses are:

1. That the interrupted vascularization of the tendon be reestablished without interfering with motion.

2. That the overall vascularization and innervation of the finger be good.

3. That the operation be followed by a period of active reeducation such that the motion obtained surgically is maintained.

4. Most important, that the patient understand and be able to cooperate fully with the prescribed program.

Six local prerequisites must additionally be observed:

1. The corresponding muscle must be functionally intact.

2. Joint mobility must be good.

3. Active and passive motion of the antagonist muscle must be free.

4. The freed tendon must be sufficiently resistant to rupture.

5. The surface of the liberated tendon must be smooth and regular in diameter.

6. The tendon bed must be free of bony spicules, surrounding fibrosis, and denuded bone.

Contraindications of tenolysis include any procedure that would prevent active early mobilization such as lengthening or shortening of a tendon, free skin grafts, and corrective osteotomy (if stable enough, osteosynthesis will permit immediate mobilization).

TECHNIQUE

It should be recognized in advance that tenolysis can be as technically difficult and as delicate as tendon grafting. Simply liberating the tendon over a short distance, as over a callus formation, is inadequate in most cases, for the adhesions often extend beyond the primary suture or graft area, even as far as the musculotendinous junction.

Tenolysis of Flexor Tendons

Tenolysis of flexor tendons is most often necessary at the digital canal and at the wrist, although it may be necessary at any level. The incisions and approach are the same as those used for tendon grafts. Because the palmar zigzag incision for the finger may inhibit immediate postoperative motion, a midlateral incision is preferred.

In the digital canal one must excise the sheath segmentally as necessary, taking care to leave appropriately placed pulleys. Alternatively one may incise the sheath at its insertion for the necessary length, as Duparc and Alnot (1970) have proposed. This approach makes possible easy mobilization of the tendon and traumatizes it less (Fig. 9–1). The sheath is then resutured securely to allow early mobilization.

For a successful result it is important to maintain as long a pulley as possible at the metacarpophalangeal joint. Complete resection of the sheath may be necessary distal to this. If so, the flexor digitorum profundus will be maintained in place by the bifurcation of the superficialis.

Every effort is made to try to preserve both tendons. The nutritive vessels for the flexor profundus at the level of the proximal phalanx traverse a vinculum arising in the region of the proximal interphalangeal joint and passing through the superficialis to reach the profundus. Removal of the superficialis tendon at this level destroys this vascularization and leads to further adhesion formation. It is recommended that these vincula be exposed and preserved whenever mobilizing the tendon.

One may at times find that the retraction of the proximal interphalangeal joint is not caused by the tendons themselves but by a thick fibrous layer behind the sheath, covering the distal two-thirds of the proximal phalanx and volar plate like a pannus. This finding necessitates complete resection to bone with partial resection of the adjoining volar plate. Full extension should be possible following this operation, although it is sometimes necessary to maintain extension with a fine oblique Kirschner wire through the joint; this wire should be removed after 10 days.

Such a fibrous pannus probably develops following primary repair when the basal pulley has been resected over a considerable distance. If the wound that severed the flexor tendons also penetrated the posterior wall of the synovial sheath, this would allow proliferation of the fibrous pannus in both directions across the volar surface of the proximal interphalangeal joint.

Following tenolysis one must determine, with a counterincision at the palm or wrist (Fig. 9–2), that selective traction on the tendon achieves the desired flexion; the fingertip must touch the palm.

TENOLYSIS OF EXTENSOR TENDONS

Dissection to free the extensor tendons may be less extensive than that of the flexor tendons because of the functional partitioning of the extensor system. For the fingers a laterally based flap is raised. In the region of the proximal interphalangeal joint and proximal phalanx it is helpful to separate the middle and lateral bands by a longitudinal incision and to identify the sliding planes in a nonadherent region. The operator then has less difficulty in the adherent zones, and the risk of deterioration of tendon function is diminished. Sometimes tenolysis must be combined with excision of the dorsal part of the ligamentous system and with release of the dorsal articular capsule of the proximal interphalangeal.

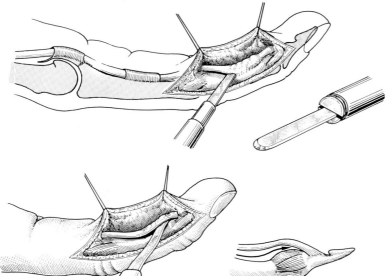

Figure 9–1. Tenolysis for adhesions after suturing the flexor digitorum profundus tendon in zone 1.

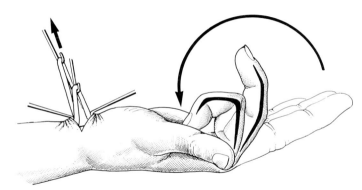

Figure 9–2. Counterincision in the wrist verifying the freedom of tendon excursion.

Across the dorsal surface of the hand and wrist, adhesions of the extensor tendons will cause a tenodesis effect, such that the fingers or wrist can be separately flexed passively but not simultaneously. For this reason one should verify at the end of the operation that complete flexion of the fingers and wrist is possible. If not, the gliding amplitude of the tendons is not sufficient. Only when complete passive flexion of all joints is obtained can one be satisfied.

ASSOCIATED OPERATIONS, TECHNIQUES, AND ALTERNATIVES

Operations that are often performed simultaneously with tenolysis include Z-plasty in cases of cutaneous contractures, excision of a scar or contracted subcutaneous fibrous tissue, removal of foreign bodies or metallic hardware, neurolysis, and resection of the lumbricals in the "lumbrical plus" syndrome (Parkes, 1970).

Collateral nerve damage, often associated with flexor tendon injury, raises the question of simultaneous neurorrhaphy and tenolysis. These operations seem incompatible; however, it is possible to combine nerve suturing and grafting with tenolysis provided full excursion of the finger is limited postoperatively by a dorsal splint for the three weeks necessary to provide satisfactory nerve healing.

If adequate tenolysis denudes a bone surface adjacent to the tendon, or if considerable scar tissue remains, the recurrence of adhesions is likely. Three techniques are useful in avoiding this recurrence:

1. Wrapping the released tendon with a sheet of tricipital paratenon. This works best for extensor tendons.

2. Interposing a thin sheet of Silastic between the liberated tendon and the bone or scar tissue. If the synthetic sheet is not held securely in place, it may become dislocated and hinder more than it helps: for this reason it should never be utilized over a joint.

3. As an alternative to tenolysis one may excise the tendon and all the sheath except for one or two pulleys and reconstruct a new sheath around a Silastic or Hunter rod and perform tendon grafting three months later.

POSTOPERATIVE CARE

The initial postoperative compressive dressing should maintain the fingers in a flexed position such that at the time of its removal 48 hours after surgery, the surgeon can passively mobilize the fingers by extending them. This maneuver breaks the first adhesions caused by clotting of blood. Subsequent dressings should allow full amplitude unless there has been a concomitant nerve suturing.

Anti-inflammatory drugs such as salicylates, butazolidine, or alpha-chymotrypsin should be used. Corticosteroids may increase the chance of tendon rupture and are likewise to be avoided.

Although young children will not be able to cooperate knowledgeably with the rehabilitative and re-education program, games supervised by their parents can easily be substituted. These should be accompanied by passive mobilization under the supervision of a physiotherapist.

COMPLICATIONS

We have seen that the freed tendon must be sufficiently strong to resist rupture. This fact is sometimes difficult to appreciate, and we have had, as is seen world-wide, some cases of rupture that have necessitated other therapeutic measures, such as tendon grafts, on a second occasion or tenodesis. It is there-fore wise not to perform a tenolysis for at least three months following a direct tendon repair or for at least six months following tendon grafting. It is, of course, necessary to maintain a full range of passive joint move-ments by suitable physiotherapy.

In those rare instances in which tenolysis is performed following suppurative synovitis of the tendon sheath, the interval between infection and operation must be at least six months. The operation must be "covered" by appropriate antibiotics, which should be continued for one week postoperatively. Reactivation of a dormant microorganism is always to be feared.

RESULTS

We completed a study in 1971 (with Craw-ford and Martini-Benkeddac) of 92 patients (64 men and 28 women) aged four to 68 years, 51 per cent between the ages of 21 and 40. Tenolysis was accomplished in 177 ten-dons in 124 fingers. Tenolysis was particularly useful in zones 1 and 2 as a follow-up pro-cedure following primary tendon surgery. Zones 6 and 7 likewise benefited from a secondary tenolysis when necessary.

Results were graded 1 to 5 as follows:

5 = Excellent. Normal flexion and exten-sion.

4 = Good. Moderate improvement of flex-ion or extension and ability to flex the finger to 2.5 cm. from the distal palmar crease.

3 = Fair. Some improvement but persist-ence of a notable deficit of flexion and exten-sion; ability to flex the finger 2.5 to 5 cm. from the distal palmar crease.

2 = Mediocre. No improvement.

1 = Poor. Deterioration, amputations.

The combined results in all 177 tenolyses of flexor and extensor tendons showed 50 per cent excellent and good results. Sixty-five per cent of patients subjectively reported excel-lent and good results. If category 3 is in-cluded, 78 per cent obtained favorable re-sults.

Tenolysis of 29 extensors sutured primarily resulted in 17 good or excellent results, only four cases showing no improvement. The latter 4 all involved juxta-articular zones 1, 3, and 5 (Verdan, 1972).

A similar analysis of 19 flexors showed 11 tenolyses in zone 1 with seven improvements

(64 per cent) and eight tenolyses in zone 2 with seven improvements (87 per cent). When all flexor zones were considered, there was an overall improvement in 81 per cent of the cases.*

In a more recent study the various param-eters that can influence the results of tenol-yses were noted (Egloff and Verdan, 1978). The parameters chosen included the age of the patient, the finger involved, the zone of the initial lesion, the etiology, associated pro-cedures, the timing of tenolyses, and the duration of the procedure. The analysis of figures for pre- and postoperative active joint mobility, taking into account the foregoing parameters, allowed several interesting con-clusions to be reached:

1. It is logical to suppose that the results of tenolyses are adversely affected by increas-ing age. Beneficial results are less certain after the age of 50.

2. The results are better for the thumb than for the other fingers. That is understand-able. There is one joint less but, equally, only one extrinsic flexor, and multiple intrin-sic muscles that are able to compensate in large measure for the function of the extrinsic musculature.

3. Study of function in the various zones revealed, above all, that tenolyses were nec-essary in zones 2 and 3 for the flexor tendons (81 per cent of the tenolyses) as well as the extensors (75 per cent of the tenolyses).

4. The type of initial trauma and the method of tendon repair have an important bearing on results. Our analysis showed that the results were better for the flexor tendons (71 cases) than for the extensor tendons (29 cases). One can add that the results of tenol-yses are superior when they follow tendon surgery alone (primary or secondary suturing, secondary grafting, two stage grafting, ten-don transfer) than when they are performed in the presence of associated bone, joint, or skin lesions (fracture, dislocation, degloving, inflammatory processes, cutaneous injury). This is true for the flexor tendons alone. We did not observe this difference in the extensor tendons.

5. An analysis of the value of associated procedures showed that ideally one should limit the procedure to tenolysis. Indeed the

---

*For complete details, refer to the original 1971 pub-lication.

difference between the results with tenolysis alone and tenolysis with other procedures was significant. We were able to distinguish between procedures that did not complicate the postoperative course following tenolysis and those that yielded unfavorable results. In the first group, those that were not unfavorable, we were able to include resection of flexor superficialis, neurolysis of one or two digital nerves, tenodesis, and arthrodesis of the distal interphalangeal joint. On the contrary, secondary suture or grafting of a digital nerve, arthrolysis, and corrective osteotomies are all procedures that markedly decrease the success of tenolysis itself. Finally, although resection of the flexor superficialis does not seem to compromise the results of tenolysis, its resection notably increases the risk of tendon rupture; of the three tendon ruptures observed, all occurred in this group.

6. We were able to show statistically that it is better to perform a tenolysis at six months. Beyond one year the improvement that can be gained is minimal.

7. Finally, when the duration of the operation exceeds one and one-half hours, the beneficial results one can expect diminish considerably.

From this study we are able to establish the following as adverse factors in tenolysis: patients older than 40 years, other procedures performed on the same finger at the same time, tenolysis performed more than one year after the preceding trauma or surgery, or after infections or inflammatory conditions, tenolysis performed after conservative treatment of a tendon injury, and prolonged surgical procedures.

If many of these factors are present, there is doubt that surgery will be successful. In hand surgery one must try to reduce the number of surgical interventions to a minimum. One should have concrete indications for surgery that can be verified statistically rather than basing surgery on subjective criteria.

SUMMARY

Tenolysis is an effective procedure to free adherent tendons, its success being dependent on early postoperative mobilization. Technical details are important, and one must be certain that the indications for operations are established in every case.

In the two studies reported here, 78 and 73 per cent of all flexor and extensor tenolyses resulted in considerable improvement. This procedure is clearly a worthwhile adjunct to tendon surgery.

REFERENCES

Carstam, N.: Effect of cortisone on the formation of tendon adhesions and on tendon healing. Acta Chir. Scand., Suppl. 182, 1953.

Duparc, J., and Alnot, V.: Personal communication.

Egloff, D., and Verdan, C.: Ann. Chir. Main. 1978.

Parkes, A.: The "lumbrical plus" finger. Hand, 2:164, 1970.

Verdan, C.: Chirurgie des Tendons de la Main. Paris, Expansion Scientifique Française, 1976.

Verdan, C.: Die Eingriffe an Muskeln, Sehnen und Sehnenscheiden. In Wachsmuth W., and Wilhelm, A.: Chirurgische Operationslehre. Heidelberg, Springer Verlag, 1972, Vol. 10. Ch. 3.

Verdan, C., Crawford, G., and Martini, Y.: Tenolysis in traumatic hand-surgery. Educational Foundation of the American Society of Plastic and Reconstructive Surgeons. Vol. 3, Symposium on the Hand. St. Louis, The C. V. Mosby Co., 1971.

Verdan, C., and Michon, J.: Le traitement des plaies des tendons fléchisseurs des doigts. Rev. Chir. Orthop., 47:285, 1961.

LESIONS OF THE EXTENSOR TENDONS

INTRODUCTION

Raoul Tubiana

The traditional distinction between lesions of the flexor tendons of the digits, considered difficult to repair and having a poor prognosis, and those of the extensor tendons, thought to be easier to treat, is in fact arbitrary.

The extensor tendons have the advantage of being extrasynovial along most of their length, which facilitates their repair. However, they are thin superficial structures lying immediately adjacent to the bones and joints, and, when damaged, they tend to adhere to these underlying tissues. Their excursion is much less than that of the flexors, and thus it is more difficult to compensate for any loss of length. Moreover, there is normally a precise length relationship between the central and lateral extensor tendons.

Together with the intrinsic muscles of the digits and the flexor tendons, the extensors make up a complex system to maintain stability while allowing independent motion of each phalanx. In fact, in our experience treatment of lesions of the extensor apparatus has probably resulted in more disappointments; however, the repercussions of failures or partial failures of treatment are usually less serious than with the flexor tendons and the sequelae are less damaging to function.

Increased understanding of the extensor mechanism has been provided by anatomical and physiological investigations (Landsmeer, 1949; Kaplan, 1959; Eyler and Markee, 1954; Stack, 1962; Tubiana and Valentin, 1964;

Littler, 1967, 1977; Harris and Rutledge, 1972). More physiological methods of repair carry better chances for success. The considerable predominance of the power of the antagonist flexor muscles must always be kept in mind.

This section of the book presents methods

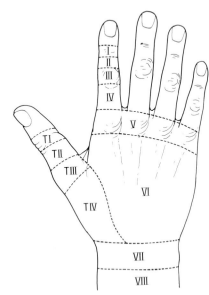

Figure 1. The extensor tendons of the fingers cross eight zones. The extensor tendons of the thumb cross six zones, four specific to the thumb, which are preceded by the letter T (thumb). Two zones are shared with the extensors of the fingers: zones VII (wrist) and VIII (forearm).

73

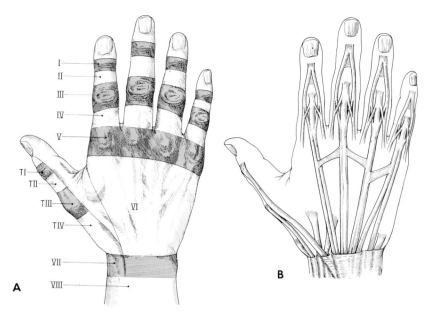

Figure 2. Extensor tendons of the hand. *A*, Division into topographical zones. *B*, Anatomy of the extrinsic extensor tendons.

for repair of the extensor apparatus of the fingers and the thumb after traumatic injury. Restoration of function after rheumatoid lesions or paralysis is discussed in separate chapters in Volume IV.

Generally the approach to treatment and the prognosis will vary according to whether the lesion is recent or not. In the case of an old lesion, disequilibrium will have had time to become fixed, resulting in deformities of the digits that must always be corrected before attempting repair of the extensor apparatus.

We have followed the division of the extensor tendons into zones, as proposed by Verdan and adapted at the Rotterdam Meet-

ing of the International Federation of Societies for Surgery of the Hand (Figs. 1 and 2). We will consider in turn lesions of the extensor tendons within the fingers, on the back of the hand, at the wrist, and in the thumb.

In view of the superficial position of the extensor tendons, their treatment following traumatic injury depends largely on the condition of the skin. Hence, in the first chapter Michel Merle discusses techniques and indications for skin coverage of the extensors.

REFERENCES

References will be found following Chapter 23.

Chapter 10

SKIN COVER FOR THE EXTENSOR APPARATUS AND INDICATIONS FOR ITS USE

MICHEL MERLE

Lesions of the extensor apparatus are erroneously regarded as benign, yet a simple lesion of the central extensor tendon can lead to a boutonnière deformity. Lesions of the tendon alone are rare: They are usually complicated by lesions of the joints and by skin loss because most injuries tend to occur when the digit is flexed. Whenever the loss of skin exposes the tendon apparatus, it is preferable to repair the lesions at one session followed by early mobilization. However, this plan presupposes familiarity with the various types of skin flaps: homodigital, heterodigital, forearm flaps, and flaps from a distant site. To simplify description of the site of the lesion, we shall use the classification proposed by Verdan (1966).

PRINCIPLES OF EMERGENCY RECONSTRUCTION OF THE EXTENSOR APPARATUS

Each digital zone poses specific problems of skin covering. To avoid repetition, we shall first review briefly the procedures usually regarded as reliable.

SNOW'S PLASTY (1976)

At the level of the proximal interphalangeal joint, it is possible to reconstruct the middle band by cutting a flap from the extensor apparatus as it runs over the shaft of the proximal phalanx. This strip with its pedicle based distally is turned about 180 degrees, threaded through the bone, and fixed to the base of the middle phalanx. Aiache et al.

(1979) have advocated a longitudinal hemisection of each lateral tendon, the two halves then being sutured edge to edge in the midline to reconstitute a central tendon.

FOLD-BACK PLASTY

When tissue loss is more extensive, especially in zones III, IV, and V, Foucher suggests the fold-back plasty (Fig. 10–1). This consists of splitting the extensor communis, which is then folded back 180 degrees on its distal insertion and used to cover the defect between the two zones.

USE OF THE EXTENSOR INDICIS PROPRIUS

In some lesions of the extensor tendons of the thumb and fingers in zones V and VI, extension can be reactivated by using the extensor indicis proprius. Flexion injuries of the metacarpophalangeal joints usually result in loss of tissue of the extensor apparatus, its retinaculum, and the metacarpal heads. Reconstruction of the extensor system then can be carried out by a folding tendon plasty or by transfer of the extensor indicis proprius tendon. Our technique for stabilization of the extensor tendon relies on a double pulley, which runs through the head of the damaged metacarpal (Fig. 10–2). If there is loss of substance in more than one digital ray (zone VI), a secondary repair is usually preferable.

Extensor tendon grafts are made easier by the insertion of a Hunter silicone rod at

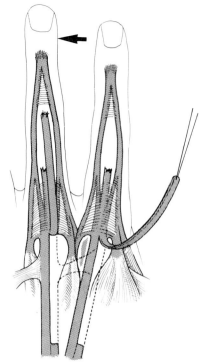

Figure 10–1. Eversion plasty of the extensor communis (after Foucher). Longitudinal hemisection of the extensor tendon in zone VI allows reconstruction in zones III, IV, and V.

emergency surgery. This technique protects the grafts against periosteal adhesions and the thinning of skin flaps.

Whenever there is a risk of adhesion between the extensor tendons and the skeleton, we use as a partition a Silastic sheet or sheets of retinaculum, which provide a good gliding surface.

All these techniques are reliable when used by surgeons who are familiar with the handling of vascularized skin flaps.

TECHNIQUES AND INDICATIONS ACCORDING TO THE LEVEL OF THE LESION (VERDAN'S CLASSIFICATION)

When the perimysium is intact, skin cover is provided by a partial or full thickness skin graft regardless of the level of the lesion. The exposed area has a good enough blood supply to feed the graft and keep it supple and elastic enough to allow the finger to move freely. The shape of the graft of course must conform to the principle of functional unity

in order to avoid formation of a retractile band, which might interfere with function.

When the perimysium is damaged, the defect is covered with skin flaps—local flaps for a limited defect and flaps from a distant site for more extensive ones.

TISSUE LOSS IN ZONE I

Skin loss in zone I is seldom limited to this zone. When the defect is isolated, it is possible to use a homodigital rotation advancement flap borrowed from the dorsal aspect of the middle phalanx.

Reconstruction of the extensor apparatus is not always necessary, because one of the two lateral bands and its terminal insertion on the distal phalanx often survives intact.

If the extensor apparatus is totally destroyed, the fibrosis that develops under the flap within four to eight weeks constitutes a good mechanical substitute for restoring the function of the distal interphalangeal joint.

TISSUE LOSS IN ZONE II

This type of injury usually consists of a multidigital dorsal abrasion over the middle phalanx: one of the two lateral bands often survives, but the phalangeal bone is left exposed. This injury requires a flap from a distant site; a Colson brachial flap has the

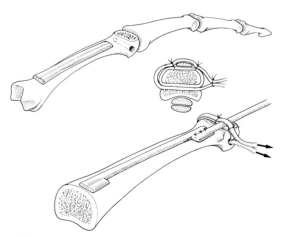

Figure 10–2. Loss of tissue in the extensor tendon in zone V with dorsal abrasion of the metacarpal head reconstructed by means of an eversion plasty of the extensor communis. To prevent subluxation, a strap is fashioned by passing the tendon of the palmaris longus through the head of the metacarpal.

advantage of keeping the hand protected in addition to providing a covering of fine supple skin. The flap is separated after two weeks. In female patients however, the brachial scar may be unacceptable.

When the area of skin loss is small and limited to one digit, it can be repaired with a translation flap taken from the side of the finger. In most cases, however, the best solution is a thinned cross finger flap, the "reversed dermis flap," as described by Pakiam (1978) (see Volume II). The procedure is simple and reliable, but the cosmetic result at both the donor and receptor sites is variable.

TISSUE LOSS IN ZONE III

Zone III is the most vulnerable. In addition to the skin loss, one often has to deal with an open joint and repair the middle band of the extensor tendon (using the techniques described earlier).

When the defect is less than 1 cm., we use a local rotation and advancement autoplasty. This requires an L shaped incision on the dorsolateral border of the proximal phalanx running transversely toward its base. The flap is carefully lifted off the perimysium of the extensor tendon. The defect at the base of the finger can be covered at once, using a full thickness skin graft (Fig. 10–3).

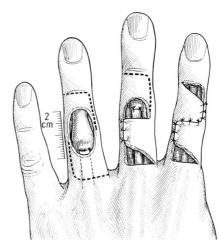

Figure 10–4. Principle of the double flap. The flap is advanced from the proximal phalanx and recessed from the middle phalanx. This type of flap can cover a defect of up to 2 cm.

This flap by itself can cover a defect 1 cm. across, with no tension or restriction of movement at the distal interphalangeal joint. It has proved highly reliable; we had no instance of necrosis in our series of 45 cases.

For defects 1 to 2 cm. in size, we combine this flap with another taken from the middle phalanx (Fig. 10–4).

The foregoing combination of flaps protects the joint and also the repaired median band of the extensor. Because tension is minimal, early mobilization is possible (Figs. 10–5 to 10–7).

Larger defects extending beyond zone III require a flag flap. It is worth remembering that flag flaps raised at the proximal phalanx are reliable, whereas those originating at the middle phalanx have a poor blood supply and are liable to become necrotic.

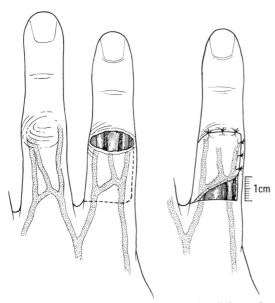

Figure 10–3. Rotation advancement flap lining a defect of less than 1 cm. at the interphalangeal joint.

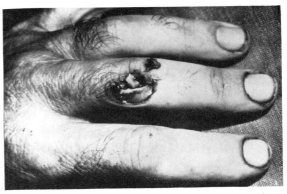

Figure 10–5. Loss of skin and tendon tissue opposite the proximal interphalangeal joint.

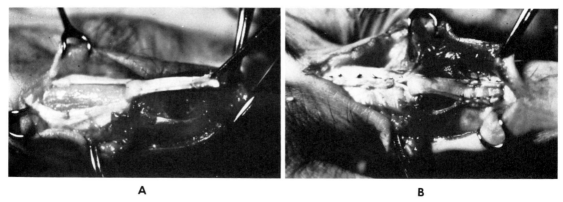

A　　　　　　　　　　　　　　　**B**

Figure 10–6. *A* and *B*, Snow's eversion plasty used in the repair of the median band of the extensor tendon.

When tissue loss is extensive on the dorsal side and a venous channel needs to be reconstructed, the same flap can be made "vein bearing," as described by Foucher et al. (1970). The flap is raised along with one or two veins, which are anastomosed to the veins draining the receptor finger. This procedure guarantees an adequate venous return and prevents postoperative stasis and edema.

TISSUE LOSS IN ZONES IV AND V

Loss of skin tissue is seldom limited to zone IV and usually involves zone V. For a relatively limited defect a cross finger flag flap is usually sufficient. In multidigital lesions there is the possibility of using flaps from a distant site to cover the proximal phalanges and metacarpophalangeal joints. Our preference is for a Colson bipedicled flap from the arm or forearm, which offers the advantage of keeping the digital chains in a protected position.

For more extensive defects involving zones V and VI as well as IV, it is advisable to use an inguinal (McGregor) flap centered on the superficial circumflex iliac artery.

At emergency repair we have now given up using free flaps, such as the dorsopedal and parascapular flaps, because of the great difficulty in assessing a recently contused vascular pedicle.

In practice, since the introduction of the forearm or Chinese flap, the indications for flaps from a distant site have decreased. Indeed the Chinese island flap, with its retrograde perfusion from the radial artery, can be used to cover all kinds of defects of the fingers and dorsum of the hand (Fig. 10–8). When this flap is used on the digital chain in zones II, IV, V, and VI, it is later disconnected and thinned prior to reconstruction of the first web space.

In multidigital lesions, a condemned digit can be justifiably amputated and used to reconstruct an adjacent one (Figs. 10–9 and 10–10).

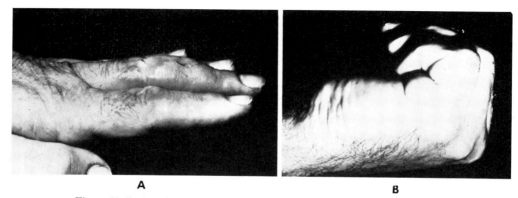

A　　　　　　　　　　　　　　　**B**

Figure 10–7. *A* and *B*, Result at six weeks of procedure shown in Figure 10–6.

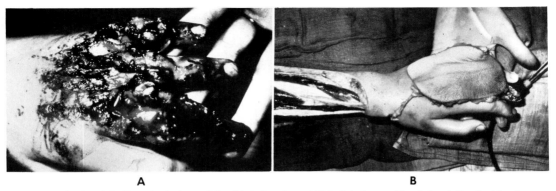

Figure 10–8. *A* and *B*, Complex lesions of the third, fourth, and fifth digital rays. The defect is lined with a forearm "Chinese flap" pedicled on the radial artery.

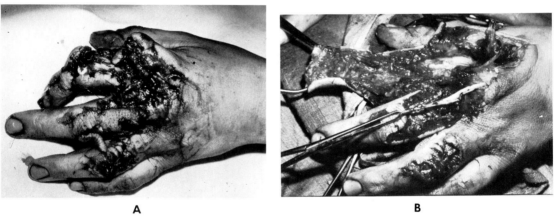

Figure 10–9. *A* and *B*, Wound of the three middle digits caused by a top. The index finger is sacrificed for reconstruction of the extensor apparatus of the middle finger and the covering of its surface. A Snow eversion plasty was performed on the ring finger.

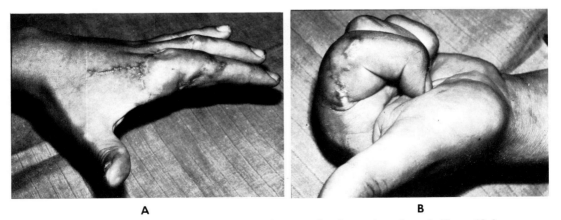

Figure 10–10. *A* and *B*, Results at three months of procedure shown in Figure 10–9.

TISSUE LOSS IN ZONE VI

In severe injuries with tissue loss, zone V is usually involved along with zone VI. The same larger types of flaps are indicated as for associated lesions of zones IV and V. Our view is that flaps from a distant site should be utilized only if a Chinese flap from the forearm proves unfeasible. However, the introduction of the composite Chinese flap, in which the flexor carpi radialis or brachioradialis is used as a vascularized tendon graft, has revolutionized the indications for flaps from distant sites and for two stage repairs of the extensor apparatus.

When the contusion or the risk of adhesions is too great to allow a safe one stage emergency repair, it is preferable to insert a Hunter silicone rod, which will be replaced by conventional tendon grafts at a later stage.

PROBLEMS SPECIFIC TO THE THUMB

The lesions of the thumb are mostly articular—the interphalangeal joint in zone I and the metacarpophalangeal joint in zone V.

Reconstruction of the extensor apparatus is relatively simple; it usually involves connecting the extensor longus to the extensor brevis or transferring the extensor indicis proprius.

Defects of 1 to 1.5 cm. in zone V usually can be covered by means of a rotation advancement flap, but care must be taken to leave a broad based pedicle at the first intermetacarpal space to avoid contracture of the first web space.

For zone I defects smaller than 1 cm. over the interphalangeal joint, the answer is a

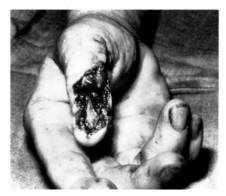

Figure 10–11. Loss of bone, skin, and tendon tissue on the dorsal aspect of the thumb.

dorsal rotation advancement flap, as described for zone III in the fingers.

For wider defects involving zone I and the shaft of the proximal phalanx, the Foucher kite flap offers a particularly elegant solution (see the chapter on kite flap in Volume II). This flap carries an artery and a vein in addition to nerve fibers; it can cover a defect of up to 4.5 by 2.5 cm. and derives its sensibility from its radial innervation (Figs. 10–11 and 10–12). This flap has good trophicity and is cosmetically excellent, and the scar on the donor zone of the index finger is acceptable provided it is covered with a thin graft and the hand is dynamically splinted as early as possible.

CONCLUSION

For a surgeon familiar with the techniques of digital skin flaps, it is now possible, even

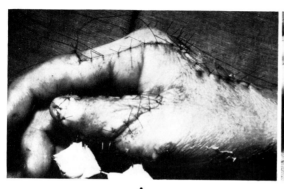
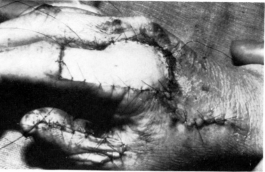

| A | B |

Figure 10–12. *A* and *B*, Kite flap in place. The donor zone is covered with a partial thickness graft.

in injuries involving more than one digit, to reconstruct the extensor apparatus and repair the overlying skin defects at one operation. Only if the perimysium is intact does one have recourse to full or partial thickness skin grafts.

Flaps from a distant site require, in addition to a long stay in hospital, the "parasitization" of the hand in a dependent position with the attendant risks of edema and stiffness. The present trend favors the use of simple or composite forearm pedicled flaps.

REFERENCES

Aiache, A., Barsky, A. J., and Weiner, D. L.: Prevention of "boutonnière" deformity. Plast. Reconstr. Surg., *46*:166–167, 1979.

Foucher, G., Braun, F., Merle, M., and Michon, J.: Le "doigt banque" en traumatologie de la main. Ann. Chir., *34*:693–698, 1970.

McGregor, I. A., and Morgan, G.: Axial and random pattern flaps. Br. J. Plast. Surg., *26*:202, 1973.

Pakiam, A. I.: The reversed dermis flap. Br. J. Plast. Surg., *31*:131–135, 1978.

Snow, J. W.: A method of reconstruction of the central slip of the extensor tendon of a finger. Plast. Reconstr. Surg., *57*:45–49, 1976.

Chapter 11

LESIONS OF THE DIGITAL EXTENSOR

RAOUL TUBIANA

Extension of the fingers is a complex movement involving both extrinsic muscles (extensor communis, extensor indicis proprius, and extensor digiti quinti) and intrinsic muscles (the interosseous and lumbrical muscles). (The physiology of extension has been reviewed in Volume I, Chapter 39.)

Injuries of the extensor apparatus of the fingers are common and their repair can be difficult. Division of the extensor tendons at various levels gives rise to many different problems. At the wrist and over the dorsum of the hand, the difficulties are not so much in the technique of repair but in the prevention of adhesions and joint stiffness. At the metacarpophalangeal joint the main complication is subluxation of the tendons.

In the fingers one is faced with lesions not so much of the extensor tendons but of the extensor apparatus, which consists of a thin fibrous sheet spread over the whole of the dorsum of the finger and which is inserted into each phalanx.

The extensor aponeurosis of the fingers is made up of the terminal fibers of the long extensor tendons and of the intrinsic digital muscles, which mingle with passive retinacular fibrous structures. This complex arrangement allows muscles that have only a small excursion to act at each phalangeal level with a large amplitude of extension.

Figure 11–1 depicts the various components of this complex and will help in recalling the nomenclature we have chosen. (For further details see Volume I, pp. 53–65, 244–254, and 389–398.) Injuries of the extensors at the hand and wrist will be discussed subsequently.

It is usual to use a topographical division to study lesions of the extensor tendons, especially at the wrist and on the dorsum of the hand, but at the level of the fingers, the three phalanges constitute a kinetic chain, and injury at one level may alter the balance of the whole finger (Fig. 11–2). Nevertheless we will use here a topographical division according to the main site of the lesion. These lesions will be discussed starting distally at the distal interphalangeal joint (mallet finger). Lesions at the proximal interphalangeal joint are discussed under two main headings—boutonnière and swan-neck deformities. In the boutonnière deformity the lesion is always at the proximal interphalangeal joint level, but the swan-neck deformity can result from lesions in any part of the digital chain.

We will conclude with a discussion of divisions of the extensor mechanism at the level of the shaft of the middle and proximal phalanges, lesions at the level of the metacarpophalangeal joints, and lesions at the level of the dorsum of the hand and wrist.

Figure 11–1. Diagram of the extensor apparatus of the fingers (front and side views). 1 = interosseous muscle, 2 = extensor communis tendon, 3 = lumbrical muscle, 4 = tendon sheath, 5 = sagittal band, 6 = intermetacarpal ligament, 7 = transverse fibers of dorsum of interossei, 8 = oblique fibers of dorsum, 9 = lateral band of extensor tendon, 10 = central or middle band of extensor tendon, 11 = central or middle band of interosseous tendon, 12 = lateral band of interosseous tendon, 13 = oblique retinacular ligament, 14 = central or middle extensor tendon, 15 = spiral fibers, 16 = transverse retinacular ligament, 17 = lateral extensor tendon, 18 = triangular ligament (or lamina), 19 = terminal extensor tendon, 20 = flexor superficialis tendon, 21 = flexor profundus tendon.

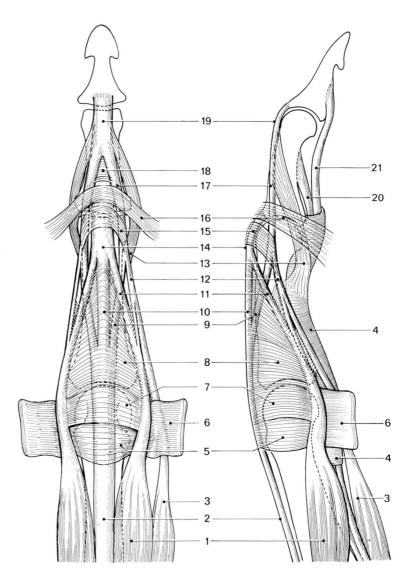

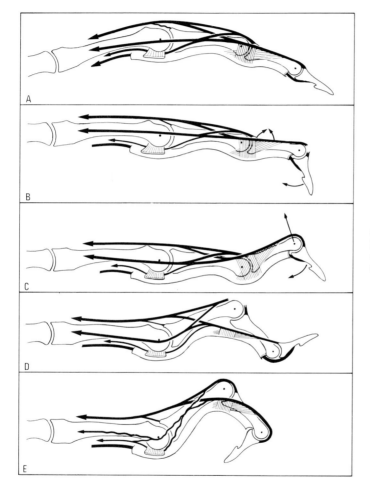

Figure 11–2. Deformities of the kinetic chain of the fingers. *A*, Normal chain. *B*, Mallet deformity. *C*, Swan-neck deformity. *D*, Boutonnière deformity. *E*, Claw-hand deformity.

Chapter 12

THE MALLET FINGER

Raoul Tubiana

The term mallet finger denotes the persistent flexion of the distal phalanx of a finger resulting from a lesion of the extensor apparatus at the level of the distal interphalangeal joint (Fig. 12–1). The inability to extend the distal phalanx is due to a variety of lesions, both traumatic and nontraumatic, of the extensor tendons. This chapter deals primarily with lesions of traumatic origin.

ANATOMY

The terminal extensor tendon, formed by the union of the two lateral extensor tendons, is inserted across most of the width of the dorsal aspect of the base of the distal phalanx. It consists of a flat tendinous expansion, which adheres to and blends with the joint capsule. The tendon has an excursion of about 4 mm. It must be remembered that extension of the distal phalanx results from the combined action of the extensor communis and the intrinsic muscles, and that the first part of the movement—i.e., between 90 and 45 degrees of flexion—is brought about passively and in conjunction with extension of the middle phalanx, by the oblique fibers of the retinacular ligament.

ETIOLOGY

Lesions of the extensor apparatus near the distal interphalangeal joint can result from a variety of injuries: lacerations, rupture, avulsion of the bony insertion of the tendon, fracture of the base of the distal phalanx, and epiphyseal detachment. The more distal and the more complete the lesion, the more marked the deformity. Thus Stack (1969) differentiates between central lesions of the terminal tendon, where the peripheral fibers arising from the oblique retinacular ligament are intact and the deformity is less than 45 degrees, and complete ruptures.

MECHANISM

The mechanism by which closed injuries cause the mallet finger has been the subject of argument for a long time. Segond in 1880 described avulsion of the bony insertion of the extensor tendon, and Schoening (1887) reported tendon ruptures without bone injury.

It would appear therefore that we must differentiate among the following:

1. Tendon ruptures, which are produced by trauma to the dorsal aspect of the extended distal phalanx, causing sudden flexion of the joint while the extensors are contracted (Fig. 12–2). Rupture occurs during the first half of flexion of the distal phalanx. Because the retinacular ligament is not under tension, its fibers are not torn (Fig. 12–3A). This type of central injury can occur following relatively minor trauma.

2. Bone avulsion, which occurs in the course of forced flexion of the distal phalanx beyond 90 degrees when the proximal interphalangeal joint is extended. Zancolli (1979) has shown in cadaver experiments that bone avulsion is due to resistance of the retinacular ligaments (Fig. 12–3B).

3. A crush fracture of the base of the distal phalanx which can be caused by a blow to the extremity of the finger.

The incidence of concomitant bone injuries varies from 24 per cent, according to Stark et al. (1962), to 40.6 per cent according to Albertoni (1977) and 41.7 per cent according to Smillie (1936).

These are three main types of bone lesions:

1. Avulsion of a small triangular fragment

85

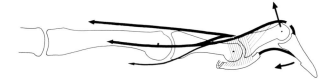

Figure 12–1. Lesion of the extensor apparatus at the distal interphalangeal joint results in a mallet deformity.

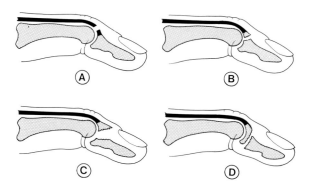

Figure 12–2. Different types of mallet finger. *A*, Tendon rupture. *B*, Avulsion of small bone fragments. *C*, Fracture of base of distal phalanx. *D*, Epiphyseal separation.

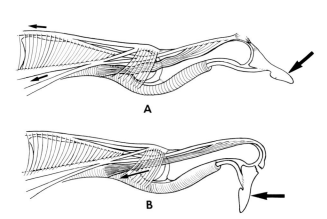

Figure 12–3. Mechanisms of closed trauma. *A*, Rupture of the central portion of the tendon. The deformity is moderate. *B*, Avulsion of a small bone fragment. This occurs when a flexion force is applied to the distal phalanx and the proximal interphalangeal joint is in full extension.

Figure 12–4. If a fracture involves more than one third of the articular surface of the distal phalanx, volar subluxation will occur.

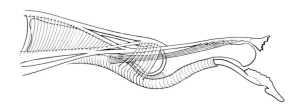

from the posterior border of the distal phalanx. The fragment usually shows little displacement but rotates posteriorly.

2. Fractures splitting off a larger fragment of the phalangeal base. If the fracture involves more than one-third of the articular surface, the phalanx will show palmar displacement (Fig. 12–4).

3. Finally there is the possibility, in children, of an epiphyseal detachment, but this deformity appears to be due most often to traction of the flexor profundus tendon, which is inserted distally, on the shaft, rather than the extensor communis, which is inserted at the base (Fig. 12–5).

NATURAL COURSE OF THE LESIONS

The natural course of the lesions is of particular interest because they are often seen at a late stage. After sectioning, rupture, or avulsion, the extensor communis tendon retracts. In complete lesions the tendon can retract up to 1 cm., in which case there is simultaneous retraction of the retinacular ligaments. This event in turn has a number of functional repercussions:

1. Inability to extend the distal phalanx. A tendinous callus is formed, and although continuity is restored, the tendon is too long to allow extension of the phalanx (Fig. 12–6A).

2. Proximal retraction of the extensor apparatus reinforces its action on the middle phalanx. If the proximal interphalangeal joint is lax, its secondary hyperextension results in a swan-neck deformity (Fig. 12–6B).

3. Retraction of the fibers of the retinaculum thwarts attempts to reposition the extensor communis tendon in patients presenting for late surgical repair.

CLINICAL FEATURES

The clinical picture is different after closed and open injuries. In the latter, further differentiation is required between the clean wound and the crush injury in which the state of the skin and the skeleton dominate the clinical picture.

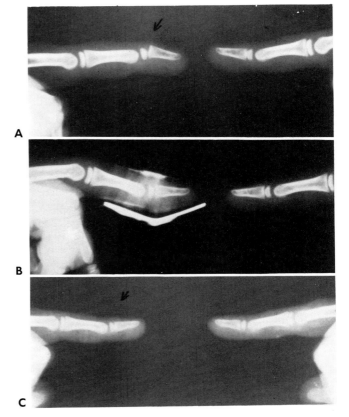

Figure 12–5. Epiphyseal separation in the distal phalanx of the long finger in a 10-year-old boy (Albertoni). *A*, Initial radiograph comparing lateral views of the slipped epiphysis in the distal phalanx. *B*, X-ray monitoring of closed reduction and immobilization in an aluminum splint. *C*, X-ray monitoring four weeks after discarding the splint.

Distal ruptures of the extensor apparatus can result from different types of injury. In some cases there is a clear history of violent trauma, e.g., in ball games. In others the injury is much less obvious, e.g., in the housewife who turns over a mattress or folds bedsheets, when the actual trauma may pass unnoticed. Any fingers may be affected, although the middle finger and ulnar fingers are most frequently involved; the thumb rarely suffers. The result is permanent flexion of the distal phalanx whatever the position of the other joints. The patient can further flex the affected phalanx but cannot extend it beyond the starting point. The extension deficit varies with the severity of the tendon lesions. Passive extension is possible at least in the early stages, but edema and fibrosis gradually restrict the mobility of the joint. Pain, when present, is minimal, and the symptoms are so benign that the patient does not seek medical advice and expects a spontaneous recovery. It is only the persistent nature of the deformity that takes him to the doctor, and this is why diagnosis is usually delayed.

Anteroposterior and lateral x-ray views are taken to detect bone avulsion and anterior dislocation of the phalangeal base. A mallet finger with little bone displacement and no joint instability requires the same treatment as pure tendon avulsion.

Among the factors that can have an unfavorable effect on the prognosis include the age of the patient (correction of the deformity and the return of mobility are less readily achieved in older patients). The percentage of successful repairs is also lower in the index

and middle fingers than in the ring and little fingers (Albertoni, 1977). We have already mentioned the unfavorable results when the severity of the deformity is greater than 45 degrees, the avulsion of a bone fragment leads to joint instability, and the proximal interphalangeal joint tends to hyperextend. Delayed repair and inadequate fixation are other such factors.

TREATMENT

The management of these apparently straightforward lesions is in fact far from simple. First a number of factors must be taken into account—the age of the lesion, the cause, the stage of the skin and skeleton, the age of the patient, his occupation, sex, and psychological status, and the finger involved. In patients who are seen late, one must also consider the functional loss, the presence or absence of pain, and the degree of passive mobility of the distal joint.

One must never forget the predominance of the flexor profundus. Also unfavorable local conditions of extensor repair require prolonged immobilization (seven to eight weeks) of the distal phalanx in extension.

Flexion of the proximal interphalangeal joint relaxes tension in the lateral extensor tendons and facilitates apposition of the divided tendon ends. However, it may be difficult to restore full extension of this joint if flexion is maintained for too long a time, particularly in the elderly. We prefer to avoid immobilization of the proximal interphalangeal joint in flexion for longer than two weeks.

We shall consider in turn the primary repair of lacerations, ruptures, and avulsions before discussing secondary repairs.

PRIMARY REPAIR

Primary Treatment of Laceration

When the wound is clean, primary suturing can be performed. Surgical repairs at this level are made difficult by the closeness of the joint and the slimness of the integuments. The skin is thin and fragile and is poorly vascularized, especially in hyperextension when it can be seen to blanch. The incision is restricted by the nail matrix. All these factors explain the potential for complications

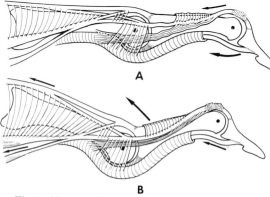

A

B

Figure 12–6. *A*, When the tendon heals with lengthening, the mallet deformity will persist. *B*, Proximal retraction of the extensor apparatus causes a swan-neck deformity, if the proximal interphalangeal joint is lax.

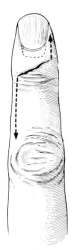

Figure 12–7. The wound is enlarged at its extremities, avoiding the formation of poorly vascularized acute angle flaps.

if the whole procedure is not conducted with the utmost care.

The skin wound is usually transverse or oblique and can be enlarged longitudinally (Fig. 12–7). The integuments are manipulated with care by means of traction sutures; distally they are only partially elevated, extension of the phalanx being usually sufficient to expose the distal end of the tendon. It is important to remember that the nail matrix extends about 5 mm. proximal to the visible part of the nail.

The tendon is extremely slender near its insertion and a suture through it is always fragile; tension can be relieved by maintaining the distal phalanx in extension. One way

to help maintain this position is to fix the distal joint in 5 degrees of hyperextension by means of a fine Kirschner wire before actually placing the suture. On the other hand, excessive hyperextension interferes with the blood supply to the integument and must be avoided. The Kirschner wire is usually introduced from the lateral border of the finger so as to pass obliquely through the joint (Fig. 12–8).

The tendon is repaired with a 4-0 or 5-0 white nylon crisscross suture, taking a supporting bite through the lateral extensor tendons. The knot, which is poorly tolerated by the thin dorsal skin, is buried as deeply as possible. Lorthioir et al. (1958) advocate a double crisscross suture passing through both lateral tendons (Fig. 12–9); other authors prefer a pull-out suture or a blocked suture.

Once the repair is completed, the finger is immobilized in a palmar splint, which maintains the distal interphalangeal joint in extension and the proximal interphalangeal joint in about 45 degrees of flexion (Fig. 12–10) to relax the tension in the lateral extensor tendons (Fig. 12–11). The palmar splint and Kirschner wire are removed after 15 days, but immobilization of the distal joint is continued with a shorter splint for another three weeks (see the following section on treatment of ruptures) after which it is worn between sessions of active mobilization for an additional two weeks.

When the circumstances do not favor primary suturing, e.g., in the presence of a contused wound, the first priority is to provide a good skin cover. The distal joint is

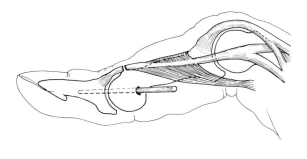
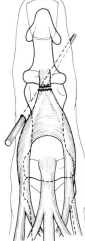

Figure 12–8. A fine Kirschner wire maintains the distal interphalangeal joint in slight hyperextension.

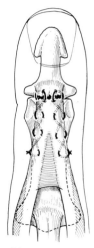

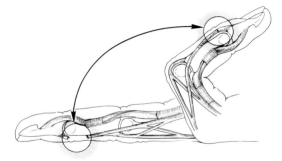

Figure 12–11. Flexion of the proximal interphalangeal joint involves relaxation of the lateral extensor tendons, which facilitates the junction between the two ends of the tendon.

Figure 12–9. Double suture of the two lateral extensor tendons.

maintained in extension for seven weeks, after which secondary repair, tendon suturing, or arthrodesis is seldom required.

Primary Treatment of Ruptures and Bone Avulsions

The distal phalanx is again immobilized in extension for seven consecutive weeks. Several methods of immobilization have been suggested.

Splinting. Producing a suitable splint is not as easy as it may seem. The splint may be made of plaster and immobilizes the proximal interphalangeal joint in slight flexion and the distal joint in extension (Smillie, 1937). The patient can be made to hold the digit in the position of correction while the plaster sets.

Circular plaster casts ensure good immobilization but unless perfectly molded, they can produce pressure sores. The nail matrix, the nail, and the dorsal aspect of the proximal interphalangeal joint must be left uncovered.

To bypass the difficulties of plaster mold-ing, some authors have suggested using mechanical or plastic splints. There are several designs available in different sizes, some malleable, others already fixed in the correcting position, with or without rubber foam lining.

Palmar splints, of whatever design, are difficult to keep in place for several weeks. They require frequent checks because they can slip and become ineffective. For this reason some models have been designed (such as that of Stack) that are partly supported on the dorsum of the middle phalanx while also supporting the pulp (Fig. 12–12). A recent modification (Stack, 1986) with two large windows has been introduced to allow evaporation of moisture and sweat more easily and to allow contact against the pulp surface of the finger.

There are also the dorsal splints, as used by Michon, supported by the nail and the dorsal aspect of the middle phalanx. The advantage is that the sensitivity of the pulp is respected.

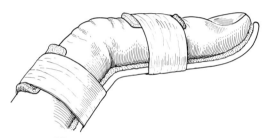

Figure 12–10. Long digital splint.

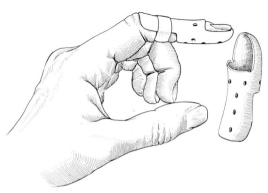

Figure 12–12. Stack splint made of polyethylene, which applies dorsal pressure on the middle phalanx.

Immobilization by Kirschner Wire. The distal joint can be immobilized by a Kirschner wire introduced about 2 mm. under the nail (Casscells and Strange, 1969). It goes without saying that the insertion of the wire must be carried out under aseptic conditions. The Kirschner wire is checked regularly and replaced by a movable splint at the first sign of inflammation. We do not use the same Kirschner wire, as suggested by Pratt (1952), to fix the distal joint in extension and the proximal joint in flexion.

We know of no infallible method for preventing infection around a transcutaneous Kirschner wire. Some surgeons advocate the use of a dressing held in place by surgical varnish, while others believe that a transpulpar longitudinal wire inserted close to the nail is protected by the growing nail (Albertoni, 1977). The risk is reduced if a splint is also worn or if the wire is buried under the skin.

Surgical Repair. In selected cases the ruptured tendon may be repaired surgically as a primary procedure, using a technique similar to that described for open injuries. Esteve (1964) has described a specific method: A nylon suture with a curved needle at both ends is tacked through the proximal extremity of the ruptured tendon; the two needles take a bite through the periosteum of the distal phalanx and emerge through the nail on either side of the lunula (Fig. 12–13). The two sutures are placed under traction to pull the tendon down and are tied under tension to produce hyperextension of the distal joint. The slow growth of the nail during immobilization helps to maintain the correct tension.

NATURE OF THE LESIONS. The more severe and the more distal the injury, the greater the deformity will be. When it is greater than 45 degrees, it may be preferable to release the traction exerted by the lateral bands of the extensor apparatus and maintain the proximal interphalangeal joint flexed for the first two weeks of treatment.

THE FINGER INVOLVED. The figures published by Albertoni (1977) emphasize the fact that the results are worse when the middle and index fingers are involved, regardless of the method of immobilization chosen.

CHOICE OF TREATMENT. The choice of treatment must also take into account the age and occupation of the patient.

It is probably fair to say that the treatment as a rule is conservative and closed. The presence of a small bone fragment, which

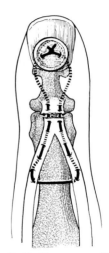

Figure 12–13. The suture of Esteve.

can be reduced by extension of the distal phalanx, in no way modifies this approach and is not in itself an indication for open surgical repair.

In the majority of cases the choice lies between use of a short splint immobilizing the distal interphalangeal joint only or a long one immobilizing both interphalangeal joints.

1. When conditions are favorable, i.e., when the index or middle finger is not involved, the deformity is less than 45 degrees, and the patient is cooperative and motivated, it may be possible just to use a splint with a dorsal component to immobilize only the distal joint for seven weeks without interruption. Because this is not cumbersome, the patient can resume most of his activities. It is kept in position by adhesive tape and reinforced as required by the patient.

2. When the conditions are unfavorable from the start, i.e., severe deformity of more than 45 degrees, involvement of the index or middle finger, or a tendency to hyperextension of the proximal interphalangeal joint, a long splint immobilizing both joints is prescribed. After two weeks the splint is replaced by a short one, which is worn continuously for a further five weeks.

In any event the position of the distal phalanx after removal of the splint must be watched. If a lack of extension persists, wearing of the splint must be continued before starting active mobilization, which must be progressive, without any attempt to achieve complete flexion of the distal interphalangeal joint for several months.

In our opinion surgery is indicated only in

rare cases in which a large bone fragment is avulsed and is irreducible by external maneuvers. In the absence of reduction, extension of the distal phalanx may remain limited and post-traumatic osteoarthrosis may develop (Green and Rowland, 1975).

A fragment including one-third of the joint surface may result in palmar subluxation of the joint. Hyperextension of the distal phalanx accentuates the displacement. Fixation of the bone fragment and correction of the articular displacement are now indicated. Reduction of the interphalangeal luxation with a Kirschner wire can render reduction of the displaced fragment more difficult. The latter maneuver therefore is carried out first, although it too can be far from easy in view of the limited joint exposure.

Immobilization of the fragment, which is usually triangular, poses another problem by reason of the small size of the fragment and the risk of splitting it if the drill or wire used is too large. If equipment of the right size is not available, it is probably safer to maintain the fragment in place by means of a transperiosteal suture. Allieu (1977) has advocated the use of barbed wire with the barb holding onto the bone fragment; the suture is passed close to the fragment, holding it down against the phalanx, and after changing to a curved needle is carried through the nail.

We have used with satisfactory results a procedure described by Blalock, modifying only the incision. A transverse incision is made away from the nail matrix with V-shaped prolongations at each end, making it possible to fold back two flaps, one proximal and one distal (Fig. 12–14). Fibrous tissue is removed from the area that is to receive the

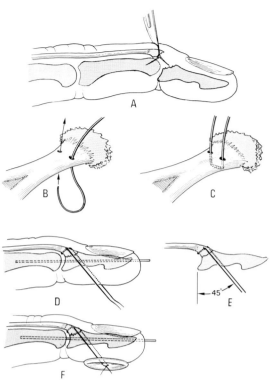

Figure 12–15. Reposition of an avulsion fracture, causing subluxation of the distal phalanx. *A*, Transverse incision. *B*, Suture of the extremity of the extensor tendon using the S. Blalock technique. *C*, The suture makes a U shape under the deep surface of the tendon at the edge of the avulsed fragment. *D*, The fragment is replaced. The subluxation is reduced and the distal phalanx is stabilized with a Kirschner wire. *E*, The suture holding the triangular bone fragment in place makes a 45 degree angle with the joint surface. *F*, The suture is tied at the end of the procedure, thereby ensuring stability.

avulsed fragment. A strong U-shaped suture is passed through the tendon from the undersurface at the edge of the bone fragment, as indicated by Blalock (1980) (Fig. 12–15). The fragment is replaced, held by the anchoring suture, which presses down on its dorsal surface. Each end of this suture is passed around either side of the distal phalanx, from a dorsal direction and through the pulp along an axis of 45 degrees to the joint surface. Before fixing the suture, a transarticular wire correcting the subluxation is inserted. The suture is then fixed by tying over a button (Fig. 12–15). Radiological control is used systematically. If the reduction of the bony fragment is not perfect, the technique of Hamas (1978) can be used. He obtains a better view of the base of the distal phalanx by dividing the extensor tendon 5 mm. from

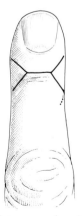

Figure 12–14. Transverse dorsal incision with V-shaped prolongations at each end.

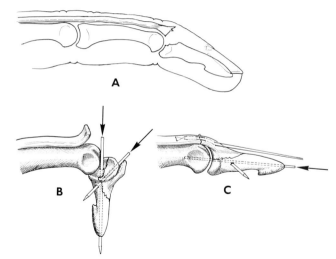

Figure 12–16. Repositioning of an avulsion of the base of the distal phalanx by the Hamas procedure. *A*, The avulsed fragment. *B*, The distal extensor tendon is divided. The fracture is reduced and maintained by an oblique Kirschner wire. A longitudinal Kirschner wire is inserted in the base of the distal phalanx. *C*, The longitudinal wire is pushed proximally and fixes the joint in extension. The extensor tendon is then sutured.

its insertion (Fig. 12–16). A fine Kirschner wire is inserted through the joint into the distal phalanx. The bone fragment is reduced under direct vision and immobilized by means of an oblique Kirschner wire. The phalanx is then extended, the subluxation reduced, and the first wire inserted backward into the middle phalanx. The divided tendon is repaired, and the wires are extracted after seven or eight weeks.

Early surgical repair can also be considered when there is a pronounced flexion deformity suggesting complete rupture and retraction of the extensor. Our surgical experience is too limited, however, to allow us to express an opinion, but we have had some good results in such cases using nonsurgical treatment.

We have never performed an arthrodesis of the distal interphalangeal joint as a primary procedure.

SECONDARY REPAIR

We group together the indications for secondary treatment of open injuries and ruptures, except for cases in which scarring makes a direct surgical approach risky.

There is some disagreement about when a rupture can be regarded as "chronic." Some authors call a lesion old (chronic) after 15 days (Albertoni, 1977; Pratt, 1952), whereas others, such as Zancolli, use the term after only eight weeks.

Is there a time limit for nonsurgical treatment? We have had good results with immobilization up to six months after the injury,

but it is also true, as shown by the data of Stark, Boyes, and Wilson (1962), that the percentage of failures increases steadily with the age of the lesion.

Protected immobilization with only a possible chance of success can be extremely inconvenient for a manual worker. Only rarely do we resort to such immobilization after two months, and then only after discussing the various possibilities with the patient.

"Inactivity" is often advocated. There is a tendency to underestimate the sequelae of the mallet finger. There is seldom much functional embarrassment, although catching the deformed finger mechanically can be a recurring nuisance. In the index and middle fingers, pulp to pulp opposition, with the distal phalanx extended, is much more commonly used than terminal pinch with the distal phalanx in flexion. Thus a fixed flexion deformity of the distal joint in some professional circumstances can cause some constraint. Pain is not uncommon and can last for a long time. Finally there is the cosmetic aspect, which can be an important one, especially in women.

To imply that the deformity improves with time is tantamount to hoping that the patient will adapt to the lesion. When we decide against treatment, it is primarily because no treatment can ensure success.

Surgical treatment is not without drawbacks, and the results are not always satisfactory. Correction of the deformity may be incomplete, flexion of the terminal phalanx is often reduced, and persistent pain is not unknown. For these reasons one should op-

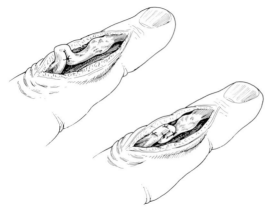

Figure 12–17. Shortening of the extensor apparatus by plication in a healthy area.

erate on mallet fingers only when they interfere with manual function or when the hyperextension of the proximal interphalangeal joint tends to increase.

A number of surgical procedures have been devised and all have yielded a proportion of good results, but the percentage of failures remains significant. The procedures described include resection of the callus and tendon suturing, shortening of the extensor tendon (by plication) in a healthy zone in conjunction with a tenolysis, and reinsertion of the tendon (Fig. 12–17). We shall only describe the techniques that we use most commonly: excision of the callus combined with a skin excision, tendon graft, tenotomy of the median extensor tendon, and arthrodesis.

SIMULTANEOUS CALLUS AND SKIN EXCISION

Brooks and F. Iselin independently have developed a technique that involves the following steps:

1. A transverse ellipse of skin, about 2 to 3 mm. wide, is excised from the dorsal aspect of the distal interphalangeal joint.

2. The tendon callus at the same level is excised, preferably without opening the capsule, a maneuver that is not always possible.

3. Four 3-0 monofilament nylon sutures are passed through the skin, tendon, and capsule on one side and then on the other. They are not tied at once, but the sutures are crossed over to check that full extension of the joint can be obtained.

4. Graner added a Kirschner wire, which

fixes the terminal phalanx in slight hyperextension.

5. The sutures are then tied en bloc.

The Kirschner wire is left in place for six weeks.*

TENDON GRAFTING

Our technique of tendon grafting is based on the method devised by Nichols. A longitudinal incision provides a good view of the extensor apparatus. The integuments are gently lifted, and care is taken not to damage the small distal neurovascular pedicles coursing to the nail matrix. The joint is fixed in 5 degrees of hyperextension with a fine oblique wire. The extensor apparatus is tenolysed on the dorsum of the middle phalanx without touching the gliding plane. Resection of the retracted oblique fibers of the retinacular ligament may be useful in facilitating distal advancement of the common extensor.

A thin strip 6 cm. long and 2 mm. wide is taken from one of the wrist flexors (palmaris longus or flexor carpi radialis). The middle part of the graft is anchored to the base of the terminal phalanx (to the fibrous tissue if it is tough enough; otherwise a small hole is drilled in the bone). The two ends of the graft are then crossed over the midline at the level of the distal joint and passed through the lateral tendons (Fig. 12–18). The proximal joint is then flexed, and the tension in

---

*Albertoni analyzes the results in old lesions repaired by this technique in Chapter 13.

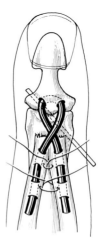

Figure 12–18. The technique of grafting used by author.

the graft is adjusted by means of several stitches (whose knots are buried), uniting the two ends of the graft. The finger is immobilized for two weeks with the proximal joint in flexion. The wire is removed after four weeks, but the distal joint is immobilized in extension with a short splint for a further three weeks (i.e., seven weeks in all).

The graft offers the advantage of reinforcing the stretched callus and of being tethered to the proximal part of the tendon, which is thus pulled distally. In addition, it tends to retract, whereas a fragile callus, submitted to continuous tension, would show a tendency to stretch.

CORRECTION OF MALLET DEFORMITY ASSOCIATED WITH A SWAN-NECK DEFORMITY

Littler's spiral tendon graft (Thompson et al., 1978) (see Chapter 16, on swan-neck deformities) permits an elegant correction of these two deformities when both joints are mobile. Another technique of reconstruction of the oblique retinacular ligament has been described by Kleinman and Petersen (1984), the tendon graft being fixed by soft tissue technique only.

TENOTOMY OF THE MEDIAN EXTENSOR TENDON

This technique, advocated by Fowler (1949), can be used only if the joints are supple and mobile. It is contraindicated in

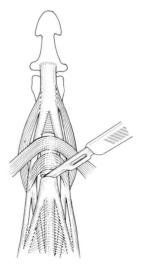

Figure 12–19. Tenotomy of the middle extensor tendon. The transverse structures are preserved. The triangular lamina and especially the spiral fibers prevent volar sliding of the lateral extensor tendons.

the presence of stiffness of the distal joint that prevents its passive correction.

Dividing the central extensor tendon only on the base of the middle phalanx allows the terminal band and fibrous callus to retract proximally (Fig. 12–19). There is little risk of a boutonnière deformity if one spares the spiral fibers and the other transverse structures that prevent the lateral tendons from pulling apart. The central tendon is divided through a small incision over its insertion (Fig. 12–20). The two interphalangeal joints are immobilized in extension for three weeks. However, the deformity is only partially corrected.

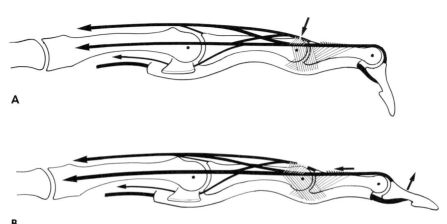

A

B

Figure 12–20. Mechanism of tenotomy. Section of the central extensor tendon involves a proximal retraction of the extensor apparatus.

This technique is usually reserved for mild rheumatoid deformities. It has the advantage of making sutures unnecessary; they are often poorly tolerated in patients with very fragile skin. Bowers and Hurst (1978) have reported good results with this technique. It can also be used for traumatic lesions in which the hand joints remain supple but hyperextension of the proximal interphalangeal joint develops rapidly. If this deformity is very pronounced, a tenodesis may be indicated.*

ARTHRODESIS

Arthrodesis is reserved for cases in which the distal joint is painful or is the site of a fixed deformity. It is also a last resort when surgery has failed to correct a deformity. If the proximal interphalangeal joint has retained its mobility, the distal joint is fixed in a position agreed upon with the patient. This will vary between 5 and 20 degrees of flexion, the ulnar fingers being flexed more than the radial ones.

SUMMARY

In a mallet finger seen more than one month after the injury, surgical correction is

---

*See Chapter 16 on swan-neck deformities.

indicated only if the deformity constitutes such a functional handicap that the patient himself demands it, or if splinting alone has failed to bring about significant improvement.

In the majority of cases of a long standing mallet finger deformity of traumatic origin, we now use the Brooks Graner technique, which by virtue of its simplicity is tending to replace other procedures.

When the extensor lag exceeds 60 degrees, exploration of the lesion seems preferable. If the tendinous callus is only a few millimeters in length, it is merely resected, with associated careful tenolysis of the extensor apparatus along the full length of the middle phalanx, allowing tendon suturing without tension. After the tendon has been freed, if the fibrous tissue providing continuity of the tendon appears to be of poor quality, risking rupture, this would necessitate a resection of 5 mm. or more when the phalanx is held straight, and thus a tendon graft would be justified.

There are special indications for tenotomy of the central extensor tendon and arthrodesis.

REFERENCES

References will be found following Chapter 23.

Chapter 13

THE BROOKS-GRANER PROCEDURE FOR CORRECTION OF MALLET FINGER

WALTER MANNA ALBERTONI

The mallet finger injury, a flexion deformity of the distal interphalangeal joint with the inability to actively extend it, is a rather common ailment. It is likely to occur in sports related and work related injuries. The terminal extensor tendon ruptures near its insertion at the base of the distal phalanx, and an avulsion fracture may also occur. Both the deformity and the resulting functional incapacity depend on the time elapsed since the injury. In older injuries, there is not only a marked drop of the distal phalanx but also an imbalance in hyperextension of the proximal interphalangeal joint is established, leading to a deformity known as the "swanneck" finger.

Although there are several procedures for correcting this deformity, none provides an invariably reliable result.

In 1961 Brooks from the Royal National Orthopaedic Hospital in London, visited São Paulo (Brazil) and described an operative procedure for treatment of the mallet finger that he had been using since 1958 with apparently good results.

The technique was simple, consisting of elliptical wedging of the soft tissues in the dorsum of the injured distal interphalangeal joint, including the skin and subcutaneous tissue and the scarred extensor tendon. The wound edges were then closed with two or three en bloc mattress sutures, resulting in a hyperextended position of the distal interphalangeal joint. The digit was then externally splinted, either in a plaster cast or in an aluminum splint, for four weeks.

Since then, Graner, in São Paulo, has used the proposed technique, with both good and unsatisfactory results, but he decided to use a thin Kirschner wire to keep the distal interphalangeal joint in hyperextension, instead of employing an external support, thus modifying Brooks' original method (Figs. 13–1

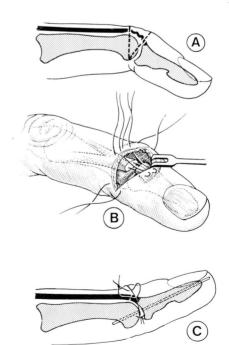

Figure 13–1. Diagram of Brooks-Graner procedure. *A*, Excision of tendon callus and skin. *B*, Suture of tendon and skin. *C*, Fixation of distal interphalangeal joint by Kirschner wire.

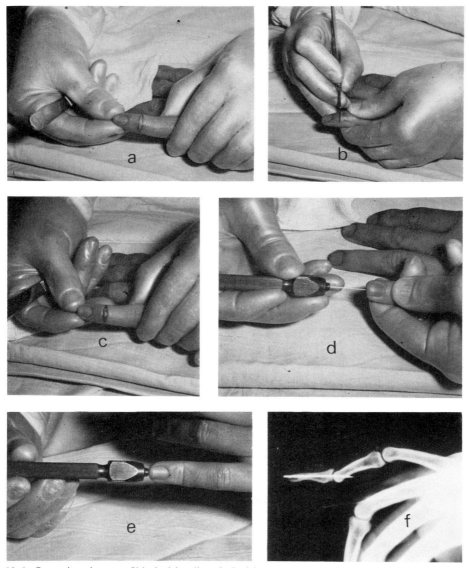

Figure 13–2. Operative views. *a*, Skin incision line. *b*, Incision on dorsal aspect of the joint. *c*, Resection of skin and tendon. *d*, The distal joint is placed in slight hyperextension. *e*, Wire in place. *f*, X-ray follow-up.

and 13–2). The Kirschner wire is left in place for 45 days. After using the modified procedure in more than 200 cases, Graner reported greater reliability of the results.

I have been interested in this procedure since 1972, when I started to write a doctoral thesis on the subject, and in 1975 the preliminary results were reported to Brooks, in London. Because the description of the technique had not been published at the time, in mutual agreement with the authors we decided to call it the Brooks-Graner procedure.

MATERIAL AND METHODS

From 1972 to 1979, 48 patients who had mallet fingers were treated with the Brooks-Graner procedure (Fig. 13–3).

The ages of the patients ranged from eight to 66 years, with the majority of patients between 20 and 30 years old.

Of the 48 patients, 30 had received no initial treatment, and most had delayed seeking treatment, for periods ranging from 18 days to one year after injury. The other 18 patients had been treated elsewhere, by other methods, with unsatisfactory results.

Detailed radiographic and photographic recordings were made of the fingers operated upon, before and after surgical treatment, in order to measure the distal phalangeal drop.

The functional result in the distal interphalangeal joint was evaluated at least 30 days after the Kirschner wire had been removed. Its measured value, in degrees, was expressed as a "deficit" in relation to the corresponding digit on the other hand (both for flexion and for extension).

In the final evaluation of the result, because active extension of the distal interphalangeal joint is the main objective, a 10 degree "deficit" of active extension is considered a satisfactory result, but when the deficit is more than 10 degrees, the result is unsatisfactory. Flexion capability is estimated after treatment; a limitation of as much as 30 degrees in that range of motion does not interfere with the result, whereas when the loss of flexion is more than 30 degrees, the result is considered unsatisfactory.

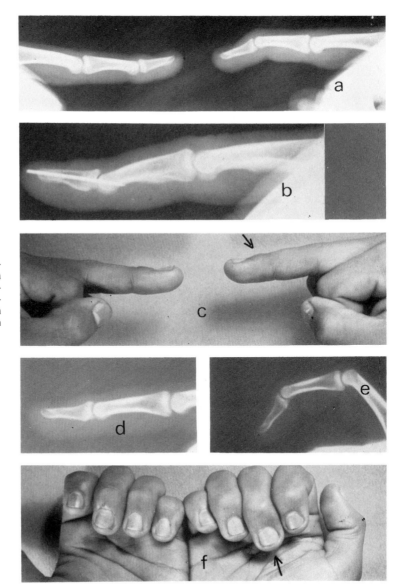

Figure 13–3. Clinical case. *a*, Preoperative x-rays comparing both hands. *b*, Wire in place. *c*, Postoperative photograph. *d*, X-ray of distal phalanx in extension. *e*, X-ray in flexion. *f*, Comparative view of both hands in flexion.

RESULTS

Of the 48 patients with previously untreated mallet finger deformities treated by use of the Brooks-Graner procedure, satisfactory results were obtained in 44, i.e., 91.6 per cent. Of the four unsatisfactory results, three were due to extension deficits of more than 10 degrees and one to a limitation of flexion of more than 30 degrees.

DISCUSSION

The good results obtained with this technique apparently reflect the fact that in old lesions of the extensor tendon, unlike the fresh rupture, there is a strong fibrous scar bridge between the insertion and the proximal ruptured part of the extensor mechanism, which acts as an elongated tendon that is unable to fully extend the joint. The wedge resection of the soft tissues in the dorsum of the distal interphalangeal joint, accompanied by en bloc mattress suturing and internal fixation of the distal interphalangeal joint in the hyperextended position, promotes shortening of the tendon, thus correcting the deformity once the extensor mechanism has been compensated for.

Several authors, including Pagani and Bilancini (1962), Rueff et al. (1967), and Ducourtioux and Pouliquen (1969), had already called attention to the characteristics of the connective tissue filling in the gap of the separated parts of the terminal extensor mechanism; 20 days after the time of injury it looks very much like the tendon itself. We performed histological studies of fragments of the interposed scars, and in the older cases a "fibrin network was found enveloping a denser one of connective tissue containing foci of osseous metaplasia."

No serious complications have been observed in using this procedure. In a few cases a purulent blister was found at the point of entry of the Kirschner wire at the pulp, which was often triggered by minor trauma to the area. This does not hamper the result of the treatment, for the infection is superficial and swiftly clears upon removal of the wire. The incidence of this complication diminished when patients were asked not to cut the nails on the affected digits, so as to develop a natural protective "bumper."

An accidental rupture of the Kirschner wire was reported by one patient who had fallen, stubbing his finger. Both portions of the Kirschner wire were removed and the operation was again performed by use of the same technique. The result was satisfactory.

In one case superficial necrosis of the skin was observed on the dorsum of the distal interphalangeal joint. Viable tissue eventually replaced it, and the patient had a satisfactory result.

The Kirschner wire is used to penetrate the volar cortex of the middle phalanx in a firm grip, after transfixing the distal phalanx. The hyperextended position is thus firmly maintained and prevents the wire from accidentally migrating proximally, necessitating a troublesome retrieval.

Iselin et al. (1977) have used a procedure for the treatment of mallet finger deformities that is similar to the one described here, including a dorsal resection of the distal interphalangeal joint, called "tenodermodesis," done in much the same way as proposed by Brooks, in which external immobilization was maintained for 35 days. The same authors reported that their method had been used since 1973, with 22 satisfactory results in 26 cases.

CONCLUSION

Because the Brooks-Graner procedure is technically simple and yields a high proportion of satisfactory results, it is an excellent method for the management of both old untreated and previously unsuccessfully treated mallet finger deformities.

REFERENCES

Albertoni, W. M.: "Mallet Finger": Techniques of Treatment. Thesis, São Paulo, Brazil, 1977.

Brooks, D. (London): Personal communication, 1976.

Casscells, S. W., and Strange, T. B.: Intramedullary wire fixation of mallet finger. J. Bone Joint Surg., 51A:1018–1019, 1969.

Ducourtioux, J. L., and Pouliquen, X.: Our experience in the treatment of mallet finger. Ann. Chir. Plast., 14:249–253, 1969.

Graner, O.: Contribuição para o tratamento do "dedo em martelo" (in press).

Iselin, F., Levame, J., and Godoy, J.: A simplified technique for treating mallet fingers: tenodermodesis. J. Hand Surg., 2:118–121, 1977.

Pagani, A., and Bilancini, G.: Le lesioni traumatiche dei tendini estensori delle dita della mano. Minerva Ortop., 13:679–684, 1962.

Rueff, F., Bedacht, R., and Pannike, A.: Clinical features of the extensor tendon at the distal end of the finger. Chirurgia, 38:317–321, 1967.

Tubiana, R.: Treatment of mallet fingers. In Verdan, C. (Editor): Lesions Tendineuses, Monographie du G.E.M. Paris, Expansion Scientifique.

Chapter 14

ANATOMY OF THE EXTENSOR APPARATUS AT THE LEVEL OF THE PROXIMAL INTERPHALANGEAL JOINT

RAOUL TUBIANA

This region is anatomically and physiologically the most complex. The extensor apparatus at this level consists of a central tendon and two lateral tendons (Fig. 14–1).

The terms "tendon" and "band" are commonly used interchangeably to describe the various structures of the extensor apparatus at this level (Fig. 14–2). In the interests of clarity here we shall reserve use of the term "tendon" to designate the terminal portion of insertion formed by junction of the bands arising from the intrinsic and extrinsic muscles.

At the level of the proximal interphalangeal joint there is one central (or middle) extensor tendon that crosses the proximal interphalangeal joint on its dorsal surface and is then inserted into the base of the middle phalanx. This tendon is formed by the junction of the central bands of the extensor digitorum and of the intrinsic muscles.

According to Stack (1962), the amplitude of movement at this level is about 8 mm. The middle tendon plays a highly important role in extension of the three phalanges. It extends the middle phalanx into which it is inserted, except when the metacarpophalangeal joint is in hyperextension; the action of extensor communis is then spent on its proximal insertion. It also acts indirectly on the other two phalanges; it contributes to the extension of the proximal phalanx by displacing the base of the middle phalanx dorsally on the head of the proximal phalanx when the proximal interphalangeal joint is flexed. It also extends the distal phalanx, at least in

the first half of the movement, through the passive coordinating action of the oblique retinacular ligament.

On the dorsolateral aspect of the joint the two lateral bands of the interosseous tendons receive lateral bands from the extensor communis to become the lateral extensor tendons. Both these fiber bands glide along the posterolateral aspect of the joint during flexion movements; the gliding is closely checked by several other fibrous structures—the triangular ligament, the spiral fibers of the extensor apparatus, and the retinacular ligaments.

The *triangular ligament* or lamina comprise the transverse fibers arising from the medial borders of the lateral extensor tendons at the level of the middle phalanx (Fig. 14–3). They form a fine triangular membrane at the apex of which the two lateral tendons unite.

The *spiral fibers* are more proximal and curl from the lateral extensor tendons to the central tendon over the proximal interphalangeal joint (Fig. 14–4). These fibers were described by Hauck in 1923 and then by Baumann and Patry in 1943, but lately they have been confused with the other transverse structures of this region, the transverse lamina and the transverse retinacular ligament (Fig. 14–5). Their action has been more recently defined by Gaul (1971) and by Van Zwieten (1980). The spiral fibers are continuations of the long extensor tendon and the interosseous tendons. They branch off the lateral margins of the lateral tendons at the distal third of the proximal phalanx and run

101

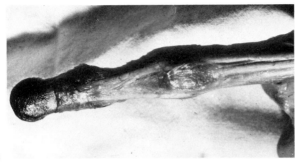

A

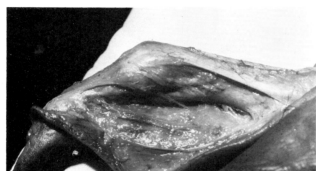

B

Figure 14–1. Anatomical preparation showing the extensor apparatus at the level of the proximal interphalangeal joint. *A*, Dorsal view. *B*, Lateral view.

Figure 14–2. Diagram showing principal anatomical features of the extensor apparatus. 1 = insertion of the middle extensor tendon on the base of the middle phalanx; 2 = spiral fibers; 3 = transverse retinacular ligament, which is inserted laterally in the dermis; 4 = triangular lamina; 5 = lateral extensor tendon; 6 = oblique retinacular ligament; 7 = terminal extensor tendon.

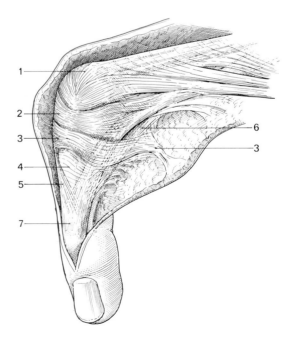

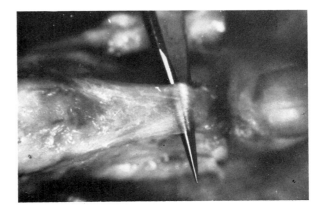

Figure 14–3. Terminal extensor tendon and triangular lamina.

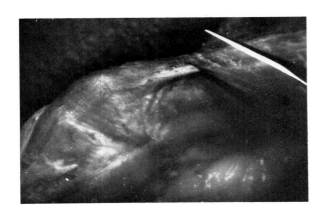

Figure 14–4. Spiral fibers running from the lateral extensor tendons to the central tendon at the proximal part of the proximal interphalangeal joint.

Figure 14–5. Transverse tendon structures at the proximal interphalangeal joint. The spiral fibers are the most proximal and the triangular lamina the most distal. The more superficial transverse retinacular ligament has been removed.

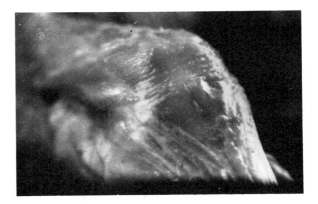

distally and medially, spiraling over the dorsal surfaces of the lateral tendons. They are arranged in two flat sheets, which join together in midline at the level of the distal part of the central tendon. These fibers prevent lateral displacement of the lateral extensor tendons.

The *oblique retinacular ligament* was identified by Weitbrecht (1742) under the name of "retinaculum tendini longi" (Kaplan, 1965) and has been described by Landsmeer (1949), who defined its function. This fibrous bundle extends symmetrically on either side of the proximal interphalangeal joint and has no muscular connection. It is inserted in one part on the volar surface of the lateral surface of the distal third of the proximal phalanx and on the fibrous flexor tendon sheath. It crosses obliquely the lateral aspect of the proximal interphalangeal joint running distally and dorsally. It progressively approaches the lateral extensor tendons, which it joins in the distal half of the middle phalanx. The fibers mingle with the fibers of the two lateral extensor tendons and form the distal extensor tendon, inserting into the base of the distal phalanx.

These ligaments coordinate the movements of the interphalangeal joints. In fact, these ligaments, which cross diagonally the axis of rotation of the proximal interphalangeal joint, are placed under tension by flexion of the distal interphalangeal joint and cause simultaneous flexion of the proximal interphalangeal joint. The ligaments are also placed under tension by extension of the proximal interphalangeal joint (caused by the central extensor tendon), which in turn causes extension of the distal interphalangeal joint.

The *transverse retinacular ligament* is non-tendinous but moves superficially and runs in the subcutaneous and subfascial spaces around the proximal interphalangeal joint (Fig. 14–6). These fibers are attached to skin and the subcutaneous layers as well as to the extensor apparatus. These fibers form a thin fibrous lamella on the lateral and dorsal surfaces of the extensor apparatus to which they adhere on either side of the joint.

Flexion of the proximal interphalangeal joint causes distal and lateral gliding of the lateral extensor tendons. This results in a reduction in tension within the lateral and terminal extensor tendons and allows the distal interphalangeal joint to be flexed by the flexor profundus. The lateral displacement is controlled by the lateral transverse structures. The triangular lamina can have only an accessory role because it is thin and situated distally. The transverse retinacular ligament is an even more fragile structure and can have such an action only when it is sclerosed and thickened in pathological situations, as in the boutonnière deformity.

It is the spiral fibers that normally play the essential role in the control of and coordination between the lateral tendons, by virtue of their obliquity, their length, their location in relation to the proximal interphalangeal joint, and their combined attachment to the lateral tendons and the central tendon. The mechanism of these displacements has been well demonstrated by Van Zwieten (1980). Any disturbance in this delicate mechanism results in a deformity of the fingers.

If the balance in the phalangeal chain is broken, three types of deformities result, each having a descriptive name:

The "clawhand" deformity is characterized by hyperextension of the metacarpophalangeal joint and flexion of the proximal inter-

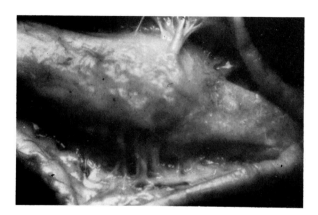

Figure 14–6. The transverse retinacular ligament is a nontendinous structure that transversely crosses the proximal interphalangeal joint and extensor apparatus and is inserted on both sides into the deep surface of the dermis.

phalangeal joint. It is the result of a paralysis of the interosseous muscles and does not come within the scope of this chapter.

We shall describe the so-called "buttonhole" or "boutonnière" and "swan-neck" deformities even though they can also have nontraumatic origins. In the boutonnière deformity the primary lesion lies in the middle extensor tendon, leading to flexion of the proximal interphalangeal joint and hyperextension of the distal interphalangeal joint.

In the swan-neck deformity the proximal interphalangeal joint is in hyperextension and the distal interphalangeal joint in flexion. The deformity can be caused by a variety of factors, which have in common excessive traction on the middle tendon inserted into the base of the middle phalanx.

REFERENCES

References will be found following Chapter 23.

Chapter 15

THE BOUTONNIÈRE DEFORMITY

Raoul Tubiana

Division, avulsion, rupture, or progressive elongation of the middle (or central) extensor tendon inserted on the base of the middle phalanx does not lead to deformity if the spiral fibers of the extensor apparatus and the triangular lamina that join the two lateral extensor tendons on the dorsum of the proximal interphalangeal joint and the middle phalanx are intact (Fig. 15–1). However, when these transverse fibers are also damaged, the lateral extensor tendons sublux (Fig. 15–2). They form a "buttonhole" or "boutonnière" through which the proximal interphalangeal joint protrudes (Fig. 15–3). This results in a zigzag deformity of the finger.

The boutonnière deformity is a progressive condition. First the middle phalanx is flexed by the now unopposed action of the flexor superficialis. Then the distal phalanx becomes hyperextended (Fig. 15–4) as a result of the increased power of extension because of proximal retraction of the central extensor tendon (Fig. 15–5). When the lateral tendons slide volarly on the sides of the proximal interphalangeal joint, they are under tension because of the width of the joint even though

their route is theoretically shorter in a sagittal plane. When the lateral tendons pass in front of the axis of rotation of the proximal interphalangeal joint, they act as primary flexors and increase the flexion of the proximal interphalangeal joint. Proximal contracture of the middle tendon sometimes can put the metacarpophalangeal joint into hyperextension because of the traction on the proximal insertions of the extensor digitorum (sagittal bands) and the insertion onto the base of the middle phalanx (Fig. 15–6).

The retinacular ligament contributes to the fixation of this deformity in two ways (Fig. 15–7): its retracted transverse fibers maintain the palmar dislocation of the lateral extensor tendons, and its oblique fibers, which are inserted distally on the lateral tendons at the level of the middle phalanx and proximally on the fibrous flexor sheath and the periosteum of the proximal phalanx, are at first relaxed by the proximal displacement of the extensor apparatus. Secondarily these oblique fibers retract, fixing the middle phalanx in flexion and the distal phalanx in extension.

Haines (1951) and Zancolli (1968) have

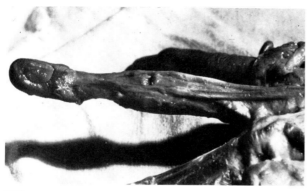

Figure 15–1. Photograph of an anatomical specimen with division of the middle extensor tendon near its insertion on the base of the middle phalanx. The lateral extensor tendons are left in place; there is no deformity.

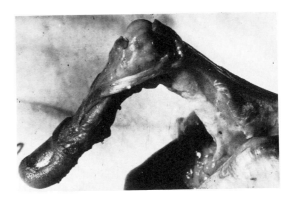

Figure 15–2. The transverse fibrous structures: the spiral fibers and the triangular lamina are ruptured. The lateral extensor tendons are subluxated volarly, creating a boutonnière.

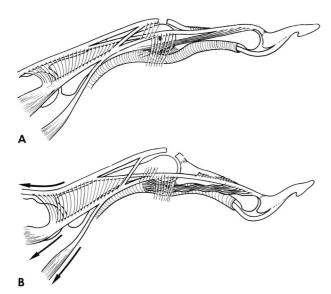

A

B

Figure 15–3. The pathological anatomy of the boutonnière deformity. *A*, Division or rupture of the middle extensor tendon. The transverse fibrous formations which unite the lateral extensor tendons are still intact. The spiral fibers and triangular ligament are in part preserved. The lateral tendons maintain their normal anatomical position. *B*, If there is a rupture of the transverse fibers, the lateral extensor tendons sublux laterally, forming a buttonhole through which the proximal interphalangeal joint herniates.

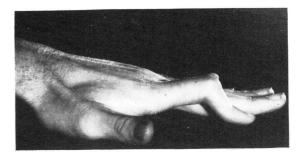

Figure 15–4. Photograph showing a zigzag deformity of the three joints of the digital kinetic chain.

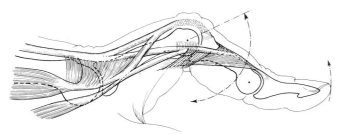

Figure 15–5. Progression of the deformity. The loss of insertion of the middle extensor tendon into the base of the middle phalanx causes a proximal retraction of the extensor apparatus. This results in hyperextension of the distal interphalangeal joint.

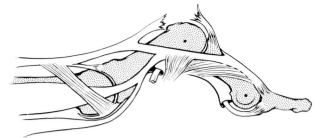

Figure 15–6. Diagram showing the proximal insertion of the common extensor tendon onto the base of the proximal phalanx, causing hyperextension of the metacarpophalangeal joint, and the contracture of the oblique and transverse retinacular ligaments, which fix the deformity.

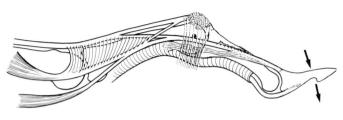

Figure 15–7. Diagram showing the progressive contracture of the oblique and transverse retinacular ligaments.

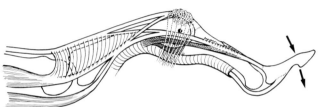

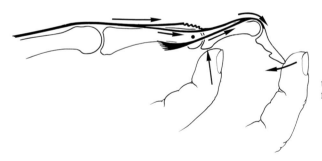

Figure 15–8. Haines-Zancolli test is negative. If the middle phalanx is maintained in extension, flexion of the distal phalanx is still possible.

Figure 15–9. Haines-Zancolli test is positive. If the middle phalanx is maintained in extension, flexion of the distal phalanx is not possible.

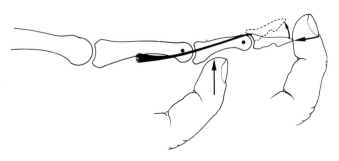

demonstrated this retraction by means of a clinical test (Fig. 15–8). In the absence of retraction of the oblique fibers, the distal phalanx can be passively flexed while the middle phalanx is maintained in extension (the retinacular test is then said to be negative). However, when these fibers are retracted, passive extension of the middle phalanx prevents flexion of the distal phalanx (and the retinacular test is termed positive) (Fig. 15–9).

ETIOLOGY

The boutonnière deformity can result from a variety of causes: injuries (division, avulsion, or rupture of the middle extensor tendon) can be associated with bony avulsion at the base of the middle phalanx. "Spontaneous rupture" may occur late after partial lacerations of the extensor tendons or after closed trauma. Burns of the dorsum of the digits and rheumatoid arthritis are other causes. A variety of problems arise in the two latter cases, which will not be considered here.*

In a series of 32 traumatic boutonnière deformities treated surgically (including 20 lacerations and 12 ruptures), we found an overall male predominance of 2:1 for both groups (Tubiana and Valentin, 1969). The average age of the patients was 39 years for the lacerations and 27 for the ruptures, figures well below those found for subcutaneous ruptures of other tendons.

The initial trauma causing the ruptures that led to the deformity was often severe. In the 12 cases of rupture there were four interphalangeal joint dislocations and five cases of violent trauma suggesting traumatic rupture of normal tendons. In that series the left hand was more often involved, as were the peripheral fingers, i.e., the index and little fingers.

---

*See chapters on burns and rheumatoid arthritis in Volume IV.

CLASSIFICATION

One can schematically classify boutonnière deformities into several clinical stages:

Stage 1: Minimal Deficiency of Extension. In these cases the lack of extension of the proximal interphalangeal joint is minimal (less than 30 degrees) and can be corrected passively with full flexion of the proximal interphalangeal joint and only slight limitation of flexion at the distal joint. This represents a moderate subluxation of the lateral tendons, which are still on the dorsal aspect of the axis of rotation of the joint. This lesion is easily reducible and produces little functional impairment.

Stage 2: Proximal Contracture of the Middle Extensor Tendon. Such proximal contracture accompanied by further subluxation of the lateral tendons that brings them in front of the axis of rotation results in an increase of flexion contracture of the proximal interphalangeal joint and of extension of the distal interphalangeal joint and slackening of the transverse and oblique fibers of the retinacular ligament. At an early stage before these deformities become fixed, the Haines-Zancolli retinacular test is negative (Fig. 15–8).

Stage 3: Contracture of Retinacular Ligaments. Fixed contracture of the oblique fibers of the retinacular ligament prevents passive flexion of the distal joint, thus giving a positive Haines-Zancolli test (Fig. 15–9). Fixed contracture of the transverse fibers of the retinacular ligament maintains the lateral tendons in the subluxed position but does not prevent passive correction of the flexion deformity at the proximal interphalangeal joint.

Stage 4: Fixed Contracture of the Proximal Interphalangeal Joint. Contracture of the volar plate, collateral ligaments, and capsule eventually leads to a fixed flexion contracture of the proximal interphalangeal joint (Fig. 15–10). A small amount of free flexion is still possible so long as the articular cartilage of the joint is not involved. The distal joint is fixed in hyperextension.

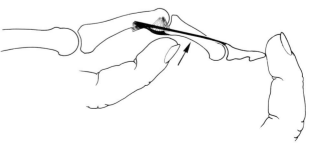

Figure 15–10. Contracture of the volar plate and the lateral accessory collateral ligaments, which become fixed, blocking passive extension of the joint.

The majority of traumatic boutonnière deformities at this stage of retraction do not progress. Some, according to Souter (1974), improve with time; others may become worse.

Possible Aggravating Factors. The deformity can be aggravated by further hyperextension of the distal interphalangeal joint, loss of the active flexion of the proximal interphalangeal joint, or fixed hyperextension of the metacarpophalangeal joint.

TREATMENT

A distinction must be made between easily reducible lesions of recent onset and chronic lesions complicated by contracture.

RECENT LESIONS

The line of treatment will be different depending on whether there is a laceration or a rupture.

Recent Lacerations

Injury to the extensor tendon on the dorsal aspect of the proximal interphalangeal joint does not lead immediately to a complete boutonnière deformity. The first symptom is the inability to actively extend the proximal interphalangeal joint, although passive extension is possible. Flexion of the distal joint is slightly limited, but hyperextension does not occur until a few days later when proximal retraction of the middle tendon occurs.

The first aim of treatment of lacerations consists of protecting the open joint against infection. The possibilities of tendon repair depend on the condition of the overlying skin. When local conditions are favorable, it is preferable to attempt direct repair to restore the normal anatomy rather than to undertake conservative treatment by splinting.

The lesions should always be systematically explored by enlarging the wound at both ends (Fig. 15–11). The proximal interphalangeal joint is fixed in the straight position by a fine wire inserted obliquely. The divided middle tendon is sutured directly (Fig. 15–12). Occasionally a small fragment of bone is avulsed with the tendon and this should be reattached or removed if it is very small and the tendon

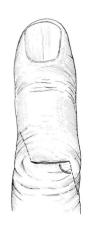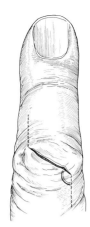

Figure 15–11. The wound is enlarged at its extremities, avoiding the formation of poorly vascularized acute angle flaps.

reinserted. The lateral tendons, if damaged, are also repaired. They are maintained in their physiological position by partially reconstructing the triangular ligament by means of a few sutures to approximate the distal parts of the lateral tendons.

A palmar splint should be used to immobilize the wrist in extension (25 degrees), with the metacarpophalangeal joint in slight flexion (20 degrees), and the distal interphalangeal joint in flexion (45 degrees) in order to relax tension on the suture line (Fig. 15–13). A Kirschner wire can be used to reinforce the splinting of the distal joint at 45

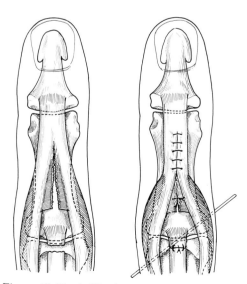

Figure 15–12. A Kirschner wire fixes the proximal interphalangeal joint in extension. The middle tendon is sutured and the lateral tendons are approximated.

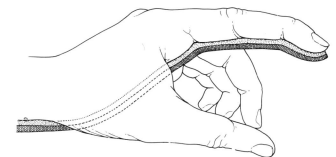

Figure 15–13. A splint immobilizing the wrist and the finger.

degrees. This wire in addition to the wire through the proximal interphalangeal joint is removed at two weeks, and the splint is removed after three weeks. Active mobilization of the metacarpophalangeal and distal interphalangeal joints is then resumed while the proximal interphalangeal joint is maintained in extension within a small circular plaster cast for two more weeks (Fig. 15–14). Then a dynamic splint of the Bunnell safety pin or Capener type is used, which keeps the proximal interphalangeal joint in extension but allows active flexion (Fig. 15–15).

The results of surgical repair in these open injuries at the proximal interphalangeal joint are usually good when the skin and tendon wounds are clean and tidy. By contrast, when the wound is contaminated or badly contused or if there is skin loss, the problem becomes difficult. One must provide an adequate skin cover for the joint. The proximal interphalangeal joint is held in extension. This causes a relatively large amount of scarring between the two tendon ends. The resulting joint stiffness is unavoidable. Physiotherapy has only minimal effect because of this scarring. A tenolysis performed a few months after the primary repair may be beneficial. However, the adhesions may be such that the freed tendinous mechanism is weakened, raising the possibility of a recurrence of the boutonnière deformity.

In order to avoid such sequelae, one should try to treat injuries involving tendon loss immediately. Snow (1973) proposed the construction of a retrograde flap of the proximal portion of the central extensor tendon that would cover the joint (Fig. 15–16). This "reverse plasty" can be extended along the extensor digitorum tendon on the dorsum of the hand (Foucher, see Chapter 10, Fig 10–1). Aiache et al. (1979) split the two lateral extensor tendons longitudinally and take the two medial bands, which are joined at the midline, to cover the joint (Fig. 15–17). A Bunnell safety pin splint maintains the proximal interphalangeal joint in extension, and mobilization of the distal interphalangeal joint is begun immediately.

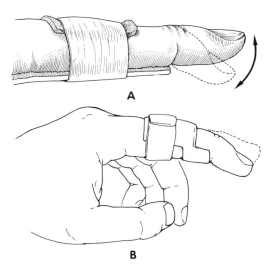

A

B

Figure 15–14. *A*, A short digital splint, leaving the distal interphalangeal joint free. *B*, A polyethylene splint can be used in the same way as the distal joint splint of Stack. It includes a distal palmar portion and a proximal dorsal portion over the proximal interphalangeal joint. These splints leave the distal joint free.

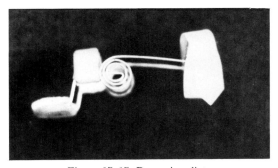

Figure 15–15. Dynamic splint.

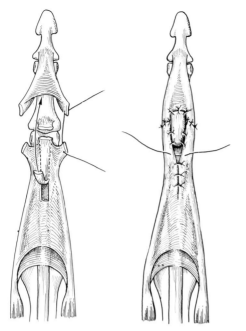

Figure 15–16. Snow procedure.

In severe injuries in which there is gross damage to the extensor mechanism, a joint arthrodesis may be indicated.

Recent Ruptures

Recent ruptures are usually successfully treated conservatively by splinting. A metal splint and a plaster cast maintain the wrist in extension, with the metacarpophalangeal joint in 20 degrees of flexion, the proximal interphalangeal joint in extension, and the distal interphalangeal joint in 45 degrees of flexion for three weeks. At the end of that time only the proximal interphalangeal joint is kept immobilized in extension by a short splint or plaster cast for another two weeks, following which a dynamic splint is worn for a further three or four weeks.

If during mobilization either after a wound or a rupture the deformity tends to recur, the distal joint must be immediately splinted in flexion to concentrate the action of the extensor apparatus on the middle phalanx.

Surgery is not indicated for the repair of recent ruptures, unless there is an associated irreducible or unstable transarticular fracture involving the base of the middle phalanx or the head of the proximal phalanx. The displaced bone fragment is reduced and fixed by means of a wire, a mini-screw, a mini-bolt

(see Vol. II), or a suture. The tendon lesions are repaired. The joint can be maintained in extension by a fine, obliquely placed Kirschner wire; the latter is left in place for two weeks following which extension of the proximal interphalangeal joint is maintained with a splint.

Chronic Lesions

Chronic boutonnière deformities secondary to either a wound or a rupture can be considered together, as they pose similar problems, although extensive scarring will obviously complicate the situation.

The results of surgical management in these cases are often disappointing, and a trial of conservative treatment is always worthwhile before embarking on surgery.

Conservative Treatment

The use of corrective splints aims at reducing the flexion contracture of the proximal interphalangeal joint and, when combined with active mobilization of the distal interphalangeal joint, causes distal traction on the extensor apparatus. As progress is made, the splint can be altered. A dynamic splint may also be used.

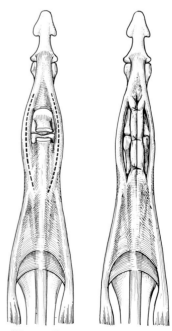

Figure 15–17. Aiache procedure.

In a few weeks one is often able to achieve a significant correction of the flexion deformity. Progress is rapid at the beginning but becomes slower with time, especially with older lesions. This treatment alone can be sufficient to correct the deformities. If correction is obtained, this is maintained with a plaster cast applied for one month, leaving the distal interphalangeal joint free. Physical therapy and splinting are then progressively restarted. There can, however, still be a residual proximal interphalangeal contracture, which is somewhat bothersome, and a flexion deficit of the distal interphalangeal joint.

If surgery is deemed necessary, physiotherapy is restarted immediately postoperatively. It is an essential factor in the ultimate success of the operation.

SURGICAL TREATMENT

If in spite of adequate conservative treatment for at least two or three months there is persistent deformity of the finger that troubles the patient, surgical treatment may be considered.

The surgical correction of a boutonnière deformity requires:

1. Recovery of passive extension at the proximal interphalangeal joint;
2. Restoration of a physiological balance between the various elements of the extensor apparatus (a) by reconstructing an active extensor to the middle phalanx, (b) by replacing the lateral extensor tendons in their physiological position, and (c) by correcting hyperextension of the distal phalanx.

These corrections can be performed in separate or combined procedures.

As a general rule, the operation includes two distinct steps: (1) the correction of deformities of the proximal and distal interphalangeal joints, and (2) the repair of the extensor apparatus.

Correction of the Deformities

One should remember that both the extension defect of the proximal interphalangeal joint and the flexion defect of the distal interphalangeal joint must be corrected. The persistence of one of these two deformities risks producing recurrence of the other. The choice of incision will depend upon the amount of preoperative passive mobility.

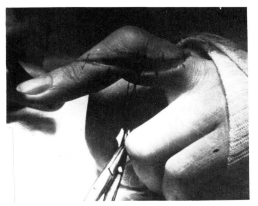

Figure 15–18. Incision used when chronic lesions can be reduced passively.

Correction of the flexion contracture of the proximal interphalangeal joint can be achieved, if it is not too severe, by freeing the extensor apparatus. Nevertheless, if in spite of physiotherapy there continues to be a marked deficit in passive extension of the joint, tenolysis of the extensor apparatus alone is insufficient, and the contracted anterior elements of the joint may have to be freed. In order to be complete, this anterior arthrolysis may require a palmar incision.

Liberation of the Posterior Structures. The incision must be extensive in order to permit wide access to the extensor apparatus (Figs. 15–18 and 15–19). One must not only free the lateral extensor tendons but also permit distal advancement of the entire extensor apparatus. This is an essential step. One begins by locating the middle extensor tendon, or more exactly, by recreating it in the sheet of fibrous tissue which covers the joint. The two lateral borders are freed beginning at their insertion for a length of about 3 cm.

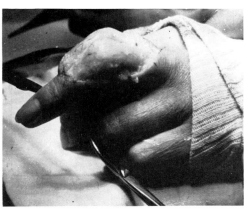

Figure 15–19. Exposure of the lesions.

(Fig. 15–20). Next, distally with respect to the insertion of the central tendon, one frees the medial aspect of the two lateral extensor tendons (Fig. 15–21A). Thus, one creates a triangular fibrous flap with a proximal base corresponding to the triangular ligament (triangular lamina), which has been stretched by the lateral displacement of the two lateral tendons. Along the length of the defect thus created, a thin spatula is introduced laterally, freeing the deep aspect of the two lateral extensor tendons, and proximally, the extensor apparatus over the dorsal aspect of the proximal phalanx, while sparing the periosteum and gliding planes (Fig. 15–22). This extensive liberation will allow the extensor apparatus to be drawn distally. In addition, the lateral tendons must be relocated dorsally. These tendons are fixed in palmar subluxation, and their lateral borders must be freed on each side of the proximal interphalangeal joint (Fig. 15–21B), extending distally as necessary and returning them to their physiological laterodorsal position. This liberation disinserts the transverse fibers as well as a portion of the oblique fibers of the retinacular ligaments. Several possibilities then exist:

1. Physiological balance of the finger is restored. The interphalangeal joints are spontaneously slightly flexed, and they can be placed passively in extension or in complete flexion. Obtaining complete passive mobility in the two interphalangeal joints is a prerequisite for a satisfactory surgical repair.

2. Passive extension of the proximal interphalangeal joint is obtained, but it is not possible to flex the distal joint when the proximal interphalangeal joint is held in extension. By contrast, it can be flexed if the proximal interphalangeal joint is flexed. The retinacular test is positive, and following the technique of Zancolli, one can resect a por-

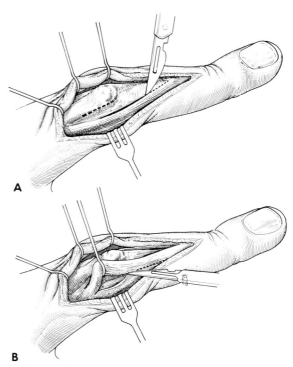

Figure 15–21. Freeing of the lateral extensor tendons. *A*, Freeing of the medial border. *B*, Freeing of the lateral border.

tion of the oblique retinacular ligament opposite the base of the middle phalanx (Fig. 15–23).

3. Passive extension of the proximal interphalangeal joint is obtained, but it is not possible to flex the distal joint, regardless of the position of the proximal interphalangeal joint. This may be caused by either adhesions in the distal part of the extensor apparatus, which must be tenolysed, or stiffness of the distal joint. In these cases it is necessary to

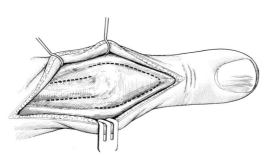

Figure 15–20. The dotted lines show the incisions on the extensor apparatus.

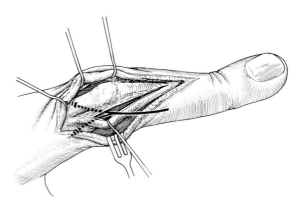

Figure 15–22. Tenolysis of the extensor apparatus.

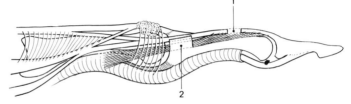

Figure 15–23. *1*, Tenotomy of the terminal tendon. *2*, Resection of the oblique lateral retinacular ligaments (after Zancolli).

free the volar plate of the distal interphalangeal joint and hold the joint in 30 degrees of flexion with a Kirschner wire.

Liberation of the Anterior Structures. In patients with very severe chronic contractures, extension of the proximal interphalangeal joint is not obtained by a simple freeing of the extensor apparatus because of interphalangeal joint stiffness and sometimes adhesions of the flexor tendons. In these cases the flexor tendons' fibrous sheath is opened at the level of the proximal interphalangeal joint. The proximal "check reins" of the volar plate are divided (Taleisnik, 1982). Sometimes this is sufficient to allow extension of the proximal interphalangeal joint. If not, one continues by dividing the accessory collateral ligament. We do not resect either the collateral ligaments or the volar plate. One must be careful in freeing the joint that excessive surgery does not lead to hyperextension of the proximal interphalangeal joint, resulting in a swan-neck deformity.

The freedom of the flexor tendons can be tested by a small palmar incision; if there are adhesions, they may need to be liberated.

When a synovitis of the flexor tendons is associated with a boutonnière deformity, regardless of its cause, a synovectomy must be done prior to repair of the extensor apparatus.

Repair of the Extensor Apparatus

The main aim here is to restore the normal anatomical conditions. This involves repairing the middle tendon, adjusting its tension, and reinserting it on the base of the middle phalanx. Numerous procedures have been described to achieve this repair.

Reconstruction of the Middle Tendon. The proximal end of the middle tendon is freed. Plication of the fibrous tendon scar has yielded poor results in our experience. The fibrous scar of the middle tendon is resected, care being taken to preserve (when it persists) the distal insertion of the tendon at the base

of the middle phalanx. At this stage one of two situations may prevail:

LIMITED TISSUE LOSS. When tissue loss is limited, it is often possible, after freeing the proximal end of the tendon, either to advance the whole extensor apparatus and reattach the tendon to the base of the middle phalanx, or to suture the stumps end to end. This is the simplest solution (Elliot, 1970; Kaplan, 1959; Pardini et al., 1979; Pulvertaft, 1970; Souter, 1967).

Zancolli (1979) combines bony fixation with suturing of the tendon ends. This increases the strength of the repair.

The author's technique is similar. We combine a moderate resection of the fibrous callus with distal advancement of the extensor apparatus, recentralization of the lateral extensor tendons, and flexion of the distal joint. The fibrous callus of the central tendon is resected for about 3 mm. toward its bony insertion (Fig. 15–24). The proximal interphalangeal joint is held in extension by an oblique Kirschner wire. The shortened central tendon is sutured and the repair is reinforced by a transosseous suture (Fig. 15–25).

It is also necessary to correct the volar subluxation of the lateral extensor tendons. The distal phalanx is flexed, advancing the

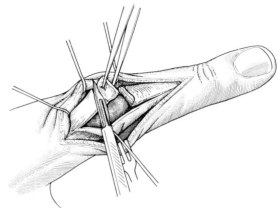

Figure 15–24. Shortening of the middle tendon by resection of the scar.

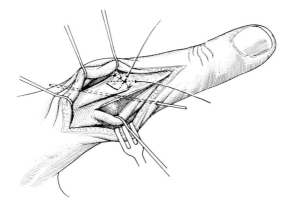

Figure 15–25. The proximal interphalangeal joint is held in extension by a Kirschner wire. The central tendon is sutured to itself and to the base of the middle phalanx.

Figure 15–26. The triangular ligament is retracted. The lateral extensor tendons are replaced in their physiological dorsal position and are sutured one to the other at their distal ends.

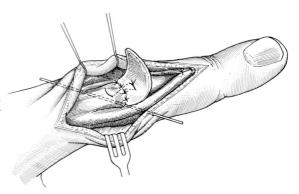

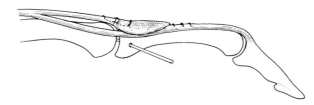

Figure 15–27. The distal phalanx is flexed to allow distal advancement of the extensor apparatus.

Figure 15–28. The triangular lamina is overlapped onto the lateral extensor tendons and secured with several sutures.

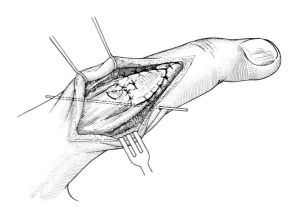

terminal extensor tendon and the entire extensor apparatus distally. The two lateral tendons are sutured together at their distal ends (Fig. 15–26). The triangular flap that has been saved is then fixed with several fine sutures to the lateral tendons, which it overlaps in part (Figs. 15–27, 15–28).

The finger is immobilized with a splint holding the proximal interphalangeal joint in extension and the distal interphalangeal joint in 40 degrees of flexion. The distal joint is moved in two weeks; the proximal interphalangeal joint is held in extension for six weeks. The Kirschner wire is removed after three weeks and is replaced with a well padded cylindrical plaster cast, leaving the distal

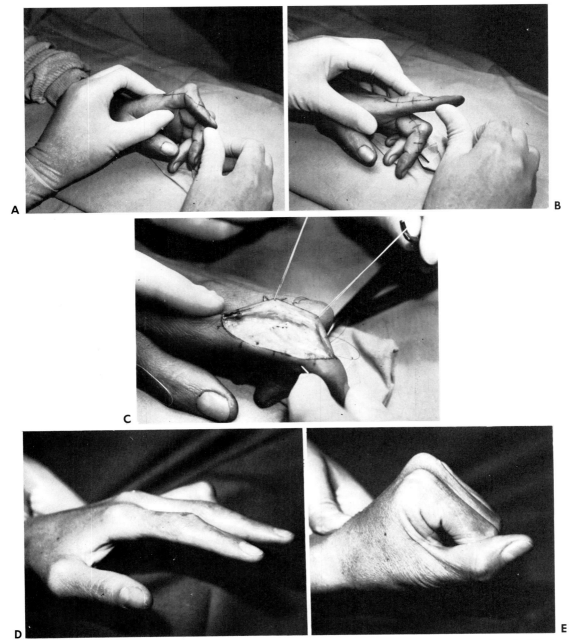

Figure 15–29. Photographs showing the procedure described. *A*, Chronic boutonnière deformity. *B*, Physical therapy and splinting allow complete passive correction. *C*, Operative view. *D* and *E*, Results. Fingers in extension and in flexion.

phalanx free. The cast is removed four weeks later. One then begins careful mobilization of the proximal interphalangeal joint. Between physical therapy sessions, the joint is protected by a short extension splint, and then later by a dynamic extension splint, for several additional weeks. Long careful follow-up is necessary to avoid recurrence of the deformity. If there is a suggestion of recurrence, one holds the distal joint in flexion with a dorsal splint. Physical therapy is continued until satisfactory mobility of the two distal phalanges is obtained (Fig. 15–29).

EXTENSIVE TISSUE LOSS. In such cases, the loss of tissue is too great at the level of the central tendon to permit repair by suturing or reinsertion. A loss of more than 5 mm. will permit distal advancement under excessive tension, risking hyperextension of the proximal interphalangeal joint. The defect can be filled with adjacent fibrous tissue and the tendon reconstructed by using a lateral tendon or even a tendon graft.

Local Fibrous Tissue. Fibrous tissue can be taken from the proximal digital segment or from the lateral side or more distally at the level of the middle phalanx (Butler, 1969; Salvi, 1969). A small, proximally based flap of extensor aponeurosis can be reflected to fill the gap between the two tendinous extremities.

Use of the Lateral Tendons. The lateral tendons can be utilized in a variety of ways. Usually, regardless of the procedure used to repair the central tendon, the lateral tendons are approximated distally in order to reconstruct the triangular ligaments. Dorsal suturing of the bands along their whole length is unphysiological and impedes flexion.

Planas (1962) divides one of the bands proximally and brings it over to the midline. He himself criticized his method when he reported that he was able to obtain flexion of the proximal interphalangeal joint but failed to obtain flexion of the distal joint. Actually flexion of that joint is possible only if the lateral tendons are able to glide over the lateral aspects of the proximal interphalangeal joint, thus allowing the terminal tendon an excursion of some 4 mm and the middle tendon, 8 mm. For this reason Matev (1964) lengthens the lateral band running to the distal joint and fixes the other to the base of the middle phalanx (Fig. 15–30). Littler (1967) uses both lateral tendons, which are tenotomized and turned over to reconstruct a middle tendon.

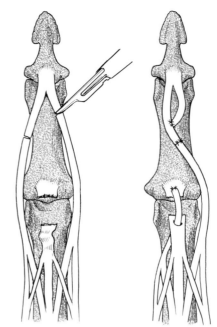

Figure 15–30. The Matev procedure. The lateral extensor tendons are divided at different levels. The tendon that is divided more proximally is passed through the proximal end of the middle extensor tendon, through which it glides, and then is fixed to the base of the middle phalanx. The other lateral tendon is lengthened by suturing it to the distal end of the previous lateral tendon.

Tendon Grafts. Several muscles can be used as motor muscles—usually the extensor communis, the interosseous muscles, or even the flexor digitorum superficialis. The middle tendon can be reconstructed by means of a single graft, a fine tendinous strip being laced through the tendon and tied to the distal stump or to the bone (Nichols, 1966). In the latter case it is attached to the site of insertion of the original tendon, on the base of the middle phalanx. When a tunnel is drilled transversely in the base of the middle phalanx, care must be taken that it is not too anterior or too broad transversely.

Fowler (1949) uses a thin graft, the middle of which he attaches to the base of the middle phalanx. He then crosses the two ends over the dorsal aspect of the proximal interphalangeal joint and sutures them laterally to the interosseous tendons at the root of the finger (Figs. 15–31, 15–32). If these mucles are not suitable, the graft is tethered to the two terminal bands of the flexor superficialis in the palm.

Tubiana Grafting Technique (Trident Graft). In an attempt to reconstruct an exten-

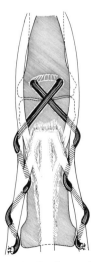

Figure 15–31. The Fowler graft procedure.

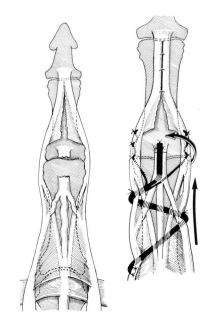

Figure 15–33. The trident graft. The graft is woven through the retracted extensor apparatus, which it pulls distally, and is fixed to the base of the middle phalanx. Two small bands are detached from the graft proximal to the joint and are fixed to the lateral extensor tendons, which are brought out on the dorsal aspect of the joint.

sor apparatus as close to normal as possible, we have used a three tailed graft (Fig. 15–33). The motor source is the tendon of the long extensor, if it is not too bound down by adhesions and can be freed sufficiently. If it is too adherent, one can use the interosseous muscle. A thin graft, for example, from the palmaris longus, is threaded several times in a zigzag fashion through the proximal part of the extensor on the dorsal surface of the first phalanx. The extensor aponeurosis is thus reinforced, and it can then be advanced distally to correct the stretching of the fibrous callus. Before crossing the joint, the graft is divided into three bands. The central one, which should be the largest, is fixed to the base of the middle phalanx at the level of the insertion of the central extensor tendon. The two lateral bands of the graft are fixed on each side of the joint to the lateral extensor tendons to prevent their palmar luxation.

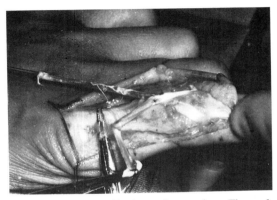

Figure 15–32. The Fowler graft procedure. The graft is passed through the interosseous tendons.

Tenotomy. Tenotomy may be performed alone or in association with reconstruction of the central tendon.

TENOTOMY ONLY. This procedure has been suggested by Fowler (1959) in an attempt to restore the balance of extensor forces at the level of the distal phalanges. By dividing the distal insertion of the extensor tendon on the distal phalanx, he corrects hyperextension at the distal interphalangeal joint and reduces the flexion of the proximal interphalangeal joint produced by the dislocation of the lateral tendons. However, if the tendon is divided more proximally so as to spare the distal insertions of the oblique retinacular ligament, extension of the distal phalanx can be partially preserved (Dolphin, 1965; Fig. 15–34).

Some surgeons make small partial incisions at different sites along the terminal extensor tendon and the lateral extensor tendons (Rousso, 1984), whereas others make step incisions (Curtis, 1983). Our own technique for isolated tenotomy in the treatment of a boutonnière deformity is as follows (Fig. 15–35):

The two lateral extensor tendons are divided obliquely, starting at the medial border at the midpoint between the two interphalan-

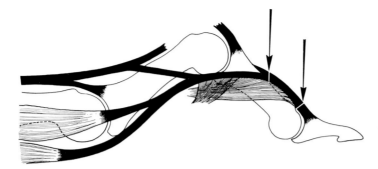

Figure 15–34. Treatment of the boutonnière deformity by tenotomy. The proximal tenotomy of the terminal extensor tendon (Dolphin) is preferable because it allows the preservation of the distal insertions of the oblique retinacular ligaments.

geal joints. The distal phalanx is progressively flexed passively; it is often not necessary to divide the lateral border of the lateral extensor tendon into which the oblique retinacular ligament is inserted in order to obtain complete flexion of the distal joint. A blunt spatula is passed under the lateral tendons on either side of the proximal interphalangeal joint to free them and under the dorsal aspect of the proximal phalanx. This tenotomy done in association with tenolysis reinforces the action of the extensor apparatus on the middle phalanx. The obliqueness of the division allows lengthening of the distal extensor apparatus without loss of contact between the ends of the divided tendon. The proximal interphalangeal joint is immobilized in extension for five weeks. Active mobilization of the distal phalanx is started after one week.

A small splint holds the interphalangeal joints in extension between exercises.

TENOTOMY COMBINED WITH RECONSTRUCTION OF THE CENTRAL TENDON. A tenotomy of the lateral tendons to flex the distal interphalangeal joint can be combined with one of the procedures aiming at reconstructing the middle tendon. Thus, Littler and Eaton (1967) advocate elective tenotomy (Fig. 15–36). They divide the lateral tendons at the level of the middle phalanx and spare the distal oblique fibers of the retinacular ligaments, which run to the terminal tendon, as well as the more peripheral portion of the radial tendon in continuity with the tendon of the lumbrical muscle. Next the divided lateral tendons are folded over themselves and fixed to the base of the middle phalanx to replace or reinforce the middle tendon

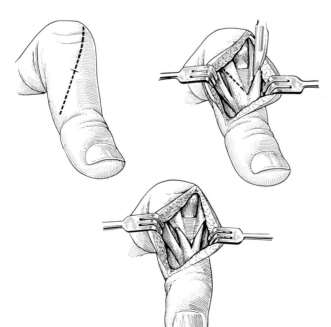

Figure 15–35. Oblique tenotomy of the lateral extensor tendons.

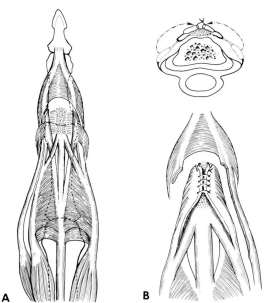

Figure 15–36. Procedure of Littler and Eaton using the lateral extensor tendons. *A*, Tenotomy of the lateral extensor tendons distal to the interphalangeal joint, conserving the lumbrical tendon. *B*, The two lateral tendons are turned over and fixed to the base of the middle phalanx.

(Fig. 15–37). In this way two extensor systems are constructed, one for each interphalangeal joint. All the active extension takes place at the proximal interphalangeal joint while the oblique retinacular ligaments exert an "active tenodesis" effect, which is reinforced by the lumbrical muscle to prevent a mallet finger deformity.

Tenotomy with Arthrodesis of the Proximal Interphalangeal Joint. A partial tenot-omy of the lateral extensor tendons can be combined with an arthrodesis of the proximal interphalangeal joint in cases of severe retraction. This permits flexion of the distal phalanx.

Arthrodesis of the Proximal Interphalangeal Joint. The indications for arthrodesis must be weighed carefully, for fixation of the proximal interphalangeal joint, if it is to be accepted by the patient, should be less crippling than the primary boutonnière deformity. Arthrodesis of the proximal interphalangeal joint can be combined with a distal tenotomy as a salvage procedure.

Arthroplasty. Arthroplasty provides another alternative when the flexors are intact and the extensor system is salvageable. The latter should be carefully reconstructed.*

THERAPEUTIC INDICATIONS

Despite this lengthy enumeration of surgical procedures, splinting and physiotherapy remain the basic treatment for the boutonnière deformity. When used from the first signs of deformity they are often sufficient for preventing the deformity and also constitute an essential step prior to any operation. At least two months must elapse before considering surgical intervention.

Surgery is therefore indicated only if the correction obtained by a trial of splinting is insufficient and the functional disability is

---

*See Chapters 61 and 110 on articular implants by Swanson and by Iselin and Pradet in Volume II.

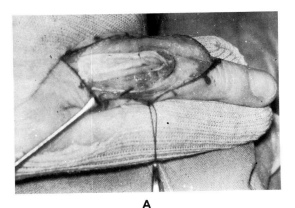

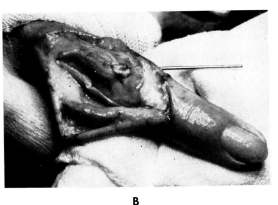

Figure 15–37. Intraoperative photographs showing the procedure of Littler and Eaton. *A*, The tenotomy is performed. A Kirschner wire fixes the interphalangeal joint in extension. *B*, The tendons are turned over and fixed to the base of the middle phalanx. The lumbrical tendon and the oblique retinacular ligament will extend the distal interphalangeal joint.

significant. These esthetically unpleasing boutonnière deformities are often well accepted
functionally when they remain supple and are
not too marked. It is difficult to evaluate how
much the deformity bothers the patient because this is measured not only by the degree
of the contracture. Other elements which
must be considered are as follows:

An occupation requiring complete extension or flexion of the fingers.

The finger injured and the location of the
contracture. An extension deficit of the middle phalanx is less bothersome in the ulnar
than the radial fingers, and it alters function
less than does a flexion defect if it remains
within acceptable limits (which differ according to the finger). The flexion deficit of the
distal phalanx can be more disabling to the
grip than the extension deficit in the proximal
interphalangeal joint, especially in the ulnar
fingers. In the index finger, however, the
flexion deficit in the distal phalanx is relatively less restricting.

Sex and esthetic considerations: the deformities are more visible in the radial fingers.

Surgical indications should take into account both the discomfort experienced by the
patient and the possibilities of repair. If this
discomfort justifies surgical intervention,
which type of operation should be proposed?
What result can one expect?

The prognosis of these tendon repairs is
influenced by:

a. The degree of the contracture in the
two interphalangeal joints. If in spite of
physiotherapy and the splinting, significant
stiffness persists, or more precisely, if the
defect in passive extension of the proximal
interphalangeal joint exceeds 40 degrees, the
chances for improvement provided by surgical repair of the extensor apparatus are
low. On the contrary, recovery of complete
passive extension and flexion of the proximal
joint has a favorable prognosis, especially if
this recovery can be obtained before the
operation.

b. Other factors negatively influence the
prognosis of surgical repair (Strickland and
Powell, 1980): patients over 45 years of age,
the presence of a joint fracture with a significant fragment, and tendon ruptures all give
poorer operative results than simple lacerations. A previous attempt at surgical repair
followed by failure considerably worsens the
prognosis.

SURGICAL TREATMENT

Surgical treatment of chronic boutonnière
deformities remains a difficult problem. Our
choice, in the presence of chronic boutonnière deformities, is adapted to the particular
clinical conditions. The choice of techniques
that we use is guided by the significance of
persistent deformity after physiotherapy.
These can be classed into four categories:

1. Complete passive extension of the proximal interphalangeal joint.

2. Deficit in passive extension of the proximal interphalangeal joint less than 30 degrees.

3. Deficit in passive extension of the proximal interphalangeal joint greater than 30
degrees.

4. Destruction of the proximal interphalangeal joint articular surfaces.

*When complete passive extension of the
proximal interphalangeal joint was obtained
before the operation.* A dorsal skin flap centered over the joint allows exposure of the
extensor apparatus (Fig. 15–38). One often
feels confused by the multitude of available
techniques. Fortunately, with experience, the
choices are more clear. The majority of repair
techniques using only the lateral extensor
tendons are no longer used except for treating
certain forms peculiar to the boutonnière
deformity, during rheumatoid arthritis, or
following burns (Joshi, 1982).

To restore active extension to the distal
phalanx in the usual forms of traumatic boutonnière deformities, most authors agree with
direct repair of the central extensor tendon.
As we have described, we resect the callus
and reimplant the central tendon associated
with distal advancement of the extensor ap-

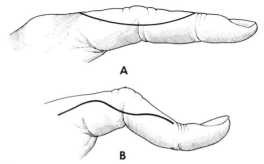

Figure 15–38. Skin incisions. *A*, Dorsal flap used when
the proximal interphalangeal and distal interphalangeal
deformities are passively corrected. *B*, Curtis incision.

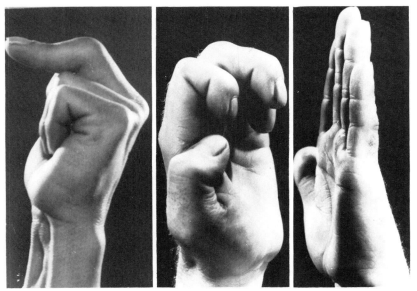

Figure 15–39. Result of a boutonnière deformity treated by a trident graft.

paratus when the proximal contracture of the central tendon is moderate.

In rare cases, we perform grafting when there is loss of tissue substance and contractures of the extensor apparatus that are difficult to correct by simply using neighboring tendinofascial materials which have become too sclerosed and full of adhesions. These grafts can provide good results (Fig. 15–39).

When there exists a deficit in passive extension of the proximal interphalangeal joint of less than 30 degrees. A mid-lateral incision on the finger permits the formation of a dorsal skin flap and eventually an approach to the anterior aspect of the joint. These moderate contractures are usually corrected by posterior liberation. However, in certain cases, it is necessary in addition to divide the proximal check-reins of the palmar plate, which may necessitate a short mid-lateral counterincision on the opposite side (Fig. 15–40).

When there exists a deficit in passive extension of the proximal interphalangeal joint greater than 30 degrees. In these forms of severe contracture, when the articular surfaces are not altered, a liberation of the anterior structures may be necessary. An anterior zigzag Bruner incision will provide wider exposure of the flexor apparatus and joint (Fig. 15–41). A posterior oblique incision opposite the middle phalanx will permit a tenotomy of the extensor apparatus. It is necessary to restore flexion of the distal phalanx while risking recurrence of the deformity. The proximal interphalangeal joint is maintained in extension for a month; then it is progressively mobilized.

If the active extension deficit of the proximal interphalangeal joint remains a problem, one could reintervene several months later, via a dorsal incision, to repair the extensor apparatus when the joints will have recovered good passive mobility.

Figure 15–40. Skin incision used when a deficit of passive extension of the proximal interphalangeal joint inferior to 30 degrees persists. *A*, Solid line = the incision; dotted line = distal extension of the incision when the distal interphalangeal joint has to be freed. *B*, Counter-incision on the opposite side of the proximal interphalangeal joint is sometimes necessary.

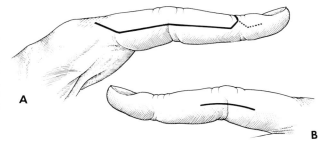

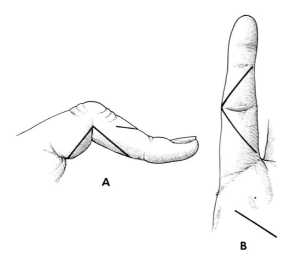

Figure 15–41. Incision used when a deficit of passive extension of the proximal interphalangeal joint persists greater than 30 degrees. *A*, Zigzag palmar incision and oblique dorsal incision for tenotomy of the lateral extensor tendons. *B*, Palmar view, showing the zigzag incision and a more proximal palmar incision to test the gliding of the flexor tendons.

When the articular surfaces of the proximal interphalangeal joint are altered after a fracture or because of chronic lesions, the choices are reduced to either an arthroplasty or an arthrodesis.

Arthroplasties with implants require flexor tendons that are in good condition, an extensor apparatus that can recover, and good cutaneous cover. The replacement of the proximal interphalangeal joint by an implant often results in only limited mobility, but in a better functional range. However, there may be insufficient lateral stability to resist thumb pressure in heavy manual workers.

Arthrodesis is the only solution when the extensor apparatus is largely destroyed.

REFERENCES

References for this chapter will be found following Chapter 23.

Chapter 16

THE SWAN-NECK DEFORMITY

Raoul Tubiana

Excessive traction on the extensor apparatus inserted on the base of the middle phalanx, due to overaction of either the extrinsic or the intrinsic muscles, causes hyperextension of the proximal interphalangeal joint, especially if that joint is lax for some reason. Regardless of its origin, this deformity causes dorsal displacement of the lateral extensor tendons toward the midline. Their line of action being thus shortened, the tendons become lax and their extensor effect on the distal phalanx consequently diminishes. At the same time the flexor profundus tendon is stretched by hyperextension of the proximal interphalangeal joint, and the distal interphalangeal joint is forced into flexion. The overall result is the so-called "swan-neck" deformity, which combines hyperextension of the middle phalanx with flexion of the distal phalanx (Fig. 16–1).

PATHOPHYSIOLOGY

The altered distribution of forces on the two distal phalanges causes imbalance of the kinetic chain formed by the three phalanges, and this in turn has several consequences:

1. The functional unity of the interphalangeal system is disorganized. Deformity of the proximal interphalangeal joint has repercussions on the distal joint, which becomes in turn progressively flexed This sets up a vicious cycle; hence, the need to correct the two deformities.

2. In theory the retinacular ligaments should prevent such a deformity because the transverse fibers check the dorsal displacement of the lateral tendons, and the oblique fibers prevent flexion of the distal interphalangeal joint when the proximal joint is extended. However, the fragility of these ligaments is such that they offer little resistance to the abnormal forces that produce the deformity. Destruction or elongation of the oblique retinacular ligament heralds a loss of coordination between the two distal joints. Reconstitution of its action is an essential step in the correction of the swan-neck deformity.

3. The pulling of the two interphalangeal joints in opposite directions has severe repercussions on the dynamics of digital movements.

We have already seen that digital flexion normally starts at the proximal interphalangeal joint.* In the swan-neck deformity the flexion cycle starts at the distal joint under the action of flexor profundus while the proximal interphalangeal joint remains blocked in hyperextension (Fig. 16–2). Only when the distal joint is fully flexed can the proximal interphalangeal joint begin to flex, and this is often accompanied by a characteristic "click" as the oblique retinacular ligament slips to a position anterior to the rotation axis of the proximal interphalangeal joint.

If the interosseous muscles are functionally shortened (one of the causes of the swan-neck deformity), they can begin to relax only when the metacarpophalangeal joint is sufficiently flexed.

ANATOMICAL CLASSIFICATION

A number of anatomical lesions can cause hyperextension of the proximal interphalangeal joint. Any lesion at any level of the kinetic chain which reinforces the action of the middle extensor tendon on the base of the middle phalanx may give rise to a swan-

---

*See the section in "Movements of the Fingers" on page 48 in Volume I.

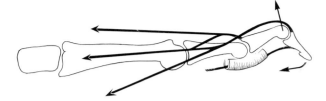

Figure 16–1. Swan-neck deformity with hyperextension of the middle phalanx and flexion of the distal phalanx.

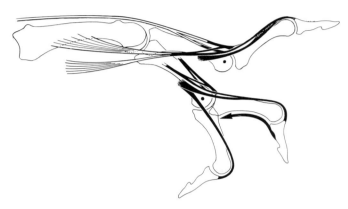

Figure 16–2. The rhythm of flexion is disordered in the swan-neck deformity. Only when the distal interphalangeal joint is flexed will the proximal interphalangeal joint begin to flex. A click occurs as the oblique retinacular ligament moves anterior to the axis of rotation of the joint (after Zancolli).

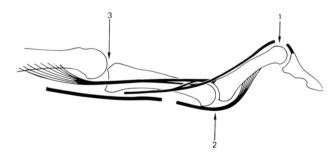

Figure 16–3. 1, Distal rupture of the extensor tendon; 2, section of the flexor digitorum superficialis tendon at the proximal interphalangeal level; 3, volar subluxation at the base of the proximal phalanx. All these lesions reinforce the action of the extensor tendon on the base of the middle phalanx.

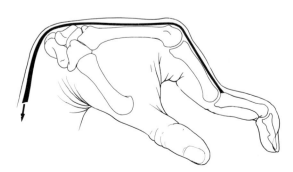

Figure 16–4. Excessive traction of the extensor on the middle phalanx can be caused by a flexion contracture of the wrist.

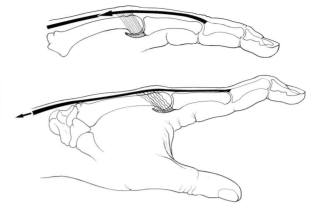

Figure 16–5. Section or lengthening of the sagittal bands that form the proximal insertion of the extensor tendon results in a reinforced extensor action on the base of the middle phalanx.

neck deformity (Fig. 16–3). Zancolli (1979) has divided these lesions into three groups:

EXTRINSIC FACTORS

"Extrinsic" factors that tend to enhance the action of the extensors digitorum on the base of the middle phalanx include flexion deformities of the wrist or metacarpophalangeal joints (Fig. 16–4), ischemic or spastic contraction of the long extensors, laxity or detachment of the proximal insertions of the extensor digitorum communis at the base of the finger (Fig. 16–5), and mallet deformity of the distal phalanx (Fig. 16–6).

INTRINSIC FACTORS

"Intrinsic" factors tend to reinforce the action of the intrinsic muscles on the proximal interphalangeal joint. One such factor is ischemic or spastic contracture of the interosseous muscles (Finochieto, 1923; Parkes, 1945; Bunnell, 1948) (Fig. 16–7). This can be tested for and we shall describe it when discussing the clinical signs (Fig. 16–1). Shapiro (1982) has suggested that the loss of carpal height, frequent in rheumatoid arthritis, may decrease the efficiency of the long extrinsic muscle tendon units crossing the wrist, thus initiating an extrinsic-minus or comparatively intrinsic-plus attitude of the fingers. Another factor is shortening of the interosseous muscles on the ulnar side in ulnar deviation of the fingers. Finally, anterior subluxation of the base of the proximal phalanx may be a cause (Fig. 16–8); this leads to the dorsal displacement of the functional axis of the intrinsic muscles and increases their extensor action on the proximal interphalangeal joint.

ARTICULAR FACTORS

"Articular" factors affect the stabilizing elements of the proximal interphalangeal joint. The structures that normally prevent hyperextension of the proximal interphalangeal joint are the volar plate, the glenoid insertions of the collateral ligaments, the fibrous flexor sheath, the flexor superficialis tendon, and the oblique retinacular ligament (Fig. 16–9).

ETIOLOGY

These lesions have a variety of etiologies.

Figure 16–6. Section of the terminal extensor tendon is accompanied by proximal retraction of the extensor apparatus, the action of which is reinforced on the base of the middle phalanx. This is why a mallet finger can cause a swan-neck deformity when the structures that oppose hyperextension of the proximal interphalangeal joint are lax.

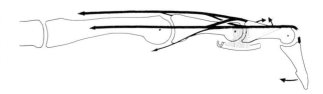

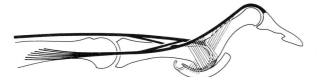

Figure 16–7. Contraction of the intrinsic muscles of the fingers causes excess traction on the base of the middle phalanx.

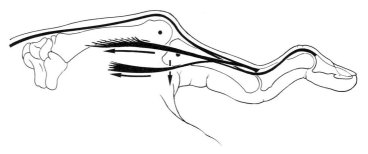

Figure 16–8. Volar subluxation of the base of the proximal phalanx has the effect of placing the interosseous tendons in a dorsal position, thus reinforcing their extensor action on the proximal interphalangeal joint.

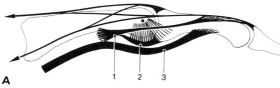

A

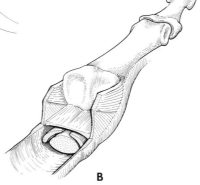

B

Figure 16–9. *A*, Structures that normally oppose hyperextension of the proximal interphalangeal joint. 1 = oblique retinacular ligament, 2 = volar plate, 3 = flexor superficialis. *B*, The proximal phalanx has been removed to show the volar fibrous structures of the joint.

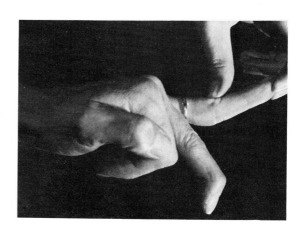

Figure 16–10. Swan-neck deformity after graft to the flexor profundus.

TRAUMATIC CAUSES

Open or closed injuries can cause division, rupture, adhesions, and deviation of the tendons, as well as fractures, dislocations, and sprains. Tears of the volar plate can result from violent trauma during hyperextension. Arthrography can be a valuable aid to diagnosis in such cases.

OTHER CAUSES

These deformities can also result from abnormal joint laxity of congenital or paralytic origin, from muscular contracture of ischemic or spastic origin, and from rheumatoid disease. Rheumatoid disease, trauma, and neurological conditions are the most common causes of the swan-neck deformity. The deformity, however, can be brought about by a variety of mechanisms (synovitis, rupture, deviation, adhesions, tendon elongation, muscular and articular lesions) that must be identified before the appropriate treatment is decided upon.*

SWAN-NECK DEFORMITY SECONDARY TO SURGERY

The swan-neck deformity is sometimes seen after flexor tendon grafting when the flexor superficialis is sacrificed and only the profundus is reconstructed (Fig. 16–10). The proximal interphalangeal joint then tends to drift into hyperextension, especially when surgical dissection has weakened the anterior articular structures and when the retinacular ligament is sacrificed together with the fibrous sheath.

Therefore, steps must be taken to prevent hyperextension of the proximal interphalangeal joint, and whenever possible one should try to preserve the bands of insertion of the flexor superficialis opposite that joint.

*See the chapters on rheumatoid arthritis in Volume IV.

A swan-neck deformity can also be produced surgically, e.g., in tendon transfers for interosseous palsy when the motor muscle used to extend the distal phalanges is too powerful, the joints are too lax, or the insertion is too distal. For these reasons Bunnell's technique of transferring the flexor superficialis tendons onto the interosseous aponeurosis is sometimes contraindicated.

CLINICAL CLASSIFICATION

A four stage classification related to the severity of the deformity is possible based on Nalebuff's technique for the correction of swan-neck deformities seen in rheumatoid arthritis (Nalebuff, 1969). This clinical classification can be of help in choosing the appropriate surgical treatment.

1. The joints retain their suppleness. Merely preventing hyperextension of the middle phalanx corrects the flexion deformity of the distal phalanx (Fig. 16–11). Full active flexion of the proximal interphalangeal joint is retained. Digital function is almost normal, but the initial flexion of the distal phalanx, which precedes that of the proximal phalanges, makes the grasping of large objects difficult.

2. Flexion of the proximal interphalangeal joint is influenced by the position of the proximal phalanx and the metacarpophalangeal joint. When the latter is held in extension, flexion of the proximal interphalangeal joint is impossible if the interosseous muscles are contracted. Flexing the proximal phalanx, however, renders flexion of the joint possible (Fig. 16–12). This test is used to detect contracture of the interosseous muscles (intrinsic = plus sign).

3. Flexion of the proximal interphalangeal joint is limited owing to retraction of tendons, skin, and joint (Fig. 16–13). The stiffness of the proximal interphalangeal joint causes severe limitation of function because it prevents the gripping of small objects between the deformed finger and the palm. The functional prognosis is worse if several fingers are affected.

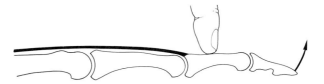

Figure 16–11. Classification of deformity: Stage I. The joints are supple. If hyperextension of the middle phalanx is prevented, flexion of the distal phalanx is corrected.

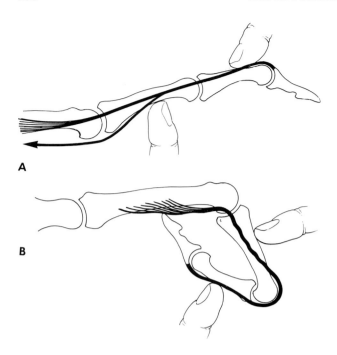

A

B

Figure 16–12. Stage II. *A*, When the proximal phalanx is maintained in extension, it is impossible to flex the middle phalanx. *B*, Flexion of the proximal phalanx allows flexion of the middle phalanx. This maneuver indicates an interosseous muscle contracture.

4. In the most severe forms of the deformity there is destruction of the articular surfaces (Fig. 16–14).

TREATMENT

The treatment of swan-neck deformities must be directed at the cause whenever possible and the deformities corrected.

The complexity of the extensor apparatus at the level of the proximal interphalangeal joint makes surgical correction difficult, and secondary contractures further complicate the problem.

We will concentrate here on the surgical correction of the deformity, but it goes without saying that treatment directed at the cause is also indicated. Etiological treatment is discussed in several chapters of this work.*

Any skeletal deviation that accompanies a swan-neck deformity must be corrected. Thus anterior dislocation of the base of the proximal phalanx or a fracture of the metacarpal neck with anterior displacement of the head must be corrected to reduce tension in the intrinsic system, which is transmitted to the distal phalanges. Similarly, an old mallet de-

---

*See chapters on sprains and dislocations of the fingers in Volume II and on contracture of the interosseous muscles, spastic hands, paralytic hands, and rheumatoid arthritis in Volume IV.

formity giving rise to a swan-neck deformity deserves correction.

Whether surgery is indicated or not, physiotherapy and the wearing of corrective splints must be prescribed. Surgical treatment aims to correct deformities, prevent their recurrence, restore mobility to a stiff proximal interphalangeal joint, or immobilize the joint in a functional position.

CORRECTION WHEN THE PROXIMAL INTERPHALANGEAL JOINT REMAINS MOBILE

If the proximal interphalangeal joint remains mobile, the treatment consists of preventing hyperextension of the joint while restoring extension of the distal joint. Several procedures have been described.

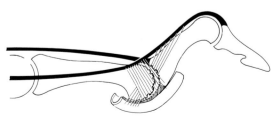

Figure 16–13. Stage III. Fixed swan-neck deformity due to soft tissue contractures.

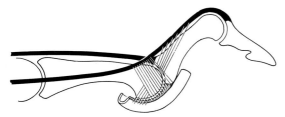

Figure 16–14. Stage IV. The articular surfaces of the proximal interphalangeal joint are destroyed.

Dermodesis, simple resection of a transverse ellipse of skin on the anterior aspect of the proximal interphalangeal joint (Swanson, 1966), helps to correct hyperextension of the proximal interphalangeal joint. However, this alone is insufficient and must be combined with some other procedure, such as capsulorraphy, as advocated by Bates (1945), or tenodesis, which is the most popular and for which several techniques have been developed.

Correction by Use of a Band of Flexor Superficialis Tendon

When a flexor tendon lesion is complicated by hyperextension of the proximal interphalangeal joint, it is possible to perform a tenodesis by fixing one of the bands of the flexor superficialis to the proximal part of the capsule with the joint in 30 degrees of flexion (Tubiana, 1960). Swanson (1960) fixes the tendinous band to the shaft of the proximal phalanx. Bossé (1981) has accurately described this technique (Fig. 16–15).

Reconstruction of the Oblique Retinacular Ligament Using a Band from the Extensor Apparatus

This procedure offers the advantage of preventing hyperextension of the proximal interphalangeal joint while extending the distal joint. Littler (1967) suggested reconstructing the oblique retinacular ligament by means of a lateral extensor tendon, preferably the medial one. The latter is divided at its proximal origin and is freed down to its distal dorsal insertion, which is left intact. It is then redirected along the axis of the oblique retinacular ligament, which crosses the lateral aspect of the proximal interphalangeal joint (Fig. 16–16). The tendinous band is passed in front of the fibers of Cleland's ligament, which form a fibrous septum between the skin and the skeleton. This makes it run anterior to the axis of rotation of the proximal interphalangeal joint because it is fixed to the fibrous flexor sheath.

Zancolli (1979) has described a similar technique in which a whole lateral extensor tendon is split into two. One strip is passed in front of Cleland's ligament. The extensor apparatus is reconstructed by suturing the oblique retinacular ligament to the tendon remnant, while the band is passed inside the flexor sheath, under a "fibrous bridge" at the level of the proximal interphalangeal joint before being sutured to the sheath (Fig. 16–17). These two authors have progressively improved their techniques.

Figure 16–15. Tenodesis of the proximal interphalangeal joint. Bossé procedure. *A* and *B,* One terminal band of the flexor superficialis is detached for about 4 cm., preserving its insertion on the middle phalanx. *C,* The distal extremity of the proximal phalanx is perforated on the opposite side. The band of the flexor superficialis is passed through this tunnel and is sutured to itself. This will have a double effect: (1) a pulley for the flexor profundus and (2) tenodesis for the proximal interphalangeal joint.

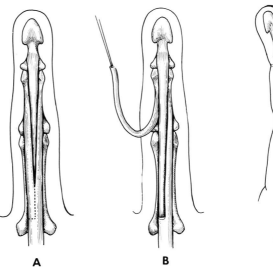
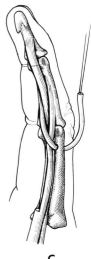

A   B   C

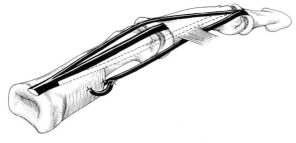

Figure 16–16. Littler tenodesis using the lateral extensor tendons, early technique.

Littler's Construction of a Spiral Anterior Ligament That Limits Extension of the Proximal Interphalangeal Joint

Littler has modified his technique for reconstructing the oblique retinacular ligament (Thomson, Littler, Upton, 1978). He constructs an anterior spiral check rein by means of a tendon graft, both of whose extremities transfix the skeleton. A slender graft (taken from the palmaris longus or the plantaris) is passed transversely through the base of the proximal phalanx from the medial to the lateral side (Fig. 16–18). Twisted on itself, it is passed across the anterior aspect of the proximal interphalangeal joint, then over the medial aspect of the middle phalanx anteroposteriorly before being implanted under tension on the middle of the base of the distal phalanx; the tension in the graft is adjusted with the proximal interphalangeal joint in slight flexion (10 degrees) and the distal pha-

lanx in extension. The two ends of the graft are tethered with a bolus or a clip.

This graft corrects both the hyperextension at the proximal interphalangeal joint and the flexion at the distal joint (Fig. 16–19). Active flexion at the proximal joint, by relaxing the graft, facilitates flexion of the distal phalanx.

Zancolli Translocation of the Lateral Extensor Tendon

Zancolli (1986) liberates the lateral extensor tendon, usually on the radial side of the finger. The lateral extensor tendon is then subluxed volarly in front of the volar plate of the proximal interphalangeal joint and is maintained in this position by fixation of the volar plate to the flexor digitorum superficialis tendon distally in relation to the proximal interphalangeal joint. The lateral extensor tendon of the opposite side consequently shifts laterally to a more normal position, and an active correction of the deformity is obtained.

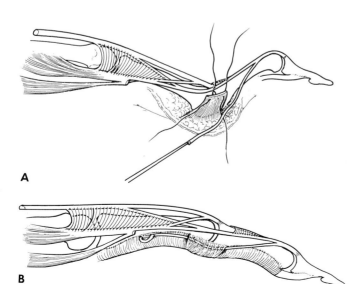

A

B

Figure 16–17. *A* and *B*, Zancolli reconstruction, early technique.

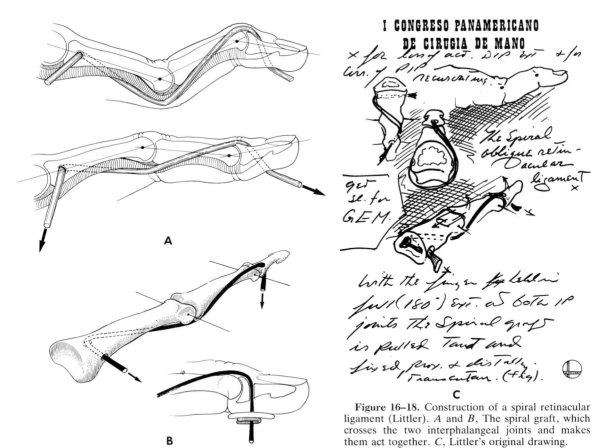

Figure 16–18. Construction of a spiral retinacular ligament (Littler). *A* and *B*, The spiral graft, which crosses the two interphalangeal joints and makes them act together. *C*, Littler's original drawing.

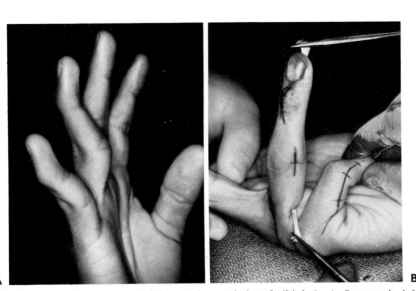

Figure 16–19. Correction of a swan-neck deformity by a spiral graft (Littler). *A*, Swan-neck deformity before correction. *B*, Adjusting the length of the graft.

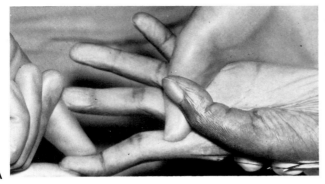
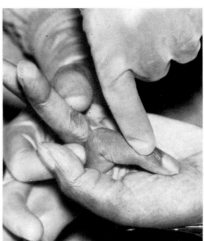

Figure 16–20. Swan-neck deformity after retraction of the intrinsic muscles. *A,* When the proximal phalanx is maintained in extension, the distal phalanges cannot be flexed. *B,* Flexion of the proximal phalanx allows flexion of the distal phalanges.

Figure 16–21. *A,* Part *a,* shows the normal location of the extensor apparatus. *b,* Central displacement of the two lateral extensor tendons in swan-neck deformity. *c,* Correction: the lateral extensor tendon of the opposite side and both oblique retinacular ligaments shift to their normal position by the effect of the "translocated lateral band." 1 = Central extensor tendon; 2 = lateral extensor tendon; 3 = oblique retinacular ligament. *B,* The lateral extensor tendon is subluxed volarly after freeing its medial border. *C,* The lateral extensor tendon is introduced between the volar plate of the proximal interphalangeal joint and the flexor digitorum superficialis tendon. The volar plate is sutured to the flexor digitorum superficialis distal to the proximal interphalangeal joint. A Kirschner wire is temporarily placed at the distal interphalangeal joint, maintaining flexion.

Figure 16–22. *A*, Resection of the oblique fibers of the interosseous hood. *B* and *C* show the operative technique. *B*, Exposure of the extensor apparatus at the level of the proximal phalanx. *C*, Triangular resection of the oblique fibers of the interosseous hood.

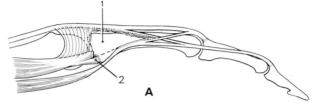

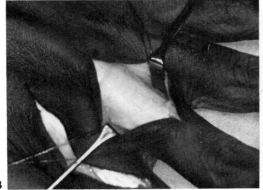

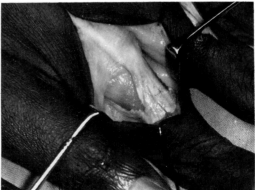

B

C

CORRECTION WHEN FLEXION OF THE PROXIMAL INTERPHALANGEAL JOINT IS INFLUENCED BY THE POSITION OF THE PROXIMAL PHALANX AND THE METACARPOPHALANGEAL JOINT

There is often contracture of the interosseous muscles (Fig. 16–20). Resection of the oblique fibers of the interosseous hood at the level of the proximal phalanx, as described by Littler, restores flexion of the proximal interphalangeal joint when the proximal phalanx is held in extension (Figs. 16–20 to 16–23).* In some cases contracture of the interosseous muscles causes such a great degree of metacarpophalangeal joint flexion that the main complaint is the inability to open the palm. In such cases Bunnell advocates surgical release and distal advancement of the interosseous muscles at the level of the metacarpal (Fig. 16–24).

CORRECTION WHEN FLEXION OF THE PROXIMAL INTERPHALANGEAL JOINT IS RESTRICTED

Whatever the position of the proximal phalanx and the metacarpophalangeal joint, the object of mobilizing surgery in improving

flexion of the proximal interphalangeal joint is to free all the shortened tissues—skin, extensor apparatus, and joint. The extensor apparatus is explored through a long curved incision. If the lateral tendons are contracted they must be freed to allow flexion.

In some cases the contracted lateral tendons and middle tendons form an adherent mass on the dorsum of the proximal interphalangeal joint. Extensive tenolysis is required to flex the joint and restore tendon

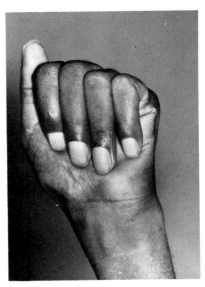

Figure 16–23. Result.

---

*See the chapter on retraction of the interosseous muscles in Volume IV.

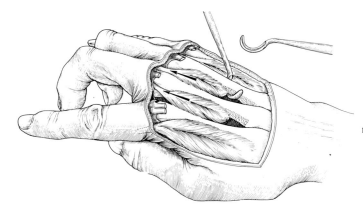

Figure 16–24. Sliding of the interosseous muscles distally (Bunnell).

balance. The middle tendon can be lengthened by dividing it obliquely by a tendon graft.

When flexion is prevented by contractures of the capsule and ligaments, these can be released using the technique devised by Curtis (1983). Freeing of all periarticular fibrous structures allows extension of the distal phalanx unless the distal joint is stiff. An arthrodesis of the distal joint may be necessary to correct the flexion deformity.

The construction of a "brake" is also necessary to prevent recurrence of the hyperextension at the proximal interphalangeal joint, and this is when Littler's spiral graft becomes useful.

There remains the problem of the skin. The incision must be designed to produce a skin flap capable of covering the proximal interphalangeal joint. The bare area created on the dorsum of the middle phalanx can be left to heal spontaneously or grafted over (Nalebuff, 1969).

Correction When the Articular Surfaces of the Proximal Interphalangeal Joint Are Damaged

When the proximal interphalangeal joint is fixed in extension and the joint surfaces are damaged, the choice lies between an arthroplasty and an arthrodesis.

POSTOPERATIVE CARE

Postoperative care plays an important part after any of these mobilizing procedures. A plaster cast is used to immobilize the wrist in slight extension and the finger in the position of correction, i.e., with the proximal interphalangeal joint in 30 degrees of flexion and the distal interphalangeal joint straight. Kirschner wires can be used to maintain the joints in the desired position; one of these is inserted obliquely through the proximal interphalangeal joint and left in place for one week, after which a dorsal splint is worn that allows flexion but prevents hyperextension. Another Kirschner wire inserted through the distal interphalangeal joint keeps it in extension for three weeks. When this is removed, a small splint is worn to keep that joint extended for a further three weeks; this serves to transfer the action of flexor profundus to the proximal interphalangeal joint. It is important that early flexion of the distal phalanx be avoided in order to relieve tension on the tenodesis and thus prevent recurrence of the deformity.

REFERENCES

References for this chapter will be found following Chapter 23.

Chapter 17

LESIONS OF THE EXTENSOR APPARATUS AT THE LEVEL OF THE SHAFT OF THE PROXIMAL AND MIDDLE PHALANGES

RAOUL TUBIANA

On the dorsal aspect of the phalanges, the extensor apparatus is very superficial. It is formed by the tendons of the extensor communis and the expansion of the interosseous and lumbrical muscles. The effect of these muscle groups is the same at this level, and they can substitute for each other to effect extension of the two distal phalanges. The extensor aponeurosis is broad at this level and partial lacerations are frequent. The prognosis is different for clean lacerations repaired with several fine sutures and wounds with tissue loss, crush injuries, and fractures.

A good skin cover is essential. When adjacent digits sustain similar injuries, it is difficult to provide a cover with flaps from neighboring digits.

Postoperative adhesions are frequent, especially with associated injuries. Thus it seems preferable to use a technique of tendon suturing with early mobilization (see Chapter 23 on protected passive mobilization).

Whatever the suture technique used, the wrist must be immobilized in extension to relax the extrinsic extensors. Loss of tendon substance must be repaired with bridge grafts.

Tenolysis is often necessary when there are associated bone lesions, but this should not be carried out before five months.

Limited adhesions of the central extensor tendon at the proximal half of the proximal phalanx can cause the "extensor-plus syndrome," to be discussed in Chapter 20.

Chapter 18

LESIONS OF THE EXTENSOR TENDONS AT THE LEVEL OF THE METACARPOPHALANGEAL JOINT

RAOUL TUBIANA

Each long extensor tendon crosses the dorsal aspect of the metacarpophalangeal joint. It is held in the axis of the digit by inconstant and rather loose insertions at the base of the proximal phalanx, and especially by the sagittal bands that cross the lateral aspects of the joint before inserting into the deep transverse intermetacarpal ligament. These bands constitute the true proximal insertions of the tendon.

The excursion of the long extensor at this level is about 15 mm. Extension of the proximal phalanx relies on two motor systems.

Direct Motor System. The insertion of the extensor digitorum communis on the base of the proximal phalanx is inconstant and is sometimes reduced to mere adhesions between the tendon and the dorsal capsule. It can act only when the proximal interphalangeal joint is extended and is relaxed by flexion of the interphalangeal joints, causing the dorsal extensor aponeurosis to slide distally.

Indirect Motor System. The pressure exerted on the head of the proximal phalanx by the base of the middle phalanx tends to push it dorsally when the proximal interphalangeal joint is flexed.

Lacerations do occur at the level of the metacarpophalangeal joint, but ruptures are exceptional. Another type of lesion seen here is lateral displacement of the tendon. At this level bite injuries are more common, and because of the proximity to the joint, this is a serious problem.

138

DIVISION OF THE EXTENSOR TENDON

Division of the extensor tendon results in loss of extension of the proximal phalanx. Extension of the distal phalanges is performed by the interosseous and lumbrical

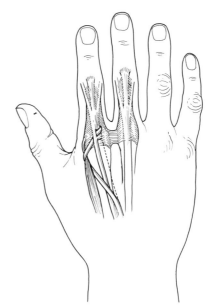

Figure 18–1. The distal end of the extensor indicis proprius tendon is divided, passed around the tendon of the first dorsal interosseous muscle, and reattached to the extensor communis tendon after the deviation has been corrected.

muscles when they are intact. Retraction of the tendinous extremities is limited by the sagittal bands and juncturae tendinum. With the tendon injury one usually finds an open joint capsule and sometimes a tear in the sagittal bands and the dorsal aponeurosis, both of which help to keep the tendon in the axis of the joint. After careful wound toilet these three structures must be carefully sutured with 5-0 nylon and immobilized for three weeks with the wrist and finger in extension and the metacarpophalangeal joint in 10 degrees of flexion to prevent retraction of the collateral ligaments.

BITES

Bites are frequent near the metacarpophalangeal joint. Injury results either from a human bite or from a blow to the mouth from a clenched fist. These are very contaminated wounds and never should be closed primarily. It is necessary to explore the wound because they often contain foreign bodies and debris from the teeth. X-ray views are useful. After cultures are taken, the wound is carefully irrigated. Administration of an antibiotic appropriate for mouth flora is begun, and the hand is immobilized.

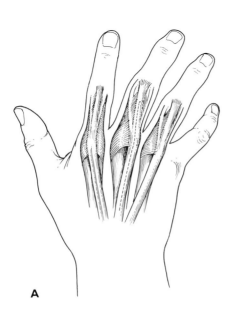

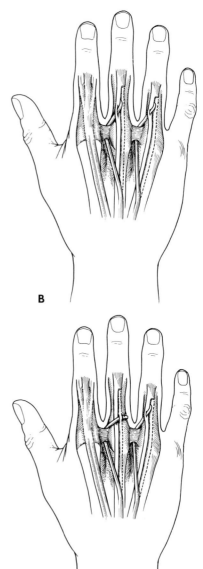

Figure 18–2. *A*, In the long finger, a long strip is detached from the ulnar border of the extensor communis tendon. *B*, It is passed under the intermetacarpal (or interglenoid) ligament, which serves as a pulley, and after correction it is fixed to the extensor communis. *C*, The transferred band is passed over the extensor tendon and is fixed to the fibrous tissue on the ulnar side of the tendon.

SECONDARY SUTURES AND GRAFTS

Secondary repair is sometimes possible, but if tissue contraction does not permit, one resorts to a graft. No primary suturing is attempted if the wound is contused or contaminated.

Ducourtioux and Pouliquen (1969) thread a thin strip of palmaris longus into the distal capsulotendinous plane. The two ends of the graft run crosswise over the dorsal aspect of the joint and are joined to the proximal end of the extensor tendon.

LATERAL DISPLACEMENT OF THE EXTENSOR TENDON

The long extensor tendon is maintained on the dorsal aspect of the metacarpophalangeal joint by the interosseous aponeurosis and its fragile proximal insertions (sagittal bands, loose adhesions of the capsule, and inconstant insertion on the base of the proximal phalanx). When these structures are torn by trauma or stretched by arthritis, the tendon, when submitted to passive tension as in flexion, tends to slide over the ulnar side of the joint. As the lesions become more severe, the tendon is displaced into the intermetacarpal valley and contributes to the maintenance of the flexion deformity and ulnar deviation of the metacarpophalangeal joint. In addition, freed from its proximal attachment, the extensor tendon exerts an even stronger pull on the middle phalanx, forcing it into hyperextension.

Such tendon displacement must be corrected, the difficulty being to maintain the tendon in its axis without impeding its gliding movement. Our experience with such tendon displacement has been chiefly in rheumatoid hands. For correction we use a band taken from the extensor communis or an extensor proprius. When the index finger is involved, the distal end of the extensor proprius is detached and passed around the tendon of the first dorsal interosseous muscle (Fig. 18–1). For the other fingers a tendon band detached from the extensor communis is passed under the intermetacarpal ligament (Helal, 1974) (Fig. 18–2). Rather than reattaching the transferred band, it is passed over the extensor tendon and is fixed to the fibrous tissue on the ulnar side of the tendon, preventing a new subluxation (Fig. 18–2C). Michon, who has been interested in this problem for a long time, discusses this subject in the next chapter.

REFERENCES

References for this chapter will be found following Chapter 23.

Chapter 19

LESIONS OF THE EXTENSOR TENDONS IN THE METACARPOPHALANGEAL ZONE

JACQUES MICHON

Clean tears of the extensor tendons in the metacarpophalangeal joint region are easy to repair. Interrupted suturing usually gives a good result. The surgical interest in this area lies with lesions of the bands that maintain the tendons over the metacarpal heads.

Stretching or rupture of a strap results in dislocation of the tendon into the intermetacarpal space during flexion. Closed ruptures are rare and usually occur in combination with sprains or dislocations of the metacarpophalangeal joint. The bands usually snap in the course of a primary disease of the joint, such as acute arthritis, arthrosis, and rheumatoid arthritis. They deserve particular attention because their rupture contributes to the subsequent ulnar deviation.

Clean tears are rare, and in the majority of cases direct suturing is not possible. In stretch lesions, which are commonly seen in rheumatoid arthritis, plication "double breasted" suturing usually restores the tendon balance.

In cases of rupture or when the band has been weakened, a plasty may be necessary. Wheeldon (1954) advocates the use of a strip of an adjacent intertendinous band. Michon and Vichard (1961) raise a pedicled strip from the tendon itself and tether its free end to the transverse ligament or to the capsule (Fig. 19–1A, B). The tension in the newly constructed strap is adjusted with the metacarpophalangeal joint flexed in order to avoid overcorrection.

THE INDEX FINGER

The radial band of the extensor system of the index finger is inserted on the neck of the

second metacarpal where it exchanges fibers with the first dorsal interosseous tendon that contribute to the lateral stability of the tendon. If the band is ruptured or weakened, the interosseous muscle slips palmarward and loses its abductor role, while the extensors fall into the space between the second and

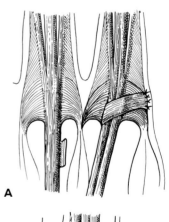

A

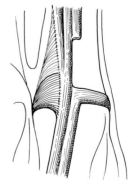

B

Figure 19–1. *A,* Wheeldon plasty. The anastomotic band is turned over the extensor tendon and sutured on the opposite side of the joint. *B,* The tendon is divided and a portion is fixed to the joint capsule.

141

third metacarpal heads. The synergistic inter-
osseous-extensor relationship (necessary in
the gesture of pointing and in the pinch) is
lost; index function is weakened and ulnar
deviation sets in.

To treat this lesion, it is necessary to restore the intertendon relationship by means
of a plasty. We prefer to use a strip of tendon,
which we wind around the interosseous tendon to make a pulley and suture it down on
the radial aspect of the joint (Fig. 19–1*B*).

THE THUMB

At the level of the metacarpophalangeal
joint, the extensor pollicis longus is held in
position by the dorsal expansions of the tendons of abductor pollicis brevis and of the
transverse head of adductor pollicis. In cases
of dislocation and of severe sprain, as occurs
in the course of rheumatoid arthritis, the
abductor expansion may be damaged and
produce medial subluxation of extensor longus, which is often associated with an avulsion of the extensor brevis from the base of
the phalanx. Here again it is important to
restore normal anatomical conditions by direct repair or by means of a plasty, with
fixation to the metacarpal or to the lateral
capsule.

LOSS OF TENDON SUBSTANCE

Trauma by abrasion against the dorsum of
the metacarpophalangeal joint is not rare and
may result in loss of tendon substance. In
such cases emergency treatment must deal
with bone repair and skin cover (details of
which are not to be discussed here).

When the time comes to carry out the
tendon graft, one must remember to reconstruct the hood. If the capsule is intact, the
transplant is simply slipped under a transverse capsular strap, which holds it down in
place (Fig. 19–2, 1). If the capsule is absent,
a hood must be constructed. This can be

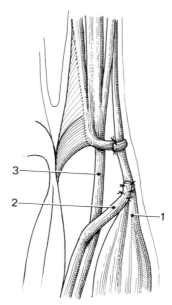

Figure 19–2. In the index finger, the extensor proprius
is divided and its two extremities are sutured to the first
dorsal interosseous tendon. 1 = first dorsal interosseous
muscle, 2 = extensor proprius of the index, 3 = extensor
communis tendon of the index finger.

done by means of a second tendon graft laid
at right angles to the first and tethered to the
extensor graft and to either side of the joint
(Fig. 19–2, 2).

CONCLUSION

In lesions of the extensor hood, the lesion
helps one to understand the traumatology
and vice versa. A study of traumatic lesions
and their functional repercussions improves
our understanding of rheumatoid lesions, especially ulnar deviation of the fingers and
deformities of the thumb.

References

References will be found following Chapter 23.

Chapter 20

EXTENSOR TENDON INJURIES ON THE DORSUM OF THE HAND AND WRIST

Raoul Tubiana

LESIONS AT THE LEVEL OF THE DORSUM OF THE HAND

The tendons of the extensor communis fan out at the wrist toward the four fingers. They often split before being reunited through the juncturae tendinum (or conexus intertendineus), which provide some degree of coordination in extension movements of the fingers (Fig. 20–1).

The proprius tendons of the index and fifth fingers are situated on the medial side of the corresponding extensor communis tendon, allowing some extra freedom of action for these border digits. When only one of the extensor tendons of the index or little finger is severed, the only functional loss is a slight lack of autonomy in extension of the proximal phalanx if the proprius tendon has been damaged. The degree of retraction of the proximal end of the extensor communis tendon on the dorsum of the hand depends partly on the site of the lesion in relation to the insertion of the juncturae, retraction being more marked in proximal lesions.

As a rule, the repair of the extensor tendons on the dorsum of the hand is easy, the conditions prevailing at that level being generally favorable. The tendons are extrasynovial except in the proximal part of the hand, and the limited excursion of the extensor (less than 1 cm. at that level) means that slight restriction of gliding will have little effect on extension of the finger.

In spite of this, complications are far from uncommon and may have severe repercussions on future function. In fact, most of these complications are due to associated lesions.* For this reason it is important that a distinction be made between simple tears of the extensor tendons and complex wounds.

Rupture of the extensor tendons on the dorsum of the hand is rare. It commonly occurs more proximally at the intrasynovial part of the tendon within the osteofibrous tunnels of the wrist.

PRIMARY REPAIR

Uncomplicated Tears

When there is a clean wound affecting only skin and tendons, repair of the extensor tendons poses no problem in itself, although the search for the proximal end may require enlargement of the wound. Downward massage along the course of the extensor communis may help to bring the tendon into view.

Approximation of the tendon ends during suturing is made easier by extension of the wrist. Several suturing techniques have been described. Bunnell (1944) advocates the figure of eight suture, which transfixes both skin and tendon.

It is also possible to use a Kessler type of locking suture or a single U suture. Jennings' barbed wire suture avoids the use of plaster immobilization but creates other problems.

In fact, tendon healing is easy to obtain. It is important, however, to avoid peritendinous adhesions and joint stiffness. Fine buried sutures should be used, and skin and tendon

---

*See chapter on wounds of the dorsal surface of the hand in Volume II.

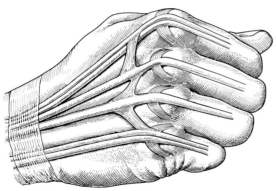

Figure 20–1. General view of the extensor tendons on the back of the hand. The extensor communis tendons are united by intertendinous connections at the distal part of the back of the hand. The extensor proprius of the index finger is situated medial to the extensor communis tendon. The extensor proprius of the little finger is doubled. In this diagram the extensor communis tendon of the little finger is not shown. It is often missing and is replaced by a tendinous band from the extensor communis tendon of the ring finger.

sutures must be separate. Joint stiffness is avoided by not immobilizing the metacarpophalangeal joint in complete extension. It is also important to relax the extensor communis by immobilizing the wrist in 45 degrees of extension for four weeks. The metacarpophalangeal joints can be lightly flexed to 15 degrees. The proximal interphalangeal joints are immobilized in extension, and movement is encouraged for the distal interphalangeal joints. It is preferable to immobilize the finger next to the injured one. If the tendon laceration is distal to the intertendinous connections, one can flex the metacarpophalangeal joint of the adjacent fingers to relieve tension on the suture line (Fig. 20–2).

Recently, Allieu et al. reported a method for passive movement of the extensor tendons comparable to that used for the flexors (see Chapter 23). At the end of the operation, a metal and elastic apparatus is placed on the dorsum of the finger operated upon and adjacent fingers. This device causes passive extension of the fingers following active flexion of the metacarpophalangeal joint. This activity has been verified with electromyography. At the end of four weeks the device is removed and active flexion and extension of the proximal phalanx are begun while the proximal and distal interphalangeal joints are kept in flexion.

The use of early passive mobilization should develop after repairs of extensor ten-

dons as well as after those of flexor tendons. It is above all useful in complex forms with concomitant lesions.

Complicated Injuries

When a tendon injury is complicated by associated lesions, the prognosis is quite different. The danger is not so much a loss of extension of the proximal phalanx (although this can be a handicap) as a flexion deficit, which together with stiffness of the metacarpophalangeal joints in extension represents the most severe functional complication. Stiffness is always a threat when there is marked dorsal edema, even in the absence of associated lesions in other tissues.

Associated Lesions. Associated lesions include extensive skin damage following crushing or avulsion, multiple tendon lesions with tissue loss, and fractures of the underlying metacarpals. In all these complicated cases the first aim of treatment is to prevent stiffness of the metacarpophalangeal joints, which sets in notoriously early if these joints are immobilized in extension. Repair of the extensor tendons, which necessitates subsequent immobilization of the metacarpophalangeal joints in extension, if combined with repair of the adjacent structures, leads inevitably to stiffness, which in turn renders the

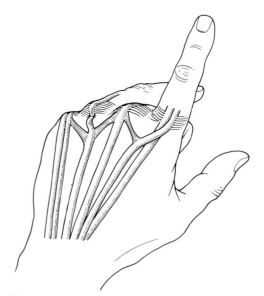

Figure 20–2. Section of the extensor communis of the ring finger distal to the conexus intertendineus. There is little retraction. The suture is relaxed by flexion of the two fingers on either side of the injured finger.

newly repaired tendons unusable. It is preferable first, therefore, to treat the fractures and soft tissue injuries and immobilize the metacarpophalangeal joints in flexion and to repair the tendons at a later stage. This precaution, however, is not an absolute requirement. If stable internal fixation of the bone is achieved, allowing early mobilization, it is reasonable to perform a tendon repair at the same session, provided good skin cover is available. This is, in fact, one of the chief indications for the barbed wire suture, which does not require subsequent immobilization. It is sometimes better in such cases to transfer the distal end of the severed extensor to an adjacent tendon to avoid suturing a tendon in scar tissue.

Extensive loss of skin substance may require a skin flap taken elsewhere. The skin of the forearm or of the contralateral arm (radial Chinese flap, Colson's flap graft) provides covering of excellent quality, but the esthetic sequelae are such that it may be preferred to take the flap from a less visible area. Loss of substance from the dorsum of the hand can be covered using a forearm ulnar flap supplied by a collateral artery of the ulnar artery. It has the advantage of not sacrificing any important artery and there is only minimal scarring (see Chapter 21).

SECONDARY REPAIRS

Secondary repairs of the extensor tendons can succeed only if the fractures are correctly reduced, the joints are mobile, and the skin covering allows free gliding of the underlying tendons. Hence, the occasional need for prior skin flaps, osteotomies, or capsulectomies.

We distinguish two types of secondary repairs—mobilizing operations, such as tenolysis and reconstruction of gliding planes, and tendon reconstruction proper using direct suturing, grafts, anastomoses, or transfers.

Mobilizing Operations

Adhesions can occur in the superficial planes or in the deeper planes. Adhesions with the skin, which is usually mobile, are of less consequence. It is preferable to approach the tendon through an incision placed away from the adhesions to prevent further adhesion formation. However, when broad cicatricial plaques are present along the course of the tendon, one may have to excise them and fill the defect by a skin flap.

Adhesions with the fixed structures have the poorest prognosis. When the adherent zone is limited, a good result is possible after tenolysis if postoperative mobilization is started early, but if extensive adhesions have formed, simple tenolysis is insufficient.

One may try to reconstruct the gliding planes, as suggested by Bunnell (1944), by means of paratenon grafts taken from the superficial aspect of the fascia lata or around the flexor carpi ulnaris. The extensor retinaculum may be transposed beneath the grafts when there is a high risk of adhesion formation. More recently, fine silicone membranes have been introduced for that purpose. These are sutured flush over the deep fascia. Two gliding planes develop in contact with the silicone membrane, in front and behind, but not at the periphery of the encapsulation. The membrane and the layer of connective tissue covering it must therefore be removed after two to three months. They are best removed after two months, when the gliding planes have re-formed. Attempts to wrap the tendon within an artificial gliding membrane are doomed to failure.

We now commonly use interposition of the dorsal retinaculum under the extensor tendon in accordance with techniques frequently used in rheumatoid arthritis surgery (Fig. 20–3). This method can be used after the repair of traumatic lesions of the extensor tendons on the proximal part of the dorsum of the hand and of the wrist. The transfer of well-vascularized gliding tissue such as the flap of the aponeurosis of the forearm pediculated on the radial artery (Ti-Sheng Chang*) or taken from the forearm or the temporal aponeurosis and revascularized by microsurgical anastomoses (Schoops et al., 1983; Wintsch and Helaby, 1985; Upton et al., 1986) probably represents the most effective means of avoiding new adhesions when extensive plaques of scar tissue are present.

Tenolysis should not be carried out too early; the best time is usually about five months after primary repair when it can be combined with a mobilizing procedure on the metacarpophalangeal joints. In such cases flexion posture splints will be worn postoperatively except during the twice daily sessions of active mobilization.

---

*See "The Forearm Flap in Reconstruction of Burns of the Hand," Chapter 74.

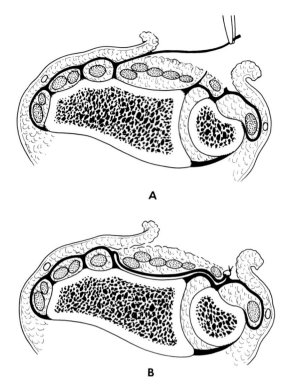

Figure 20-3. Transposition of the extensor retinaculum underneath the extensor tendons of the fingers. *A,* The retinaculum is divided at its ulnar border. *B,* The retinaculum is transposed beneath the extensor tendons of the fingers.

Tendon Repairs

Delayed suturing remains feasible for a long time, especially in distal lesions, because the juncturae tendinum prevent retraction of the proximal end. Delayed repair, however, is not indicated in more proximal lesions because of the tension on the suture lines resulting from tendon retraction. It is preferable to suture the distal tendon to a neighboring extensor and use a tendon graft or tendon transfer.

Anastomosis to an adjacent tendon is the simplest solution, which of course necessitates the presence of a viable motor muscle. The anastomosis should lie in healthy (i.e., unscarred) tissue.

Finally, tendon transfers represent an excellent method of reactivating the digital extensors, an adjacent tendon of sufficient length being the first choice. When available, the extensor indicis proprius provides the ideal transfer because it can reactivate the extensor tendons of one or two fingers. One can also use a part of the extensor digiti

minimi when there is duplication of this tendon. One does not use the whole tendon because of the risk of leaving extension of the little finger weak. The tendons of the flexor and extensor carpi ulnaris are not usually long enough to be anastomosed to the distal stumps of the digital extensors when the lesion lies at the level of the dorsum of the hand. If utilized, they must be lengthened by a graft. There is also the possibility of using the flexor superficialis, which possesses enough length and power to be transferred to three or four extensors.* In all these procedures the movements of the wrist assist the action of the transfer considerably.

Grafts

Segmental tendon grafts are used when tendon transfers are not possible. They permit reconstruction in multiple injuries, the advantage being that the sutures can be placed in a healthy zone. Ideally the proximal suture should lie at the musculotendinous junction in the forearm, where the subcutaneous ridge is better concealed, than at the wrist or dorsum of the hand. The grafts are passed superficial to the retinaculum. The most common sources of grafts are the palmaris longus, plantaris, and extensor digitorum of the toes. When the graft must lie in a scarred bed, it is best to carry out a two-stage procedure. The first stage consists of preparing a gliding surface with a silicone rod. This technique permits one to place an extensor graft beneath the extensor retinaculum and even beneath a skin graft (Bevin and Hothem, 1978).

Extensor-Plus Syndrome

Among the many secondary complications of extensor tendon lesions on the dorsum of the hand and proximal phalanx, it is important to single out the extensor-plus syndrome (Kilgore et al., 1975). The syndrome probably results from either shortening of the tendon or adherence of the tendon to the first part of the proximal phalanx at the extensor hood. It results in the inability to flex the proximal interphalangeal and metacarpophalangeal joints simultaneously, although each joint can be flexed normally individually. The clinical test demonstrating this state

*These operations are described in detail in the chapter on rheumatoid arthritis in Volume IV.

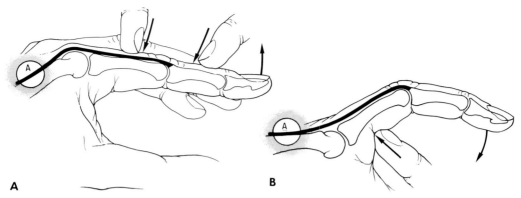

Figure 20–4. Test showing the presence of a retraction of the extensor tendons (extensor-plus syndrome). *A*, Flexion of the proximal phalanx prevents flexion of the distal phalanx. *B*, Release of the tension in the extensor tendon is obtained by hyperextension of the proximal phalanx. This permits flexion of the distal phalanges.

is the opposite of the intrinsic-plus. Flexion of the metacarpophalangeal joint prevents flexion of the proximal interphalangeal joint. If, on the contrary, one flexes the proximal interphalangeal joint, the metacarpophalangeal joint goes into hyperextension (Fig. 20–4). If in spite of physiotherapy the condition persists, surgery may be indicated.

If the tendon is adherent, treatment consists of using a tenolysis. If the tendon is shortened, tenolysis is not sufficient. Kilgore

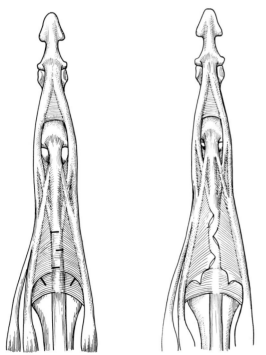

Figure 20–5. Correction of the extensor-plus syndrome by partial tenotomies (Kilgore).

(1977) suggests lengthening the extensor tendon and sagittal bands by stepcutting (Fig. 20–5).

Littler (1977) bases surgical correction of this problem on the concept of the double action of the extrinsic extensors and intrinsic muscles on extension of the distal phalanges. Because either group of muscles can act alone, he proposes the following: in cases of shortening of the intrinsic muscles resection of the oblique fibers of the extensor hood and in cases of shortening of the central extensor tendon resection of that portion of the central tendon overlying the proximal end of the proximal phalanx (Fig. 20–6). Burton (1982) suggests doing the operation under digital block (not a wrist block, which paralyzes intrinsic motor function), permitting the patient to flex the digit so that the surgeon can monitor the extent of resection necessary.

Physiotherapy is begun immediately, and a splint holding the proximal interphalangeal joint in extension is used.

LESIONS AT THE LEVEL OF THE WRIST

At the level of the wrist the extensor tendons pass under the extensor retinaculum along osteofibrous compartments separated by fibrous septa that connect the ligament to the radius. There are six such tunnels within which the tendons run inside their synovial sheaths. From the lateral side one finds the sheaths of the abductor pollicis longus, extensor pollicis brevis, extensor carpi radialis longus and brevis, and extensor pollicis longus, the common sheath of the extensor digitorum

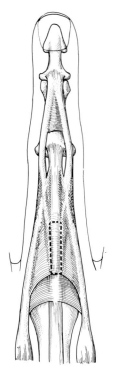

Figure 20–6. Resection of the central extensor tendon in the adherent zone at the level of the proximal phalanx (Littler).

procedure, the annular ligament being partially resected opposite the suture. The wrist is immobilized in extension with the metacarpophalangeal joint in slight flexion, but the interphalangeal joints are left free.

Ruptures. Tendon ruptures can occur after a fracture or a dislocation of the wrist, but they are most common in rheumatoid arthritis. The most vulnerable tendons are the extensors of the little finger at the level of the distal extremity of the ulna. Such a rupture may then be followed by tendon rupture of the ring and middle fingers. For that reason, when extension of the little finger is lost, early surgical intervention is indicated to protect the other extensors.

Old Lesions. In treated old injuries, mobility may be restricted by adhesions, although the fingers can be partially extended by flexion of the wrist through a tenodesis effect. If the limitation constitutes a handicap, a tenolysis is justified; the extensor retinaculum is divided medially and passed under the tendons.

In nontreated old injuries and old ruptures, the possibility of tendon grafts or transfers can be considered, as on the dorsum of the hand.

Lesions of the Extensor Tendons of the Wrist

Tears of the wrist extensors, like those of the thumb extensors (which will be discussed in Chapter 21), can be associated with lesions of the digital extensors. In wounds involving the lateral part of the wrist, systematic exploration should include the extensor carpi radialis tendons; in medial wounds the extensor carpi ulnaris should be carefully examined. Primary suturing followed by four weeks' immobilization usually ensures good results.

When the lesions are old, delayed suturing is often prevented by contractures, and the choice of treatment rests between tendon grafts and transfers. Restoring the action of the extensor carpi radialis brevis is a priority, because this muscle, by reason of its location, is the most important extensor of the wrist.*

and extensor proprius indicis, that of the extensor digiti minimi, and finally that of the extensor carpi ulnaris. The excursion of the digital extensor tendons at this level is about 5.5 cm., and the problem of gliding here is of primary importance.

TREATMENT

The presence of tight osseofibrous tunnels and of synovial sheaths and the importance of tendon excursion make tendon repairs at this level more difficult.

Lesions of the Digital Extensors

Recent Lesions. An extensor lag of only the middle and ring fingers can be due to tearing of the extensor communis tendons, in which the extensor proprius tendons take over extension of the index and little fingers. The state of the four tendons therefore should be systematically checked.

The primary repair depends on the state of the skin. A suture protected against traction, such as that used for the flexors in the digital canal, often can be used as a primary

REFERENCES

References will be found following Chapter 23.

---

*The technique of tendon transfer is dealt with in detail in the chapter on paralysis of the extensors of the wrist in Volume IV.

Chapter 21

THE ULNAR FLAP

CORINE BECKER
AND ALAIN GILBERT

Several types of local flaps have recently been described that may be used to cover large areas of soft tissue deficit in the hand. These have subsequently reduced the need to utilize distant flaps. Unfortunately, many of these flaps sacrifice a major arterial axis of the upper limb. However, the ulnar flap does not present this disadvantage because it is based upon a collateral branch of the ulnar artery.

ANATOMY

Forty dissections in the region of the wrist were carried out. Following injection of the ulnar artery with latex, it could be demonstrated that a constant collateral branch of this artery originates between 2 and 4 cm. proximal to the pisiform and runs medially beneath the flexor carpi ulnaris tendon (Fig. 21–1). This common trunk is 3 to 7 cm. in length and 1 to 1.5 mm. in diameter. Beneath the tendon, the trunk divides into several branches: a branch supplying the flexor carpi ulnaris muscle, a branch vascularizing the pisiform, and finally a cutaneous branch supplying the skin of the medial wrist that further divides into ascending and descending branches. The ascending branch runs along the ulnar border of the forearm for 15 to 20 cm., while the descending branch vascularizes the dorsal aspect of the hand and also supplies a branch to the abductor digiti minimi. The zone vascularized by this flap is situated on the medial aspect of the ulnar side of the forearm and measures up to 20 cm. by 5 by 9 cm. in size (Fig. 21–2).

Venous drainage is ensured by the venae comitantes and large subcutaneous veins.

The dorsal branch of the ulnar nerve originates about 2 cm. proximal to the ulnar artery and runs toward the dorsal aspect of the wrist. It is vascularized by this same artery.

This anatomical arrangement is found in 75 per cent of cases. In an appreciable number of cases (24 per cent), there are two separate arteries, one of which supplies the pisiform and the other a more proximal musculocutaneous branch. In a few cases, the three branches originate separately.

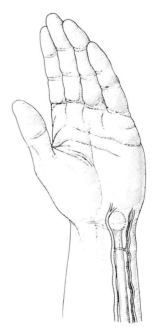

Figure 21–1. The ulnar cutaneous flap. The cutaneous branch arises from the ulnar artery and passes under the flexor carpi ulnaris.

149

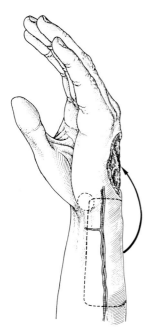

Figure 21–2. The flap is centered on the cutaneous vessels.

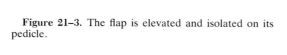

Figure 21–3. The flap is elevated and isolated on its pedicle.

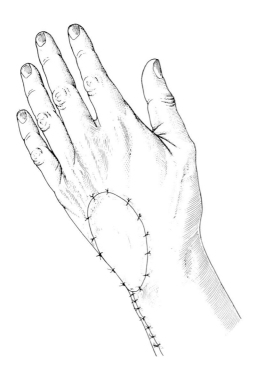

Figure 21–4. The defect is covered by the flap.

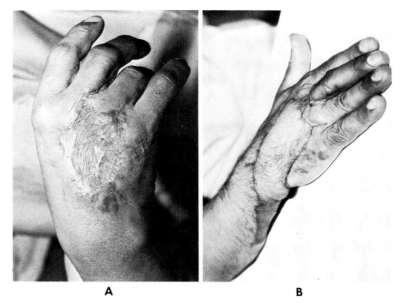

Figure 21–5. *A*, Traumatic lesion of the back of the hand involving the skin and the extensor tendons of the three ulnar fingers. *B*, Repair of the skin defect and of the extensor tendons using an ulnar skin flap.

A   B

SURGICAL TECHNIQUE

The flap is drawn on the dorso-ulnar aspect of the forearm. A dorsal incision is made first. It is necessary to design the length of the flap in relation to the axis of rotation, which is approximately 2 cm. proximal to the pisiform. The artery does not need to be dissected, but when the flap is raised, care must be exercised as the dissection approaches the pisiform so that the pedicle of the flap is not damaged. The fascia does not need to be included with the flap because the course of the artery is entirely subcutaneous (Fig. 21–3). Next, the distal pedicle of the flap is raised and may be rotated either anteriorly or posteriorly on the wrist. A complete rotation of 180 degrees is possible. The cutaneous pedicle should then be divided, preserving only the vascular pedicle to allow rotation of the flap.

The donor defect may be closed primarily if the width of the flap does not exceed 3 or 4 cm. Otherwise, it is necessary to cover the defect with a skin graft.

CLINICAL USE

We have used this flap in a variety of clinical situations with a diversity of indications: the reconstruction of a large area of soft tissue loss on the dorsum of the hand (Figs. 21–4 and 21–5), the surgical excision of a hand tumor, the correction of a dorsal contracture of the wrist, and the covering of the median nerve after repeated neurolyses or nerve grafts. This flap provides a simple means of providing good-quality coverage in a zone that has already been operated upon and become fibrosed.

CONCLUSION

The ulnar flap provides a new method of soft tissue coverage in the hand. When a moderate amount of tissue has been lost, it may be used without sacrificing a major arterial axis. Because the flap is not innervated, it cannot be used as a sensory flap.

Chapter 22

LESIONS OF THE EXTENSORS OF THE THUMB

Raoul Tubiana

Extension of the thumb differs from that of the other fingers in several respects. The mechanism of phalangeal extension is simpler because only two phalanges are concerned. Each phalanx has its own extrinsic extensor (the extensor pollicis brevis for the proximal and the extensor pollicis longus for the distal). Like the interosseous muscles for the fingers, the intrinsic thenar muscles also contribute to phalangeal extension through their dorsal expansions, but here they act only on the distal phalanx. Their action at the proximal phalanx is more one of flexion.

The main difference between extension of the thumb and that of the fingers is at the level of the metacarpals. Although the finger metacarpals are virtually fixed, the movements of the first metacarpal control the action of the column of the thumb. To talk in terms of flexion and extension here would be a misleading analogy. The movements are far more complex and are better described in terms of opening and closure combined with rotation.* Opening of the first metacarpal results from the action of both the extrinsic (abductor pollicis longus and extensor pollicis brevis) and the intrinsic (abductor brevis and opponens) muscles. The extensor pollicis longus, whose course is quite different from that of the other extrinsic muscles because it is reflected around Lister's tubercle, adducts the first metacarpal while extending the phalanges, its action reinforcing that of the extensor brevis on the first phalanx (Fig. 22–1). It is an antagonist of the thenar muscles at the level of the metacarpal, yet it has the same action as the latter on the distal phalanx. Such complex actions require an excur-

sion of 5 cm., i.e., much greater than that of the other dorsal extrinsic tendons of the thumb (namely, the abductor longus and extensor brevis).

TREATMENT

Repair of the extensor apparatus of the thumb depends on the nature of the injury, the timing of the operation, and the site of the lesion.

INJURY AT THE LEVEL OF THE INTERPHALANGEAL JOINT

The lesion may be a division, rupture, or avulsion of the long extensor tendon. The situation is similar to that prevailing at the distal interphalangeal joints of the fingers. The antagonistic action of the long flexor produces a flexion deformity of the distal phalanx.

Primary Repair

Division of the tendon on the dorsal aspect of the joint is common. The joint capsule is usually damaged by the injury. Retraction of the proximal stump is minimal because of the pull exerted by expansion of the intrinsic muscles. It is preferable to repair the capsule and tendon in two distinct layers. If the distal stump of the tendon cannot hold a strong suture, one can insert the proximal end directly into the distal phalanx. A wire inserted obliquely through the extended joint and left in for three weeks will protect the new insertion. In addition the interphalangeal and

---

*See chapter on movements of the thumb in Volume I.

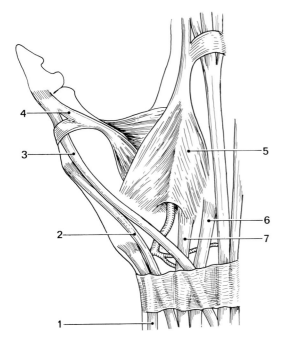

Figure 22–1. The extensor tendons of the thumb. 1 = abductor pollicis longus, 2 = extensor pollicis brevis, 3 = extensor pollicis longus, 4 = expansion of the adductor on the extensor pollicis longus, 5 = first dorsal interosseous, 6 = extensor carpi radialis brevis, and 7 = extensor carpi radialis longus.

metacarpophalangeal joints are immobilized in extension in a plaster cast. After removal of the wire, immobilization with plaster alone is continued for another week.

Tendon ruptures, producing mallet "thumb," are much less common. The tendon may rupture flush with the bony insertion, sometimes avulsing the posterior edge of the base of the distal phalanx. A wire is used to hold the joint in extension, and the thumb is immobilized in plaster for five weeks. If the bone fragment is relatively large and displaced, an open reduction and a transfixion wire running through the fragment may be necessary.

Delayed Repair

If the joint has retained its mobility, a delayed tendon repair may be attempted. If, on the other hand, the joint has become fixed in flexion, arthrodesis may be indicated, especially if it is the dominant hand. Thumb–index finger pulp pinch with the distal phalanx of the thumb in extension is more commonly used than the terminal grip between opposing flexed phalanges. In fact, when the

distal interphalangeal joint of the thumb is stiff, precision is lost, since this implies a constant adaptation to the volume of the object, which requires a mobile joint.

INJURY AT THE LEVEL OF THE BASE OF THE FIRST PHALANX AND METACARPOPHALANGEAL JOINT

The broad dorsal tendinous sheet at this level consists of the tendons of the long and short extensors as well as the expansions of the adductor and of the thenar muscles. The sheet is usually only partially damaged; retraction is minimal and suturing of individual structures is made easier.

Clinically one should take care not to ignore an injury to the extensor pollicis longus when the distal phalanx retains some extension through the action of the interosseous muscles, or injury to extensor brevis when the metacarpophalangeal joint can still be extended by the action of the extensor pollicis longus. The extensor pollicis brevis allows independent extension of the first phalanx regardless of the position of the distal phalanx. If an injury to that tendon is neglected, the thumb inevitably loses some freedom of movement. Secondary suturing, even at a late stage, is often possible.

INJURY AT THE LEVEL OF THE FIRST METACARPAL AND THE WRIST

The situation here is quite different. The tendons form into two groups, which border the anatomical snuffbox—laterally the abductor longus and extensor brevis and medially the extensor pollicis longus, which crosses superficially over the extensor carpi radialis longus and brevis before being reflected around Lister's tubercle. Each group of tendons runs into a separate fibro-osseous compartment at the lower end of the radius, clothed in its own synovial sheath.

Primary Repair of Tendon Divisions

An important precaution in this situation is to spare the sensory branches of the radial nerve. Primary suturing should be carried out before the retraction of the proximal tendon stump becomes permanent. If the suture is placed close to the fibro-osseous compartments, these should be laid open in order to avoid later constrictions. Tenosynovitis producing a true de Quervain syndrome can develop, especially after suturing of the abductor pollicis longus. One should be aware of the various anatomical anomalies in this area: thus, the abductor longus tendon may be split and the extensor brevis tendon may travel in a separate tunnel.

The extensor pollicis longus tendon at this level reflects around Lister's tubercle. A suture should not be placed at this point of reflection. If the tendon is rerouted outside its fibro-osseous tunnel, it will act as a radial abductor of the thumb. To keep its action of retroposition and adduction of the first ray, one should reconstruct another pulley, with a strip of the dorsal retinaculum, just lateral to Lister's tubercle.

Delayed Repair

Delayed repair is indicated not only to restore mobility but also (and quite often) to free adhesions that may restrict the movements of the thumb. Late suturing is seldom possible, except in the case of the abductor longus tendon when retraction of the proximal end has been prevented by the insertion of an aberrant tendon. When retraction is marked, a tendon graft or transfer is indicated. The excursion of the extensor pollicis longus is twice that of the abductor pollicis longus and extensor pollicis brevis, so it is clear that a single tendon transfer fixed into these three tendons would greatly restrict movement of the extensor pollicis longus. One should therefore use one transfer for the abductor longus and extensor brevis (e.g., flexor carpi radialis or palmaris longus) and one for the extensor longus. As we shall see, use of the extensor proprius indicis constitutes a very appropriate transfer.

RUPTURE OF THE EXTENSOR POLLICIS LONGUS

These ruptures deserve special consideration because their etiology and treatment have been the subject of much argument. We shall consider here only ruptures of the proximal part of the tendon that pose special problems. Ruptures and avulsions of the distal end have already been dealt with.

Since 1876, when Duplay reported the first case of tendon transfer, numerous articles have been published about this lesion, especially in Germany. These ruptures first were found to occur with some frequency in drummers (Dums, 1896; Zander, 1891). Later others noted that a high proportion of these ruptures were preceded by fractures of the lower end of the radius (Axhausen, 1929; Hauck, 1923; Trevor, 1950). Advances in the treatment of the rheumatoid hand brought to light an increasing number of such lesions.

Etiology

Rupture can occur without any preceding trauma. Occasionally there is evidence of synovitis. At one time the presence of "sago" granules was regarded as indicating an attenuated form of tuberculosis. In other cases rupture seems to occur "spontaneously," and if the patient is female, there is often a link with a rheumatoid condition. Possible causes of tendon rupture include attrition against a bony ridge, invasion of the tendon by a diseased synovium, and degenerative changes, which may be due to disturbances of tendon vascularization. Local injections of steroids are not without risk.*

In a number of cases, excessive use of the wrist at work has been blamed, e.g., in elderly army drummers, carpenters, woodcutters, and polishers; most patients in this group are male. It is believed that repeated minor trauma may with time induce tendon degeneration.

One relatively important group of cases is that in which the tendon rupture follows an injury to the wrist. In fact, post-traumatic ruptures are relatively rare—two ruptures in 800 fractures of the radius according to Oppolzer (1934), and three in 1250 wrist injuries in the series reported by Stapelmohr (1936), who noted that ruptures are not necessarily more common after major injuries than after minor ones. Some ruptures occur after displaced fractures that have been immobilized in plaster after incomplete reduction. In other cases rupture follows correctly reduced or undisplaced fractures, or even fractures that have been missed and discovered radiologically by chance at the time of the tendon rupture.

There is an enormous variation in the time gap between injury and rupture. Immediate rupture is rare: the interval can be a few days (Lapeyre, 1932), more commonly a few

---

*All these causes are discussed in the chapter on the rheumatoid hand in Volume IV.

months or even years, or even 10 years (Mouchet, 1940).

For half a century opinions have differed as to the causes of rupture of the extensor pollicis longus after fractures of the lower end of the radius. Mechanical erosion at the fracture site and primary vascular lesions of the tendon have been suggested. In the latter case the ischemia is induced by avulsion of the mesotendon at the level of the fracture, as was demonstrated microscopically at operation by Freilinger and Zacheil (1970).

A modified form of the avascular necrosis theory has been exposed by Enkvist and Lundborg (1979): in an undisplaced fracture of the distal end of the radius there may be bleeding or effusion within the intact fibrous sheath which will increase the pressure inside the tunnel, causing impairment of the nutrition of the already poorly vascularized tendon segment close to Lister's tubercle.

Helal et al. (1982) believe that there is a higher risk that the tendon of extensor pollicis longus will rupture in undisplaced Colles' type of fracture than in those which are displaced. In displaced fractures, the extensor retinaculum is torn from the bone and thus allows the tendon to escape.

Clinical Features

The rupture can be sudden and may be accompanied by acute pain. Sometimes the symptoms are so minor that the diagnosis is made only when the patient complains of a weakened thumb. One should take care not to be misled by the presence of extension movements at the distal phalanx because these can be produced by the thenar muscles when the proximal phalanx is flexed. On the contrary, with his hand flat on a table, the patient cannot move the thumb into retroposition. Comparison with the contralateral hand shows an absence of contraction of the extensor longus tendon on the medial border of the anatomical snuffbox, and on the lateral border the extensor brevis and abductor longus tendons produce a sharp ridge. This sign is less obvious with the thumb in adduction; hence, the need to carry out this test with the thumb well abducted.

Treatment

Exploration is effected through a curved longitudinal incision. The proximal end of the tendon usually has retracted up to the wrist so that end to end suturing is impossible. The two choices then are a tendon graft or a tendon transfer.

Tendon Grafting. Tendon grafting is the more physiological procedure. The palmaris longus, when present, is the best source of the graft. The proximal anastomosis is made at the musculotendinous junction and the distal anastomosis at the level of the shaft of the first metacarpal. Any rough bony ridge should of course be excised or filed. The thumb is immobilized in plaster in extension and retroposition with the wrist extended. Hamlin and Littler (1977) regard tendon grafting as the procedure of choice.

Tendon Transfer. Several tendons can be considered for transfer. Many authors advocate the use of the extensor carpi radialis brevis and longus, which run nearby, and it is possible that these may yield a satisfactory, if only partially successful, result. We prefer to preserve the extensor carpi radialis brevis, which we regard as one of the most important muscles of the upper limb. These two carpal extensors have an excursion that is much more limited than that of the extensor pollicis longus, and the patient will need to flex the wrist in order to activate the long thumb extensor. Also it will be difficult to flex the thumb with the wrist in flexion.

The extensor pollicis brevis also has an insufficient excursion, but it has a favorable axis of traction and is sometimes used.

The tendon of the extensor proprius indicis appears to be ideal for transfer (Trevor, 1950) by reason of its appropriate length, direction, and excursion. It is taken on the dorsal aspect of the metacarpophalangeal joint of the index finger through a curved incision, which raises a laterally based skin flap such that the incision does not cross the path of the extensor tendons. The extensor proprius indicis, which runs medial to the extensor communis, is divided at the level of the joint line and its distal stump is sutured to the extensor communis (Fig. 22–2).

Another more lateral incision is made starting at Lister's tubercle; it runs obliquely inferolaterally toward the first metacarpal and curves slightly away from the tendon. Through it the divided tendon of extensor proprius can be drawn upward, the distal stump of the extensor pollicis longus can be identified, and the sensory branches of the radial nerve are retracted. Finally the tendon of extensor proprius indicis is drawn along a straight line from its exit at the fibrous tunnel

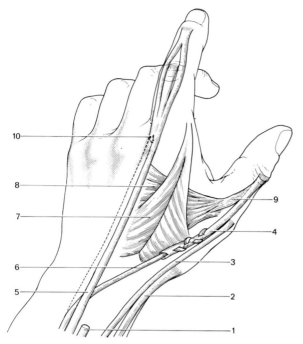

Figure 22–2. Transfers of the extensor proprius indicis to the distal end of the extensor pollicis longus. 1 = retracted proximal end of extensor pollicis longus, 2 = abductor pollicis longus, 3 = Extensor pollicis brevis, 4 = distal end of extensor pollicis longus, 5 = extensor communis indicis, 6 = transfer of the extensor proprius indicis tendon to the distal end of the extensor pollicus longus, 7 = first dorsal interosseus muscle, 8 = adductor pollicis, 9 = dorsal expansion of adductor on extensor pollicis longus, 10 = distal expansion of the extensor proprius indicis sutured to the extensor communis.

of the wrist down to the distal stump of the extensor pollicis longus.

A transfixing suture, allowing accurate adjustment of the tension, is used in the transfer and tied with the motor tendon at half the distance of its excursion, the wrist being kept straight and the thumb in extension and full retroposition. Anteposition of the thumb should be possible when the wrist is passively extended. Immobilization is ensured by a plaster cast maintaining the wrist in extension and the thumb in retroposition and extension for four weeks. However, transfer of the extensor proprius indicis may be contraindicated in patients whose occupation requires independent movements of the index, e.g., in typists and musicians.

REFERENCES

References for this chapter will be found following Chapter 23.

PROTECTED PASSIVE MOBILIZATION AFTER SUTURING OF THE EXTENSOR TENDONS OF THE HAND:
A Survey of 120 Cases

Yves Allieu,
Gérard Asencio,
and Jean-Claude Rouzaud

In 1971 we published our results over five years with the use of Jenning's barbed wire in suturing extensor tendons without post-operative immobilization (Allieu and Romieu, 1971; Lapeyrie et al., 1966). We found that this material allowed relatively active mobilization of the tendon thanks to the assisting suture. In 1977 we pointed out the risk of infection with the use of this material (two instances in 78 cases) if the technique is not perfect (Allieu, 1977). We observed that the widespread use of this material in all emergency surgery centers might yield less satisfactory results than those reported by ourselves and by other specialized centers that have adopted this technique (Nancy and Strasbourg; Foucher et al., 1977; Merle et al., 1976).

In 1972 we started protecting the barbed wire suture with a dynamic appliance. Active mobilization thus became assisted passive mobilization. This method, which allowed immediate mobilization, was used in our department until 1979. It then occurred to us that the protection afforded by the appliance was such that we could abandon the barbed wire and replace it by a fine atraumatic suture. The dynamic element of the appliance has been improved over the years. It is our new technique, as practiced since 1980 (Allieu, 1984), which we shall review in this chapter.

Our technique is essentially that advocated by Kleinert for the flexor tendons, which we have adapted to use with the extensors. Laboureau and Renevey in 1980 reported the method of Kleinert et al. (1973) applied to the extensor apparatus using a "crab" type of segmental dynamic appliance. The forearm-to-palm splint maintains the wrist in hyperextension, but the authors gave no details of the technique or of the results. In 1982 Frere, reporting 75 cases, described the advantages of early post-operative relative mobilization (using Levame's apparatus) in the repair of fresh traumatic lesions of the extensors of the fingers. More recently Evans and Burkhalter (1983) emphasized the merits of this method for complex lesions of the extensor tendons.

TECHNIQUE

The tendon is repaired with a square suture of 4–0 proline. Repair is completed under magnification by approximation of the epitendon using a continuous suture of absorbable material. The overlying skin is closed, with eversion of the subcutaneous tissues to avoid adhesions between skin and tendon. The patient is immobilized for 48 hours in a temporary splint, which maintains the wrist and fingers in extension. In our series all patients (except for nine children) were operated upon under regional anesthesia (intravenous anesthesia or axillary block). In 76 cases the repair was carried out as an emergency procedure and in 16 after a delay of 24 hours; the emergency procedure was "delayed" when there was no associated vascular problem.

The appliance consists of a dynamic extension splint, which maintains the wrist in dorsiflexion and in 30 to 40 degrees of extension, depending on the patient. The metacarpophalangeal joints are left free. The splint is molded directly on the patient's limb and designed for his use only (Fig. 23–1). Our first splint proved too cumbersome, especially when the patient attempted to dress.

To compensate for these inconveniences we have tried to construct a splint using a calibrated and measurable motor: the gauged spiral spring. This allows us to know the exact force that we applied. We have at our disposition an assortment of 12 gauged springs from 50 gm. to 1000 gm. that are color coded. The stretch is fixed at 50 gm. (Fig. 23–2).

The advantage in using a gauged dynamic assistance is the adaptability for each individual, the variations in pathology, and in the chronology of treatment. That allows us to modify forces according to progression of scar

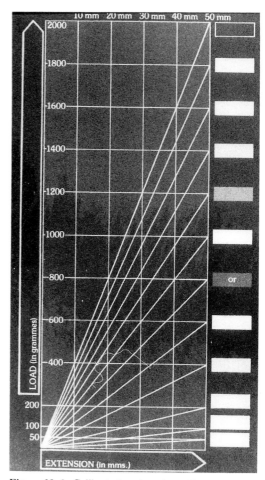

Figure 23–2. Calibrated springs from 50 to 1000 gm.

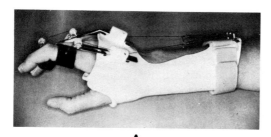

A

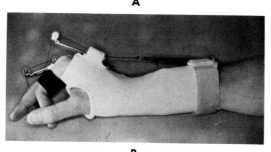

B

Figure 23–1. *A* and *B*, Postoperative dynamic extension splint. The digits are mobilized on the third day. The wrist is immobilized in extension.

tissue. The gauge guarantees a mechanical fidelity along with strength.

The return mechanism is assured by return pulleys, which are fixed on the proximal part of the splint. This technique allows a transmission of the applied forces with negligible friction.

In case of lesions of the extensor tendons on the dorsal part of the hand to the metacarpophalangeal joint, we use a straight plate positioned above the middle first phalanx of the affected finger. This system allows us to effect a premature mobilization and protects the suture of the extensors starting 48 hours postoperatively. We are able to attain a range of motion of 70 degrees in the flexion of the metacarpophalangeal joint during the two weeks after surgery, and about 90 degrees at the end of the fourth week. The final result is obtained by the fifth week in simple cases.

In case of lesions of extensor tendons above the proximal interphalangeal joint, we use a curved plate (45 degrees) with an adjustable stop pad counter propper against P1. The recall is done under P2 by using two pulleys fixed on the plate.

Their minimal obstruction allows us to position simultaneously four plate supports in case of pluritendinous lesions with different anatomic situations and even in case of a narrow metacarpal palette.

This system can also be applied in lesions of the extensors of the thumb. It suffices to place the plate support radially. One must bend the plate slightly to obtain a hyperextension of the column of the thumb.

According to our background studies, the middle forces used are: 800 to 400 gr for men, from 600 to 300 gr for women in case of lesions of extensors according to the affected finger. The middle forces according to the anatomic situations are from 500 to 600 gr in zone 5 and from 200 to 300 gr in zone 3 (Fig. 23–3).

MOBILIZATION OF THE SUTURED TENDON

Mobilization of the sutured tendon is effective. We were able to demonstrate this radiologically after placing a small radio-

Middle Forces According to Extensors

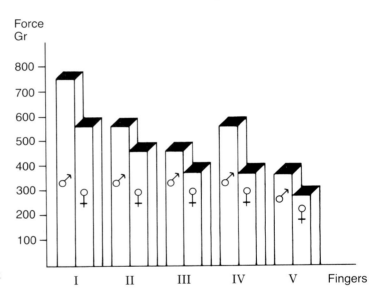

Figure 23–3. Middle forces according to extensors.

Middle Forces According to Localization (Extensors)

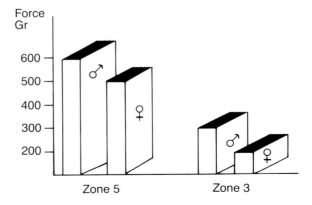

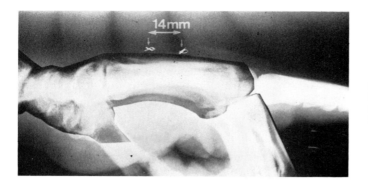

Figure 23–4. Superimposed radiographs of splinted fingers in flexion and in extension. Because of the metallic marker, the suture (zone VI) can be seen to move 14 mm.

paque marker at the site of the repair. Up to 14 mm. of displacement is achieved over the dorsum of the metacarpal (Fig. 23–4).

Electromyographic studies have also shown that mobilization is obtained with no tension on the suture. Immobilization of the wrist in dorsiflexion is essential in order to neutralize the extensors. When the patient actively flexes his fingers, a lack of electromyographic activity in the extensors is obtained only if the wrist is extended (Fig. 23–5). Thus, in extension there is no resistance from the extensors and the suture line is mobilized without tension. In extension the suture is also mobilized without tension, displacement being achieved with the help of the dynamic extension splint.

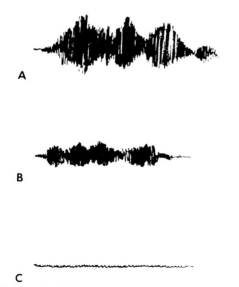

A

B

C

Figure 23–5. Electromyogram of the extensors during active flexion of the fingers. Extension of the wrist results in electromyographic silence, indicating relaxation of the extensors and tension-free mobilization of the suture. *A,* Wrist in complete flexion. *B,* Wrist in neutral position. *C,* Wrist in extension (dorsiflexion).

The system used is the same as that advocated by Kleinert for flexor tendons, the two basic necessities being fine atraumatic suturing and assisted passive mobilization of the sutured tissue. As with the technique described by Kleinert et al. (1973) for the flexors, the key element is the position of the wrist.

CLINICAL MATERIAL

Since 1979 we have treated 100 fingers in 92 patients, a total of 120 lesions of the extensor tendons. The fingers and zones (17) involved are summarized in Figure 23–6. The average age of our patients was 34, ranging from 10 to 74 years. We wish to emphasize that only 17 per cent of our cases resulted from injuries sustained at work, the majority of our patients being victims of domestic accidents. Thus 72 per cent of the patients in our series presented with clean lacerations caused by a knife (15 cases) or by broken glass (27 cases), lesions that have a favorable prognosis. However, in 17 cases a joint was opened (the proximal interphalangeal joint in 7 and the metacarpophalangeal joint in 10 cases), and in 24 cases there was an associated fracture (the proximal phalanx in 4 cases, the middle phalanx in 8, and the metacarpal in 9). We were never faced with loss of cutaneous tissue. Thus in our series 80 per cent of the wounds were simple and involved a single digit. It is clear that this method of management is unsuitable in multidigital lesions, in complex lesions, and in cases of tissue loss.

RESULTS

The results of treatment are summarized in Table 23–1. Our system of evaluation takes

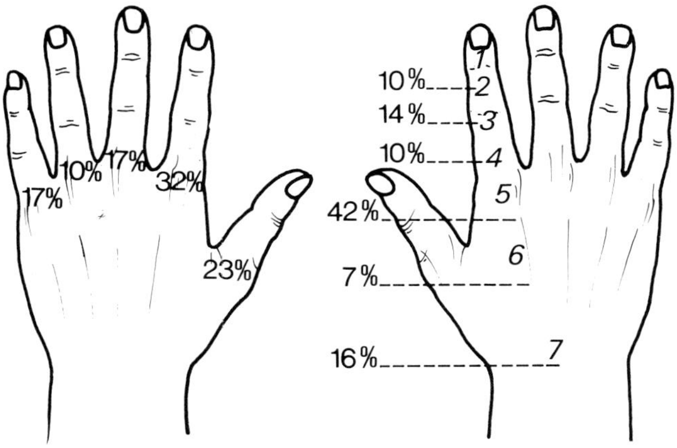

Figure 23–6. Distribution of extensor lesions of the fingers according to the different zones (of Verdan).

into account the extension achieved as well as the loss of flexion secondary to the tenodesis effect. The loss of extension is measured for the whole digit, i.e., for the three joints. A result is graded excellent only when full active extension is obtained with the wrist in flexion and in extension. As for the thumb, we included only sections of the extensor pollicis longus because extensor brevis function is difficult to assess individually. The results are shown in Table 23–2.

FINGERS

Fifty patients were followed for five months to three years; the rest were lost to follow-up. The results at the last visit were satisfactory but not accurately graded. The results for these 50 cases are summarized in Table 23–3; 84 per cent were good or excellent.

EXTENSOR POLLICIS LONGUS

Nineteen cases were followed, with the results shown in Table 23–4. Of the four patients with poor results, two had a double tendon lesion and another was complicated by a phalangeal fracture.

ANALYSIS OF RESULTS

The results were also analyzed according to the zone involved and associated lesions. The best results were obtained with lesions in zones V, VI, and VII (17; 92 per cent graded good or excellent), i.e., proximal to the metacarpophalangeal joint. The prognosis was clearly worse for lesions in the fingers (50 per cent good and excellent results), but it is relevant that associated lesions, especially fractures, are much com-

Table 23–1. EVALUATION OF RESULTS FOR THE FINGERS

Excellent	Full extension (Metacarpophalangeal + proximal interphalangeal + distal interphalangeal)	Wrist held straight Wrist in extension
	Full flexion	*PPC + PDPCD 0
Good	Extension deficit	15°
	Flexion	PPC + PDPCD 15 mm.
Mediocre	Extension deficit	30°
	Flexion	PPC + PDPCD 35 mm.
Poor	Extension deficit	30°
	Flexion	PPC −

*PPC, pulp to palm contact. PDPCD, pulp to distal palmar crease distance.

Table 23–2. EVALUATION OF RESULTS IN THE THUMB

Excellent	Full extension	(CM + metacarpophalangeal + metaphalangeal)
	*CTPM5	0
Good	Loss of extension	15°
	DTPM5	20 mm.
Mediocre	Loss of extension	30°
	DTPM5	40 mm.
Poor	Extension loss	30°

*CTPM5, contact thumb pulp to head of fifth metacarpal. DTPM5, distance between thumb pulp and head of fifth metacarpal.

moner with tendon lesions distal to the metacarpophalangeal joint.

The percentage of good results drops appreciably when there are associated articular or bone lesions (56 per cent good or excellent). Without discussing the details of individual complications, we can say that the prognosis is always worse when the tendon lesion is distal and when there are associated lesions.

COMPLICATIONS

In this series we had no infections, and it is worth comparing this method with that making use of Jenning's barbed wire, which emerges from the skin and can be a point of entry for infection.

In three cases tendon sutures gave way; twice this occurred within 48 hours after surgery and before splinting. The reason was an inadequate immobilization and postoperative monitoring by the nursing staff. One suture loosened on the thirtieth day; it was on the extensor pollicis longus in zone V. The extensor pollicis longus is notoriously fragile and four weeks is the bare minimum for safe recovery of repair. All three tendons were resutured by the same technique and the result was good in all three.

We performed only two minimal secondary tenolyses. Both were in zone V and involved limited adhesions between skin and tendon. In our opinion a tenolysis was not indicated in the 13 patients with mediocre or poor results (eight in the fingers and five in the thumb).

DISCUSSION

The advantages of protected passive mobilization of tendon sutures have been highlighted in both experimental (Gelberman et al., 1981; Matthews, 1973) and clinical studies (Duran and Houser, 1975; Strickland and Glogovác, 1980). Passive assisted mobilization aids tendon healing, reduces the formation of adhesions, and hastens the molding of callus. Although all these studies dealt with the flexor tendons, it seems logical to assume that the findings would be similar for the extensors.

Our own experience has shown that this technique constitutes a genuine step forward. It is safe and reliable and can be used by most surgeons even as an emergency procedure. By contrast, the manufacture of the splint is more sophisticated. It must be carefully designed and constantly adjusted, and the patient must be under constant observation. If the later proves impossible, the technique should not be used.

Table 23–3. RESULTS IN THE FINGERS
(50 Cases Followed for Five Months
to Three Years)

Excellent	24
Good	18
Mediocre	7
Poor	1

Table 23–4. RESULTS IN EXTENSOR
POLLICIS LONGUS (19 Cases Followed
for Five Months to Three Years)

Excellent	8
Good	6
Mediocre	1
Poor	4

We have used this method in children but in none under the age of 10. In younger children and uncooperative patients it is preferable to have recourse to standard immobilization. Complicated wounds make it difficult to fit a dynamic splint and often constitute a contraindication to the method.

The present series includes only tendon injuries with relatively simple wounds, but recently Evans reported good results with this technique in repairs complicated by skin and bone lesions (Evans and Burkhalter, 1983). The design of the splint is then more complex and close observation of the limb is essential.

This technique is indicated primarily for tendon lesions in zones IV, V, VI, and VII; for more distal lesions, standard immobilization and short dynamic splints are still preferable. The technique is reliable and readily teachable and yields highly satisfactory results in lesions of the extensor tendons at and proximal to the metacarpophalangeal joint. Immediate mobilization eliminates the risk of stiffness attendant upon immobilization in extension (Stuart, 1985). However, a suitable dynamic splint, constant reappraisal of its position, and regular supervised postoperative exercising are all prerequisites for success.

REFERENCES

Allieu, Y.: L'utilisation du barb wire de Jenning en chirurgie de la main. Note de catamnèse. Ann. Chir., *31*:359–361, 1977.

Allieu, Y., and Romieu, C.: L'utilisation du "barb wire" de Jenning dans les sutures tendineuses. Absence d'immobilisation post-operatoire. Ann. Chir., *25*:987–994, 1971.

Allieu, Y., Asencio, G., Gomis, R., Teissier, J., and Rouzaud, J. C.: Suture des tendons extenseurs de la main avec mobilisation assistée. A propos de 120 cas. Rev. Chir. Orthop., *70*:68–73, 1984.

Duran, R. J., and Houser, R. G.: Controlled passive motion following flexor tendon repair in zones 2 and 3. *In* AAOS Symposium on Tendon Surgery in the Hand. St. Louis, The C. V. Mosby Company, 1975, pp. 105–114.

Evans, R. B., and Burkhalter, W. E.: Early passive motion in complex extensor tendon injury. Communication, Second International Meeting of American Society of Hand Therapists, Boston, October 19, 1983.

Foucher, G., Merle, M., and Michon, J.: Traitement "tout en un temps" des traumatimes complexes de la main avec mobilisation précoce. Ann. Chir., *31*:1059–1063, 1977.

Frere, G.: Intérêt d'une mobilisation relative par appareil de Levame en post-opératoire immédiat des lésions traumatiques récentes de l'appareil extenseur des doigts longs. Presentation (Société Française de Chirurgie de la Main), Lyon, May 21–22, 1982.

Gelberman, R. H., Amifl, D., Gonsalves, M., Woo, S., and Akeson, W. H.: The influence of protected passive mobilization on the healing of flexor tendons. A biochemical and microangiographic study. Hand, *2*:120, 128, 1981.

Jenning, E. R., and Yeager, G. H.: Tendon suturing with barbed wire. Arch. Surg., *70*:566–569, 1970.

Kleinert, H. E., Kutz, J. E., Atasoy, E., and Stommo, A.: Primary repair of flexor tendons. Orthop. Clin. North Am., *4*:865–876, 1973.

Laboureau, J. P., and Renevey, A.: Utilisation d'un appareil personnel de contention et de rééducation segmentaire élastique de la main type "crabes." Ann. Chir., *25*:165–169, 1980.

Lapeyrie, M., Pous, J. G., and Allieu, Y.: Un procédé simple de suture tendineuse appuyée évitant l'immobilisation post-opératoire. Montpellier Chir., *12*:333–339, 1966.

Matthews, P.: The pathology of flexor tendon repair. Hand, *3*:233–242, 1978.

Merle, M., Foucher, G., and Michon, J.: La technique de Kleinert dans les réparations primaire des tendons fléchisseurs dans le "no man's land." Ann. Chir., *30*:883–887, 1976.

Strickland, J. W., and Glogovac, S. V.: Digital fixation following flexor tendon repair in zone II: a comparison of immobilization and controlled passive motion techniques. J. Hand Surg., *5*:537–543, 1980.

Stuart, D.: Durée de l'immobilisation après réparation des tendons extenseurs à la main. J. Bone Joint Surg., *47B*:72–79, 1965.

Tubiana, R.: Surgical repair of the extensor apparatus of the fingers. Surg. Clin. North Am., *48*:1015–1031, 1968.

Verdan, C.: Primary and secondary repair of flexor and extensor tendon injuries. *In* Flynn, J. E. (Editor): Hand Surgery. Baltimore, The Williams & Wilkins Company, 1966.

GENERAL REFERENCES ON EXTENSOR TENDON INJURIES

Aiache, A., Barsky, A. J., and Weiner, D. L.: Prevention of boutonniere deformity. Plast. Reconstr. Surg., *46*:164–167, 1979.

Albertoni, W. M.: Mallet finger. Techniques of treatment. Thèse, São Paulo, Brazil, 1977.

Allieu, Y.: L'utilisation du barb wire de Jenning en chirurgie de la main. Note de catamnèse. Ann. Chir., *31*(4):359–361, 1977.

An K. N., Chao, E. J., Cooney, W. P., and Linscheid, R. L.: Normative model of human hand for biomechanical analysis. J. Biomechanics, *12*:775–788, 1979.

Anson, B. J., Wright, R. R., Ashley, F. L., and Dykes, J.: The fascia of the dorsum of the hand. Surg. Gynec. Obstet., *81*:327, 1945.

Axhausen, G.: Die Spätrutur der Sehne des Extensor pollicis longus bei typischer Radiofractur. Brun's Beitr. Klin. Chir., *133*:78, 1925.

Bates, J. T.: Operation for the correction of locking of the proximal interphalangeal joint in hyperextension. J. Bone Joint Surg., *27*:142–144, 1945.

Baumann, J A., and Patry, G.: Observations microscopiques sur la texture fibreuse et la vascularisation de l'ensemble tendineux extenseur du doigt et de la main, chez l'homme (considérations fonctionnelles). Rev. méd. Suisse Romande, *63*:900–912, 1943.

Bevin, A. G., and Hothem, A. L.: The use of silicone rods under split-thickness skin grafts for reconstruction of extensor tendon injuries. Hand, *10*:254–258, 1978.

Blue, A. I., Spira, M., and Hardy, S. B.: Repair of extensor tendon injuries of the hand. Am. J. Surg., *132*:128–132, 1976.

Boyes, J. H.: *Bunnell's Surgery of the Hand.* 5th ed. Philadelphia, J. B. Lippincott, 1970.

Bowers, W. H., and Hurst, L. C.: Chronic mallet finger. The use of Fowler's central slip release. J. Hand Surg., *3*:373–376, 1978.

Bunnell, S.: *Surgery of the Hand.* Philadelphia, J. B. Lippincott, 1944.

Bunnell, S., Doherty, E. W., and Curtis, R. M.: Ischemic contracture, local, in the hand. Plast. Reconstr. Surg., *3*:424, 1948.

Burton, R. O.: Extensor tendons. Late reconstruction. In Green, D. P. (Ed.): *Operative Hand Surgery.* Edinburgh, Churchill Livingstone, 1982, pp. 1465–1505.

Cantero, J., and Chamay, A.: Les plaies des tendons extenseurs sur le dos de la main et du poignet. In Verdan, C. (Ed.): *Chirurgie des Tendons de la Main.* Paris, Expansion Scientifique. 1976.

Casscells, S. W., and Strange, T. B.: Intramedullary wire fixation of mallet finger. J. Bone Joint Surg., *51A*:1018, 1969.

Chao, E. Y., Opgrande, J. D., and Axmaer, F. E.: Three-dimensional force analysis of finger joints in selected isometric hand functions. J. Biomechanics, *9*:387–396, 1976.

Curtis, R. M., Reid, R. L., and Provost, J. H.: A staged technique for the repair of the traumatic boutonniere deformity. J. Hand Surg., *8*(2):167–171, 1983.

Dolphin, J. A.: The extensor tenotomy for chronic boutonniere deformity of the finger. J. Bone Joint Surg., *47A*:161–164, 1965.

Doyle, J. R.: Extensor tendons. Acute injuries. In Green, D. P. (Ed.): *Operative Hand Surgery.* Edinburgh, Churchill Livingstone, 1982, pp. 1441–1464.

Ducourtioux, J. L., and Pouliquen, X.: Experience dans le traitement des "mallet finger." Ann. Chir. Plast. Surg., *14*:249–253, 1969.

Dums, F.: Trommlerlähmung. Dtsch. Militärärztl. Z., *25*:145, 1896.

Duplay, M.: Rupture sous-cutanée du tendon du long extenseur du pouce de la main droite au niveau de la tabatière anatomique. Bull. Mém. Soc. Chir. Paris, *2*:788, 1876.

Elliott, R. A.: Injuries to the extensor mechanism of the hand. Orthop. Clin. North Am., *1*:335–354, 1970.

Elliott, R. A.: Splints for mallet and boutonniere deformities. Plast. Reconstr. Surg., *52*:282–285, 1973.

Engkvist, O., and Lundborg, G.: Rupture of the EPL after fracture of the lower end of the radius. The Hand, *11*:176–185, 1979.

Entin, M. A.: Repair of extensor of the hand. Surg. Clin. North Am., *40*:275, 1960.

Esteve, P.: Traitement de la rupture distale des tendons extenseurs. Entretiens de Bichat, Chirurgie. Expansion Scientifique. Paris, 201, 1964.

Eyler, D. L., and Markee, J. E.: Anatomy of the intrinsic musculature of the fingers. J. Bone Joint Surg., *36A*:1–9, 1954.

Flatt, A. D.: *The Care of Minor Hand Injuries.* 4th ed. St. Louis, C. V. Mosby, 1979.

Fowler, S. B.: Extensor apparatus of the digits. J. Bone Joint Surg., *31B*:477, 1949.

Fowler, S. B.: The management of tendon injuries. J. Bone Joint Surg., *41A*:579–580, 1959.

Freilinger, G., and Zacherl, H.: Zur Ruptur der langen Daumenstrecksehne nach Radiusfraktur. Handchirurgie, *2*:76, 1970.

Frere, G., Moutet, F., Sartorius, C., and Vila, A.: Mobilisation contrôlée post-opératoire des sutures des tendons extenseurs des doigts longs. Ann. Chir. Main, *3*:139–144, 1984.

Gama, C.: Results of the Matev operation for correction of boutonniere deformity. Plast. Reconstr. Surg., *64*:319–324, 1979.

Gaul, J. St.: The ratio of motion of the interphalangeal joints. Unpublished report, 1971.

Green, D. P., and Rowland, S. A.: Fractures and dislocations of the hand. *In* C. A. Rockwood and D. P. Green (eds.): Philadelphia, J. B. Lippincott, 1975.

Haines, R. W.: The extensor apparatus of the finger. J. Anat., *85*:251–259, 1951.

Hamas, R. S., Horrell, E. D., and Pierret, G. P.: Treatment of mallet finger due to intra-articular fracture of the distal phalanx. J. Hand Surg., *3*:361–363, 1978.

Hamlin, C., and Littler, J. W.: Restoration of the EPL tendon by an intercaleted graft. J. Bone Joint Surg., *59A*:412–414, 1977.

Harris, C., and Rutledge, G. L.: The functional anatomy of the extensor mechanism of the finger. J. Bone Joint Surg., *54A*:713–726, 1972.

Hauck, G.: Die Ruptur der Dorsalaponeurose am ersten Interphalangealgelenk; zugleich ein Beitrag zur Anatomie und Physiologie der Dorsalaponeurose. Arch. Klin. Chirurgie, *123*:197–232, 1923.

Helal, B.: The reconstruction of rheumatoid deformities of the hand. Br. H. Hosp. Med., *617*:226, 1974.

Helal, B., Chen, S. C., and Iwegbu, G.: Rupture of the E.P.L. in undisplaced colles fracture. The Hand, *14*:41–47, 1982.

Iselin, F., Levame, J., and Godoy, J.: A simplified technique for treating mallet fingers: tenodermodesis. J. Hand Surg., *2*:118–121, 1977.

Iselin, F., and Pradet, G.: Traitement des lésions anciennes des extenseurs en boutonnières invétérées par résection arthroplastique avec implant. Ann. Chir. Main, *1*:11–17, 1982.

Kaplan, E. B.: Anatomy, injuries and treatment of the extensor apparatus of the hand and fingers. Clin. Orthop., *13*:24–41, 1959.

Kaplan, E. B.: *Functional and Surgical Anatomy of the Hand.* 2nd ed. Philadelphia, J. B. Lippincott, 1965.

Kettlekamp, D. B., Flatt, A. D., and Moulds, R.: Traumatic dislocation of the long finger extensor tendon. A clinical, anatomical, and biomechanical study. J. Bone Joint Surg., *53A*:229–240, 1971.

Kilgore, E. S., Jr., Graham, W. P., Newmeyer, W. L., and Brown, L. G.: The extensor plus finger. Hand, *7*:159–165, 1975.

Kilgore, E. S., and Graham, W. P.: *The Hand. Surgical and Nonsurgical Management.* Philadelphia, Lea & Febiger, 1977.

Kleinman, W. B., and Peterson, D. P.: Oblique retinacular ligament reconstruction for chronic mallet finger deformity. J. Hand Surg., *9A*:369–404, 1984.

Laine, V. A. I., Sairanen, E., and Vainio, K.: Finger deformities caused by rheumatoid arthritis. J. Bone Joint Surg., *39A*:527–533, 1957.

Landsmeer, J. M. F.: The anatomy of the dorsal aponeurosis of the human finger and its functional significance. Anat. Rec., *104*:31–44, 1949.

Landsmeer, J. M. F.: A report on the coordination of the interphalangeal joints of the human finger and its disturbance. Acta Morphologica Neerlando-Scandinavica, 2:59–84, 1958.

Littler, J. W., and Eaton, R. G.: Redistribution of forces in correction of boutonniere deformity. J. Bone Joint Surg., 49A:1267–1274, 1967.

Littler, J. W.: The finger extensor mechanism. Surg. Clin. North Am., 47:415–432, 1967.

Littler, J. W.: Principles of reconstructive surgery of the hand. In Converse, J. M. (Ed.): Reconstructive Plastic Surgery. 2nd ed. Philadelphia, W. B. Saunders, 1977, pp. 3126–3127.

Littler, J. W.: Restoration of the oblique retinacular ligament for correcting hyperextension deformity of the proximal interphalangeal joint. In La Main Rhumatismale. GEM. Paris, Expansion scientifique, 1966.

Lorthioir, G., Evrard, H., and Van der Elst, E.: Le traitement des traumatismes récents de la main. Acta Orthop. Belgica, 24(Suppl. 1):157, 1958.

Maisels, D. O.: The middle slip of boutonniere deformity in burned hands. Br. J. Plast. Surg., 18:117, 1965.

Mann, R. J., Foffeld, T. A., and Farmer, C. B.: Human bites of the hand. Twenty years experience. J. Hand Surg., 2:97–104, 1977.

Mannerfelt, L.: Surgical treatment of the rheumatoid wrist. Clin. Rheum. Dis., 10:549–570, 1984.

Matev, I.: Treatment of long-standing boutonniere deformity of the fingers. Br. J. Plast. Surg., 17:281, 1964.

Michon, J., and Vichard, P.: Luxations latérales des tendons extenseurs en regard de l'articulation M.P. Rev. Méd. Nancy, 86:595–601, 1961.

McCoy, F. J., and Winsky, A. J.: Lumbrical loop operation for luxation of the extensor tendons of the hand. Plast. Reconstr. Surg., 44:142–146, 1969.

McFarlane, R. M., and Hampole, M. D.: Treatment of extensor tendon injuries of the hand. Can. J. Surg., 16:366–375, 1973.

Montant, R., and Baumann, A.: Rupture luxation de l'appareil extenseur des doigts au niveau de la première articulation interphalangienne (physiologie et clinique). Revue Orthop. Chir. App. moteur, 25:5–22, 1938.

Nalebuff, E. A.: Surgical treatment of finger deformities in the rheumatoid hand. Surg. Clin. North Am., 49(4):833–846, 1969.

Nichols, H. M.: Manual of Hand Injuries. 2nd ed., Chicago, Year Book Publishers, 1966.

Pardini, A. G., Costa, R. D., and Morais, M. S.: Surgical repair of the boutonniere deformity of the fingers. Hand, 11:87–92, 1979.

Parkes, A.: Traumatic ischemia of peripheral nerves with some observation on Volkmann's ischaemic contracture. Br. J. Surg., 32:403, 1945.

Planas, J.: Buttonhole deformity of the fingers. The Second Hand Club, Réunion de Paris, 21–22, 1962.

Pratt, R. R.: Internal splint for closed and open treatment of injuries of the extensor tendon at the distal joint of the finger. J. Bone Joint Surg., 34A(4):785–788, 1952.

Ranney, D. A.: The superficialis minus deformity and its operative treatment. Hand, 8:209–214, 1976.

Rothwel, A. G.: Repair of the established post traumatic boutonniere deformity. Hand, 10:241, 1978.

Saffar, Ph.: La réparation secondaire du long extenseur du pouce. Annales Chir. Main, 1986.

Salamanca, F. E. de: Swan-neck deformity: mechanism and surgical treatment. Hand, 8:215–221, 1976.

Salvi, V.: Technique for the buttonhole deformity. Hand, 1:96, 1969.

Schoofs, M., Bienfait, B., Calteux, N., Dachy, C., Vandermaeren, C. and de Coninck, A.: Le lambeau aponévrotique de l'avant-bras. Ann. Chir. Main, 2:197–201, 1983.

Shrewsbury, M. M., and Johnson, R. K.: A systematic study of the oblique retinacular ligament of the human finger: its structure and function. J. Hand Surg., 2:194–199, 1977.

Smillie, I. S.: Mallet finger. Br. J. Surg., 24:438–445, 1937.

Smith, R. J.: Nonischemic contractures of the intrinsic muscles of the hand. J. Bone Joint Surg., 53A:1313–1331, 1971.

Snow, J. W.: Use of a retrograde tendon flap in repairing a severed extensor tendon in the P.I.P. joint area. Plast. Reconstr. Surg., 51:555–558, 1973.

Spoor, C. W., and Landsmeer, J. M. F.: Analysis of the zigzag movement of the human finger under influence of the extensor digitorum tendon and the deep flexor tendon. J. Biomechanics, 9:561–566, 1976.

Souter, W. A.: The boutonniere deformity. J. Bone Joint Surg., 49B(4):710–721, 1967.

Stack, H. G.: Muscle function of the fingers. J. Bone Joint Surg., 44B:899–909, 1962.

Stack, H. G.: Buttonhole deformity. Hand, 3:152, 1971.

Stack, H. G.: Mallet finger. The Hand, 1:83–89, 1969.

Stack, H. G.: A modified splint for mallet finger. J. Hand Surg., 11B:263, 1986.

Stark, H., Boyes, J., and Wilson, J.: Mallet finger. J. Bone Joint Surg., 44A:1061, 1962.

Steichen, J. B., Strickland, J. W., Call, W. H., and Powell, S. G.: Results of surgical treatment of chronic boutonniere deformity: an analysis of prognostic factors. In J. W. Strickland and J. B. Steichen (eds.): Difficult Problems in Hand Surgery. St. Louis, C. V. Mosby, 1982, pp. 62–69.

Stewart, I. M.: Boutonniere finger. Clin. Orthop., 23:220, 1962.

Randell, G.: Post-traumatic rupture of the extensor pollicis longus. Pathogenesis and treatment. Survey based on 207 cases, including 14 personal cases. Acta Chir. Scand., 109:81–96, 1955.

Swanson, A. B.: Surgery of the hand in cerebral palsy and the swan-neck deformity. J. Bone Joint Surg., 42A:951–964, 1960.

Swanson, A. B.: Pathomechanics of the swan-neck deformity. J. Bone Joint Surg., 47A:636, 1965.

Taleisnik, J.: Boutonniere deformity. In J. W. Strickland, and J. B. Steichen (Eds.): Difficult Problems in Hand Surgery. St. Louis, C. V. Mosby, 1982, pp. 54–61.

Thompson, M.: Tendon transfers for defective long extensors of the wrist and finger. Scand. J. Plast. Surg., 3:71–78, 1969.

Thomson, J. S., Littler, J. W., and Upton, J.: The spiral oblique retinacular ligament (SORL). J. Hand Surg., 3:482–487, 1978.

Trevor, D.: Rupture of the extensor pollicis longus tendon after Colles fracture. J. Bone Joint Surg., 32B:370, 1950.

Tubiana, R.: Greffes des tendons fléchisseurs des doigts et du pouce. Rev. Chir. Orthop. 46:191–214, 1960.

Tubiana, R., and Valentin, P.: Anatomy of the extensor apparatus and the physiology of finger extension. Surg. Clin. North Am., 44:897–906, 907–918, 1964.

Tubiana, R.: Surgical repair of the extensor apparatus of the fingers. Surg. Clin. North Am., 48(5):1015–1031, 1968.

Tubiana, R., and Valentin, P.: Les déformations en boutonnière des doigts. Revue Chir. Orthop. Répar. App. moteur, 55:111–124, 1969.

Tubiana, R.: Lésions traumatiques de l'appareil: extenseur au niveau des doigts. *In* Verdan, C. (Ed.): Monographie GEM. Paris, Expansion Scientifique, 1976.

Tubiana, R.: Injuries of the extensor apparatus on the dorsum of the fingers. *In* Verdan C. (Ed.): *Tendon Surgery of the Hand*. Edinburgh, Churchill Livingstone, 1979, pp. 119–128.

Tubiana, R., and Grossman, J. A. I.: The management of posttraumatic boutonniere deformity. Bull. Hosp. Joint Dis. Orthop. Inst., 4(2):542–551, 1984.

Upton, J., Rogers, C., Durham-Smith, G., and Swartz, W.: Clinical applications of free temporo-parietal flaps in hand reconstruction. J. Hand Surg., *11A*:475–483, 1986.

Urbaniak, J. R., and Hayes, M. B.: Chronic boutonniere deformity. An anatomic reconstruction. J. Hand Surg., 6:379–383, 1981.

Verdan, C.: Primary and secondary repair of flexor and extensor tendon injuries. *In* J. E. Flynn (Ed.): *Hand Surgery*. Baltimore, Williams and Wilkins, 1966, p. 220.

Weeks, P. M., and Wray, R. C.: *Management of Acute Hand Injuries. A Biologic Approach*. 2nd ed. St. Louis, C. V. Mosby, 1978, p. 314.

Wheeldon, F. T.: Recurrent dislocation of extensor tendons in the hand. J. Bone Joint Surg., *36B*:612–617, 1954.

Wilhelm, A.: *Verletzungen der Strecksehnen Handchirurgie*, Vol. II, Chapter 29. H. Nigst, D. Buck-Gramcko, and H. Millesi (Eds.). New York, Thieme, 1983.

Wintsch, K., and Helaby, P.: Further experience with the gliding tissue free flap. Communication Congrès Intern. de Microcirurgie, Paris, 1985.

Zancolli, E.: *Structural and Dynamic Bases of Hand Surgery*. 2nd ed., Philadelphia, J. B. Lippincott, 1979.

Zancolli, E.: Swan-neck deformity (flexible). Translocation of the lateral band. Personal communication, 1986.

Zander, A.: Trommlerlähmung, Zit. nach W. Weigeldt, Diss. Berlin, 1981.

Zwieten, K. J. van: The spiral fibres (Hauck) in the extensor assembly of the human finger. Acta Morphologica Neerlando-Scandinavica, *16*:143–144, 1978.

Zwieten, K. J. van: The extensor assembly of the finger in man and non-human primates. Thèse: Leiden, 1980.

Section 3

INJURIES OF THE FLEXOR TENDONS

Chapter 24

TRAUMATIC LESIONS OF THE FLEXOR TENDONS OF THE FINGERS AND THE THUMB

RAOUL TUBIANA

Lesions of the flexor tendons are particularly serious, for they can jeopardize the prehensile function of the hand. Repair is always difficult because it requires both a strong tendon callus to resist traction of a powerful muscle and, even more difficult to obtain, functional gliding planes capable of ensuring the mobility of tendons having an unusually long excursion.

We review in this chapter traumatic lesions of the extrinsic flexor tendons of the thumbs and fingers, i.e., the flexor pollicis longus and flexors digitorum superficialis and profundus.

ANATOMY AND PHYSIOLOGY

The topographical anatomy and physiology of flexion have been studied in the first volume of this work. We shall mention here only some essential points.

Unlike their extensor counterparts, the flexor tendons of the thumb and fingers run an almost entirely intrasynovial course; this course eases their gliding but renders surgical repair more difficult for a number of reasons: The tendons are unusually long, they act on several joints, they have a lengthy excursion, they transmit considerable force during a power grip; and the deep and superficial tendons have an intricate gliding relationship.

The flexor tendons have a precarious blood supply, especially at the level of the digital sheaths. Lundborg et al. (1977) have demonstrated the presence of several vascularly deprived zones—an "avascular segment" of the flexor superficialis just proximal to the chiasma, and two "avascular segments" of the flexor profundus, proximal and distal to vinculum longus (Fig. 24–1). In addition, at the level of the proximal interphalangeal joint the flexor profundus tendon is vascularized only along its dorsal aspect. The anterior 1 mm. of the tendon, on which considerable pressure is exerted, is "avascular."

This segmental supply system, clearly inadequate in some areas, explains the difficulties of surgical repair and emphasizes the importance of the nutritional role of synovial fluid (Figs. 24–2 and 24–3).

167

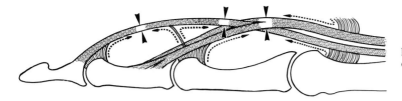

Figure 24–1. The three "avascular segments" of the flexor tendons of the fingers (after Lundborg).

TOPOGRAPHICAL REGIONS AND SURGICAL ZONES

The variation in the blood supply and the proximity of the fixed anatomical structures account for the influence that the site of the lesion plays in flexor tendon repair.

There exists some confusion between the anatomical regions that flexor tendons cross and the arbitrary "surgical zones" that permit therapeutic criteria to be established. Different numbering systems for topographical regions further complicate these classifications. These tendons, some of which exceed 20 cm. in length in the adult, cross different topographical regions. Anatomically the flexor tendons of the fingers cross five well defined regions, which are, from proximal to distal, the wrist, the carpal tunnel, the part of the palm extending from the exit of the carpal tunnel to the entrance of the fibrous flexor sheath suspended from the volar plate of the

metacarpophalangeal joint, the portion of the osseofibrous canal of the fingers (digital canal) that is common to the deep and superficial flexor tendons and reaches halfway down the middle phalanx, and the distal segment of the same tunnel, which transmits only the flexor profundus tendon (Figs. 24–4 to 24–8).

The tendon of flexor pollicis longus also crosses five regions—the wrist, the carpal tunnel, the palmar region (or more accurately, the thenar eminence), the digital canal extending from the entrance of the proximal pulley at the volar plate of the metacarpophalangeal joint down to the exit of the "oblique pulley" halfway down the proximal phalanx (Doyle and Blythe, 1975), and the distal segment, which reaches the insertion of the tendon on the base of the distal phalanx.

Anatomical relations in these various zones make it clear that the danger of adhesions to

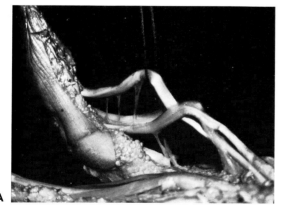

A

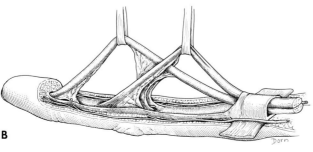

B

Figure 24–2. *A* and *B*, The vincula of the flexor tendons in the digital sheath. It can be seen that complete removal of the flexor superficialis tendon may devascularize the flexor profundus tendon.

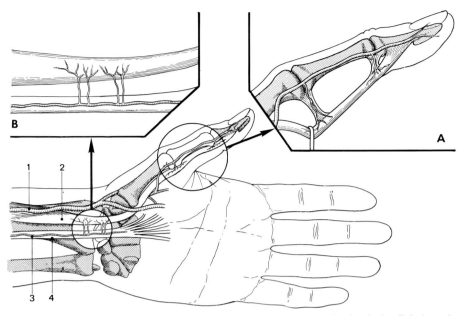

Figure 24–3. The flexor pollicis longus tendon also has a segmental vascularization in its digital portion. *Inset A*, In the distal portion, the vascularization comes from the vincula. *Inset B*, In its proximal portion, the tendon receives ˙branches from the median nerve artery. 1 = radial artery, 2 = flexor pollicis longus, 3 = median nerve artery, and 4 = median nerve.

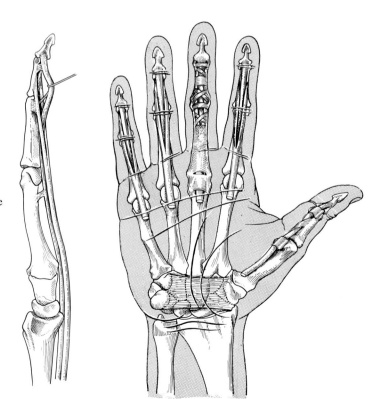

Figure 24–4. Flexor tendons and the pulley system.

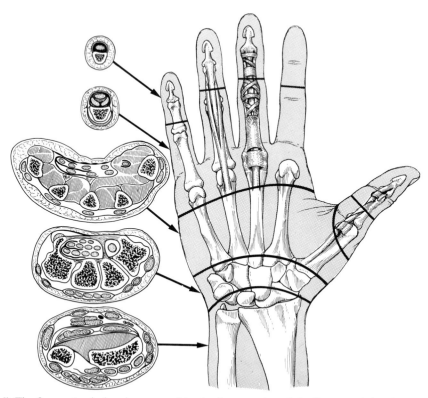

Figure 24–5. The five anatomical regions crossed by the flexor tendon of the fingers and thumb. The sections show the anatomical relations of the tendons.

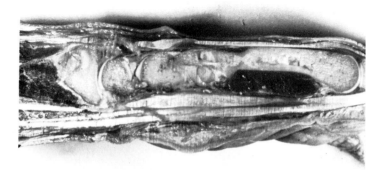

Figure 24–6. Axial section of the palm of the hand and wrist showing the relations of the flexor tendons.

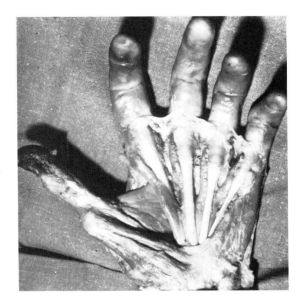

Figure 24–7. The flexor tendons in the palm.

the fixed structures is greater where the tendon runs within a fibrous sheath and also that multiple tendon injuries tend to occur in regions where the tendons are bundled together, i.e., in the wrist and the carpal tunnel.

This topographical classification provokes several observations.

1. Parallels no doubt exist between the topographical regions crossed by the flexor tendons of the fingers and those of the thumb. Verdan's classification (1952) groups the terminal portions of the flexor digitorum profundus and flexor pollicis longus in zone 1; (Fig. 24–9). It then distinguishes a metacarpophalangeal (zone 3) and a thenar zone (zone 4) for the thumb. Kleinert et al. (1975) use a similar classification for the fingers with different numbering, as do the classifications of Paneva-Holevich (1977) and Nigst (1976).

The Committee on Tendons of the International Federation of the Hand Societies has standardized these demarcations in a new classification (Fig. 24–10). The regions crossed by the long flexor of the thumb are preceded by the letter T.

2. The classification into anatomical regions can be extended by the introduction of subdivisions: Thus, the digital canal corresponding to the so-called "no man's land" has been further subdivided by Boyes and Stark (1971) into three portions: the distal portion where complete sectioning of the flexor profundus is usually accompanied by a partial lesion of superficialis; the middle portion, which corresponds to the pulley inserted on the shaft of the proximal phalanx (A_2); and the proximal portion extending from the distal palmar crease to the root of the finger (Fig. 24–11).

These subdivisions are of interest in analyzing results of treatment. For example, failure of union has proved more common after primary suturing in the middle part of the digital canal than in the other two portions

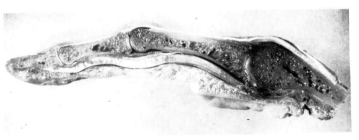

Figure 24–8. Axial section of a finger showing the anatomical relations of the flexor tendons.

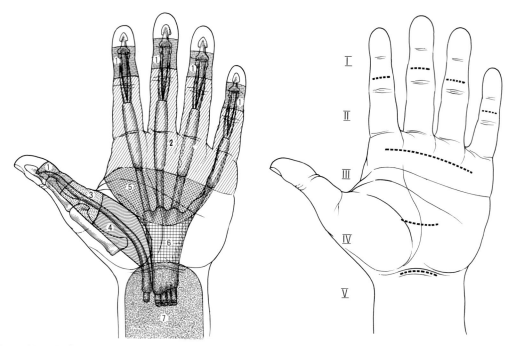

Figure 24–9. *Left*, The topographical classification of Verdan and Michon. *Right*, The topographical classification of Kleinert.

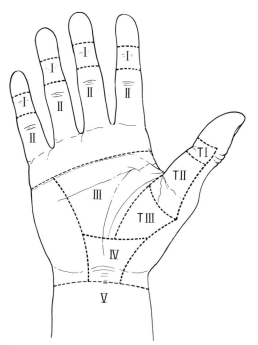

Figure 24–10. Topographical classification adopted by the International Federation of Societies for Surgery of the Hand. Only the regions crossed by the flexor pollicis longus tendon are preceded by the letter T (thumb).

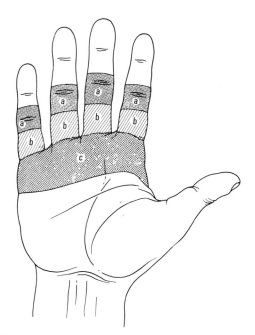

Figure 24–11. Subdivision of "no man's land" into three parts.

of the same zone (Duran and Houser, 1975). This has been confirmed by the results obtained by Tsuge et al. (1977).

In regard to indications for treatment, however, a surfeit of topographical subdivisions can prove cumbersome. Our tendency is to simplify this classification.

The Surgical Zones

Although the flexor tendons travel through several anatomical regions, surgical indications can be discussed with reference to only three main zones. (Fig. 24–12):

The Distal Zone. The distal zone (zone 1) is distal to the insertion of the flexor superficialis tendon and has specific characteristics in that only one tendon is present (the flexor profundus), the insertion of the tendon is nearby, and the functional sequelae are limited.

The Intermediate Zone. The intermediate zone (zone 2), the former "no-man's land," corresponds to the fibro-osseous canal (Fig. 24–13). This zone poses the most difficult problems and the most controversial solu-

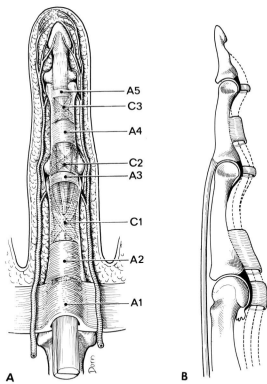

A　　　　　　　　　　**B**

Figure 24–13. The distal fibro-osseous canal. *A*, General view. A1 to A5, The five annular portions (pulleys) of the fibrous flexor tendon sheath. C1 to C3, The three cruciform portions where synovial fluid is accumulated and the configuration changes with motion of the phalanges. Small arterial transverse branches from the digital palmar arteries penetrate the flexor sheath at the level of the cruciform portions. They continue into the flexor tendon vincula. *B*, The digital pulley is formed by dense inextensible transverse fibers. There is often an interruption between pulleys A1 and A2.

tions because of the close association of two tendons within a common fibrous sheath, the proximity of fixed anatomical structures, and the poor blood supply.

The Proximal Zone. The proximal zone (zone 3) includes the palmar, carpal, and wrist regions. Although the anatomical relations are different, certain factors account for the fact that the surgical attitudes to the tendons are similar: First, the blood supply of the tendons is good, and the prognosis for the repair is better. Second, the tendons are close together, and this accounts for the frequency of multidigit injuries. Third, differences in treatment in various regions of this zone are not due to the tendinous injuries per se but to associated injuries, in particular to those of the nerves and vessels. For these

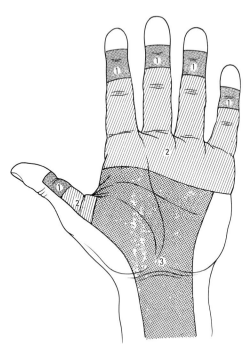

Figure 24–12. The three surgical zones from a therapeutic standpoint. A distinction is made for the flexor tendon of both the fingers and the thumb: a distal zone, or zone 1; an intermediate zone, or zone 2; and a proximal zone, or zone 3.

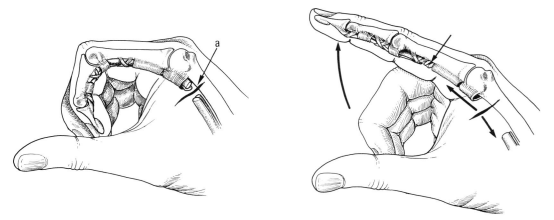

Figure 24–14. Influence of the position of the fingers on the site of the divided tendon extremities. The wound being in the distal part of the palm, if the finger is flexed, extension of the finger draws the tendon extremities distally in the digital sheath.

tendons, primary suturing when possible is the accepted treatment of choice.

In clinical practice the limits between zones is never so clear cut as anatomical diagrams suggest. To start with, the relations between the digital canals, the tendons, and the skin vary with movement. This explains why a flexor tendon injury in the distal part of the palm occurring when the digit is flexed becomes digital in extension. Thus the position of the finger at the time of the injury determines whether the tendon wound coincides with the skin wound (Figs. 24–14, 24–15). Any tendon repair that requires surgical entry into the narrow part of the digital canal runs the risks attendant to that particular zone. For this reason this zone should be extended.

This classification into three surgical zones also holds good for the flexor pollicis longus

tendon. Here again the intermediate or middle zone (zone 2), corresponding to the narrow digital canal opposite the metacarpophalangeal joint (Fig. 24–16), poses difficult surgical problems, the solution to which sometimes lies with a tendon graft.

There is, however, an important difference between lesions of the flexor tendons of the fingers and that of the thumb. The flexor pollicis longus runs alone within its sheath because the thumb has only two phalanges and needs only one extrinsic flexor, whereas the fingers have three phalanges and require two extrinsic flexors. The flexor superficialis and flexor profundus, which run together in close apposition, move in a piston-like fashion within a tight common sheath and glide next to one another. For too long surgeons have undervalued the importance of the

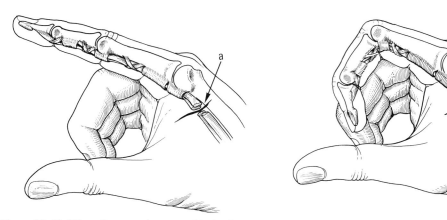

Figure 24–15. When the wound occurs with the finger in extension, the distal extremities of the tendons remain in the palm.

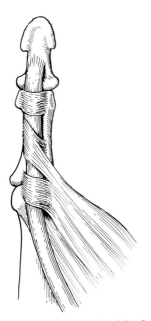

Figure 24–16. The fibrous sheath of the flexor pollicis longus has two annular pulleys, one proximal and one distal, with an oblique pulley between them.

flexor superficialis tendon, which they have readily sacrificed. Formerly when the two flexor tendons were injured, the teaching was to repair the flexor profundus and resect the flexor superficialis in order to "make room."

Resection of the flexor superficialis tendon can give rise to serious anatomical and physiological disorders: the strength and autonomy of the finger are significantly reduced, the stability of the proximal interphalangeal joint is put at risk, and a swan-neck deformity may develop.

Finally, removing the superficialis tendon can interfere with the blood supply of the profundus and promote the formation of adhesions. When the superficialis must be sacrificed for suturing or grafting, it is important to preserve the vincula longus, which at the level of the proximal interphalangal joint contributes to the blood supply of both flexor tendons.

PATHOLOGY

Although it is true that flexor tendon lesions are usually caused by open injury, closed rupture can occur. Traumatic rupture is far less common in the flexors than in the extensors. Some pathological processes, such as rheumatoid arthritis, can weaken the flexor tendons of fingers and thumb, particularly in the digital tendon sheath, and lead to so-called "spontaneous" rupture by friction at the wrist or at the palm.

Terminal avulsion of the flexor digitorum profundus after a violent effort or blow has been reported, mostly in athletes. It is seen in rugby and football players when, in grabbing an opponent's shirt, the distal phalanx of the finger is passively hyperextended while the phalanges of the other fingers remain flexed. These injuries are seen predominantly in the ring finger. Manske and Lesker (1978) have shown that the insertions of the flexor profundus tendon are weaker in the ring than in the middle finger.

Another possible anatomical explanation as to why these lesions are more common in the ring finger than in the index or middle finger is based on the anatomical arrangement of the extensor tendons. When the metacarpophalangeal joints of the middle and little fingers are flexed 90 degrees, the ring finger cannot be fully extended because the extensor tendon of the ring finger is pulled distally by the intertendinous connections (Leddy and Packer, 1977). The index finger is less susceptible because the muscle body of the flexor profundus is independent. These avulsions can also accompany a fracture at the base of the distal phalanx. When there is a large bone fragment, it is caught by the A4 pulley. If the fragment is small, it retracts proximally. The distal phalanx can be dorsally dislocated when the bony avulsion is large. Sometimes there are many bone fragments and the tendon may remain attached to a fragment.

The tendon of the flexor profundus is made up of superficial and of deep fibers (Fig. 24–17). The former are divided into two bundles, which diverge from the midline to insert on either side of the base of the distal phalanx. The deeper fibers are visible when the superficial ones are pulled apart; they are inserted more distally in the middle of the palmar aspect of the shaft of the same phalanx (Wilkinson, 1953). According to Robins and Dobyns (1975), this dual insertion explains the variable size of the avulsed fragment, its size depending on whether it is pulled off by the superficial or the deep fibers, or by both. The tendon also can become detached from the avulsed fragment. The treatment depends on the anatomical findings as well as on the

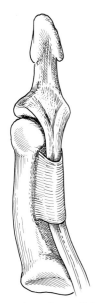

Figure 24–17. Insertion of superficial and deep fibers of the flexor profundus tendon on the base of the distal phalanx.

degree of retraction. The latter is relevant because limited retraction will not pull off the vinculum longum so that retraction into the palm gives rise to marked devascularization.

Leddy and Packer (1977) distinguish three principal types of lesions:

Type 1. The vincula are torn and the tendon retracts into the palm. The tendon loses a large part of its vascularization.

Type 2. This is the most common injury. The tendon does not retract past the proximal interphalangeal joint, leaving the vinculum longum intact. The prognosis is better.

Type 3. There is a large bone fragment, which must be reattached.

CLINICAL SIGNS

The clinical signs of division or rupture of the flexor tendons are not always obvious, for we must remember that the extrinsic flexor tendons are not solely responsible for flexing the fingers and the thumb. The intrinsic muscles contribute to flexion of the metacarpophalangeal joints of the fingers and to flexion-adduction of the thumb. In the thumb the flexor pollicis longus contributes to flexion of the metacarpophalangeal joint, but it is the only one capable of flexing the interphalangeal joint. In the fingers, interruption

of both flexor tendons makes active flexion of the two distal phalanges impossible. By contrast, lesions of either tendon alone make diagnosis much more difficult.* The flexor profundus acting alone can flex all the finger joints, but it is the only one that can flex the distal phalanx when the middle phalanx is held in extension. The profundus tendons have a common muscle body, whereas the superficialis tendons arise from independent muscle heads. This anatomical arrangement explains why the flexor profundus cannot flex one digit if the others are extended. It also means that the action of each superficialis tendon can be tested separately: the flexor superficialis, which is independent, can flex the proximal interphalangeal joint of a finger while the other fingers are held in extension in order to suppress the action of flexor profundus.

A thorough clinical examination usually indicates the diagnosis, but errors are still not uncommon, for several reasons. The examination may be restricted because of pain, or a tendon lesion may be missed when the skin wound is small and there is no sensory loss. Or a rupture may be overlooked in the absence of an open wound. Any wound overlying a flexor tendon should be explored systematically to detect even a partial tendon tear, which may necessitate surgical treatment. When no skin wound is present, persistent pain and restricted flexion after trauma should arouse suspicion: a history of injury should be sought, the clinical examination repeated, and avulsed bone fragments looked for on x-ray views.

EVOLUTION OF SURGICAL TREATMENT

FLEXOR TENDON HEALING

The problems of healing in tendons are reviewed at length in the first volume of this work by Peacock as well as in the preceding chapters of this volume. Reference to these chapters will help the reader to understand the evolution of surgical treatment.

Primary suturing, which used to give acceptable results in the so-called proximal and distal zones, was almost always doomed to failure in the intermediate zone, i.e. the

*See Chapter 58, "The Clinical Examination of the Hand," in Volume I.

digital canal. Although the tendon callus was usually satisfactory, adhesions were so extensive that tendon mobility was nil. In the face of these consistently poor results following primary suturing in what he called the "no man's land," Bunnell in 1922 gave this advice: "Close the skin, wait for the wound to heal, then perform a secondary repair as follows: excise the two flexors and graft the profundus tendon alone from the lumbrical to the digital extremity."

This teaching was held as dogma by generations of surgeons for the treatment of lesions within the "no man's land." However, the results of delayed grafts were unpredictable, and some surgeons, following the example of Verdan (1952), returned to primary suturing using atraumatic techniques and blocked sutures.

Is it now possible, in the light of their respective results, to advocate one method in preference to the other? This is probably the wrong way of looking at the problem, because both grafts and sutures have yielded excellent results in operations performed by highly specialized surgeons. But as Verdan (1976) has pointed out, "When a primary suture is performed with inadequate material and technical conditions . . . the result can be far from ideal. We can all bear witness to the fact that a badly performed primary repair can jeopardize the whole hand. This is why I sometimes wonder whether I was right in setting primary suture as a dogma or if my contradictors had visualized the problem more accurately."

The problem of repair of the flexor tendons is still not fully solved and will probably never be solved by a sterile and bigoted rivalry between those who favor one method or the other. Only a better appreciation of the relative indications for each technique will enable us to reduce significantly the functional sequelae of these lesions.

We shall begin therefore by mentioning the theoretical advantages of grafts and of sutures, and in the chapter on Surgical Indications we shall try to give more precisely the indications for each method.

ARGUMENTS FAVORING SUTURING AND GRAFTING

These arguments can be grouped as follows:

Biological Factors

We know that adhesions are proportional to the extent of the injury to the tendons and to the gliding surface, whether traumatic or surgical. We also know that the more the tendon is tethered by adhesions to the fixed structures (e.g., fibrous sheaths, bone, palmar fascia, retinaculum), the more its mobility will be restricted.

From this, we can make the following deductions: The site of the repair depends entirely on the location of the wound. Adhesions are often the result of poorly placed sutures.

A tendon graft necessitates a wide exposure, with the attendant risk of more extensive adhesions. These will be greatest at the two extremities of the graft, but at least the fixation points can be chosen so that the adhesions will cause the least amount of interference.

Other Arguments Are Related to the Method Used

Some favor direct suturing. In regard to the assessment of tension, only by primary suturing of an otherwise intact tendon can one restore the functional musculotendinous unit to its original length. The length of a graft is at best an approximation. Suturing obviously does not require the sacrifice of a tendon for grafting. Repair of both the profundus and superficialis tendons restores normal anatomy, but only one can be repaired by grafting when both have been severed.

Others favor grafting, for a graft can make up for loss of tendon substance. Moreover, the suture lines are not under tension, and the sutures can be placed in zones where adhesions will be least crippling. The main argument of those who favor secondary grafting is that if primary suturing fails, the damage will be much greater than if the skin has only been closed while awaiting delayed repair. It goes without saying that the damage would be even greater after failure of primary grafting.

These arguments in favor of each technique must all be weighed in the light of recent progress. Thus the surgical trauma caused by direct suturing has diminished considerably in recent years. A smaller area of access is required, resection of the fibrous sheath is more limited, and the flexor superficialis is not resected systematically. The use of magnifying devices (loupe or microscope) means that sutures as fine as 6-0 can be used. On the other hand, the results of tendon grafting have improved with the introduction of a two stage repair in difficult cases, a silicone implant to restore the gliding plane being inserted prior to grafting.

Economic Arguments

Finally a series of economic arguments must be considered that take into account the following factors:

First one must consider the number of operations necessary to obtain a useful functional result. Primary suturing in theory requires only one operation, whereas delayed grafting is preceded by a stage of debridement and closure of the skin wound.

Tenolyses tend to be more common after primary suturing than after delayed grafting. But then two stage grafts imply an extra operating session.

The duration of incapacity is of considerable economic importance. Primary suturing, when successful, reduces the amount of time lost. If it fails, however, delayed grafting becomes necessary, preceded by the insertion of a silicone implant, i.e., three stages in all. The incapacity in such cases often exceeds one year.

Finally, the possibilities of application and general usage of each method must be considered. Although both require the same care and precision, suturing is easier to teach than grafting, but there is a risk associated with this advantage.

CONCLUSIONS

We can conclude this introduction to the treatment of flexor tendon injuries with the concept that there is no single standard method of treatment, but a series of techniques, to be amplified in subsequent chapters. These must be adapted to each case. The results of these tendon repairs are too often imperfect. It is hoped that progress will result from a better understanding of the biological phenomena of healing, improved techniques of repair, and most importantly improved organization of emergency services.

In the following chapters on the treatment of traumatic lesions of the flexor tendons, the main surgical techniques will be discussed: sutures, one stage grafts, two stage grafts, anterior tenoarthrolysis, and composite grafts of the whole flexor apparatus. Finally we will try to evaluate the results of repair and give the indications for each technique described.

REFERENCES

Azar, C. A., Culver, J. E., and Fleegler, E. J.: Blood supply of the flexor pollicis longus tendon. J. Hand Surg. 8:471–475, 1983.

Boyes, J. H., Wilson, J. N., and Smith, J. W.: Flexor tendon ruptures in the forearm and hand. J. Bone Joint Surg., 42A:637, 1960.

Boyes, J. H.: Bunnell's Surgery of the Hand. 5th ed. Philadelphia, J.B. Lippincott, 1970.

Boyes, J. H., and Stark, H. H.: Flexor tendon grafts in the fingers and thumb. J. Bone Joint Surg., 53A:1332–1342, 1971.

Buck-Gramcko, D.: Benhandlung. Nigst H., Buck-Gramcko, D., and Millesi, H. (Editors): Handchirurgie, Vol. 2. New York, Thieme, 1983.

Bunnell, S.: Repair of tendons in the fingers. Surg. Gyn. Obstet., 35:88–97, 1922.

Caplan, H. S., Hunter, J. M., and Merklin, R. J.: The intrinsic vascularisation of flexor tendons in the human. In Proceedings, American Society of the Hand. J. Bone Joint Surg., 57A:726, 1975.

Carroll, R. E., and Match, R. M.: Avulsion injury of the long flexor tendons. J. Trauma, 10:1109, 1970.

Doyle, J. R., and Blythe, W.: The finger flexor tendon sheath and pulleys: anatomy and reconstruction. Symposium on Tendon Surgery in the Hand. St. Louis, The C.V. Mosby Co., 1975.

Duran, R. J., and Houser, R. G.: Controlled passive motion following flexor tendon repair in zones two and three. In AAOS Symposium on tendon surgery in the hand. St. Louis, The C.V. Mosby Co., 1975, p. 105.

Kleinert, H. E., Kutz, J. E., Atasoy, E., et al.: Primary repair of flexor tendons. Orthop. Clin. N. Am., 4:865, 1973.

Kleinert, H. E., Kutz, J. E., and Cohen, M. J.: Primary repair of zone 2 flexor tendon lacerations. In AAOS Symposium on tendon surgery in the hand. St. Louis, The C.V. Mosby Co., 1975, p. 91.

Kleinert, H. E., Forshew, F. C., and Cohen, M. J.: Repair of zone 1 flexor tendon injuries. In AAOS Symposium on tendon surgery in the hand. St. Louis, The C.V. Mosby Co., 1975, p. 115.

Leddy, J. P., and Packer, J. W.: Avulsion of the profundus tendon insertion in athletes. J. Hand Surg., 2(1):66–69, 1977.

Leffert, R. D., Weiss, C., and Athanasoulis, C. A.: The vincula. J. Bone Joint Surg., 56A:1191–1198, 1974.

Lundborg, G., Myrhage, P. D., and Rydevik, B.: The vascularisation of human flexor tendons within the digital synovial sheath region. Structural and functional aspects. J. Hand Surg., 2(6):417–427, 1977.

Manske, P. R., and Lesker, P. A.: Avulsion of the ring finger flexor digitorum profundus tendon: An experimental study. Hand, 10:52, 1978.

Mansat. M.: Avulsion du fléchisseur commun profond et pratique du rugby: "Jersey finger." Ann. Chir. Main, 4:185–196, 1985.

McGrouther, D. A.: Flexor tendon excursion in no-man's land. Hand, *13*:129, 1981.

Nigst, H., Buck-Gramcko, D., and Millesi, H. (Editors): Handchirurgie. New York, Thieme, 1983.

Paneva-Holevich, E.: Reconstructive surgery of the flexor tendons in the hand. Med. Fiz Kult. Sofia, 1977.

Peacock, E. E.: A study of the circulation in normal tendons and healing grafts. Ann. Surg., *149*:415, 1959.

Robins, P. R., and Dobyns, J. H.: Avulsion of the insertion of the flexor digitorum profundus tendon associated with fracture of the distal phalanx. *In* AAOS Symposium on tendon surgery in the hand. St. Louis, The C.V. Mosby Co., 1975, p. 151.

Smith, J. W.: Blood supply of tendons. Am. J. Surg., *109*:272, 1965.

Tsuge, K., Ikuta, Y., and Matsuishi, Y.: Repair of flexor tendons by intratendinous tendon suture. J. Hand Surg., *2*(6):436–440, 1977.

Tubiana, R.: Les voies d'abord dans la chirurgie des tendons de la main. Ann. Chir. Plast. (Semaine des Hôpitaux), *5*(2):100–109, 1960.

Tubiana, R.: Le traitement des plaies des tendons de la main. Ann. Chir., *14*:117–118, 1093–1106, 1960.

Tubiana, R., and Malek, R.: Plaies des tendons de la main. E.M.C., *44*:395, 1966.

Verdan, C.: Chirurgie réparatrice et fonctionnelle des tendons de la main. Paris, Expansion Scientifique Française, 1952.

Verdan, C., and Michon, J.: Le traitement des plaies des tendons fléchisseurs des doigts. Rev. Chir. Orthop., *47*:287, 1961.

Verdan, C.: Chirurgie des tendons de la main. Monographie du G.E.M. Paris, Expansion Scientifique Française, 1976.

Wilkinson, J. L.: The insertions of the flexors pollicis longus and digitorum profundus. J. Anat., *87*:75, 1953.

Chapter 25

BIOLOGICAL DETERMINANTS IN THE RESULTS OF DIGITAL FLEXOR TENDON REPAIR

PHILLIP MATTHEWS

Much controversy still surrounds the management of the cut digital flexor tendon, and most surgeons would agree that treatment cannot yet be regarded as ideal. Although the initial soft tissue wounds in these injuries are often remarkably small, the operative procedures required for reconstruction are complex, and rehabilitation is usually slow, so that incapacity for work is often prolonged. If the results of treatment were uniformly good, this would be less important, but unfortunately this is not the case. The failure of surgery to restore active finger movement is all too common, and, worse, the finger may be converted to a semirigid hook, which proves a constant nuisance to the patient.

The results of treatment vary from one center to another, but even in the most specialized hand units there will still be some cases in which treatment will fail. Surgical expertise in selecting and carrying out the operative procedure will increase the chances of success, but even then it cannot be guaranteed. Surgical skill alone, it seems, does not hold the solution to the problem, and it is becoming apparent that our difficulties arise as a result of biological factors, only some of which are under our control. The functional demands on the flexor tendons are great, and their anatomical and physiological arrangements have become adapted to meet them. At the same time, this leaves the tendons uniquely vulnerable not only to injury but also to certain elements in surgical treatment. The effects that they produce may often be quite subtle, but they may be crucial in determining the outcome of surgery. An understanding of the pathophysiology of

flexor tendon injuries is needed by all those actively involved in their treatment and is essential if further advances are to be made in improving the prognosis.

Whereas the treatment of injuries to the extensor tendons of the fingers is usually rewarded by excellent return of movement, it was long ago realized that in the case of the flexor tendons, simple methods of suturing were rarely successful in restoring function. It was, indeed, disillusion with the results of tendon repair as practiced in his time that led Sterling Bunnell to introduce delayed tendon grafting as an alternative method of treatment. The marked discrepancy between the results of repairs in extensor and flexor tendons can be related to their respective functions and the manners in which the tendons are adapted for them. To achieve their required effect, the extensors need only a comparatively short range of motion, so that a paratenon type of arrangement is quite satisfactory. The flexor tendons, by contrast, have a much larger amplitude of motion in relation to the fixed fibro-osseous structures, and in pursuing their course they must undergo repeated acute angular deformations. To allow for this, the sublimis and profundus tendons are disposed within a highly specialized, synovial fluid lined fibrous sheath, which enables them to move freely not only in relation to the skeletal structures but also in relation to each other. Although this arrangement is ideal under normal conditions, its reconstruction after injury presents formidable problems. During the repair phase after surgical suturing, adhesion formation and a massive fibroblastic response are difficult to avoid. Whereas in the extensor tendons this may have virtually no effect on movement, the presence of scar tissue between the flexor tendons and the surrounding tissues restricts the sliding motion of the tendon, which is essential for normal transmission of muscle force, and active flexion is no longer possible.

The frequency of adhesion formation during flexor tendon repairs and the disastrous effect it has on finger movement have stimulated much basic research into the healing processes in tendons. Perhaps the main point of contention arising from this has been the source of the cells responsible for bringing about repair, and in regard to this subject there have been several schools of thought. Although some have maintained that the tendon tissue itself is involved, others have believed that the tissues around the tendon are more important; yet another school has believed that both elements are necessary at different stages in the process. In 1962 the debate came to a temporary halt with the publication by Potenza of the results of his detailed experimental studies of the mode of healing in canine flexor tendons. By meticulous research he was able to prove beyond doubt that divided tendons repaired by crisscross suturing and then splinted heal entirely by the ingrowth of fibroblastic tissue originating outside the tendons. Throughout his experiments the tendon cells remained inactive and appeared to play no part in the process. Potenza inferred from this that tendon cells were inert as regards repair, speculating that they might be too highly differentiated to participate in the healing process.

Potenza's report met with wide acceptance. Its clinical implications were clear. If the tendon itself were inert, it must, of necessity, rely for healing on the formation of adhesions, and however undesirable they might be in terms of function, such adhesions were, nevertheless, essential before continuity could be restored. The thesis amply explained why the results of tendon repair had been so poor and was powerful supporting evidence in favor of tendon grafting as the preferred treatment for these injuries.

In recent years the proposition that tendon tissue is inert has come under reappraisal. There had been some difficulty in explaining why tendon, which is a living vascularized tissue, should be so totally lacking in repair properties, and if this really were so, it became impossible to explain certain clinically observed features of its behavior. It had been found that when the flexor tendons were cut within the finger, the most usual sequel was that the stumps retreated into an undisturbed portion of the sheath and became smoothly rounded off, to lie there free, bathed in synovial fluid. Although this "rounding off" was earlier thought of as being due to simple atrophy, it much more closely resembles an active remodeling process (Furlow, 1976; Richards, 1977). Surgeons had also been aware that although incomplete tendon injuries are sometimes seen, they seldom pose any problem in treatment, for healing seems to take place without restrictive adhesions. Phenomena such as these would defy explanation if tendon tissue were truly inert.

Prevailing opinion at the present time is that tendon tissue is not entirely inert but, on the contrary, may be shown under carefully controlled conditions to possess a definite intrinsic potential for repair and remodeling. This change has come about as a result of experimental work on the healing of tendons that have been only incompletely transected so that there was not the total loss of continuity (Matthews and Richards, 1974; McDowell and Synder, 1977; Fig. 25–1). This technique thus avoided the need for either sutures or splintage, which had been a necessary part of the earlier studies. In addition, the method of exposing the tendon was planned so that at the end of the operation the zone of tendon traumatization was able to slide back into an intact portion of the synovial sheath (Fig. 25–2). Under these conditions it was found, on killing the experimental animals, that healing took place without adhesion formation and by a process originating from the tendon itself. After an initial phase during which the cut tendon edges became swollen and retracted, the defect began to fill in with a firm semitransparent reparative tissue, which was adherent to the underlying intact tendon (Fig. 25–3). During the weeks that followed, the defect slowly became obliterated, so that by the end of the experiment the area of the cut could no longer be distinguished.

Histological examination revealed that within a few days after the injury there was a morphological change in the tendon cells in the vicinity of the cut toward a more active "tenoblast" form (Figs. 25–4, 25–5). Progressive proliferation of these tenoblasts was followed by synthesis of new collagen fibrils, which eventually matured and took on the characteristics of normal tendon fibers (Fig.

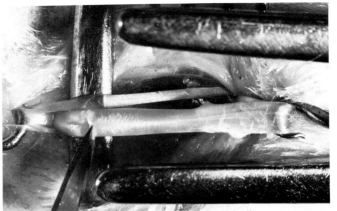

Figure 25–1. Incomplete transection experiment. The intrasynovial part of the profundus tendon has been drawn proximally out of its sheath by traction on the hook to the right. While supported from behind by the dissector, it is then cut most of the way through, but not all the way, by a sharp scalpel. The sublimis tendon, relatively slender in the rabbit, lies parallel to the profundus and more toward the top of the photograph.

Figure 25–2. Illustration of the principle behind incomplete transection experiments. The figures represent longitudinal sections through the digits. *A*, Through a short incision (arrow) in the "palm" area at the level of the proximal pulley, the profundus tendon is exposed. The synovial reflection is then opened and, by strong proximal traction on the tendon accompanied by full flexion of the digit, part of the intrasynovial portion of the tendon is exposed. The tendon is then cut across transversely, leaving just enough tissue intact to preserve its continuity. *B*, On releasing the traction on the tendon, the traumatized zone (*arrow*) slides back to life within an undisturbed area of the sheath. For purposes of clarity, the sublimis tendon is not shown.

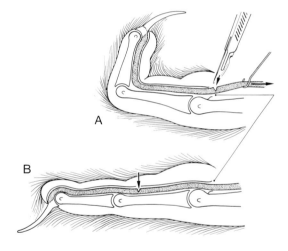

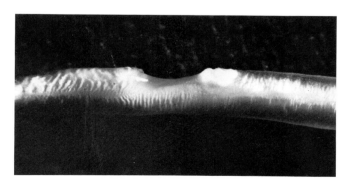

Figure 25–3. Healing tendon three weeks after the incomplete division. The cut fibers have retracted for a short distance to each side of the original site of division. The resulting gap is filling with a semitranslucent repair tissue, which is densely adherent to the underlying tendon.

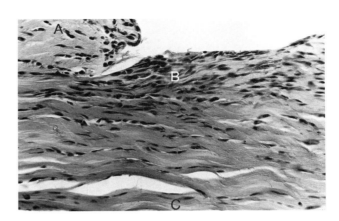

Figure 25–4. Longitudinal section through the healing tendon eight days after operation. The divided tendon fibers (A) have retracted a short distance from the point of the original injury. Note the zone of active cellular proliferation (B) in the floor of the cut and the intact tendon fibers (C) in the lower part of the photograph. Hematoxylin and eosin, ×220.

25–6). Throughout this sequence the sheath and perisheath tissues were unchanged and adhesions did not develop.

These "incomplete transection" experiments have been very useful in demonstrating the existence of a capacity for repair and remodeling in the tendon itself. It is important that this finding be viewed in perspective, however, for one must appreciate that the observations were made in an experimental, not to say artificial, situation. It would be wrong to assume from the results that a clinically severed flexor tendon could join without adhesions, and there are valid reasons why this might not be a practical possibility.

Assuming that the tendon possesses the potential for regeneration, it is pertinent to inquire why healing by adhesions is such a frequent occurrence in clinical tendon injuries, and why also it was so constant a feature in the experimental study by Potenza. The development of the adhesions cannot be attributed to the initial injury to the tendon, for, as we have seen, the most usual response after injury is for the stumps to separate, round off, and lie free within the digital sheath. The adhesive response seems, somehow, to be related to surgical repair, and the indications are that in most cases it is induced by factors that are integral parts of the operative and postoperative treatment program. Although there is much variation in the techniques of clinical tendon repair, three elements are common to all: the ends of the cut tendon have to be exposed by laying open or even excising the sheath, the stumps must be apposed by sutures or some similar device, and finally the anastomosis must be protected from excessive tension during healing, usually by plaster splintage.

Earlier experimental work, in particular that of Lindsay and Thomson (1960), had suggested that such "iatrogenic" factors might be implicated in the production of adhesions, and this has been confirmed in more recent studies. Evaluation of the individual effects of these various elements of tendon repair has presented some difficulty, in that when the experimental model involves

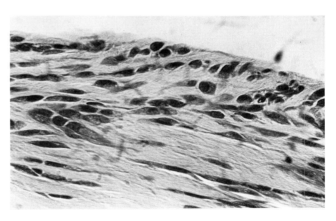

Figure 25–5. High-power view through an area of tendon regeneration 10 days after injury. In the more superficial layers there is a change in the morphological configuration of the tendon cells toward an active tenoblast form, capable of bringing out reconstitution of the defect. Hematoxylin and eosin, ×458.

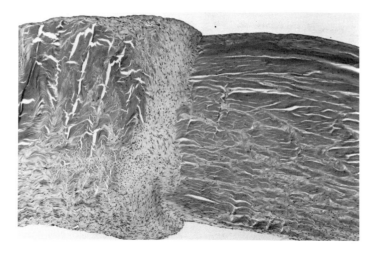

Figure 25–6. Healing tendon at eight weeks. The gap between the cut tendon fibers has been filled in with a cellular reparative tissue consisting of proliferating fibroblasts and newly synthesized collagen fibers. With progressive maturation this tissue later takes on the appearance of normal tendon. Hematoxylin and eosin. (Reproduced by kind permission of Dr. Charles L. McDowell and Dr. David M. Snyder.)

complete sectioning of the tendon, all three conditions must be present if healing is to take place. In an attempt to overcome this problem, Matthews and Richards (1976) utilized their earlier incomplete-transection model, because it offered the advantage that although the tendon was cut, it retained its continuity. The various factors under study could thus be introduced either separately or in combinations and their effects analyzed. This device, although not strictly comparable to the clinical injury, has provided information that would be unobtainable in any other way. It was found that when all three variables—that is, a Bunnell suture, digital sheath excision, and splintage—were applied simultaneously, the traumatized area of tendon became enveloped in dense adhesions derived from the perisheath layer. Within the tendon itself there was no indication of repair activity, the cells remaining inert and many, indeed, showing evidence of degenerative change (Fig. 25–7). The appearances were comparable to those described by Potenza, and in the same way healing was achieved through the ingrowth of fibroblastic tissue from outside the tendon itself. On analyzing the findings in the different groups of experiments there was no doubt that, of the factors studied, tendon suturing was the main culprit in provoking the adhesive response. Nevertheless the most profuse and most restrictive adhesions were found when all three factors were present simultaneously, and it was concluded that sheath excision and immobilization also play significant complementary roles in encouraging adhesion formation or determining their quality.

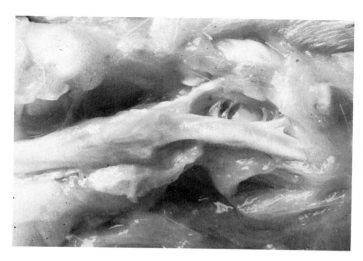

Figure 25–7. Healing of the profundus tendon in the presence of suture and splintage and after the overlying digital sheath has been excised. The repaired tendon is densely adherent to the surrounding tissues, and no useful movement is possible.

At the present state of our knowledge, it seems that flexor tendon possesses a definite capacity for repair and remodeling that is independent of other tissues. For healing of a severed tendon, however, a prerequisite is that its ends be exposed and then held in apposition, and it is unfortunate that the means of achieving this are themselves likely to suppress tendon cell activity and to promote the formation of adhesions. At this point it is appropriate to consider in more detail some of the factors that may influence the outcome in flexor tendon repair.

THE TENDON CIRCULATION— THE EFFECTS OF INJURY

As a living tissue, tendon is characterized by a low but definite metabolic rate, and in consequence certain nutritional requirements must be met. For the most part these needs are served by the circulation of blood through minute vascular channels in the tendon, although, as might be expected, the actual rate of blood flow per unit volume of tendon is very slow (White et al., 1964). Extensive study has been made of the vascular anatomy of the digital flexor tendons, and extrinsic and intrinsic circulatory pathways have been described in detail. In response to the specialized function of the tendons, the arrangement of the circulation is such as to allow nourishment and movement to take place simultaneously, and the tiny vessels running in the vincula are regarded as playing a particularly important role.

Although the blood supply to the flexor tendons is perfectly adequate under normal conditions, there is reason to suspect that it is vulnerable to injury, and that even simple sectioning of the tendon can sometimes lead to alterations in blood flow that have far-reaching effects. It was earlier stressed that in most cases in which the flexor tendons are divided, the cut ends retract from each other, lying free within the sheath and retaining a normal or even increased blood supply (Fig. 25–8). This is not invariably the case, however, and in a small minority of instances the outcome is quite different.

Injection studies in animals have shown that after closed tenotomy of the flexor tendons, a relatively small number of the cut ends appear to lose their blood supply (Matthews, 1977; Fig. 25–9). At a later stage of the experiment a similar number of stumps were noted to have become adherent to the surrounding tissues Fig. 25–10), and leashes of new blood vessels were visible running into the tendon (Fig. 25–11). The presumption was that the stumps had been rendered ischemic as a result of the tenotomy and had become adherent in an effort to pick up a new blood supply. The same type of phenomenon is sometimes apparent clinically when, at the time of a delayed repair or graft, one or the other of the stumps is found to have become adherent to the floor of the digital canal, and may also show faint yellow discoloration and degenerative changes.

Embarrassment of the circulation to the cut end of a tendon could come about in a variety of ways. It is conceivable that because of the low flow rate in the small vessels, retrograde thrombosis might occur. The slender vincula could be kinked or even torn as a result of the proximal muscle pull on the

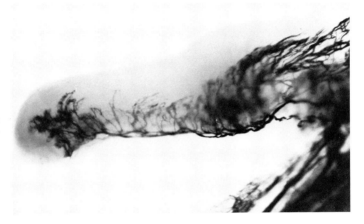

Figure 25–8. Injection study, showing the vascular pattern within the distal stump of a profundus tendon eight days after simple tenotomy. The tendon end is rounding off, and there is a marked increase in the vascularity in this region. Colloidal silver iodide technique.

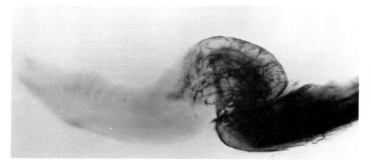

Figure 25–9. Four days after closed tenotomy, this severed profundus tendon shows complete failure of vascular filling at the cut end. Colloidal silver iodide technique.

tendon. Finally, since the circulation in the tendons is segmental (Smith, 1965; Young and Weeks, 1970), the possibility exists that their sectioning would result in diversion of blood flow away from the cut end. If we assume that this last explanation is correct, the precise level of the division may be a critical factor in determining the outcome of surgical repair.

The existence of a small group of tendon injuries in which the stumps will adhere by reason of ischemia has far-reaching clinical implications. There would seem no way of overcoming this tendency by any of the available methods of repair, and such tendons would therefore appear doomed to adhere regardless of the technical excellence of the operation. This would explain why the results of tendon repair are unpredictable, and means too that there may be a finite limit to the results obtainable from this procedure. There is a natural tendency to assume that progressive refinement of the techniques of repair could ultimately lead to consistently good results, but there may be valid biological reasons why this would be impossible.

MAINTENANCE OF TENDON APPOSITION DURING HEALING

A necessary first step in obtaining healing of most tissues is that the cut edges be brought into close apposition. This is particularly so in the case of the flexor tendons, since the cut ends separate widely from each other as a result of proximal muscle pull. In clinical practice, by far the most common method of securing stump apposition involves the insertion of some form of tendon suture. While serving this purpose well enough from the purely mechanical standpoint, sutures unfortunately suffer from the grave disadvantage that they are a potent factor in stimulating the formation of adhesions between the tendon and the surrounding tissues.

To give the best possible chance of success in flexor tendon repair, it is mandatory to use suture material that does not excite an exaggerated foreign body response. Studies have shown that several readily available materials, such as silk and catgut, provoke intense tissue reactions, and they should be abandoned in tendon suturing for this reason

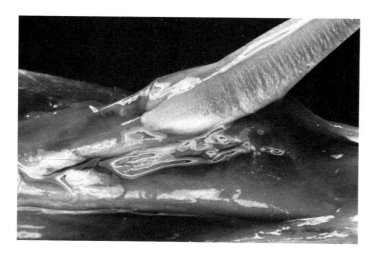

Figure 25–10. After simple tenotomy this tendon stump has become densely adherent to the sheath and the adjacent phalanx.

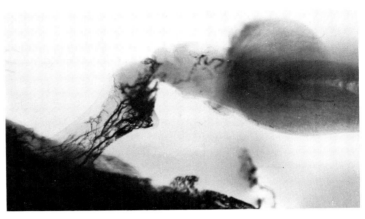

Figure 25–11. Injection study showing the appearance within a tendon stump that has become adherent. Many new blood vessels are coursing through the adhesion toward the tendon, while the latter is almost totally devoid of patent blood vessels. Colloidal silver iodide technique.

(Srugi and Adamson, 1972). Being less reactive, stainless steel and the synthetic fibers are to be preferred for the purpose. Nevertheless, even when these inert materials are used, adhesion formation still occurs, and it cannot, therefore, be solely attributed to foreign body reaction. Instead it is now believed that most of the harm resulting from suturing is due to its strangulating effect on the tendon circulation. In microradioangiographic studies Bergljung (1968) was able to show that the presence of a Bunnell suture within the Achilles tendon is enough to cut off the circulation to the areas of tendon grasped by the suture. In the synovial fluid covered flexor tendons also, research has shown that the blood supply is vulnerable, and that the stumps may be rendered ischemic as a result of suturing (Matthews, 1977; Fig. 25–12). At later stages of these experiments, adhesions carrying many new blood vessels were found to have developed between the tendons and the surrounding tissues, and the impression was that they had developed in order to revascularize the ischemic area (Fig. 25–13). It would seem from this that circulatory impairment is mainly responsible for adhesion

formation, and it also makes understandable certain other features of the behavior of the sutured tendon ends.

Several authors have reported that after suturing, tendon ends have microscopic features suggesting diminished viability, with degeneration of cells and reduced cellularity (Flynn and Graham, 1962; Matthews and Richards, 1976; Skoog and Persson, 1954; Fig. 25–14). This could arise through nutritional deprivation, and in such circumstances it is hardly surprising that the tendon cells would be incapable of participating in any healing process. Indeed much of the original tendon within the limits of the suture is probably so ischemic as to be damaged beyond recovery, since at a later stage it is replaced by new connective tissue.

Although there can be little doubt that sutures are intimately concerned in the pathogenesis of adhesions, it is difficult to see how they could be dispensed with if the stumps are to be maintained in apposition for healing. Although various alternative methods, such as "barbed" wire, blocking techniques, and "suturing at a distance," have been described, they have not sup-

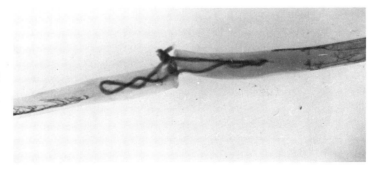

Figure 25–12. Three days after open tenotomy and repair by Bunnell suture, injection studies demonstrate failure of filling of the blood vessels within the area of suture. Colloidal silver iodide technique.

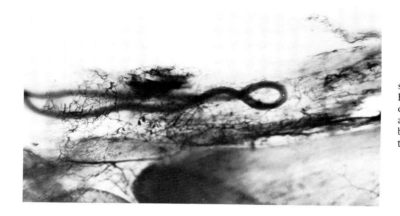

Figure 25–13. Injection study of a sutured profundus tendon two and a half weeks after operation. The area of repair has become enveloped in adhesions containing many fine new blood vessels. Colloidal silver iodide technique.

planted orthodox suturing, and it can only be presumed that they have disadvantages that are just as great. Perhaps the most that we can expect in the future is that the design of sutures will take into account their effect on tendon circulation as well as their mechanical properties.

SURGICAL EXPOSURE AND THE SIGNIFICANCE OF THE DIGITAL SHEATH

In any operative procedure to repair the digital flexor tendons, a prerequisite is that sufficient exposure be obtained to allow access to the tendon ends for insertion of the suture. Provided the basic principles underlying hand surgery are adhered to, the type of skin incision chosen is not critical, although it would seem preferable to limit its extent to the minimum necessary. When it comes to the matter of the incision into the digital sheath, however, opinion is divided. In the

past the sheath has been credited with little significance, and many authors have recommended that it be widely excised over the site of repair in the belief that if adhesions form, it is better that they be attached to relatively mobile subcutaneous tissue than to the rigid theca.

This attitude has been questioned in the light of a new awareness of the importance of the synovial fluid in the physiology of the flexor tendons. It has been recognized that, in addition to its primary role as a lubricant, the synovial fluid is intimately concerned in the nutrition of the tendon (Eiken et al., 1975; Matthews, 1976; Potenza, 1964). This being so, it has been suggested that the preservation of this synovial pathway during surgical repair might be beneficial in providing an alternative source of nutrients when the blood flow to the tendon is already embarrassed by sutures. A further theoretical advantage of retaining the digital sheath is that its presence as an intact mesothelial layer between the repaired tendon and the peri-

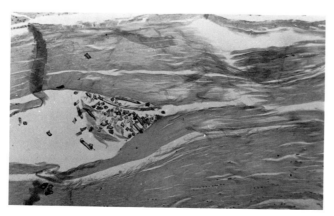

Figure 25–14. Histological appearance of the inside of a flexor tendon four days after insertion of a Bunnell suture of braided Dacron. The tendon in the immediate proximity of the suture has become completely acellular, and even those cells more remotely placed show changes of reduced viability, suggesting nutritional impairment. Hematoxylin and eosin, × 130.

sheath wound may constitute an isolating barrier and limit adhesion formation. It has been pointed out that where the sheath is excised, the cut in the tendon becomes but one part of a larger pool of repair involving the whole of the soft tissue wound, so that as healing progresses, some adherence is inevitable (Peacock, 1964).

As part of clinical tendon repair, the difficulties of preservation and reconstruction of the digital sheath are not to be underemphasized, and their performance requires considerable skill and patience. Nevertheless both Miller (1971) and Richards (1977) have reported good results in their series of cases, and it is certainly a promising technique that deserves further application.

POSTOPERATIVE SPLINTAGE AND ITS EFFECTS ON TENDON REPAIR

It is only natural to assume that if, after a flexor tendon has been repaired, active movements are commenced at an early stage, adhesions will be unable to form during the healing phase and restoration of normal function will be assured. There is, furthermore, experimental evidence that rigid immobilization of the repaired tendon is one of the factors that contributes to its becoming incarcerated in scar tissue (Matthews and Richards, 1976). Despite this, clinical experience over the years has repeatedly shown that encouraging early active movement does not improve the results of tendon repair, and indeed is likely to lead to even more adhesions than when the digit is splinted. This state of affairs, although at first glance contradictory, becomes more comprehensible when it is considered in the wider context of flexor tendon repair.

It was earlier explained that the tendency for adhesions to occur during healing arises as an attempt to revascularize tendon stumps that have become ischemic, as a result of either the injury or the surgical treatment. If this is accepted, it follows that active tendon movement cannot prevent adhesions, although it has other important effects. When active movements are encouraged, the repeated muscle contraction necessarily produces an increase in tension along the tendon, and this in turn is transferred to the suture itself. The increased tension in the thread can only aggravate the tissue strangulation induced by the suture and also encourages

the formation of a gap at the site of repair. Both these factors are potent stimuli to the production of adhesions.

When the experimental evidence is examined more critically, it seems clear that the effect of mobilization per se is not on the quantity of adhesions formed during repair, but rather on their quality, directing the deposition of the fibrous tissue elements in such a way as to allow motion to continue. If this is so, it may be inferred that provided the evil influence of excessive suture tension can be avoided, movement of the tendon during healing is an aim to be desired. It may be no coincidence that Kleinert, who has reported most impressive results from primary flexor tendon repair, achieves this objective precisely by utilizing a technique of passive tendon movement by elastic traction, the flexor muscle itself being reflexly inhibited.*

Although the earlier concepts of tendon healing have now had to be amended to admit the existence of intrinsic properties of regeneration by the tendon, it is still evident that there are major obstacles to prevent us from reaching our goal of achieving repair without adhesions. Although for the majority of flexor tendon injuries this would seem at least a theoretical possibility, various elements implicit in the surgical treatment program are themselves capable of combining to provoke an adhesive response. Some of these are under our control, but others are not, and we may have to accept the fact that the problem of adhesions may never be entirely eliminated in flexor tendon repair. It is fair, indeed, to pose the question whether adhesions are ever eliminated, but even this is incapable of a direct answer. Certainly successful restoration of movement may follow tendon repair, but in such cases there is no way of telling whether adhesions are absent or, alternatively, have developed in such a way as to permit useful motion. As Peacock (1965) has rightly emphasized, the mere presence of adhesions between the tendon and its surroundings is not necessarily a disaster, provided their configuration is such as to allow longitudinal motion. In these "favorable" adhesions, the repair tissue has become reorganized so that the fiber bundles have a loose areolar configuration similar to that of paratenon. The process of secondary remodeling of scar is without doubt an important

---

*See Chapter 28.

determinant factor in the results of tendon surgery, but we still have little understanding of how it is controlled.

The intensive research studies that have been undertaken in the field of tendon physiology and healing have added greatly to our knowledge and clarified the problems that face us in the management of flexor tendon injuries. That they have provided no clear solution may reflect not so much a lack of understanding as the unique nature of the biological predicament that this injury presents.

ACKNOWLEDGMENTS

I am indebted to the Clinical Research Committee of the Welsh Office for substantial grants to support continuing investigations in this field. I would like to give particular thanks to Mr. Harold Richards, F.R.C.S., for many years Consultant-in-Charge of the Hand Unit at Cardiff Royal Infirmary, who first stimulated my interest in tendon healing and has been a constant source of help and inspiration. I am most grateful to Miss Jayne Gambold for secretarial assistance in the preparation of the manuscript for this article.

REFERENCES

Bergljung, L.: Vascular reactions after tendon suture and tendon transplantation, a stereo-micro-angiographic study on the calcaneal tendon of the rabbit. Scand. J. Plast. Reconstr. Surg., Suppl. 4, 1968.

Eiken, O., Lundborg, G., and Rank, F.: The role of the digital synovial sheath in tendon grafting. Scand. J. Plast. Reconstr. Surg., 9:182, 1975.

Flynn, J.E., and Graham, J.H.: Healing following tendon suture and tendon transplants. Surg. Gynecol. Obstet., 115:467, 1962.

Furlow, L.T.: The role of tendon tissue in tendon healing. Plast. Reconstr. Surg., 57:39, 1976.

Lindsay, W.K., and Thomson, H.G.: Digital flexor tendons: an experimental study. Part I—The significance of each component of the flexor mechanism in tendon healing. Br. J. Plast. Surg., 12:289, 1960.

Matthews, P.: The fate of isolated segments of flexor tendon within the digital sheath—a study in synovial nutrition. Br. J. Plast. Surg., 29:216, 1976.

Matthews, P.: Vascular changes in flexor tendons after injury and repair: an exprimental study. Injury, 8:227, 1977.

Matthews, P., and Richards, H.J.: The repair potential of digital flexor tendons. J. Bone Joint Surg., 56B:618, 1974.

Matthews, P., and Richards, H.J.: Factors in the adherence of flexor tendon after repair. J. Bone Joint Surg., 58B:230, 1976.

McDowell, C.L., and Snyder, D.M.: Tendon healing: an experimental model in the dog. J. Hand Surg., 2:122, 1977.

Miller, R.C.: Flexor tendon repair over the proximal phalanx. Am. J. Surg., 122:319, 1971.

Peacock, E.E.: Fundamental aspects of wound healing related to the restoration of gliding function after tendon repair. Surg. Gynecol. Obstet., 119:241, 1964.

Peacock, E.E.: Biological principles in the healing of long tendons. Surg. Clin. N. Am., 45:461, 1965.

Potenza, A.D.: Tendon healing within the flexor digital sheath in the dog: an experimental study. J. Bone Joint Surg., 44A:49, 1962.

Potenza, A.D.: The healing of autogenous tendon grafts within the flexor digital sheath in dogs. J. Bone Joint Surg., 46A:1462, 1964.

Richards, H.J.: Digital flexor tendon repair and return of function. Ann. R. Coll. Surg. Engl., 59:25, 1977.

Skoog, T., and Persson, B.H.: An experimental study of the early healing of tendons. Plast. Reconstr. Surg., 13:384, 1954.

Smith, J.W.: The blood supply of tendons. Am. J. Surg., 109:272, 1965.

Srugi, S., and Adamson, J.E.: A comparative study of tendon suture materials in dogs. Plast. Reconstr. Surg., 50:31, 1972.

White, N.B., Ter-Pogossian, M.M., and Stein, A.H., Jr.: A method to determine the rate of blood flow in long bone and selected soft tissues. Surg. Gynecol. Obstet., 119:535, 1964.

Young, L., and Weeks, P.M.: Profundus tendon blood supply within the digital sheath. Surg. Forum, 21:504, 1970.

Chapter 26

ENLARGEMENT PLASTY OF THE PROXIMAL PULLEYS

ADALBERT I. KAPANDJI

We know from our biomechanical studies that the efficacy of the tendons in the hand, especially the flexors, depends on their running in close apposition to the skeleton. If a tendon bowstrings away from the osteoarticular chain, it undergoes a relative lengthening, which results in a corresponding loss of power at its terminal insertion. When the fingers are flexed, the osteoarticular chain (metacarpal and phalanges) forms a deeply concave curve, and it is only the osteofibrous groove of the digital canal that keeps the tendons and their synovial sheaths in intimate contact with the skeletal arc. The system of pulleys has only recently been described in its most minute details (Doyle and Blythe, 1974). An important component is the proximal pulley over the metacarpal neck, the volar plate of the metacarpophalangeal joint, and the proximal portion of the proximal phalanx.

How then do we explain the lack of deference with which this proximal pulley is divided at the slightest excuse, starting with the humble trigger-finger, which results from an intratendinous nodule? When performing an extensive tenolysis, many authors now advocate reconstruction of the pulley by means of a tendon graft or a fragment of the extensor retinaculum. Yet nothing replaces the pulley better than the pulley itself.

TECHNIQUE OF ENLARGEMENT PLASTY

Two situations can arise depending on whether the pulley is intact or has been severed along with the tendon.

PLASTY ON AN INTACT PULLEY

Dividing the Pulley

Here lies the secret of the enlargement plasty—a pulley should be divided diagonally and never longitudinally (A and A'; Fig. 26–1). Once the upper and lower borders of

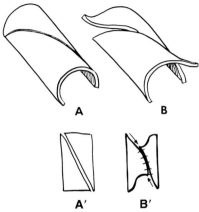

Figure 26–1. *Simple plasty.* First the pulley is divided diagonally (A and A') so as to produce two triangular flaps (B) whose common hypotenuse is the line of section. In the next stage, the edges are moved in opposite directions (B and B') and resutured with 8-0 monofilament.

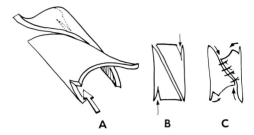

Figure 26–2. *Plasty with "opening."* To achieve further widening of the pulley, each flap is partially disinserted along a line from the long side of the right-angled triangle (A and B) toward the small side. This "opening" allows further sliding of the hypotenuses (C), which are then resutured.

the pulley have been identified, a diagonal cut is made with the knife across the middle part—without damaging the tendon. It is then completed above and below with fine scissors until the tendon and its nodule (if any) are widely exposed.

Creating the Plasty

The plasty operation can be done in one of two ways:

1. Sliding the two edges of the diagonal section, which are then sutured with four or five monofilament (8-0) stitches;

2. If further widening is required, the pulley is opened as already described, and a short cut is made at the base of each flap flush with the bone, at the point of insertion of the free border of the right-angled triangle (Figs. 26–2 and 26–3). The flaps are then allowed to slide and are resutured. The pulley is now reconstructed and is sufficiently enlarged to allow insertion of the tip of the scissors between pulley and tendon (Fig. 26–4).

Plasty on a Severed Pulley

When the pulley has been injured along with the tendon, it is usually divided along a transverse or short oblique line. One of the main difficulties in simultaneous repair of both flexor tendons has been the increase in caliber of the tendons, which meant that the pulley had to be left open. It is now possible to reconstruct the pulley and enlarge it sufficiently to allow the tendon sutures to glide through (Fig. 26–5).

Dividing the Pulley

The pulley, having already been cut transversely, now requires not one but two diagonal sections. From one extremity of the traumatic division, a first diagonal section is started with the knife and completed with scissors. From the other extremity, a second diagonal cut is carried out parallel to the first. The two flaps thus produced (both in the shape of a right-angled triangle) are now reflected to open up free access to the ten-

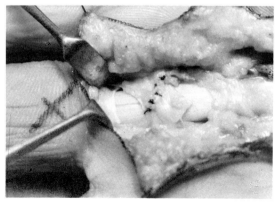

Figure 26–3. *Plasty with "opening" completed.* Here we can see the suture line as well as the two "openings," especially the one in the lower field.

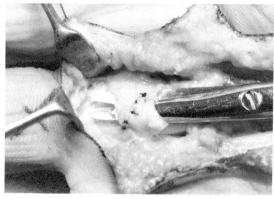

Figure 26–4. *Enlargement.* This plasty, with an opening at the base of the flaps, produces sufficient enlargement for the scissors to be inserted between the tendon and the reconstructed pulley.

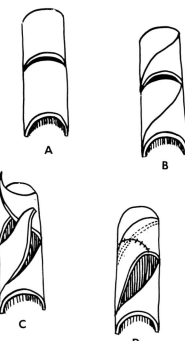

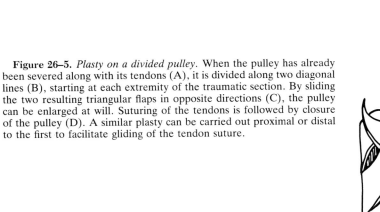

Figure 26–5. *Plasty on a divided pulley.* When the pulley has already been severed along with its tendons (A), it is divided along two diagonal lines (B), starting at each extremity of the traumatic section. By sliding the two resulting triangular flaps in opposite directions (C), the pulley can be enlarged at will. Suturing of the tendons is followed by closure of the pulley (D). A similar plasty can be carried out proximal or distal to the first to facilitate gliding of the tendon suture.

dons. When necessary, the exposure can be enlarged by raising two more similar flaps proximally over the digital canal. If the adhesion between tendon and pulley can be freed, a tenolysis, followed by reconstruction of the canal, becomes feasible.

Creating the Plasty

The plasty operation is even simpler than in the previous situation. The small sides of the right angled triangles are slid and resutured according to the degree of enlargement required. Successive plasties are sutured along the same lines.

POSTOPERATIVE COURSE

No immobilization is required. Active flexion-extension movements, without effort, are started as soon as the patient is awake. A useful range of movement is restored within a few days.

REFERENCE

Doyle, J. R., and Blythe, W.: Macroscopic and functional anatomy of the flexor sheath. J. Bone Joint Surg., *56A*:1094, 1974.

Chapter 27

PRIMARY REPAIR OF FLEXOR TENDONS IN THE DIGITAL CANAL

CLAUDE E. VERDAN

In 1960 we described a technique for the primary repair of flexor tendons in zones 1 and 2 in the fingers and zones 1 and 3 in the thumb. It can be summed up as follows:

1. The tendon sheath is resected together with part of the corresponding pulley over a length equal to the expected range of gliding of the future tendinous callus.

2. The muscle traction to which the proximal end of the tendon is submitted is relieved by semiflexion of the wrist and transverse transfixion of the tendon by means of a metal pin, which unites it to the sheath and to the skin.

3. The distal and proximal segments are approximated by passive flexion of the digital extremity and maintained in that position either by transversely transfixing the tendon, as just discussed if the distal end is long enough, or by transarticular block if it is short.

4. The surfaces of the tendon ends are accurately approximated and joined by four fine, accurately placed, horizontal mattress epitendinous sutures similar to epineural nerve sutures.

5. The digit is immobilized for three weeks.

Figures 27–1 and 27–2 present the technical details.

We thought at first that when the two flexor tendons were cut, the superficialis should be systematically resected to make room for the profundus and only the latter sutured (Bunnell, 1948). In 1968 we started suturing both tendons because the vascularization of the tendinous segments concerned depends essentially on the vincula and mesotendons (Verdan, 1972, 1979; Verdan and Crawford,

194

1971). However, the vinculum that supplies the segment of the flexor profundus overlying the proximal phalanx arises from the anterior aspect of the proximal interphalangeal joint and crosses over the decussation of the superficialis before penetrating the profundus (Fig. 27–2).

Whether the vinculum is avulsed or remains intact depends on the site of the injury, the degree of flexion or extension of the finger, and the force exerted by the patient at the time of injury. If the vinculum has been spared, it would be unfortunate to destroy it by careless surgery. Yet if the superficialis is extracted through a palmar incision, the vinculum is inevitably avulsed; the precious blood supply is lost and suturing is performed under unfavorable conditions.

This was confirmed by work carried out on the dog by Potenza (1979). In primary suturing of the flexor profundus, postoperative adhesions were far more extensive when the superficialis had been resected. If superficialis had been severed by injury, adhesions were less if its distal end was left in situ.

It is preferable, therefore, to leave the tendons in their sheaths. Through a transverse palmar incision one should try to gently nurse them distally while massaging the forearm musculature downward with the wrist flexed. Once they reach the digital wound, the tendons are tethered with an atraumatic suture and pinned at a distance through the intact sheath either in the metacarpal region or at the wrist, or even by a traction suture fixed to the skin (Duparc and Alnot, 1973). This offers the advantage of not traumatizing the sheath and the tendons in the digital canal where there would be a risk of further

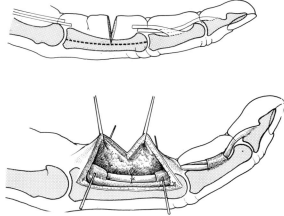

Figure 27–1. Mid-lateral incision above and below the traumatic wound on the side where a collateral nerve has been injured. (If both nerves have been injured, the incision is made on the side on which nerve repair is more important.) The flexor profundus tendon or both tendons are brought into the wound, transfixed with a 0.7 mm. wire, and sutured with 6-0 Polydek, as described in the text. Finally, the collateral nerve is sutured with 9-0 nylon. Vascular microsurgery under microscopic control allows suturing of the collateral artery. The finger is immobilized in plaster for three weeks.

unwanted adhesions. Once the two tendons have been transfixed and immobilized, they are sutured separately, at slightly different levels if possible. The lateral bands of the superficialis require only one or two approximating stitches.

When, as is common, the finger has been injured in flexion, the suture should be distal to the skin wound. If irreversible adhesions were to form around the callus, they would overlie the middle rather than the proximal phalanx. The proximal phalanx would then move with the residual gliding of the tendons and some extra flexion would have been gained.

In the thumb the same method of pinning and suturing is used, the difference being that here only one tendon is involved. Suturing therefore is simpler. However, if the suture were to lie within zone 3 and necessitate total resection of the pulley, there would be an indication for immediate lengthening of the tendon at the musculotendinous junction over the wrist and for placing the suture more distally in zone 1 where the prognosis is better.

Finally, if the pulley and metacarpal ring are destroyed, it is possible to approximate the bodies of the two muscle heads· of the flexor brevis over the midline in order to create a new pulley.

TENOLYSIS AFTER SUTURING OF THE FLEXORS IN ZONE 2

This is an essential part of the treatment and the patient should be forewarned (Verdan and Milhon, 1961). In about one-third of the cases partial or total tendon block occurs, which necessitates a secondary procedure.* We advocate a delay of three to six months after flexor tendon suturing before embarking on a tenolysis (Egloff and Verdan, 1979). If performed earlier, the latter carries a risk of tendon rupture during the period of functional re-education.

RESULTS OF TENDON SUTURES IN THE DIGITAL CANAL

If we take into account the marked improvement that can be obtained with secondary tenolysis, the results of suturing in zone 2 are at least as good and probably fractionally better than those achieved with grafts.

---

*See Chapter 9 on tenolysis.

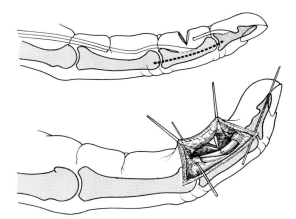

Figure 27–2. The technique described in Figure 27–1 is the same for more distal wounds in zone 1. However, as the distal end of the flexor profundus is too short to be pinned transversely within its sheath, the distal interphalangeal joint is immobilized in semi-flexion by an axial or oblique transarticular wire. In both cases we have used the following precautionary steps for several years: The wrist is maintained in semi-flexion to relax the muscle bodies. The other healthy fingers are extended, a maneuver that puts traction on the bodies of the common flexors and relaxes the severed tendon. At the end of the operation, the nail of the involved finger is tethered to the palm by means of a large nylon thread in order to avoid the risks of involuntary traction on the delicate suture, e.g., during sleep and when the dressing is being changed. The plaster cast and wires are removed after three weeks.

In 1971 we reported the results in 36 fingers, 31 of them in patients who were followed up (Verdan and Crawford, 1971).

In 14 cases both tendons were repaired. In 11 cases the flexor profundus alone was sutured and the superficialis resected. In six cases the profundus alone was involved in zone 2. All six patients were able to flex the finger and touch the palm at a distance of 2.5 cm. between the pulp and the distal palmar crease. In the 25 cases in which both tendons had been severed, the best results were obtained when both were resutured: 90 per cent of fingers could reach to within 2.5 cm. or less of the distal palmar crease.

INDICATIONS

In view of the alternatives available, it would reek of dogmatism to state that suturing is the only acceptable primary treatment and grafting the only acceptable secondary treatment. Tendon grafting certainly has an important part to play and is often justified, but it remains biologically a last resort (Boyes and Stark, 1979). We should mention that during the same period that we performed 35 primary repairs, our unit carried out 65 flexor tendon grafts.

If we consider all cases, including those with severe tendinous lesions and associated lesions at the onset, good results were obtained in about 55 per cent.

It should be remembered that when tendon suturing has failed, grafting is still possible provided the finger has remained passively mobile and the primary repair has not rendered the operation field impracticable.

Boyes and Stark (1979) have shown that grafts performed after the failure of primary suturing yield worse results than those performed as a primary procedure.

The choice of repair must take into account the following factors: the time elapsed since the accident, the type of wound (contusion precludes primary suturing), the quality of emergency care, the age of the patient, his professional requirements, the technical possibilities and equipment available, and, last but not least, the experience of the surgeon.

Recent improvements in the quality of suture materials, which now combine strength and resilience with a small caliber, have enabled Kleinert and Weiland (1979) to make a further step forward in the field of primary suturing: a "shoe lace" suture (Polydek 5-0) together with an epitendinous continuous suture (6-0) is strong enough to allow removal of the transfixing pin at the end of the operation provided the wrist is held in flexion and the nail is tethered with an elastic band to the plaster cast rather than the skin. These precautions give the patient a slight range of mobility, for as he extends the finger, the flexor tendons relax and the strain on the tendon suture is minimal. This method of relative immobilization in fact allows some slight degree of "protected" mobilization, which may well have contributed to the good results obtained by these authors. We have now adopted this technique, although it is too early to assess the results.

Our belief today is therefore to use an analogous technique. This is based on an analysis of the published experimental works concerning the details of the vascularization of the flexor tendons in their sheath, their healing process, and, notably, the role of the synovial fluid (Caplan et al., 1975; Hunter and Jaeger, 1975; Lindsay, 1979; Lundborg and Rank, 1980; Matthews and Richards, 1976; Peacock, 1959; Potenza, 1979; Richards, 1979; Winckler, 1979).

As we have noted, study of the blood supply of the tendons indicates that it is necessary to repair both tendons without exteriorizing them. Moreover, the tendon suture must not be inserted in the dorsal part of the tendon, along which the nutrient artery runs. The role of the synovial fluid has been elucidated by Lundborg and Rank (1980); it is not only a lubricant to facilitate tendon gliding but also a nutritional medium—similar to a tissue culture—which permits the passage and free circulation of fibroblasts from the parietal layer toward the site of the tendon suture and also the local proliferation of tenocytes at the tendon ends (Potenza, 1979). But in the latter case it is necessary that the two leaves of the synovial sheath be intact. With this knowledge, the method of healing of the intrasynovial suture can be better understood.

This healing process, considered by some to be axial (Paget) and by others to be peripheral (Adams), perhaps truly does vary depending on whether the tendon sheath is intact or not. This integrity of the sheath is a biological phenomenon, since it provides an environment that is like a culture medium. This type of environment is seldom met in the trauma situation. In the presence of even minimal infection, the defense mechanisms of the organism come into action, with the production of extensive vascular fibrous tissue and dense adhesions. The opening of the tendon sheath by accidental trauma and then by surgery itself puts the tendon in a biological environment in which the tenoblastic proliferation that thrives in a synovial fluid "tissue culture" medium will be uncertain if not impossible. Healing would then be able to occur only if there were an adequate vascular and lymphatic circulation to carry the necessary nutrients required by the proliferating cells. The vascularity or ischemia of the divided tendon ends thus becomes the most important factor. If the intrinsic vascular supply is adequate to nourish the tendon ends, healing will occur with the aid of fine vascular adhesions. If the intrinsic blood supply is absent, the healing of the ischemic tendon can be achieved only by the formation of dense vascular adhesions. In the first instance the discrete adhesions will be resorbed and lengthened by active and passive mobilization. In the second instance gross restriction of tendon gliding can be expected.

In conclusion, therefore, all other factors being equal, reparative surgery must include the following three points: respect and preservation of the tendinous blood supply, early mobilization, and restoration of the integrity of the synovial sheath. The first two factors to a large part have been resolved, but it is the third factor that must concern us in the future. If possible, surgical incisions into the tendon sheath should be placed away from the traumatic incision, which should be sutured. The tendon suture line should be protected by ensuring that it lies in an area of intact synovium, by flexing or extending the digit, depending on the position of the digit at the time of injury. The surgical incision in the tendon sheath should then be sutured.

If the tendon sheath has been destroyed, one can aid its reconstruction by the insertion of a Silastic prosthesis (Hunter and Jaeger, 1975). Used in secondary suturing, this prosthesis can be associated with collateral nerve repair and pulley reconstruction, the integrity of which is essential for free digital function. This argument adds strength to the precedent for restoring the tendon sheath.

REFERENCES

Adams, W.: *In* Boyes, J. H., 1976.

Boyes, J. H.: On the Shoulders of Giants. Notable Names in Hand Surgery. Philadelphia, J. B. Lippincott Co., 1976.

Boyes, J. H., and Stark, H.-H.: Flexor tendon grafts in the fingers and thumb. *In* Verdan, C. E., 1979a.

Bunnell, S.: Surgery of the hand. Ed. 2. Philadelphia, J. B. Lippincott Co., 1948.

Caplan, H. S., Hunter, J. M., and Merklin, R. J.: Intrinsic vascularization of flexor tendons. *In* Symposium on Tendon Surgery in the Hand. St. Louis, The C. V. Mosby Co., 1975.

Duparc, J., Alnot, Y., et al.: Plaies récentes des tendons fléchisseurs au doigt. Ann. Chir., 27:467, 1973.

Duran, R. J., and Houser, R. G.: Controlled passive motion following flexor tendon repair in zones 2 and 3. *In* Symposium on Tendon Surgery in the Hand. St. Louis, The C. V. Mosby Co., 1975.

Egloff, D. V., and Verdan, C. E.: Valeur des ténolyses des tendons fléchisseurs. Ann. Chir., 33:663–667, 1979.

Hunter, J. M., and Jaeger, S. H.: The active gliding tendon prosthesis: progress. *In* Symposium on Tendon Surgery in the Hand. St. Louis, The C. V. Mosby Co., 1975.

Kleinert, H. E., and Weiland, A. J.: Primary repair of flexor tendon lacerations in zone II. *In* Verdan, C. E., 1979a.

Lindsay, W. K.: Tendon healing: a continuing experimental approach. *In* Verdan, C. E., 1979a.

Lundborg, G., and Rank, F.: Experimental studies on cellular mechanisms involved in healing of animal and human flexor tendon in synovial environment. Hand, 12, No. 1, 1980.

Matthews, P.: Biological factors in the management of flexor tendon injuries. *In* McKibbin (Ed.): Recent Advances in Orthopaedics. Edinburgh, Churchill Livingstone, 1979.

Matthews, P., and Richards, H.: Factors in the adherence of flexor tendon after repair. J. Bone Joint Surg., 58B:230, 1976.

Paget, J.: *In* Boyes, J. H., 1976.

Peacock, E.: A study of the circulation in normal tendons and healing grafts. Ann. Surg., 3:149, 1959.

Potenza, A. D.: The healing process in wounds of the digital flexor tendons and tendon grafts. An experimental study. *In* Verdan, C. E., 1979a.

Richards, J. R. (1979): The role of primary suture in injuries to the flexor tendon. *In* McKibbin (Ed.): Recent Advances in Orthopaedics. Edinburgh, Churchill Livingstone, 1979.

Strickland, J. W., and Glogovac, S. V.: Digital function following flexor tendon repair in zone II. Presented at 35th Annual Meeting, A.S.S.H., Atlanta, Georgia, February 4, 1980.

Verdan, C. E.: Chirurgie réparatrice et fonctionnelle des tendons de la main. Paris, Expansion Scientifique Française, 1952.

Verdan, C. E.: Primary repair of flexor tendons. J. Bone Joint Surg., 42A:647–657, 1960.

Verdan, C. E.: Die Eingriffe an Muskeln, Sehnen u. Sehnenscheiden. *In* Wachsmuth, W., and Wilhelm, A.: Allgemeine und spezielle Chirurgische Operationslehre. Springer Verlag, Heidelberg, 1972, Vol. 10, Ch. 3.

Verdan, C. E.: Tendon Surgery of the Hand. Edinburgh, Churchill Livingstone, 1979a.

Verdan, C. E.: Historische Entwicklung der Beugesehnen-Chirurgie und "Detaillierte Beschreibung einer primären Beugesehnennaht im Digitalkanal." Frankfurt, Kongress der Deutschsprachigen Arbeitsgemeinschaft für Handchirurgie, 1979b.

Verdan, C. E., and Crawford, G.: Flexor tendon suture in the digital canal. Transactions of the Fifth Congress, IPRS. Melbourne, Butterworths Pty. Ltd., 1971.

Verdan, C. E., Crawford, G., and Martini, Y.: Tenolysis in traumatic hand surgery. *In* Symposium on the Hand. St. Louis, The C. V. Mosby Co., 1971, Vol. 3.

Verdan, C. E., and Michon, J.: Le traitement des plaies des tendons fléchisseurs des doigts. Rev. Chir. Orthop., 47:285, 1961.

Winckler, G.: Normal anatomy of the flexor and extensor tendons of the hand. *In* Verdan, C. E., 1979a.

Chapter 28

PRIMARY REPAIR OF FLEXOR TENDONS

Harold E. Kleinert
Timothy Gill
and Bruce Schlafly

Primary repair of flexor tendons is not only routinely accepted but is also the present day preferred method of treatment for the majority of these injuries. Good results can be achieved in most cases with primary repair; however, by no means can these injuries be regarded as routine and straightforward. Primary flexor tendon repair demands the highest level of concentration and care from the surgeon, both intraoperatively and postoperatively. There is little margin for error. The large number of flexor tenolyses and other secondary tendon procedures required on an active hand surgery service attests to the difficulties encountered in flexor tendon surgery.

The term "primary repair" of a lacerated flexor tendon indicates tendon repair at the time of injury. It is subdivided into "early" (within 24 hours) and "delayed" (extends to the point when wound edges can still be bluntly separated). It is futile to predetermine treatment for patients with flexor tendon injuries based on the exact number of hours or days elapsed since injury. Each case must be judged on its own merits, considering the nature of the injury, appearance of the wound, and degree of contamination and other factors; however, the longer the interval from injury to repair, the more difficult it is to obtain a good result. Eventually because of irreversible changes in the injured extremity, the point is reached at which good results are impossible to achieve by direct flexor tendon repair and a secondary method of reconstruction, such as a tendon graft, must be employed. In most cases delay beyond one month will require secondary reconstruction.

We prefer to repair flexor tendon injuries as early as possible, ideally within hours from the time of accident. Not all patients, however, are candidates for immediate primary tendon repair, and some are never suitable. For example, local wound infection must be treated prior to dealing with the tendon injury. The additional wound manipulation and dissection necessary for primary repair, which also includes postoperative mobilization, thus precludes early primary repair in the presence of infection.

Loss of significant local tissue, whether it be skin, tendon, pulley, bone or cartilage, often precludes the possibility of primary tendon repair. Fractures, neurovascular injuries and extensor tendon lacerations do not necessarily contraindicate flexor tendon repair but may produce less favorable results. Even in these circumstances, the results of primary repair are often better than those obtained by delayed reconstruction.

ANATOMY

Surgical technique and expected results vary with the location of the flexor tendon injury. Therefore, it is conventional to use the anatomical divisions of flexor tendons established by the International Federation of Societies for Surgery of the Hand (Kleinert and Verdan, 1983). These divisions, or zones, reflect the important anatomical differences in the regions traversed by the flexor tendons (Fig. 28–1).

In the forearm and palm, the flexor tendons lie loosely in surrounding soft tissue. In the carpal tunnel and digits, unyielding fi-

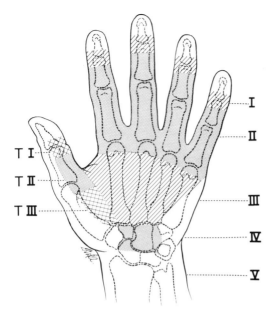

Figure 28–1. Zones of the flexor tendons. (From Kleinert, H. E. and Verden, C.: Report of the committee on tendon injuries. J. Hand Surg. *8(5)*:794–798, 1983.)

brous bands constrain the tendon relatively tightly against the skeleton. By preventing so-called bowstringing of the tendons, these restraining bands or "pulleys" ensure that a normal contractile excursion of the muscle-tendon unit will produce a full range of flexion of the finger joints. Their presence, however, leaves little margin for error in tendon repair (Fig. 28–2).

Nowhere is this more true than in the fingers proximal to the insertion of the superficialis tendons (zone II). The profundus and bifurcating superficialis tendons slide within a confined fibro-osseous tunnel (much

as a piston in a cylinder), which extends from the metacarpophalangeal joint to the middle phalanx. The tunnel has a synovial sheath constrained by a number of areas of fibrous thickenings or pulleys, the strongest of which are annular (A) pulleys. The annular pulleys are located over bony phalanges and the cartilaginous volar plates. The cruciate (C) pulleys contract and expand and are located where maximum joint motion occurs.

Biomechanical studies have demonstrated that the two most critical pulleys for maintaining full range of motion of the finger joints are A2 and A4, over the proximal and middle phalanges, respectively (Doyle and Blythe, 1976). This is also the portion of the sheath that is most difficult to surgically repair, because these pulleys tightly encircle the tendons, and sutures tend to pull out of their transversely oriented fibers. The analogous pulley in the thumb is the oblique pulley over the proximal phalanx (Doyle and Blythe, 1977).

The challenge of zone II flexor tendon injuries is to achieve strong union of up to three tendons (the bifurcated superficialis and the profundus) all in one finger, while at the same time maintaining both their normal excursion and their mechanical efficiency.

PHYSIOLOGY

Recent research on flexor tendon nutrition and healing has provided us with information that has important implications for the hand surgeon.

Studies support the theory that flexor tendons have the capacity to heal by means of intrinsic collagen synthesis without the in-

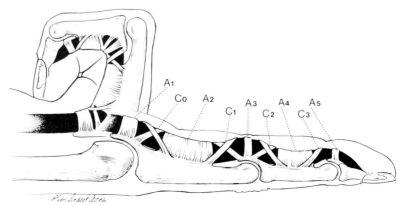

Figure 28–2. The flexor tendon pulley system. A = annular, C = cruciate. (From Lister, G. D.: The Hand, Diagnosis and Indications. Ed 2, Edinburgh. Churchill Livingstone, 1984.)

growth of granulation tissue from the surrounding environment (Gelberman, 1985). Such ingrowth of granulation tissue, of course, results in tendon adhesions. These external adhesions were previously regarded as a necessary evil in tendon repair—necessary because the intrinsic healing capability of tendons was not appreciated, and evil because the adhesions resulted in permanent loss of motion. In order to permit tendon healing by means of external adhesions, it was customary to immobilize the tendons in the initial postoperative period. In addition, there was no advantage in maximum preservation of the flexor tendon sheath, since its presence might restrict the ingrowth of external adhesions.

Laboratory evidence that flexor tendons can heal solely by intrinsic means without external adhesions supports the clinical observation that results of tendon repair are superior if the tendons are moved early and frequently in the early postoperative period (Manske et al., 1984; Lister et al., 1977; Strickland and Glogovac, 1980). Such movement reduces or eliminates adhesions, which are now regarded as both unnecessary and evil (Gelberman et al., 1983).

Intrinsic tendon healing requires adequate nutrition independent of external granulation tissue. The sources of flexor tendon nutrition in zone II include blood vessels in the synovial membrane reflections, the distal osseous attachment, the vinculae, and the synovial fluid contained in the synovial sheath. Of these, the last one is probably the most important (Manske and Lesker, 1982; Lundborg and Rank, 1978). The importance of synovial nutrition favors the concept of repairing the synovial sheath after primary tendon repair. It has not yet been demonstrated that this additional step improves the clinical result (Lister and Tonkin, 1986).

The vinculae play an important role in providing blood supply to the flexor tendons in zone II. Disruption of the vinculae is a factor in producing poor results in primary flexor tendon repair (Amadio et al., 1985). This is one reason to repair rather than resect the superficialis tendon, since resection destroys the vinculum longum to the profoundus.

DIAGNOSIS

The diagnosis of injury to the flexor tendon system is not always obvious and may result in harmful delay of appropriate treatment. Furthermore, since repair of a flexor tendon injury demands muscle relaxation, the surgeon should correctly diagnose these injuries in the emergency room so that arrangements are made for adequate operating room anesthesia.

Complete division of both the superficialis and profundus tendons results in an extended finger posture and the diagnosis is obvious even in the uncooperative patient. If only one of the two finger tendons is lacerated or avulsed, the deformity is less apparent to the untrained observer. Careful testing of individual flexor digitorum superficialis and profundus and flexor pollicis longus function should eliminate mistakes such as overlooking an avulsed profundus tendon, which is usually more common in the ring finger. The profoundus of the index finger is relatively independent of its companions in the other fingers, and blocking the latter in extension will not block function of the index finger profundus. Therefore, one must specifically check for index finger superficialis action by assessing pulp to pulp pinch with the thumb with index finger proximal interphalangeal joint flexion and distal interphalangeal joint extension. The small finger also presents diagnostic difficulties because some patients cannot independently flex this digit using only the superficialis tendon.

A complete flexor tendon laceration may continue to transmit partial motion to a joint if the vincular connections are preserved. Thus, the examiner must qualitatively assess the strength and degree of motion of the tendons tested, looking for weakness and incomplete motion. Similarly, the partially lacerated flexor tendon will still function, but active flexion against resistance is usually accompanied by increased pain and decreased strength.

Lack of patient cooperation hinders accurate diagnosis and is commonly seen in the frightened child and the intoxicated adult. Directly probing the unanesthetized wound in the emergency room rarely yields additional information even in those instances in which it is possible. Therefore, such practice is discouraged. Inspection of the wound may reveal a lacerated tendon sheath with apparently intact tendon visible through the opening in the sheath. Lacerations through the sheath commonly involve the underlying tendon, at least in part.

By detailed questioning, attempts must be

made to learn the position of the hand and digits at the time of injury. Digits fully flexed during the accident have tendon lacerations distal to the skin and sheath wound, whereas fully extended digits have proximal tendon lacerations. Thus, partial tendon laceration is usually not visible in the original sheath wound and only by full finger excursion is the tendon laceration demonstrated. Repair of complete lacerations when the fingers are injured in the extremes of motion requires extension of the wound. Obtaining a correct history from the patient as a preliminary procedure aids the surgeon in determining the exposure likely to be required.

SURGICAL TECHNIQUE

In no area of hand surgery is precise surgical technique of more importance than in primary flexor tendon repair. It requires a capable surgeon working in an operating facility with good lighting and fine, delicate instruments, and appropriate loupe magnification. Surgery must be performed in a bloodless field and with motor and sensory anesthesia of the extremity. A pneumatic tourniquet on the upper arm requires that anesthesia extend proximally to the shoulder.

Because of these requirements, more distal blocks such as metacarpal, wrist, or intravenous regional block are unacceptable for primary flexor tendon repair. In the vast majority of our cases, axillary block is employed. The anesthesiologist should be skillful in this technique and the patient cooperative. The lack of either may necessitate general anesthesia. Repair in the intoxicated adult is delayed for a few hours until the alcohol blood level falls and the patient can cooperate with the physician. Although we have successfully used axillary block with sedation in children less than one year old, inevitably some will require general anesthesia.

When using the axillary block technique, one should be wary of partial blocks. For example, an axillary block that does not fully include the ulnar nerve will leave residual muscle tension in the ulnar half of the flexor digitorum profundus. This muscle tension will upset the normal resting cascade of the fingers in which each finger is slightly less flexed than its ulnar neighbor. A repair of the profundus of the ring finger in such circumstances will appear too tight because the finger will assume an excessively flexed posi-

tion. Unless this anesthesia problem is appreciated the surgeon may think he failed to restore the anatomy correctly.

After the prerequisites for anesthesia have been fulfilled, the surgeon can proceed with the repair (Fig. 28–3). Adequate surgery requires adequate exposure of the involved anatomy, dissecting through skin to tendon sheath to expose the injured tendon ends and to allow preservation and closure of the tendon sheath as well as to avoid or eliminate longitudinal skin scars following the tendon repair. Skin lacerations are incorporated into volar zigzag Bruner incisions (Bruner, 1967). When additional sheath exposure is necessary, incisions in the A2 and A4 pulleys are to be avoided because these pulleys are more important for function and more difficult to anatomically repair. Incisional flaps in the sheath are based in the cruciate pulleys, which after repair create funnels that facilitate passage of the tendon repair beneath an otherwise unyielding tight edge of the open pulley (Fig. 28–4).

Distal and proximal tendon ends are located, and provided that the proximal end has not retracted outside the A1 pulley into the palm, this end can be delivered into the distal wound by maneuvers such as compressing the proximal (not distal) forearm, flexing the wrist and digits, and grasping the cut tendon end with a fine hemostat. The tendon should be handled only by its cut ends and ideally never by the epitenon. Blind attempts to grasp the end of the tendon increase trauma and are to be avoided. Repeated clamping frays the tendon ends, requiring further sharp débridement.

If the proximal tendon end is in the palm and not in the A1 pulley, that is, outside the fibro-osseous canal, it is often impossible to return the tendon into the sheath by closed manipulation, and a second incision is required in the palm. In flexor tendon lacerations of the thumb attempts to blindly grasp the flexor pollicis longus in the thenar region risk damaging the recurrent branch of the median nerve. It is safer to retrieve the flexor pollicis longus tendon by a direct incision in the thenar region. Retrieval of the proximal tendon at the wrist as is commonly practiced (particularly for lacerations of the thumb) further interrupts tendon nutrition by removing the proximal tendon from its normal synovial bursae and thus increases scarring. Therefore, this maneuver is to be avoided.

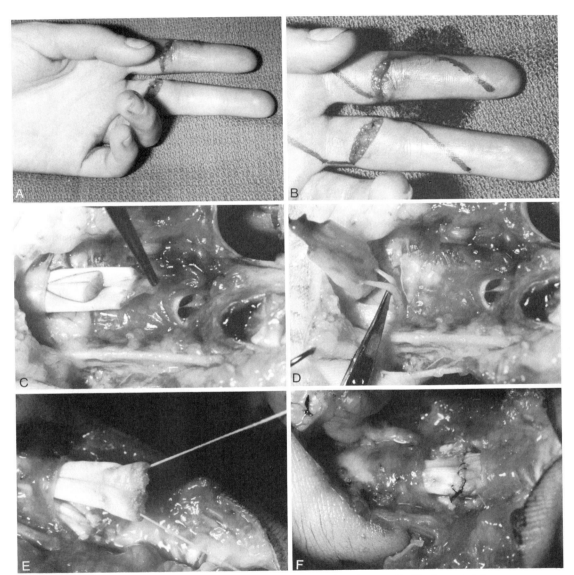

Figure 28–3. *A*, Lacerated flexor profundus and superficialis tendons in zone II. The lacerated fingers assume an extended position rather than the partially flexed position of the normal, uninjured fingers. *B*, Zigzag incision outlined for extension of the wound. *C*, Retrieval of the proximal end of lacerated superficialis and profundus. *D*, Instruments demonstrate that tendon retraction is limited by the intact vinculae. *E*, Placement of the core suture in the tendon end. *F*, Tendon repair is completed with a running circumferential suture.

Illustration continued on following page

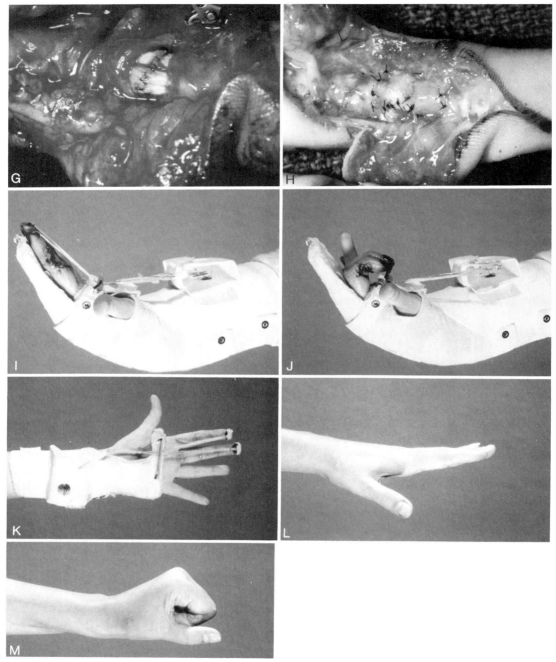

Figure 28–3 *Continued G*, Profundus and superficialis repaired. *H*, Following tendon repair the sheath is closed. *I and J*, Immediate postoperative dynamic splinting with lever arm to avoid a constant increasing tension from the rubber bands as the fingers extend. *K*, The splint is modified at three and one-half weeks to permit metacarpophalangeal joint extension. *L and M*, Flexion and extension four months postoperatively. (*A, F,* and *H* from Kleinert H. E., et al.: Surgery of the hand. In Monaco, A. P. (Ed.): Textbook of Surgery. New York, The Macmillan Book Company, in press. *B, E, G, I–M* from Kleinert, H. E., et al.: Hand injury. In Mattox, K. L. (Ed.): Trauma. New York, Appleton-Century-Crofts, 1987.)

Figure 28–4. L-shaped windows cut in the tendon sheath facilitate repair. (From Lister, G. D.: Infections and techniques for repair of the flexor tendon sheath. Hand Clin., *1(1)*:85–95, 1985.)

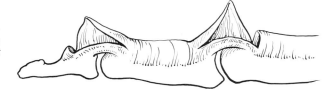

Once the tendon ends are retrieved, a 25 gauge hypodermic needle is placed transversely through the proximal tendon, and the finger is positioned so that the distal end is coapted, ensuring that the repair is accomplished without tension.

The goal is precise end-to-end approximation of the tendon ends. A Kirchmayr core suture of 4-0 nonabsorbable braided polyester is placed in the volar half of the tendon to avoid compromising the intratendinous blood vessels located more dorsally (Kirchmayr, 1917). Of importance is the relationship of the transverse to the longitudinal limbs of the core suture. As Pennington (1979) has explained, and as one can demonstrate with a string around the finger, for the sutures to grasp the tendon the transverse limbs at each end should lie in a position that is superficial or volar to the longitudinal limb in order to lock onto a group of tendon fibers (Fig. 28–5). Placement of the core suture requires that at least 1 cm. of each tendon end protrude from beneath the pulley. The suture is tied with five tight square knots to prevent slippage.

The circumferential suture of 6-0 monofilament nylon, in addition to providing increased strength, serves to smooth out the tendon repair site (Fig. 28–6). This suture is designed to catch the epitenon to produce a smooth juncture and its success is nearly impossible if the tendon ends are ragged. Frayed ends are therefore trimmed prior to suturing, avoiding removal of more than 1 cm. of tendon. The surgeon must avoid further iatrogenic injury as he manipulates the ends during the repair.

To correctly place the core suture and circumferential suture in a tension free position while preserving the A2 and A4 pulleys, one must manipulate the tendon ends back and forth under the pulleys so that the best exposure can be obtained (Lister, 1983). Usually this means placing the core suture in one tendon and then moving it to a different location in the sheath to join it to the other tendon end.

Superficialis tendon lacerations present unique considerations of their own. The orientation of the profundus and superficialis tendons changes near the base of the finger, and lacerations of both tendons at this level can be confusing. Correct identification and orientation of the tendon is made by accurately matching up the cut ends and checking for free gliding. Because of the sharply spiraling nature of each superficialis tendon slip, considerable care is taken to approximate the ends of each divided slip in the correct, rather than a reversed 180 degree, orientation. Usually a laceration of the superficialis immediately distal to its bifurcation leaves two tendon slips, each requiring repair.

Once the superficialis divides into two tendinous slips, they are smaller, flat structures, not suitable for the standard Kirchmayr suture. A figure eight suture is employed distal to the chiasm with the knot positioned dorsally to avoid impingement on the profundus. Proximal to the chiasm the flat semicurved superficialis is repaired with a central core

Figure 28–5. Kirchmayr suture for profundus repair. (From Kleinert, H. E., et al.: Surgery of the hand. In Monaco, A. P. (Ed.): Textbook of Surgery. New York, The Macmillan Book Company, in press.)

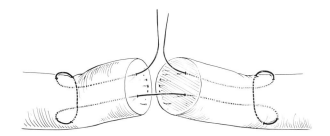

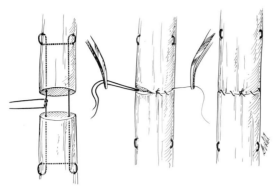

Figure 28–6. After placement of the core suture, the peripheral running suture is placed. (From Kleinert, H. E., et al.: Flexor tendon injuries. Surg. Clin. North Am., *61*:267–286, 1981.)

suture and a posterior/anterior running suture for a smooth juncture (Fig. 28–7).

Partial flexor tendon lacerations are treated according to the percentage of cross-sectional area of tendon involved. Very small lacerations, 10 to 20 per cent of the tendon or less, may simply be rounded off by resecting the small flap. Lacerations involving greater than 50 per cent of the tendon are repaired with a core and circumferential suture, placing the suture through only the injured part of the tendon and not through intact tendon. Lacerations that fall in between these groups are repaired with only a circumferential approximating suture.

The sheath is repaired with 6-0 or 8-0 monofilament nylon suture, and this repair can be as difficult as repair of the tendons. Sheath closure restores the anatomy for maximum nutrition of the tendons from synovial fluid and eliminates an edge upon which the tendon repair may snag, thereby decreasing

the diameter of the sheath as it is dragged forward, further limiting tendon excursion. If closure of the sheath produces constriction on the tendon, a sheath graft may be necessary. The superficial fascia of the wrist or a portion of the extensor retinaculum of the wrist or ankle is suitable for this purpose (Lister, 1979). After sheath repair or graft, testing is performed for free tendon gliding within the sheath, through a full range of wrist or finger excursion. The tourniquet is released at the conclusion of the repair prior to skin closure to ensure hemostasis.

Avoiding the nail bed and pulp, a double loop of 5-0 nylon suture is placed in the fingernail for dynamic traction. Wounds are dressed and a dorsolateral plaster splint is applied, maintaining the wrist and metacarpophalangeal joints in about 30 to 40 degrees less than maximum flexion, but permitting full interphalangeal joint extension. A rubber band is attached between the loop in the fingernail and the splint at the wrist so that the digit is gently held in flexion but is capable of full interphalangeal joint extension. Since 1984 we have employed a splint modification with a roller bar and spring loaded lever arm attached to the rubber band, which advances and retracts with finger flexion and extension, thereby providing a reasonably constant tension force on the finger. The rubber band glides beneath the roller in the palm, providing both distal and proximal interphalangeal joint motion, which facilitates differential profundus and superficialis tendon gliding. Results appear to be better and complications less with this splint modification (Fig. 28–8).

Zone I tendon lacerations involve only the profundus tendon. If the laceration leaves a distal stump at least 1 cm. in length, standard

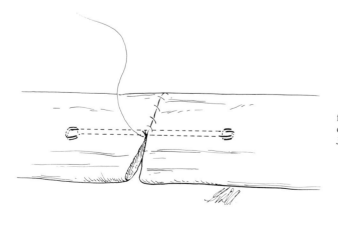

Figure 28–7. Central core suture for the superficialis. (From Kleinert H. E., et al.: Current state of flexor tendon surgery. Ann. Chir. Main., *3(1)*:7–17, 1984.)

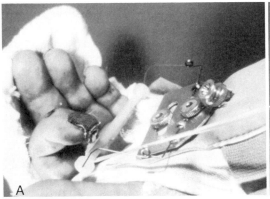
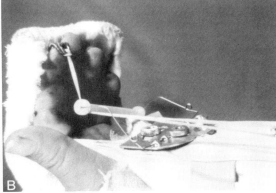

Figure 28–8. *A* and *B*, The spring-loaded roller bar is demonstrated. It retracts with finger flexion and advances with finger extension, facilitating proximal interphalangeal and distal interphalangeal joint motion, and further eliminates undue rubber band tension with extension.

suture repair may be performed. If not, the profundus can be advanced and attached to the distal bony phalanx with a pullout suture.

Closed avulsions of the profundus tendons from the distal bony phalanx may occur with such force that vinculae rupture and the tendon retracts and coils into the palm. Early diagnosis within 7 to 10 days before tendon swelling and necrosis become advanced from loss of both sources of nutrition (i.e., blood supply and synovial fluid) permits tendon reinsertion through the sheath to the distal bony phalanx attachment. A thin walled silicone rubber catheter facilitates reinsertion of the tendon in its proper location in the fibro-osseous canal (Fig. 28–9).

Zone III and zone V tendon lacerations are repaired with a suture technique similar to those used in profundus lacerations in zone II. Repair is simplified by the absence of the fibro-osseous tunnel.

Repair of *zone IV* lacerations in the carpal tunnel may require partial release of the transverse carpal ligament to provide adequate exposure. However, since the wrist is immobilized in flexion postoperatively, the ligament must be kept partially intact or restored to prevent prolapse of the flexor tendons and median nerve into the superficial subcutaneous tissue.

Primary repair of flexor tendons in small children requires less modification of the surgical technique than does the postoperative management. Intraoperatively one simply uses smaller instruments and sutures as indicated. For example, one might transfix the tendon with a 27 gauge needle and repair it with a 5-0 core suture. The circumferential suture and sheath repair will probably be performed with 8-0 instead of 6-0 nylon. A long arm plaster splint with elbow, wrist and metacarpophalangeal joint flexion may be

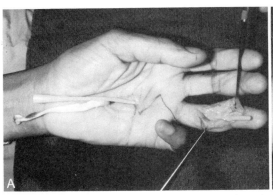
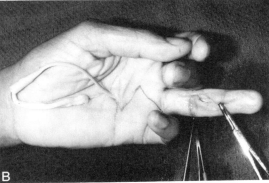

Figure 28–9. *A* and *B*, Disruption of the insertion of profundus tendon ring finger. The distal end was located in the A1 pulley. The proximal tendon is thickened, necessitating the catheter retrieval technique to place the swollen tendon anatomically through the chiasm of the superficialis and the fibro-osseous sheath.

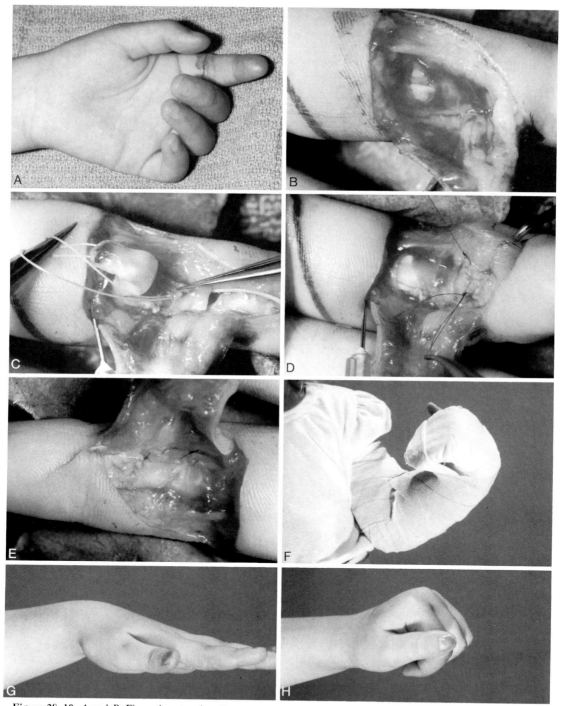

Figure 28–10. *A* and *B*, Finger in extension. Lacerated profundus resulting from an injury with the finger in flexion. This necessitated a combined repair on either side of the A4 pulley. *C* and *D*, Placing the Kirchmayr suture in the proximal end proximal to the A4 pulley and completing the repair distal to the A4 pulley with a running 6-0 suture. *E*, Completed sheath repair. *F*, Postoperative splint with the wrist and metacarpophalangeal joints in flexion, allowing full interphalangeal joint extension. In a child, rubber band traction is not necessarily used. *G* and *H*, Extension and flexion three months postoperatively.

applied. A dynamic splint is not necessarily required (Fig. 28–10).

POSTOPERATIVE MANAGEMENT

Postoperative management is as important as the intraoperative technique. A dorsal splint with dynamic rubber band traction is applied for tendon repair in all five zones. The patient is encouraged to extend and then relax the digits several times daily after the first postoperative day. The rubber band acts to passively flex the digit when the patient relaxes the extensor muscles. The problem of inadequate passive flexion of the distal interphalangeal joint is corrected by adding a distal palmar pulley to the splint to alter the vector of the rubber band force on the finger. Excessive tension on the rubber band is prevented by attaching it proximally to a coiled lever arm that advances and retracts, thereby maintaining uniform tension so that complete interphalangeal joint extension is easily accomplished. The patient is seen at least once a week for the first four weeks to ensure proper motion and to modify the splint as needed.

Patients with poor motion are started earlier on active unprotected flexion than are those with excellent motion, for these are the cases more likely to experience rupture of the repair.

About four weeks postoperatively, the dorsal splint is removed and active flexion of the fingers is started If there is excellent finger motion, dynamic traction continues for an additional two to three weeks with the rubber band attached to a wrist cuff, which permits the patient to move the wrist yet provides further protection of the repair sites. More forceful flexion with blocking of proximal joints to facilitate tendon pullthrough or distal gliding is permitted at about five weeks. If needed, passive extension exercises can also begin at five to six weeks, particularly if done with the wrist flexed. At 12 weeks the patient is released for regular work and use of the hand.

Because the preceding protocol requires patient cooperation, postoperative management in the young child is substantially modified. Fortunately most children do well in spite of the compromises that must be made. The safest postoperative course in the young child is to immobilize the wrist and metacarpophalangeal joints in partial flexion as described for the adult and to block the interphalangeal joints, allowing nearly full extension. A plaster cast is applied and maintained for three weeks. When the cast is removed, the child is permitted active motion of the digits while wearing a dorsal splint for another three weeks. The splint blocks full extension of the wrist and metacarpophalangeal joints to additionally protect the repair.

COMPLICATIONS

Despite the surgeon's best efforts, complications may arise in the care of flexor tendon injuries, especially those in zone II, and one must be prepared to modify treatment accordingly. Flexor tendon injuries are often associated with neurovascular laceration, joint disruption, fracture, extensor tendon laceration, skin loss and even complete amputation.

Neurovascular repairs do not preclude flexor tendon repair. However, they may require a dorsal blocking splint on the finger to prevent full extension of one of the interphalangeal joints. The decision to use this splint is made in the operating room by evaluating tension on the neurovascular anastomoses with the wrist and metacarpophalangeal joints partially flexed and with full extension of the interphalangeal joints.

Associated fractures are internally stabilized, when possible, to permit early joint motion.

Extensor tendon disruptions are repaired, but they preclude use of a dynamic flexor tendon splint. When both flexor and extensor tendon are repaired, as in replantation, a program of limited active flexion and extension without resistance is employed in the immediate postoperative period.

Loss of skin will necessitate skin graft or flap for wound coverage. This may require postoperative immobilization, which can compromise the result of the flexor tendon repair. Primary repair will be contraindicated in some of these cases.

Crushing injuries often produce flexor tendon disruptions with ragged, untidy tendon ends. Excision (or advancement as in zone I) of more than 1 to 1.5 cm. of tendon to obtain normal tendon ends may produce a permanent flexion contracture of the finger; therefore, primary repair in crushing injuries may be contraindicated. Some cases will be borderline and if after primary suture the repair is somewhat untidy, postoperative management should be modified. Maintenance of full interphalangeal joint motion should be emphasized using passive flexion and extension if necessary in the standard dorsal block splint. Motion is maintained even at the risk of rupturing the repair. One should never allow a significant flexion contracture to develop trying to protect a tenuous repair. It is better to maintain passive motion, obtain wound healing and later reconstruct the tendon with a graft.

Isolated partial tendon lacerations are at the other extreme of flexor tendon injuries. Since the patient can demonstrate full flexion in the emergency room, one may be tempted to leave these injuries untreated; however, failure to treat partial flexor tendon lacerations runs the risk of developing entrapment, rupture, or triggering of the tendon (Schlenker et al., 1981). These injuries should be explored and treated in the operating room as previously outlined. To prevent possible rupture, partial lacerations involving more than 30 per cent of the tendon should be protected postoperatively with the same dynamic traction splint used for complete lacerations.

As in any hand operation, hematoma and wound infection may occur. A serious wound infection will ruin any tendon repair, no matter how precise it is. Obviously the surgeon must adhere to the standard principles of hand surgery during tendon repair, such as thorough wound toilet, adequate débridement, atraumatic technique, control of bleeding after release of the tourniquet, and appropriate use of antibiotics. Postoperative infection does require immobilization and always compromises the result.

It is often tempting to try to improve exposure for zone II tendon repairs or to increase excursion after such repairs by removing some or, tragically, all of either the A2 or A4 pulleys. Such temptation must be completely resisted because these pulleys are essential to prevent bowstringing of the tendons with resultant loss of both flexion and extension. Although partial resection of a pulley to increase tendon excursion does cause less bowstringing than complete resection, it generally is of little benefit, since the finger flexors require a long excursion of

about 7 cm. and the repair can still catch on the exposed pulley edge. If this occurs or is demonstrated at operation, the solution is to restore the continuity of the sheath and pulley using a graft when necessary and to avoid resection of the pulley. If the repair is still too untidy to pass into the pulley, one must question whether the primary repair is acceptable. Again, in borderline situations, the emphasis should be on maintaining range of motion postoperatively. If the repair fails to glide adequately in the sheath intraoperatively, it is unlikely the situation can be salvaged by a later tenolysis, and it may be prudent to insert a silicone rod to facilitate tendon graft later. These procedures will be considerably more complicated if the pulleys have been sacrificed during the primary procedure.

The most common complications seen after primary flexor tendon repair are attenuation or elongation of the repair, rupture of the repair, adhesions at the repair site and tendon bowstringing from inadequate pulleys.

Elongation without complete rupture of the repair has been shown to occur by using radiopaque markers in the tendon ends. Clinically, elongation results in a decrease in active flexion. Seradge (1983) showed that the amount of elongation correlated with the need for tenolysis, that is, all repairs with elongation of 4 mm. or more required tenolysis. Elongation is observed less with the modified Kirchmayr suture than with the crisscross suture.

Complete rupture may occur suddenly or may represent the end stage of gradual progressive elongation. Sudden rupture occurs most commonly in the first two weeks when the tendon repair is weakest; however, it can occur later, even six weeks postoperatively, when the patient is moving the digit well with little pain and attempts to do heavy, forceful work. The treatment for rupture is exploration and repeated repair.

Failure to treat a ruptured profundus will not only leave the patient with loss of active distal interphalangeal joint flexion but also may create a lumbrical plus finger, which is likely to interfere with flexion of the proximal interphalangeal joint.

Adhesions were the frequent and usual complication of flexor tendon repairs previously treated by immobilization, and this stimulated the development of dynamic traction splinting. Although postoperative dynamic traction has markedly reduced the incidence of this complication, it has not been entirely eliminated. Adhesions occur for a variety of reasons: extensive initial damage to the tendon or its sheath, failure to achieve complete gliding of the tendon repair through the pulleys at the time of the repair, hematoma, infection, inadequate postoperative supervision, or poor patient compliance. Frequently, no single factor can be identified. It may be difficult to clinically distinguish adhesions from elongation or rupture of the repair until the tendon is re-explored. One often finds both adhesions and breakdown or elongation of the repair in these cases.

The treatment for adhesions with unacceptable loss of active flexion is tenolysis. Usually this is not done until six months after surgery or until a plateau in function is reached. This trial of physical therapy allows adequate healing of the tendon and other soft tissues prior to tenolysis. If the repair site is elongated by more than 4 mm. of scar tissue and tenolysis is performed, the tendon is again protected using the rubber band dynamic splint. If the tendon itself is unsatisfactory, a one or two staged tendon graft will be necessary. Successful tenolysis requires good patient cooperation and physician supervision postoperatively to maintain active motion. Such cooperation cannot be expected in a young child. Thus following unsuccessful primary flexor tendon repair in a child the stiff contracted finger is more difficult to salvage and will likely require a staged tendon graft procedure.

By itself the problem of adhesions limiting gliding of the flexor tendon in its sheath can usually be overcome in the cooperative adult. The presence of a superimposed flexion contracture of the proximal interphalangeal joint, however, compounds the situation. Tenolysis combined with capsulectomy requires meticulous surgical technique and tedious postoperative management or the result will be less successful.

Dynamic rubber band traction can produce flexion contractures unless the physician maintains close supervision of the patient, thereby ensuring finger extension postoperatively. This is the principal reason for not using dynamic traction in young children. If a flexion contracture starts to develop, the splint is modified even to the point of discontinuing the dynamic traction and placing the patient in a protective static splint, if necessary.

The best treatment for flexion contracture is prevention. One must be especially watchful for this complication if the initial injury also included trauma to the volar plate or collateral ligament of a joint. Flexion contractures are minimized by avoiding excessive tension on the rubber band as the spring loaded lever arm attachment to the rubber band does, or by blocking the metacarpophalangeal joint in nearly full flexion and constantly encouraging the patient to fully extend the interphalangeal joints. This is best accomplished by placing a sponge rubber block dorsal to the proximal phalanx to facilitate full proximal interphalangeal joint finger extension.

Bowstringing of the flexor tendon is avoided by maintaining the fibro-osseous sheath. If necessary, pulleys such as the A2 or A4 have been destroyed they are replaced in the acute situation with a strip of retinaculum that is passed around the bony phalanx and flexor tendon, overlapped and doubly sutured (Lister, 1979). The Weilby weave technique of restoring a pulley is suitable only in the chronic situation (Kleinert and Bennett, 1981).

SUMMARY

Primary flexor tendon repair still challenges the most skillful surgeons. A successful result with almost full finger motion can be obtained in most cases by adhering to certain principles and to methods outlined in this chapter. The possibility of complications accompanies any surgical procedure. It is the surgeon's responsibility to minimize complications, although they cannot always be eliminated.

REFERENCES

Amadio, P. L., Hunter, J. M., Jaeger, S. H., Wehbe, M. A., and Schneider, L. H.: The effect of vincular injury on the results of flexor tendon surgery in zone 2. J. Hand Surg., *10A*:626–632, 1985.

Bruner, J. M.: The zig-zag volar digital incision for flexor tendon surgery. Plast. Reconstr. Surg., *40*:571, 1967.

Doyle, J. R., and Blythe, W. F.: The finger flexor tendon sheath and pulleys: Anatomy and reconstruction. In AAOS Symposium on Tendon Surgery in the Hand. St. Louis, The C.V. Mosby Company, 1976, pp. 81–87.

Doyle, J. R., and Blythe, W. F.: Anatomy of the flexor tendon sheath and pulleys of the thumb. J. Hand Surg., 2:149–151, 1977.

Gelberman, R. H.: Flexor tendon physiology: tendon nutrition and cellular activity in injury and repair. In AAOS Instructional Course Lectures, Vol. 34. St. Louis, The C.V. Mosby Company, 1985, pp. 351–360.

Gelberman, R. H., Vande Berg, J. S., Lundborg, G. N., and Akeson, W. H.: Flexor tendon healing and restoration of the gliding surface. An ultrastructural study in dogs. J. Bone Joint. Surg., 65A:70–80, 1983.

Kirchmayr, L.: Zur technik der Sehnennaht. Zentralbl. Chir., 44:27–52, 1917.

Kleinert, H. E., and Bennett, J. B.: Digital pulley reconstruction employing the always present rim of the previous pulley. J. Hand Surg., 3:267, 1981.

Kleinert, H. E., and Verdan, C.: Report of the Committee on Tendon Injuries. J. Hand Surg., 8:794–798, 1983.

Lister, G. D.: Reconstruction of pulleys employing extensor retinaculum. J. Hand Surg., 4:461–464, 1979.

Lister, G. D.: Incision and closure of the flexor sheath during primary tendon repair. Hand, 15:123–135, 1983.

Lister, G. D., and Tonkin, M.: The results of primary flexor tendon repair with closure of the tendon sheath. Presentation to American Society for Surgery of the Hand, New Orleans, Louisiana, Feb. 19, 1986.

Lister, G. D., Kleinert, H. E., Kutz, J. E., and Atasoy, E.: Primary flexor tendon repair followed by immediate controlled mobilization. J. Hand Surg., 2:441–451, 1977.

Lundborg, G., and Rank, F.: Experimental intrinsic healing of flexor tendons based upon synovial fluid nutrition. J. Hand Surg., 3(1):21, 1978.

Manske, P. R., and Lesker, P. A.: Nutrient pathways of flexor tendons in primates. J. Hand Surg., 7:436–444, 1982.

Manske, P. R., Gelberman, R. H., Vande Berg, J. S., and Leske, P. A.: Intrinsic flexor tendon repair. A morphological study in vitro. J. Bone Joint Surg., 66A:385–396, 1984.

Pennington, D. G.: The locking loop tendon suture. Plast. Reconstr. Surg., 63:648–652, 1979.

Schlenker, J. D., Lister, G. D., and Kleinert, H. E.: Three complications of untreated partial laceration of flexor tendon—entrapment, rupture, and triggering. J. Hand Surg., 6:392–396, 1981.

Seradge, H.: Elongation of the repair configuration following flexor tendon repair. J. Hand Surg., 8:182–185, 1983.

Strickland, J. W., and Glogovac, S. V.: Digital function following flexor tendon repair on zone II: A comparison of immobilization and controlled passive motion technique. J. Hand Surg., 5:537–543, 1980.

Chapter 29

THE BEVEL (BECKER) TECHNIQUE FOR FLEXOR TENDON REPAIR

HILTON BECKER
AND JOHN A. I. GROSSMAN

The aim in primary repair of flexor tendon injuries in the hand is the achievement of full function. Adhesion formation is often the limiting factor in reaching this goal, and since early active motion seems to increase tendon healing and to maintain gliding, it seems reasonable to employ a method of tendon suturing that respects these two concepts (Becker et al., 1981; Furlow, 1976; Lundborg and Rnak, 1978). Such a method should allow the tendons to heal by intrinsic processes, respecting the fascicular pattern of the cut ends and limiting the formation of adhesions on the interface between the cut ends.

Several reports indicate that a "bevel" technique for flexor tendon repair coupled with early active motion satisfies these requirements and, when properly performed, can provide consistently good results (Becker, 1978; Becker et al., 1979; Pribaz et al., 1981). This method is applicable in all cases in which primary or delayed primary repair of lacerated flexor tendons in the hand is indicated. Our current technique for this repair differs in several ways from that originally described by the senior author (Becker, 1978; Becker et al., 1979).

TECHNIQUE

The operation is always done with a tourniquet. Antibiotics are always given prophylactically. It is essential that both the surgeon and his first assistant operate with the aid of magnification (3.5 to 4.5×), using fine forceps and scissors.

The tendon sheath is exposed and, where necessary, the pulley(s) opened by a step incision that allows a closure creating a pulley of a larger diameter (Fig. 29–1). A wide exposure is essential to allow performance of the repair. Both tendons are repaired if possible.

The tendon ends are carefully brought into the wound and held in position with Keith needles. Great care is taken to protect and preserve the vincula.

The two tendon ends are beveled on reciprocal surfaces for approximately 0.75 cm. This can be done either with fine curved iris

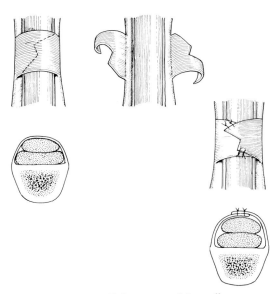

Figure 29–1. Enlargement of the pulley.

213

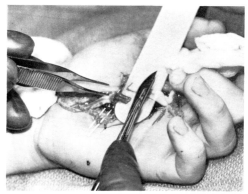

Figure 29–2. The tendon ends are beveled.

overlapping ends of unbeveled tendon and continues distally past the bevel before being woven back. Originally stay sutures were placed laterally to hold the tendon ends. We now routinely avoid using them, and if a stay suture is necessary, we remove it after the weave is completed. This reduces the amount of suture material in the repair. In addition, the knot on each side is buried between the beveled flaps of tendon. The step incision on the pulley is closed, the Keith needles are removed, and the digit is passively flexed and extended completely to ensure free movement of the tendon within the fibro-osseous canal.

The strength of the repair is immediately obvious. As a result of the suture technique, when tension is applied, longitudinal forces are converted into horizontal compressive forces.

The tourniquet is released and complete hemostasis obtained. The skin is carefully closed with 5-0 nylon simple sutures. The hand is placed in a large bulky gauze dressing with a dorsal block splint extending past the fingertip. The wrist is flexed 25 to 30 degrees and the metacarpophalangeal joints to 80 degrees.

scissors or with a fresh number 20 blade and a tongue depressor (Fig. 29–2). At certain levels (e.g., distal sublimis) where the two tendon ends are quite flat, it is unnecessary to bevel them.

The two beveled ends are overlapped, and a running stitch of 4-0 or 5-0 Prolene is woven along the edge (Fig. 29–3). Neither suture line approaches the midaxis of the tendon, thus protecting the vessels. The stitch starts at least several millimeters proximal to the

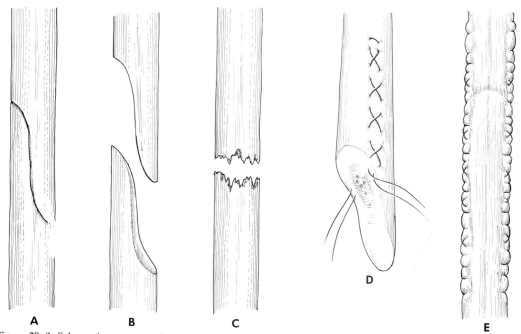

Figure 29–3. Schematic representation of the repair. The cut tendon is beveled if necessary (*A, B*) and overlapped for approximately 0.75 cm. (*C*). The weaving suture is done along the edge of the tendon to respect the vascularity and is continued proximally and distally to the bevel for about 5 mm. (*D, E*).

POSTOPERATIVE MANAGEMENT

Immediately postoperatively, under the supervision of the physician or therapist, the patient is encouraged to actively move his distal phalanx. He is instructed to stop when any pain occurs. Over the course of the following three weeks small amounts of gauze are removed from the dressing, and the patient is encouraged to increase his movement within the pain-free range.

Most patients can touch the palm within 15 days. Skin sutures are removed at three weeks. A dorsal block splint with the wrist at 25 degrees is maintained for six weeks, and all movement against resistance is forbidden. Close supervision by the hand therapist is mandatory.

In 60 patients (130 tendons) followed for an average of two months, results were graded according to the criteria of Lister et al. (1977). Good to excellent results were achieved in 75 per cent. There was an overall 10 per cent incidence of rupture. These results compare favorably with those obtained by other groups using this technique.

COMPLICATIONS

There is the possibility of several varieties of complications with this technique. Attention to the technical details of the procedure and awareness of this potential constitute the best prevention. Rupture occurred in 10 per cent of the cases. It results from disregard of the limits imposed on postoperative active motion and inadvertent cutting of the sutures

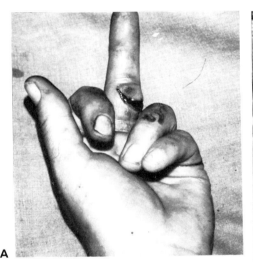

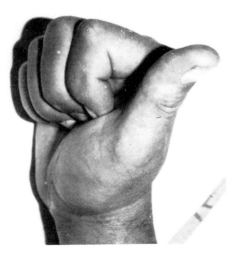

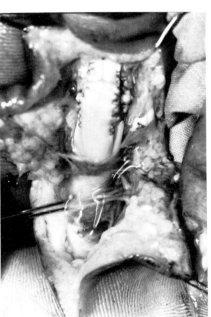

Figure 29–4. Clinical example. *A*, Section of the flexor tendons of the middle finger at the level of the proximal phalanx. *B*, Suture by the bevel technique. *C*, Results.

during the weaving process. Uncooperative patients should be closely followed and their range of motion carefully and slowly increased by reducing the bulky dressing over a longer time period. We now use 4-0 or 5-0 Prolene on a small tapered needle to avoid cutting the suture, an occurrence in two cases. Originally 6-0 or 7-0 Prolene on a cutting needle was employed. In cases of rupture, immediate reoperation using the same bevel technique is mandatory. A good to excellent result can be expected.

We are currently experimenting with a new nonabsorbable suture with a very high tensile strength (7-0 size) and low reactivity that cannot be damaged with a cutting needle, as this is the ideal instrument for the repair. In addition, some of the newer absorbable sutures show promise for use in flexor tendon surgery.

The breakdown of the skin incisions with early motion can be avoided by limiting motion to only the distal phalanx for five days and using a careful everting wound closure. As with all flexor tendon repairs, some prolonged stiffness and a slow return of extension can be expected in a number of cases. As the experience of the surgeon and therapist increases with this technique, these problems will be minimized.

There is no perfect method for flexor tendon repair. The advantages of the bevel technique with early active motion are both the-oretical and functional. The repair is strong enough to permit patients to actively obtain a good range of motion very early (10 days) and to touch the palm in two to three weeks (Fig. 29–4). Moreover, a return to work is hastened. The strength of the repair has encouraged us to apply it to extensor tendon injuries, tendon grafts, tendon transfers, and for shortening of an elongated tendon in tenolysis.

REFERENCES

Becker, H.: Primary repair of flexor tendons in the hand without immobilization—preliminary report. Hand, *10*:37, 1978.

Becker, H., and Davidoff, M.: Eliminating the gap in flexor tendon surgery. Hand, 9:306, 1977.

Becker, H., Graham, M., Cohen, I., and Diegelmann, R.: Intrinsic tendon cell proliferation in tissue culture. J. Hand Surg., 6:616, 1981.

Becker, H., Orak, F., and Duponselle, E.: Early active motion following a beveled technique for flexor tendon repair—report on fifty cases. J. Hand Surg., *4*:454, 1979.

Furlow, L. T.: The role of tendon tissues in tendon healing. Plast. Reconstr. Surg., 57:39, 1976.

Lister, G., Kleinert, H., Kutz, J., and Atasoy, E.: Primary flexor tendon repair followed by immediate controlled mobilization. J. Hand Surg., 2:441, 1977.

Lundborg, G., and Rnak, F.: Experimental intrinsic healing of flexor tendons based upon synovial fluid nutrition. J. Hand Surg., *3*:21, 1978.

Pribaz, J., Morrison, W., and MacLeod, A.: Primary repair of flexor tendons in no man's land using the Becker repair. Plast. Surg. Forum, *4*:122, 1981.

Chapter 30

FLEXOR TENDON GRAFTS IN THE HAND

RAOUL TUBIANA

The aim in using flexor tendon grafts is to restore active flexion of the fingers when end to end repair of the divided tendons is risky or impossible. Such grafts offer two advantages: They allow repair without excess tension, and the sutures can be placed optimally away from fixed fibrous structures.

The earliest attempts at tendon grafting were made about 1880, but it was only after publication of the work of Biesalski (1910) and Lexer (1912) that this procedure became accepted. Even today the results are often far from perfect, especially when local conditions are not optimal because of associated lesions that alter the gliding structures. In these cases it appears to be preferable to proceed with two stage reconstruction; the first stage is devoted to reconstructing a new tendon sheath as a bed for the graft, which is introduced in the second stage.

The technique and results of two stage tendon grafting are discussed in Chapter 32 by Hunter. We shall deal here with flexor tendon grafting accomplished in one stage.

Until only a few years ago one stage flexor tendon grafting was the most frequently used method for repairing flexor tendon injuries in the "no man's land" area. They have been used less frequently since the "rediscovery" of primary suturing and the development of two stage techniques.

PRINCIPLES OF THE TECHNIQUE

Watching experienced surgeons in Europe and the United States, one is struck by the diversity of technique. Often a surgeon stresses the importance of a technical detail that is neglected by others with a similar proportion of successful results. As we shall see, few axioms are universally accepted.

A variety of skin incisions are used. Some surgeons use short interrupted palmar incisions; others prefer a large digitopalmar approach. In the finger, some incise anterior, and others posterior, to the neurovascular bundle. The flexor profundus is usually reconstructed, but reconstruction of the flexor superficialis offers some advantages.

The sources of the graft are as varied as the methods of fixation of the extremities of the graft.

It is agreed that suture material should be fine, nonirritating, and resistant, but some use silk whereas most prefer steel wire or nylon.

The duration of immobilization has been the subject of lengthy discussion. Pulvertaft (1956), however, following a comparative trial, showed that his results were the same with early motion and after three weeks of immobilization with the wrist and fingers flexed.

Which principles are in fact universally accepted? There are indeed very few, but they are important.

1. Only one flexor is grafted per digit because of the risk of adhesions. Reconstitution of the normal anatomical features, i.e., two flexor grafts as used by Lexer (1924), is now avoided. In a few selected cases the flexor profundus may be grafted in the presence of an intact flexor superficialis.

2. However, under no circumstances should an intact superficialis tendon be removed to replace a profundus.

3. The extremities of the graft should be sutured in zones where adhesion to neighboring structures does not compromise mobility.

4. As much of the flexor pulley system as possible should be preserved.

5. The length of the graft should be carefully adjusted in each case.

6. There should be no tension at the suture lines.

7. Finally, the one common factor among all surgeons who achieve success in this field is meticulous surgical technique. Careful suturing, good hemostasis, and scrupulous postoperative care are essential for a good prognosis. In addition to conforming to these broad principles, each operative stage must be adapted to individual circumstances.

We shall first consider the usual method of graft replacement of the flexor profundus in the fingers. Next we shall review the techniques for reconstructing the flexor superficialis when both flexors have been destroyed, the flexor profundus when the superficialis is intact, and the flexor pollicis longus.

METHOD OF GRAFTING DIGITAL FLEXOR TENDONS

INCISIONS

Interrupted incisions, which were once popular, necessitated difficult subcutaneous tunneling. It seems paradoxical to advocate the use of short stepped incisions in the hand to dissect in difficult anatomical areas while using long incisions in the leg or forearm to obtain grafts. It appears that the latter can be extracted through limited incisions without adversely affecting the ultimate result. By contrast, a long continuous digitopalmar incision provides a much better exposure (Fig. 30–1).

In the fingers, a lateral W incision is preferable to the Bruner anterior zigzag (Fig. 30–2), since it is easier to suture with the finger flexed and the scar does not overlie the tendons. In practice the pre-existent scars are often used in part.

If tendon lesions are present in adjacent digits, only one digital incision is extended into the palm. A small subcutaneous tunnel can be formed at the base of one of the fingers (Fig. 30–3).

EXPOSING THE LESIONS

In operating upon the fingers some surgeons prefer to pass in front, and others behind, the neurovascular bundle. The important points are to protect the bundles and not to alter sensation in the digit.

The bundles are safe if the skin approach remains posterior to Cleland's ligament, which connects the skin to the lateral aspects of the phalanges—but then all the dorsal neurovascular branches are divided, and this may be a severe handicap if the opposite

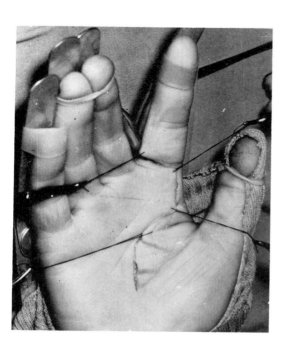

Figure 30–1. Sinuous digitopalmar approach to the index finger. It is preferable to situate the digital incision of the index finger on the ulnar surface, which is not a grip area (whereas the radial surface is a greatly used grip area.)

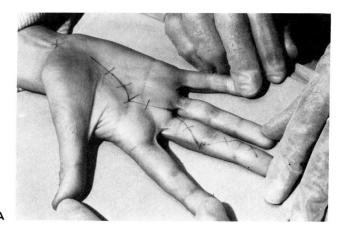

Figure 30–2. Zigzag incisions. *A*, Bruner anterior zigzag incision. *B*, Zigzag incision with W-lateralization in finger, which we now prefer as the approach to the flexor tendons. Suturing is easier at the end of the operation, with the finger flexed, and, above all the scar does not overlie the tendons.

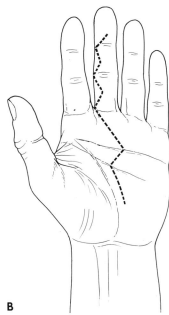

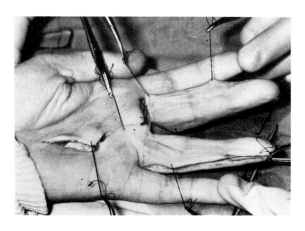

Figure 30–3. Tendon lesions in adjacent fingers; only one of the digital incisions is extended into the palm.

bundle has already been damaged (Fig. 30–4). When scar tissue makes dissection difficult, it is preferable to expose the neurovascular pedicles in proximal healthy tissue and follow their course. When a midlateral incision is used (Fig. 30–1), the approach to the neurovascular pedicles is volar in the proximal portion of the finger in order to preserve the dorsal branches, then passes dorsally at the distal half of the middle phalanx in order to preserve the branches to the pulp. A zigzag cutaneous incision allows an approach which remains volar to the pedicles throughout their course.

If associated nerve lesions exist, they are repaired only after fixation of the tendon graft.

The palmar fascia, which is a possible source of adhesions, is resected in the area that will come into contact with the graft.

PREPARING THE GRAFT BED

A broad exposure facilitates preparation of the graft bed. At this stage one must consider the amount of tendon and sheath to remove.

The Sheaths

The attitude toward the fibrous and synovial flexor sheaths has changed considerably in recent years. For a long time the tendency was to resect as much of the sheaths as possible and to preserve only narrow pulleys. The reasoning was that the sheaths formed a barrier against vascularization of the graft

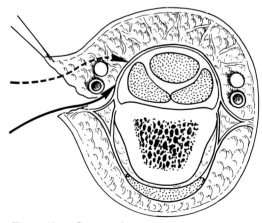

Figure 30–4. Cross section at the base of a finger. The neurovascular bundles are anterior to Cleland's fascia.

and that there was a risk of the graft's becoming adherent to a fixed structure. However, the mechanical action of the fibrous sheath is now better understood, as are the important repercussions of extensive sheath resection.

In effect, the opening of the fibrous sheath at the level of the metacarpophalangeal joint (A_1 pulley) has an important directional influence in the transverse plane. Loss of the A_1 pulley does not prevent complete finger flexion, but flexion of the metacarpophalangeal joint precedes that of the interphalangeal joints. (Advancement of the pulley is a procedure used in the treatment of paralyses of the intrinsic muscles.)

The A_3 pulley has a strategically important position but is not as strong as the A_2 and A_4 pulleys, which insert directly along a broad area on the shaft of the two proximal phalanges. The persistence of only these two pulleys (A_2 and A_4) can suffice for complete flexion of the phalanges, but the graft is not closely applied to the skeleton opposite the proximal interphalangeal joint, and in the retrotendinous space, scar tissue accumulates and may produce a flexion contracture of the joint (Fig. 30–5).

Experiments on cadavers, however imprecise because of differences in tissue resistance, demonstrated that the persistence of only either the A_2 or the A_4 pulley does not permit complete finger flexion. The A_2 pulley is the most useful and most resistant, followed by, in order of importance, the A_4, A_3, and A_1 pulleys. An effective pulley system must conserve or reconstitute A_2, A_4, and A_3. Finally, it is necessary to note that the skin, especially if scarred, can (very imperfectly) supply a pulley-like action.

In practice, the condition of the fibrous sheaths must also be taken into account.

Favorable Cases. Areas where the sheath is permeable and appears normal are not disturbed, while fibrous adherent segments are resected. In any case one strives to preserve or reconstruct flexion pulleys (Fig. 30–6).

When adhesions are few, three segments of the pulley system can be preserved. These are the thickened shinier areas of the sheath, opposite the metacarpophalangeal joint, and the shafts of the proximal two phalanges (A_1, A_2, A_4; Fig. 30–7).

Intermediate Cases. In the numerous cases in which the adhesions are such that pulleys cannot be preserved at the foregoing sites,

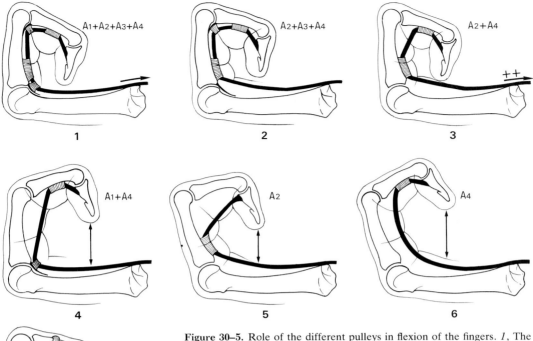

Figure 30–5. Role of the different pulleys in flexion of the fingers. *1*, The four normal pulleys ensure complete flexion of the phalanges. *2*, Elimination of A_1 does not prevent complete flexion of the fingers. *3*, Despite the elimination of A_1 and A_3, complete flexion of the finger remains possible by the presence of A_2 and A_4 only, but the force which the tendon must exert is greater. *4*, Persistence of the two pulleys A_1 and A_4 does not permit flexion of the finger. *5*, Persistence of pulley A_2 only; flexion of the finger is incomplete. *6*, Persistence of pulley A_4 only; the deficit is even greater. *7*, The three most useful pulleys which must be preserved and reconstructed are A_2, A_4, and A_3 (or a pulley just proximal to the proximal interphalangeal joint).

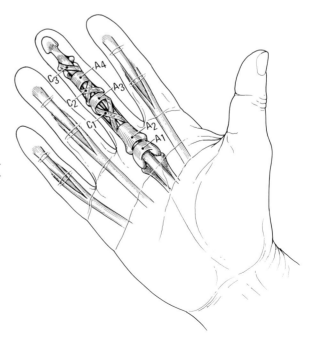

Figure 30–6. Diagram of the fibrous sheaths consisting of four annular portions and three cruciform portions (after Doyle and Blythe).

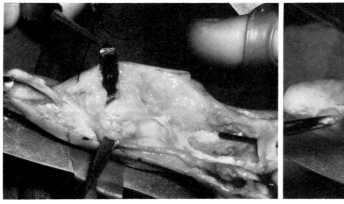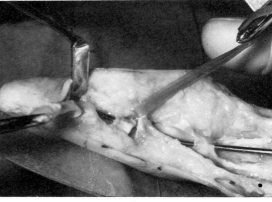

A   B

Figure 30–7. The flexor tendons are extirpated and cut into sections as needed, in such a way as to preserve the principal pulleys. *A*, A metal rod is passed through pulley A_2 at the proximal part of the proximal phalanx. *B*, The rod is passed beneath a pulley situated at the distal part of the phalanx just proximal to the proximal interphalangeal joint and beneath pulley A_4. The neurovascular bundle is retracted by a rubber vessel loop.

an attempt should be made to preserve at least one or two bands in a healthy segment. This site is determined by approaching the sheath transversely at several different levels. Incising the sheath blindly in its longitudinal axis produces unjustified mutilation.

When A_2 and A_1 cannot be conserved, but the sheath can be kept in good condition at the level of the middle phalanx, the choice is a difficult one. One is tempted, to gain time, to perform a graft and to construct a pulley at the same time, but this is not without risk. The alternative, as in unfavorable cases, consists of constructing a pulley around an implant as a first stage.

Unfavorable Cases. Sometimes the fibrous sheath cannot be salvaged and no pulley can be preserved. A new pulley could be constructed from a segment of tendon and solidly fixed to the bone, but the risk of adhesions to the underlying graft is so great that it is safer not to attempt immediate reconstruction of a pulley (see following section). Artificial pulleys made from synthetic materials have been suggested (Bader and Curtin, 1971), but seem to be seldom used because of fear of rupture of the underlying tendon. Prior to the era of two stage techniques using silicone implants, such cases posed a difficult surgical problem. The graft was usually placed in its bed after total resection of the sheaths with the hope that the skin would prevent excess bowstringing of the grafted tendon. Pulley reconstruction could be envisaged as a secondary procedure, but one usually settled for diminished flexion. The results

were so mediocre after extensive resection of the sclerotic sheaths that some authors preferred to insert the graft by tunneling in front of the fibrous sheath directly under the skin, all done through limited incisions.

The introduction of silicone implants made it possible to remove the tendon and its adherent sheaths as a first stage and to reconstruct pulleys by means of tendon grafts placed around the implant. Two to three months later the graft is slid into its new sheath by attaching it to the implant, which is then withdrawn without incising the new sheath.

PULLEY RECONSTRUCTION. Pulley reconstruction is fraught with numerous difficulties: First, the pulleys must resist considerable pressure from the tendon during flexion of the finger. Second, they must adapt strictly to the caliber of the flexor tendon without strangulation or interference with gliding. Third, they must not develop adhesions to the underlying tendon.

It is not possible to reconstruct the entire fibrous sheath, but it is preferable for mechanical reasons to reconstruct the most important pulleys at the level of the proximal and middle phalanges. Numerous techniques have been proposed. The most favorable site for a pulley, mechanically speaking, is as close as possible to the joint, distal to it. Bunnell and Boyes (1970) constructed a circular pulley around one phalanx. Riordan preferred to fix the graft with horizontal drill holes in the base of the proximal phalanx (Doyle and Blythe, 1975).

The technique we use differs when we reconstruct a pulley simultaneously with a graft, around a silicone implant, or as a secondary procedure after a graft.* In the first case one uses an intact tendon to reconstruct the pulley to limit the risk of adhesions—the palmaris longus or part of an extensor or the plantaris or a strip of the wrist dorsal retinaculum. Around an implant, on the contrary, one can use a piece of the resected flexor tendon, any tendon split lengthwise, or a strip of fascia lata. When we reconstruct a pulley for the proximal phalanx, we introduce a thin graft in a transverse bone tunnel made in the base of the proximal phalanx with a 2.5 mm. drill bit. The graft is then wrapped around the remnants of the fibrous sheath, which are attached to the bone, in such a manner that it makes two or three passes in front of the flexor tendon graft (or the implant). We do not cross the graft through the proximal phalanx twice, which would weaken it too much, we make a transosseous suture by using a fine drill permitting the passage of a suture which is tied over a button. This distal fixation being assured, the pulley tension can be adjusted by pulling the graft into its proximal osseous tunnel (Fig. 30–8). One flexes the digit to adjust the tension of the new pulley with the help of small mattress sutures between the graft and the remnants of the fibrous sheath.

This helical graft wrapped several times around the tendon provides the best mechanical advantage and best resists the pressure

*See discussion on the complications of grafts on page 225.

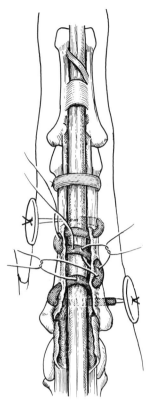

Figure 30–8. Diagram of the reconstruction of a pulley at the base of the finger using a graft of palmaris longus, fixed to the bone at both ends to reconstruct A_2. A circular graft at the distal part of the proximal phalanx reconstructs A_3.

of flexion (Fig. 30–9). The two extremities, firmly fixed in bone, allow passive mobilization (or active in the case of a tenolysis), thus diminishing the risk of adhesions. Because

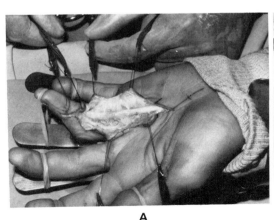

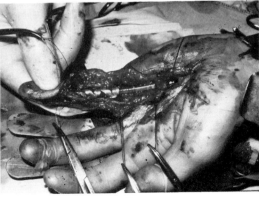

A   B

Figure 30–9. Reconstruction of a pulley at the base of the ring finger. *A*, Sequelae of flexor tendon lesion already operated upon twice. The finger is contracted, the tendons are adherent, and the pulleys are destroyed. *B*, The tendons have been extirpated and the contracture corrected. A broad proximal pulley is reconstructed from a palmaris longus tendon graft around a Silastic rod.

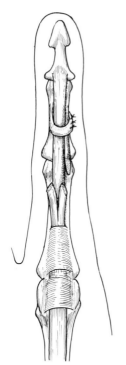

Figure 30–10. Reconstruction of a pulley at the level of the middle phalanx using insertion band of the flexor superficialis.

Excision of Injured Tendons and Evaluation of Passive Joint Motion

When the fibrous sheath is widely excised, it is relatively easy to remove even adherent tendons under direct vision. A narrow tenotome blade is preferable to a blind stripper. Some precautions must be taken during the dissection, especially at the level of the joints. One must make every effort to avoid damaging articular structures. Volarly the joints are often closely adherent to the flexor profundus at the metacarpophalangeal and distal interphalangeal joints or the flexor superficialis at the proximal interphalangeal joint. Opening the joints leads to stiffness. Detachment of the volar plate tends to produce instability in hyperextension, especially at the proximal interphalangeal joint. In some patients this joint is normally lax in hyperextension, whereas in others laxity follows division of the insertions of the flexor superficialis. In the absence of an active superficialis, the presence of laxity in hyperextension may lead to flexion difficulties (to be described).

The other fingers should always be tested for hyperextension. If they show unusual laxity, the insertion bands of the flexor superficialis at the proximal interphalangeal joint of the injured finger should not be resected (Fig. 30–11). Generally we do not detach these bands unless their adhesions prevent the correction of extension of the joint. If extension of the proximal interphalangeal joint is normal after excision of the flexor profundus, we preserve the distal part

the graft crosses several times, a tendon length of about 10 cm. (the total length of the palmaris longus tendon in an adult) is required.

Lister (1979) has recommended the use of a band taken from the dorsal retinaculum of the wrist to reconstruct the proximal pulley. He passes a band 6 to 8 cm. long and 8 mm. in width for one pulley around the proximal phalanx and the flexor tendons and deep to the neurovascular bundles and superficial to the extensor apparatus. The two ends of the band are crossed over and sutured. This material, which is wide and solid, has been used around grafts and Silastic implants. It permits immediate mobilization after tenolysis.

For the middle phalanx the simplest technique consists of using one of the bands of insertion of the superficial flexors while conserving its bony insertions (Tubiana, 1960; Fig. 30–10). We now use this procedure only around an implant. If the insertion of the superficial flexor is not usable, a graft, or a band from the dorsal retinaculum is necessary.

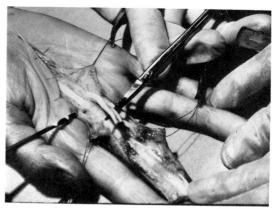

Figure 30–11. The insertion bands of flexor superficialis are preserved in front of the proximal interphalangeal joint except when their adhesions prevent the correction of the contracture. The flexor superficialis tendon is removed under the pulley.

of the flexor superficialis because its removal allows hyperextension of the joint and, as shown by Potenza (1979), promotes the formation of adhesions with the graft.

The passive mobility of all the joints of the finger can be improved by the removal of adherent flexor tendons. Marked stiffness of the metacarpophalangeal or proximal interphalangeal joint is normally a contraindication to grafting. In contrast, stiffness of the distal interphalangeal joint is not, but as we shall see later, the superficialis rather than the profundus can then be reconstructed.

CHOICE OF THE MOTOR MUSCLE

The flexor profundus is commonly used as a motor muscle because of its long excursion and because it receives the insertion of the lumbrical muscle. However, these advantages are only theoretical. We shall see that the presence of a lumbrical muscle can be detrimental. Also the independent bellies of the flexor superficialis enjoy greater freedom of movement.

In practice one should carefully free the proximal portion of the tendons, strip them of their fibrotic coverings, and test the excursion of each muscle by pulling on its tendon. The one with the longest excursion is chosen as the motor muscle. It is known that the course of the flexor tendons can exceed 6 cm. at the wrist. However, when these secondary repairs are studied, contractions of the motor muscles show an excursion of only 2.5 to 3 cm. in the palm. Nevertheless, this course is sufficient for obtaining complete flexion of the grafted finger when wrist movements are normal. Supplementary contributions from wrist extension makes up for the deficit in amplitude of the flexor muscle. Patients having flexor tendon grafts in the presence of wrist stiffness risk having less than perfect results. In the little finger the flexor profundus is a safer choice than the superficialis, which is usually much weaker. Some surgeons try to reinforce their actions by suturing the two muscles, but in practice the one with the shorter excursion restricts the other.

CHOICE OF THE GRAFT

We have had no experience with homografts and have always used autografts to replace flexor tendons. Our choice in order of preference is as follows:

Palmaris Longus. The palmaris longus tendon, which is accessible in the same operative field, can supply a graft long enough to run from the tip of the finger to the proximal part of the palm. We take it through two oblique small incisions at the wrist and on the forearm (Fig. 30–12); these can be extended if necessary. The distal extremity of the tendon is first divided and a traction suture is passed twice through the tendon in planes perpendicular to each other. The distal extremity often adheres to the fascia and is freed by subcutaneous dissection for 3 or 4 cm. Traction on this end allows the muscle to be palpated beneath the skin. A short oblique incision 1.5 cm. long is made about 12 to 13 cm. proximally in the forearm of an adult male. The tendon usually receives its

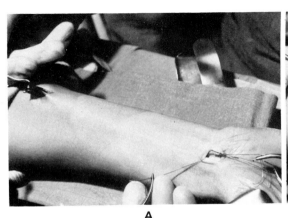
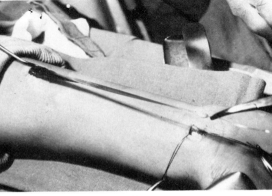

| A | B |

Figure 30–12. *A* and *B*, Removal of the tendon of the palmaris longus via two short oblique incisions.

more distal muscle fibers at this level. A second traction suture is passed through this end of the tendon, which is freed from its muscle fibers. The tendon is then divided and pulled. The graft can also be taken using a Brand stripper (Fig. 30–13).

Plantaris. The plantaris is useful for a long graft (finger tip to wrist), for providing two grafts, or for a single thin tendon graft to replace the flexor profundus when the flexor digitorum superficialis is intact. However, unlike the palmaris longus, its presence cannot be ascertained preoperatively.

We usually proceed as follows: The ipsilateral lower limb is prepared for surgery whenever it appears that the plantaris may be required, i.e., in cases already mentioned in which the plantaris is preferable, when the palmaris longus is absent, and when a graft is required for the middle finger and the palmaris longus may be too short.

A tourniquet is placed around the thigh but is not inflated until needed. The limb is prepared with antiseptic and wrapped in sterile stockinette. Only after the hand lesions have been exposed and confirmed should an assistant start on the leg. The cuff is then inflated and the medial border of the tendo-Achilles is exposed. If the plantaris is present, it is usually excised by the surgeon himself only when the graft bed is ready for its reception. For a long time we used Brand's blunt stripper. Later we extracted the tendon through a second incision in the upper part of the leg (Fig. 30–14) without the stripper to try to reduce the damage to the epitenon. An incision 6 cm. long is made at the superomedial portion of the calf, two fingerbreadths behind the medial aspect of the tibia. The fascia is incised; a slender plantaris tendon is found deep in the space between the soleus and medial head of the gastrocnemius.

Our results do not seem to have been influenced by the technique used to obtain the graft. We preserve a thin membrane of areolar tissue around the graft. Excess paratenon is excised.

Flexor Superficialis. We rarely use a flexor superficialis tendon for grafting except for short bridge grafts, but this graft is preferred by certain surgeons including Littler. In cases of tendon lesions in more than one finger, however, it has proved possible to use the

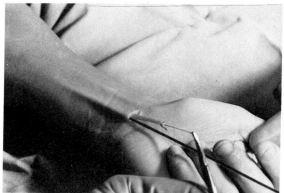

A

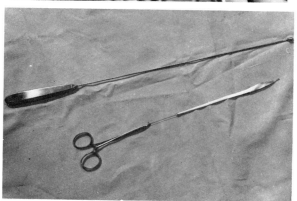

B

Figure 30–13. *A* and *B*, Graft taken using a Brand stripper. The stripper is rarely used to obtain the palmaris longus tendon, the proximal extremity of which is superficial. It is mostly used to obtain the tendon of plantaris, the proximal extremity of which is deep.

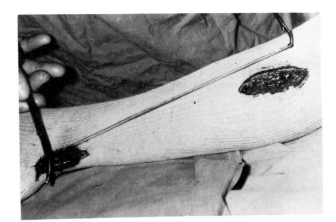

Figure 30–14. Taking a long graft of plantaris via two medial incisions on the leg.

discarded superficial flexor of a longer finger as a graft for the shorter one. End to end suture economizes on tendon graft length. In the little finger the flexor superficialis tendon, which is always slender, can be used as a graft.

Extensor Digitorum of the Toes. The extensor digitorum tendons (of the toes) are used when the foregoing grafting material is not available. After the plantaris, however, it is the tendon of choice to replace a first stage silicone implant. We then remove the extensor of the fourth toe or several extensors when there exist multiple tendon lesions requiring several grafts. On the other hand, the toe extensors are presently used in cases in which the graft is placed secondary to a silicone implant. We try to take them by using a stripper or by making several short separate incisions on the dorsum of the foot (Fig. 30–15), but often we are obliged to unite these incisions to liberate the extensor tendons, which have frequent interconnections. We have always used each tendon separately, and although it is anatomically possible to fashion a many tailed graft when the extensor is taken high up at the ankle, we have had no experience with this.

Whatever type of graft is used, it is always immediately placed in its digital bed without soaking it in saline. It is passed under the pulleys by means of traction threads and sutured at one of its extremities.

FIXATION OF THE GRAFT AND DETERMINATION OF ITS TENSION

Some surgeons prefer first to fix the proximal end of the graft and find it easier to adjust its tension distally.* For similar reasons we prefer to tether the distal end first on a fixed bony point. The skin of the finger can then be sutured before the tension is adjusted (because it constitutes an important element in the regulation of the tension). However, regardless of whether the proximal or distal end is sutured first, the important point is to insure the correct adjustment of tension in the graft.

Distal Fixation

The following points are important when the distal end is fixed: First, fixation should be firm, and this can be achieved by keeping the extremity of the tendon in contact with decorticated bone. For the graft to function at its best mechanical advantage, it must be inserted at the anatomical site. Finally, the graft should not be bulky, because the anastomosis might interfere with movement at a nearby joint.

Our method of fixation is basically that devised by Bunnell (1944)—a transosseous pullout suture combined with a suture joining the graft to the stump of the profundus tendon (Fig. 30–16).

The residual stump of the flexor profundus tendon, which has been preserved to a length of less than 1 cm., is divided along its midline to its insertion. A small osteoperiosteal flap is raised from the bone to receive the graft. The bone at this point is perforated with an awl or a drill in the middle of the nail distal to the lunula to avoid damaging the matrix.

The graft is fixed to the bone by means of a pullout suture of 3-0 nylon. Depending on

---

*This method is discussed by Pulvertaft in Chapter 31.

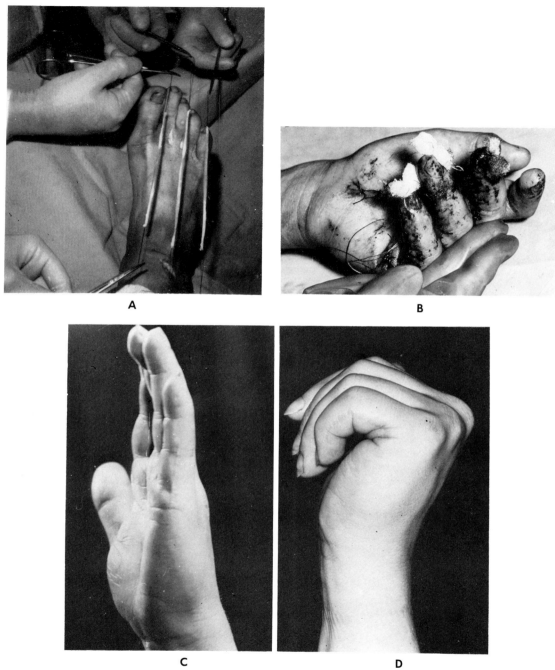

Figure 30–15. Graft of the three ulnar fingers. *A,* The extensor digitorum tendons of the toes are obtained using a stripper. *B,* Position of the three grafted fingers. *C* and *D,* Result.

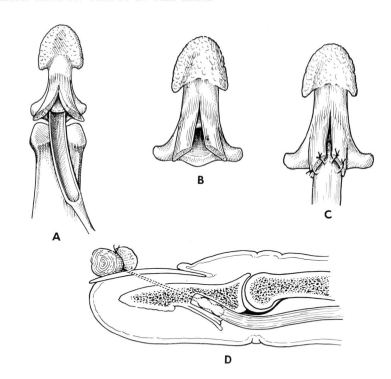

Figure 30–16. Distal fixation of the graft. *A*, The distal extremity of the flexor profundus tendon is divided in the midline. A small gouge raises a osteoperiosteal flap beneath the tendon. *B*, View of the small bone niche into which the tip of the graft will be inserted. *C*, The extremities of the flexor profundus tendon are sutured to the graft to hold it in its niche. *D*, Views of the final arrangement showing the tip of the graft in its niche and its transosseous anchoring suture perforating the nail attached over a small pad (or a button). The small bone flap raised by the gouge is reapplied over the graft.

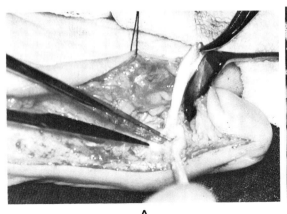

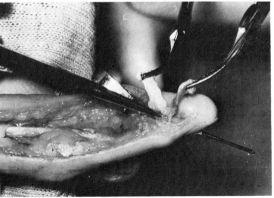

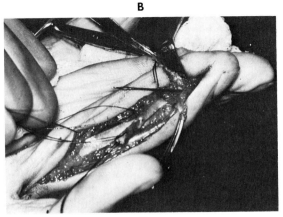

Figure 30–17. Different stages of distal fixation. *A*, A small area of bone is raised and excavated at the site of the insertion of the flexor profundus tendon, which has been split in two longitudinally. A small osteoperiosteal flap is raised using a small gouge, and the bone underneath is perforated with a bradawl or drill. *B*, This bradawl passes through the bone and nail obliquely, distal to the lunula. *C*, A straight needle is passed in a retrograde direction through the bony tunnel starting at the nail, since it is easier to first insert the blunt end through the ungual orifice than the point which catches in the bone.

the mode of fixation, one or both ends of the
suture are threaded through a large straight
needle, which transfixes the distal phalanx
(in practice, it is easier to pass the needle
blunt end first from the nail side) (Fig. 30–
17). The graft is then held in place by suturing
it to the residual stump of the flexor profundus. A fine 4-0 suture is used and should be
kept separate from the transosseous stitch.
The heavy 3-0 transosseous stitch is then tied
without tension on the nail or over a button.
It is removed four weeks later. It is important
that this suture be pulled out distally because
traction in the proximal direction might dis-
lodge the suture (Fig. 30–18).

When the graft is first fixed proximally, the
tension is adjusted distally. A small graft is
passed through the distal segment of the
flexor digitorum profundus tendon, then in
contact with the anterior surface of the distal
phalanx with the aid of a rongeur. The graft
traverses the skin at the tip of the pulp under
the nail. The length is then adjusted (Fig.
30–19). The graft is fixed over the dorsal face
of the nail and is attached to it.

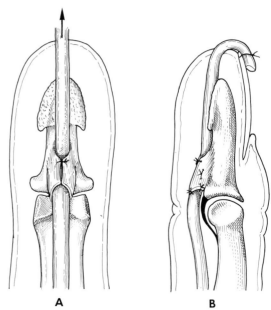

Figure 30–19. Secondary proximal fixation. *A*, When
the graft is first fixed proximally, it is passed through the
distal insertion of flexor digitorum profundus. The palmar surface of the distal phalanx is abraded along its
whole length using a small gouge. The tension of the
graft is adjusted by pulling it distally. *B*, Once suitable
tension is obtained, the graft is fixed to the distal end of
flexor profundus and to the nail.

Adjusting the Tension

This is a vital stage of the operation. Unfortunately there are no objective criteria for
adjusting the length of the graft to the contractility of the motor muscle. For greater
accuracy, some surgeons suggest that the
operation not be performed under general
anesthesia and that, with the cuff deflated,
the length of the graft be adjusted while the
patient actively flexes and extends the finger.
Others prefer to apply a standard faradic
stimulus to the synergistic muscles to induce
contraction of the unit formed by the motor
muscle and the graft (Omer, 1965).

These methods, however ingenious, are
not free from error. Frequently the motor
muscle has not functioned for a prolonged
period of time. Besides such methods may
complicate and prolong an already lengthy
surgical procedure. Like most surgeons, we
rely on more empirical means of assessment.

Once the distal fixation is finished, the skin
of the finger is sutured. When a lateral incision has been used, we first insert several
nylon stitches into the digital fascia and scar
tissue to prevent significant bowstringing of

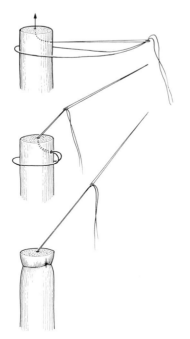

Figure 30–18. Planas technique for transosseous fixation over a button or a small bundle of padding by a
pull-out suture. The suture is removed by distal traction,
which is an advantage over the pull-out suture of Bunnell
in which extraction has the risk of pulling the extremity
of the graft proximally.

the graft when a large part of the fibrous flexor sheath has been resected. We then supplement these as required with stitches in the skin. This is an indispensable preliminary step to the correct adjustment of tension in the graft. Next we test the excursion of the motor muscle by pulling its tendon with the aid of a traction suture. Once the mobility range has been determined, we immobilize the motor tendon halfway through its course by a needle transfixing the skin and the motor tendon transversely, the wrist being held in the neutral position.

Clearly the shorter the excursion of the motor muscle, the more difficult it is to adjust its length. The length of the graft is such that with the wrist held in neutral, the grafted finger is flexed 15 degrees more than in a normal position of function, the fingers on the ulnar side being, as is physiologically correct, more markedly flexed than those on the radial side.* The graft is then provisionally sutured to the motor tendon to maintain this position. The needle uniting the motor tendon to the skin is removed, and with the wrist in about 40 degrees of flexion, it should be possible to fully extend the grafted finger. Full wrist extension should carry the pulp of the flexed finger to within 3 or 4 cm. of the palm. A landmark stitch is used to indicate the correct length of the graft.

Proximal Fixation

A malleable splint or an assistant holds the finger in a relaxed position while the tendon is being sutured proximally. The site and mode of the proximal fixation pose a number of problems that do not apply with the distal suture. Although the distal end is fixed at a point where by definition the flexor tendon has no mobility, the proximal suture lies at or near the point of greatest excursion. Adhesions between the tendon and the fixed structures, beneficial distally, must be avoided at all costs at the proximal suture line.

The Site. The proximal suture should lie in a zone where the tissues are mobile, away from the fixed fibrous structures (osteofibrous flexor tunnel) to which it might become adherent. This constitutes one of the main advantages of the graft. There are two favorable

*See the chapter on positions of immobilization in Volume II.

sites—the proximal part of the palm and the wrist.

Which of the two should one choose? The wrist is physiologically preferable. The most likely adhesions are to the adjacent tendons, which are mobilized at the same time anyway. However, most grafts are sutured in the palm because this requires a shorter graft length; only a plantaris graft is long enough to reach the wrist. Some surgeons used to wrap the lumbrical muscle around the suture line, but this is not without risk. We usually suture the graft at the proximal part of the palm. When this region appears too extensively scarred, the graft is sutured above the wrist, but we then prefer to use a two-stage graft technique.

The Mode of Fixation. The mode of fixation depends on the type of graft used. If the graft has a caliber similar to that of the motor tendon, an end to end crisscross suture or a grasping suture of the Mason-Kessler type is used. If, as occurs most commonly, the graft has a smaller caliber, we prefer the interlacing technique, developed by Pulvertaft, which compensates for the difference in caliber (Fig. 30–20). The slender tendon graft transfixes the motor muscle at two or three points in different planes beginning about 1 cm. from its extremity. Fixation is then completed by a row of small interrupted sutures. The end of the tendon is partially split and opened out in such a way as to ensheath the graft. The whole junction is then modeled into a spindle by means of a few very fine stitches (Fig. 30–21).

Admittedly this transfixion method creates a bulkier junction and requires a longer graft, but the fixation is then more secure and the bare ends of the tendons are not exposed.

There is as yet no conclusive evidence that the risk of adhesions is significantly reduced if the suture is "sheathed." Isolation by means of artificial sheaths cannot yet be advocated, and in the hand, sheathing the suture within the lumbrical runs the risk of producing a lumbrical retraction syndrome.

Brand's method of sheathing the suture by splaying out the extremity of the graft is readily feasible when the plantaris is used, and it is esthetically pleasing, but we are not convinced that it reduces the chance of adhesions. The same applies to the technique whereby a thin collarette of paratenon is folded back over the suture in the extrasynovial zones above the wrist.

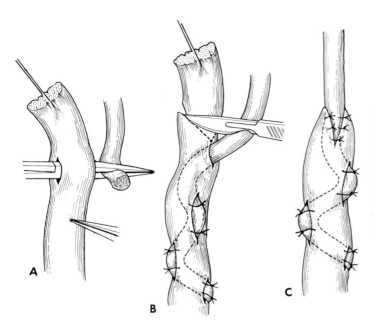

Figure 30–20. Diagram of proximal fixation. The interlacing technique of Pulvertaft may be used to compensate for the difference in caliber between the graft and the flexor tendon. *A*, The motor tendon is transfixed using a finely pointed tendon forceps. Successive transfixions are in different planes, perpendicular to each other. *B*, The end of the motor tendon is cut into two valves between which the graft is placed. *C*, Modeling of the anastomosis.

HEMOSTASIS, CLOSURE, AND DRESSINGS

Hemostasis

Meticulous hemostasis is necessary for success, for a hematoma may jeopardize the result. Depending on the time taken for the dissection, we release the cuff after the distal fixation is completed and before closing the digital skin. The proximal fixation can be carried out without the tourniquet. If the dissection has not been prolonged, the cuff is kept inflated until the two extremities of the graft have been sutured, the digital skin having been closed only temporarily to help adjust the tension.

Closure

To promote rapid primary healing, the skin is closed with carefully placed, fine interrupted sutures.

Dressings

The hand is molded in an elastic compressive dressing that includes all the fingers with only the tips protruding. It is kept immobilized for three weeks to avoid tension at the suture lines and to allow for revascularization. The wrist and fingers are maintained in a relaxed position by a dorsal plaster splint. This position should be carefully chosen,

being different from that adopted during adjustment of the graft. In children and young adults we do not hesitate to maintain the wrist in 40 degrees of flexion. In older patients wrist flexion should be less. However, tension can be relieved by holding the metacarpophalangeal joints in about 70 degrees of flexion; less flexion is applied to the interphalangeal joints where the recovery of extension is notoriously slow. The proximal interphalangeal joints are flexed to about 30 degrees and the distal interphalangeal joints are almost totally extended.

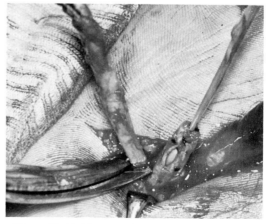

Figure 30–21. Photographs of proximal fixation. The unused flexor superficialis tendon is excised.

POSTOPERATIVE CARE AND RE-EDUCATION

The operated limb is kept elevated. Mobilization of the finger following flexor tendon repair poses different problems after suturing, after one-stage tendon grafting, or after a two-stage graft. Indeed, the conditions of nutrition are different, depending upon whether or not there is a sheath and on the length of the devascularized tendon. The precarious condition of the nutrition of a one-stage graft whose sheath has been largely resected requires great care when movements are restarted. Although a technique of early passive mobilization is used after suturing or two-stage grafting, it seems preferable, for fear of tendon rupture, to maintain a one-stage graft immobilized in the relaxed position for 10 days. Then, with the wrist and metacarpophalangeal joints still immobilized by a dorsal splint, passive mobilization of the operated finger is undertaken by manipulation or elastic traction. The amplitude of passive movements is greatly limited by the dressing.

The splint is removed after 25 days, but contraction against strong resistance risks rupturing the sutures, particularly at the more fragile distal junction, for several more weeks. For this reason, the distal suture is left in place for another week after the splint is removed.

The period that follows, during which motion is begun, is critical for the future of the graft. The surgeon should personally supervise all stages of re-education and see the patient every week at least for the first month after the plaster cast is removed.

Re-education after flexor tendon grafting is considered in detail in another chapter,* but we shall briefly outline the principles of physical therapy with which every hand surgeon should be familiar (Tubiana, 1974). The aim is to recover, first, passive flexion, and then active flexion without resistance, active extension, passive extension, and finally active flexion against resistance. This is a generalization, which must be adapted for each of the joints (Table 30–1).

The re-education program for the first week after removal of the plaster cast begins with work on passive flexion in all joints. It is not wise at this stage to try to recover complete passive extension, but one must not allow

---

*See the chapter on renabilitation in Volume IV.

Table 30–1. PROGRAM OF REHABILITATION AFTER ONE-STAGE FLEXOR TENDON GRAFTING

Between the tenth and twenty-fifth days: passive flexion with splint
First week after removal of splint: passive flexion of finger
Second week after removal of splint: active flexion without resistance
Fourth week after removal of splint: passive extension
Fifth week after removal of splint: flexion against resistance.

---

contractions to occur, for they might be difficult to correct subsequently. To achieve this, with the wrist and metacarpophalangeal joints in passive flexion, the distal interphalangeal joint is passively extended while the proximal interphalangeal joints are mobilized in 30 to 90 degrees of passive flexion. To avoid initiating a swan-neck deformity, which may occur in the absence of the flexor superficialis, the proximal interphalangeal joint should not be fully extended even with the metacarpophalangeal joint flexed. During the same period one must strive to obtain some degree of active flexion of the proximal interphalangeal joint with the metacarpophalangeal joint maintained in extension. An external ring 1 cm. wide is placed around the proximal phalanx to reinforce the pulley. This early active flexion is difficult to obtain at first because of the patient's apprehension, discomfort, and loss of voluntary control. It may be helpful to encourage the patient to simultaneously contract the neighboring fingers as well as the corresponding finger of the opposite hand.

During the second week after removal of the plaster cast, the pullout wire and the button are removed. Active contractions at the proximal interphalangeal joint without resistance are continued, and extension of the same joint is encouraged without trying to achieve complete extension.

Active flexion-extension movements of the distal interphalangeal joint are continued until full extension is obtained with metacarpophalangeal joints flexed.

During the third week after removal of the plaster cast, active flexion of the distal interphalangeal joint is started with the proximal interphalangeal joint in extension (Fig. 30–22) using a precut wood block. Active flexion of the proximal interphalangeal joint is continued. Simultaneous flexion of the interphalangeal joints is practiced progressively, but

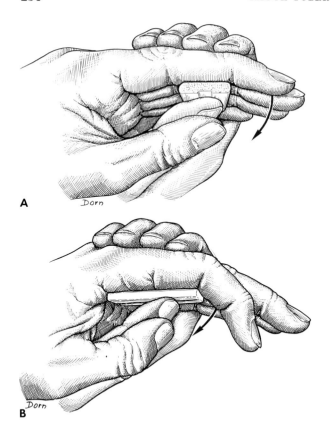

A

B

Figure 30–22. Active flexion exercises using a precut wood block. *A*, Flexion of the proximal interphalangeal joint of one finger. *B*, Flexion of the distal interphalangeal joints of all the fingers (flexor profundus being common to all).

flexion of the metacarpophalangeal joint is restrained to prevent abnormal action of the intrinsic muscles, which may be difficult to overcome later.

Even at this stage one should guard against unphysiological movements of the extensor system such that the grafted finger remains extended when the others are flexed. The active part played in this syndrome by the lumbricals has been well demonstrated by Parkes (1971), but this deformity has been known to occur even in the absence of the lumbrical. It is a protective reflex, which urges the patient to contract the extensors when the injured flexors are flexed. The surgeon and physiotherapist will find that the patient requires gentle and continuous persuasion. His cooperation is essential. In some cases local anesthesia of the ulnar nerve at the wrist, by suppressing flexion of the interosseous muscles at the metacarpophalangeal joints, may help the patient to understand the function of the graft. At the same time one must work at obtaining full extension of all the joints with the help of elastic traction splints or successive corrective plaster casts

between exercises, as advocated by Wynn Parry (1973).

During the fourth week after removal of the plaster cast, flexion-extension exercises against resistance are started. By now, full active and passive extension should be possible; occupational therapy adapted to each case can be extremely useful.

In his own interest the patient should resume partial professional activities after two months of therapy, even if, as is usually the case, flexion has not yet been fully recovered. The stage of intensive re-education in a specialized center is now completed, but the patient should continue exercises on his own with a weekly check at the center. The surgeon should see the patient on a monthly basis.

Flexion will continue to improve for four to six months and re-education must be pursued. Too early cessation of exercises may hinder his progress, especially if the patient is not achieving full flexion. This applies mostly to the index finger in which full active flexion is less commonly required than in the ulnar digits.

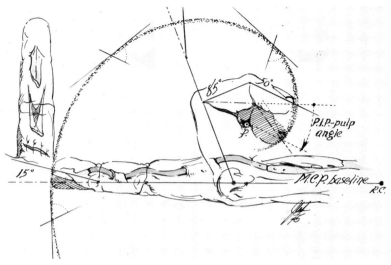

Figure 30–23. Diagram of flexor profundus tendon graft. *Left*, Preoperative state. Flexion of the finger shows the result obtained (Littler).

SPECIAL TECHNIQUES FOR GRAFTING FLEXOR TENDONS

GRAFT TO RECONSTRUCT ONLY THE FLEXOR SUPERFICIALIS

One should not attempt to replace a severed superficialis tendon when the profundus is intact. In the present stage of tendon graft surgery, the risk of interfering with such an essential tendon is too great. In certain cases, however, it may be preferable to reconstruct the superficialis rather than the deep flexor when both tendons have been injured (Figs. 30–23, 30–24). Osborne in 1960 pointed out that restoring flexor power at the level of middle phalanx is more useful in difficult cases than a vain attempt at restoring articular mobility in all the joints of a finger. Inserting a graft on the middle phalanx mobilizes the proximal interphalangeal joint, and the result is much more predictable than insertion on the distal phalanx.

This is just what we do when the distal interphalangeal joint is stiff, when the distal phalanx has been partially amputated and mobility of the distal joint would serve no useful purpose, in difficult cases in which previous repairs have failed, and when the only graft available is too short to reach the distal phalanx.

The technique on the whole is similar to that used for grafting the flexor profundus, but before fixing the distal extremity of the

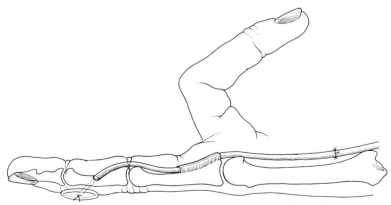

Figure 30–24. Graft reconstructing the flexor superficialis tendon only.

graft, the position of the distal phalanx must be adjusted. If the latter is fixed (usually in excessive flexion), its position must be corrected; otherwise it may interfere with the future function of the grafted finger. This can usually be achieved by release of the flexor profundus tendon, combined if necessary with an arthrolysis. Arthrodesis of the distal joint is rarely necessary. The phalanx is held by an oblique Kirschner wire in a position that varies with the occupation of the patient and the affected finger.

The graft is implanted on the proximal third of the middle phalanx at least 1 cm. from the proximal interphalangeal joint so as not to interfere with mobility. The phalanx is drilled obliquely from front to back and from proximal to distal. The small tunnel thus produced is broadened volarly to receive the extremity of the graft; its distal part only transmits the transosseous suture and the phalanx should not be weakened by excessive drilling. The transfixion suture transfixes the bone, the extensor apparatus, and the skin with the distal interphalangeal joint in extension and is tied over a small bolus dressing or a button. Transfixion of the extensor apparatus assists in fixation by tenodesing the distal joint.

GRAFTING THE FLEXOR PROFUNDUS TENDON IN THE PRESENCE OF AN INTACT FLEXOR SUPERFICIALIS

The lesion may consist of a division of the flexor profundus tendon or more rarely an avulsion of its distal extremity but without damage to the superficialis. In some favorable cases (usually young patients) one may elect to perform a tendon graft. The graft should be thin (the plantaris is ideal) and should be placed in close contact with the flexor superficialis within the fibrous sheath. The site where the profundus perforates the superficialis, which lies proximal to the division of superficialis, is exposed. When surgical repair has been delayed, this orifice is often obliterated, and it is better to route the graft alongside the superficialis tendon and not through it, because it might then injure the mesotendon, which carries the blood supply, and thereby produce adhesions (Fig. 30–25). Resection of one of the terminal bands of the superficialis to create more space for the graft has been advocated by some authors (Harrison, 1959), but this is not necessary.

The proximal and distal extremities of the graft are fixed as previously described, and the tension is carefully adjusted to prevent residual retraction. This adjustment is carried out with the wrist and metacarpophalangeal and proximal interphalangeal joints straight and the distal interphalangeal joint in 40 degrees of flexion. When the graft is fixed, the finger is not immobilized in this position. The wrist and the metacarpophalangeal joint are maintained in flexion by a dorsal splint, as used after a normal tendon grafting when both flexor tendons have been divided with the wrist flexed at 30 degrees and the metacarpophalangeal joint at 70 degrees. The two interphalangeal joints are placed in slight flexion. A little passive flexion is allowed at the distal interphalangeal joint.

After one week, active flexion of the proximal interphalangeal joint, metacarpophalangeal joint, and wrist is started while the

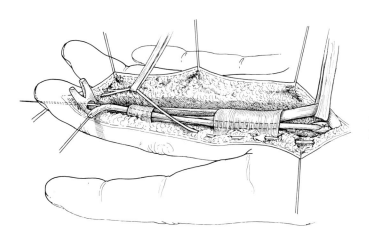

Figure 30–25. Flexor profundus graft with flexor superficialis tendon kept in place.

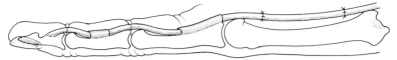

Figure 30–26. Bridge graft in the palm.

distal interphalangeal joint is maintained in extension. After three weeks, active flexion of the distal interphalangeal joint is allowed, while the proximal interphalangeal and metacarpophalangeal joints remain flexed; however, the dorsal splint and pullout suture fixing the graft to a button are removed, only after a total of four weeks. At the fifth week, the distal phalanx is actively flexed, with the middle phalanx maintained in extension.

Some authors (Versaci, 1970; Honner, 1975; Wilson et al., 1980) prefer to graft the deep flexor tendon in two steps, the tendon graft being preceded by the placement of a silicone implant. Such an attitude does not always appear to be required, as shown by the satisfactory results in a large series of one-stage grafts (Pulvertaft, 1960; Stark et al., 1977; McClinton et al., 1982). It would be useful if a pulley reconstruction or liberation of a stiff joint was required.

BRIDGE GRAFTS

Bridge grafts are designed to span a gap in the tendon at some distance from both the proximal origin and the distal insertion (Fig. 30–26). This type of graft is usually only several centimeters in length. It is used in the palm when the proximal and distal stumps are free of adhesions. If adhesions exist or a tenolysis is needed, it is advisable to fabricate a standard terminal graft.

GRAFTING THE FLEXOR POLLICIS LONGUS TENDON

The technique is similar to that described for flexor grafts of the fingers. The operation is performed through a long digitopalmar incision. Distal fixation and surgical treatment of the fibrous sheaths are the same, and one should strive to preserve a flexion pulley opposite the proximal phalanx (Fig. 30–27). Adjusting the tension of this graft must be done with the wrist held straight, the first metacarpal in anteposition with respect to the second and a spreading angle of 30 degrees,

the metacarpophalangeal joint flexed at 15 degrees, the interphalangeal joint flexed at 45 degrees, and the motor tendon fixed halfway along its course. When the proximal stump of the tendon is found in the thenar eminence, the graft may be short (Fig. 30–28); if not, it is passed through the carpal tunnel and sutured at the wrist at a safe distance from the tunnel. The palmaris longus tendon usually provides a suitable graft, but in some cases the plantaris may be needed for extra length.

Good stability of the metacarpophalangeal joint with the absence of hyperextension is necessary to obtain satisfactory flexion of the distal phalanx (Fig. 30–29).

PEDICLED TENDON GRAFT

Paneva-Holevitch (1977) has devised a two stage technique for a pedicled tendon graft.

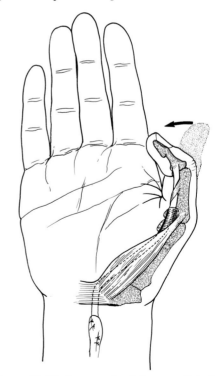

Figure 30–27. Long graft of flexor pollicis longus. Proximal fixation is at the level of the wrist.

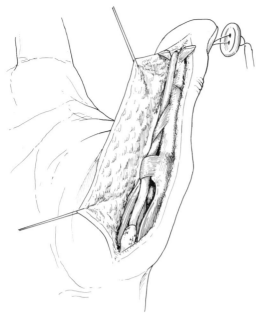

Figure 30–28. Short graft of flexor pollicis longus.

In the first stage, which usually coincides with the primary repair of the digital wound, a small cutaneous flap is raised on the palm. The superficial and deep flexor tendons of the injured finger are divided at the level of the lumbrical, and the proximal ends are sutured to each other.

One month later the distal extremities of the tendons are resected. The flexor superficialis tendon is divided near the fleshy belly in the forearm, passed under the pulleys, and fixed on the distal phalanx. Movements are resumed on the fifth postoperative day.

This technique has been adapted to flexor tendon injuries in the thumb. The proximal end of the long thumb flexor is sutured to the distal end of the palmaris longus, which subsequently functions as the graft. A similar technique of pedicle graft with palmaris longus may be used for the fingers.

The author believes that the good results obtained are due to the absence of traction on the primary suture which has been rested for a month and to the longitudinal revascularization as in pedicled nerve grafts.

RESULTS AND COMPLICATIONS

The results of flexor tendon grafting are not consistently satisfactory (Figs. 30–30, 30–31). Most of the figures reported show a significant proportion of failures or poor results with the pulp remaining at a distance from the palm. This is not entirely surprising when one realizes that the surgical repair is far from physiological. Flexion of the fingers is a complex mechanism involving the movement of two tendons with different excursions

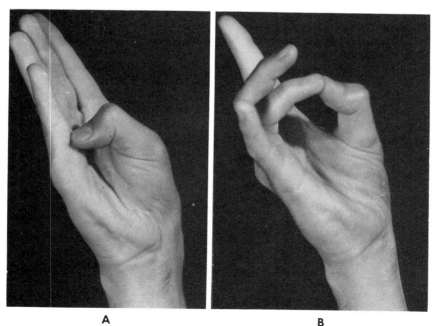

A   B

Figure 30–29. *A* and *B*, Results of a long graft of the flexor pollicis longus.

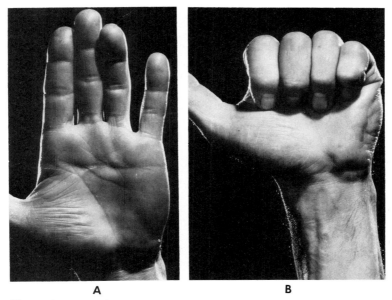

Figure 30–30. *A* and *B*, Result of a graft of the flexor tendon of the ring finger.

gliding freely within a tight fibrous sheath lined with a synovial membrane. The trauma and ablation of the severed tendons destroy the synovial sheath and a large proportion of the fibrous sheath. Additionally only one tendon is reconstructed when normal anatomy requires two.

Factors Influencing Results

In addition to the mechanical and technical problems, the function of the tendon graft depends on the intensity of the healing reaction and the adhesions it engenders.

An assessment of the results of flexor tendon grafting must take into account the site of the lesions and the preoperative state of the finger. It is well known that tendon grafts in the thumb are more successful than in the fingers. This is understandable because here the graft replaces a single tendon.

There is little doubt also that associated lesions, such as contracted scars, joint stiffness, nerve and bone lesions, and multiple

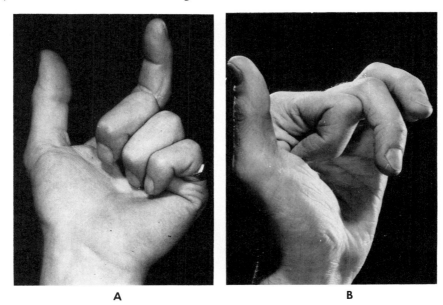

Figure 30–31. *A* and *B*, Result of a graft of the flexor tendon of the index finger.

tendon injuries, can have an adverse effect on the results of tendon grafting. Similarly unsuccessful attempts at primary suturing also worsen the prognosis.

Boyes and Stark (1977) have classified the preoperative state of fingers requiring flexor tendon grafts into five categories. In this important study of the factors influencing results of flexor tendon grafting they concluded that the most important factor was the preoperative state of the digit. Hence in cases classified as category 1 (tissues in good condition), excluding factors such as age, sex, affected finger, and site of donor graft, in 23 per cent of the cases the extremity of the grafted finger reached the distal palmar crease, 64 per cent flexed within 1 to 2 cm. and 13 per cent reached to 2 to 5 cm. from the distal palmar crease. In category 2 (scarred tissues) and the proportion of excellent results diminished to 9 per cent. In categories 3 (joint stiffness) and 4 (destructive lesions or previous infections), no finger could reach the distal palmar crease.

In category 5 (multiple tendon injuries affecting several digits) an excellent result was obtained in 9 per cent of the digits (Fig. 30–32). After reclassifying this category according to the conditions of each finger, the results parallel closely those of its corresponding category, showing that it is the state of each finger that determines the final result.

This study also dealt with other factors capable of influencing the results. Thus an associated single collateral nerve lesion rarely influences the postoperative degree of flexion obtained, but injuries to both digital nerves do. The study of results according to age showed that the best results are obtained in patients between 11 and 15 years of age. Before age six and after 40 years of age the percentage of good results decreases.

If one takes into account the finger involved, the best results (excluding the thumb) are obtained in the fifth finger and the worst in the index finger whose flexion is least frequently required and whose function is independent. Secondary tendon grafting has a better chance of success following a failed tendon suture than a failed tendon grafting.

DOES THE TIMING OF THE GRAFTING INFLUENCE THE RESULT?

It would seem logical to assume that early grafting, prior to the establishment of contracture and sclerosis, would be technically easier to perform and more likely to succeed. However, early operations may be more predisposed to infection. For this reason and because of the difficulty for a specialist to

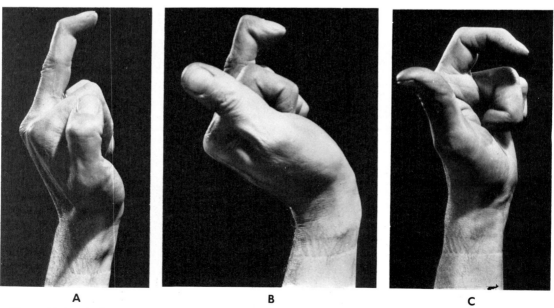

A   B   C

Figure 30–32. *A*, Swan-neck deformity following flexor profundus tendon graft with persistent flexion of distal phalanx. *B*, Flexion of the finger starts at the level of the distal phalanx, which flexes from 70 to 90 degrees. *C*, The proximal interphalangeal joint then flexes with a click.

make himself available for an emergency grafting, few results have been published. The scanty figures available relating to emergency repairs by grafting argue in favor of secondary grafting (Harrison, 1958; Thompson, 1967).

According to Harrison, the risk of infection is reduced after a few days. Tissue reactions in a clean wound regress rapidly. He therefore advocates delayed primary grafting, which in his series was performed on the average on the ninth day following injury. Despite the good results (the pulp of the finger reached the palm in 83.4 per cent of the cases compared with 66.6 per cent of the cases in emergency grafts and 74.5 per cent after secondary grafts), most surgeons continue to be in favor of the late repair. Peacock (1977) believes, on biological grounds, that the best time for grafting is six to 12 weeks after the injury. Pulvertaft (see Chapter 31), who has had abundant experience with late grafting, prefers to wait for at least six months before the repair.

Delay appears to have little relevance. This is borne out by Pulvertaft's surprisingly good results in selected cases in which grafting was carried out two to 18 years after the injury. It is the condition of the hand, much more than the time elapsed, that matters.

In cases involving clean wounds that have healed by first intention, we admit the patient to the hospital for grafting two months after the injury. We wait longer, however, if the wound is contused, or if there is persistent edema, stiffness, or contracted scars. A long delay is not a contraindication to tendon grafting provided the joints are supple and sensibility sufficient to justify the reconstruction is present.

COMPLICATIONS OF TENDON GRAFT SURGERY

The commonest causes of failure are invasion of the gliding planes by adhesions, ruptures of the sutures, and errors of fixation.

Some complications, such as infection or dehiscence, can be blamed on a technical error, and others, such as absence of pulleys, hyperextension of the proximal interphalangeal joint, and retraction of the lumbrical muscle, are due to mechanical problems. The former are avoidable and the latter can be corrected, but we are helpless in the presence of adhesions, which to a certain extent are part of the repair mechanism.

Suture Disruption. Sutures disrupt most often at the distal insertion of the graft. This is more likely to occur when the tendon is not closely applied to the bone, the area of contact is too small, some other structure intervenes, or necrosis of the distal end of the graft results from too tight a suture. Dehiscence of the proximal junction is rare with transfixion methods but occurs frequently after end to end suturing, especially under tension. Synthetic monofilament sutures are very slippery and readily come undone if not properly tied. Five knots should be used.

Dehiscence is suspected when active flexion is suddenly lost during the re-education period. One should reoperate as soon as possible in the hope of repairing the graft before retraction sets in.

Adhesions. Adhesions are the commonest complication and the most difficult to treat. Active flexion is minimal or completely lost after a few months. The prognosis varies according to whether passive flexion persists or disappears, being much worse in the latter case.

Reoperation should be delayed. Michon and Verdan (1961) have shown that early tenolysis (before the fifth month) may result in rupture. It is best to wait until edema and pain have decreased and the joints and soft tissues are supple. In some cases the adhesions are localized, preventing complete extension of the finger, but limited active flexion is still possible and passive flexion of the proximal joints allows extension of the distal joints. It is in these cases that one can hope for a good result from tenolysis. Too often, however, adhesions are widespread, the graft becomes stuck to the pulleys, and there seems to be little hope of restoring mobility by a simple tenolysis. Silastic implants now appear to be the best available solution.

Bowstring Effect. The bowstring effect is due to the absence of pulleys, the graft becoming dislocated anteriorly like the string of a bow. The grafted tendon remains capable of slightly flexing the finger, especially when the object grasped presses on the base of the finger but flexor power remains weak. Bunnell (1966) suggested that the patient be advised to wear a ring, but this ingenious device is often not enough and one may have to reconstruct a pulley. This operation is

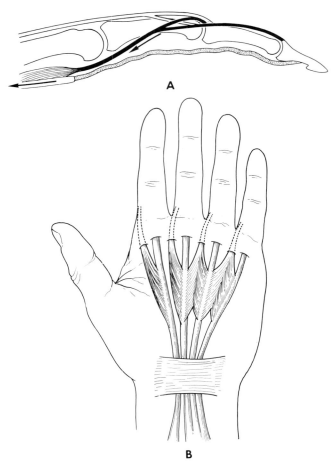

A

B

Figure 30–33. *A*, Lumbrical plus syndrome when the flexor profundus tendon graft is too long. *B*, This syndrome occurs above all with the index and middle fingers. The bicipital insertion of the lumbricals of the ring and little fingers usually limits their retraction.

delicate because the pulley must be close enough to the graft to strap it down without, however, becoming adherent to it. In these secondary procedures, one must respect the gliding planes that have been reconstituted around the graft. Early motion without resistance is advisable.

Abnormal Flexion Due to the Absence of the Flexor Superficialis. Removal of the flexor superficialis is not a surgical step to be taken lightly. In the normal finger the middle phalanx is flexed before the distal one under the pull of the flexor superficialis. Reconstruction of the profundus alone may lead to a swan-neck deformity. The balance between the flexor and the extensor apparatus is disturbed, the proximal interphalangeal joint going into hyperextension and the distal joint into flexion. The flexion arc of the finger is distorted, the distal phalanx flexes before the middle phalanx, and the latter finally goes into flexion with a painful snap (Fig. 30–32). Fortunately the swan-neck deformity is rare, and it is indeed surprising that it does not

occur more frequently after flexor tendon grafting. The reason may lie in the imperfection of our results such that, because of the residual stiffness in the interphalangeal joints, full extension of the proximal joint is prevented and only limited movement of the distal joint occurs. The graft glides least near its distal insertion, and the limitation of movement allows the graft to flex more efficiently at the middle than at the distal phalanx. This swan-neck deformity is more likely to occur if the proximal interphalangeal joint is lax and tends to drift into hyperextension. Therefore this tendency, as we have mentioned, must be controlled while the graft bed is being prepared.

The treatment of this deformity consists essentially in preventing hyperextension of the proximal interphalangeal joint. Reconstruction of an oblique retinacular ligament seems to be well adapted to this purpose.*

---

*See Chapter 16, "The Swan-neck Deformity."

Complications Due to Retraction of the Lumbrical. Parkes (1971) has described a syndrome of retraction of the lumbrical muscle that he calls the "lumbrical plus" syndrome. It is due to traction on the proximal attachment of the lumbrical when the profundus tendon is severed or avulsed distal to this attachment. The same phenomenon occurs when the graft designed to replace the tendon defect is too long. The lumbrical during its action as an extensor of the digital phalanges is then not counterbalanced by the flexor (Fig. 30–33). The ulnar two lumbricals having two heads arising from the adjacent deep flexors of the ring and little fingers retract less, usually preventing this deformity. It is commonest in the index and middle fingers. When the patient is asked to flex all the fingers, paradoxically he extends the grafted finger. Flexion can be restored by dividing the lumbrical muscle in the palm. To avoid retraction of the lumbrical, one should refrain from burying the proximal anastomosis in this muscle.

In addition to the causes of failure we have already mentioned, individual healing factors, about which we know little, can affect the results of grafting procedures. However, there is little doubt that unfavorable preoperative conditions and traumatic or incorrect surgery also have an adverse effect.

Technique remains an essential determinant of prognosis, but although there is still room for improvement, it is doubtful that the explanation for the usual 30 per cent of poor results lies in technique alone. Other solutions have been proposed, which will be described.

REFERENCES

References for this chapter will be found following Chapter 38.

Chapter 31

FLEXOR TENDON GRAFTING AFTER LONG DELAYS

ROBERT GUY PULVERTAFT*

From time to time a patient is seen several years after a tendon has been divided within the digital theca. The finger or thumb may be in good general condition, with normal mobility and sensibility, but lacking active flexion. Previous surgery may have failed, or the patient may have been advised that there was no effective treatment for the injury. The disability has been accepted until, for some reason, further advice is sought. Function can be restored in a high proportion of these cases, and the surgeon experienced in this work need not hesitate to advise reconstruction.

The object in this chapter is to examine the results of treatment in these cases, describe the technique, and discuss the indications and the prognosis. To this end a review has been made of all cases of patients operated upon during the course of 29 years—1942 to 1970 inclusive—in which the delays from injury to tendon grafting have been more than two years.

It has become accepted practice to evaluate the results of flexor tendon grafting by the method adopted by Boyes (1950). Flexor tendon action in the finger is recorded by measuring the distance by which the finger tip fails to reach the distal crease of the palm (Fig. 31–1A). It is assumed that extension is complete unless otherwise stated. Boyes was not concerned with the restoration of profundus action alone in the presence of a normal sublimis tendon, and for these cases an additional assessment is needed. The range of active motion in the distal interphalangeal joint is measured with the finger in semiflexion (Fig. 31–1B). For the thumb the active motion in the interphalangeal joint is ex-

pressed either as an absolute figure or as a percentage of the passive range (Fig. 31–1C).

The preoperative assessment used by Hunter (1971) was followed, and only those cases that fell into grades 1 and 2 are considered here. Grade 1 (good) indicates good soft tissues, supple joints, and no significant scarring. Grade 2 (fair) indicates a deep cicatrix, resulting from injury or previous surgery, as well as slight soft tissue contractures, which in a few instances were severe enough to necessitate preliminary plastic procedures. Grades 3, 4, and 5 indicate limitation of joint movement sufficient to necessitate mobilization by traction, nerve damage with trophic changes in addition to tendon bed scarring and joint stiffness, and multiple digit injuries with scarring and joint changes, sometimes complicated by palmar involvement.

An overall total of 527 tendon grafting operations were performed for flexor tendon division in the digits. In 77 cases the delay between injury and operation was more than two years. Seven cases that fell into grade 3 have been excluded. Of the remaining 70 cases, there were 12 for which the records were inadequate; these have also been excluded, leaving a total of 58 cases for analysis.

FLEXOR DIGITORUM PROFUNDUS

For late treatment of the isolated profundus injury the choice lies between acceptance of the disability, which to some persons is not particularly disturbing; arthrodesis or tenodesis of the distal joint; or restoration of tendon action by tendon grafting (Pulvertaft, 1960). The operation is quite complex and should not be advised unless the patient is

*Deceased.

244

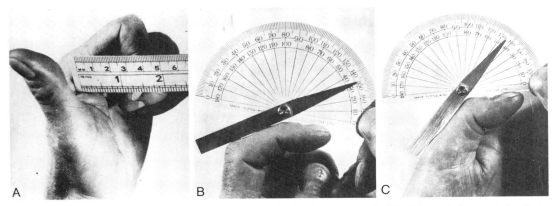

Figure 31–1. Measurements. *A*, Pulp of finger tip to distal palmar crease. *B*, Distal interphalangeal joint flexion with the finger in semiflexion. *C*, Thumb interphalangeal joint flexion.

determined to seek perfection and the surgeon is confident of his ability to offer a reasonable expectation of success without undue risk of doing harm.

There were five cases in this group. There had been no previous operative treatment. The average delay had been four years, and the average age of the patients at operation was 19 years. Subsequent tenolysis was not needed. One operation failed because of graft rupture, and the distal joint was arthrodesed. Of the remaining four patients, two had complete extension and the other two had 10 degree and 12 degree losses of extension. Including the treatment failure (zero), the average distal interphalangeal flexion range attained was 48 degrees, and the average tip-to-distal-crease distance was 1.5 cm., or 0.6 inch (Fig. 31–2). The number of cases is too small to warrant a graph.

FLEXOR DIGITORUM SUBLIMIS AND FLEXOR DIGITORUM PROFUNDUS

The choice between primary tendon suturing and secondary tendon grafting for the acute injury is controversial, and no doubt the matter will be disputed for years to come, but for the late case the only reasonable treatment is tendon grafting, either by the standard method or preceded by a prosthetic implant. Grafting is successful only when the digit is in reasonably good condition, with an adequate passive range and no severe scarring, and with at least one sensory digital nerve intact (grades 1 and 2). Hunter (1971) has shown how it is possible to restore function to fingers with more extensive damage by the preliminary use of a silicone-dacron implant.

Figure 31–2. The flexor profundus tendon of the index finger was severed when this patient was 12 years old. A plantaris graft was attached to the flexor profundus two years and eight months later. Thumb interphalangeal joint extension is minus 12 degrees; flexion, 60 degrees. Proximal interphalangeal joint extension is minus 5 degrees; flexion, 90 degrees. The distance from the finger tip to the distal crease is 0.6 cm.

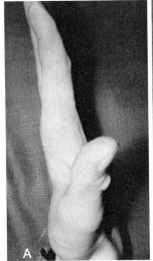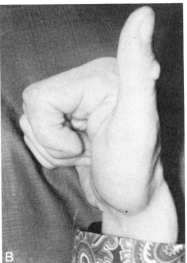

There were 42 cases in this group. In six cases there had been a previous failed suturing operation, and in seven cases there had been a previous failed tendon grafting. The average delay was five years, and the average age of the patients at operation was 14 years. In seven cases tenolysis was subsequently performed. There were two complete operative failures—one due to rupture of the graft and the other caused by gross adhesions. If one includes these two cases in the analysis, the average distance by which the finger tip failed to reach the distal crease was 1.8 cm., or 0.7 inch. The proximal interphalangeal joint had 30 degrees of flexion contracture in two cases and 20 degrees of contracture in three cases. The distal joint had 40 degrees of contracture in one case, 30 degrees in

three cases, and 20 degrees in one case (Figs. 31–3 to 31–6).

FLEXOR POLLICIS LONGUS

The normal range of motion at the interphalangeal joint varies between 75 and 90 degrees, but an active range of 40 degrees is adequate for most purposes.

There were 11 cases in this group. In one case there had been a previous failure of suturing. The average delay was five and one half years, and the average age of the patients at operation was 18 years. Subsequent tenolysis was not necessary. In one case the active range was only 25 degrees, and in two cases, 35 degrees. If one includes these indifferent

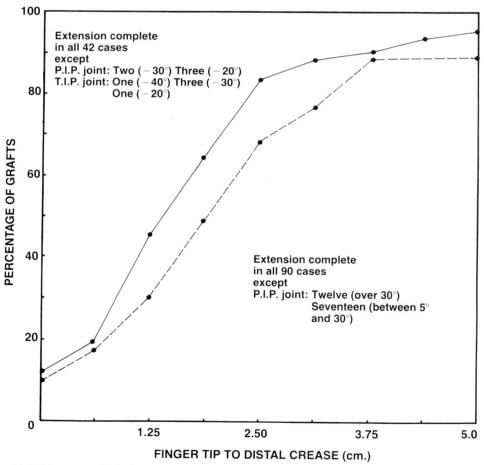

Figure 31–3. Treatment of injuries of the flexor sublimis and flexor profundus tendons: results in cases in which treatment was delayed at least two years compared with results in an earlier series in which there was no significant delay in the majority of cases. Continuous = results in 42 delayed cases (1942 to 1970), broken line = results in all 90 cases (1942 to 1954).

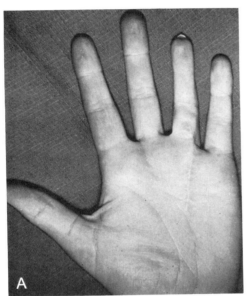

Figure 31–4. Both flexor tendons of the ring finger were severed when the patient was one and one half years old. A plantaris graft was attached to the flexor sublimis tendon 11 years later. Thumb interphalangeal joint extension is minus 10 degrees; flexion, 90 degrees. Proximal interphalangeal joint extension is 0 degrees; flexion, 100 degrees. The finger tip touches the distal crease. Note the imperfect development. A palmar scar from the previous operation can be seen.

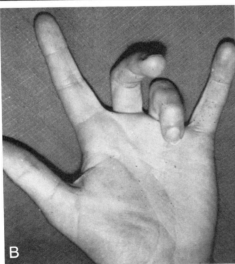

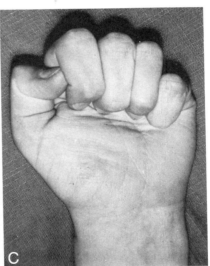

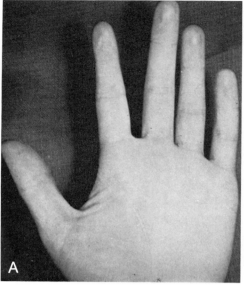 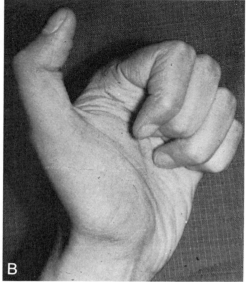

Figure 31–5. Both flexor tendons of the index finger were severed when the patient was nine years old. A plantaris graft was attached to the flexor profundus four and one half years later. Thumb interphalangeal joint extension is minus 5 degrees; flexion, 50 degrees. Proximal interphalangeal joint extension is 0 degrees; flexion 100 degrees. The distance from the finger tip to the distal crease is 0.6 cm.

results, the average active joint range was 64 degrees (Figs. 31–7, 31–8).

SOURCE OF THE GRAFT

A palmaris longus tendon is present in approximately 90 per cent of the population (Wood-Jones, 1920). It is usually, but not invariably, of good quality and of a convenient size. It is just long enough to reach from the finger tip to the proximal palm. It is removed through 2.5 cm. transverse incisions at the wrist and in the upper forearm. The distal end is divided and the tendon is drawn out through the proximal incision. Withdrawn in this manner, it comes out ensheathed in its delicate mesentery and has no paratenon attached to it.

The plantaris tendon, present in approximately 93 per cent of the population (Wood-Jones 1920), is a more slender tendon and sufficiently long to serve as two grafts. Occasionally it is very thin and unsafe to use. It is of particular value for the replacement of the flexor profundus in the presence of a normal sublimis tendon, for it will slip easily through the sheath without embarrassing the sublimis. Two small incisions are needed, one on the medial side of the Achilles tendon and

the other three fingerbreadths behind the medial border of the tibia in the upper calf, where the tendon lies between the gastrocnemius and soleus muscles. It is drawn out in the same manner as the palmaris longus tendon.

The extensor digitorum longus tendon may be used if neither of the other tendons mentioned is present. It can be removed cleanly only by open dissection, and a long curved incision reaching from the base of the toes to the ankle is necessary. For a single graft, the tendon of the fourth toe is selected, but a leash of four tendons may be removed if needed.

OPERATIVE TECHNIQUE

A pneumatic tourniquet is used at a pressure of 220 mm. Hg for an adult or 180 mm. Hg for a child after preliminary exsanguination with an Esmarch bandage. The hand is supported in a Fisk lead hand splint. The finger is exposed by an exact midlateral incision down to the fibrous sheath and passing posterior to the vessels and nerve. Excellent access is obtained, and healing occurs with an almost imperceptible scar. This approach has been used in all cases and is preferred to

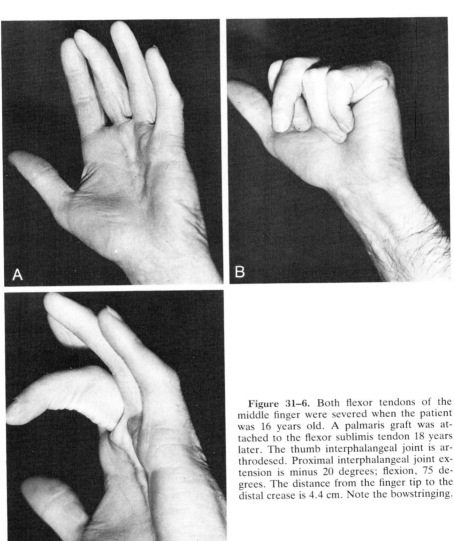

Figure 31–6. Both flexor tendons of the middle finger were severed when the patient was 16 years old. A palmaris graft was attached to the flexor sublimis tendon 18 years later. The thumb interphalangeal joint is arthrodesed. Proximal interphalangeal joint extension is minus 20 degrees; flexion, 75 degrees. The distance from the finger tip to the distal crease is 4.4 cm. Note the bowstringing.

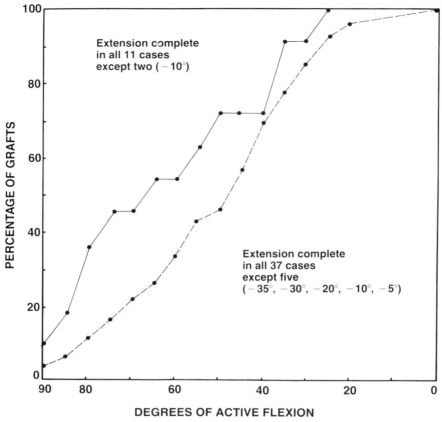

Figure 31–7. Treatment of injuries of the flexor pollicis longus: results in cases in which treatment was delayed at least two years compared with results in an earlier series in which there was no significant delay in the majority of cases. Continuous line = results in 11 delayed cases (1942 to 1970); broken line = results in all 37 cases (1942 to 1954).

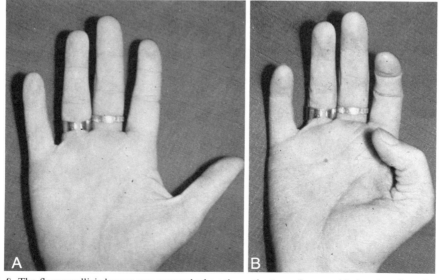

Figure 31–8. The flexor pollicis longus was severed when the patient was 8 years old. A palmaris graft was attached to the flexor pollicis longus eight years later. Extension is 0 degrees; flexion, 65 degrees.

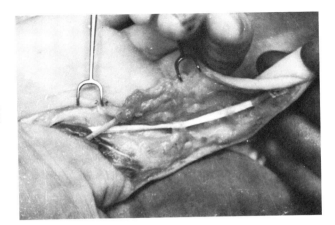

Figure 31–9. Exposure of the little finger, showing the tendon graft, the slings, and the digital nerve.

the anterior zigzag incision. The palm is opened by an incision in the appropriate skin crease that is continuous with the finger incisions in the index and little fingers (Figs. 31–9, 31–10). The middle and ring finger incisions may be joined with the palmar incision when it is necessary to expose the proximal part of the sheath, but this is not always necessary (Fig. 31–11). Because the proximal graft juncture is performed just distal to the flexor retinaculum, a second proximal exposure is needed, except for the index finger, in which the incision follows the course of the thenar crease for the required length. When the sublimis has been chosen as the motor muscle and a long graft (plantaris) is available, the proximal junction may be made above the wrist, but this does not appear to offer any significant advantage. Three incisions are used for the thumb—

midlateral on the radial side of the thumb, on the thenar crease, and above the wrist (Fig. 31–12A). The thenar crease incision facilitates removal of the divided tendon and correct placement of the graft (Fig. 31–12B). There are important structures in this area that must be avoided, namely, the digital nerve to the radial side of the index finger, the two digital nerves to the thumb between which the flexor tendon lies, and the median motor branch.

In the fingers the flexor tendons pass through a fibro-osseous canal that holds the tendons close to the bones and the finger joints. This canal is lined by synovial membrane, which suspends the tendons in a mesentery. The sheath is strengthened opposite the middle of the proximal and middle phalanges by transverse bands. The entire sheath is removed except for the transverse ligaments, which are retained as slings (Fig. 31–9). A sling is also retained in front of the

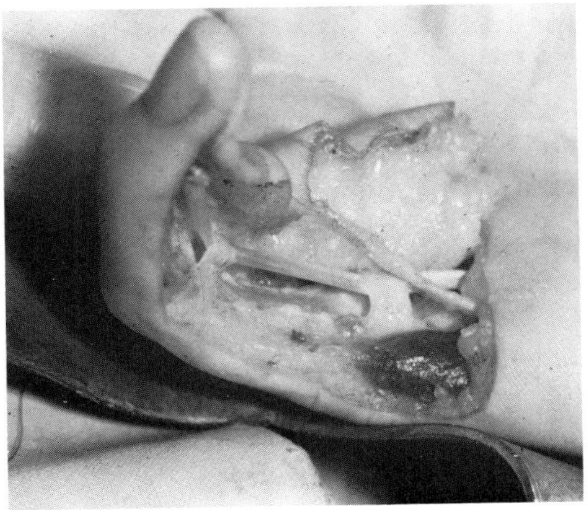

Figure 31–10. Exposure of the little finger, showing the tendon graft, the slings, and the digital nerve, which has been sutured.

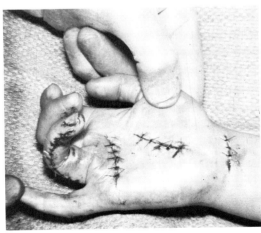

Figure 31–11. Incisions for the ring finger.

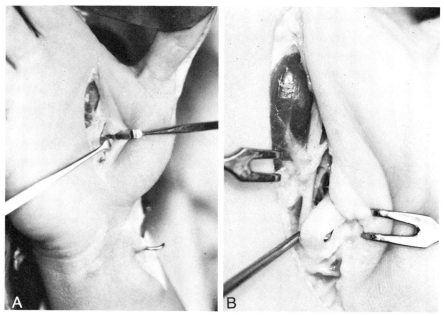

Figure 31–12. *A*, Incision for the thumb. *B*, The flexor pollicis longus tendon, one digital nerve of the thumb, and the digital nerve to the radial side of the index finger are shown.

metacarpophalangeal joint. It is not always possible to follow this ideal arrangement when the sheath is severely scarred, and modifications are necessary. When circumstances will permit the retention of only two pulleys, one should be situated just proximal to the proximal interphalangeal joint and the other in front of the metacarpophalangeal joint (Fig. 31–10). Occasionally new slings have to be formed from a short length of graft, which is attached to either side of the fibrous sheath.

The injured tendon or tendons are removed by precise dissection, leaving no fragments and avoiding damage to the remaining sheath. A small tag of tendon is left attached to the distal phalanx. The palmar portions of the tendon are removed and the ends drawn out through the proximal palmar incision. They are tested for excursion, the better of the two being chosen and the other cut back. At the wrist level the normal functional length of the flexor profundus varies between 3 cm. for the index finger and 4.5 cm. for the ring finger. The flexor sublimis is 0.5 to 0.75 cm. shorter than the corresponding profundus tendon. The functional length of the flexor pollicis longus ranges from 5.5 to 6 cm. (Kaplan, 1965). It is unusual to find excursions as great as these, for some muscle shortening will have occurred. When the am-

plitudes of movement of the sublimis and profundus tendons are equal, there appears to be no special advantage to either for repair of the index finger. For the middle and ring fingers the sublimis tendon has some advantage, because the muscle has an independent action, whereas the flexor profundus to the middle, ring, and little fingers is a conjoined muscle; when the sublimis tendon is used, there exists the possibility of natural adjustment of length should the graft tension be inaccurate. For the little finger, the profundus is preferable, because the sublimis muscle of this finger is usually less effective than is the profundus muscle.

The proximal suturing of the graft is performed by use of a modification of the interlacing technique (Fig. 31–13*A*). The tendon is slit with a tenotome near its end and the graft is passed through the slit. It is passed back through a second slit placed in the opposite plane. Transverse mattress sutures are inserted, and finally the end of the tendon is split and the fishtail thus formed is stitched to and embraces the graft. When profundus tendon is used, the junction is covered by the lumbrical muscle. Care is taken at the completion of the distal suturing to make sure that normal flexion movement takes place through the graft and not through the lumbrical tendon. Should the latter occur, a

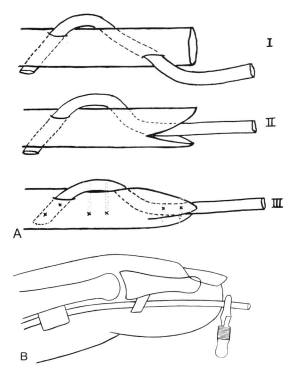

Figure 31–13. *A*, The proximal suture. *B*, The distal suture.

paradoxical action will develop, causing extension of the proximal interphalangeal joint—the lumbrical plus syndrome (Parkes, 1971).

The distal attachment is made in either of two ways, by the Bunnell pullout stitch, emerging through the finger pulp and tied over a small wool pack, or by a method that has proved particularly helpful for determining the final tension of the graft (Fig. 31–13*B*). The graft is drawn through the finger pulp with a Reverdin needle and the protruding part is clasped by an arterial clip; the tension can be adjusted with precision by allowing the graft to slip back or by withdrawing it a little farther, as needed. The graft is stitched to the profundus tag, through which it has passed before entering the pulp; the end is then cut off and allowed to fall back into the finger.

The ideal suture material is determined by its strength, ease of use, and the tissue response it evokes. Since this work was started, synthetic materials have been developed that fulfil these requirements, but in this series stainless steel wire (0.1 mm.) was used throughout. It is attached to a 2.5 cm. needle having a thin bayonet shape. The needle is malleable and can be bent as desired to facilitate insertion. In no case has harm resulted from the permanent presence of the wire. A standard overhand knot is used, and the wire is cut off as short as possible using the ends of fine scissors.

The tension at which the graft is set is clearly of the utmost importance. The muscle of the divided tendon shortens as it adapts itself to the inevitable retraction. It is not unreasonable to assume that some return toward normal may occur on subsequent use. For this reason the tension under which the graft is placed should be a little greater than would appear to be normal at the time of operation. This tension can be estimated by comparison with the other fingers, the index finger being flexed the least and the little finger the most (Fig. 31–11).

Hemostasis is secured by high elevation of the limb when the tourniquet is released. After some minutes most of the bleeding ceases. Vessel ligation or bipolar diathermy is used until the wound is completely dry. A dressing of tulle gras is applied, and the palm is filled by a pack of steel wool with the digits in moderate flexion. Finally the hand and forearm are supported by a copious wool and crepe bandage. Compression dressings are not used.

AFTERCARE

Splintage is maintained for three weeks. During this time the dressings are not disturbed. For a further week, or two weeks in the case of young children, the finger is held in slight flexion by an adhesive elastic check-rein strap stretching from the finger to the forearm (Fig. 31–14). This permits flexion movements and prevents extension strain.

This check-rein strap is not suitable for the thumb, which is better controlled by wool and bandage splintage, permitting slight movements. Subsequently, free active movements are encouraged and are assisted when necessary by a physiotherapist. In this series all patients were cared for in this manner except six in whom movements were commenced during the first postoperative week.

PROGNOSIS

The results of treatment for tendons divided within the digital theca are notoriously

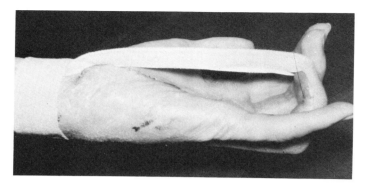

Figure 31–14. The check-rein strap.

uncertain, whether the tendon is sutured primarily or replaced later by a free tendon graft. The expectation of success when grafting is performed after a delay of years is subject to the same uncertainty, but there is sufficient evidence to justify late grafting, provided the digit is in good general condition. It is of interest that the results in this series of delayed cases were slightly better than results obtained in those reported in 1956 (Pulvertaft): in the majority of cases (87 per cent) the operation was performed within a few months after injury (Figs. 31–3, 31–7). The improved results in the delayed treatment cases can be explained in part by the fact that only grades 1 and 2 were analyzed, whereas in the 1942 to 1954 series other grades were included. The operative techniques were identical in all essential details. In all cases in both series the muscle of the injured finger or thumb was used, although, on reflection, it would have been more profitable in some cases to have used the flexor sublimis of an uninjured finger. The flexor profundus was used in cases of isolated profundus division; the profundus or sublimis, whichever had the better amplitude of movement, was used in cases of combined division, and the flexor pollicis longus was used for the thumb.

It is clear that muscle shortening does not occur as often or as severely as might be expected, retraction being prevented by local adhesions. This applies to children as well as to adults, for the attachment ensures that the muscle develops normally with growth. Nevertheless the functional length of the muscle should be carefully assessed, and if it is judged to be insufficient, another muscle, preferably the sublimis of an adjacent finger, should be used as the motor source. This possibility should be discussed with the patient and permission given for its use should it be found necessary.

In these cases the tendon and the sheath distal to the division were usually found to be in good condition when the injury had occurred in adult life. In children there is no stimulus to development, and the tendon and sheath remained as they had been at the time of injury. There may also be some general lack of finger development in children (Fig. 31–4). It may be necessary under these circumstances to remove the distal sheath completely and construct new slings to retain the tendon graft in the correct position to prevent bowstringing.

The delays before treatment in the 58 cases reported here ranged from two to 18 years and were due to exceptional circumstances. It appears that the delays were not harmful in the majority of cases, and there may be a positive advantage in deferring surgery until the tissues have completely recovered from the original trauma. It has, in fact, become standard practice in recent years to allow a minimum of six months to elapse between injury and reparative treatment.

REFERENCES

Boyes, J. H.: Flexor-tendon grafts in the fingers and thumb. J. Bone Joint Surg., *32A*:489, 1950.

Hunter, J. M.: Flexor-tendon reconstruction in severely damaged hands. J. Bone Joint Surg., *53A*:829, 1971.

Kaplan, E. B.: Functional and Surgical Anatomy of the Hand. Ed. 2. Philadelphia, J. B. Lippincott Co., 1965.

Parkes, A.: The "lumbricalis plus" finger. J. Bone Joint Surg., *53B*:236, 1971.

Pulvertaft, R. G.: Tendon grafts for flexor tendon injuries in the fingers and thumb. J. Bone Joint Surg., *38B*:175, 1956.

Pulvertaft, R. G.: The treatment of profundus division by free tendon graft. J. Bone Joint Surg., *42A*:1363, 1960.

Pulvertaft, R. G.: The results of tendon grafting for flexor tendon injuries in fingers and thumb after long delay. Bull. Hosp. Joint Dis., *21*:317, 1960.

Wood-Jones, F.: The Principles of Anatomy as Seen in the Hand. London, J. & A. Churchill, Ltd., 1920.

Chapter 32

TENDON RECONSTRUCTION WITH IMPLANTS

James M. Hunter
Scott H. Jaeger
Daniel I. Singer
and Evelyn J. Mackin

The injured flexor and extensor tendon systems can present difficult problems for the hand surgeon. Although primary repairs may yield good results, the outcome is not consistently satisfactory. In addition, certain clinical circumstances may contraindicate primary repair. In these acute situations and in complex soft tissue problems, alternative techniques are required. Free tendon grafting may be indicated, but unless the anatomical bed into which the graft is placed is minimally scarred or not scarred at all, the result may be less than satisfactory. Staged tendon grafting using Hunter tendon implants can be employed as an alternative in most of these difficult cases. When patients are selected wisely and the technique is used correctly, the results can be predictably successful.

HISTORICAL BACKGROUND

Since the advent of flexor tendon reconstruction, surgeons have been plagued with the problem of adhesions. The modern era of flexor tendon grafting was initiated by Konrad Biesalski of Berlin, who in 1910 described the problem of adhesions in tendon transfer. He used autogenous sheaths of paralyzed tendons to avoid adhesions. Since then, many attempts have been made to avoid the adhesions that occur when a tendon is grafted into an injured bed. These attempts can be categorized into three groups: (1) adhesion blocking devices, (2) interposition implants, and (3) inert gliding implants that produce a pseudosynovial sheath.

The use of the blocking concept involved the interposition of foreign material between the tendon and the surrounding tissue in an effort to block scar invasion. Early attempts described the use of tensor fasciae latae or veins. These attempts were all unsuccessful and at times increased the adhesions around the tendon. Other artificial substances were subsequently used, for example, a cargile membrane was used, and although it did not increase adhesions it also did not solve the problem. Wheeldon, in 1939, attempted to utilize cellophane as a permanent tendon sheath; this also was unsuccessful.

The second group of investigators attempted to avoid scars by interposing foreign material, such as an artifical tendon. In 1900, Lange worked with a silk tendon. Then there was a lag of many years until new material, such as braided tantalum wire, was introduced. A dual material concept using nylon fishing line through two polyethylene tubules was introduced in 1956 by Sarkin, with early success reported. Since then other materials have been used with varying degrees of success. Wire or silk covered with polyethylene tubes, Teflon rods, nylon and tetron, arterial tissue and nylon thread have all been tried with limited success. Materials that are too stiff cannot be used because they block passive digital motion, thereby increasing joint stiffness. Tubes pose a continual threat of a dead space in which fluid, blood, and bacteria can collect. They are subjected to excessive functional wear and tend to kink in extremes of flexion. The idea of using an implant made of a durable but flexible inert material was not introduced until the 1960s.

The concept of a psuedosynovial sheath was a major advancement in overcoming the problem of resrictive adhesions. Many investigators attempted to use foreign material implants to induce the surrounding scar to form a pseudosynovial sheath. This method takes advantage of the tendency of a scar to layer and form a mesothelium-like membrane as it matures around the inert surface. Leo Mayer in 1936 made possible our understanding of the concept of a pseudosynovial sheath in his classic experiments with celloidin tubes. Unfortunately he was unable to find a flexible inert material and abandoned this method. Mayer's concepts remained dormant for many years until Carroll and Basset (1959) used silicone rods to induce pseudosheath formation. Silicone is durable, chemically inert, flexible, and elastic. However, it lacks strength and tear resistance. Therefore, silicone by itself lacks the properties necessary for a suitable method of juncture to surrounding connective tissues.

In 1960 an implant was developed for limited clinical use, which possessed the necessary qualities for a successful passive gliding tendon implant. A woven Dacron core molded into silicone rubber provided the necessary combination of inertness, firmness, and flexibility, as well as the smooth glistening surface required to ensure ease of insertion and free passive gliding throughout the finger, palm and forearm.

SCIENTIFIC BACKGROUND

The basic concept of the pseudosynovial sheath technique of staged tendon grafting is that an implant is used to prepare the tendon bed for subsequent replacement by a tendon graft. The survival and the gliding properties of the tendon graft are enhanced by characteristics of the sheath. The usual cellular response to a static surgical implant is the formation of a fibrous capsule. However, the capsule can be modified by the reactivity of the implant and the physical demands at the implant bed interface. Hunter tendon implants have a woven Dacron core and are coated with a smooth silicone rubber surface (Fig. 32–1). Controlled gliding of the implant is the key factor in the production of the capsule that has the characteristics of a pseudosynovial sheath. When the sheath is formed in response to a biologically inert gliding structure (the implant), the cells adapt so that they can effectively accept another gliding structure (the tendon graft).

Early in the production of the pseudosynovial sheath, there is a proliferation of mesenchymal cells, probably perivascular fibro-

A

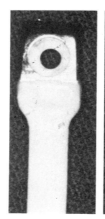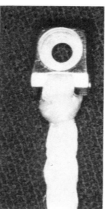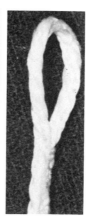

B

Figure 32–1. Hunter tendon implants. The implant is composed of a woven Dacron core coated with silicone rubber. *A,* Passive tendon implant (proximal). *B,* Active tendon implant of high tenacity Dacron braid. *Middle,* Silicone mold covered. Attached to metal plate. *Left,* proximal loop before silicone cover is added *(right).*

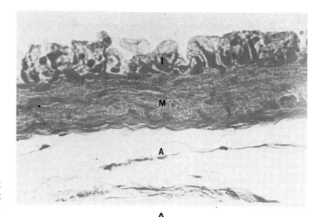

A

Figure 32–2. Pseudosynovial sheath in primate at four months. *A*, Pseudosynovial sheath, early (eight weeks). *B*, Pseudosynovial sheath, mature (16+ weeks). This photomicrograph of a mature pseudosynovial sheath demonstrates the three distinct layers: the inner intima (I), the middle media (M), and the outer adventitia (A).

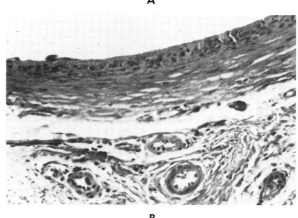

B

cytes, which differentiate into a stable coherent structure in about 12 weeks. After 12 weeks, there is little change in the sheath (Fig. 32–2). The pseudosynovial sheath is composed of three distinct layers, and these layers contribute to the maintenance and efficiency of the gliding system.

The mature intima is composed of cuboidal cells, which provide a smooth, slippery interface for the gliding of the implant. In addition, a periodic acid-Schiff (PAS) positive material is found on the surface of the layer and in vacuoles within the cells. This mucin-like glycosaminoglycan acts as a lubricant for the passive tendon. This substance may have characteristics and functions similar to those of synovial fluid and therefore may contribute to the early nutrition of the tendon graft through mechanically assisted diffusion.

The medium is a dense array of fibrocytes within a collagen matrix. This layer provides the structural integrity of the pseudosynovial sheath. Furthermore, its vascularity can provide a nutrient bed for the tendon graft. This layer remains stable for long periods and does not demonstrate a tendency to contract longitudinally or form a cicatrix.

The adventitial layer is composed of a loose arrangement of vascular fibrous tissue. It acts as an interface between the sheath and the surrounding tissue. This interface layer demonstrates a number of clefts or gliding planes that allow various degrees of motion in relation to the immobile surrounding structures.

A gliding tendon implant can transform the scattered confusion of a severely injured flexor system and its bed into an organized coherent predictable structure. This pseudosynovial sheath provides a gliding interface, lubrication, diffusible nutrients, and an organized vascular system. This aids in the survival of the tendon graft with a minimum of adhesion formation.

FLEXOR TENDON RECONSTRUCTION

Reconstruction of a damaged flexor tendon mechanism can be a complicated and, at times, perplexing problem. The surgeon must be aware of a great number of factors that enter into the decision making process. Many of these parameters, although appearing insignificant, may contribute greatly to the success or failure of the reconstruction, and they will be emphasized.

INDICATIONS

Staged tendon grafting is most often indicated when a primary tendon repair has failed and one stage tendon grafting is contraindicated. One stage tendon grafting is often compromised in a severely scarred tendon bed or when pulley reconstruction and joint releases are required concurrently.

Replantation surgery is becoming more common, with good results in regard to digit survival. However, the functional results are less satisfying. One major deficit is in flexor tendon function after replantation. In a digital replantation, both the flexor and the extensor tendons must be required and rehabilitated. This presents an especially difficult problem for the hand therapist because both tendon repairs are in proximity to a healing bone defect. In selected cases, the primary use of a passive flexor tendon implant can make the rehabilitation of the digit less of a problem and the ultimate tendon function more satisfying.

There are other instances in which primary passive tendon implants may be indicated. A flexor tendon laceration in zone II associated with an unstable phalangeal fracture that cannot be fixed well enough to allow early controlled motion is one indication. However, any zone II tendon laceration associated with a bone, joint, or extensor tendon injury that can interfere with a program of early controlled flexor tendon mobilization may be best treated by a tendon implant. This concept represents a departure from the traditional view. However, when basic principles of wound débridement and antibiotic coverage have been adhered to, infection has been minimal.

CONTRAINDICATIONS

Active infection and an uncooperative or unreliable patient are absolute contraindications for staged tendon grafting.

A digit with poor vascularity or an insensate digit that cannot be made to perceive sensation by appropriate nerve repair or grafting is a relative contraindication for staged tendon grafting. In a child less than five years of age, tendon implant insertion is not contraindicated, but stage II surgery should be delayed until the patient can cooperate.

PREOPERATIVE CARE FOR STAGE I SURGERY

Patient Education

Once the patient is considered a candidate for staged tendon grafting, it is extremely important that he understand the importance of the patient's role in the success of the procedure. The success of the technique rests largely on the patient's intelligent cooperation. The patient should be aware that frequent postoperative sessions with a hand therapist will be required to ensure the success of the procedure. The decision to perform staged reconstruction should be delayed until after the patient has successfully completed a regimen of preoperative hand therapy to determine his psychological suitability for the procedure.

Hand Therapy

A successful result in two staged tendon reconstruction is largely dependent upon the pre- and postoperative hand therapy program. The hand surgeon should communicate the goals of reconstruction to the hand therapist so that there is a full understanding of the nature of the surgical procedure. The therapist must be familiar with the anatomy and biomechanics of the hand. The intelligent participation of the surgeon, therapist, and patient often determines the difference between a good and a poor result.

Prior to surgery, the therapist carefully evaluates the digit. Ideally, the finger should passively flex fully with no loss of active extension. More commonly, when staged grafting is indicated the digit is severely scarred. Limited passive flexion, joint contractures, poor skin condition, and decreased sensation and vascularity can often be improved by therapeutic techniques such as splints, massage, exercise, and sensory re-education. Flexion contractures are a tenacious problem because if they are present preoperatively they often recur postoperatively if not vigorously treated throughout the reconstruction program.

OPERATIVE TECHNIQUE STAGE I

Stage I Surgery Versus Tenolysis Versus Free Tendon Grafting

Often the definitive surgical treatment required for a digit is not known prior to exploration of the flexor canal. Depending on the condition of the tendon and the retinacular pulley system, a tenolysis, a free tendon graft, or a tendon implant may be indicated. A Brunner zigzag incision is the preferred initial exploratory incision (Fig. 32–3). This incision gives the best exposure and has the least deleterious effect on the vascular supply of the flexor system. Tenolysis is best performed under neuroleptanalgesia so that the patient can actively flex and extend the fingers upon the surgeon's command. This permits an accurate immediate evaluation of the completeness and likely success of a tenolysis. However, the anesthesia staff should be prepared to institute general anesthesia if the decision is made to perform a free tendon graft or a tendon implant. Success with a tenolysis requires that the flexor tendon be intact with adequate pulleys because early postoperative active motion is required. Success with a one stage tendon graft requires

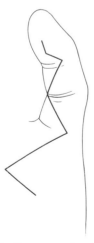

Figure 32–3. In finger, a volar zigzag incision popularized by Brunner is the incision of choice.

that the anatomical and functional aspects of the digit, including the pulley system, the flexor canal, and joint mobility, be intact. If after exploration, any of these anatomical or functional parameters are suboptimal, a tendon implant should be considered. Although the use of an implant necessitates a second procedure, it improves the probability of overall better active digital motion. By using an implant, the surgeon can reconstruct the pulley retinacular system, release stiff joints, and repair nerves without the danger that these procedures will interfere with optimal postoperative care.

Choice of Implant. There are four types of tendon implants commercially available if this proves to be the procedure of choice: (1) cylindrical pure silicone rods, (2) ovoid pure silicone rods (Swanson-Hunter design), (3) Dacron reinforced ovoid silicone rods inserted with only a distal juncture (Hunter passive implant), and (4) Dacron reinforced ovoid silicone rods with proximal and distal junctures (Hunter active implant). At present, Dacron reinforced silicone rods are preferred because the juncture between rod and tendon is stronger. If an implant juncture breaks and the implant becomes loose, synovitis frequently results, which impairs the overall result.

The passive Dacron implant coated with silicone rubber is available in two forms. One form is designed to be secured to bone by suturing techniques (Hunter design), whereas the other implant has a metal endpiece designed to be secured to bone using a screw (Hunter-Hausner design). The suture technique is indicated when bone is inadequate or in skeletally immature patients in order to preserve the growth plate. The screw technique is otherwise indicated because the fixation is more secure.

The active implant is constructed of a woven Dacron tubular twill core within a silicon coating (Fig. 32–4). The implant terminates in a loop proximally and a metal plate distally. It has a tensile rating greater than 100 lb. The implant is available in a 4 mm. diameter, a 2 mm. thickness, and lengths of 16, 18, 20, and 22 cm. A specially designed implant holder is available and maintains tendon length during autoclaving.

The indications for a passive versus an active implant are individualized. The active implant has the advantage of unrestricted use of the digit for extended periods prior to

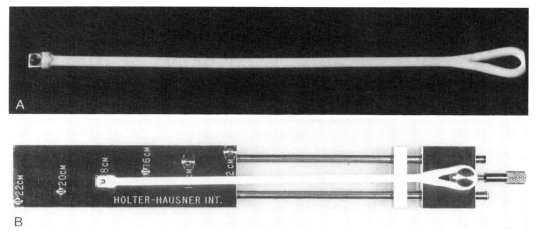

Figure 32–4. *A*, Active tendon implant with metal plate distally and loop proximally. *B*, Active implant held in tension on its holder.

replacement with a tendon graft. In elderly patients, it can be left in place indefinitely. The ultimate improvement in total active motion after a passive or an active implant is comparable and appears to be related more to the preoperative condition of the digit than to the type of implant used.

Technique of Implantation

PASSIVE IMPLANT. The retinacular pulley system is preserved in this procedure, but all scar tissue should be meticulously excised. The entire system from the proximal edge of the A1 pulley to the distal phalanx should be exposed and explored. All remnants of the flexor tendons should be excised through multiple transverse incisions in the retinacular pulley systems. A curvilinear incision is made on the volar ulnar aspect of the forearm. The flexor tendons are explored and the original motor muscles to the involved digit are identified. If these muscles appear to be functional, they should be preserved by suturing them to an adjacent intact tendon. If the origin motor muscle has been maintained by being scarred in the palm, these adhesions can be left intact. A muscle that is maintained in a stretched position will keep its capacity to contract and can be used as a motor source in stage II of the procedure. The implants are available in four sizes—3, 4, 5, and 6 mm. *The implant size should be chosen with the expected size of the future tendon graft in mind* rather than the size of the tendon being replaced. The 3 mm. implant is indicated in children. The 4 mm. implant is indicated when the plantaris or palmaris longus is the

expected graft material. The 5 and 6 mm. implants are used if a large tendon is to be used in stage II of the procedure.

The implant should be long enough to extend into the forearm. This ensures that the implant will glide smoothly with passive motion of the digit. If the end of the implant ends in the palm, mechanical obstruction can cause kinking and synovitis can result. Furthermore, when the implant extends into the forearm, at stage II surgery the proximal juncture can be at this point, which is preferable to a juncture in the palm. Because tissue planes are more mobile in the forearm, restrictive adhesions and flexion contractures are less likely when the proximal junction is located here.

The implant is placed in the retinacular pulley system from a distal to a proximal direction. At the proximal A1 pulley, the implant can be passed through the palm into the forearm with either a Bunnell or a Carroll tendon passer.

Great care should be used in handling the implant. Silicone rubber carries a significant static electrical charge, which causes it to attract lint and dust. These contaminants can cause severe synovitis. The implant should be kept immersed in an antibiotic saline solution until it is ready for use and then it should be handled only with smooth jawed forceps. If any contact occurs with gloves or drapes, the implant should be returned to the solution.

The distal juncture can be created by either suture techniques or screw fixation. Suture

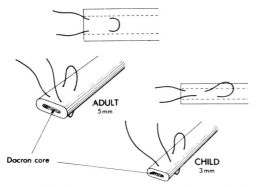

Figure 32–5. Distal juncture suture placement in implant. The sutures should be placed in the implant in such a way that they pass through the Dacron core.

techniques are preferred in the skeletally immature patient or when the bone stock of the distal phalanx is insufficient. The key points are that a stump of the flexor digitorum profundus be preserved for fixation and that the sutures be placed in the implant in such a way that they pass through the Dacron core (Figs. 32–5 and 32–6). A suture of multifilament 3-0 or 4-0 Dacron or monofilament wire is preferred.

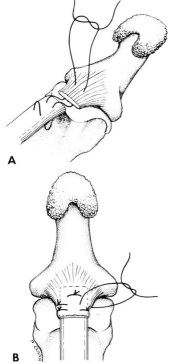

Figure 32–6. Fixation suture technique, distal juncture. *A*, The implant should be secured to the remaining stump of the flexor tendon. *B*, Additional sutures should be used to ensure proper fixation of the implant.

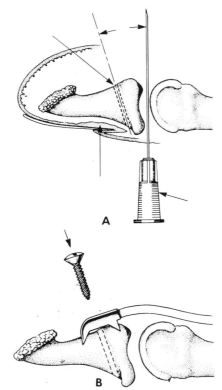

Figure 32–7. Distal juncture fixation screw technique (for passive and active tendons). *A*, A 27 gauge needle is inserted into the joint to confirm joint position and alignment. A 1.5 mm. hole is drilled at a 30 degree angle to the needle. Care should be taken to avoid the nail bed. *B*, A 2 mm. self-tapping screw is used to secure the implant. Care should be taken to avoid use of a screw that extends through the dorsal cortex more than 1 mm. (Note: Extraction forces are on metal plate, the screw holds the plate to the bone only.)

The screw fixation technique is more secure and this method is preferred in skeletally mature patients. This technique is demonstrated in Figure 32–7.

After the distal juncture is completed, a tunnel is bluntly dissected in the forearm to allow unimpeded proximal excursion of the implant with full flexion of the wrist and digits. Any constrictions in the path of the implant that could cause kinking with passive gliding should be dilated with a curved hemostat.

Traction should be placed on the proximal end of the implant and the amount of excursion as well as the maximal digit flexion should be recorded. The implant should be examined for any significant areas of bowstringing resulting from an inadequate retinacular pulley system. If the retinacular pulley system is adequate, skin closure is performed. Drains normally are not necessary. Short-term prophylactic antibiotic treatment is indicated.

ACTIVE IMPLANT. Active implants follow the same general guidelines for insertion as passive implants using the same incisions. The motor tendon unit in the forearm is exposed and tested for excursion. The profundus of the injured digit or digits is the preferred choice, but if excursion is insufficient, another available motor tendon unit is chosen. A superficialis motor unit can be chosen if necessary but its excursive potential is less than that of an intact profundus. The length of the implant is estimated by measuring the distance from the distal phalanx to the motor tendon unit in the forearm. The implant is threaded from palm to distal phalanx beneath the pulley system. The A4 pulley must be released to allow passage of the plate and is subsequently resutured. The distal juncture is prepared in the same manner as demonstrated in Figure 32–6 for the passive implant. Proximally, the motor tendon unit is placed through the loop and woven back on itself in a Pulvertaft weave under appropriate tension.

Retinacular Pulley Reconstruction

One of the major advantages of the passive staged tendon graft technique is that the surgeon can reconstruct the retinacular pulley system without fear of adhesions or disruption of the reconstructed system with active tendon excursion. An adequate intact retinacular pulley system is essential for good tendon function. Tendon bowstringing robs the flexor system of the longitudinal excursion required for angular excursion. Also, bowstringing can lead to flexion contractures as a result of the maldirection of tendon forces. Therefore, when the retinacular pulley system is inadequate and bowstringing is noted, reconstruction of the system is indicated (Fig. 32–8).

The prime function of the retinacular pulley system is to maintain the position of the tendon close to the bone, especially at the distal portion of the proximal and middle phalanges. These areas correspond to the distal portions of the A2 and A4 pulleys. When bowstringing exceeds 2 to 3 mm. in these areas, pulley reconstruction is indicated.

Various biological materials are available for pulley reconstruction; however, we prefer free tendon grafts. These materials can be used in a number of ways: they can be sutured to the residual rim of the retinacular system, passed through a drilled hole in the bone, and passed around the bone. We use either a portion of an excised flexor tendon or the palmaris longus. Our preferred technique is to pass the tendon graft around the bone twice and then suture it to itself with multiple multifilament Dacron sutures. The tendon is passed under the neurovascular bundle, deep to the extensor tendon mechanism at the proximal phalanx and superficial to the extensor tendon mechanism at the middle phalanx. The dissection is done with a right-angled hemostat and a Swanson designed suture passer. After the suturing has been completed, the site of juncture is rotated to the lateral aspect of the digit. This technique provides a tight pulley that has good tensile strength and does not interfere with bone

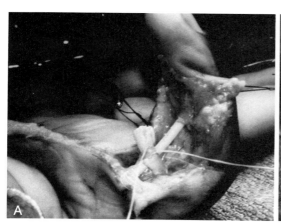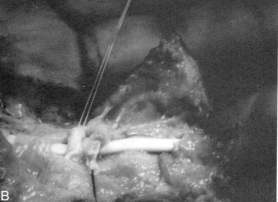

Figure 32–8. *A,* Building a pulley over a bowstring tendon. *B,* Double-wrapped tendon graft pulley at A$_2$ level.

integrity. The key points are to make the pulley wide by passing the tendon graft around the bone twice and to balance the reconstructed pulley system. The A2 and A4 pulleys are essential for flexor tendon function.

Skin Coverage

Often a flexion contracture is present in the digit at the time of the stage I operation. When the flexion contracture is released, skin coverage can present a significant problem, as the focus of injury has resulted in a firm scar bed and reduced digital nutrition.

A number of techniques are available to overcome this problem. The most applicable method involves advancing the zigzag flaps of the Brunner incision. The skin incisions are planned so that all the flaps of the Brunner zigzag are of equal size and have 90 degree angles. When the contractures are released, the flaps can be advanced in a V to Y fashion, thus providing full-thickness skin coverage of a fully extended digit.

If the skin deficit is too great to be corrected by advancing V-Y flaps, local transpositional flaps can be used. Defects in the mid-digit can be covered by cross finger flaps and flag flaps. Skin defects at the base of the digit can be covered by local rotational flaps on the palm. These local flaps prevent early controlled motion, but lack of adhesions with the staged tendon graft technique allows the use of a number of sophisticated reconstructive techniques in association with the staged method. Therefore, when there are severe skin coverage problems, even distant pedicle flaps can be used without fear of compromising the success of the staged tendon graft. The real problem is a return of the contracture, because the basic segmental vascular nutrition of the digit is poor. Experience over the past 20 years has shown that under circumstances such as this, a superficialis tendon finger has given the best results for the patient (Fig. 32–9). The major skin problem can be corrected by shifting the skin to cover the proximal phalanx. The distal interphalangeal

joint undergoes arthrodeses or tenodesis in a functional position and the implant's distal insertion is into the base of the middle phalanx. Skin grafting the remaining defect distal to the insertion of the implant can be performed if required.

Ancillary Procedures

Owing to the lack of adhesions to the silicone rubber coated tendon implant, other ancillary procedures can be performed during stage I that do not interfere with the final result of staged reconstruction. These include osteotomies, joint releases, neurorrhaphies, extensor tenolysis, and silicone joint replacements. Sufficient healing time and gentle early mobilization can be started immediately postoperatively without fear of implant adhesions or disruption. Extensor tenolysis is often required after joint releases, and silicone replacement arthroplasties can be performed with the knowledge that a postoperative therapy program can be followed that will encapsulate the joint replacement appropriately.

Dressings

The postoperative dressings are important to permit appropriate early hand therapy. We have preferred less bulky hand dressings so that complete digital flexion is permitted within the dressing. A dorsal splint is applied to extend 2 cm. beyond the fingertips with the wrist flexed to 30 degrees and the metacarpophalangeal joints flexed to 60 to 70 degrees. It is essential that the splint allow full extension of the proximal and distal interphalangeal joints.

POSTOPERATIVE THERAPY AFTER STAGE I SURGERY

Passive Implant

The splint is left in place for three weeks. Light protected function, initiated in the first week, consists of gentle passive flexion and

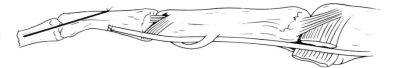

Figure 32–9. Superficialis finger. The distal end of the implant is set into the middle phalanx. The distal phalanx is either tenodesed or arthrodesed.

light finger trapping. If a proximal or distal interphalangeal joint flexion contracture existed prior to stage I surgery, it is likely to recur postoperatively. The hand therapist must be certain that the patient can fully extend the interphalangeal joints. If the contractures begin to recur, they should be treated aggressively with passive extension splints and gentle manual passive extension of the contracted joints.

The postoperative splint is removed after three weeks, and programmed activity is begun. Whirlpool baths and massage are initiated, as is the use of a Velcro finger trapper. The trapper incorporates the involved finger into useful function. Intensive therapy is required for the first six weeks. At six weeks, with the use of the trapper, some patients may be able to return to some type of employment during the period before stage II tendon grafting.

The goals of hand therapy for the period between the stage I and stage II operations are to obtain good mobility of joints, passive flexion of the digit to the distal palmar crease (or motion equal to that obtained at stage I surgery), correction of flexion contractures, and a viable gliding system. The patient's hand should be in its best possible condition prior to stage II surgery. Radiographs to visualize the tendon implant are taken at six weeks and again one day prior to stage II surgery.

Active Implant

The patient's hand is maintained in the protective dorsal splint applied at surgery. Therapy begins the first postoperative day. The first exercise, performed 10 times hourly, involves passive elastic band flexion and active extension of the proximal interphalangeal and distal interphalangeal joints. The tension of the elastic band must be carefully adjusted to assure that the patient is capable of fully extending the interphalangeal joints against its force. Full passive hold exercises are also begun. This exercise involves passive placement of the reconstructed digit in the flexed position and active maintenance of this position. Ten repetitions are performed three or four times a day. Both exercises ensure early gliding of the implant while minimizing tensile stresses.

To assure full digital flexion, the exercise program includes gentle manual full passive flexion of the digits, 10 repetitions three times a day.

The protective dorsal splint is generally removed six weeks postoperatively. The exercise program of passive elastic band flexion and active extension of the interphalangeal joints is continued for an additional two weeks with the elastic band attached to a wristlet.

Active flexion is begun eight weeks postoperatively; however, at four weeks the patient may gently squeeze a piece of foam rubber, ten repetitions several times a day, within the dorsal splint. Resistive flexion is started 10 weeks postoperatively. After three months no restrictions are placed upon the digit. The preceding timetable for therapy is adjustable depending upon the active restoration of motion. We have been more aggressive in therapy when motion has been poor and have held back when early motion has been rapidly obtained. Also, the timetable is modified depending upon the surgeon's assessment of the security of the junctures.

Reconstructed pulleys are protected in the early postoperative period by a pulley ring or by having the patient apply direct digital

---

Figure 32–10. A 23-year-old with right hand dominance sustained a crushing injury to the long finger and an amputation to the index finger of his right hand from a log splitter. Revascularization and tendon grafting were followed by a tenolysis. Two years later, however, severe tendon adhesions limited hand function. He became a candidate for superficialis finger reconstruction using an active tendon implant.

A, Stage I of the two stage tendon reconstruction using a Hunter active tendon implant. Radiographs show the metal endpiece secured into the base of the middle phalanx. The distal interphalangeal joint undergoes arthrodesis.

B–D, Passive hold exercise initiated the first postoperative day. The exercise involves passive placement of the digit in the flexed position and active maintenance of this position. Ten repetitions are performed three or four times a day. When rapid improvement in active flexion occurs, elastic band traction is initiated (passive flexion/active extension). Passive hold exercises are continued; however, the elastic band traction adds protection.

E, Wristlet with elastic band traction applied six weeks postoperatively. Reconstructed pulleys (A_1 and A_2) protected with thermoplastic pulley rings. The forceful early training program often requires that direct digital pressure with the uninvolved hand be applied over the reconstructed A_1 pulley as an additional reinforcement.

F, Resistive flexion eight weeks postoperatively. Depending on the job description, there are generally no restrictions placed on the digit after three months.

G, Hand therapy after stage II is essentially the same.

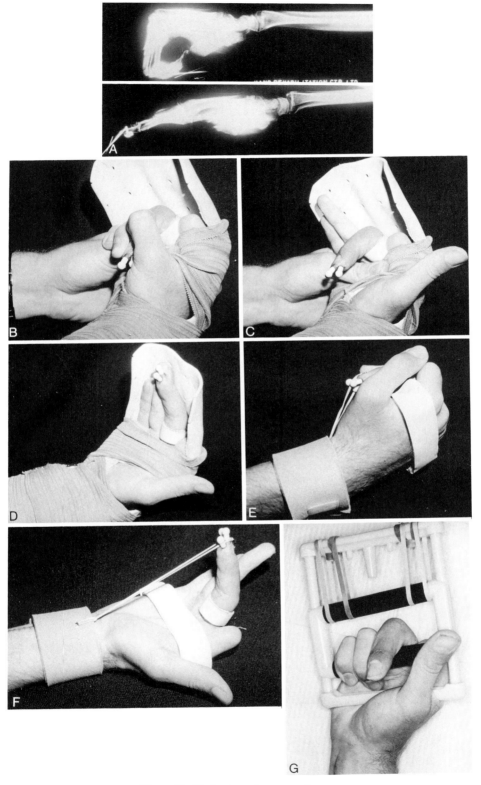

Figure 32–10. *See legend on opposite page*

pressure over the reconstructed pulley with the uninvolved hand. A Velcro and felt pulley ring can be fabricated, and the patient can progress to a molded thermoplastic ring as swelling recedes. A metal ring can replace the thermoplastic ring and can be used until six months after the pulley reconstruction (Fig. 32–10).

COMPLICATIONS FOLLOWING STAGE I SURGERY

The three most common complications after stage I surgery are sterile synovitis, loosening of the juncture, and infection. In general, these complications are uncommon if meticulous implantation technique is followed.

Sterile synovitis may develop any time between stage I and stage II surgery. It presents as a diffuse swelling of the digit (Fig. 32–11). If untreated, enough fluid can be produced to lead to bursa formation in the forearm. A focus of open drainage may develop. The fluid is initially sterile but can become secondarily contaminated after open drainage occurs. The synovitis is caused either by contamination of the surface of the static electricity charged implant or to abnormal mechanical factors. Contamination by foreign material can be prevented by care in the handling of the implant prior to implantation. This includes keeping the implant moist and handling it only with wet smooth forceps. *It is imperative that the implant not come in contact with gloves or drapes.* Mechanical factors that can cause synovitis include loosening of the distal juncture (Fig. 32–12), kinking of the implant during digital flexion, and twisting of the implant. These problems can be prevented by correct implantation technique and ensuring unrestricted gliding of the implant prior to skin closure. Usually, loosening only of the distal juncture in the active implant causes synovitis. Loosening of

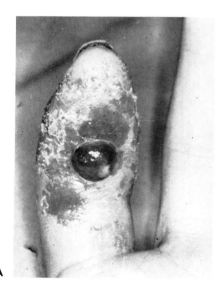

A

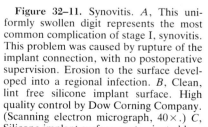

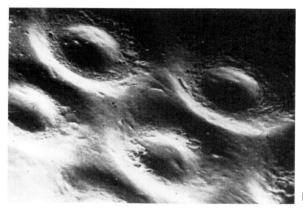

B

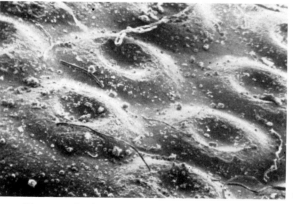

C

Figure 32–11. Synovitis. *A*, This uniformly swollen digit represents the most common complication of stage I, synovitis. This problem was caused by rupture of the implant connection, with no postoperative supervision. Erosion to the surface developed into a regional infection. *B*, Clean, lint free silicone implant surface. High quality control by Dow Corning Company. (Scanning electron micrograph, 40×.) *C*, Silicone implant surface contaminated by contact with surgeon's glove and operating room drapes—a cause of synovitis. (Scanning electron micrograph, 40×.)

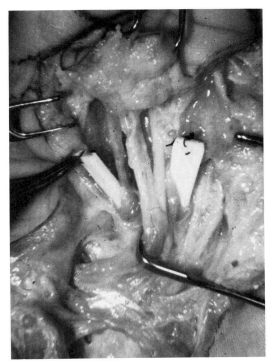

Figure 32–12. Stage I synovitis, palm. Here the sterile synovitis was due to implant loosening. This patient required removal of the implant and revision of stage I.

the proximal juncture of the active implant does not seem to cause synovitis.

If sterile synovitis occurs, the treatment is rest and splinting. This usually alleviates the inflammation, after which the hand therapy program can be resumed. If the synovitis recurs repeatedly, the options include revising stage I versus completion of stage II. The decision depends on the time that has elapsed since stage I surgery and the suppleness of the joints. If four weeks have passed since stage I surgery and the joints are supple, stage II surgery can be safely performed. However, if it is premature to carry out stage II surgery, the implant can be removed, the pseudosheath irrigated, mechanical factors corrected, and a new implant inserted.

Loosening of the distal juncture in the passive implant has been uncommon since the development of the Hunter-Hausner implant with screw fixation. However, the active implants ultimately will fail at either the proximal or the distal juncture. Therefore, it is important to obtain frequent radiographs after stage I surgery to anticipate juncture loosening (Fig. 32–13). If no synovitis is present after distal loosening, and migration of the implant does not occur proximal to the

middle phalanx, the hand therapy program can be continued.

True septic synovitis after stage I surgery is extremely rare. Initial treatment is antibiotics and immobilization. If the infection continues, the implant should be removed. After resolution of the infection, stage I surgery can be safely attempted once again.

OPERATIVE TECHNIQUE STAGE II

After three months of passive and active gliding, the tendon implant will have led to the development of a mature pseudosynovial sheath that can nourish an autogenous free tendon graft without adhesions. One of the advantages of the staged tendon graft technique is that at the time of stage II tendon grafting, the incisions and dissection required are minimal. Only the most distal portion of the digital incision and the volar forearm incision need be reopened (Fig. 32–14). Then, through careful dissection, the distal and proximal ends of the implant are identified.

Choice of Tendon Graft

The surgeon should not impair the final result by using a suboptimal tendon graft.

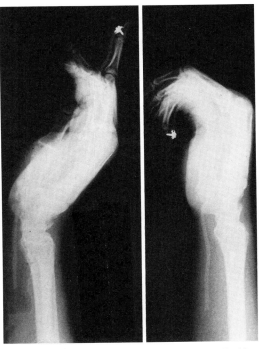

Figure 32–13. X-ray, postoperative, stage I. Note extension and flexion excursion of implant.

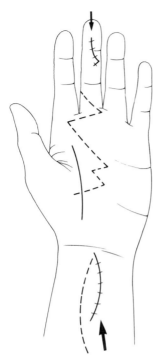

Figure 32–14. Stage II of surgery. Only the most distal portion of the digital incision and the volar forearm incision need be reopened.

The palmaris longus and plantaris have proved to be the best tendon grafts in our experience. A superficialis tendon left in the proximal palm may be freed and used as a tendon graft. The diameter of this tendon graft is large, but if the tendon bed has been prepared by a large 5 or 6 mm. tendon implant, a superficialis tendon can be a useful source for a tendon graft. The palmaris longus is the easiest to harvest but may be too short for the index, middle, or ring fingers. The plantaris is longer but often is too thin or is absent, precluding its use. If these tendons are absent or inadequate, the long extensors to the second, third, or fourth toes are chosen. These tendons are always available, but owing to the difficulty in harvesting them their quality is uneven.

Bunnell referred to the paratenon as "slippery stuff" and transferred the paratenon with the tendon graft. We prefer to carefully remove all paratenon, because it is believed to contribute to adhesion formation. After the graft has been harvested and cleaned, it is placed in a wet sponge. It is essential that the graft remain moist.

Choice of Motor Muscle

The motor muscle must have adequate excursion capabilities and strength. When using a passive implant, the motor muscle should be tentatively selected at the time of stage I surgery. The best motor muscle is the original flexor digitorum profundus of the affected digit. Appropriate measures should be taken during stage I surgery to preserve the function of this muscle. This requires that the muscle be maintained in a condition of stretch, either by suturing it to an adjacent profundus or by leaving it scarred in the palm.

If the original flexor digitorum profundus is not adequate or available, the tendon graft can be sutured to an adjacent profundus muscle. The flexor digitorum superficialis muscle is an alternative, although its excursion capability is limited compared with a profundus tendon.

The motor muscle selected to receive the tendon graft should be prepared with as little dissection as possible, but scar tissue should be excised at the site of the tendon juncture.

Distal Juncture

The distal end of the implant is identified and exposed, preserving the stump of the profundus tendon. The distal fixation (either screw or suture) is removed and the implant is freed. The tendon graft is sutured to the distal end of the implant and the implant is removed proximally, drawing the tendon graft into the pseudosynovial sheath. If at any time the tendon graft is accidentally removed from the pseudosynovial sheath, the implant can be moistened and reinserted into the sheath. If there is difficulty in passing the original implant, the next smaller size will pass through the sheath canal with ease.

The preferred method to secure the tendon graft to the distal phalanx is as follows: The site of tendon graft contact should be prepared by dissecting scar and periosteum from the bone. A broach can be used to drill a shallow hole in the volar cortex of the phalanx. A Keith needle is used to pass the suture through the bone and nail, but care must be taken to avoid the germinal matrix of the nail. After the suture is tied over the button and petrolatum gauze has been wrapped under the button to reduce button movement and slippage, additional 4–0 multifilament Dacron sutures are used to secure the tendon graft to the profundus tendon stump (Fig. 32–15). The digital incision is closed prior to creating the proximal juncture to muscle.

Proximal Juncture

When dissecting the motor tendon unit after an active implant has been inserted at stage I surgery, care should be taken to disturb the tendon bed minimally if gliding has been adequate. This prevents devascular-

ization of the proximal tendon and ultimately proximal rupture. Use of a Pulvertaft inter-woven suture is the preferred technique for the proximal juncture in both active and passive implants. Tension is of greatest importance, and it should be tested after the first weave is completed. The tension should be slightly tighter than that in adjacent digits. Testing is accomplished after preliminary suturing by passively flexing and extending the wrist and observing the tenodesis effect. In selected patients the stage II operation can be performed under neuroleptanalgesia,

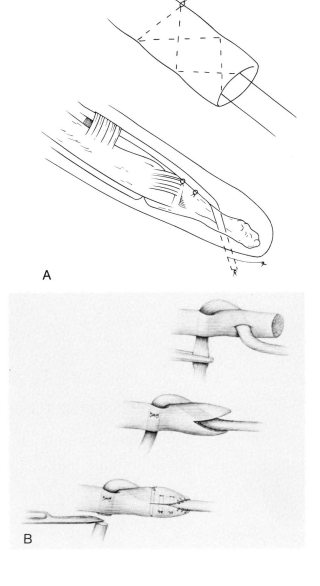

Figure 32–15. *A*, After the suture is tied over the button, additional 4-0 multifilament Dacron sutures are used to secure the tendon graft to the profundus tendon stump. *B*, The Pulvertaft inter-weave as applied at the lumbrical level in the palm is similarly applied in the forearm, preferably at the profundus, or at the superficialis muscle tendon juncture. *Top*, Profundus tendon is divided, leaving lumbrical muscles and tendon free in proximal palm. *Top Middle*, After distal end of tendon graft is attached, the proximal end is drawn into the profundus tendon. *Bottom Middle*, Tendon graft passes in and out of the profundus at 90 degree angles. *Bottom*, Graft is fixed to the profundus with multiple wire sutures.

which allows for active muscle excursion to test the tension of the tendon graft. After the tension is set, at least two more 90 degree weaves of the tendon should be completed. It may be helpful to use several stainless steel sutures in the proximal juncture in order to assess excursion radiographically in the postoperative period.

Dressings

After the forearm wound is closed, a 4–0 monofilament suture is placed through to the distal aspect of the fingernail for supervised elastic band control. The dressings are essentially the same as those used in the stage I operation.

HAND THERAPY

Elastic Band Traction. Hand therapy after stage II active or passive tendon implantation is essentially the same. The patient is seen by the hand therapist on the first postoperative day to begin tendon gliding and contracture control. As already expressed, the concept behind the two stage tendon reconstruction system is to carry out all the ancillary reconstructive procedures at the stage I operation. The surgeon has created a system that will create fluid and is designed to move. A tendon graft at stage II surgery does not require immobilization postoperatively. Biologically, at stage II the tendon graft must be moved early, with controlled movement carefully supervised by the hand therapist. The use of early mobilization in primary tendon repair has improved tendon gliding. The program should be applied to patients undergoing staged tendon grafting.

The patient's hand is maintained in a protective dorsal splint applied at surgery. The dressing applied to the fingers is partially removed so that passive digital flexion to the palm is possible within the confines of the splint. When the dressing is removed, the splint may not fit as securely. Adhesive tape should be applied across the forearm, wrist, and palm to ensure that the patient's hand will not slip within the splint, putting tension on the newly sutured junctures.

One advantage of elastic band traction is that it facilitates tendon and joint movement without requiring active pull on the flexor tendon. Another advantage is that it protects

against sudden injury. If the patient jerks the hand during sleep or if he falls, the elastic band will protect the juncture from the stress of active flexion. Although the monofilament suture is placed through the distal fingernail at surgery for elastic band traction, we prefer to wait until the patient first comes to therapy so that the quality, positioning, and tension of the elastic band can be accurately established. The elastic band should be placed 3 to 4 inches proximal to the wrist crease on the volar aspect of the forearm dressing with the finger in its normal alignment. The tension of the rubber band is important. It should be adjusted so that the rubber band pulls the finger into flexion at rest and yet permits the antagonist muscles to actively extend the finger completely within the limits of the dorsal splint so that flexion contractures will not develop.

We have found that the commercially available graded rubber bands are never quite right. If the elastic band holds the finger in the appropriate flexion at rest, it often does not allow the patient to actively extend his finger fully against the tension of the elastic band. Failure to completely extend the proximal and distal interphalangeal joints will result in flexion contractures. The elastic that best suits our purpose is elastic thread.* It may be used as a single strand, and as the patient becomes stronger the strands may be doubled, increasing the tension.

When the finger is flexed and at rest, there should be very little tension on the elastic band. With careful positioning in the splint and with light tension on the elastic band, the patient may actively extend the finger and permit the elastic band to passively flex the finger 10 times each hour. In addition, gentle passive full flexion of the proximal and distal interphalangeal joints is carried out 10 times, 3 or 4 times a day. Manual passive flexion of the joints must be done carefully. Previous operations and too much passive cranking may cause attenuation of the extensor tendon; thus as we strive to get passive distal interphalangeal joint flexion, we also emphasize active distal interphalangeal joint extension.

Early attention to beginning flexion contractures is of primary importance, because

---

*Available from Elastic Thread, #7034 Alimed, 68 Harrison Ave., Boston, MA 02111.

patients who have difficulty with contractures prior to stage I and stage II surgeries are likely to develop recurrent contractures. If the dorsal splint does not allow full extension of the proximal interphalangeal joint, the patient must be instructed to passively flex the metacarpophalangeal joint of the involved finger to facilitate active extension of the interphalangeal joints.

When the surgeon and the therapist are alerted to the development of proximal or distal interphalangeal flexion contractures, passive extension of the interphalangeal joints may be initiated as early as the first week. No "tendon tension" passive extension may be initiated. Tension is taken off the tendon by flexion of the adjacent joint. With the dorsal splint supporting the wrist and the metacarpophalangeal joints in flexion, the therapist may support the metacarpophalangeal joint in flexion and gently extend the proximal interphalangeal joint passively to improve extension. If the distal interphalangeal joint shows a beginning contracture, the therapist may support the metacarpophalangeal and proximal interphalangeal joints in flexion and gently extend the distal interphalangeal joint passively. Passive extension effected by this technique decreases the tension at the tendon juncture. These passive extension exercises should be included in the patient's home program.

Persistent flexion contractures may require a proximal joint wedge or a proximal interphalangeal passive extension splint. An AlumaFoam splint that positions the metacarpophalangeal joint in greater flexion and

gently pulls the contracted interphalangeal joint into extension is custom fitted within the dorsal splint (Fig. 32–16). This splint should be worn intermittently during the day. The exact schedule depends upon the "feel" of the contracture, that is, whether it will quickly or slowly respond to stretching. With this technique of passive stretching we have found that problems with flexion contractures can be minimized and overall tendon function enhanced.

Full excursion of the tendon graft occurring within the first three to four postoperative weeks indicates minimal adhesion formation. In such a case, the tendon junctures are at greater risk of rupture if stressed. We have found this to be especially true when active tendon implants have been inserted, in which the flexor system is already geared up for active motion after stage I surgery. If the tendon graft is gliding well, and if measurements taken by the surgeon and hand therapist indicate rapid improvement in active flexion to the distal palmar crease, the patient is maintained in the dorsal splint for six weeks. The button is removed at five to six weeks. When the dorsal splint is removed, the patient's hand is maintained in a wristlet with elastic band traction. The wristlet permits full active extension of the interphalangeal and metacarpophalangeal joints with the wrist in a neutral position. The elastic band pulls the fingers back into flexion at rest. Wrist dorsiflexion may be done with the fingers resting in flexion.

At 8 to 10 weeks, the wristlet is removed and the patient begins active flexion exer-

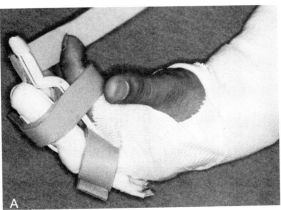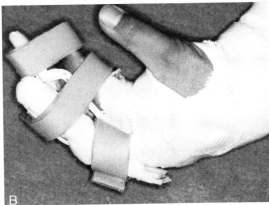

Figure 32–16. *A*, Persistent flexion contractures may require a proximal interphalangeal passive extension splint. *B*, An AlumaFoam splint fitted within the dorsal splint is used to position the metacarpophalangeal joint in greater flexion and gently pull the contracted interphalangeal joint or joints into extension.

cises. The initiation of active exercise depends upon the restoration of active motion. When adhesions seem to be restricting motion, we begin active flexion earlier and have held the patient back when active flexion is excellent. Finger blocking, tendon gliding exercises, and the use of putty may be initiated at this time. Whirlpool therapy may be started again. Fingers that have been stiff prior to stage I surgery may require softening with lanolin massage. At 10 weeks the patient may begin light supervised woodworking (sanding, filing). Progressive weight resistance exercises and heavy resistance exercises are not permitted until three months postoperatively.

Early Motion. In certain circumstances, depending on the condition of the tendon bed and the strength of the graft and its junctures, active flexion may be initiated following stage II tendon grafting without the use of an elastic band, even as early as the first postoperative week. We begin with a passive hold exercise within the dorsal splint. The splinting guidelines for this method of early motion are essentially the same as those discussed for early motion using elastic band traction, that is, dressing applied at surgery is pulled away from the fingers and adhesive tape is applied across the palm, wrist, and forearm to secure the splint firmly.

The passive hold exercise is performed in the following manner. The patient rolls the finger or fingers into the palm with the uninvolved hand, releases the uninvolved hand, and tries to hold the finger or fingers in flexion with his own muscle power (Fig. 32–

17). It takes less force to maintain a flexed finger in flexion than to actively pull the finger into flexion from an extended position, whereas tendon excursion is similar and ensured. We ask the patient to carry out this exercise in full flexion and at two levels of partial flexion. Three repetitions at each level are performed three to four times a day. In addition, gentle flexion of the interphalangeal joints is performed several times a day within the dorsal splint. If the patient begins to glide the tendon very early and excellent tendon pullthrough is demonstrated, we slow him down at two weeks by applying elastic band traction. The patient can still do the passive hold exercise; however, the elastic band traction program adds protection.

The 6 to 12 week postoperative program is essentially the same as that described earlier. Careful attention is also given to the prevention of flexion contractures.

SPECIAL CONSIDERATIONS

Pulley Reconstruction

Testing the strength and integrity of the pulley system is an important part of stage I surgery. Weak or absent pulleys may have to be reconstructed. Before wound closure, the free proximal end of the implant is grasped and pulled, the finger being brought from extension to flexion. If the finger does not fully flex to the distal palmar crease, it may be necessary for the surgeon to modify the pulley system or to accept the reduced active

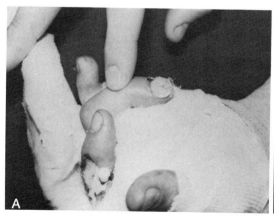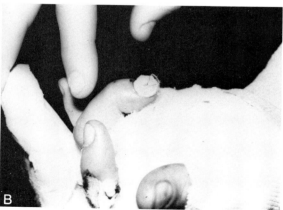

Figure 32–17. "Passive hold" exercise. *A,* The patient rolls his finger or fingers into the palm with the uninvolved hand. *B,* He then releases the uninvolved hand and holds his finger or fingers in flexion with the most delicate amount of muscle power possible.

potential as a final result after stage II surgery. This predicted potential is measured and recorded. When active implants are used, the pulley system is constantly being tested between stage I and II surgeries and can be reconstructed prior to stage II surgery if inadequate. Reconstructed pulleys of stage II (passive tendon implant) and stages I and II (active tendon implant) must be protected in the early postoperative period. As explained earlier, the patient may apply direct digital pressure over the reconstructed pulley with the uninvolved hand or wear a pulley ring. Initial rings can be fabricated from Velcro and felt and from a thermoplastic material such as Aquaplast* when swelling recedes. A metal ring can eventually replace the thermoplastic ring. Reconstructed pulleys should be protected for six months postoperatively.

Moleskin Sling

When a nylon suture cannot be attached to the tip of the fingernail at surgery (e.g., because of absence of the fingernail), a sling of moleskin may be used to provide elastic band traction around the button and pullout wire. A segment of moleskin about 3 inches long and ½ inch wide is folded in half and an eyelet is punched through at the folded end. An S hook, made from a paperclip, is hooked through the eyelet opening, and an elastic band is attached from it to a safety pin on the volar surface of the forearm dressing or, when the protective splint is no longer required, to a wrist cuff. Tincture of benzoin applied to the finger helps the moleskin adhere.

Adhesions

Each patient is unique, and postoperative treatment must always be modified and changed according to the patient's progress. If active flexion improves steadily each week, the program is not changed. If the formation of adhesions is limiting active motion, the dorsal splint should be discarded at four weeks and a more active exercise program initiated earlier, beginning with finger blocking and progressing to resistive exercise with a Bunnell wood block and putty exercises at five weeks. Squeezing a household sponge in the whirlpool followed by massage will help to soften the tissues. Light sustained grip

*Aquaplast available from WFR/Aquaplast Corp., P.O. Box 635, Wyckoff, NJ 07481

activities (e.g., woodworking) are instituted at six weeks, progressing to heavy resistance exercise by the 12th postoperative week.

Tendon Gliding Exercises

When active flexion of the involved digit or digits is permitted, tendon gliding exercises are an important part of postoperative management. Differential tendon gliding is an important factor in controlling the formation of adhesions between and around tendons following hand injury and disease (Fig. 32–18).

Bunnell Wood Block

The Bunnell wood block is ¼ inch thick and about the size of a cigarette pack. The metacarpophalangeal joint is supported firmly against the block with the fingers and thumb of the opposite hand when flexing the proximal interphalangeal joint. Similarly, the patient may block the metacarpophalangeal and proximal interphalangeal joints when flexing the distal interphalangeal joint. Blocking facilitates isolated superficialis and profundus action.

COMPLICATIONS AFTER STAGE II SURGERY

The most frequent complications after stage II surgery are rupture of the tendon graft, infection, and adhesions. Infection is extremely uncommon. The signs and symptoms are those of septic tenosynovitis, and the four signs of Kanavel are present. Once the condition is diagnosed, cultures are obtained and the pseudosynovial sheath is flushed with antibiotic solution. Wide spectrum antibiotics should be administered intravenously until specific microorganisms are cultured. Often these measures can salvage the tendon graft. Tendon grafts can survive infection as long as they remain moist under tension.

Rupture of the tendon graft is diagnosed when the digit loses its normal cascade. Often the patient reports a "snap" during exercise or sudden, accidental hyperextension of the digit. The treatment depends on the correct identification of the site of the tendon rupture. The rupture usually occurs at the distal juncture, although it can occur at the proximal juncture. Exploration of the sheath is begun in the mid-palm. At this level the

TENDON GLIDING EXERCISES

This exercise program is a very important part of your treatment.

There are three ways of making a fist:

  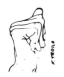

Straight   Hook   Fist   Straight Fist

1. Start with your fingers straight every time.

2. Make each type of fist ten times.

3. Curl your thumb down in your palm as much as possible then stretch it out as far as possible. Repeat ten times.

4. Do these exercises at least three times every day.

Figure 32–18. Anatomical, clinical, and electromyographic studies demonstrate that the profundus and superficialis tendons glide over each other maximally in the hook position; the profundus glides most in respect to bone in the fist position, and the superficialis reaches its maximum excursion in respect to bone when assuming the straight fist position.

tendon graft can always be found and the site of the rupture identified. If the rupture is re-explored early, it is often possible to reinsert the tendon graft. If this is impossible, a tendon implant can be used as an obturator to pass a new tendon graft with no additional incisions or exploration.

In some instances salvage of the entire flexor system may not be indicated. In this case the concept of the superficialis digit is applicable (see Fig. 32–19). The distal interphalangeal joint undergoes either tenodesis or arthrodesis and the tendon graft is fixed to the middle phalanx. This form of salvage can yield a satisfying functional result.

Occasionally, despite good care by the surgeon and the hand therapist and cooperation by the patient, adhesions can develop that interfere with tendon excursion. If after six months the digit shows little progress, tenolysis is indicated. The tenolysis should be performed with neuroleptanalgesia, and a postoperative anesthetic catheter should be used.

EXTENSOR TENDON RECONSTRUCTION

The use of the staged tendon grafting technique in flexor tendon reconstruction is well known, but the use of the tendon implant in

the extensor system is less familiar. However, the staged tendon graft technique can yield significant benefit in the reconstruction of a severely damaged extensor tendon system.

INDICATIONS

Simple lacerations of extensor tendons can be easily repaired with consistently good results. However, in severe avulsion injuries and burns in which a significant loss of extensor substance and loss of skin occurs, tendon implants can be useful. Another indication is in replantation surgery in which the amputation is proximal to the metacarpal heads and distal to the musculotendinous junction of the extensors. In this case repair of both the flexors and the extensors poses difficult problems in hand therapy. The flexors can be repaired and passive extensor tendon implants can be used. The patient can be fitted with a dynamic extensor splint and the initial hand therapy program can be directed to rehabilitation of the flexors.

OPERATIVE TECHNIQUE STAGE I

The extensor system is approached through a lazy S incision, and the extensor insertion on the extensor hood is identified. A 4 mm.

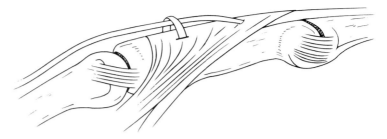

Figure 32–19. Implant centralized with a pulley near the metacarpophalangeal joint level.

tendon implant is sutured to the insertion with a 3–0 multifilament Dacron suture; the proximal ends of the implants are passed under the extensor retinaculum to the area of the extensor musculotendinous junctions. If a flap is necessary for skin coverage, the implants are well tolerated by the flap tissue. The implant should be centralized with a pulley near the metacarpalphalangeal joint level (Fig. 32–19).

HAND THERAPY

Passive gliding is necessary for the production of an adequate pseudosynovial sheath. This can be accomplished by passive range of motion exercises and with dynamic splints. A dorsal outrigger with rubber band slings provides dynamic extension with active flexor activity.

After one to two months it may be noted that the patient has regained some active extension. This phenomenon was first noted by one of the authors (JMH) early in the course of active tendon research. Prototype active tendon implants had been used to replace the wrist extensors in dogs, with apparent success. However, after the active implants had been removed for analysis, the dogs continued to have good extensor function. It was found that the pseudosynovial sheath that formed in response to the active implants became fixed to adjacent tissue to reproduce extensor tendon function. This is possible because the bed of the extensor system is quite different from that of the flexor system, and gliding planes can develop between the pseudosynovial sheath and the surrounding fixed tissues to allow excursion of the pseudosynovial sheath. This sometimes alleviates the need for stage II tendon grafts when the implant is removed.

OPERATIVE TECHNIQUE STAGE II

Three months after implantation, the extensor tendon implants are exposed, with care being taken not to interfere with the pseudosynovial sheaths. The tendon grafts should be passed through the pseudosynovial sheaths and woven into the extensor hood distally and the extensor tendons proximally. The tension is determined by observing the tenodesis effect with passive flexion and extension of the wrist. If the extensor motor muscles are absent or inadequate, flexor digitorum superficialis tendons can be transferred through the interosseous membrane, and the tails of split tendon can be passed through the pseudosynovial sheaths to the extensor hoods.

HAND THERAPY

A dynamic extensor outrigger splint is used in the postoperative period. The splint allows

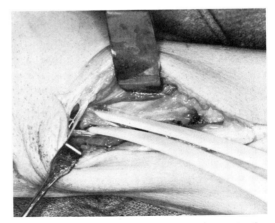

Figure 32–20. Transinterosseous membrane tendon transfers, forearm. Two 6 mm. implants can be used at stage I to prepare a sheath for later tendon transfers through the interosseous membrane.

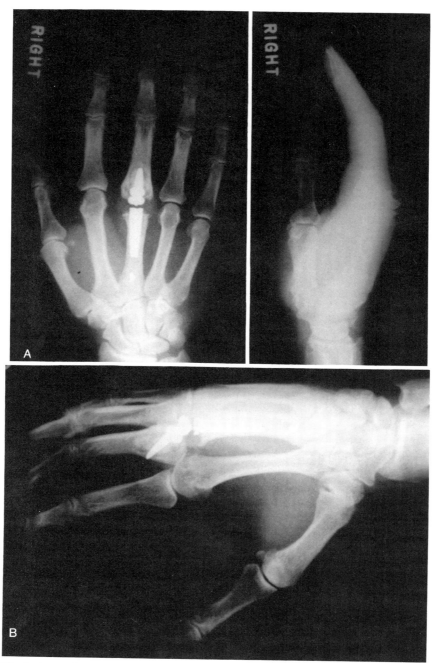

Figure 32–21. Active tendon program. *A* and *B*, A 54 year old man with right hand dominance underwent a metallic implant arthroplasty for degenerative arthritis. Approximately four years after surgery he lost motion and pain developed in the digit. He was referred to the Hand Center for evaluation. The implant had fractured and perforated the proximal phalanx volarly, with rupture of the flexor digitorum profundus and flexor digitorum superficialis tendons of the long finger.

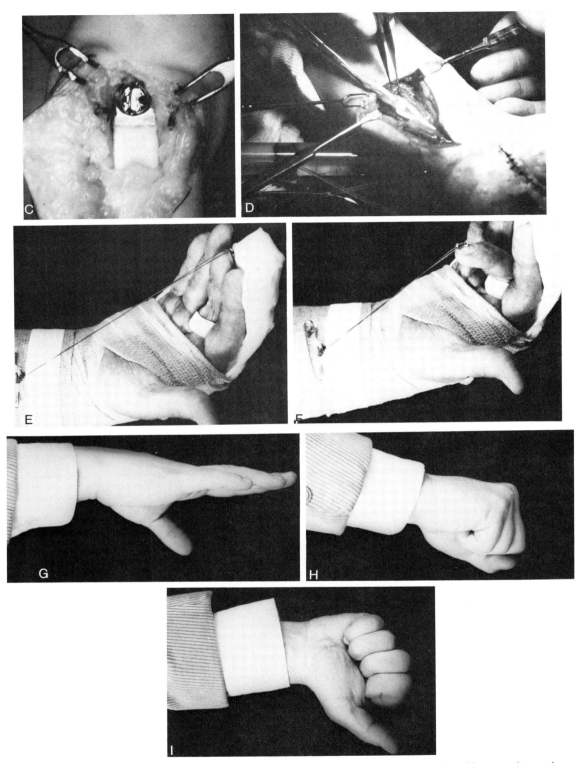

Figure 32–21 *Continued C*, Stage I of the two stage tendon reconstruction procedure using a Hunter active tendon implant. The metal endpiece is secured distally to bone using screw fixation (Hunter-Hausner design). *D*, Active implant proximal silicone-coated Dacron loop for motor tendon unit juncture. The appropriate motor capsule is chosen and pulled through the loop to set the tension. *E*, Dorsal protective splint and rubber band traction. Early mobilization in primary tendon repair has improved tendon gliding and should be used in staged tendon reconstruction, with gentle active extension. *F*, Pulley ring supports reconstructed A₂ pulley. *G*, Final result after metacarpophalangeal implant arthroplasty and staged tendon reconstruction using a Hunter active tendon implant. Extension. *H* and *I*, Flexion.

277

active range of motion but protects the reefed pseudosheath or tendon graft junctures until sufficient healing occurs.

OTHER USES OF TENDON IMPLANTS

In addition to the use of tendon implants in the reconstruction of damaged flexor and extensor systems, the tendon implant has other applications.

STAGED OPPONENSPLASTY

The staged tendon graft technique can be applied to opponensplasty when there has been significant scarring at the base of the thumb. The tendon can be sutured to the appropriate site on the thumb and passed subcutaneously around a fixed pulley point and into the forearm. The flexor digitorum superficialis of the ring finger or tendon graft can be used three months later to provide opposition with few adhesions and rapid recovery.

RADIAL NERVE PALSY TENDON TRANSFERS

The transfer of the flexor digitorum superficialis of the middle and ring finger tendons through the interosseous membrane to provide extension is a mechanically sound procedure. However, adhesions to the interosseous membrane can severely hinder excursion. Therefore, the procedure can be staged, a pseudosynovial sheath being formed through the membrane prior to tendon transfer (Fig. 32–20).

CONCLUSION

Tendon implants can be a powerful tool for the hand surgeon. However, in order to obtain reliable, satisfying results, the surgeon must understand the concepts of the technique and the biology of repair. Most important, success in these procedures requires the cooperative effort of the surgeon, the hand therapist, and the patient (Fig. 32–21).

REFERENCES

Biesalski, K.: Ueber Sehnenscheidenauswechslung. Dtsch. Med. Wochenschr., 36:1615–1618, 1910.

Biesalski, K., and Mayer, L.: Die physiologische Sehnenverpflanzung. Berlin, Springer Verlag, 1916.

Brand, P.: Principles of free tendon grafting, including a new method of tendon suture. J. Bone Joint Surg. 41B:208, 1959.

Brunner, J. M.: The zig-zag volar digital incision for flexor tendon surgery. Plast. Reconstr. Surg., 40:571–574, 1967.

Carroll, R. E., and Bassett, A. L.: Formation of tendon sheath by silicone rod implants. J. Bone Joint Surg. 45A:884–885, 1963.

Doyle J. R., and Blythe, W.: The finger flexor tendon sheath and pulleys: anatomy and reconstruction. In American Academy of Orthopedic Surgeons: Symposium on Tendon Surgery in the Hand. St. Louis, The C. V. Mosby Company, 1975.

Hunter, J. M.: Artificial tendons: early development and application. Am. J. Surg. 109:325–338, 1965.

Hunter, J. M.: Artificial tendons: early development and application. J. Bone Joint Surg. 47A:631–632, 1965.

Hunter, J. M.: Two-staged tendon reconstruction using gliding tendon implants. In Rob, C., and Smith R. (Eds.): Operative Surgery. Sevenoaks, Kent, Butterworth & Company, Ltd., 1978, pp. 601–616.

Hunter, J. M., and Amadio, P. C.: Two-stage tendon reconstruction using gliding tendon implants. In Dudley, H. and Carter D. (Eds.): Operative Surgery, Ed. 4. Seven Oaks, Kent, Butterworth & Company, 1984, pp. 149–167.

Hunter, J. M., and Jaeger, S. H.: The active gliding tendon prosthesis: progress. In American Academy of Orthopaedic Surgeons: Symposium on Tendon Surgery in the Hand. St. Louis, The C. V. Mosby Company, 1975.

Hunter, J. M., and Jaeger, S. H.: Tendon implants; primary and secondary usage. Orthop. Clin. North Am., 8:473–489, 1977.

Hunter, J. M., and Salisbury R. E.: Use of gliding artificial implants to produce tendon sheaths: techniques and results in children. Plast. Reconstr. Surg., 45:564, 1970.

Hunter, J. M., and Salisbury R. E.: Flexor tendon reconstruction in severely damaged hands. J. Bone Joint Surg., 53A:829, 1971.

Hunter, J. M., Salem, A. W., Steindel, C. R., and Salisbury, R. E.: The use of gliding artificial tendon implants to form new tendon beds. J. Bone Joint Surg., 51A:790, 1969.

Hunter, J. M., Schneider, L. H., and Mackin, E. J.: Tendon Surgery in the Hand. St. Louis, The C. V. Mosby Company, 1987.

Hunter, J. M., Schneider, L. H., Mackin, E. J., Callahan, A.: Rehabilitation of the Hand, Ed. 2. St. Louis, The C. V. Mosby Company, 1984.

Hunter, J. M., Singer, D. I., Mackin, E. J., and Jaeger, S. H.: Active Tendon Implants in Flexor Tendon Reconstruction. Presented at the Annual Meeting of the American Society for Surgery of the Hand, New Orleans, Feb. 1986.

Hunter, J. M., Steindel, C., Salisbury, R., and Hughes, D.: Study of early sheath development using static non-gliding implants. J. Biomed Mater. Res., 5:155, 1974.

Hunter, J. M., Subin, D., Minkow, F., and Konikoff, J.: Sheath formation in response to limited active gliding implants (animals). J. Biomed Mater. Res., 5:163, 1974.

Kanavel, A. B.: Infections of the Hand. Ed. 7. Philadelphia, Lea & Febiger, 1939, Ch. III, pp. 39–50.

Lange, F: Ueber Periostale Schninverpflanzuagen bei Lahmunger. 47:486–490, 1900.

Matsui, T., Miyaji, T., Merklin, R., and Hunter, J. M.: A study of vascularization of the flexor tendons of the hand. Orthopaedics 28:1315–1318, 1977.

Mayer, L., and Ranshoff, N.: Reconstruction of the digital tendon sheath. A contribution to the physiological method of repair of damaged finger tendons. J. Bone Joint Surg., 18:607–616, 1936.

Ochiai, N., Matsui, T., Miyaji, T., Merklin, R., and Hunter, J. M.: Vascular anatomy of flexor tendons. I. Vincular system and blood supply of the profundus tendon in the digital sheath. J. Hand Surg., 4:321–330, 1979.

Pulvertaft, R. G.: Tendon grafts for flexor tendon injuries in the fingers and thumb: a study of technique and results. J. Bone Joint Surg., 38B:175, 1956.

Pulvertaft, R. G.: Experiences in flexor tendon grafting in the hand. J. Bone Joint Surg., 41B:629, 1959.

Rayner, C. R. W.: The origin and nature of pseudosynovium appearing around implanted Silastic rods: an experimental study. Hand, 8:101, 1976.

Sarkin, I. I.: The plastic replacement of severed flexor tendons of the fingers. Br. J. Surg., 44:232–240, 1956.

Urbaniak, J. R., Bright, D. S., Gill, L. H., and Goldner, J. L.: Vascularization and the gliding mechanism of free flexor tendon grafts inserted by the silicone rod method. J. Bone Joint Surg., 56A:473, 1974.

Wehbé, M. A., and Hunter, J. M.: Flexor tendon gliding in the hand. Part I. In vivo excursions. J. Hand Surg., 10A(4):570–574, 1985.

Wehbé, M. A., and Hunter, J. M.: Flexor tendon gliding in the hand. Part II. Differential gliding. J. Hand Surg., 10A(4):575–579, 1985.

Wheeldon, T.: The use of cellophane as a permanent tendon sheath. J. Bone Joint Surg., 21:393–396, 1939.

Chapter 33

LATE REPAIR OF ZONE II FLEXOR TENDONS IN UNFAVORABLE CASES (PEDICLE TENDON GRAFT)

E. Paneva-Holevich

In 1965 we reported a small series of flexor tendon injuries in zone II in which a new technique for secondary reconstruction was employed to which we have given the name "two stage tenoplasty" (Paneva-Holevich, 1965). Essentially the operation involves use of the superficial flexor of the respective finger as a pedicled graft after suturing it at an earlier operation to the deep flexor at the lumbrical muscle level (Paneva-Holevich, 1969).

Hunter et al. (1969) described a two stage procedure using a silicone rod for preliminary preparation of a pseudosheath. His first publication referred to long implants reaching proximally up to the carpal canal. However, in a few cases with lesions involving zone II, short silicone rods were employed in preparing only the sheath of the digit (Hunter and Salisbury, 1971). During the last decade both these methods have been used by various authors (Arakaki, 1972; Bäuerle and Reil, 1976; Pernet et al., 1969, 1970; Verdan and Simonetta, 1975; Vračevic, 1976; Wenstein et al., 1976).

Van der Meulen (1969) suggested a combination of the two procedures, and thereafter a number of reports were published (Alnot et al., 1980; Brug and Stedtfeld, 1979; Chaplinsky and Popik, 1975; Chong, 1972; Fujita et al., 1977; Geldmacher, 1980; Iketani et al., 1977; Ito et al., 1975; Kessler, 1972; Rozovskaya, 1977; Winspur et al., 1978). It is in zone 2 that these techniques were especially used. Since both methods are performed in two stages, some authors use the term "pedicled tendon graft" instead of "two stage tendon plasty" (Kessler, 1972).

This chapter outlines our experience with the use of pedicled tendon grafts both as a separate procedure and in combination with the preliminary formation of a sheath by the temporary implantation of a silicone rod when this additional step was considered necessary.

TWO STAGE TENDON PLASTY USING A PEDICLED TENDON GRAFT FROM THE SUPERFICIAL FLEXOR

We have employed this technique in 428 cases, of which 139 were rated unfavorable according to the initial clinical condition. However, only the long term results in 58 unfavorable and unselected cases (42 patients) with a detailed follow-up are discussed here.

Preliminary Data

The patients ranged in age from eight to 57 years; most of the patients were in the third (26) and fourth (11) decades of life.

The time interval between injury and surgery ranged from one month to six years. Most of the patients presented after a time interval of up to six months following injury.

According to universally accepted criteria, the cases were classified as belonging to either the "scar" or the "joint" group, although it was not possible to make a strict distinction between them. Unlike other authors who consider all multiple lesions to belong to the group of "unfavorable" cases, our experience demonstrates that the factor of "multiple" injuries itself does not necessarily carry this connotation (Paneva-Holevich, 1972). In cases in which there is no significant scar, joint stiffness, or damage, the degree of repair does not differ significantly from that in injuries to single digits. For that reason only patients with fingers suffering "multiple" injuries who in addition had scarring and joint stiffness were included in the "unfavorable" lesion group. Denervated fingers were not classified into a separate group because as a rule they also had adhesions and joint stiffness or damage. Thus, the distribution of our cases is as follows:

Extensive Scarring and Adhesion Formation ("Scar"). In this group there were 18 digits (15 patients), three of them with severe flexion contractures exceeding 90 degrees, eight with moderate flexion contracture, and seven fingers without contracture and extensive scars of the skin and deeper tissues. Four digits had impaired sensation. In most of the patients in this group, the adhesions were caused by abortive primary suturing.

Joint Stiffness or Damage ("Joint"). In this group there were 40 digits (27 patients). The cases in this group were characterized by cicatricial changes associated with restricted mobility in one or both interphalangeal joints owing to intra-articular derangements (e.g., shortened lateral ligaments, intra-articular fractures, preceding Sudeck atrophy). Depending on the severity of stiffness, the cases could be classified into severe (four patients: passive movements in both interphalangeal joints totaling less than 80 degrees), moderate (20 patients: passive movements in both interphalangeal joints totaling up to 120 degrees), and mild (16 patients: passive movements in both interphalangeal joints exceeding 120 degrees). Seven of the digits assigned to this particular group had impaired sensation and five had malunited fractures. One or more neighboring fingers had been amputated in four patients.

OPERATIVE TECHNIQUE

First Stage

This minor operation is performed under local or regional intravenous anesthesia; general anesthesia is resorted to only in children. A small inverted L incision is made along the course of the distal palmar and thenar creases. After dissection of the flap, the underlying part of the palmar fascia is excised. In this way an adequate approach is gained to the tendons of one of the triphalangeal digits or to the tendons of several digits. The deep flexor is cut at the level of the respective lumbrical muscle and the superficial flexor is cut a little more distally. The paratenon of the proximal stump of the superficial flexor is retracted 0.5 cm. and the stripped tendon end is removed. Then the proximal cut ends of the deep and superficial flexors are sutured end to end. Three mattress sutures (5-0) are inserted, involving not more than 2 to 3 mm. of the tendon ends. The sutures are covered by the dissected paratenon of the superficial flexor (Fig. 33–1). In case of rupture of the paratenon a portion of the muscle belly of the respective lumbrical is used. When the fifth finger is involved and its superficial flexor is appreciably thinner than the deep one, we use a crisscross suture. Next the skin wound is closed and a moderate compression bandage is applied. Immobilization is unnecessary. We advise our patients to use the hand as early as possible as well as to perform repeated passive movements of the joints of the injured digits throughout the day. The latter is of utmost importance in patients with joint stiffness.

In some of the patients, during the first stage of the plasty with the pedicled tendon graft, correction of the digital contracture was carried out by excising the scars and resurfacing the volar aspect with a pedicled flap (one case), lengthening the longitudinal scar by exchanging opposite triangular flaps (four cases), surgery of the ligaments of the proximal interphalangeal joint (two cases), or removing the deep scars and the distal cicatricial fragments of the tendons (two cases).

Second Stage

The second stage of the operation is performed at least 30 days after the first stage. This operation is usually carried out under regional intravenous or plexus anesthesia (in children, under general anesthesia). The approach in the palm follows the course of the old incision. Thereafter it is continued proximally and runs along the thenar crease and volar aspect of the forearm, extending

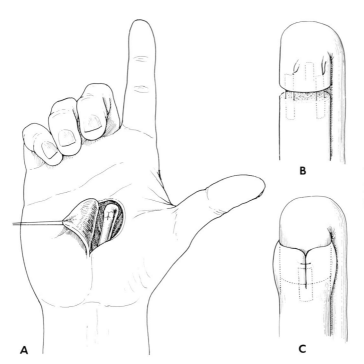

Figure 33–1. First stage of tenoplasty with a pedicled graft. *A*, General schema. *B* and *C*, Details of the suture between the proximal stumps of the superficial and deep flexors.

7 to 8 cm. At the wrist level it bends slightly in a transverse direction (Fig. 33–2*A*). The carpal canal is opened, and the superficial flexor is identified and severed at its musculotendinous junction. Then the pedicled graft is stripped together with its epitenon in the area of the carpal canal and with the paratenon in the forearm (Fig. 33–2*B*). The pedicled graft is rotated distally and is slightly stretched to test the strength of union between the tendon ends and the contractile capacity of the muscle. When adhesions in the area of the tendon loop are present and interfere with tendon movements, they are excised.

The pedicled graft can be stripped using a stripper, without opening the carpal area, through a small incision on the palm and forearm only. The more extensive approach described is preferred because it is less traumatic and the risk of damage to the neighboring tendons and median nerve is avoided.

With a separate incision along the midlateral line of the digit, observing the principles postulated by Tubiana (1960), access is gained to the osteofibrous canal. The remnants of the distal fragments of the tendons are removed, conserving only several millimeters of the distal end of the deep flexor. When possible, the annular ligaments are preserved. The pedicled graft is passed under

the superficial arterial arch, through the intact proximal portion of the sheath, and under the annular ligaments. The skin wound is sutured up to the level of the proximal interphalangeal joint. Then the end of the pedicled graft is fixed under physiological tension to the distal phalanx, using a pullout wire suture in the fashion shown in Figure 33–2*C*. Between the deep flexor remnants and the graft we apply an additional 4-0 suture, attaching the graft to the distal stump of the deep flexor tendon. The remaining part of the skin incision is sutured.

In cases with marked adhesions it is often necessary to broaden the original approach by resorting to full excision of the anterior wall of the osseofibrous canal with reconstruction repair of the annular bands, extending the incision over the distal part of the palm in the manner described by Tubiana (1960) and exposing the entire osseofibrous canal using a zigzag incision on the volar aspect of the finger method recommended by Bruner (1967) and others (Fig. 33–3).

POSTOPERATIVE TREATMENT

A moderate compression bandage is applied. The wrist and fingers are immobilized

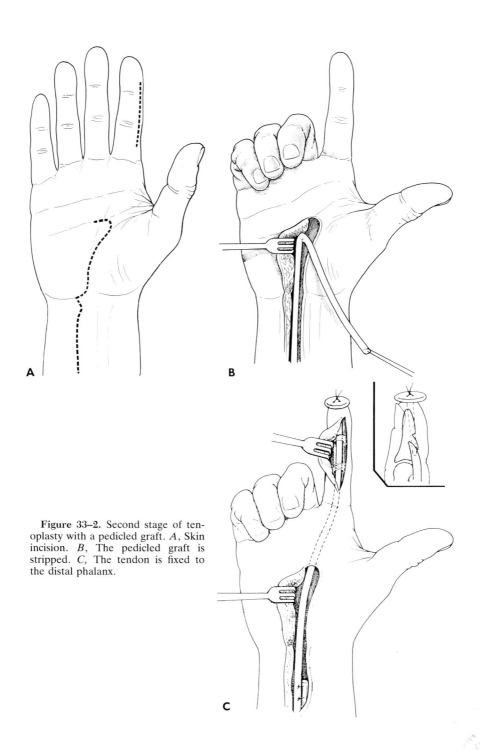

Figure 33–2. Second stage of tenoplasty with a pedicled graft. *A,* Skin incision. *B,* The pedicled graft is stripped. *C,* The tendon is fixed to the distal phalanx.

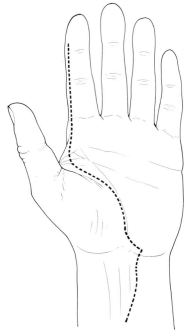

Figure 33–3. Extended incision and approach to the whole sheath with marked adhesions.

in semiflexion for five days. The splint does not allow full extension of the digits that have been operated upon, but it does not interfere with active flexion of the interphalangeal joint. On the sixth day the plaster splint is removed and a light dressing is applied. We encourage the patient to perform movements without undue strain, avoiding full extension of the wrist. The pullout wire suture is removed on the thirtieth day and then physiotherapy is undertaken. In some cases there is a tendency for the flexion contracture to recur after the second month, and here a dynamic splint is employed. Assessment of the end results is made at least six months after the operation.

RESULTS

We use the criteria suggested by Boyes (1955). For easy orientation, cylinders with appropriate diameters are used (Fig. 33–4). As suggested by White (1956), the limitation of extension of the finger is also considered. In persisting flexion contracture ranging from 20 to 40 degrees (total for both interphalangeal joints of the digit), we reduced the rating suggested by Boyes (1955) by 1 degree and in contractures ranging from 40 to 80 degrees

by 2 degrees. In contractures exceeding 80 degrees, the outcome of the treatment is evaluated as poor regardless of the distance between the pulp of the finger tip and the distal palmar crease during flexion.

The final outcome in this series of patients in presented in Table 33–1.

COMPLICATIONS

Transient drainage from the wound after the second stage of the operation was observed once. In another case, on the fifteenth day after the operation during attempted passive extension of the finger, the distal insertion of the graft was avulsed, necessitating reintervention. The final outcome was good. In two patients, because of an unsatisfactory range of active movement, tenolysis

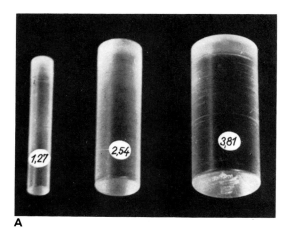

A

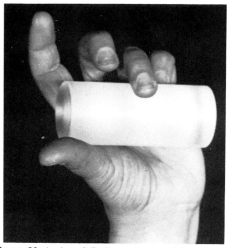

B

Figure 33–4. A and B, Prompt recognition regarding the degree of active flexion using plastic cylinders of different sizes.

Table 33–1. FINAL RESULTS

Preoperative Condition	Total	Very Good	Good	Fair	Poor
Extensive adhesions	18	3(16.6%)	10(55.5%)	3(16.6%)	2(11.1%)
Joint damage and stiffness	40	2(5.0%)	16(40.0%)	12(30.0%)	10(25.0%)
Total	58	5(8.7%)	26(34.4%)	15(26.0%)	12(20.7%)

was performed within three months after the operation. A favorable result was recorded in only one of them.

Three illustrative cases from this group are shown in Figures 33–5 to 33–7.

TWO STAGE TENDON PLASTY WITH A PEDICLED GRAFT FROM THE SUPERFICIAL FLEXOR AND PREPARATION OF THE PSEUDOSHEATH BY TEMPORARY SILICONE ROD IMPLANTATION

Since 1977, we have used this method for secondary reconstruction of the flexor tendons in zone II in "unfavorable" cases. Our experience comprises 47 fingers in 37 patients. The results were verified in 35 fingers (26 patients).

PRELIMINARY DATA

The ages varied from eight to 58 years. Most of the patients (20) were in the third decade of life. The interval from injury to surgery ranged from two months to three years. Depending on the preoperative condition, the distribution pattern was the following:

Extensive Scarring and Adhesion Formation ("Scar"). In this group there were 21 fingers, of which two had severe contracture, eight moderate, and 11 none.

Joint Stiffness and Damage ("Joint"). In this group there were 14 fingers, four of which had marked restriction of movements, six moderate restriction and three slight restriction. Two fingers in this group were denervated, and in three of the patients there were concomitant bone lesions and amputation of adjacent digits.

OPERATIVE TECHNIQUE

First Stage

Surgery is carried out under regional intravenous or plexus anesthesia. Both flexors are exposed and cut at the level of the lumbrical muscle. Their proximal stumps are sutured to each other in the fashion already described. Then the volar aspect of the finger is exposed through a zigzag incision (Fig. 33–8A). When the cicatricial changes involve the distal portion of the palm or the tendon fragments are tightly adherent within the sheath, the incision is enlarged and connected with the one on the palm. The scarred tissues are excised and the tendon remnants are removed, conserving only 0.5 cm. of the distal end of the deep flexor. When possible, the annular ligaments were preserved but in most of the cases under review their reconstruction was mandatory.

A silicone rod of suitable size is chosen (thicker if possible but allowing free gliding of the implant under the annular ligaments—usually 4 or 5 mm. in thickness for the second to fourth fingers and 3 or 4 mm. in thickness for the fifth finger). The distal end of the silicone rod is cut obliquely. This facilitates its passage beneath the annular ligaments and helps reduce the strain from the mass of tissues and suture material at the level of the distal insertion. After moistening the silicone rod it is passed through the sheath and under the annular ligaments. Its distal end is fixed under the tendon remnant of the deep flexor using a strong 4-0 suture. By pulling the implant from the palmar aspect we test the strength of the suture and the range of motion in the interphalangeal joints. When the prosthesis has an adequate thickness and the annular ligaments have been preserved or reconstructed, the interphalangeal joints can be flexed fully or to the extent of the passive movements present. When the digit is extended, the implant glides freely distally. Finally the proximal end of the silicone rod is divided at the level of the lumbrical muscles with the finger bent. This gives an optimal length to the implant so that it can move freely within the sheath when the digit is in extension and flexion (Fig. 33–8B).

After suturing of the skin wound a moderate compression bandage is applied. It is replaced by a lighter one on the third day,

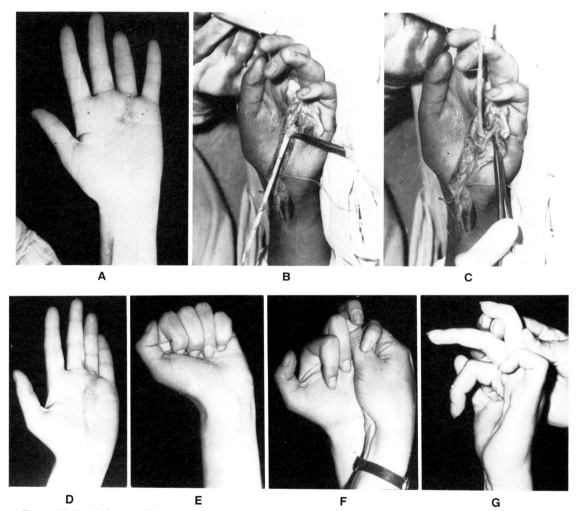

Figure 33–5. A 25-year-old female patient. *A*, Preoperative condition—adhesions with a slight contracture in the metacarpophalangeal joint are present after an abortive primary suture. *B* and *C*, Operative view of the second stage of the pedicled tenoplasty. *D* to *G*, Results.

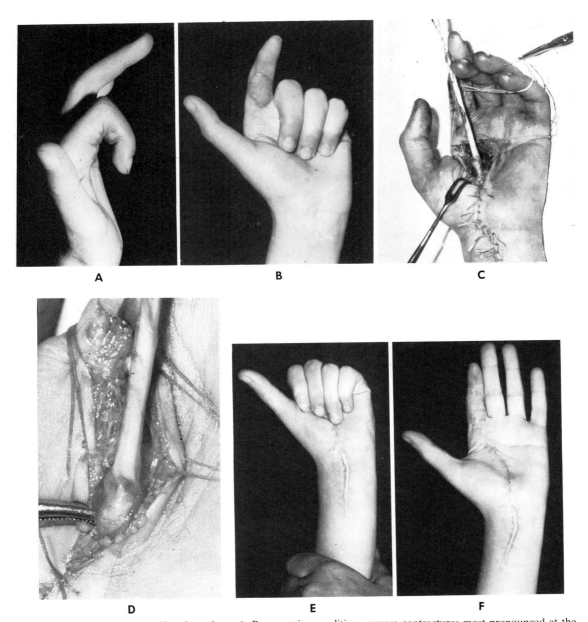

Figure 33–6. A 10-year-old male patient. *A*, Preoperative condition—severe contractures most pronounced at the proximal end of the interphalangeal joint after abortive primary suture. *B*, After the first stage of tenoplasty and correction of the contracture (using a distant skin graft). *C*, Operative view of the second stage of tenoplasty with a pedicled graft. *D*, The site of suture between the proximal stumps of the superficial and deep flexors. *E* and *F*, Results.

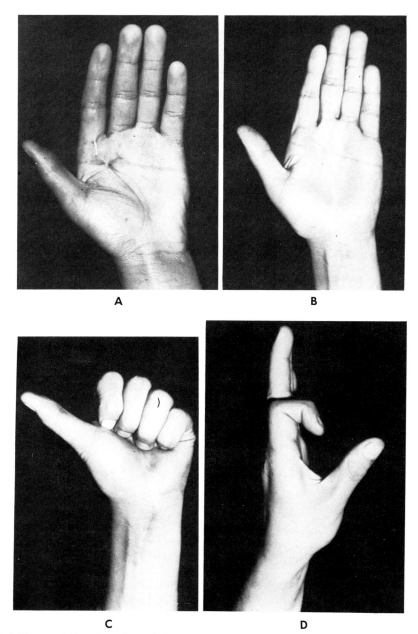

Figure 33–7. A 21-year-old female patient. *A*, Preoperative condition—adhesions on the base of the phalanx. *B* to *D*, Results.

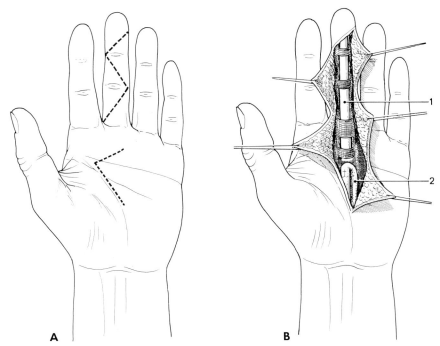

Figure 33–8. First stage of combined two-stage tenoplasty. *A*, Diagram of the skin incision. *B*, Diagram of the suturing of the proximal stumps of the superficial and deep flexors and implantation of a silicone rod.

and the patient is advised to perform passive movements of the digital joints. After wound healing and removal of the sutures, the passive exercises are carried out for not less than two to three months.

Second Stage

In our patients the second stage of the operation is performed two to three months after the first stage. Probably the longer waiting period after the first stage (as recommended by Hunter) contributes to the formation of a better pseudosheath, but this would prolong the treatment time. However, earlier exercising of the respective muscle would contribute to its more rapid restoration.

Following adequate anesthesia, the proximal skin incision over the palm and the distal part of the forearm and the dissection of the pedicled tendon graft are carried out according to the technique for our two stage tenoplasty already described. By flexing the digit, the proximal end of the silicone implant is exposed. Usually it ends in a blind cul de sac, which must be opened. The end of the pedicled graft is temporarily sutured to the silicone rod using strong thread. A small

lateral incision is made at the level of the distal phalanx. The distal end of the implant is identified, and the thread with which it is sutured to the deep flexor remnants is cut. The silicone rod is pulled carefully through the canal until the end of the pedicled tendon graft emerges in the wound. The flexor retinaculum is restored and the palmar and forearm wounds are sutured. The distal end of the pedicled graft is fixed to the distal phalanx under physiological tension by the method described for the two stage tenoplasty (Fig. 33–9).

POSTOPERATIVE TREATMENT

Postoperative treatment is the same as in the two stage tenoplasty without a silicone implant.

RESULTS

The results obtained following the combined two stage procedure (pedicled graft and preliminary formation of a pseudosheath), rated according to the criteria already described, are presented in Table 33–2.

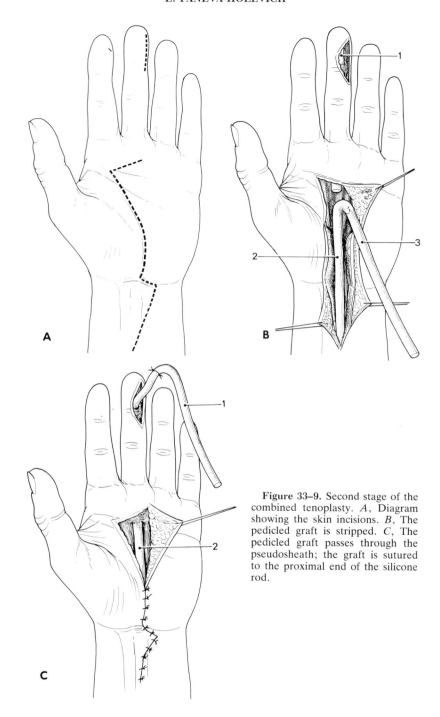

Figure 33–9. Second stage of the combined tenoplasty. *A*, Diagram showing the skin incisions. *B*, The pedicled graft is stripped. *C*, The pedicled graft passes through the pseudosheath; the graft is sutured to the proximal end of the silicone rod.

Table 33–2. RESULTS WITH THE COMBINED TWO STAGE PROCEDURE

Preoperative Condition	Total	Very Good	Good	Fair	Poor
Extensive adhesions	21	10(47.6%)	7(33.3%)	2(9.5%)	2(9.5%)
Joint damage and stiffness	14	—	7(14.3%)	9(65.0%)	3(21.2%)
Total	35	10(28.1%)	9(25.7%)	11(31.4%)	5(14.3%)

COMPLICATIONS

Sinus formation occurred in two patients in this group at the level of the distal suture of the implant after the first stage. This necessitated its removal. Within two months the second stage tenoplasty was performed using a pedicled graft. In another two cases the digit was edematous for a prolonged period of time. During the second stage of the operation a clear secretion free of microorganisms was discharged from the pseudosheath. The result in these four patients with complications was fair. In two cases tenolysis had to be performed without any significant improvement in results. Four illustrative cases from this group are shown in Figures 33–10 to 33–13.

DISCUSSION

In our experience in cases classified as "unfavorable" because of the preoperative condition ("scar" or "joint"), the two stage tenoplasty using a pedicled graft alone or combined with the preliminary formation of a pseudosheath by the temporary insertion of a silicone rod probably has certain advantages

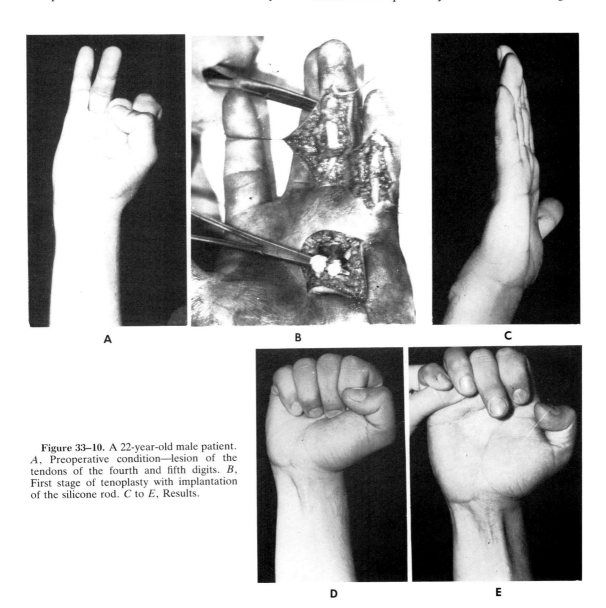

Figure 33–10. A 22-year-old male patient. A, Preoperative condition—lesion of the tendons of the fourth and fifth digits. B, First stage of tenoplasty with implantation of the silicone rod. C to E, Results.

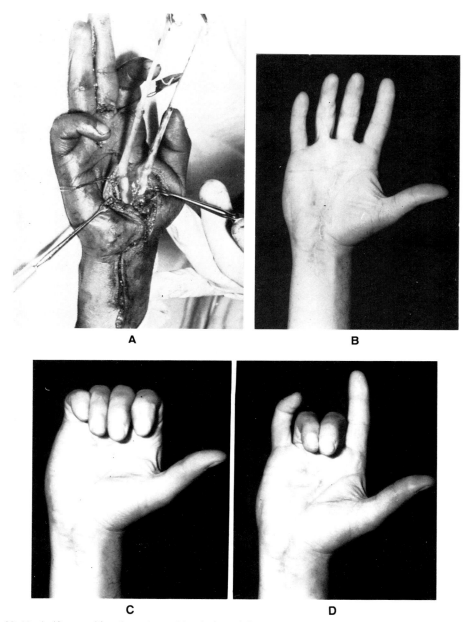

Figure 33–11. A 48-year-old male patient with a lesion of the tendons of the third and fourth digits. *A*, Operative view of the second stage of tenoplasty, showing how the tendons pass through the pseudosheath by pulling the silicone rod. *C* to *D*, Results.

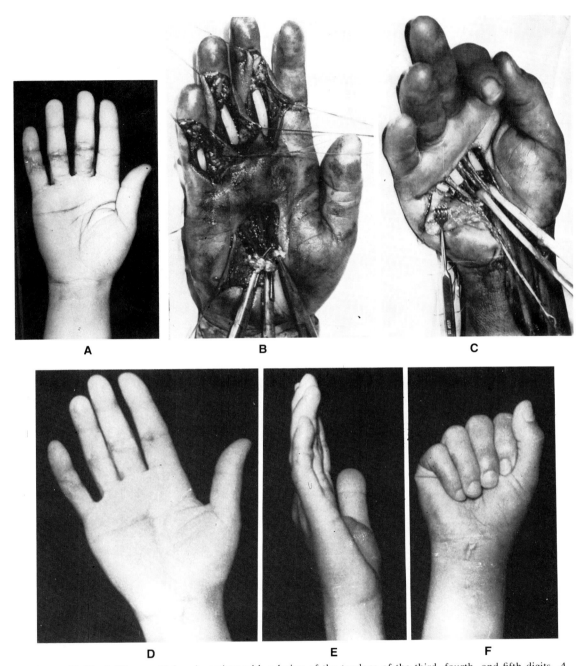

Figure 33–12. A 30-year-old female patient with a lesion of the tendons of the third, fourth, and fifth digits. *A*, Preoperative condition. *B*, First stage of tenoplasty with implantation of the silicone rod. *C*, Second stage of the tenoplasty. *D* to *F*, Results.

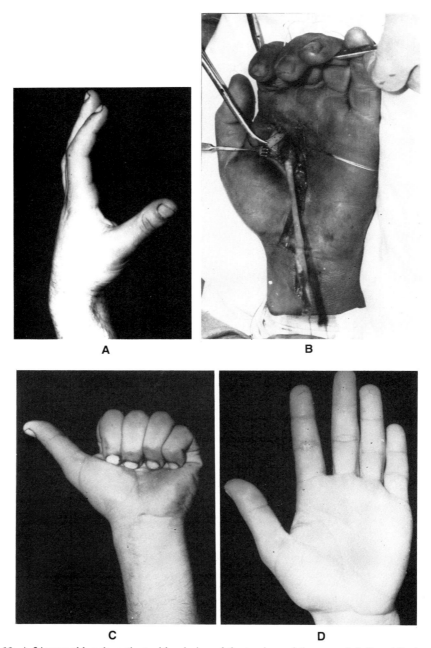

Figure 33–13. A 24-year-old male patient with a lesion of the tendons of the second digit and flexion contracture. *A*, Preoperative condition. *B*, Formation of the loop between the deep and superficial flexors and implantation of the silicone rod. *C* and *D*, Results.

over the classic method of free tendon grafting. Nevertheless the results remain greatly inferior to those seen in "favorable" cases. Our data relating to the two stage tenoplasty with a pedicled graft, already published, indicate that excellent and good results were attained in 95 per cent (73 per cent excellent and 22 per cent good) of the cases considered "favorable" according to the preoperative condition (Paneva-Holevich, 1975). The outcome of the use of this procedure in "unfavorable" cases was much more modest (7 per cent excellent and 50 per cent good results).

As compared with the "joint" cases, a considerably better outcome was attained in "scar" cases regardless of the method employed (Paneva-Holevich, 1970, 1971). This is readily explicable when one considers that the passive movements of the finger joints before operation were more or less restricted. At best, the active movements in those patients barely reached the level of passive movements before operation.

Our experience is in disagreement with Hunter's observations claiming rather good results in such "joint" cases. It is difficult to make a comparative study since the degree of joint stiffness and the level of injury are by no means comparable. The longer period of treatment following the first stage carried out by Hunter may explain the results obtained.

It would be of interest to compare the results achieved in "scar" and "joint" cases following both the methods we used. Unfortunately a strictly objective comparison is impossible because of the varying preoperative state of the digits. When we employed the first procedure, the number of "joint" cases was greater. Nevertheless it is worth noting that when employing the first of the methods described, the percentage of very good and good results reached 43.1 per cent and with the combined technique, 53.8 per cent. This difference is more significant if comparison is made between only the "very good" results (8.7 and 28.1 per cent).

These observations coincide in part with the results reported by other authors. Having employed the combined procedure in "unfavorable" cases, Geldmacher (1980) attained 45 per cent very good and good results; Iketani et al. (1977), 61 per cent (26 cases); Winspur et al. (1978), 75 per cent (11 cases); Chaplinsky and Popik (1975), 70 per cent (16 cases); Rozovskaya (1977), 50 per cent (59 cases); Alnot et al. (1980), 58 per cent (17 cases); and Brug and Stedtfeld (1979), 23 per cent (17 cases).

When using the original two stage plasty as adapted by Paneva-Holevich, Arakaki (1972) reported 45 per cent very good and good results (11 cases). We would like to draw attention to the observations of Fujita et al. (1977). They employed the unmodified two stage tenoplasty in eight cases and the combined method in seven. The movements in the combined procedure series had a greater range within the first two months following the operation, and the long term results of reconstruction using a pedicled graft proved to be better.

On the basis of our limited series it is difficult to establish a relationship between the results obtained in the unfavorable group and additional factors such as age, time interval following injury, anatomical peculiarities, patient's collaboration, and the like. Undoubtedly such a correlation exists, but it is manifested much more conspicuously in the "favorable" cases.

The rather modest results obtained in the "joint" cases pose the question of whether the efforts at secondary reconstruction are justified. Our observations and the questionnaire used in a group of patients in regard to their personal assessment give us sufficient reason to assume that often the regaining of active movements, even in a modest range, improves the overall prehensile capacity of the hand and is thereby positively evaluated by the patient, who states that the finger has ceased troubling him. The positive assessment by the patient is particularly emphasized when several digits are involved.

SUMMARY

Our experience with the late repair of zone II flexor tendons in unfavorable ("scar" and "joint") cases is reported. The following two methods were employed:

1. Two stage plasty with a pedicled graft. The results obtained and assessed according to Boyes' criteria in 58 cases ("scar," 18, and "joint," 40) were as follows: very good—5, good—26, fair—15, and poor—12.

2. Combined plasty with a pedicled tendon graft and formation of a pseudosheath by temporary insertion of a silicone rod. The results assessed in 35 cases ("scar," 21, and

"joint," 14) using the same criteria were as follows: very good—10, good—9, fair—11, and poor—5.

Comparison of the results in both groups favors the combined surgical procedure. A completely objective comparison is not possible because the cases were of different severity. The "joint" cases dominate the first group, and according to our observations, there is considerably less hope for their satisfactory repair when compared with the "scar" cases.

REFERENCES

Alnot, J. J., Dujour, G., and Augereau, B.: Flexor tendon grafts with modification of Hunter's technique. Proceedings of the First Congress, International Federation of Societies for Surgery of the Hand. Rotterdam, 1980, p. 199.

Arakaki, T.: Tenoplastia en dois estagios nas seccoes traumaticas dos tendoes flexores dos dedos da mao dentro da bainha fibrosa. Sao Paulo, 1972.

Bäuerle, E., and Reil, P: Ergebnisse und Erfahrungen nach 100 Beugesehnentransplantationen unter Verwendung des Silistikstabes. Unfallheilkunde, 79:513–521, 1976.

Boyes, J. H.: Evaluation of results of digital flexor tendon grafts. Am. J. Surg., 89:1116–1119, 1955.

Brug, E., and Stedtfeld, H. W.: Experience with a two-stage pedicled flexor tendon graft. Hand, 11:198–205, 1979.

Bruner, J. M.: The zig-zag volar digital incision for flexor-tendon surgery. Plast. Reconstr. Surg., 40:571–574, 1967.

Chaplinsky, V. V., and Popik, E. I.: Two-stage primary repair of severely combined injuries with impaired flexor tendons of the fingers. Ortop. Travinatol. Protez., 9:43–46, 1975.

Chong, J. K.: Combined two-stage tenoplasty with silicone rods for multiple flexor tendon injuries in "no man's land." J. Trauma, 12:104–121, 1972.

Fujita, S., et al.: Two-staged U-procedure for the flexor tendon injuries in the hands. Proceedings of the Twentieth Annual Meeting, Tokyo, 1977, pp. 33–34.

Geldmacher, J.: Tendon grafts. Proceedings of the First Congress, International Federation of Societies for Surgery of the Hand. Rotterdam, 1980, p. 24.

Hunter, J. M., Aalem, A., Steindel, C. R., and Salisbury, R. E.: The use of gliding artificial tendon implants to form new tendon beds. J. Bone Joint Surg., 51A:790, 1969.

Hunter, J., and Salisbury, R.: Flexor-tendon reconstruction in severely damaged hands. J. Bone Joint Surg., 53A:829–858, 1971.

Iketani, M., et al.: Treatment results on the rupture of flexor tendons within no man's land. Proceedings of the Twentieth Annual Meeting Tokyo, 1977, pp. 32–33.

Ito, T., et al.: Clinical studies on flexor-tendon repair under bad conditions (on our combined two-stage tenoplasty). Proceedings of the Eighteenth Annual Meeting, Morioka, 1975.

Kessler, F.: Use of pedicled tendon transfer with silicone rod in complicated secondary flexor tendon repairs. Plast. Reconstr. Surg., 49:439–443, 1972.

Paneva-Holevich, E.: Two-stage plasty in flexor tendon injuries of finger within the digital synovial sheath. Acta Chir. Plast., 7:112–124, 1965.

Paneva-Holevich, E.: Two-stage tenoplasty in injury of the flexor tendons of the hand. J. Bone Joint Surg., 51A:21–32, 1969.

Paneva-Holevich, E.: Two-stage tenoplasty in "ciatricial" cases. Proc. Postgrad. Med. Inst. (Sofia), 17:213–217, 1970.

Paneva-Holevich, E.: Influence of different factors on the results of the two-stage tendon plasty. Proc. Postgr. Med. Inst. (Sofia), 18:165–172, 1971.

Paneva-Holevich, E.: Résultats du traitement des lésions multiple des tendons fléchisseurs des doigts par greffe effectuée en deux temps. Rev. Chir. Orthop. Repar., 58:481–487, 1972.

Paneva-Holevich, E.: Tenoplastie de fléchisseurs des doigts effectuée en deux temps chex 184 cas (234 tendons). Arch. Union Med. Balkanique, 13:415–417, 1975.

Pernet, A., Campos, W. A., and Gama, C. C.: Comentarios sobre a enxertia tendinosa pela tecnica de Paneva-Holevich. Bol. Sul. Am. Cir. Mao, 2B:3–13, 1970.

Pernet, A., Freitas, E., and Campos, W. A.: Pedicle tendon graft—Paneva-Holevich method. Bol. Sul. Am. Cir. Mao, 18:48, 1969.

Rozovskaya, T. P.: Invertebrate injuries of the flexor tendons of the fingers and their treatment. Ortop. Traum. Protez., 4:68–70, 1977.

Tubiana, R.: Les voies d'abord dans la chirurgie des tendons de la main. Ann. Chir. Plast., 5:99–109, 1960.

Van der Meulen, J. C.: Tendon healing in relation to different methods of treatment. Ann. Chir. Plast., 14:168–175, 1969.

Verdan, C., and Simonetta, C.: Les greffes de tendons fléchisseurs apres implantation provisoire d'une tige en silicone. Med. Hyg., 33:402–404, 1975.

Vračevic, D.: Tenoplasty of the flexor tendons in the zone between the distal palmar crease and the proximal interphalangeal joint after the method of Paneva-Holevich. Acta Ortop. Jugoslav., 137–142, 1976.

Wenstein, S., Sprague, B. L., and Flatt, A.: Evaluation of the two-stage flexor tendon reconstruction in severely damaged digits. J. Bone Joint Surg., 58A:786–791, 1976.

White, W. L.: Secondary restoration of finger flexor by digital tendon grafts. An evaluation of seventy-six cases. Am. J. Surg., 91:622–668, 1956.

Winspur, I., Dennis, D. B., and Boswick, J. A.: Staged reconstruction of flexor tendons with a silicone rod and a "pedicled" sublimis transfer. Plast. Reconstr. Surg., 61:756–761, 1978.

Chapter 34

TOTAL ANTERIOR TENOARTHROLYSIS

P. Saffar

Repeated operations on a finger, in particular after sectioning of the flexor tendons in zone 2, result in progressive retraction of the skin, of the whole flexor apparatus, and in particular of its sheath, the floor of which is formed by the periosteum and the glenoid plates of the proximal and distal interphalangeal joints.

Combined treatment involving tenolysis of the flexor tendons and arthrolysis of the interphalangeal joints does not provide very good results when the finger has a fixed flexed deformity.

A different approach consists of detaching the entire sheath en bloc from the underlying skeleton, a method that after partial division of the collateral ligaments allows straightening of the finger. This is total anterior tenoarthrolysis. This operation is thus limited to fingers that have retained a degree of active flexion.

The sector of mobility is transferred by the operation to a more favorable sector, and mobility at the proximal interphalangeal joint is sometimes increased.

Proximal sliding of the finger soft tissue exposes the bone at the distal end to some extent, and special techniques are often necessary to preserve an adequate pulp.

The prognosis depends on careful examination of the digit. The extent of likely improvement should be clearly indicated to the patient, who must retain the willpower necessary for re-education.

EXAMINATION

The skin is examined thoroughly, care being taken to note sites of scarring or areas of skin already grafted and the presence of fibrous bands. In judging the adequacy of the blood supply, one notes trophic changes, color, sensitivity to cold, and unrepaired old injuries to collateral arteries: an arteriogram may prove useful. The sensibility of the fingers is evaluated. The mobility of each tendon segment is recorded. The joints, especially the proximal interphalangeal joint, are assessed radiologically. One also should try to find out about the patient's motivation and about his habits.

CONTRAINDICATIONS

A stiff finger with no flexion or extension ability constitutes a contraindication to operation as are severe trophic changes, especially those of vascular origin, or an anesthetic finger. Insufficient motivation on the part of the patient may also be a contraindication. Destruction of the proximal interphalangeal joint is another.

TECHNIQUE

The surgical approach is carried out from the lateral side at the junction of the palmar and dorsal skin, always choosing the side previously incised (Fig. 34–1). The incision extends from the middle of the proximal phalanx to the end of the distal phalanx and is located several millimeters below the extensor tendon. One need not modify the incision because of the presence of previous incisions or grafts on the anterior surface of the phalanges. After traversing the subcutaneous tissue, one makes direct contact with the phalangeal diaphysis. No attempt is made to dissect upward or downward; one goes

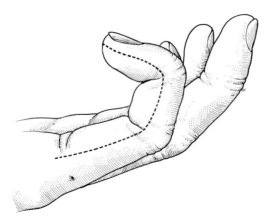

Figure 34–1. Mid-lateral incision for total anterior tenoarthrolysis.

directly to the bone. It is necessary to avoid damaging the dorsal digital artery, which courses obliquely, distally and backward, and takes its origin from the palmar artery in the middle part of the proximal phalanx. It supplies part of the dorsum of the finger.

Next, one incises the periosteum of the proximal two phalanges on their lateral sides. The incision is continued over all the anterior surface of the proximal two phalanges. With a straight periosteal elevator the periosteum on the anterior surface of the proximal two phalanges is detached (Fig. 34–2). The release of the periosteum begins on the lateral surface of the phalanx on the side of the incision. It must be done very carefully as this is one of the most important steps. This release must be done slowly, evenly, and without tearing; if the periosteum separates well, the periosteal elevator suffices. If it adheres too closely, a small scalpel can help, always staying in contact with the bone. A curved periosteal elevator enables one to detach the periosteum from the lateral sur-

face of the opposite side of the bone. Two retractors are used to raise the part separated by the periosteal elevator, forming a bridge at the proximal interphalangeal joint.

The fascia covering the lateral ligaments is incised, exposing them. Then the volar fibers of the lateral ligaments are cut, detaching the volar plate from the lateral ligaments (Fig. 34–3). This plate is in continuity with the raised periosteum. In this way the volar plate is freed from its bony attachments and is raised, forming one piece with the periosteum. This step is carried out at the proximal and distal interphalangeal joints. All the elements of the anterior surface of the proximal two phalanges are then detached from the bony skeleton.

If one then tries to straighten the finger, the lateral ligaments of the proximal interphalangeal joint are tensed and prevent full extension. If necessary, they are sectioned under direct vision while trying to preserve their posterior part. With the scalpel one sections the ligaments from front to back, alternating sides, and progressing slowly, all the time trying to extend the finger after each partial section. One stops whenever adequate extension is possible. Generally, it is possible to preserve the posterior part of the ligaments. However, in some cases the ligaments must be totally sectioned. There is then instability of the joint during the course of the operation but this should not be worrisome, for it always disappears postoperatively.

At times, part of the lateral ligaments of the distal interphalangeal joint must also be sectioned. If the finger is straightened, one sees that extension is possible, but flexion of the distal interphalangeal joint occurs. This is a cause of recurrence of the "hook" and explains the frequent failure of arthrolysis limited to the proximal interphalangeal joint.

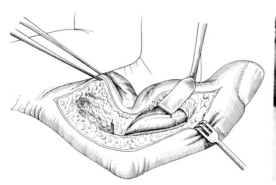
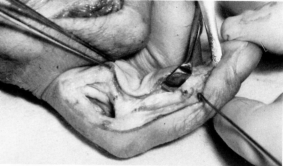

Figure 34–2. Detaching the periosteum.

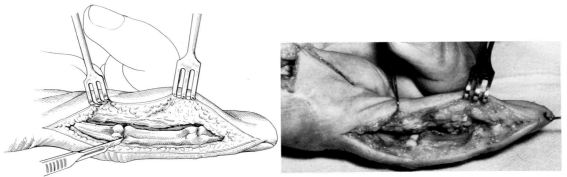

Figure 34–3. Cutting the volar fibers of the lateral ligaments detaches the volar plate.

To effect release of the finger, the flexor digitorum profundus tendon must be sectioned. This sectioning is also an important part of the technique. At times this is not necessary if release of the finger can be effected without it. If sectioning is necessary (which is the case most often), it is done in the following manner: because there is no periosteum on the distal phalanx, the cut is made flush with the bone. One starts from the lateral surface and goes through all the elements inserted on it, i.e., the pulp and the tendon of the flexor digitorum profundus, without any dissection in order to leave the tendon united to the tissues surrounding it. When there has already been surgery on the tendon, one sometimes sees only fibrous tissue.

Once all the pulp is detached, the finger is extended. It is sometimes necessary to continue the incision around the pulp. The finger is then straightened, and all the anterior tissues slide proximally along the bone, exposing the distal part of the skeleton. The sliding is in proportion to the severity of the "hook finger." The condition of the cartilage of the proximal and distal interphalangeal joints is noted.

Using this technique, one can always completely straighten the finger, but it is not always desirable to obtain complete straightening; this must be judged in relation to the preoperative flexion. The suturing is entirely cutaneous (Fig. 34–4). The sliding displacement of the tissues uncovers the distal part, which remains exposed and which consists of bone and pulp remnants. The area of tissue loss is generally small and is left to heal by secondary intention. It is dressed with a petrolatum dressing under a compression bandage, with the finger in the desired position of extension.

POSTOPERATIVE CARE

The first dressing is changed on the fourth day when the patient is allowed to perform a few flexion movements. Two splints are molded—one in extension and the other in complete flexion—and are worn alternately for periods of 12 hours. At the end of the first week, active flexion is started.

The splints are worn for about two months, alternation depending on the progress achieved. An extension splint may have to be worn at night for up to six months.

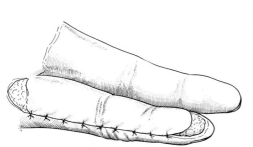
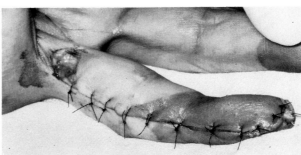

Figure 34–4. Total anterior tenoarthrolysis completed with skin suturing.

DISTORTION OF THE PULP

One important problem involves the pulp. When the clawing is moderate (no worse than a stage II Dupuytren contracture), distal gliding is very limited and one can either close the distal incision or, if the bare area is no more than 0.5 cm. in length, leave it to cicatrize spontaneously. With severe clawing, however, several maneuvers may be necessary to preserve the shape and function of the pulp.

Several solutions are possible:

1. To cover the area of skin loss over the pulp, a transverse incision can be made along the digitopalmar skin crease with undermining of the skin, and the skin can be moved distally. This maneuver will cover most of the pulp loss, and the secondary defect at the base of the finger can be covered by a full thickness graft. In the little finger the incision can be made either at the digitopalmar level or at the distal palmar crease.

The usual incision can be extended proximally and a Z-plasty performed, which will provide a little extra length.

2. Because in these fingers the distal interphalangeal joint is almost invariably stiff, there is the possibility of performing a shortening arthrodesis at that level. If this is done, however, the flexor profundus tendon should not be detached because of the risk of devascularization of the distal phalanx. This technique should be reserved for severe cases with a stiff distal interphalangeal joint, and one must keep in mind the risk of distal ischemia.

3. If there seem to be tendon adhesions within the palm, an incision can be made at the level of the distal palmar crease either in

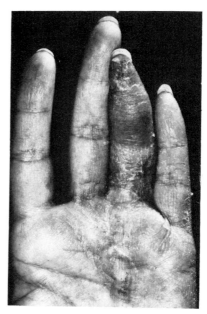

Figure 34–6. Distortion of the pulp when there has been excessive proximal displacement.

continuity with the initial incision or as a separate incision. The state of the metacarpophalangeal pulley, the extension of the tendons, and their action on digital flexion can be assessed. A tenolysis can be performed as necessary (Fig. 34–5).

All these maneuvers are designed to safeguard the sensitivity and nutrition of the pulp and to avoid hyperextension of the distal interphalangeal joint, which may follow excessive proximal migration of the anterior structures (Figs. 34–6 to 34–8).

RESULTS

On the skin, subcutaneous bands may stretch or disappear. This operation remains a possibility even in cases of severe scarring or in the presence of skin grafts or flaps.

Improvement in mobility can be expected between six weeks and two months. When preoperative flexion is good and the pulp touches the transverse palmar crease, digital mobility will be improved. When the pulp does not reach the palm preoperatively, improvement is obtained only in a more functional range of motion.

At the proximal interphalangeal joint, there is an increase in mobility and in the force of flexion of the middle phalanx. Im-

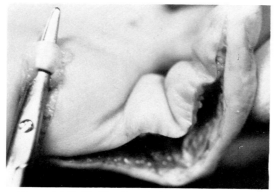

Figure 34–5. Verification of the action of the flexor tendon by proximal incision in the palm.

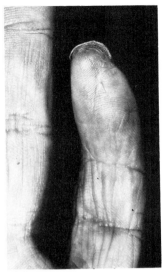

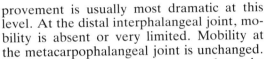

Figure 34–7. Moderate amount of pulp displacement gives intermediate results.

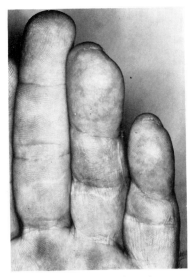

Figure 34–8. Good results.

provement is usually most dramatic at this level. At the distal interphalangeal joint, mobility is absent or very limited. Mobility at the metacarpophalangeal joint is unchanged.

Full extension of the finger can always be obtained but should not be attempted when flexion is restricted. The overall result may be improved during the period of re-education so as to obtain mobility within the most useful sector, depending on the finger involved and the patient's profession (Fig. 34–9).

DISCUSSION

It is possible to preserve the continuity of the floor of the flexor sheath, which is formed by the periosteum of the first two phalanges and the volar plates of the proximal and distal interphalangeal joints.

Repeated surgery on the finger induces overall contraction, especially at the level of the proximal interphalangeal joint which all the structures cross over. From the anatomical point of view, only the retinacular ligament is incised. The displacement of the flexor apparatus in relation to the skeleton is after all quite limited. Excessive gliding is the result in skin complications, which must be dealt with separately.

Instability of the joints, which is sometimes seen at the end of the operation, always disappears in time.

Two points remain to be discussed:

1. Division of the flexor digitorum profundus usually results in loss of mobility of the distal interphalangeal joint with a tenodesis effect. Although this joint has little mobility preoperatively, the situation should not be aggravated by creating stiffness in hyperextension at that level, as happened to us at the beginning of our experience in cases in which the pulp moved proximally.

2. Scarring of the pulp must be avoided.

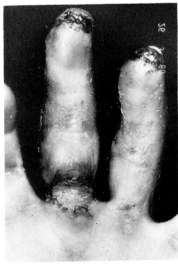

Figure 34–9. The long finger and the ring finger have been operated on. Full-thickness skin graft has been used at the base of the long finger. There is moderate distortion of the pulp.

Pulp function must be preserved by repairing the skin as already mentioned.

INDICATIONS

The classic indication for total anterior tenoarthrolysis is the finger that has already been operated upon and continues to exhibit evidence of tendon, articular (proximal interphalangeal joint), and skin deformities: flexion is full and extension restricted.

The desirable sector of mobility is different for the index finger and the little finger.

CONTRAINDICATIONS

The digit is stiff without flexion or extension.

Significant trophic problems especially with vascularization or insensitivity.

Lack of patient cooperation.

Destruction of the proximal interphalangeal joint.

CLINICAL EXPERIENCE AND RESULTS

The results obtained by standard methods of arthrolysis and tenolysis of the flexor tendons combined with arthrolysis are given first. The mean gains in extension, according to the finger, were as follows: index finger, 24 degrees; middle finger, 9 degrees; ring finger, 16 degrees; little finger, 21 degrees. There was a mean loss of flexion of 13 de-grees, as follows: preoperatively, 55 to 79 degrees; postoperatively, 37 to 66 degrees.

RESULTS WITH TOTAL ANTERIOR TENOARTHROLYSIS

The following figures are generally accepted as defining the useful sector for each finger: index finger, 30 to 60 degrees; middle finger, 30 to 90 degrees; ring finger, 40 to 90 degrees; little finger, 40 to 100 degrees.

The following criteria were adopted:

Greatly improved: Fingers with improvement in mobility of the proximal interphalangeal joint greater than 35 degrees and a gain in extension of 35 degrees in the useful sector.

Improved: A gain in extension in a better sector of mobility or better mobility in the useful sector.

Unchanged: A change of plus or minus 10 degrees.

Worsened: Decreased mobility, mobility in a less useful sector, or amputation.

Seventy-three fingers have been operated upon, with a follow-up period of more than six months, since January 1976. Twenty-one (29 per cent) were greatly improved, and 31 (42 per cent) were improved. Thus, 71 per cent were improved or greatly improved. In 15 cases (20 per cent) function was unchanged, and in six (8 per cent) function was poorer. The mean gain in extension in the 73 cases was 35 degrees (Fig. 34–10).

The results may be summarized as follows:

1. The fingers: The index finger almost always yields a poor result. Fair results are obtained with the ring finger. The best results are obtained with the little finger and the middle finger.

2. Etiology: Repair of lesions of the flexor

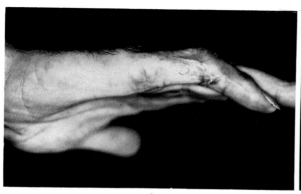
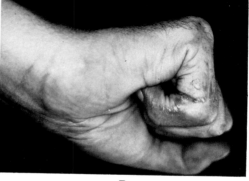

A   **B**

Figure 34–10. *A* and *B*, Complex retraction of the finger and results after one year: good flexion.

tendons in zone 2 with stiff proximal interphalangeal joints in flexion gives the best results. Results are good in Dupuytren's contracture (without sectioning of the flexor digitorum profundus). Poor results are obtained in cases of finger fracture or malunion and in cases of stiff proximal interphalangeal joints secondary to detachment of the volar plates.

3. Sectioning or nonsectioning of the flexor digitorum profundus: In 25 per cent of the cases the flexor digitorum profundus was not divided; two-thirds of the cases yielded poor results.

4. Preoperative evaluation of flexors in the palm of the hand: The result was improved in four-fifths of the cases when there was preoperative evaluation of the course of the flexor tendons in the palm.

Finally, it should be borne in mind when assessing these results that the fingers concerned had already been operated upon on an average two to three times.

Chapter 35

TENDON HOMOGRAFTS*

John T. Hueston

The successful transfer of tendons from one human body to another with the restoration of function and virtually no later evidence of any difference between the homografted tissue and the host tissues is now an accepted accomplishment in hand surgery.

This success, of course, is possible because of the simple fact that it is the collagenous framework in which we are interested, and not survival of the donor cells. Thus, the complexities of tissue cell typing are avoided. It makes no difference whether the cells in the donor tendon homograft are viable at the time of transfer—as they are in some circumstances—or dead, and indeed specifically killed by chemical preparation of the homograft. The viable cells will all be dead within two weeks after the transfer, and both types of homografts will then be in the same relationship to the host, namely, awaiting repopulation by new host cells, which will assume control of the local matrix turnover and the production, resorption, and remodeling of the collagenous pattern within the tendon homograft. Function follows.

Once any real difference between living and dead tendon homografts has been eliminated, however, it is necessary to distinguish between the two, which are so fundamentally different that their consideration together would be irrational.

The free "simple" tendon homograft is taken with a minimum of paratenon in the same way most autografts are taken. The free "composite" tendon homograft, by contrast, includes the entire intact synovial sheath of the tendon, so that the digital segment of the grafted tendon is literally not seen during transfer, being enclosed in this capsule of highly specialized synovium. The difference between the complexities of these two groups of tendon homografts is fundamental.

With a simple tendon graft, adhesion of the host tissue must take place if vascularization and cellular repopulation, and hence survival, are to occur. The restriction on early excursion of this adherent tendon is the same as when autografts of the same anatomical simplicity are used, with the same direct dependence on universal host contact for survival.

In the case of the composite flexor tendon homograft the same need for universal adhesion to the host tissue exists, but occurs outside the fibrous flexor sheath, and a synovial compartment is left intact with no direct contact between its enclosed tendons and the host tissues. Survival of these enclosed tendons occurs by vascularization along the pre-existing vascular channels of the vincula (Hueston et al., 1967), with the vascular circumferential extrasynovial adhesions providing the source of this new blood supply.

In each type of homograft the cells of the tendon disappear within two weeks and are then slowly replaced over six weeks by new host fibroblasts. The synovial lining cells, of course, are not exempt from this process and likewise disappear early, but the extraordinarily rapid spread of a layer of mononuclear cells around first the parietal and then the visceral layer of this cavity within less than one week—long before the enclosed tendon is repopulated—probably is the reason for the lack of adhesions between these two early reconstituted surfaces. Being unopened, and hence uninjured during transfer, even the reconstituted synovial lining is capable of retaining its integrity without adhesion formation. This immunity from adhesion production, a feature of the normal intact syn-

*This technique is perhaps now of historical and biological interest only.

ovium, is easily lost after even the most minor breach.

PRESERVED TENDON HOMOGRAFTS

If it is accepted that all viable (and for that matter all nonviable) cellular elements must be eliminated from a tendon homograft before its progressive repopulation by host cells, it is logical to expect some delay while an immune inflammatory response to the donor cells occurs and autolysis is completed. This phase must be associated in many instances with an initial increase in the normal vascular response in the immediate host tissues and the production of more adhesions than even a normal homograft (Seiffert, 1971). I have seen painful swelling of the fingers operated on, slight fever, and regional lymph node enlargement 12 to 14 days after multiple fresh composite grafting of more than one finger, consistent with this phase of rejection and cellular clearance.

Thus the transfer of cell free tendons has a more than theoretical advantage, in that one would expect less initial adhesion and a smoother, less delayed reconstitution of a normal cellular and vascular pattern within the tendon itself.

For more than two decades Iselin (1963) has advocated the use of such preserved—and hence dead acellular—tendons for free grafts, on the basis of both convenience and his mature assessment that the functional results are at least as good as those obtained by the use of fresh tendon autografts.

The mercurial solution (sodium 2-ethylmercurithiobenzoxazole-5-carboxylate; Cialit) that Iselin used for tendon preservation has more recently been studied by Seiffert and Schmidt (1971), who confirmed the clinical value of these tendons. They have also shown, by studies with ^{14}C labeled proline, that the collagen of tendon homografts is replaced by "creeping substitution" within six to eight weeks, although morphologically the vascular and cellular elements of the homografted tendons are indistinguishable from autografts within two to three months.

SIMPLE TENDON HOMOGRAFTS

Whether preserved by chemical destruction of their cells, preserved by deep freezing without immediate destruction of their cells, or transplanted directly from a recent cadaver under sterile conditions, the fate of a simple tendon homograft is cellular repopulation after cellular clearance. For this to occur, universal adhesions are necessary to provide universal cellular and vascular contact with the new host bed, in exactly the same way as we depend on the identical situation to allow survival of any free autograft, be it skin, nerve, bone, cartilage—or tendon.

The same prognosis is therefore to be expected from these free, preserved simple tendon homografts as from autografts—with perhaps additional early adhesion around those still containing cells capable of initiating an early immune inflammatory response, as Seiffert has indicated.

The use of Silastic rods to prepare a bed for the subsequent introduction of these preserved grafts has been a logical step in this area and is planned, as in the use of autografts, to lessen the restriction on subsequent excursion of the tendon graft (Seiffert and Schmidt, 1971).

While the lesser inflammatory reaction is recognized, some authors such as Geldmacher (1971), who have had experience with Cialit preserved tendons, point to the need for longer immobilization and the possibility of subsequent ruptures after implantation of these preserved tendon homografts. They caution against too ready acceptance of what can only be regarded as a free collagen transplant—admittedly already arranged and organized for function.

COMPOSITE TENDON HOMOGRAFTS

Inspired by the immunity of an intact synovial sheath from adhesion formation, and recognizing the fundamental freedom of most collagen and connective tissue elements from immunological responses, Peacock and Madden (1967) conceived the brilliant procedure of transferring the intact synovial sheath.

The contents of the sheath, of course, are both the flexor digitorum sublimis and the flexor digitorum profundus, and its walls are composed of not only the entire fibrous flexor sheath anteriorly but also all the phalangeal periosteum and the volar plates of the interphalangeal joints posteriorly. The fundamental concept, however, was the transfer of an

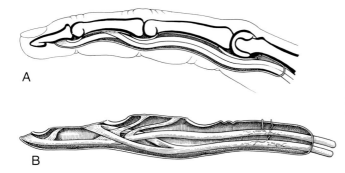

A

B

Figure 35–1. *A*, Flexor apparatus of the fingers. *B*, The flexor apparatus is taken in total with the synovial sheaths intact, including the fibrous flexor sheath in front and the periosteum and volar plates of the joints behind.

intact synovial sheath (Fig. 35–1). Only by this means could adhesions to the transplanted tendons be entirely eliminated. After practice, first experimentally, and subsequently by clinical application to patients in both the practice of Peacock and the present author's practice in Melbourne, this logical but giant stride in tendon grafting has proved to be successful. Only by such a composite transfer can tendons be freely grafted without the universal adhesions to the tendon seen after simple free tendon grafting.

Universal adhesions, of course, must occur around a composite graft if it is to survive, but they occur on the outside of the grafted complex whose walls have just been defined. The proximal anastomosis of the flexor digitorum sublimis and flexor digitorum profundus, whether in the palm or at the wrist, must be associated with adhesions if any biological union is to occur, but the crucial range of tendon length within the digital theca is preserved entirely free of adhesions.

The indications for this type of elaborate replacement of the entire flexor tendon complex are now rare, since the introduction of Silastic rods to reconstitute potential gliding spaces in otherwise hopeless graft beds. The concept, however, remains entirely valid.

Technically the most elaborate phase is the removal of the tendon complex from the cadaver, which often takes twice the time needed to introduce it into the recipient bed, in view of the need to avoid any perforation of a synovial sheath. This is particularly difficult in the elevation of the periosteum from the volar aspect of the proximal and middle phalanges of the digit.

The technique of transfer is simple after complete clearance of everything except the neurovascular bundles and the volar plates from the front of the injured finger (Hueston

et al., 1967; Peacock and Madden, 1967). Postoperatively, independent movement of the flexor digitorum sublimis can be demonstrated.

The cadavers used as a source of fresh composite grafts have been fresh cadavers being used for renal transplants, but deep freezing for as long as one week has not lessened the quality of results in these otherwise hopeless fingers—namely, those in which no sheath or tendon could otherwise be retained or reconstituted and amputation seemed inevitable. Patients with such injuries are often young, and in any event the procedure is worthy of consideration.

Immunosuppressive drugs are not given, because the cells are expected to die and to be replaced without jeopardizing the surgical results.

An interesting extension of this concept of transferring the entire synovial system in order to avoid adhesions to the tendons within the digital theca has been commenced by Dr. P. B. Chacha of Singapore (personal communication). In the mixed Asian population of Singapore it is difficult, mainly on cultural and religious grounds, to obtain cadaver material, and yet this surgeon has sought to replace the entire flexor system in selected cases of flexor tendon injury. He has used composite autografts from the foot. When measurements are made of the phalangeal length and tendon excursions, this may at first seem unreasonable, but his careful selection of the longest toe and its use as a donor for the shortest two fingers have produced results worthy of commendation. Some residual flexion deformity is usual in his cases, but because the ring and little fingers are those in which it is most important to regain full flexion for restoration of the power grip, this can be accepted. The possible practical applications of this concept, initially proposed by Peacock, are clearly still far from being fully exploited.

REFERENCES

Chacha, P. B.: Personal communication, 1969.

Geldmacher, I.: Prevention of adhesions in free flexor tendon grafting. *In* Transactions of the Fifth International Congress of Plastic Surgeons. London, Butterworth & Co. (Publishers) Ltd., 1971, p. 503.

Hueston, J. T., Hubble, B., and Rigg, B.: Homografts of the digital flexor tendon system. Aust. N.Z. J. Surg., *36*:269, 1967.

Iselin, M., Delaplaza, F. A.: Surgical use of homologous tendon grafts, preserved in Cialit. Plast. Reconst. Surg., *32*:401, 1963.

Peacock, E. E., and Madden, J. W.: Human composite flexor tendon allografts. Ann. Surg., *166*:624, 1967.

Seiffert, K.: Preserved grafts in reconstructive surgery. *In* Transactions of the Fifth International Congress of Plastic Surgeons. London, Butterworth & Co. (Publishers) Ltd., editor, J. T. Hueston, 1971, p. 766.

Seiffert, K., and Schmidt, K. P.: Preserved tendon grafts in hand surgery. *In* Transactions of the Fifth International Congress of Plastic Surgeons. London, Butterworth & Co. (Publishers) Ltd., editor, J. T. Hueston, 1971, p. 511.

Chapter 36

EVALUATION OF RESULTS AFTER FLEXOR TENDON REPAIR

RAOUL TUBIANA
STANLEY GORDON
JOHN A. GROSSMAN
AND PETER McMENIMAN

An ideal system for the evaluation of the results of flexor tendon repairs should be easy to interpret and should take into account the preoperative mobility of the fingers; moreover the results also should be easily comparable with the results in other series of cases. At present there is no internationally accepted system of evaluation. Each investigator presents his results using his own criteria. In an issue of the *Journal of Hand Surgery* (June 1977) containing numerous articles dealing with flexor tendon injuries, four different methods for the evaluating of results were used by various authors. Even in this book several different assessments are used.

EVALUATION OF FLEXOR TENDON FUNCTION IN THE FINGERS

Boyes in 1950 proposed a method for evaluating finger flexion by measuring the distance between the pulp of the distal phalanx and the distal palmar skin crease (Fig. 36–1). His results were presented graphically, plotting the percentage of tendon grafts against the flexion deficit. The range of active flexion of the interphalangeal joint was used to assess thumb function.

This method was adopted by a group of specialists at the Congress of SICOT in Bern in 1954. Using these criteria, Pulvertaft presented his results in flexor tendon grafting in

1956. He added an evaluation of the range of motion of the distal interphalangeal joint in this assessment. However, he did not account for loss of extension of the fingers. We have evaluated our results of tendon grafts in 1960 according to this method (Fig. 36–2).

White (1956), by contrast, evaluated his results in flexor tendon surgery by a combination of total angular flexion and pulp–distal crease measurements. Extension contractures were taken into consideration by summating the total extension loss for all the joints. The thumb was assessed in terms of a percentage of the range of motion of the interphalangeal joint of the contralateral extremity—70 per cent or more being considered excellent.

Lister (1977) also used pulp to palm measurements to evaluate the results of controlled mobilization after flexor tendon repair. Extension deficits were evaluated by measuring the angle between the distal phalanx and the metacarpal, i.e., summating the extension deficits.

Subsequently Stark et al. (1977) altered their system to include the total angular motion and the pulp-palm distance. They believed that following repair the distal interphalangeal joint must have at least 20 degrees of active flexion and less than 30 degrees of fixed flexion deformity in the proximal interphalangeal joint and flex to within 3.2 cm. of the midpalmar crease in order for the result to be rated as satisfactory.

Verdan and Michon (1961) classified their

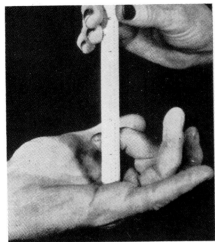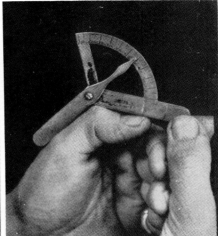

Figure 36–1. *Left*, Measurement of the distance between the fingertip and the distal palmar flexion crease. *Right*, Measurement of the amplitude of flexion of the interphalangeal joint of the thumb.

cases with reference to active flexion to the palm. Their cases were subdivided according to whether flexion was achieved within 2.5 cm. of the distal palmar crease (categories I and II) or to within 2.5 cm. of the palm (categories III and IV). Each 45 degree lack of extension was penalized one category. Assessment of thumb function was based on the recovery of 50 per cent or more of the motion of the distal interphalangeal joint.

The Committee for Evaluation of the American Society of Hand Surgery (1976) recommended the use of a formula comparing the total passive mobility to the total active mobility:

Total passive mobility = total passive flexion (metacarpophalangeal + proximal interphalangeal + distal interphalangeal) − lack of passive extension (metacarpophalangeal + proximal interphalangeal + distal interphalangeal).

Total active mobility = total active flexion (metacarpophalangeal + proximal interphalangeal + distal interphalangeal) − lack of active extension (metacarpophalangeal + proximal interphalangeal + distal interphalangeal).

This method is simple and has the advantage of being usable in other situations as well as after tendon surgery. However, it lacks precision and implies an equal functional value for each of the three joints.

Buck-Gramcko (1971) proposed a method that takes composite flexion, pulp to palm distance, and extension deficit into consideration. (He pointed out that the measurements should be performed with slight extension of the wrist without supporting the metacarpophalangeal joints in extension.) Measurements were used to obtain the following values:

1. Composite flexion—the sum of the angular measurements of flexion of all three joints.
2. Extension deficit—the sum of the angular measurements of loss of extension of all three joints.
3. Total active motion—the difference between the composite flexion and extension deficits.
4. The flexion deficit—the distance between the finger and the distal palmar crease.

A functional system was then formulated by assigning points to each of these measurements and totaling the values (Tables 36–1

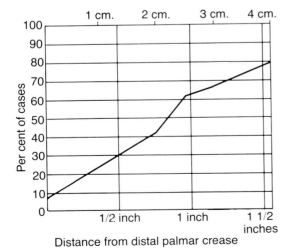

Figure 36–2. Results of flexor tendon grafts according to Boyes (R. Tubiana, 1960).

and 36–2). Duparc and Alnot (1978) only take account of the mobility of the interphalangeal joints.

DISCUSSION

These systems detail the exact change in the range of motion of each joint as a result of surgery. Such analytical evaluations are probably necessary for each case. However, with the exception of Buck-Gramcko's method, these detailed analytical measurements lack functional expressions for meaningful comparisons. Tables composed of large numbers of different angular values are difficult to interpret and use to derive comparative statistics and do not provide an evaluation of the functional state of the finger.

These systems must be supplemented by functional assessments for comparative purposes. Such a system should be accurate and easy to apply and interpret. Several factors need to be taken into account in any system of evaluation of flexor tendon repairs:

1. It is necessary to avoid subjective assessments which are not based on articular measurements. An evaluation of the movement of each joint is necessary in every case.

Table 36–1. POINT SYSTEM AND CLASSIFICATION FOR INDEX, MIDDLE, RING, AND LITTLE FINGERS*

Distance finger pulp – distal composite flexion crease†	0–2.5 cm.	≥ 200°	6 points
	2.5–4 cm.	≥ 180°	4 points
	4–6 cm.	≥ 150°	2 points
	>6 cm.	< 150°	0 points
Extension deficit		0–30°	3 points
			2 points
		51–70°	1 point
		> 70°	0 points
Total active motion		≥160°	6 points
		≥140°	4 points
		≥120°	2 points
		< 120°	0 points

Classification
  Excellent: 14–15 points
  Good: 11–13 points
  Satisfactory: 7–10 points
  Poor: 0–6 points

*Results of flexor tendon grafts according to Boyes graph (Tubiana, 1960).

†Buck-Gramcko means by "distal composite flexion crease" the fold formed by the distal transverse flexion crease on the ulnar side of the palm and the proximal transverse flexion crease on the radial side.

Table 36–2. POINT SYSTEM AND CLASSIFICATION FOR THE THUMB*

Flexion in the interphalangeal joint	50–70°	6 points
	30–49°	4 points
	10–29°	2 points
	< 10°	0 points
Extension deficit	0–10°	3 points
	11–20°	2 points
	21–30°	1 point
	>30°	0 points
Total active motion	≥40°	6 points
	30–39°	4 points
	20–29°	2 points
	<20°	0 points

Classification
  Excellent: 14–15 points
  Good: 11–13 points
  Satisfactory: 7–10 points
  Poor: 0–6 points

*Buck-Gramcko.

In addition, it is necessary to standardize the method by which these measurements are made, as this will influence the results. With the wrist in neutral position and the wrist joint in pronation and then in supination, the patient is asked to make a fist and then extend the fingers. One then measures the maximum flexion and extension of the three joints of each finger. The measurements to evaluate flexion of each joint must be made with the closed fist without maintaining the proximal segment of the joint to be measured in extension. In fact, the measurement of the individual joint movements, with the proximal joint held in extension, is much greater than the total combined range of movements for all joints flexing simultaneously. The limbs of the goniometer must be short enough not to impede movement. The goniometer is placed on the dorsum of the digit, as it is difficult to place it laterally on the central digits. One measures successively the active and passive mobility. Cantero (1983) has described a goniometer to measure all three joints together, formed by four articulated segments of adaptable length, allowing measurements in flexion and extension.

However, these measurements must be of functional value to allow meaningful comparison of results. The tables, which consist of a great number of measured angles, are difficult to interpret and difficult to use for comparative statistics, and they do not provide a useful evaluation of the functional state of the digit.

2. The sum of the movement of flexion of all three joints is not sufficient. Flexion of the metacarpophalangeal joints depends in part on the intrinsic muscles, whereas flexion of the intraphalangeal joints depends entirely on the long flexor tendons. The addition of the total range of flexion may give a misleading impression of the results of flexor tendon surgery. However, the evaluation of the movements of the interphalangeal joints is insufficient alone, as the function of the fingers also depends on movements of the metacarpophalangeal joints.

3. Measurement of pulp-palm distances may also be misleading, e.g., when the interphalangeal joints have a full range of motion and the metacarpophalangeal joints are stiff in extension or one of the interphalangeal joints is in fixed flexion.

4. The postoperative total active motion value must be compared with the preoperative value and may be an indication for tenolysis. It is insufficient, however, to allow evaluation of the function of the finger.

5. For the result to be satisfactory, the lack of extension must not be more than 30 degrees at either interphalangeal joint, and the total lack of extension must be no more than 45 degrees.

6. The range of movement in the proximal interphalangeal joint has the greatest functional value and reflects most accurately the action of the two long flexors. But it is also necessary to take into account in a lesser degree the active mobility of the metacarpophalangeal joint and distal interphalangeal joint.

METHODS USED BY THE AUTHORS

For all these reasons, we have advocated (Tubiana et al., 1979) a method of evaluation of flexor tendon repairs which includes specifically a method of assessment of proximal interphalangeal joint function.

This is easily found by determining the relationship between the long axes of the middle phalanx and the metacarpal (Fig. 36–3).

A separate assessment of the flexion deficit and the extension deficit is made, after which a composite assessment is used to determine the functional value. The method of assessment proposed in 1979 has been slightly modified and now includes a supplementary grade "normal."

Flexion Deficit

The flexion deficit is graded as follows:
Grade I (F1): Complete active flexion.
Grade II (F2): The line of the middle phalanx is parallel to the metacarpal with full active flexion, and the distal joint has at least 45 degrees of active flexion.
Grade III (F3): The middle phalanx forms an angle 0 to 30 degrees with the metacarpal with full active flexion, and the distal interphalangeal joint has at least 30 degrees of active flexion.
Grade IV (F4): The middle phalanx forms an angle of 30 to 60 degrees with the metacarpal with full active flexion, and the distal interphalangeal joint has at least 15 degrees of active flexion.
Grade V (F5): The middle phalanx forms an angle of 60 to 90 degrees with the metacarpal with full active flexion.

If distal interphalangeal joint flexion is less than 45 degrees for grade I, 30 degrees for grade II, or 15 degrees for grade III, the result is dropped one grade.

Extension Deficit

The extension deficit is estimated by adding the active extension deficit in each of the three joints.
Grade I (E1): Complete active extension.
Grade II (E2): The angle between the distal phalanx and the metacarpal is less than 15 degrees.
Grade III (E3): The angle is less than 45 degrees, with no more than 30 degrees deficit in any one joint.
Grade IV (E4): The extension deficit is between 45 and 90 degrees and is no more than 45 degrees in any one joint.
Grade V (E5): The extension deficit is greater than 90 degrees.

If the extension deficit in any joint is more than 15, 30, or 45 degrees, the result is dropped one grade.

Combined Assessment

The combined assessment is expressed by utilizing the grades of flexion deficit and extension deficit, for example, F1, E2.

Since a flexion deficit is more important

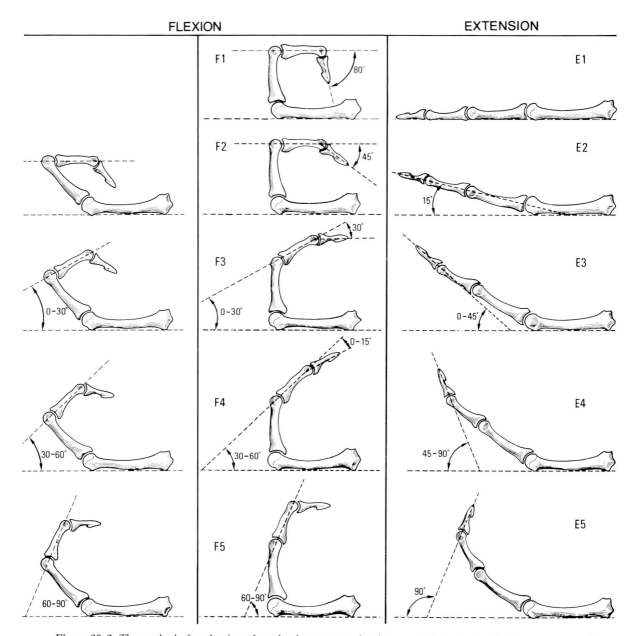

Figure 36–3. The method of evaluation of results that we use takes into account the flexion deficit as represented by the angle between the middle phalanx and the metacarpal (which we consider most important) as well as the different degrees of metacarpophalangeal flexion (note the difference between columns 1 and 2), distal intercarpophalangeal flexion, and extension deficit (column 3).

than an extension deficit, a scoring system similar to the one used by Buck-Gramcko assigning greater weight to active flexion is proposed (Table 36–3).

We agree with Stark (1977), who stated that the use of such terms as excellent, good, fair, and poor is misleading. However, every author uses these terms to express results. If required, a point system and classification for the index, middle, ring, and little finger could be established by adding active flexion and extension deficit. For example, perfect results would be 10 points, very good results would be 8 to 9 points, good results would be 7 to 6 points, fair results would be 5 to 4 points, and poor results would be 0 to 3 points. (Table 36–3).

EVALUATION OF SURGERY ON THE LONG FLEXOR TENDON OF THE THUMB

Evaluation of the results of the flexor tendon surgery in the thumb must be considered from a slightly different perspective. Flexor pollicis longus flexes the distal phalanx, but this action depends in part on the stability of the metacarpophalangeal joint. In normal conditions, the flexion of the joint approaches 90 degrees; however, a good result can be obtained with a lesser degree of flexion, if this flexes within the functional range. On the other hand, the extension deficit of the distal phalanx impedes function more than a lack of extension in another digit. A deficit of more than 15 degrees extension reduces

Table 36–3. COMBINED ASSESSMENT OF RESULTS FOR THE FINGERS

Active Flexion	
Grade I (F1)	7 points
Grade II (F2)	6 points
Grade III (F3)	4 points
Grade IV (F4)	2 points
Grade V (F5)	0 points
Extension Deficit	
Grade I (E1) and Grade II (E2)	3 points
Grade III (E3)	2 points
Grade IV (E4)	1 point
Grade V (E5)	0 points
Classification of Results	
Perfect	10 points
Very Good	8 to 9 points
Good	7 to 6 points
Fair	5 to 4 points
Poor	3 to 0 points

Table 36–4. COMBINED ASSESSMENT OF RESULTS FOR THE THUMB

Active Flexion	
Grade I (F1)	5 points
Grade II (F2)	3 points
Grade III (F3)	2 points
Grade IV (F4)	1 point
Extension Deficit	
Grade I (E1)	2 points
Grade II (E2)	1 point
Grade III (E3)	0 points
Classification of Results	
Perfect	7 points
Very Good	5 to 6 points
Good	4 points
Fair	3 points
Poor	2 to 0 points

pulp to pulp contact and efficiency of thumb-index pinch.

Flexion Deficit

Grade I (F1): Complete active motion (compared with the opposite side).

Grade II (F2): The distal interphalangeal joint has at least 60 degrees of active flexion.

Grade III (F3): The distal interphalangeal joint has at least 30 degrees of active flexion.

Grade IV (F4): The distal interphalangeal joint has less than 30 degrees of active flexion.

Extension Deficit

Grade I (E1): The angle between the proximal and distal phalanges is less than 15 degrees.

Grade II (E2): The angle between the proximal and distal phalanges is less than 30 degrees.

Grade III (E3): The angle between the proximal and distal phalanges is greater than 30 degrees.

Each of the foregoing values is recorded with the thumb in anteposition so that the final functional assessment is more meaningful. No method can be both simple and exact at the same time. The foregoing system of functional evaluation is a compromise.

REFERENCES

Boyes, J. H.: Flexor tendon grafts in the fingers and thumb. An evaluation of end results. J. Bone Joint Surg., *32A*:489–499, 531, 1950.

Boyes, J. H., and Stark, H. H.: Flexor tendon grafts in the fingers and thumb. J. Bone Joint Surg., *53A*:1332–1342, 1971.

Buck-Gramcko, D., Dietrich, F. E., and Gögge, S.: Bewertungskriterien Nachuntersuchungen von Beug'esehnenwieder-Herstellungen. Handchirurgie, *8*:65–69, 1976.

Cantero, J.: Proposition d'une méthode d'évaluation objective apres réparation du tendon fléchisseurs. Ann. Chir. Main, *2*:258–263, 1983.

Committee for Evaluation of the American Society of Hand Surgery: Report, March 10, 1976.

Doyle, J. R., and Blythe, W.: The finger flexion tendon sheath and pulleys: anatomy and reconstruction. *In* AAOS Symposium on Tendon Surgery of the Hand. St. Louis, The C. V. Mosby Co., 1975, p. 81.

Duparc, Y.: Communication, GEM Congres annual, Paris, 1978.

Duran, R. J., and Houser, R. G.: Controlled passive motion following flexor tendon repair in zones two and three. *In* AAOS Symposium on Tendon Surgery in the Hand. St. Louis, The C. V. Mosby Co, 1975, p. 105.

Kleinert, H. E., Kutz, J. E., Atasoy, E., and Stormo, A.: Primary repair of flexor tendons. Orthop. Clin. N. Am., *4*:865, 1973.

Lister, G. D., Kleinert, H. E., Kutz, Y. E., and Atasoy, E.: Primary flexor tendon repair followed by immediate controlled mobilization. J. Hand Surg., *2*:441, 1977.

Paneva-Holevich, E.: Reconstructive Surgery of the Flexor Tendons of the Hand. Sofia, Medicina i Fizkultura, 1977.

Pulvertaft, R. G.: Tendon grafts for flexor tendon injuries in fingers and thumb. A study of technique and results. J. Bone Joint Surg., *38B*:175–194, 1956.

Stark, H. H., Zemev, N. P., Boyes, J. H., and Ashworth, C. R.: Flexor tendon graft through intact superficialis tendon. J. Hand Surg., *2*:456, 1977.

Strickland, J. W.: Results of flexor tendon surgery in Zone II. Symposium on flexor tendon surgery. Hand Clin., *1*:167–179. Philadelphia, W. B. Saunders Co., 1985.

Tsuge, K., Ikuta, Y., and Matsuishi, Y.: Repair of flexor tendons by intratendinous tendon suture. J. Hand Surg., *2*:436–440, 1977.

Tubiana, R.: Greffes des tendons fléchisseurs et du pouce. Technique et résultats. Rev. Chir. Orthop., *46*:191–214, 1960.

Tubiana, R., McMeniman, P., and Gordon, S.: Evaluation des résultats après réparation des tendons longs fléchisseurs des doigts. Ann. Chir., *33*:659–662, 1979.

Verdan, C., and Michon, J.: Le traitement des plaies des tendons fléchisseurs des doigts. Rev. Chir. Orthop., *47*:285–425, 1961.

White, W. L.: Secondary restoration of finger flexion by digital tendon graft. An evaluation of seventy-six cases. Am. J. Surg., *91*:662–668, 1956.

Chapter 37

RESULTS OF FLEXOR TENDON SURGERY IN ZONE II

James W. Strickland

The restoration of tendon gliding sufficient to produce functionally adequate digital motion following flexor tendon interruption in zone II has historically been a difficult challenge for the hand surgeon. The serious student of flexor tendon repair and reconstruction is frustrated by the many variations in the methods of measurement and classification of results he encounters in the literature. Despite the efforts of many authors to introduce evaluation methods that would best demonstrate the efficacy of various procedures, no universally accepted system has evolved. This lamentable absence makes it virtually impossible for the surgeon to compare the reported results of methods of repair and reconstruction with each other or with those that he has achieved.

A widely accepted method of evaluating finger performance following flexor tendon grafting involves the measurement of the distance between the pulp of the distal phalanx and the distal palmar skin crease, as proposed by Boyes (1950). White (1956) assessed his results by using a combination of total angular flexion and distal pulp to palm measurements. His method also included consideration of flexion contractures by summating the total extension loss for all digital joints. Verdan and Michon (1961) also used a distal pulp to palm method and categorized their results accordingly, with each 45 degree extension deficit resulting in the penalization of that result by one category. Lister et al. (1977) combined pulp to palm measurements with the summation of angular extension deficits in evaluating their results in primary repair of lacerated flexor tendons in zone II. Buck-Gramcko et al. (1976) described a method combining composite digital joint flexion, pulp to palm distance, and extension

deficit in a functional system that assigned points to each of these measurements, which were then summed to provide a value for classification. Stark et al. (1977) altered their original method to include total angular motion and pulp to palm distance in assessing the results of flexor tendon grafting carried out through an intact superficialis tendon.

In 1976 the American Society for Surgery of the Hand (1976) recommended to its membership the use of a formula to measure digital function. This method consists of a summation of the active or passive angular flexion of the metacarpophalangeal and proximal and distal interphalangeal joints minus any extension deficit. One can then determine the total passive motion and the total active motion of a given digit, and meaningful comparisons between preoperative and postoperative motion can be made.

More recently Tubiana et al. (1979) developed a scoring system that assigns point values for the distal pulp to distal palmar crease distance, extension deficits, and total active motion and classifies the results according to the sum of these points. An extension of that system was presented at the Congress of the International Federation of Hand Societies in Boston, Massachusetts, in October 1983 by Tubiana and associates. In its latest form the system takes into account the patient's own interpretation of the performance of the involved digit.

Although most of these assessment methods have some features in common, the diversity among the techniques of evaluating and classifying digital performance following flexor tendon surgery makes meaningful comparison difficult. Most of these methods have one or more features that tend to distort their accuracy and negate their scientific significance. Measurement of the distance from the distal phalangeal pulp to the distal palmar crease is subject to considerable error because of the variations in measurement techniques and in the selection of anatomic reference points by individual examiners. Inclusion of measurements of metacarpophalangeal joint motion also has a strong falsifying influence on the assessment of digital function following flexor tendon surgery.

In our studies of the techniques of flexor tendon repair and reconstruction, we have almost never encountered significant alterations in metacarpophalangeal joint performance. In the absence of damage to the extensor system and with continued strong flexion produced by the intact intrinsic musculature, there is rarely any meaningful loss at that joint. Inclusion of the normal performance of the metacarpophalangeal joint in any assessment system therefore unfairly influences the final result. In the total active motion (TAM) system, for example, normal metacarpophalangeal joint motion contributes at least 30 per cent of the total digital motion and should not be included because it is not dependent on long extrinsic flexor tendon function. Those systems that fail to include joint extension deficits, which occur not infrequently following flexor tendon surgery, also fail to adequately document digital performance. Further, we believe that it is appropriate to take into account the preoperative passive range of motion of the joints of a given digit as a limiting influence on the potential performance of any reconstructive procedure carried out on the flexor tendon system.

The purpose in this chapter is to review the results of flexor tendon procedures in a single hand surgery practice utilizing simplified assessment formulas. Although the results may be at some variance with those reported by others, they represent an honest appraisal of the performance of different procedures in a fairly large patient population. A consistent system of analysis is utilized with minor variations based on factors unique to that procedure. Finally, an effort will be made to utilize the information gained from the individual study of these procedures to predict the final performance of 100 consecutive digits that sustained zone II flexor tendon interruption managed by single or multiple repair and reconstructive techniques, according to the outcome of each procedure.

METHODS AND MATERIALS

The assessment formulas utilized in this chapter to study the results of flexor tendon surgery were established in an effort to provide simple, objective, and clinically meaningful information. The rationale for these methods evolved from the published recommendations of the Assessment Committee of the American Society for Surgery of the Hand (1976) and from valued conversations with Doctors Raoul Tubiana, Claude Verdan, and Richard Eaton. As with any other assessment techniques, the reliability of the methods presented here depends on the proper completion of the examination, including accurate measurements by the surgeon or therapist and honest cooperation by the patient. Although these techniques are not devoid of the potential for inaccuracy and misinterpretation, we believe that they can provide useful information with regard to the performance of various procedures utilized in an effort to restore satisfactory flexor tendon performance.

To a great extent the formulas we have employed to assess digital performance following flexor tendon surgery are derived from the recommendations for determining total active motion and total passive motion as recommended by the Assessment Committee of the American Society for Surgery of the Hand (1976). Metacarpophalangeal joint motion is omitted in order to remove the falsifying influence of this measurement on the assessment of true flexor tendon performance. For reconstructive procedures the formulas include the total preoperative passive motion of the proximal and distal interphalangeal joints as a limiting factor when assessing the motion that can be achieved. When evaluating tenolysis, the percentage of passive preoperative motion in comparison with the percentage of active motion achieved postoperatively is considered to be the best indicator of the effectiveness of this technique.

It is important to emphasize that proximal and distal interphalangeal joint flexion measurements must be made while the patient is attempting to make a complete fist, including flexion at the metacarpophalangeal, proximal interphalangeal, and distal interphalangeal joints (Fig. 37–1). This requirement reflects the fact that less tendon excursion is required to produce middle and distal joint flexion

A. PIP AND DIP FLEXION
WHILE MAKING A FIST

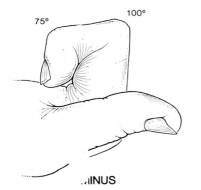

75°   100°

MINUS

B.
EXTENSION
DEFICIT   10°   20°

Figure 37–1. Technique for measuring digital motion to be used in determining total active and total passive motion (TAM and TPM) of the proximal and distal interphalangeal joints. *A*, Measurement of flexion at the proximal interphalangeal joint and distal interphalangeal joint while the patient attempts to make a complete fist. *B*, Measurement of extension deficit at the proximal interphalangeal joint and distal interphalangeal joint. The combined extension deficit of the two joints is subtracted from the combined flexion to give the total active motion (TAM). Passive manipulation of the digits is carried out and the same formula used to determine the total passive motion (TPM).

$$\text{TAM OF PIP} + \text{DIP} = (75° + 100°) - (20° + 10°)$$
$$= 175° - 30°$$
$$= 145°$$

with the metacarpophalangeal joints held in full extension than with all three joints in composite flexion. The true measurement of flexor tendon performance therefore requires that the patient attempt to actively flex all three joints simultaneously.

With these guidelines three formulas were developed for the assessment of digital performance following flexor tendon repair (see equations below):

With these formulas the results are expressed in percentages of the passive motion in excess of any active motion present prior to the tendon repair or reconstructive procedure. These percentage results are then classified as shown in Table 37–1.

In order to maintain the purest possible clinical sample, all procedures in these studies were personally carried out by the author or by his associates, whose practices are totally

1. Tendon repair

$$\frac{\text{Active PIP} + \text{DIP flexion} - \text{extension deficit}}{175 \text{ degrees}} \times 100 = \% \text{ of normal active PIP and DIP motion}$$

2. Staged flexor tendon reconstruction

$$\frac{\text{Postop. active PIP} + \text{DIP flexion} - \text{extension deficit}}{\text{Preop. passive PIP} + \text{DIP flexion} - \text{extension deficit}} \times 100 = \begin{array}{l}\% \text{ of preoperative passive motion} \\ \text{actively achieved by staged flexor} \\ \text{tendon reconstruction}\end{array}$$

3. Tenolysis

$$100 - \frac{\text{TPM}_1 - \text{TAM}_2}{\text{TPM}_2 - \text{TAM}_2} \times 100 = \begin{array}{l}\% \text{ of preoperative passive motion} \\ \text{in excess of active motion actively} \\ \text{achieved by tenolysis.}\end{array}$$

Where
TPM_1 = total passive motion (PIP + DIP − extensor deficit) before surgery.
TAM_1 = total active motion (PIP + DIP − extensor deficit) before surgery.
TAM_2 = total active motion (PIP + DIP − extensor dificit) after surgery.

Table 37–1. CLASSIFICATION OF FLEXOR
TENDON RESULTS

Group	Percentage of Return
Excellent	75 to 100
Good	50 to 74
Fair	25 to 49
Poor	0 to 24

centage of a normal 175 degree motion at these two joints was determined with the use of the following formula:

$$\frac{\text{Active PIP + DIP flexion − extension lag}}{175 \text{ degrees}} \times 100$$
$$= \% \text{ of normal active PIP and DIP motion}$$

For that study a very strict classification system was utilized and is shown in Table 37–2.

The performance of 50 digits in 37 patients was analyzed following flexor tendon repair in zone II. Twenty-five digits were managed with three and one-half weeks of protected immobilization prior to the initiation of a gradual motion program, and 25 additional digits were managed by a carefully selected regimen of intermittent passive motion initiated within the first five postoperative days according to a modification of the method described by Duran and Houser (1975). The results of that study are shown in Table 37–3.

There were four tendon ruptures (16 per cent) in the digits in the immobilization category, compared with a single rupture (4 per cent) in the early passive motion group. If one excludes the rupture cases, the average total active motion of all three joints of the immobilized digits was 168 degrees compared with 213 degrees in the mobilized fingers.

In the immobilization category there were no excellent results, 12 per cent good results, and 40 per cent in the good or fair category. When poor results were combined with the cases of rupture, there was an overall 60 per cent failure rate. In the early passive motion digits there was a 56 per cent incidence of excellent or good performance, with 72 per cent in the excellent, good, or fair categories and 28 per cent in the poor or rupture groups. The 56 per cent excellent and good results of the passive motion group were statistically significant ($p \leq 0.005$) when compared with the 12 per cent in the immobilized group.

devoted to surgery of the hand. All flexor tendon lacerations occurred in zone II and resulted from sharp trauma with minimal associated injuries. Flexor tendon severance with concomitant phalangeal fracture, severe skin loss, excessive contamination, or severe crushing were excluded, although digital nerve interruption did not result in deletion of that digit from the study. Results of conventional free tendon grafting are not included in this chapter because of insufficient numbers. The classic article by Boyes and Stark (1971) reviewing 1000 consecutive free flexor tendon graft procedures stands as the definitive documentation of the performance of that technique.

FLEXOR TENDON REPAIR

Although there has been almost universal conversion to primary flexor tendon repair within the digital fibro-osseous canal, controversy still exists as to the benefit of early mobilization techniques designed to control or modify adhesion formation. In 1980 we published the results of a study designed to assess digital function following flexor tendon repair in zone II with a comparison of postoperative immobilization and controlled passive motion techniques (Strickland and Glogovac, 1980). The assessment of digital performance in that study was carried out using a combination of existing classifications and the total active motion system recommended by the American Society for Surgery of the Hand. Because metacarpophalangeal joint motion was normal in all cases, this measurement was thought to bias a true assessment of tendon function as reflected at the proximal interphalangeal joint and distal interphalangeal joint levels. We therefore elected to use the sum of the proximal interphalangeal joint flexion and the distal interphalangeal joint flexion (fist position) minus the extensor deficit at these joints in order to compute the total active motion. The per-

Table 37–2. CLASSIFICATION SYSTEM FOR
FLEXOR TENDON REPAIRS

Group	PIP + DIP Return (%)	PIP + DIP Minus Extensor Loss (Degree)
Excellent	85–100	150+
Good	70–84	125–149
Fair	50–69	90–124
Poor	<50	<90

Table 37–3. TOTAL RESULTS

	Excellent	Good	Fair	Poor	Rupture	Total
Immobilization	0(0%)	3(12%)	7(28%)	11(44%)	4(16%)	25
Early passive motion	9(36%)	5(20%)	4(16%)	6(24%)	1(4%)	25

The excellent, good, and fair results for the passive motion group (72 per cent) and the immobilization group (40 per cent) were also significant (p≤0.05).

Results following zone II severance of the profundus alone produced one good and two fair results in the immobilization group. Five excellent results and one each in the good, fair, and poor categories followed early motion.

In an attempt to refine the comparison between the immobilization and passive early motion groups, all isolated profundus repairs or those repairs of the profundus tendon in which the superficialis tendon was excised were deleted; only those cases in which both the profundus and superficialis had been repaired were studied. The same criteria for evaluation were utilized; the results are shown in Table 37–4.

The results in 41 per cent of the 17 combined profundus and superficialis repairs managed by immobilization fell into either the good or fair category; 59 per cent were considered failures. Of the 15 fingers treated by early passive motion following repair of both tendons, either excellent or good results were achieved in 53 per cent; 66 per cent fell into the excellent, good, or fair category. Thirty-four per cent of this group of operations were considered failures. The excellent and good results in the passive motion group (53 per cent) and in the immobilized group (6 per cent) were significant (p≤0.01).

Five digits were treated by profundus tendon repair and superficialis tendon excision in the immobilization group; four of the operations yielded a poor result and in one case rupture occurred. Two digits in the early passive motion group were managed by profundus repair and superficialis excision, resulting in one excellent and one good result.

We believe that this study provided a meaningful comparison between the results with the early postoperative mobilization and immobilization methods. It gave strong support to early passive motion as an effective adhesion-limiting technique that could substantially improve the results of flexor tendon repairs in this troublesome area. The reduced rupture rate in the mobilized tendons was thought to substantiate the tensile strength studies of Mason and Allen (1941), which indicated that a tendon repair gains strength when submitted to stress at the repair site.

Unfortunately an accurate comparison of these data and previously reported studies is almost impossible because of the wide variation in surgical techniques and the great diversity of assessment methods. The results did tend to corroborate those reported by Duran and Houser (1975) utilizing the passive technique and those of Lister et al. (1977) employing early active extension.

Subsequent to our study the classification system was modified because it was thought to be too rigid by many others involved in the investigation of flexor tendon performance. In addition, we decided that identical classification systems should be utilized in each of the categories of flexor tendon surgery, i.e., repair, grafting, staged reconstruction, and tenolysis, in order to create a more standardized approach that would allow for meaningful comparison of the procedures. The revised classification system is shown in Table 37–5.

By utilizing the same formula for assessment and the revised classification system, our experience with digital function following zone II flexor tendon repair was revised to include 71 cases in 58 patients. The results for combined profundus and superficialis repairs and the results following repairs of both

Table 37–4. PROFUNDUS AND SUPERFICIALIS REPAIRED

	Excellent	Good	Fair	Poor	Rupture	Total
Immobilization	0(0%)	1(6%)	6(35%)	9(53%)	1(6%)	17
Early passive motion	3(20%)	5(33%)	2(13%)	4(27%)	1(7%)	15

Table 37–5. REVISED CLASSIFICATION
SYSTEM FOR TENDON REPAIRS

Group	PIP + DIP Return (%)	PIP + DIP Minus Extensor Loss (Degrees)
Excellent	75–100	132+
Good	50–74	88–131
Fair	25–49	44–87
Poor	<25	<44

the profundus and superficialis are displayed in Table 37–6 and Figures 37–2 and 37–3.

The results of this updated analysis utilizing a larger patient population do not differ greatly from those of our earlier report. Although the percentage of excellent results in the total study is lower (25 versus 36 per cent), the finding that 56 per cent fell in the excellent or good group is identical with the results of the original work. The change in classification systems is probably responsible for the decrease in the poor results from 24 to 13 per cent; the incidence of rupture remained 4 per cent.

When one compares the updated results with those of the original study for digits in which both the profundus and superficialis tendons were repaired, the results were again similar. The 56 per cent incidence of excellent or good results of the expanded study compares favorably with the 53 per cent in the earlier report, although, again, the slight downgrading of the classification system may be responsible for this change. There was a decrease in the percentage of poor results (17 versus 27 per cent), and the rupture incidences were similar (5 versus 7 per cent).

Although the improved performance produced by early passive motion in flexor tendon repairs in zone II is encouraging, the 22 per cent incidence of poor results in our most recent study continues to emphasize that we are still far short of the desired objectives. Additional studies investigating the effect of technical advances, including primary repair of the flexor tendon sheath, are necessary together with continuing work to determine the best postoperative mobilization method. The use of pharmacologic agents to modify adhesion formation following flexor tendon repair may also have much to offer with regard to future improvements in flexor tendon performance.

STAGED FLEXOR TENDON RECONSTRUCTION

Staged reconstruction of the flexor tendon system has become an accepted technique for repair of the badly damaged digit. The principles and methods for implantation of silicone rods and their subsequent replacement with free tendon grafts have been well documented (Hunter, 1979; Hunter and Salisbury, 1970, 1971; Hunter and Schneider, 1975; Schneider, 1978). This technique has the additional benefit of permitting other procedures, such as joint contracture release and pulley reconstruction, to be carried out concomitantly with rod implantation.

Although our experience lent credence to the report of Hunter and Salisbury (1971) that the two stage technique was the best reconstruction option for the severely damaged digit, we were aware that our results did not appear to be as good as those reported in their initial series. For that reason we conducted a clinical investigation of the results of our experience with the staged flexor tendon reconstruction procedure and published those findings in 1983 (LaSalle and Strickland, 1983). The method of evaluation was similar to that employed for the assessment of the results following flexor tendon repair, with consideration given to the limitations of ultimate digital performance resulting from alterations in the available passive range of motion in the digital joints prior to the second stage (tendon graft) of the reconstructive sequence. A comparison of preoperative passive interphalangeal joint motion with postoperative active interphalangeal joint motion was carried out utilizing the formula at the bottom of this page.

Again a classification system was utilized that would be consistent with the revised methods of analysis for each area of flexor tendon surgery (Table 37–7).

The results of 43 two stage flexor tendon reconstructions carried out by the same surgeon in 39 patients were reviewed. In all fingers both flexor tendons were severed in zone II, and reconstruction was carried out utilizing the technique described by Hunter (Hunter, 1979; Hunter and Salisbury, 1971; Hunter and Schneider, 1975). Our results are shown in Table 37–8 and Figure 37–4.

$$\frac{\text{Postoperative active PIP + DIP flexion} - \text{extensor deficit}}{\text{Preoperative passive PIP + DIP flexion} - \text{extensor deficit}} \times 100 = \begin{array}{l}\text{\% passive motion (before second} \\ \text{stage) actively achieved by two} \\ \text{stage flexor tendon reconstruction}\end{array}$$

Table 37–6. RESULTS OF ZONE II FLEXOR TENDON REPAIR WITH
CONTROLLED PASSIVE MOTION

	Excellent	Good	Fair	Poor	Rupture	Total
All repairs	18(25%)	22(32%)	19(27%)	9(13%)	3(4%)	71
Repairs of profundus and superficialis	7(17%)	16(39%)	9(22%)	7(17%)	2(5%)	41

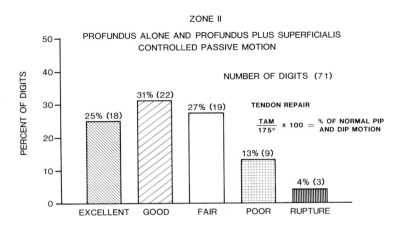

Figure 37–2. Percentage results of the various classification groups following repair of the flexor profundus and superficialis in zone II.

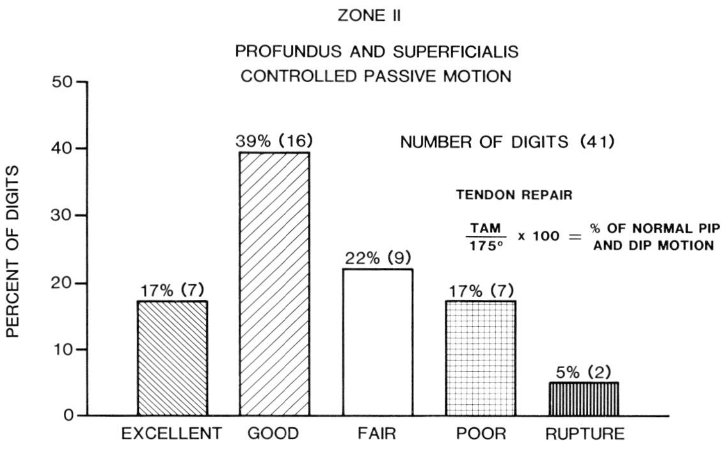

Figure 37–3. Percentage results of the various classification groups following repair of the flexor profundus and superficialis in zone II.

Table 37–7. CLASSIFICATION SYSTEM FOR
STAGED FLEXOR TENDON
RECONSTRUCTION

Group	PIP + DIP Return (%)
Excellent	75–100
Good	50–74
Fair	25–49
Poor	0–24

Table 37–8. RESULTS OF TWO STAGE
FLEXOR TENDON RECONSTRUCTION

Category	Number	Percentage
Excellent	7	16
Good	10	23
Fair	11	26
Poor	12	28
Ruptures	3	7
Total	43	100

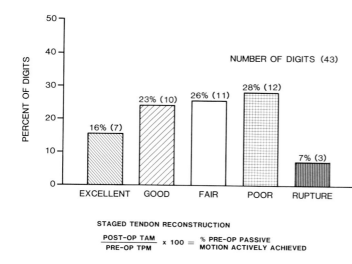

Figure 37–4. Percentage results of the various classification groups following staged flexor tendon reconstruction.

All 43 digits had some flexion deformity at either the proximal or distal interphalangeal joint, or both. The 12 digits in the poor category had the following problems: reflex dystrophy (1), infection (1), graft sloughing secondary to poor skin (1), and active motion less than 25 per cent of preoperative passive motion (9). There were no significant differences in the results of the grafts that involved proximal tendon junctures in the palm (4) and those that involved junctions in the distal forearm (39). Further, we could not measure any difference between the performance of the different donor grafts (palmaris longus, 25; plantaris, 12; toe extensor, 3; and extensor indicis proprius, 1).

The results of this study indicate that in 40 per cent of the digits subjected to two stage flexor tendon reconstruction one can anticipate more than 60 per cent recovery of the preoperative passive proximal and distal interphalangeal joint motion. The procedure, however, still incurs an extremely high incidence of failure; in over one-third of the cases less than 12 per cent of the preoperative passive motion returns. We could not demonstrate that early mobilization of tendon grafts significantly influenced final performance, nor could we determine that a specific rod design or material was best. Further, we could not glean any meaningful information as to the most optimal interval between stage I and stage II or whether the superficialis or profundus was the best motor tendon.

Tenolysis was carried out in 20 (47 per cent) of the digits in this study and resulted in the upgrading of the results in 12 digits to a higher category. The preoperative and postoperative categorizations of those digits that underwent tenolysis are compared in Figure 37–5, and the effect of the procedure on performance in the entire staged reconstruction group is shown in Table 37–9.

In our series a 47 per cent incidence of tenolysis was considerably greater than that reported by Hunter and Salisbury (1971; 6.7

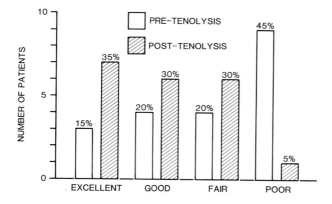

Figure 37–5. Results of tenolysis following staged flexor tendon reconstruction. Changes in the number and percentage of digits in each of the classification groups following tenolysis of adherent tendon grafts (20 digits) after two-staged reconstruction.

Table 37–9. RESULTS OF STAGED FLEXOR TENDON RECONSTRUCTION FOLLOWING
TENOLYSIS OF 20 (47%) DIGITS

	Excellent	Good	Fair	Poor (Includes Ruptures)	Total
Pretenolysis	7(16%)	10(23%)	11(26%)	15(35%)	43
Posttenolysis	11(26%)	12(28%)	13(30%)	7(16%)	43

per cent) and Chamay et al. (1979; 27 per cent). In neither of these studies did the authors define their indications for tenolysis, nor did they record the impact of the procedure on their final results. We found that most adhesions occurred between the graft and the pseudosheath formed by the tendon spacer rather than at the proximal tendon juncture as reported by Hunter and Salisbury (1971). In our series, tenolysis was an effective procedure that significantly improved the digital performance in digits with adherent tendon grafts. We conclude that it is probably appropriate to refer to the technique as "staged flexor tendon reconstruction" rather than "two stage flexor reconstruction."

Despite the relatively high percentage of poor results (16 per cent) following staged flexor tendon reconstruction, it remains the best available procedure for the reconstruction of flexor tendon function in badly damaged digits. Refinements of materials and techniques will undoubtedly lead to improvements in the performance of these techniques.

TENOLYSIS

Surgical mobilization of adherent flexor tendons or flexor tendon grafts in the digital canals is recognized as an important technique for restoring digital function. Despite some early pessimism as to the efficacy of this technique (Brooks, 1970; Bunnell, 1948; Peacock and Van Winkle, 1970; Rank et al., 1973), tenolysis has emerged as a valuable procedure when carried out properly with appropriate emphasis on postoperative maintenance of the improved tendon excursion achieved at surgery (Fetrow, 1967; Schneider and Hunter, 1975; Verdan and Michon, 1961; Whitaker et al., 1977).

In 1977 we reviewed our results with flexor tenolysis in zone II in which a technique utilizing thorough delicate release of all restraining adhesions and immediate motion was used (Whitaker et al., 1977). In assessing

the results of this procedure, it was believed to be important to determine the preoperative active and passive ranges of motion of the digital joints and to assess the postoperative changes in those measurements. It was recognized that the results of this procedure could not be evaluated by comparison with the function of a normal finger. Rather one must take into account the preoperative limitations of ultimate function as determined by the passive range of motion that was present. Therefore, any system that accurately evaluates the results of tenolysis should be expressed as the percentage of the difference between the preoperative active and passive ranges of motion actively achieved by the procedure. The formula we employed at the time of that study was based on the total passive motion and total active motion values, as advocated by the American Society for Surgery of the Hand. Subsequent to publication of that report we elected to omit the falsifying influence of the metacarpophalangeal joint and again limited the evaluation to the composite flexion at the proximal and distal interphalangeal joints while the patient attempts to make a fist, minus extension deficits at those joints. The resultant formula, which we currently use for flexor tenolysis evaluation, is as follows:

$$100 - \frac{TPM_1 - TAM_2}{TPM_1 - TAM_1} \times 100$$
= % of preoperative passive motion in excess of active motion achieved by tenolysis

Where

TPM_1 = total passive motion (PIP + DIP − extensor deficit) before surgery.

TAM_1 = total active motion (PIP + DIP − extensor deficit) before surgery.

TAM_2 = total active motion (PIP ± DIP − extensor deficit) after surgery.

The concept of evaluating tenolysis is demonstrated in Figure 37–6. Subsequent to our initial report we added cases of tenolysis in flexor tendon repairs or flexor tendon grafts (single stage or two stage) and determined the results of the procedure utilizing the

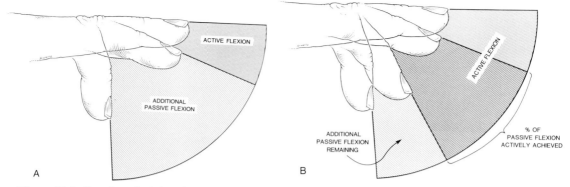

Figure 37–6. Drawings depicting the method used in determining the percentage improvement of active motion following flexor tenolysis. *A*, Diagram of the passive flexion in excess of active flexion prior to tenolysis. *B*, The postoperative change in active motion following tenolysis, indicating the percentage of the available passive flexion that was actively achieved by the procedure.

revised formula and a classification system compatible with that employed for other flexor tendon procedures (Table 37–10).

The results of flexor tendon repair and flexor tendon grafting are shown in Table 37–11 and in Figures 37–7 and 37–8.

These findings indicate that tenolysis can be expected to return at least 50 per cent of the preoperative discrepancy between active and passive ranges of motion at the proximal and distal interphalangeal joints in 65 per cent of the digits that undergo the procedure. In an additional 15 per cent fair function returned and 20 per cent failed to benefit appreciably from the operation. An incidence of rupture of 8 per cent remains disconcerting and is a calculated risk that must be explained to the patient prior to surgery.

In our early study we advocated the local injection of triamcinolone at the conclusion of the tendon mobilization, an adjunct we have largely abandoned in recent years. Although we have not specifically studied the results of lysis with or without the addition of local steroid injection, we do not believe that there has been any appreciable difference.

It should be emphasized that tenolysis is a major surgical undertaking requiring a thorough division of all restraining adhesions until one can adequately demonstrate that full passive motion can be achieved either by proximal traction on the freed tendon or, preferably, by the active cooperation of the patient under local anesthesia, as advocated by Schneider and Hunter (1975). The initiation of vigorous supervised digital motion within the first 12 hours after the operation is also an extremely important part of the protocol, and the judicious use of such modalities as transcutaneous nerve stimulation and electrical muscle stimulation also may be beneficial. In general, the results of flexor tenolysis have been gratifying. Improvement in digital flexion has been consistent, often with the restoration of nearly normal function. Moreover, the incidence of tendon rupture, infection, and delayed wound healing has been low.

COMBINED FLEXOR TENDON PROCEDURES

It can be seen from the results of flexor tendon repair, staged reconstruction, and tenolysis that restoration of satisfactory digital performance following flexor tendon severance is often very difficult. Despite continued improvements in materials and techniques, a disturbingly high percentage of flexor repairs or reconstructions yield fair or poor results or result in tendon rupture with unsatisfactory return of digital motion. It is therefore frequently necessary for the hand surgeon to

Table 37–10. CLASSIFICATION SYSTEM FOR FLEXOR TENOLYSIS

Group	Percentage Preoperative TPM − TAM Actively Regained (%)
Excellent	75–100
Good	50–74
Fair	25–49
Poor	0–24

Table 37–11. RESULTS OF TENOLYSIS

	Excellent	Good	Fair	Poor	Rupture	Total
Tendon repair (zone II)	29(51%)	8(16%)	7(17%)	5(10%)	4(8%)	49
Flexor tendon grafts (single and two stage)	10(38%)	7(27%)	4(15%)	3(12%)	2(8%)	26

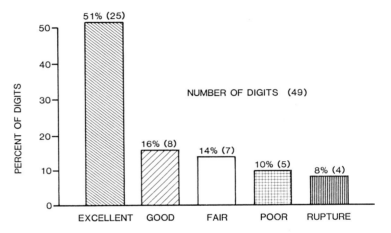

Figure 37–7. Percentage results of the various classification groups following tenolysis of flexor tendon repairs in zone II.

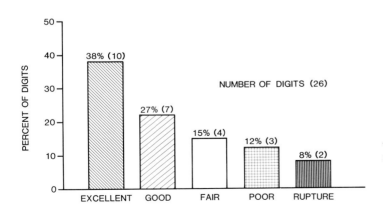

Figure 37–8. Percentage results of the various classification groups following tenolysis of flexor tendon grafts.

Table 37–12. THEORETICAL RESULTS OF 100 CONSECUTIVE FLEXOR TENDON
REPAIRS IN ZONE II (%)

	Excellent	Good	Fair	Poor	Ruptures
1. Tendon repair (profundus and profundus and superficialis + controlled passive motion)	25	31	27	13	4
2. Tenolysis of repairs (fair and poor from category 1)	46	37	6	4	7
3. Two stage reconstruction (fair, poor, and rupture from category 2)	49	41	4	5	1
4. Tenolysis of grafts (fair and poor from category 3)	52	44	1	1	2

carry out one or more additional reconstructive surgical procedures in an effort to restore or improve flexor tendon performance. Although multiple procedures may often be frustrating to the patient in terms of time and effort, the end result may be gratifying. It is extremely important that the patient be well informed and highly motivated throughout the reconstructive course. The maintenance of a good passive range of digital motion is an absolute prerequisite to the ultimate success of any reconstructive effort.

Study of results of various procedures as discussed in this chapter not only serves to determine the efficacy of those procedures but also allows the surgeon to predict the probability of success with a given procedure. This information should be shared with the patient, who must be made to realize the possibility of failure and the possible need for additional operative procedures. To that end it would be useful to combine the performance data for each of the flexor tendon procedures in an effort to determine the likelihood of achieving a satisfactory final result if appropriate reconstructive efforts were carried out in patients whose initial results were not good.

In Table 37–12 and Figure 37–9 we have indicated the percentage of excellent, good, fair, and poor results and the number of tendon ruptures that might occur following 100 flexor tendon severances in zone II if one were to carry out primary repair and proceed with appropriate reconstructive procedures in patients whose initial results were unsatisfactory. Our results from the study of the individual operative methods used in each

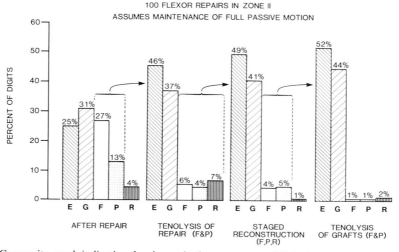

Figure 37–9. Composite graph indicating the change in the percentage of digits in each classification in a theoretical analysis of the performance of 100 flexor tendon repairs in zone II. The results of initial flexor tendon repair are shown on the left followed by the changes in the percentages in each group following tenolysis of those in the fair and poor categories. The third set of bars indicates the changes in the classification of the total group following two stage flexor reconstruction of those remaining in the fair, poor, or rupture category following tenolysis. The final bars on the right indicate the percentage of digits in each category following a final tenolysis of those digits in the fair or poor category following staged reconstruction.

step of the reconstructive process were utilized to make these predictions, and it must be assumed that all patients are willing to undergo all procedures deemed necessary to restore flexor tendon function and that a full passive range of motion can be maintained in the involved digits throughout the reconstructive course.

The results of this theoretical analysis of the potential results in 100 flexor tendon grafts following multiple procedures indicate that if the patient is well motivated and a nearly normal passive range of motion is maintained in the involved digit, approximately 96 per cent of all fingers can be returned to an excellent or good status. This would leave only 4 per cent in the fair, poor, or rupture category, and in those cases additional procedures such as tenodesis, arthrodesis, or, on occasion, digital ablation might be appropriate for the digits. Obviously this schema is an oversimplification, and many potential pitfalls may interrupt the progression of these reconstruction efforts and unfavorably affect the final results. Infection, poor skin quality, and, perhaps most important, digital joint stiffness are not infrequent complications of flexor tendon procedures and have a profoundly detrimental effect on the final digital joint range of motion that can be achieved. Nonetheless these figures do provide an overall optimistic outlook as to the potential recovery of flexor tendon performance in ideal situations

SUMMARY

In this chapter we have attempted to analyze the results of zone II flexor tendon

Table 37–13. PERCENTAGE OF RETURN

Excellent	75 to 100%
Good	50 to 74%
Fair	25 to 49%
Poor	0 to 24%

repair, staged flexor tendon reconstruction, and tenolysis based on cases taken from a single hand surgical practice. Formulas have been offered to determine the percentage return of motion at the proximal and distal interphalangeal joints utilizing total active and passive range of motion measurements. Variations in the formulas for each procedure are necessitated by the preoperative active and passive motion and are shown in the equation at the bottom of this page.

A common classification system based on the percentage return following each procedure has also been utilized (Table 37–13).

By employing these assessment methods for the digits of our patients who underwent flexor tendon repairs, we found the following results:

1. In digits undergoing primary flexor tendon repair in zone II with postoperative controlled passive motion techniques there was a 56 per cent incidence of excellent or good function, with 13 per cent in the poor category and 4 per cent resulting in tendon rupture.

2. Staged flexor tendon reconstruction produced 40 per cent excellent or good results, with 66 per cent categorized as excellent, good, or fair; 28 per cent remained in the poor classification, with a 7 per cent incidence of rupture. These results were substantially upgraded by tenolysis of the tendon

1. Tendon Repair

$$\frac{\text{Active PIP + DIP flexion} - \text{extensor lag}}{175 \text{ degrees}} \times 100 = \% \text{ of normal active PIP and DIP motion}$$

2. Free tendon grafts and staged flexor tendon reconstruction

$$\frac{\text{Postop. active PIP + DIP flexion} - \text{extensor deficit}}{\text{Preop. passive PIP + DIP flexion} - \text{extensor deficit}} \times 100 = \frac{\% \text{ of preoperative passive motion}}{\text{actively achieved}}$$

3. Tenolysis

$$100 - \frac{\text{TPM}_1 - \text{TAM}_2}{\text{TPM}_1 - \text{TAM}_1} \times 100 = \% \text{ of preoperative passive motion in excess of active motion actively achieved by tenolysis}$$

Where
TPM_1 = total passive motion (PIP + DIP − extensor deficit) before surgery.
TAM_2 = total active motion (PIP + DIP − extensor deficit) before surgery.
TAM_2 = total active motion (PIP + DIP − extensor deficit) after surgery.

grafts following stage II in 47 per cent of all digits.

3. Tenolysis was an effective procedure following a repair or graft and was found to yield 67 per cent excellent or good results when carried out for adherent tendon repairs, with 10 per cent in the poor category and an 8 per cent incidence of rupture. Excellent or good return of function followed tenolysis of flexor tendon grafts in 65 per cent of the cases, with 12 per cent judged poor and an 8 per cent incidence of rupture.

An analysis of the theoretical results of 100 zone II flexor tendon repairs following multiple procedures for digits in which the initial results were unsatisfactory indicated that under ideal circumstances as many as 96 per cent of all digits might be expected to show a return of flexor performance in the excellent or good category.

The author acknowledges that the results of flexor tendon procedures are strongly influenced by a wide array of factors, including patient age and motivation, the preoperative status of the digit, surgical technique, and postoperative management. An effort has been made here to minimize the variables by including patients taken from a single hand surgical practice and managed to a large extent by the same surgeon. The formulas utilized for the evaluation of results do not accurately assess all the parameters of digital function and are subject to error in measurement and recording. They are, however, believed to be fairly accurate indicators of the recovery of digital joint performance following flexor tendon surgery and, it is hoped, eliminate some of the less objective and falsifying features of other methods.

Obviously the results obtained in a single hand surgical practice do not necessarily reflect the experience or findings of other individuals or groups, and the material presented here must be interpreted in conjunction with the published reports of the results obtained with these techniques by others. We hope that the information imparted in this chapter will be useful to other hand surgeons in evaluating their own results and gaining an appreciation of the predictable results of these procedures.

REFERENCES

American Society for Surgery of the Hand: Clinical Assessment Committee Report, March 10, 1976.

Boyes, J. H.: Flexor tendon grafts in the finger and thumb. An evaluation of end results. J. Bone Joint Surg., 32A:488–499, 531, 1950.

Boyes, J. H., and Stark, H. H.: Flexor tendon grafts in the fingers and thumb. J. Bone Joint Surg., 53A:1332, 1971.

Brooks, D. M.: Problems of restoration of tendon movements after repair and grafts. Proc. R. Soc. Med., 63:67, 1970.

Buck-Gramcko, D., Dietrich, F. E., and Gogge, S.: Bewertungskriterien bei Nachuntersuchungen von Beugesehnenwieder herstellungen. Handchirurgie, 865, 1976.

Bunnell, S.: Surgery of the Hand. Ed. 2. Philadelphia, J. B. Lippincott Company, 1948.

Chamay, A., Verdan, C., and Simonetta, C.: The two-stage graft: a salvage operation for the flexor apparatus (a clinical study of 28 cases). In Verdan, C. (Editor): Tendon Surgery of the Hand. London, Churchill Livingstone, 1979, pp. 109–112.

Duran, R. J., and Houser, R. G.: Controlled passive motion following flexor tendon repair in zones 2 and 3. In AAOS Symposium on Tendon Surgery in the Hand. St. Louis, The C. V. Mosby Company, 1975, pp. 105–114.

Fetrow, K. O.: Tenolysis in the hand and wrist. J. Bone Joint Surg., 49A:667, 1967.

Hunter, J. M.: Two stage flexor tendon reconstruction: a technique using a tendon prosthesis prior to tendon grafting. In Verdan, C. (Editor): Tendon Surgery of the Hand. London, Churchill Livingstone, 1979, pp. 100–108.

Hunter, J. M., and Salisbury, R. E.: Use of gliding artificial implants to produce tendon sheaths: techniques and results in children. Plast. Reconstr. Surg., 45:564, 1970.

Hunter, J. M., and Salisbury, R. E.: Flexor-tendon reconstruction in severely damaged hands: a two-stage procedure using a silicone-Dacron reinforced gliding prosthesis prior to tendon grafting. J. Bone Joint Surg., 53A:829, 1971.

Hunter, J. M., and Schneider, L. H.: Staged flexor tendon reconstruction: current status. In AAOS Symposium on Tendon Surgery in the Hand. St. Louis, The C. V. Mosby Company, 1975, pp. 271–274.

LaSalle, W. B., and Strickland, J. W.: An evaluation of the two-stage flexor tendon reconstruction technique. J. Hand Surg., 8:263, 1983.

Lister, G. D., et al.: Primary flexor tendon repair followed by immediate controlled mobilization. J. Hand Surg., 2:441, 1977.

Mason, M. L., and Allen, H. S.: Rate of healing of tendons: an experimental study of tensile strength. Ann. Surg., 113:424, 1941.

Peacock, E. E., Jr., and Van Winkle, W., Jr.: Surgery and Biology of Wound Repair. Philadelphia, W. B. Saunders Company, 1970.

Rank, B. K., Wakefield, A. R., and Hueston, J. J.: Surgery of Repair as Applied to Hand Injuries. Ed. 4. Baltimore, The Williams & Wilkins Company, 1973.

Schneider, L. H.: Staged flexor tendon reconstruction using the method of Hunter: a personal series involving 57 flexor tendons. J. Hand Surg., 3:287, 1978.

Schneider, L. H., and Hunter, J. M.: Flexor tenolysis. In AAOS Symposium on Tendon Surgery in the Hand. St. Louis, The C. V. Mosby Company, 1975, pp. 157–162.

Stark, H. H., Zemel, N. P., Boyes, J. H., and Ashworth,

C. R.: Flexor tendon graft through intact superficialis tendon. J. Hand Surg., *2*:456, 1977.

Strickland, J. W., and Glogovac, S. V.: Digital function following flexor tendon repair in zone II: a comparison of immobilization and controlled passive motion techniques. J. Hand Surg., *5*:537, 1980.

Tubiana, R., and McMeniman, P., and Gordon, S.: Evaluation des résultats après reparation des tendons longs fléchisseurs des doigts. Ann. Chir., *33*:659, 1979.

Verdan, C., and Michon, J.: Le traitement des plaies des tendons fléchisseurs des doigts. Rev. Chir. Orthop., *47*:285–425, 1961.

Whitaker, J. H., Strickland, J. W., and Ellis, R. K.: The role of flexor tenolysis in the palm and digits. J. Hand Surg., *2*:462, 1977.

White, W. L.: Secondary restoration of finger flexion by digital tendon graft. An evaluation of seventy-six cases. Am. J. Surg., *91*:662, 1956.

Chapter 38

SURGICAL INDICATIONS IN FLEXOR TENDON INJURIES

RAOUL TUBIANA

PARTIAL LACERATIONS OF FLEXOR TENDONS

First we shall discuss the treatment of partial divisions of flexor tendons. These lesions can cause three potential types of complications—ruptures, nodules with triggering, and flap tears that block tendon gliding at the site of entrance of a pulley or in an opening of the fibrous sheath. If a partial laceration of a flexor tendon is discovered on wound exploration, there is a natural temptation to repair the division in the hope of preventing delayed rupture of the tendon. This approach is controversial, however, especially if one immobilizes the finger following surgery. There is then a risk of adhesion formation limiting the excursion of the tendon.

Based on experimental work with chicken flexor tendons and on their clinical experience, Wray et al. (1977, 1980) proposed not repairing partial lacerations. Instead, they institute early active movement with the finger protected by a dorsal block splint for three weeks. They only suture the partially severed tendon at one or two small points when the tendon is obliquely lacerated. When the tendon flap is small, they prefer to excise it. Wray et al. report excellent results without secondary rupture. Other surgeons prefer to repair partial lacerations and begin early passive motion as in a lesion involving complete severance (Schlenker et al., 1981).

One can summarize the approach to this problem as follows:

1. It is essential to explore all potential cases of flexor tendon injury. A partial lesion of the flexor tendon would be suspected when the tendon sheath is found to contain a he-matoma, even though active flexion is possible.

2. The repair of partially severed tendons does not significantly increase the strength of the tendon but can facilitate its gliding.

3. One may not need to repair many partial divisions of the flexor tendon when more than one third of the transverse diameter of the tendon remains intact.

4. When the partial division results in a flap that potentially can become trapped, it is better to excise the flaps that are smaller than one third of the diameter of the tendon and repair all others.

5. Early mobilization is necessary in all cases. This motion can be active if the division is less than half the diameter of the tendon. However, in these cases it is necessary to protect the tendon with a dorsal extension block splint with the wrist and metacarpophalangeal joints in a flexed position. Early mobilization is started by strapping the injured digit to its neighbor. All movement against resistance is prohibited for four weeks. If the division is greater than half the tendon diameter, early passive mobilization is preferable, as in that following a primary tendon repair.

COMPLETE DIVISION OF FLEXOR TENDONS

In the preceding chapters we have seen that various types of surgical treatment are available for flexor tendon injuries. These can be classified as follows:

1. Operations that attempt to restore the function of the flexor tendons

a. Primary suture
b. Delayed suture
c. Advancement and reinsertion of the proximal end of the divided tendon
d. Tendon grafts, which can be terminal or bridging, one stage or two stage (the actual grafting being preceded by insertion of a silicone rod)
e. Pedicle tendon grafts
f. Composite grafts of the whole flexor apparatus, which can be allografts (taken from a cadaver) or autografts (using a toe flexor apparatus)
g. Tenolysis
h. Tenoarthrolysis
2. Palliative operations
a. Tenodesis
b. Capsulodesis
c. Arthrodesis
d. Tendon transfer
e. Artificial tendons
3. Amputations

We shall now try to precisely define indications for each procedure, taking into account the following factors: the timing of the tendon repair, the existence of associated lesions, the characteristics of the patient, the surgical conditions, and the location of the lesion.

TIMING OF THE OPERATION

Indications for surgery are influenced by the time interval between the injury and the repair. One can distinguish early primary, delayed primary, and late repairs, but we must define what these terms mean, as they vary from one author to another. The Committee on Tendon Injuries of the International Federation of Societies for Surgery of the Hand has adopted the following definitions (Kleinert and Verdan, 1983):

Primary repair: Repair done within the first 24 hours following injury.

Delayed primary repair: Repair between one and 14 days following injury.

Secondary repair: Repair done after the second week following injury. *Early secondary repair* is undertaken between the second and fifth week, when direct suture repair can usually be done, and *late secondary repair* is done after the fifth week, when tendon grafting is generally the rule.

It seems to us that the distinction made between delayed primary repair and early secondary repair is rather arbitrary. Thus we

will continue to distinguish only three periods of repair rather than using the preceding classification: *primary repair*—repair within the first 24 hours, *secondary repair*—repair within five weeks, and *late repair*—repair after five weeks.

PRIMARY REPAIRS

When the patient is treated as an emergency, the decision as to how to manage the tendon will depend primarily on the state of the wound.* The quality of the skin cover plays a large part in this decision. One will attempt a tendon repair only if the wound is likely to heal primarily. This precludes primary flexor tendon repairs in contused wounds in which there is a problem of adequate skin coverage. Contaminated wounds, especially bites, run a high risk of becoming infected and are a definite contraindication to primary repairs.

In this early phase the tendon retraction is not fixed and suturing of the tendon ends is possible if there is no loss of tendon substance. Primary tendon suturing therefore is often feasible.

For a long time, great importance was attached to the time elapsed between injury and repair. Six hours was the limit, beyond which the wound was regarded as inevitably infected and no tendon repair would be attempted. Iselin (1967) showed that delay in repair could be safely prolonged, provided the wound was clean, the hand immobilized, and the patient placed on antibiotics. This concept of "delayed emergency" has been put into practice in a number of hospitals when surgical conditions were not initially favorable. Thus a number of tendon repairs were carried out after a delay of one or several days. Although this approach has proved to be useful in many instances, we do not encourage its routine use.

When surgical conditions are favorable, the repair should be done as soon as possible. If for some reason early tendon repair is not possible, one should treat the wound locally and close the skin if this is appropriate, thereby limiting the degree of contamination.

SECONDARY REPAIRS

Secondary repair is carried out when the injury is seen late or when the primary repair

---

*See chapter on hand wounds in Volume II.

was not possible because of wound contamination or associated lesions. This type of repair is possible when the wound is clean as a result of previous debridement, repeated irrigations, and use of antibiotics and if there is adequate soft tissue coverage.

Secondary repair can be done within several weeks following the injury. This is facilitated if immediately following the injury the wrist and metacarpophalangeal joint have been maintained in flexion, which limits the proximal retraction of the tendon and the destruction of the vincular network.

In practice, secondary repair of injuries distal to the wrist can be carried out within three to five weeks in adults and even later in children. A xerogram may be helpful in localizing the severed tendon ends. When the proximal tendon end is retracted in the forearm, shortening and scarring will make tendon suturing difficult. Some authors have found the results of this approach as good as those of primary tendon repair (Tsuge et al., 1977; Schneider et al., 1977). For other authors the results following secondary repair are less favorable (Verdan, 1972; Geldmacher, 1986).

Early grafting or "delayed primary flexor tendon graft" (Harrison, 1969) is also possible soon after injury (see chapter on Flexor Tendon Grafts), but most surgeons prefer to wait several weeks until inflammation, edema, and stiffness have subsided. As Pulvertaft has clearly pointed out in Chapter 31, the state of the hand is more important than the time factor.

LATE REPAIRS

At this stage, retraction has become fixed and the choice is between a tendon graft or other procedures described later in this chapter.

ASSOCIATED LESIONS

The existence of associated lesions will influence the indications as well as the prognosis for flexor tendon repairs. In 1950, Boyes clearly demonstrated the influence of these lesions on the results of flexor tendon grafting. He classified them into five groups: (1) good—optimal condition, (2) cicatrix—presence of scar tissue, (3) joint dam-

age—stiffness of the interphalangeal joints, (4) nerve damage—associated division of the digital nerves, and (5) multiple damage—multiple fingers involved or multiple lesions in a single finger. In 1971, the term "salvage" was added to classify those digits that sustained devastating injury requiring much preliminary work.

We agree in principle with the above classification and we would like to extend it to include early, intermediate, and late repairs. When flexor injuries are present in more than one finger, the condition of each finger will be assessed separately (Boyes and Stark, 1971).

Group I: Clean Wounds of the Skin and Flexor Tendons

1. *Early:* Primary repair of the flexor tendons is indicated.

2. *Intermediate:* Secondary repair is usually possible.

3. *Late:* If the condition of the wound is satisfactory with no associated lesions and with good joint mobility, a "one stage" tendon graft can be performed, except when pulley reconstruction is necessary.

Group II: Clean Wounds of the Skin and Flexor Tendons with Associated Neurovascular Lesions

1. *Early:* In the presence of a clean wound involving the flexor tendon and one neurovascular bundle, primary suture of the tendon is performed togther with a primary repair of the divided digital nerve. When both neurovascular pedicles are divided, at least one artery should be repaired if possible, in addition to the nerves and tendon.

2. *Intermediate:* Nerves are repaired but not vessels. Tendons are repaired by suturing if possible.

3. *Late*: When the neurovascular bundle has been divided in addition to the flexor tendons, a secondary repair or nerve graft is performed at the same time as the tendon graft. However, when the injury to the neurovascular bundles is bilateral, the results following intermediate and late tendon and nerve repairs are compromised owing to the poor vascularity of the digit.

Group III: Tendon Division Associated with Bone or Joint Lesions

1. *Early:* If the fracture is stable or if stability can be achieved by fixation devices without altering the gliding planes, primary suturing of the tendon is possible, assuming soft tissue coverage is adequate. If the stabil-

ity is not satisfactory or if there is a comminuted fracture, the fracture must be treated primarily and the tendon injury treated secondarily.

2. *Intermediate:* A patient with an unstable fracture necessitating open reduction may sometimes be reoperated on during the intermediate period for direct tendon suturing. However, it is usually best to avoid another procedure so soon after the initial open reduction, and a later tendon graft is preferable. A silicone rod can be placed at the time of the bone repair, in order to preserve the fibrous tunnel.

3. *Late:* Old injuries usually involve nonunion, malunion, or, most commonly, joint stiffness. Any necessary bone or joint procedures must be performed before attempting tendon reconstruction. During reconstructive bone or joint procedures it may be possible to prepare the finger for later tendon grafting by placing a silicone rod or doing the first stage of a pedicled graft. It is imperative that a functional range of passive movement is regained by physiotherapy or by an initial procedure to help restore mobility prior to tendon grafting.

Group IV: Tendon Injuries Associated with Bone and Soft Tissue Damage

1. *Early:* When there is significant skin and subcutaneous tissue destruction, the tendon repair must be delayed until adequate skin cover is obtained. With severely contused skin and contamination, the treatment is directed to the wound. The repair of the tendon must then be done secondarily. When the injury involves division of the tendon plus a combination of injuries to neurovascular pedicles, bone, joint, and skin, the question of amputation arises. The decision as to what treatment is indicated is complex and will depend on many factors, including the experience of the surgeon, the age and occupation of the patient, and the state of the rest of the hand.

2. *Late:* This group includes cases in which there is a significant amount of scar tissue or joint stiffness as a result of soft tissue damage, infection, or previous operative procedures. It also includes complex cases involving multiple injuries, i.e., to tendon, nerve, bone, joint, or skin. Tendon repair in such cases often gives poor results, and simpler procedures, such as arthrodesis or even amputations, should therefore be considered.

THE PATIENT

The age, general condition (physical and psychological), and occupation of the patient should all be taken into consideration. Whatever the patient's age, a primary suture is indicated for clean, noninfected lesions of the flexor tendons.

The results of tendon repairs are on the whole better in the young patient. If grafting is a consideration, the age of the child will determine his ability to cooperate. Pulvertaft avoids tendon grafting in children less than six years old.

The best results following tendon suturing and tendon grafting are obtained in patients between 6 and 25 years of age. The results are much less satisfactory after the age of 40. This should be kept in mind when planning the more ambitious procedures, reserving them for the younger patient.

Poor general health or severe systemic disease precludes multi-stage repairs.

The psychological state of the patient is important, as his cooperation is essential. Ambitious repairs are ruled out in poorly motivated patients whose cooperation cannot be expected. For psychological reasons, a primary tendon repair is preferable in cases of attempted suicide.

The patient's occupation also influences indications for surgery; for example, active digital flexion is important for a precision worker or a musician. An arthrodesis might be considered in a laborer for power, or in a patient who does not want to take the time off from work for multiple procedures and subsequent therapy.

SURGICAL CONDITIONS

Surgical facilities and the experience of the surgeon have a marked influence on the results of tendon surgery and are often inadequate at the time of primary repair. The requirements are: (1) a fully equipped aseptic operating room, as that used for bone surgery, and adequate instrumentation; and (2) a surgeon experienced in tendon surgery. The latter is probably the most important requirement. Tendon suturing and tendon grafting are two extremely delicate procedures, and only a surgeon familiar with both is able to assess the prevailing conditions and to make the right surgical decisions. The surgeon called to treat an emergency tendon injury must be appropriately trained to deal with associated lesions as well. He must be able to provide appropriate skin coverage and perform bone fixation and even microscopic vascular or nerve repair when necessary.

We can now consider the proper surgical management of traumatic lesions of the flexor tendons of the fingers and thumb, discussing in turn the three surgical zones (distal, inter-mediate, and proximal) previously defined.*

LESIONS OF THE FLEXOR DIGITORUM TENDONS

IN THE DISTAL ZONE

At this level only the flexor digitorum profundus is present; it can be divided or avulsed.

Distal Avulsion of the Flexor Digitorum Profundus

The avulsed tendon should be reattached whenever possible. The treatment should take into account the degree of retraction and the anatomical lesions (as described in Chapter 24) and the timing of the repair. When there is no avulsed bone fragment, the tendon is sutured directly to the bone, the technique being the same as that for the distal insertion of a tendon graft.

When the tendon is avulsed with a frag-ment of bone, the fragment should be re-placed to restore the action of the tendon and stabilize the joint. If the fragment in-cludes a large proportion of the articular surface, the joint becomes subluxed dorsally. Reduction of the dislocation is accomplished easily within the first few days, before re-traction becomes fixed. Obliquely crossing Kirschner wires maintain the reduction and fix the distal interphalangeal joint in about 15 degrees of flexion. Accurate replacement of the fragment may be difficult but is worth while for injuries of the articular surface. Fixation is obtained with a fine Kirschner wire, an intra-osseous suture, or a barbed wire.

Such reattachment is only possible in fresh

injuries. After a few days, it is usually im-possible to reinsert a tendon that has re-tracted into the palm and in which tendon vascularity is compromised. When the tendon has not retracted past the proximal interpha-langeal joint and the vinculum longus remains intact, it can be reinserted after even several weeks in young patients (Leddy et al., 1977). A xerogram can be useful in helping to lo-calize the tendon ends. Tendon grafting is not usually used in cases of rupture of the profundus tendon with an intact superficialis except for the little finger, in which the su-perficialis is often inadequate. Rather than grafting, Foucher et al. (1984) have proposed improving flexion of the proximal interpha-langeal joint of the little finger after division or avulsion of the profundus tendon by per-forming a lateral anastomosis between the profundus and superficialis at the level of the wrist accompanied by stabilization of the dis-tal interphalangeal joint by tenodesis or ar-throdesis. However, this location of injury is not common, as most of these injuries occur on the ring finger because of the anatomical reasons already discussed.*

Finally, tenolysis of the superficial flexor tendon, associated with resection of a poorly vascularized profundus tendon, is indicated in old injuries with painful flexion of the proximal interphalangeal joint, especially if synovitis is present.

Division of the Flexor Profundus Alone

Numerous types of repair can be used. Some aim at restoring tendon function and include reinsertion, primary or secondary su-turing, or grafting of the flexor profundus.

Others are directed at stabilizing the distal interphalangeal joint and include tenodesis, capsulodesis, and arthrodesis. Finally, there is the possibility of improving flexion at the proximal interphalangeal joint by a tenolysis of the flexor tendons.

Primary Repairs. *Reinsertion* is possible when the division lies within 1 cm. of the insertion (Malerich et al., 1987). In young adults, a slightly greater advancement is pos-sible, but one should guard against excessive traction, which may result in residual fixed flexion and can even restrict flexion of the profundus tendons of the other fingers (Ver-dan's "Syndrome of the Quadriga," 1960). It

---

*See Chapter 24 on Traumatic Lesions of the Flexor Tendons.

---

*See Chapter 24.

is preferable to keep at least a portion of the A4 pulley; if not, the flexion of the distal phalanx will be limited. The tendon is fixed to the bone by means of a pull-out suture that runs through the distal phalanx and the nail before being tied over a button or a bolus. The distal segment of the tendon is split lengthwise and the two halves are sutured to the proximal tendon end, as for the fixation of a graft (Chaper 30). The fibrous sheath is resected at the level of the distal interphalangeal joint. The wrist and the corresponding metacarpophalangeal joint and proximal interphalangeal joint are maintained in flexion at 40, 70, and 35 degrees, respectively, but the distal interphalangeal joint is held in almost total extension by a small distal palmar splint while passive mobilization of the proximal interphalangeal joint is started during the first few days. The splint and pull-out sutures are removed after four weeks.

The *tendon is sutured* when the division lies more than 1 cm. from the insertion but distal enough so that suturing the flexor digitorum profundus avoids the chiasma of the flexor digitorum superficialis in order not to interfere with its mobility. The degree of retraction of the proximal segment will determine which procedure to use.

When there is little retraction, the vinculum longum opposite the proximal interphalangeal joint is preserved and the conditions are favorable for suturing (Fig. 38–1). When the proximal end has retracted into the palm, the mesotendon is torn off and the prognosis

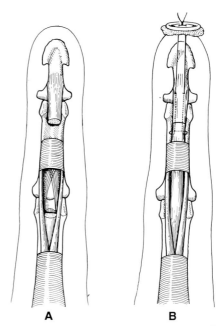

A   **B**

Figure 38–1. Suture of the flexor digitorum profundus. *A*, Retraction of the proximal end is moderate. *B*, A grasping suture is inserted through the proximal end. The tendon is passed beneath pulley A₄, which is preserved. The suture may be anchored to a button at the tip of the finger. This procedure is used primarily in the child.

is less favorable. Nonetheless, repair of the tendon may be attempted. A small soft catheter can be passed through the wound opening and down the tendon sheath in a proximal direction. This serves as a guide when the profundus tendon is pulled distally (Fig. 38–2). In many situations, it is preferable not

Figure 38–2. The passage of the retracted proximal end of the flexor profundus tendon, through Camper's decussation of the flexor superficialis tendon, is facilitated by the prior placement of a small catheter. The catheter must be placed from distal to proximal in order to find its way through the division of the superficialis tendon. One half of the grasping suture can be placed on the proximal end of the tendon and inserted into the catheter, which serves as a guide. The tendon may then be drawn distally, as illustrated here.

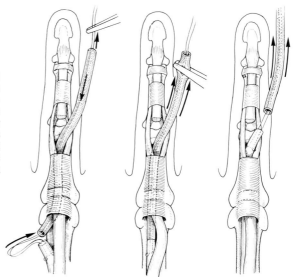

to repair the flexor digitorum profundus because of the risk of interfering with the flexor digitorum superficialis. Palliative treatment can be considered at some later time. In the little finger, however, function of the flexor digitorum profundus should be restored because the flexor digitorum superficialis is often deficient.

Secondary Repairs. Tendon surgery is delayed when the type of wound (e.g., crush injury) or the risk of infection precludes an immediate repair. The deficit in flexion resulting from a flexor digitorum profundus injury is minimal when the flexor digitorum superficialis has retained normal mobility and the distal joint is stable; however, the absence of the flexor digitorum profundus significantly diminishes the strength of the finger. In such cases, a surgical repair is not necessary unless the patient's occupation depends upon it. If so, one of five procedures is selected:

1. *Secondary tendon suturing.* This sometimes remains possible for a month or so in adults, and in children one can often wait longer.

2. *Secondary reinsertion of the tendon.* This is possible when the flexor digitorum profundus tendon glides normally alongside the flexor digitorum superficialis tendon and can be fixed without excessive tension. If extensive adhesions are present or if the camper's chiasma is blocked, this procedure is not feasible. *In no circumstances should an intact flexor digitorum superficialis tendon be sacrificed to repair the profundus.*

3. *Secondary grafting of the flexor profundus.* This procedure can be considered when conditions do not permit secondary repair. Restoration of active flexion of the distal phalanx by grafting is worth attempting in a young, active, cooperative patient. It is utilized in the ulnar fingers for restoring power grip and in the radial fingers for precision grip. The results of tendon grafting are considerably influenced by age and many authors will attempt this only in young patients (Goldner and Conrad, 1969; Stark, 1977). However, McClinton et al. (1982) showed that good results can be obtained in patients over 40 years of age. Local conditions also have a considerable influence on results of tendon grafting, and must be excellent: good skin condition, complete passive mobility of both distal and proximal interphalangeal joints. (The technique for these slender grafts

has already been described in Chapter 30 on Flexor Tendon Grafts.)

4. *Procedures aimed at stabilizing the distal interphalangeal joint.* When the first three procedures to restore the mobility of the flexor digitorum profundus are not indicated, it may be necessary to stabilize the distal interphalangeal joint if this joint is unstable and tends to go into hyperextension during grip. The joint sometimes becomes stable spontaneously as a result of the adhesions that form around the end of the tendon. Stabilizing operations on the distal interphalangeal joint (tenodesis, capsulodesis, arthrodesis) are indicated only if flexion of the flexor digitorum superficialis remains satisfactory. Tenodesis has its place when the distal end of the flexor digitorum profundus is long enough to be tethered to the fibrous sheath (A4) or, even better, to the shaft of the middle phalanx. If the section lies too distal, capsulodesis may be possible. In either case, the distal interphalangeal joint is maintained by a Kirschner wire in 15 to 25 degrees of flexion (depending on the finger) for five weeks. The inevitable stretching of the tenodesis leaves the injured finger in a more functional position. These procedures have the advantage of maintaining passive flexion of the joint, while preventing hyperextension. Arthrodesis provides excellent stability but passive flexion is lost. The position will vary from 5 to 20 degrees of flexion according to which finger is involved.

5. *Tenolysis of the flexor tendons.* When pain persists in the palm or active flexion of the proximal interphalangeal joint is restricted, the lesions must be explored.

The flexor digitorum superficialis tendon is tenolysed. The proximal segment of the flexor digitorum profundus, which is retracted and often adheres to the tendons of the adjacent fingers owing to an inflammatory reaction, is freed and resected high in the palm. It can be sutured to the tendon of the flexor digitorum superficialis if the latter is weak, especially in the little finger. The distal phalanx can be stabilized at the same operation.

When the flexor digitorum profundus has not been repaired, a lumbrical-plus deformity may occur because of proximal retraction of the lumbrical muscle originating from the proximal end of the divided profundus tendon. This results in extension of the proximal interphalangeal joint and can be treated by dividing the lumbrical muscle or its tendon.

IN THE INTERMEDIATE ZONE

The intermediate zone is the part of the digital canal where the profundus and superficialis tendons run in close contact (zone II). It extends from the insertions of the flexor digitorum superficialis to well into the palm. It is in this zone, which corresponds to Bunnell's "no man's land," that tendon repairs create the most difficult problems and the choice of treatment is the most difficult. For a long time primary suture and secondary grafting were strongly defended by their respective advocates (the advantages and disadvantages of both procedures have been discussed at length in Chapter 24). The arguments are now largely irrelevant, as the validity of both methods has been confirmed by their results. Thus Boyes and Pulvertaft, who prefer grafts, as well as Verdan and Kleinert, who advocate primary suturing, have been able to report satisfactory results in 80 per cent of cases when the initial conditions were suitable. One must admit, however, that for the majority of surgeons the results are much less acceptable. The two methods should not be regarded as rival but rather as complementary procedures. Suturing has technical advantages and is preferable economically, but the advantages resulting from the time gained should not put the future of the hand at risk. It is probably fair to say that grafting should be used only when primary suturing is contraindicated, but these contraindications must not be minimized.

Primary Repairs

Primary suturing in this difficult zone is enjoying renewed popularity. Contrary to general belief, it is an extremely delicate procedure. Primary suturing in this area should be limited to favorable cases (Table 38–1).

Both Verdan and Kleinert, the two main advocates of this method, have stressed the limits of primary suturing in this zone, which, they say, should only be carried out if:

1. After debridement, the wound can be expected to heal by primary intention.
2. The associated lesions are compatible

Table 38–1. CONTRAINDICATIONS TO PRIMARY TENDON REPAIR IN ZONE II

1. Infection + +
2. Crush injuries
3. Loss of skin coverage
4. Associated lesions
   a. Loss of two neurovascular bundles
   b. Unstable fractures
   c. Articular lesions compromising motion
5. Inadequate surgical facilities + +

with rapid mobilization. Lesions of both neurovascular pedicles of a finger, unstable fractures, and articular damage are definite contraindications to primary suturing. A primary tendon repair is justified if only one digital pedicle has been damaged, but the nerve should be repaired at the same procedure. Similarly, a fracture that can be stabilized by internal fixation does not exclude the possibility of primary tendon suturing, provided the gliding planes are not altered. The presence of flexor tendon lesions in several fingers calls for primary repair.

3. Surgical conditions are excellent. To quote Kleinert et al. (1975): "The absence of adequate personnel and facilities to perform this surgery is an absolute contraindication to primary repair. Despite its potential advantages, primary repair may have catastrophic results if careful case selection is waived. This is not a procedure for the surgeon who occasionally performs hand surgery but for one especially trained in this technique."

The technique of primary repair has continued to progress toward greater respect for the tissues and a more accurate anatomical reconstruction. The most commonly utilized techniques have been described by the authors in the preceding chapters. *They consist of six well-defined stages:*

Extension of the skin wound
Opening of the sheath
Apposition of the cut ends of the tendon
Suturing of the tendon
Closure of the wound
Postoperative care

Each stage must be adapted to suit the needs of the individual clinical case. An atraumatic technique with magnification and avoidance of tension of the suture repair are essential.

The skin wound is extended proximally for lesions which occur in extension and distally for those which occur in flexion (Fig. 38–3). The wound is elongated at its extremities

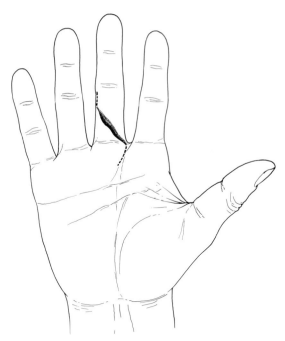

Figure 38–3. The skin wound is enlarged at its extremities, especially the proximal part when the tendon section has occurred with the finger in extension and distally for sections in flexion.

along the lateral aspect of the digit so that acute angles on the skin flaps are avoided.

The sheath is preferably opened in its membranous portion for the tendon repair. If the wound is at the level of an annular pulley and is not wide enough to allow suturing of the tendon, it is better not to extend it but to make another opening in the first or second cruciate portion of the sheath (Buck-Gramcko, 1983; Lister, 1983).

Apposition of the cut ends of the tendon: Exposure of the distal cut end of the tendon can usually be accomplished by flexing the finger joints (Fig. 38–4). The proximal ends are more difficult to expose. This may sometimes be accomplished by flexing the wrist and "milking" the palm. When there is marked retraction a soft catheter can be inserted through the wound and along the digital canal to locate the site of the palmar counterincision. Geldmacher has designed a special flexible pilot-probe to retrace retracted tendon (1986).

The tendon extremities are exteriorized and are first inspected, as their blood supply will influence subsequent management.

The irregular ends of the tendons should

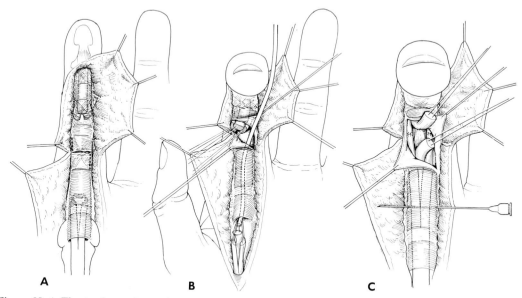

| A | B | C |

Figure 38–4. The tendon ends are drawn into the opening in the cruciform part of the tendon sheath. *A,* In this case, the C1 is opened, raising two opposite small flaps. *B,* The distal tendon stump is introduced into the opening by flexing the distal joint. A supple catheter is introduced into the proximal part of the sheath and abuts against the retracted tendons. If necessary, a skin incision is made at the level of the retracted tendon, and the tendon stumps are sutured to the catheter. *C,* The catheter is withdrawn with the attached tendons. The tendons are transfixed by a proximal transverse needle to avoid their retraction. The superficialis tendon is flat at this level and repair is by mattress sutures. When the division of the tendon is more distal, the opening of the sheath can be done at the level of C2. The sheath can be opened at both C2 and C3, and grasping sutures can be placed in each tendon end.

be converted to a clean lesion without resecting more than 5 mm. One-half of the grasping tendon suture can be placed at this time and inserted into the catheter which serves as a guide (Fig. 38–2). It is especially important to assure the normal anatomical relationship between the flexor digitorum superficialis and the flexor digitorum profundus, for an error of orientation may prevent excursion of the flexor digitorum profundus (Fig. 38–5). A straight needle transfixing both the tendons and the sheath relieves tension on the tendon during the repair.

Suture of the tendons: Although relaxation obtained by flexion at the wrist and metacarpophalangeal joints is probably more important than the strength of the suture, suture technique must not be neglected. The "grasping" suture of the Mason-Kessler or Tsuge's type, is now replacing the Bunnell criss-cross suture, as it is stronger and results in less compression and devascularization of the tendon. The suture should be placed in the palmar aspect of the tendon so that it does not interfere with the longitudinal intratendinous vessels in the dorsal portion of the tendon. A strong 3-0 or 4-0 synthetic suture is used. The knot is preferably buried in the proximal tendon end (see Chapter 8). When this is not possible, at the flattened distal portion of the superficialis tendon, a figure-of-eight suture is used (Fig. 38–6; Fig. 38–7).

The addition of a fine 6-0 peripheral run-

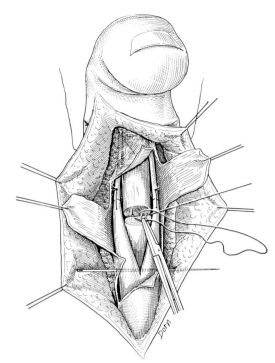

Figure 38–6. Suture of the two flexor tendons. The tendons should be sutured at two different levels when possible. At the level of the proximal phalanx the flexor digitorum superficialis is sutured first. A figure-of-eight suture is used to repair the distal flat portion of the superficialis tendon. Flexion of the distal joint brings the distal end of the flexor profundus tendon into contact with the proximal end. The posterior half of the running suture is inserted first, as it is often difficult to turn the tendon over within the confines of the sheath.

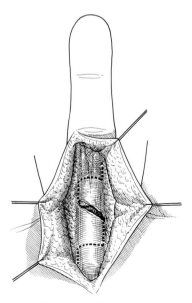

Figure 38–5. Opening of the flexor tendon sheath by fashioning flaps with opposing bases (Jones).

ning suture was advocated by Kleinert in order to produce a smooth tendon junction. The posterior half of this is done by inverting the tendon. This may be difficult to perform within the confines of the tendon sheath. One possible solution is to place the dorsal portion of the running suture via the interior of the tendon before the grasping suture is inserted (Foucher, 1984) which avoids the need to turn it over (Fig. 38–6). However, when the lesion is within one of the avascular segments of the tendon we prefer to omit the running suture on the dorsal aspect as it risks causing further devascularization of an already compromised tendon.

When the division is oblique, one may be tempted to use the beveling technique of Becker.

Closure of the sheath has the theoretical advantage of separating the healing tendon from the surrounding tissue and may affect tendon gliding by altering the nature of the

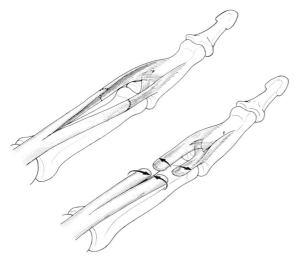

Figure 38–7. The bands of flexor superficialis spiral around the tendon of flexor profundus. If these bands are divided at the level of the proximal phalanx, the opposing bands may spiral but in different directions. If the ulnar band is sutured to the radial band, the tunnel for the profundus will be obliterated. (From Lister, G. D.: Hand Clin., *1*:1, 1985.)

adhesions that form after primary tendon surgery. Closure of the sheath after primary flexor tendon repair does not appear to be necessary for tendon nutrition (Peterson et al., 1986).* Therefore, when this may be accomplished without undue difficulty it should be attempted. Trying to close it at any price can produce complications by narrow-

---
*See Chapter 4.

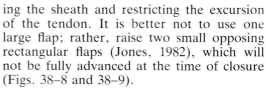

ing the sheath and restricting the excursion of the tendon. It is better not to use one large flap; rather, raise two small opposing rectangular flaps (Jones, 1982), which will not be fully advanced at the time of closure (Figs. 38–8 and 38–9).

Management of Division of One and of Both Flexor Tendons

SECTION OF THE FLEXOR DIGITORUM SUPERFICIALIS. If the flexor digitorum superficialis alone is divided and the profundus is intact, the decision as to repair is difficult. Kleinert suggests suturing followed by early semi-active mobilization, which has given good results. This is the solution adopted when local conditions are favorable. Many surgeons prefer not to repair the flexor digitorum superficialis alone, believing that the functional deficit resulting from the loss of power is preferable to the risk of adhesions restricting the mobility of the profundus tendon.

A dorsal splint is used to maintain the wrist in 40 degrees of flexion, the metacarpophalangeal joint in 60 degrees of flexion, and the proximal interphalangeal joint at 15 degrees to limit the vascular damage resulting from the retraction of the proximal end of the sectioned flexor tendon. The interphalangeal joints are actively mobilized, and the splint will prevent the proximal interphalangeal joint from going into hyperextension and producing a swan-neck deformity as a result of the division of the flexor digitorum superficialis. The same treatment applies to partial lesions of the superficialis tendon.

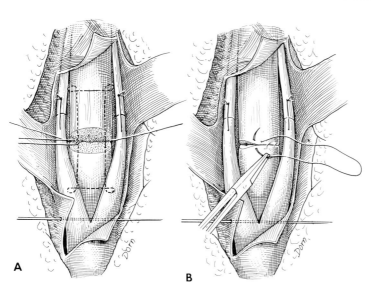

Figure 38–8. *A*, Mason-Kessler type grasping suture. We now prefer to bury the knot proximally (see Chapter 8, Fig. 8–9) and not between the two tendon ends. *B*, Anterior half of continuous suture is placed last.

A

B

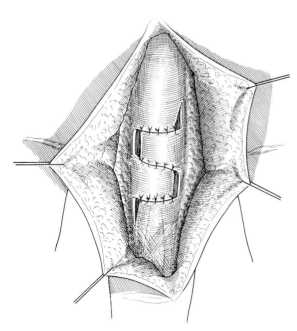

Figure 38–9. Closure of the flexor tendon sheath. The flaps elevated during exposure are not fully advanced on closure. They are sutured together to their sides. The extremities of the flaps are not sutured. A gap is left to avoid any constriction at the suture site. The triangular gaps left at each extremity of the opening in the sheath allow a progressive enlargement of the sheath and facilitate the passage of the tendon.

SECTION OF THE FLEXOR DIGITORUM PROFUNDUS. The flexor digitorum profundus is sutured at this level only if conditions are favorable, in order to avoid interfering with the mobility of the flexor digitorum superficialis. As in the distal zone, one may consider a tenodesis of the distal interphalangeal joint when this joint is unstable and goes into hyperextension or, in younger patients, a graft of the flexor digitorum profundus alone.

Of course an intact flexor superficialis tendon should *never* be resected on the pretext of repairing the profundus.

SECTION OF BOTH FLEXOR TENDONS. This is the most difficult problem to solve. The old method of systematically resecting the flexor superficialis tendon in order to repair the profundus only now is being discarded. The present tendency is to suture both tendons despite the increased risk of adhesions, as this procedure is more satisfactory physiologically. It is justified: (1) when sections are clean, (2) when the surgeon has perfected the tendon suturing technique, (3) when excision of the proximal end of superficialis

tendon (if this is divided distally) would tear off the vinculum longum at the level of the proximal interphalangeal joint, and (4) when the two tendons can be sutured at different levels. The two flexor tendons are sectioned at different levels when the injury occurs in a flexed hand, but are at the same level when the injury occurs in a straightened hand.

Repairing both tendons better maintains the vascularity provided by the vincula, theoretically assures independent flexion of each phalanx and thus greater flexion strength, and reduces the risk of hyperextension of the proximal interphalangeal joint, which is often seen after resection of the flexor superficialis.

It is preferable to suture one tendon only when the damage to the two tendons is not equal. As the tendon ends are freshened, a difference in length results that is difficult to compensate for when it is more than 1 cm. As a rule, the profundus is repaired and the proximal segment of superficialis, which occupies the digital canal, is resected. The distal end is preserved. Complete resection of the flexor superficialis tendon would destroy the vinculum longum, thus increasing the problem considerably.

Postoperative Care

We do not immobilize the wrist in full flexion but in semiflexion, i.e., about 40 degrees. If the wrist is fully flexed, complete flexion of the metacarpophalangeal joint is difficult. The dorsal splint immobilizes the wrist and extends over the dorsal surface of the proximal phalanges to hold the metacarpophalangeal joint flexed at 70 degrees. In children, the splint must extend to the elbow.

Postoperative care should not be applied in the same manner for all patients after tendon repair. Early postoperative passive motion has improved the results of flexor tendon repairs in this side zone, as shown by Strickland (1985) in two personal comparative series (see Chapter 37).

POSTOPERATIVE CARE

The influence of early mobilization is now beyond doubt. There are three methods of early postoperative mobilization: *active mobilization*, considered possible by certain surgeons with stronger tendon suture procedures (Mantero, 1976; Brunelli, 1982; Becker,

1978). These must nevertheless be accompanied by splintage holding the joints proximal to the suture in flexion in order to decrease muscle tension. Although this method has yielded some very good results, there are not yet large studies confirming its reliability.

The method of *semi-active mobilization* enabling passive flexion of the fingers by elastic traction and active extension by the preserved extensor apparatus was described by Young and Herman (1960) and widely popularized by Kleinert (1973), who confirmed its considerable usefulness. It should be said from the onset that the excellent results obtained by Kleinert and his school (Lister et al., 1977) are based not only on postoperative care but on all the various operative stages as well as the very careful technique of a team specialized in microsurgery (see Chapter 28). However, there is a definite increase in morbidity as a result of the widespread use of this technique when it is not used with care or is used inappropriately.

The direction of the tendon toward the scaphoid tubercle must be respected. This is done by using a reflection pulley in the palm of the hand to allow for complete rolling up

of the finger after the repair of the flexor profundus tendon (Fig. 38–10). The reflection pulley should be placed at the level of the scaphoid tubercle after the repair of a flexor superficialis tendon (Allieu, 1986). The extensor apparatus must be intact to allow for active extension, and thus, this method is contraindicated after digital replantation. The precise amount of tension is difficult to regulate, and too often, the elastic traction, when insufficiently regulated, does not allow for complete rolling of the fingers or maintains the proximal interphalangeal joint in flexion, leaving the digit at risk for compromised extension. This has led to the development by Allieu and Rouzaud (1986) of a system of calibrated springs, the strength of which is selected on the basis of the digits involved and the sex of the patient (Fig. 38–10).

Allieu-Rouzaud Orthesis. The principle of dynamic assistance by calibrated springs is used for flexor tendon lesions according to the Kleinert technique. The spring is attached to the anterior and proximal part of the orthesis. The traction wire reaches the damaged finger after running under a reflection pulley (technique already described by M.

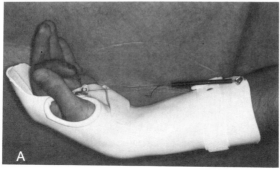
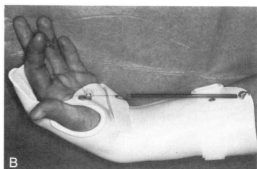
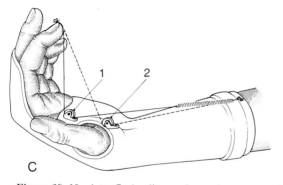
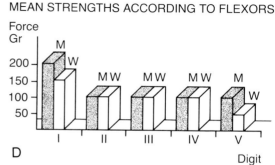

Figure 38–10. *A* to *C*, Appliances for early postoperative passive mobilization after modification of the Kleinert technique (see text). *D*, Graph of mean strengths according to flexors.

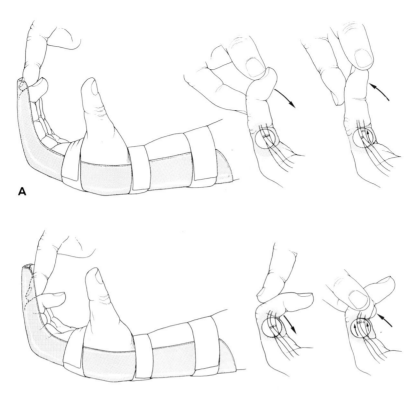

Figure 38–11. The technique of early passive motion of Duran and Houser. A dorsal splint immobilizes the wrist at 40 degrees and the metacarpophalangeal joints at 70 degrees of flexion. The interphalangeal joints are maintained in extension. Velcro bands are used to attach the splint. The method consists of mobilizing passively the proximal and distal interphalangeal joints individually, four or five times daily. *A*, Passive mobilization of the distal phalanx displaces the suture of the profundus tendon 3 to 4 mm away from that of the superficialis. *B*, The Velcro band that holds the fingers is removed to permit passive mobilization of the proximal interphalangeal joint. Both tendon sutures are moved in relation to the surrounding fixed structures.

Romain et al., 1981). The latter is positioned in the distal palmar crease for a flexion profundus lesion or overlying the scaphoid tubercle for a superficialis lesion (Fig. 38–10*C*). A low strength spring is selected on the basis of the digit involved and the sex of the patient and can be changed during the course of rehabilitation. Mean force used varies from 200 to 100 g in men and from 150 to 50 g in women according to the digit involved (Fig. 38–10*D*).

The method of semi-active mobilization should be reserved for cases in which the sutures are secured, there are no associated lesions of the extensors, and the patient is cooperative and is followed regularly.

The method of analytic *purely passive mobilization* developed by Duran and Hauser (1975) can be used to individually mobilize the proximal and distal interphalangeal joints and to move superficial and deep flexor tendon sutures in relation to each other (Fig.

38–11). It seems to have less risk of complications, in particular retraction of the proximal interphalangeal joint, than the semiactive method. The results may also be excellent but we are unaware of any comparative study of the two methods.

Are there particular indications for one or another method? Possibly in a patient who is cooperative but who cannot be seen regularly for geographic or other reasons, the method of Duran might be preferred because it is easier to teach and to carry out by the patient himself than the use of elastic traction, which is difficult to adjust. In rehabilitation centers it is possible to combine analytic passive mobilization of the distal phalanges and elastic traction. This combination seems particularly useful when there are concomitant lesions of the tendon bed.

Whichever method of early mobilization is adopted, it must be explained carefully to the patient, and the patient's exercise technique must be monitored at least once a week during the first month. In difficult, agitated, and uncooperative patients, it would be preferable to accept loss of the advantages of early passive mobilization.

The duration of dorsal protection must be adapted to each particular case. Protection is usually required for four weeks, but if the lesions were in an avascular portion of the tendon or if systematic examination of the vincula during the repair reveals the system to be widely disrupted, this protection should be extended to five or six weeks. A splint immobilizing the metacarpophalangeal joints in flexion concentrates the flexor tendon activity on the proximal and distal interphalangeal joints.

Delayed Repairs

When the conditions are unsuitable for primary suturing, treatment will be restricted to skin debridement and, if possible, skin closure. The wrist and the finger are immobilized in flexion. The tendon repair is postponed and will consist of:

1. Early secondary suturing when the conditions have improved within two to three weeks of the injury. In the child, one can afford to wait longer,

2. A secondary graft or

3. The insertion of a silicone rod to recreate a gliding space.

The timing of these procedures remains open to discussion. While they are usually postponed for two months for reasons of safety and optimal rehabilitation, it would seem that the silicone rod can be inserted at the time of the primary operation when the risk of sepsis is low. This avoids collapse of the pulleys.

Late Repairs

There are a number of different situations in which late repairs are indicated:

1. When a primary or delayed primary repair has not been attempted, a tendon graft is usually used to re-establish flexion.

2. If active and passive mobility is absent or minimal three months after a tendon suture, this may be due to a broken suture or to tight adhesions. The decision between a tenolysis and a tendon graft will depend on the findings at exploration.

3. When after primary repair active flexion

of the interphalangeal joints returns slowly and is limited while the passive range of motion is significantly greater. After treatment for five months with physiotherapy, tenolysis is considered. Several conditions must be met if tenolysis is performed: (1) good condition of the tendon, (2) good passive mobility of the joints, (3) supple soft tissue, and (4) a well motivated and cooperative patient. Preferably, tenolysis is done under regional anesthesia so the patient can actively move the tendons during the course of the operation. It might also be necessary to reconstruct the pulleys at this time.*

4. After primary repair, one can also encounter the problem of a fixed flexion deformity. If there is no active flexion, a two-stage tendon graft is undertaken after correction of the contraction. If there is active flexion of more than 40 degrees, one hesitates to sacrifice this for a tendon graft. More often than not, the patient has already undergone one or more tenolyses.

If in spite of vigorous physiotherapy the contracture remains a problem and if the patient desires correction of the deformity, an anterior tenoarthrolysis can be considered. This can change the existing mobility to a more useful range of motion. It is an operation that requires good neurovascular status of the digit, good articular surfaces at the proximal interphalangeal joint level, a functioning extensor apparatus, and a very cooperative patient.

Indications for a Tendon Graft in the Intermediate Zone

At this level a graft is used to reconstruct the flexor profundus only, from the proximal half of the palm to the distal phalanx. The proximal and distal limits of the graft are open to discussion; it can be extended into the wrist when suturing in the palm seems unsuitable. The distal end can be sutured to the middle phalanx if the distal interphalangeal joint is stiff or local conditions negate a more ambitious repair (Table 38–2).

One-Stage Graft. Secondary grafting is indicated when the condition of the wound, the risk of infection, and the presence of inadequate surgical conditions preclude primary repair by suturing. We have already reviewed

---

*See section on reconstruction of pulleys in Chapter 30 on Flexor Tendon Grafts.

Table 38–2. INDICATIONS FOR A FLEXOR DIGITORUM SUPERFICIALIS TENDON GRAFT

1. Stiff distal interphalangeal joint
2. Amputated distal phalanx
3. Swan-neck deformity
4. Failed flexor digitorum profundus graft
5. Tendon for grafting is too short

these factors, which can be diversely interpreted. The graft can be completed in one stage if the state of the hand is satisfactory (i.e., good wound healing, supple tissues, full passive mobility) and if at least one functional pulley remains at the level of the proximal phalanx (Table 38–3). In our practice, we utilize more one-stage than two-stage grafts.

Salvage Procedures

TWO-STAGE GRAFT. The two-stage graft (Fig. 38–12) is in reality a three-stage procedure, as it involves

1. Preoperative re-education. One attempts to achieve maximal passive mobility of the joints and suppleness of soft tissue.

2. Excision of fibrous tissue, insertion of a silicone rod and pulley reconstruction in their optimal position.

3. Placement of graft. After two to six months, the graft is placed in the fibrous sheath formed around the implant.

One of the chief advantages of this two-stage procedure is that only the ends of the sheath are disturbed when the graft is placed in position. The main disadvantage is that it involves two operations and a longer delay before the return of function (Table 38–4).

The two-stage graft is reserved for the following cases: (1) when large areas of scar tissue have formed in the path of the tendon, (2) when passive mobility remains limited after resection of the tendons, and (3) when the pulleys have been destroyed.

REOPERATION AFTER GRAFT FAILURE. Early reoperation is indicated when one suspects that one end of the graft has come loose.

Table 38–3. INDICATIONS FOR ONE-STAGE TENDON GRAFT

1. Good healing
2. Supple soft tissue
3. Complete passive mobility
4. Absence of pain
5. Good sensibility

When the graft is capable of active mobilization but active flexion is much more limited than passive flexion, adhesions or inadequate pulley function may be the cause. If pressure on the volar aspect of the proximal phalanx increases active interphalangeal function, the pulley function may be the root of the problem. In this case, one must wait at least six months after the graft before reoperating. The procedure used is *tenolysis* with conservation, if possible, of the most important pulleys. Otherwise, one can proceed with pulley system reconstruction.*

We have adopted the regional anesthesia technique at the wrist level recommended by Schneider and Mackin (1984), which permits the patient to actively cooperate during the operation.

If active flexion is absent or minimal but passive flexion is preserved, it is reasonable to consider a new graft provided that technical conditions are better than those at the time of the previous operation. In such cases, one will usually be content with *replacing the flexor digitorum superficialis* by fixing the graft to the middle phalanx.

When there is no active flexion and passive flexion is absent or minimal, arthrodesis of the proximal interphalangeal joint or amputation can be considered. *Arthrodesis* is preferred when the metacarpophalangeal joint is mobile and, apart from absent flexion at the interphalangeal joints, the finger remains functionally and cosmetically acceptable. By contrast, *amputation* is justified for a stiff, cold, painful, insensitive finger, especially in manual workers.

Other Procedures and Perspectives for the Future

PEDICLE TENDON GRAFTS. Pedicle tendon grafts in two stages have been described by Paneva-Holevitch (1972, 1977) for lacerations of both tendons in zone II in adults. The procedure is recommended by this author because it requires less time than the two-stage graft of Hunter when local conditions preclude primary suturing. However, if the pulleys are destroyed, it seems safer to reconstruct them around an inert implant by combining the two procedures.

TENDON TRANSFERS. Flexor digitorum superficialis transfers from an intact finger are rarely indicated for fresh injuries as the donor digit will lose its independence of flexion.

---

*See Chapter 30 on Flexor Tendon Grafts.

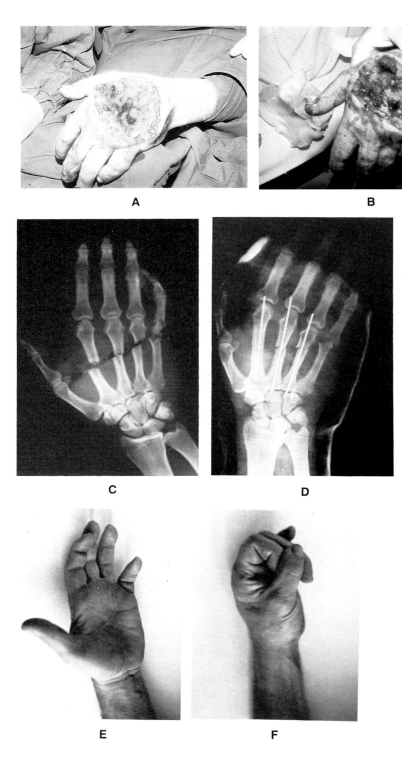

Figure 38–12. Circular saw injury of the left hand in February 1981 in a man aged 44 years. *A*, Dorsal view. *B*, Palmar view—nearly complete amputation. *C*, Radiograph showing the fractures of all metacarpals to the fingers. The thumb is intact. *D*, As on emergency, the fractures were stabilized with Kirschner wires and both wounds were sutured.

The patient was sent to us in May 1981; the fractures were united. The fingers were stiff in extension with no active movement and complete anesthesia of the fingers. Intensive physiotherapy was started. On September 16, 1981, the divided digital nerves were grafted and at the same time Silastic rods were inserted. On December 9, 1981, flexor tendon grafts were inserted into the index, middle, and ring fingers. The little finger, which was still stiff, was not grafted. *E* and *F*, Result at six months. Protective sensation in all fingers was improving. The patient had returned to work as a mason.

Table 38–4. INDICATIONS FOR TWO-STAGE TENDON GRAFT

1. Extensive scarring
2. Limitation of passive mobility
3. Pulley distribution

However, if multiple digits are involved, one can consider transferring the proximal end of the divided tendon to act as a motor for another digit that has tendon divisions if the level of the injury is appropriate.

In old injuries, tendon transfers are rarely used for flexor tendon lacerations in zone II. The tendon must have sufficient length to reach the end of the digit, and such tendons are rarely available except in cases where one is using the flexor of a digit that is going to be amputated for other reasons. The transfer of a tendon from a healthy finger should not be undertaken lightly. Tendon transfers are no guarantee against adhesion formation.

TENDON PROSTHESES. Hunter's current practice of fixing the two ends of the implant—the distal end in the bone and the proximal end in the motor tendon—constitutes a true tendon prosthesis. This prosthesis is, as yet, temporary because it is bound to rupture sooner or later. Still, it permits not only a new sheath for the secondary graft but also active flexion of the finger and continued function of the muscle motor.

COMPOSITE GRAFTS OF TENDONS AND SHEATH. These are scientifically interesting but of little practical use. They could become an ultimate recourse for a finger that has maintained its joint mobility and active extension (Peacock and Madden, 1967) (see Chapter 35).

FREE TRANSPLANTATION OF A VASCULARIZED TENDON WITH MICROSURGICAL REATTACHMENT (Morrison and O'Brien, 1985). The first cases of these tendon grafts taken on the back of the foot yielded very good results. This method is completed in one operation, but is very sophisticated; thus, it would have to be reserved for very select cases.

IN THE PROXIMAL ZONE

Although the tendons cross several different topographical regions, the anatomical conditions are usually at all levels suitable for a primary or early secondary repair.

Primary Repairs

Suturing of both the profundus and the superficialis tendon is often possible. In multiple tendon lesions, the younger the patient, the greater the chances of recovery and the more one should try to perform a primary repair on all the tendons. In older patients or following extensive trauma, one may have to be content with repairing only the profundus tendons. In this zone, the site of the lesion does not alter the modality of treatment of the tendon itself. On the contrary, the anatomical relationship of the tendons with the adjacent structures will determine the nature and extent of the associated lesions. Thus, on the anterior aspect of the wrist, the tendons, arteries, and nerves are relatively superficial and unprotected by the skeleton. This explains the high incidence in this region of multiple lesions to the flexor tendons of the wrist and fingers that are often associated with vascular and nerve lesions. Priority must be given to vascular and tendon repairs. If the circumstances are favorable (clean wound, adequate equipment), primary suturing of all tendons, including the wrist flexors, is justified. For the mixed (sensorimotor) nerve trunks at the wrist, some authors prefer a secondary repair because of better aseptic conditions and convenience. This problem will be discussed in the section on peripheral nerve repair. However, we feel that when conditions are favorable one should carry out primary nerve suture.

Within the carpal tunnel and in the palm the nerves are no longer mixed but are uniquely sensory or muscular. They are preferably sutured at the time of the initial repair as well.

When treating lesions of the wrist flexors or tendon lesions in the carpal tunnel or proximal part of the palm, the carpal flexor retinaculum is always released at its ulnar fixation. The wrist will be immobilized in only moderate flexion (10 degrees) to keep the flexor tendons from subluxating anteriorly in the absence of the flexor retinaculum pulley (bow-string effect). The metacarpophalangeal joints should be totally flexed in this instance.

Secondary Repairs

An early secondary repair is indicated whenever doubt persists as to the degree of asepsis of the initial wound.

Fixed retraction and loss of substance constitute an indication for a secondary graft. Only one tendon, usually the profundus, is repaired. The graft may be bridging or it can be extended to the tip of the finger if adhesions are present along the tendon.

INJURIES TO THE FLEXOR POLLICIS LONGUS

Although the anatomical conditions of this solitary tendon make its repair less difficult than that of the corresponding digital flexors, the choice of method and timing of the repair must be decided according to the site of the lesion. As with the flexor digitorum tendons, the course of the tendon, which crosses five topographical regions, is divided into three surgical zones.

Distal Zone (T1)

This includes the distal phalanx and the distal half of the proximal phalanx.

Primary Repair. When the distal end of the severed tendon is less than 1.5 cm. long, the proximal end can be reinserted on the distal phalanx. The flexor pollicis tendon can be advanced farther than the flexor tendons of the fingers because of the independence of the tendon and the absence of the lumbrical muscle. Thus, there is no risk of reducing the flexor power of adjacent digits by producing the "charioteer's syndrome." Excessive advancement must be avoided, especially in the older patient, as it might produce a fixed flexion deformity of the distal phalanx. The presence of tendinous connections between the flexor pollicis longus and the flexor digitorum profundus, particularly of the index finger (already noted by Fahrer [Vol. I, Chap. 40], and by Linburg [1979] in 31 per cent of his cases), obstructs advancement of the pollicis tendon. Early passive mobilization of the repaired tendon is the same as for that of the fingers.

Secondary Repair. Reinsertion remains feasible if retraction and adhesions are not too extensive. Otherwise, some other method must be tried, such as tendon lengthening, tendon grafting, or palliative surgery.

Intermediate Zone (T2)

This is the zone (the digital fibro-osseous tunnel) in which the tendon is most often divided. Whenever possible, one should try to preserve part of the proximal annular pulley opposite the metacarpophalangeal joint or of the oblique pulley opposite the proximal phalanx. Mobility of the metacarpophalangeal joint of the thumb varies from one individual to the next; the greater the mobility, the greater the role of the pulleys.

With early postoperative mobilization using Kleinert's technique, the pulley for the elastic traction is placed opposite the thumb on the hypothenar region.

Primary Repair. The tendon is sutured away from the fibrous sheath. This can be done by resecting part of the distal end and by flexing the joints, which keeps the suture away from the pulley. Suturing the two heads of the flexor pollicis brevis can, to a certain extent, palliate the absence of a pulley (El Bacha).

When the surgical conditions are favorable, one can split the tendon, as described by Rouhier (1950), at the junction of the fleshy and tendinous fibers above the wrist (Fig. 38–13). When the section is not too proximal, 2.5 to 3 cm. can be gained, which allows reattachment of the proximal end to the distal phalanx. The wrist and metacarpophalangeal joint are flexed to avoid tension, but the metacarpophalangeal joint is maintained in extension. This procedure is reliable and rarely results in secondary rupture; therefore, it is the procedure of choice in the distal and sesamoid zones (Raimbeau et al., 1985).

Secondary Repair. This same technique of lengthening and reattachment has been advocated as a secondary procedure, but we prefer a graft when the proximal end is retracted, thickened, and adherent and can barely glide along its sheath.

When the A1 pulley is destroyed, it should be repaired to avoid bow-stringing of the tendon. Le Viet and Ebelin (1982) have described a procedure for the reconstruction of this pulley. They use a 6 mm. wide strip of the adductor pollicis tendon starting at the sesamoid (Fig. 38–14). This strip must be taken as far distal on the phalanx as possible to ensure an adequate length of at least 2.5 cm. It is passed under the ulnar insertion of the volar plate and over the tendon and is fixed on the radial side of the phalanx. Post-

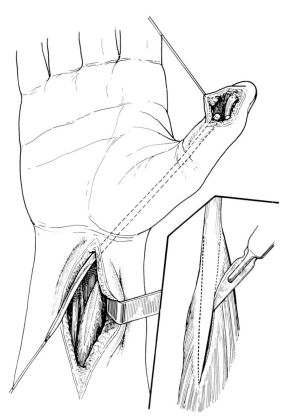

Figure 38–13. Rouhier's technique for lengthening the flexor pollicis longus tendon. The tendon is divided obliquely at the level of the musculotendinous junction, allowing lengthening of the tendon of up to 2.5 to 3 cm.

operatively, the tendon at the level of the A1 pulley is supported by an external metal splint in the shape of a semicircular metal ring 1 cm. wide. This ring allows rapid mobilization and is worn for four weeks.

PROXIMAL ZONE (T3–T4–T5)

Primary Repair. In the thenar eminence, the carpal region, and the wrist, the anatomical conditions usually allow a primary or early secondary repair by suturing. However, one should insist upon good visualization of the cut tendon ends to avoid damaging the many branching nerves in this area.

Secondary Repair. The results of grafting of the flexor pollicis longus are good when the joints are supple and the tension is precisely gauged. The tendon of the palmaris longus provides a suitable graft that can run

from the wrist, above the carpal tunnel, to the distal phalanx.

When local conditions are unfavorable, a two-stage graft can be used, which allows one to remake the pulleys around a Silastic implant. It is also possible to anastomose the proximal end of the long flexor tendon to the palmaris longus using the Paneva-Holevich method.

Palliative Procedures. When the muscle body of the flexor pollicis longus has been damaged beyond repair, the action of this muscle can be successfully replaced by transferring a superficialis tendon (preferably the fourth) on the distal phalanx of the thumb.

Arthrodesis of the interphalangeal joint of the thumb provides stable thumb-finger grip when the thenar muscles are intact, but it

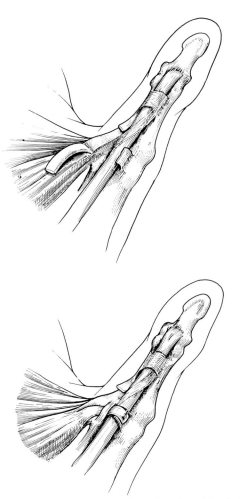

Figure 38–14. Reconstruction of pulley A1 of the flexor pollicis longus using a strip taken from the adductor pollicis tendon (after Le Viet and Ebelin).

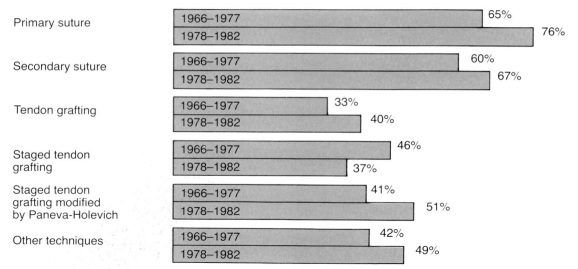

Figure 38–15. Results of flexor tendon reconstruction (University of Erlangen, Department of Hand Surgery and Plastic Surgery). 1966–1977, total of 476 fingers (52 per cent very good and good results); 1978–1982, total of 345 fingers (60 per cent very good and good results).

implies the loss of active mobility of the interphalangeal joint, which is necessary for precision grip and is thus an important part of the adduction power of the thumb.

COMPLICATIONS OF REPAIRS OF THE LONG FLEXOR OF THE THUMB

Although most authors report good results in the majority of patients after repair of the long flexor of the thumb when the surgical procedure has been chosen correctly (Urbaniak and Goldner, 1973; Sakeliarides, 1974), a certain number of complications persist, namely, stiffness, malposition, or limitation of movement (Ebelin, 1984). These malpositions are often characterized by metacarpophalangeal flexion and lack of flexion of the interphalangeal joint. The stabilization of the metacarpophalangeal joint in extension allows rehabilitation and recovery of flexion of the interphalangeal joint. Apfelberg et al.

	VERY GOOD	GOOD	SATISFACTORY	POOR	TOTAL
primary	60% (80)	16% (21)	7% (9)	17% (23)	133
SUTURES	56% (103)	18% (33)	11% (21)	15% (28)	185
secondary	44% (23)	23% (12)	23% (12)	10% (5)	52
LATE RECONSTRUCTIONS	26% (42)	19% (30)	18% (29)	37% (59)	160
TOTAL	42% (145)	18% (63)	15% (50)	25% (87)	345 (100%)

Figure 38–16. Results of flexor tendon reconstruction, 1978–1982 (University of Erlangen, Department of Hand Surgery and Plastic Surgery).

(1980) have described this situation, which they call "interphalangeal flexor lag," caused by three separate factors. First, there may be suturing under tension with functional shortening of the muscle tendon, which may need to be lengthened. Second, loss of the digital pulley mechanism may occur and should be repaired by pulley reconstruction. Third, there may be adhesions of the tendon at or distal to the metacarpophalangeal joint, for which tenolysis is indicated.

EVOLUTION OF THE INDICATIONS

As a conclusion of this chapter, we would like to present the comparative results of flexor tendon reconstruction of two successive comparative series presented by J. Gelmacher at the Third Congress of the International Federation of Societies for Surgery of the Hand, Tokyo, 1986. The assessment of results has been classified according to the Buck-Gramcko method (Figs. 38–15 and 38–16).

GENERAL REFERENCES ON FLEXOR TENDON REPAIR

Allieu, Y., Asencio, G., Bahri, H., Pascal, M., Gomis, R., and Louchahi N.: La reconstruction des fléchisseurs en deux temps (technique de Hunter) dans le traitement des doigts en crochet. Ann. Chir. Main, 2:341–344, 1983.

Allieu, Y.: Etat actuel de la réparation tendineuse en chirurgie de la main. S.O.F.C.O.T. Réunion annuelle, Nov. 83, Suppl. Rev. Chir. Orthop., 70: 1984.

Apfelberg, D. B., Maser, M. R., Lash, H., and Keoshian, L.: "I. P. flexor lag" after thumb flexor reconstruction. Causes and solution. Hand, 12:167–172, 1980.

Alnot, J. Y., and Duparc, J.: Plaies récentes des deux tendons fléchisseurs aud doigt. Rev. Chir. Orthop., 60:531–547, 1974.

Alnot, J. Y., and Dufour, G.: La réparation des lésions anciennes des tendons fléchisseurs. Ann. Chir., 45:675–682, 1980.

Becker, H.: Primary repair of flexor tendons in the hand without immobilization. Preliminary report. The Hand, 10:37, 1978.

Boyes, J. H., and Stark, H. H.: Flexor tendon grafts in the fingers and thumb. A study of factors influencing results in 1,000 cases. J. Bone Joint Surg., 53A:1332–1342, 1971.

Boyes, J. H., and Stark, H. H.: Les greffes de tendons fléchisseurs dans les doigts et dans le pouce. In: Chirurgie des Tendons de la Main. Monographie du G. E. M., Paris, Expansion Scientifique Française, 1976.

Brunelli, G., and Monini, L.: Technique personnelle de suture des tendons fléchisseurs des doigts avec mobilisation immédiate. Ann. Chir. Main, 1:92–96, 1982.

Bruner, J. M.: The zig-zag volar digital incision for flexor tendon surgery. Plast. Reconstr. Surg., 40:571, 1967.

Buck-Gramcko, D.: Verletzungen der Beugesehnen. In H. Nigst, D. Buck-Gramcko, and H. Millesi (eds.): Hanchirurgie. Vol. II, Chap. 28. Stuttgart, Thieme, 1983.

Bunnell, S.: Repair of tendons in the fingers and description of two new instruments. Surg. Gynecol. Obstet., 26:103, 1918.

Bunnell, S.: Repair of tendons in the fingers. Surg. Gynecol. Obstet., 35:88–97, 1922.

Bunnell, S.: Surgery of the Hand. Philadelphia, J. B. Lippincott, 1944.

Cameron, R. R., Conrad, R. N., Sell, K. W. et al.: Freeze-dried composite tendon allografts: an experimental study. Plast. Reconstr. Surg., 47:39, 1971.

Caplan, H. S., Hunter, J. M., and Merklin, R. J.: The intrinsic vascularization of flexor tendons in the human. J. Bone Joint Surg. (Am.), 57:726, 1975.

Carroll, R. E., and Match, R. M.: Avulsion of the profundus tendon insertion. J. Trauma, 10:1109, 1970.

Chang, W. H., Thoms, O. J., and White, W. L.: Avulsion injury of the long flexor tendons. Plast. Reconstr. Surg., 19:35, 1972.

Doyle, J. R., and Blythe, W. F.: The finger flexor tendon sheath and pulleys: anatomy and reconstruct. In: AAOS Symposium on Tendon Surgery in the Hand. St. Louis, C. V. Mosby, 1975.

Doyle, J. R., and Blythe, W. F.: Anatomy of the flexor tendon sheath and pulleys of the thumb. J. Hand Surg., 2:149–151, 1977.

Duparc, J., Alnot, J. Y., Nordin, J. Y., and Pidhorz, L.: Plaies récentes des tendons fléchisseurs au doigt. Ann. Chir., 27:467, 1973.

Duran, R. J., Houser, R. G., Coleman, C. R., et al.: A preliminary report in the use of controlled passive motion following flexor tendon repair in zones II and III. J. Hand Surg., 1:79, 1976.

El Bacha: Personal communication.

Ebelin, M.: Réparation secondaire du long fléchisseur du pouce: résultats comparatifs à propos de 46 cas. Thèse Faculte de Médecine Necker-Enfants Malades. Paris, 1984.

Flynn, J. E., and Graham, J. H.: Healing with tendon suture and tendon transplants. In: Flynn, J. E. (ed.): Hand Surgery. 3rd ed. Baltimore, Williams and Wilkins, 1982.

Foucher, G., and Merle, M.: La suture des tendons fléchisseurs selon la technique de Kleinert. Ann. Chir. Main, 3:170–172, 1984.

Foucher, G., Braun, F. M., Merle, M., and Van Genechten, F.: Amélioration de la flexion interphalangienne proximale du 5° doigt dans les plaies ou avulsions du tendon fléchisseur profond. Ann. Chir. Main. 3:269–270, 1984.

Foucher, G., Merle, M. Hoang, G.: Suture du tendon fléchisseur profond au niveau de la partie distale du "no man's land." Un artifice utilisé dans 23 cas. Rev. Chir. Orthop., 72:227–229, 1986.

Furlow, L. T.: The role of tendon tissues in tendon healing. Plast. Reconstr. Surg., 57:39, 1976.

Geldmacher, J.: Some helpful details in flexor tendon surgery. Difficulties in obtaining an objective evaluation of collective results—statistics. The Third International Congress I.F.S.S.H., Tokyo, Nov. 1986.

Goldner, J. L., and Coonrad, J. W.: Tendon grafting of flexor profundus in presence of completely or partially intact flexor sublimis. J. Bone Joint Surg. (Am.), 51:527, 1969.

Harrison, S. H.: Delayed primary flexor tendon grafts of the fingers. A comparison of results with primary and secondary tendon grafts. Plast. Reconstr. Surg., 43:366–372, 1969.

Honner, R.: The late management of the isolated lesion of the flexor digitorum profundus tendon. J. Hand Surg., 7:171, 1975.

Hunter, J. M.: Artificial tendons. Early development and application. Am. J. Surg., 109:325, 1965.

Hunter, J. M., and Salisbury, R. E.: Flexor-tendon reconstruction in severely damaged hands: a two-stage procedure using a silicone-dacron reinforced gliding prosthesis prior to tendon grafting. J. Bone Joint Surg., (Am.), 53:829–858, 1971.

Hunter, J. M., Schneider, L. H., and Fieti, V. G., Jr.: Reconstruction of the sublimis finger. J. Hand Surg., 4:282, 1979.

Iselin, M., and Iselin, F.: Traité de Chirurgie de la Main. Flammarion, 1967.

Jones, F.: Personal communication, 1982.

Kleinert, H. E., Kutz, J. E., Atasoy, E., and Stormo, A.: Primary repair of flexor tendons. Orthop. Clin. North Am., 4:865–876, 1973.

Kleinert, H. E., and Bennett, J. B.: Digital pulley reconstruction employing the always present rim of the previous pulley. J. Hand Surg., 3:297–298, 1978.

Kleinert, H. E., Kutz, J. E., and Cohen, M. J.: Primary repair of zone 2 flexor tendon lacerations. In: AAOS Symposium on Tendon Surgery in the Hand. St. Louis, The C. V. Mosby Co., 1975, p. 91.

Kleinert, H. E., and Verdan, C.: Report of the Committee on tendon injuries. J. Hand Surg., 8:794–798, 1983.

Kleinert, H. E., and Lubahn, A.: Current state of flexor tendon surgery. Ann. Chir. Main, 3:1, 1984.

Langlais, F., Gibon, Y., Canciani, J. P., and Thomine, J. M.: Etude critique de la réparation primaire des tendons fléchisseurs du canal digital. Ann. Chir. Main, 3: 1986.

Leddy, J. P., and Packer, J. W.: Avulsion of the profundus tendon insertion in athletes. J. Hand Surg., 2:66–69, 1977.

Le Viet, D., and Ebelin, M.: Un procédé de reconstruction de la poulie annulaire métacarpo-phalangienne du pouce. Rev. Chir. Orthop. 68:347–350, 1982.

Lexer, E.: Die freien transplantationen. Enke, Stuttgart, 1924.

Linburg, R. M., and Comstock, B. E.: Anomalous tendon slips from the flexor pollicis longus to the flexor digitorum profundus. J. Hand Surg., 4:79, 1979.

Lister, G. D.: Reconstruction of pulleys employing extensor retinaculum: J. Hand Surg., 4:461–467, 1979.

Lister, G. D.: Incision and closure of the flexor sheath during primary tendon repair. Hand, 15:123–135, 1983.

Lister, G. D.: Pitfalls and complications of flexor tendon surgery. Hand Clin., 1:1, 1985.

Lister, G. D., Kleinert, H. E., Kutz, J. E., and Atasoy, E.: Primary flexor tendon repair followed by immediate controlled mobilization. J. Hand Surg., 2:441–451, 1977.

Lunn, P. G., Lamb, D. W.: Rugby finger. Avulsion of profundus of ring finger. J. Hand Surg., 9B:69–71, 1984.

McLinton, M. A., Curtis, R. M., and Shaw Wilgis, E. F.: One hundred tendon grafts for isolated flexor digitorum profundus injuries. J. Hand Surg., 7:224–229, 1982.

Madsen, E.: Delayed primary suture of flexor tendons cut in the digital sheath. J. Bone Joint Surg., (Br.): 52:264–267, 1970.

Malerich, M. M., Baird, R. A., McMaster, W., and Erickson, J. M.: Permissible limits of flexor digitorum profundus tendon advancement. J. Hand Surg., 12A(1):30–33, 1987.

Mansat, M., and Bonneviaille, P.: Avulsion traumatique du fléchisseur commun profond. A propos de 19 cas. Ann. Chir. Main, 4:1–12, 1985.

Mantero, R., and Bertolotti, P.: La mobilisation précoce dans le traitement des lésions des tendons fléchisseurs au canal digital. Ann. Chir., 30:889–896, 1976.

Mason, M. L.: The immediate and delayed tendon repair. Surg. Gynecol. Obstet., 15:449–457, 1936.

Matev, I. B.: Tendons fléchisseurs des doigts. Suture primaire retardée des tendons fléchisseurs coupés dans la gaine digitale. Hand, 12:158–162, 1980.

Merle, M., Foucher, G., and Michon, J.: La technique de Kleinert pour la réparation primaire des tendons fléchisseurs dans le "no man's land." Ann. Chir., 30:883–887, 1976.

Morrison, W., and O'Brien, B.: Les transplantations de tendons vascularisés. Communication at the Congrès International de Chirurgie, Paris, 1985.

Nalebuff, E. A.: Le superficial intact. In: Chirurgie des Tendons de la Main. Monographie du G. E. M. Expansion Scientifique Française, Paris, 1976, pp. 102–111.

Omer, G. E., and Vogel, J. A.: Determination of physiological length of a reconstructed muscle-tendon unit through muscle stimulation. J. Bone Joint Surg., 47A:304–312, 1965.

Osborne, G. V.: The sublimis tendon replacement technique in tendon injuries. J. Bone Joint Surg., 42B:647, 1960.

Osborne, G. V.: The sublimis grafting for flexor tendon injuries. In: Stack, H. G. and Bolton, H. (eds.): Proceedings of the Second Hand Club, 9th Meeting. Glasgow 1960. The British Society for Surgery of the Hand, London 1975.

Paneva-Holevich, E.: Two stage tenoplasty in injury of the flexor tendon of the hand. J. Bone Joint Surg., 51A:21–32, 1969.

Paneva-Holevich, E.: Résultats du traitement des lésions multiples des tendons fléchisseurs des doigts par greffe effectuée en deux temps. Rev. Chir. Orthop., 58:481–489, 1972.

Paneva-Holevich, E.: Reconstructive surgery of the flexor tendons of the hand. Med. Fizkult., Sofia, 1977.

Parkes, A.: The "lumbrical plus" finger. J. Bone Joint Surg., 53B:236–239, 1971.

Peacock, E. E., and Madden, J. W.: Human composite tissue tendon allografts. Ann. Chir., 166:624, 1967.

Peacock, E. E.: Some biologic and technical considerations in the repair of long tendons. Orthop. Clin. North Am., 8:449–474, 1977.

Peterson, W. W., Manske, P. R., and Lesker, P. A.: The effect of flexor sheath integrity on nutrient uptake by primate flexor tendons. J. Hand. Surg., 11A(3): 413–416, 1986.

Peterson, W. W., Manske, P. R., Lesker, P. A., Kain, C. C., and Schaefer, R. K.: Development of a synthetic replacement for the flexor tendon pulley. J. Hand Surg., 11A(3):403–410, 1986.

Potenza, A. D.: The healing process in wounds of the digital flexor tendons and tendon grafts. An experimental study. In: Verdan, C. (ed.): Tendon Surgery of the Hand. Edinburgh, Churchill-Livingstone, 1979, pp. 40–54.

Pulvertaft, R. G.: Repair of tendon injuries in the hand. Ann. Roy. Coll. Surg. England. pp. 3–14, 1948.

Pulvertaft, R. G.: Tendon grafts for flexor tendon injuries in the fingers and thumb. J. Bone Joint Surg., 38B:175–194, 1956.

Pulvertaft, R. G.: The treatment of profundus division by free tendon graft. J. Bone Joint Surg. (Am.), 42:1363–1380, 1960.

Pulvertaft, R. G.: Suture materials and tendon junctures. Am. J. Surg., 109:346–352, 1965.

Raimbeau, G., Condamine, J. L., and Lebourg, M.: Réparation primitive du long fléchisseur du pouce. A propos de 60 cas. Ann. Chir. Main, 4, 1985.

Reef, T. C.: Avulsion of the flexor digitorum profundus, an athletic injury. Am. J. Sports Med., 5:281, 1977.

Richards, H. J.: Digital flexor tendon repair and return of function. Ann. Roy. Coll. Surg. England, 59:25–32, 1977.

Romain, M., Pellegrin, R., Allieu, Y., Lizlik, C., Durand, P. A., and Dupuy, S.: Rééducation après sutures primitives des tendons fléchisseurs selon la technique de Kleinert. Ann. Méd. Phys., 4:399–409, 1981.

Rouchier, F.: La restauration du tendon long fléchisseur du pouce, sans sacrifice du tendon primitif. J. Chir., 66:8–9, 1950.

Ruby, L. K.: Common hand injuries in the athlete. Orthop. Clin. North Am., 11:819–833, 1980.

Saffar, P., and Rengeval, J. P.: La tenoarthrolyse totale antérieure. Technique du traitement des doigts en crochet. Ann. Chir., 32:579–582, 1978.

Sakellarides, H. T.: The treatment of lacerated flexor tendons of the fingers and thumb in no-man's land by tendon grafting. Rhode Island Med. J., 57:55–59, 1974.

Salvi, V.: Delayed primary suture in flexor tendon division. Hand, 3:181–183, 1971.

Schneider, L. H., and Hunter, J. M.: Flexor tenolysis. In: AAOS Symposium on Tendon Surgery in the Hand. St. Louis, The C. V. Mosby Co., 1975, pp. 157–162.

Schneider, L. H., Hunter, J. M., Norris, T. R., and Nadeau, P. O.: Delayed flexor tendon repair in no man's land. J. Hand Surg., 2:452–455, 1977.

Schneider, L. H., and Mackin, E. J.: Tenolysis: Dynamic approach to surgery. In Hunter, J. et al. (eds.): Rehabilitation of the Hand, 2nd ed. St. Louis, C. V. Mosby, 1984, pp. 280–287.

Schlenker, J. D., Lister, G. D., and Kleinert, H. E.: Three complications of untreated partial laceration of flexor tendon—entrapment, rupture and triggering. J. Hand Surg., 6:392–396, 1981.

Stark, H. H., Zemel, N. P., and Boyes, J. H., Ashworth, C. R.: Flexor tendon graft through intact superficialis tendon. J. Hand Surg., 2:456–461, 1977.

Strickland, J. W., and Glogovac S. V.: Digital function following flexor tendon repair in zone II: A comparison of immobilization and controlled passive motion techniques. J. Hand Surg., 5:537–543, 1980.

Strickland, J. W.: Symposium on flexor tendon surgery. Hand Clin., 1:1, 1985.

Tsuge, K., Ikuta, Y., and Matsuishi, Y.: Repair of flexor tendons by intratendinous tendon suture. J. Hand Surg., 2:436–440, 1977.

Tubiana, R.: Greffes des tendons fléchisseurs des doigts et du pouce. Technique et résultats. Rev. Chir. Orthop., 46:191–214, 1960.

Tubiana, R.: Incisions and technics in tendon grafting. Am. J. Surg., 109:330–345, 1965.

Tubiana, R.: Complications of flexor tendon grafts. Orthop. Clin. North Am., 4:877–883, 1973.

Tubiana, R.: Post-operative care following flexor tendon grafts. Hand, 6:152–154, 1974.

Tubiana, R.: Les réparations des tendons fléchisseurs dans la zone 2. Ann. Chir., 32:619–626, 1978.

Tubiana, R., and Beveridge, Y.: Flexor tendon injuries of the hand. Curr. Orthop., 7:91–99, 1986.

Urbaniak, J. R., and Goldner, J. L.: Laceration of the flexor pollicis longus tendon. Delayed repair by advancement, free graft or direct suture. A clinical and experimental study. J. Bone Joint Surg., 55A:1128–1148, 1973.

Verdan, C.: Syndrome of the quadriga. Surg. Clin. North Am., 40:425, 1960.

Verdan, C., Crawford, G., Martini, Y.: Tenolysis in traumatic hand surgery. Educational Foundation of the American Society of Plastic and Reconstructive Surgeons. Vol. 3, Symposium of the Hand. St. Louis, The C. V. Mosby Co., 1971.

Verdan, C.: Chirurgie des Tendons de la Main. Monographie du G. E. M., Expansion Scientifique Française, Paris, 1976.

Verdan, C.: Half a century of flexor-tendon surgery. J. Bone Joint Surg., 54A:472–491, 1972.

Versaci, A. D.: Secondary tendon grafting for isolated flexor digitorum profundus injury. Plast. Reconstr. Surg., 46:570, 1970.

Weeks, P. M., Wray, R. C., and Stromberg, B. V.: The rate of functional recovery after flexor tendon grafting. J. Hand Surg., 1:75, 1976.

Wenger, D. R.: Avulsion of the profundus tendon insertion in football players. Arch. Surg., 106:106–145, 1973.

Wilson, R. L., Carter, M. S., Holdeman, V. A., and Lovett, W. L.: Flexor profundus injuries treated with delayed two-staged tendon grafting. J. Bone Joint Surg. (Am.): 5:74, 1980.

Wray, R. C., Holtmann, B., and Weeks, P. M.: Clinical treatment of partial tendon lacerations without suturing and with early motion. Plast. Reconstr. Surg., 59:231–234, 1977.

Wray, R. C., and Weeks, P. M.: Treatment of partial tendon lacerations. Hand, 12:163–166, 1980.

Whitaker, J. H., Strickland, J. W., and Ellis, R. K.: The role of flexor tenolysis in the palm and digits. J. Hand Surg., 2:462–470, 1977.

Wynn Parry, C. B. W.: Rehabilitation of the hand. 3rd Ed. London, Butterworth and Co., 1973.

Chapter 39

PRIMARY REPAIR OF FLEXOR TENDONS IN CHILDREN

A. GILBERT

AND A. MASQUELET

ETIOLOGY

In dealing with children, the clinical examination, the operation, and the possibilities of re-education after flexor tendon lesions are all quite different from the situation encountered in adults. Indeed the differences are such that these lesions deserve to be studied separately, the more so because few such studies exist in the literature.

The treatment of these lesions remains controversial despite the many publications advocating immediate suturing of both tendons (Kleinert, 1967).

In 1964 Wakefield, on the strength of his personal experience, recommended suturing of the flexor profundus only and stressed his reluctance to carry out early repairs of the flexors at the digital canal.

Even though ideas have changed over the years, it should still be possible in the light of personal experience to compare the results of modern techniques with those of older, and of more recent, publications.

From our own experience we have learned that although the surgical techniques are similar to those used in adults, the ultimate result depends on a meticulous preoperative clinical examination, an uneventful postoperative course, the age of the child, and the cooperation of the child himself and his parents.

THE INITIAL EXAMINATION

This first examination can be extremely deceptive in view of the impossibility of persuading a two-year-old child to perform a series of complex voluntary movements. Sensation itself is notoriously difficult to assess. At best one can try to determine the cause of the injury, which usually turns out to be a piece of broken glass or a knife blade. The slightest skin wound may well conceal total sectioning of a tendon.

The prime rule therefore is to carry out a full surgical exploration, under general anesthesia, of every suspicious wound of the palmar aspect of the hand. This first piece of advice may sound superfluous, and yet it happens only too often that a perfunctory examination having revealed no major injury, the wound is closed with a few superficial stitches and the child returned to its parents. The true nature of the injury is discovered only days or even weeks later. Thus, 20 per cent of our tendon repairs were carried out because of lesions that had been overlooked in the first instance.

Our first rule of systematic exploration, however, does not obviate the need for a thorough clinical examination whenever possible. In a cooperative seven- or eight-year-old child, the examination can be extremely helpful and may even uncover an associated nerve lesion. It may be worthwhile to find out whether the injury occurred in flexion or in extension, for this information may help in choosing the most suitable surgical approach.

THE SURGICAL REPAIR

With the exception of the more unusual multiple extensive lesions (crush, amputation, burns) in which repair can be justifiably delayed, our policy is to repair all divided tendons as soon as possible and regardless of the site of the section. We do this under general anesthesia, except in older children when local or regional anesthesia is sometimes possible.

The wound is extended according to the rules of hand surgery, and we try to make a full assessment of the lesions. Lesions of the nerves and vessels are searched for systematically. They are uncommon in the fingers and much more frequent in the palm and wrist.

It is usually possible, by acutely flexing the finger, to get the distal extremity of the tendon to herniate through the wound where it is marked with a traction suture. At no stage should the tendon be gripped by forceps. Identification of the proximal stump is much more difficult, for a sectioning proximal to the vincula or avulsion of the latter results in the tendon's retracting back into the palm.

If full flexion of the wrist combined with gentle manual expression fails to produce the tendon, one should resist the temptation to introduce an instrument into the sheath. It is much safer to fetch the tendon through a counterincision in the palm and fix it to a piece of silicone tubing, which is then threaded down the digital canal.

In cases of sectioning through the palm, the flexor profundus is pinned down by the lumbrical, but the superficialis often retracts back to the wrist. There again the search should be continued through an extended incision or a counterincision.

Once all the damaged structures have been identified, the tendon is reconstructed by means of square sutures with the knots buried. Our preference is for double ended atraumatic sutures with short straight needles (diameter: 1.5 for older children and 1.0 for babies). Suturing should aim at approximating the tendon ends without any pucker. The suturing is made easier if the two extremities are temporarily immobilized (in the digital canal) by means of intradermal needles. The anastomosis is completed with a running 6–0 nylon suture. The suturing should be as meticulous as possible and should be carried out with the help of magnifying loupes.

IMMOBILIZATION

Unless immobilization is carefully thought out, the child will get rid of the dressing within the first few days. The plaster cast should include the arm as well as the forearm.

We follow Kleinert's method of mobilization but with certain provisos—only in children over three years of age if they are cooperative. Re-education is started on the first postoperative day, and the child is discharged home only when he has learned to perform the movements correctly. If this proves unfeasible after 48 hours, the elastic straps are removed and the plaster cast is completed.

Mobilization of the fingers, we recall, must be carried out with the elbow and wrist flexed and the metacarpophalangeal joints bent to 60 degrees over a lumbrical prop. If only the index finger is involved, the elastic strap is fixed to that digit only. If another finger is involved, however, all three medial digits are splinted.

POSTOPERATIVE COURSE

The splint and the dressing are removed after 25 days. The stiches are taken out, and a new splint is fitted, which includes the forearm, palm, and fingers. This is worn for one week but is removed daily for active exercising. Only then is passive reeducation started. This concentrates on digital flexion. If at the end of three to four weeks an extension deficit persists, extension splints are worn at night.

RESULTS

We reviewed the cases of 50 children with a total of 100 lesions of the flexor tendons in the hand or wrist. The follow-up in all cases was longer than one year. We used the scale advocated by Tubiana for assessing the results.

Table 39–1 shows that these lesions are rare in children under three years of age.

Table 39–2 shows a fairly even distribution between the various zones of the hand:

Table 39–1. FRESH LESIONS OF THE FLEXOR TENDONS IN CHILDREN ACCORDING TO AGE GROUP

3 years	4
3–6 years	10
6–9 years	10
9–12 years	14
12–15 years	12

Table 39–2. FRESH LESIONS OF THE
FLEXOR TENDONS IN CHILDREN
ACCORDING TO SITE

Wrist	31 tendons	(10 patients)
Palm	21 tendons	(9 patients)
Zone 1	16 tendons	(16 patients)
Zone 2	30 tendons	(15 patients)

1. For lesions at the wrist the results were excellent in all cases, and the results were achieved within a few months.

2. For palmar lesions the problem is somewhat complicated by the frequent association of lesions of the nerves, vessels, and muscles (five patients of nine). Our results here were: three very good, two good, and four average. It may be that there would be a place in this group for early mobilization whenever possible.

3. In the thumb the results were all very good for the four sections of flexor pollicis longus.

4. For the 12 repairs carried out in zone 1, we obtained five very good results, two good, and four average. It is worth pointing out that in three of the five patients in whom

Table 39–3. FRESH LESIONS OF FLEXOR
TENDONS: RESULTS IN ZONE 2

Very good	4
Good	7
Average	4
Reoperated	1

results were rated as very good, mobilization was instituted early.

5. In zone 2 the proportion of good and very good results was high (Table 39–3). It is significant that of the three average results, two patients underwent repair at 10 and 12 days, the tendon lesion having been missed at the first examination.

We had one patient with a rupture in whom reoperation was performed after two years. Only the profundus tendon was sutured, and the end result was rated as excellent.

We must stress that although simple mobilization led to "good" results, all the "very good" results followed early mobilization, which seems to justify this form of treatment whenever the repair is solid. No secondary tenolysis was necessary.

Three cases are illustrated in Figures 39–1 to 39–3.

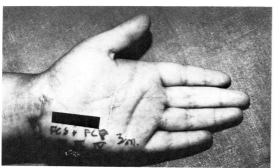

A

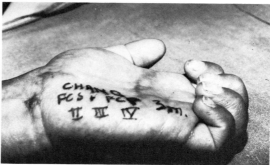

B

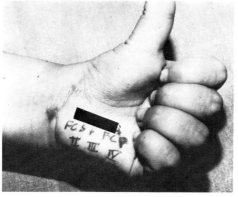

C

Figure 39–1. Wound of the palm in a four-year-old child. Section and repair of profundus and superficialis tendons of the index, long, and ring fingers. Results at three months.

Chapter 40

LATE TREATMENT OF INJURIES OF THE FLEXOR TENDONS IN CHILDREN

JULIEN GLICENSTEIN
AND CAROLINE LECLERCQ

Although hand injuries are common in children, their etiology is usually different from that in adults—grasping a sharp object, catching a hand in a household electrical or mechanical device, crushing by a door. Sectioning of one or more flexor tendons usually results from a clean laceration and is seldom associated with a complex injury involving a gaping wound, a fracture or a crush injury. A simple piece of glass can slice a tendon through an almost punctiform wound that bleeds but little and heals rapidly. This explains the high percentage of such lesions that are missed, especially in children under 10 years of age (Bell et al., 1958; Entin, 1965, 1975; Iselin and Alfonsi, 1968; Posch, 1955).

CLINICOANATOMICAL STUDY

Our study comprised 19 patients, all of whom were seen over one month after the initial injury.

The structure of the flexor tendons undergoes changes with age. Before the age of five years, the two tendons of each finger consist of a slender, flat, and delicate lamina, which tears easily when sutured. The mesotendons and vincula are also extremely fragile; hence, the high incidence of palmar retraction after tendon sectioning in the digital canal. The lesion is almost invariably found in the distal part of the palm or at the proximal phalanges (Arons, 1974; Bell et al., 1958; Iselin and Alfonsi, 1968).

Examination of the hand is often difficult, either because the child is too young to understand which active movements he is asked to carry out, or because he flexes all his fingers simultaneously. The very fact that an injury has occurred is sometimes missed if the wound has healed with little or no trace.

The examination of a young child must follow a somewhat different pattern (Bell et al., 1958; Lindsay, 1976; Posch, 1955; Williams, 1977). It should take place in peaceful surroundings, in the presence of the parents, and with the help of toys to gain the child's confidence.

A diagnosis, albeit partial, is often made just by observing the hand at rest when the injured finger is in full extension while all the others are semiflexed. This may well be confirmed when the hand is seen with the child asleep (Fig. 40–1).

The motor deficit is harder to detect during spontaneous movements of the fingers, because the injured finger is "assisted" by the adjacent fingers and appears to move actively. In some cases the finger is not utilized and is simply "ignored": this suggests a lesion dating back to early childhood, and there may well be a problem of cortical reintegration after a surgical repair.

Passive mobilization of the digit is used to demonstrate the mobility of the joints, which is usually preserved. Passive mobilization of the wrist is a useful diagnostic test, the injured finger remaining extended when the wrist is placed in extension (Lindsay, 1976).

Active mobilization is difficult to obtain in the very young. In the older child it confirms the extension deficit but does not reveal the

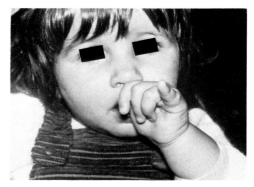

Figure 40–1. At rest and during movement, the injured finger remains extended.

extent of the damage. Not uncommonly some flexion of the proximal interphalangeal joint can be detected clinically, which at exploration is found to result from the tenodesis effect of secondary adhesions.

Associated lesions, especially of the nerves, are always looked for but may be impossible to diagnose clinically in children under five years of age.

CASES STUDIED

Our experience is based on the treatment of 19 fingers in 15 children, of which 15 cases (in 12 children) were followed. All the lesions were diagnosed more than one month after the injury, and one only four years later. In 17 of the 19 sectionings the two flexors of the fingers were severed (15 in the digital canal and two in the palm). In the remaining two the flexor pollicis longus was involved. The little finger was the digit most commonly involved.

TREATMENT

At operation the fingers are found to be freely mobile and well healed, and preoperative re-education is usually not required. Surgery is invariably carried out under general anesthesia using an inflatable cuff blown up to 180 to 250 mm. Hg, depending on the age of the child.

The incision runs along the initial scar and is prolonged if necessary, as described by Brunner (1967). As the child grows, scars tend to straighten and to move nearer the midline (Littler, 1971). If the scar cannot be found, the tendon is widely exposed, starting

with the digital canal at the proximal phalanx and distal part of the palm. The proximal end of the tendon has often retracted into the palm and in the case of flexor pollicis, into the forearm.

In such late repairs, blind counterincisions to locate an adherent proximal segment are not justified: the whole tendon track must be exposed to allow detection of associated (nerve) lesions and excision of scar tissue. Once the proximal end of the tendon has been located and immobilized, the callus is resected. Any one of three situations may now be obtained:

1. The two ends are relatively close; the callus is minimal and restricted to a fibrous bridge. Moderate traction is enough to approximate the ends, which are joined by direct suturing.

2. The proximal end of the tendon (or tendons) is markedly retracted, suggesting avulsion of the vinculum. Once the callus has been resected, the two ends lie too far apart for direct suturing. A two stage graft, using Hunter's technique (1971), is indicated for reasons that will be discussed later.

3. In the third situation the tendon is wrapped inside a mass of fibrous tissue from which it cannot be dissected. A tenolysis is pointless because the residual cord has lost both its blood supply and its biomechanical properties. Instead the whole fibrous zone is resected, and here again a tendon graft is carried out.

At this point in the discussion certain technical points should be stressed:

1. The tendon ends must be solidly tethered to each other. A square suture of 4-0 monofilament is reinforced by one or two continuous sutures of 6-0 or 7-0 monofilament joining the edges. Suturing remains possible even under a great deal of tension provided the digital and wrist joints are flexed. As the excursion of the muscle is restored with re-education, the finger will extend progressively. Both the superficialis and the profundus tendons are repaired (Fig. 40–2).

2. Tendon grafts are always carried out in two stages, as described by Hunter (1970). In the first stage the digital canal is freed of its tendon remnants and fibrous tissue, and the tendon ends are freshened. A fine silicone rod (number 2) is laid down in its place and sutured to the distal end of the tendon with nonresorbing material. The proximal end of one of the tendons selected as the motor source (usually the profundus) is not tethered

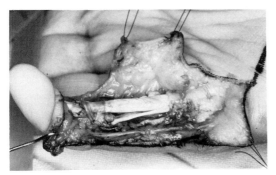

Figure 40–2. In case of secondary rupture, the two flexor tendons and their pulleys must be repaired.

to the silicone, but it is advisable to run a suture through it to serve as a landmark for the second stage, when it may be difficult to identify.

Repair of the pulleys is essential. As a result of the work of Doyle and Blythe (1975) we know that the annular pulleys must be repaired (A2 at the base of P1 and A4 over the head of P2). Simple suturing of adjacent fibrous structures is usually sufficient. Alternatively a tendon fragment is sutured to the periosteum, for transosseous fixation of the tendon graft is not feasible in the child.

The actual tendon grafting is carried out at a second sitting, after 10 days of immobilization and two months of passive re-education, which aims at restoring mobility to the joints. The graft (usually taken from the plantaris) is fixed proximally to the motor tendon using the Pulvertaft (1975) lacing procedure. The distal end of the graft transfixes the distal insertion of the flexor profundus and is sutured to it. The tension is adjusted by pulling the graft through the pulp; the length of the graft varies with the site of the lesion. The distal insertion is always at the distal phalanx, but the proximal attachment should lie at the lumbrical insertion for a digital lesion and above the wrist level for a palmar lesion.

3. Repair of associated lesions of the collateral nerves should always be attempted.

4. Postoperatively, the hand is immobilized with a large compressive bandage including the elbow. Four to six days later this is replaced by a plaster cast immobilizing the elbow in 90 degrees of flexion. The cast should be bulky but carefully molded with only the pulps emerging. This allows for observation of the digital extremities but discourages the child from discarding the plaster cast (Fig. 40–3). Early mobilization is best

avoided except for the older, more cooperative child. Immobilization must be continued longer than in adults—at least four or five weeks to reduce the risk of the suture's "giving" after removal of the plaster cast (Bell et al., 1974; Littler, 1977). Close observation is important during immobilization, as are the two to six months of physiotherapy.

RESULTS

Of the 15 children who underwent surgery, 12 (15 fingers) were followed up for over one year. The results were quantified using the criteria defined by Tubiana (1979). Flexion and extension were evaluated separately for each finger by adding for each the loss of flexion (F1 to F4) and the loss of extension (E1 to E4). By combining the F and E values, the results were placed in four groups—excellent, good, average, and poor. Using this system, we assessed the results of five tendon sutures, eight two stage tendon grafts, and two tenolyses. For the five tendon sutures we recorded three excellent and two good results. For the eight tendon grafts the results were: one excellent, three good, three average, and one poor. The tenolyses yielded one average and one poor result.

DISCUSSION

Wakefield (1964), Entin (1975), Pulvertaft (1956), and Williams (1977) advocate conservative management for lesions diagnosed late in children under five or six years and recommend a one stage grafting repair after that age. The reasons put forward are the tech-

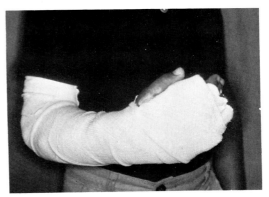

Figure 40–3. The plaster cast immobilizes the elbow in 90 degrees of flexion and the wrist in very slight flexion.

nical difficulties and the lack of cooperation in the very young. In our series the results in children under the age of six were: one excellent (tendon suture), two good, and one poor (grafting).

Along with a number of other authors, however (Bell et al., 1958; Hage & Dupuis, 1965; Iselin and Alfonsi, 1968; Lindsay, 1976; Littler, 1977; Posch, 1955), we believe in early repair, for several reasons:

1. Interruption of the flexor system results in progressive musculotendinous atrophy and degeneration of the pulleys (Littler, 1977).

2. The growth of all the digital tissues, including the skeleton, is affected.

3. A finger left inactive for long is finally ignored. It appears that the longer the gap between injury and repair, the more difficult the reintegration of the digit into the body image.

Some interesting observations can be made from an analysis of our results. Despite the small number of cases reviewed, it would seem that direct suturing yields better results than grafts; hence, the importance of immediate repairs. Once a tendon graft is deemed necessary, there remains the choice between the one stage and the two stage procedures. We prefer the latter, with the interim insertion of a silicone cord. The destruction of the pulleys and invasion of the digital canal by fibrous tissue hardly favor immediate grafting. We know that in children prolonged immobilization in plaster is not detrimental to joint mobility.

Further technical points that deserve consideration are the choice of donor tendon and the repair of the pulleys. The following tendons have been advocated by various authors: the flexor superficialis (Entin, 1965; Littler, 1977), the extensor digitorum communis of the toes (Bell et al., 1958; Entin, 1975; Posch, 1955), and the plantaris (Entin). The latter appeals to us most because it is slender and resistant. It appears that this flat slim graft has a greater chance of survival during the initial period of nutrition by imbibition of synovial fluid.

The pulleys can be made more efficacious if a ring is worn (Fig. 40–4); if worn day and night on the proximal phalanx for several months, it helps to mold the peritendinous connective tissue.

Hage and Dupuis (1965) have raised the problem of tendon graft growth in the growing child. In the absence of demonstrable evidence (such as radiopaque landmarks), it

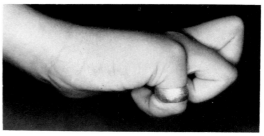

Figure 40–4. Wearing a broad finger ring reinforces the action of the proximal pulley.

might be rash to state that the graft grows with the finger. However, we never observed any delay in growth of the finger operated upon as compared with its contralateral homologue. It is possible that a combination of stretch and growth occurs in the muscle body.

CONCLUSION

Any previously overlooked flexor tendon injury demands surgical exploration as soon as the diagnosis is made, regardless of the age of the child. If the severed extremities are widely separated, if a fibrous callus has formed, and if the pulleys have been destroyed, a two stage tendon graft repair is indicated.

The results of direct suturing are usually good, although the results of grafting are somewhat less predictable. Prolonged immobilization is essential. Rupture of the tendon suture is more to be feared than joint stiffness.

REFERENCES

Arons, M. S.: Purposeful delay of the primary repair of cut flexor tendons in "some man's land" in children. Plast. Reconstr. Surg., 53(6):638, 1974.

Bell, J. L., Mason, M. L., Koch, S. L., and Stromberg, W. B.: Injuries to flexor tendons of the hand in children. J. Bone Joint Surg., 40A:1220–1229, 1958.

Entin, M. A.: Flexor tendon repair and grafting in children. Am. J. Surg., 109:287, 1965.

Entin, M. A.: Flexor tendon surgery in children. A.A.O.S. Symposium on Tendon Surgery in the Hand. St. Louis, C.V. Mosby Co., 1975, p. 132.

Hage, J., and Dupuis, C. C.: The intriguing fate of tendon grafts in small children's hands and their results. Br. J. Plast. Surg., 18:341, 1965.

Hunter, J. M., and Salisbury, R. E.: Use of gliding artificial implant to produce tendon sheaths. Plast. Reconstr. Surg., 18:341, 1965.

Iselin, F., and Alfonsi, P.: Plaies des tendons fléchisseurs des doigts chez les enfants. Ann. Chir. Plast., 13:197, 1968.

Lindsay, K. W.: Hand injuries in children. Clin. Plast. Surg., *3*:65, 1976.

Littler, J. W.: The digital extensor-flexor system. *In* Converse, J. M., and Littler, J. W. (eds.): Reconstructive Plastic Surgery. Vol. IV, 2nd ed. Philadelphia, W. B. Saunders, 1977, p. 3191.

Posch, J. L.: Injuries to the hand in children. Am. J. Surg., *89*:784, 1955.

Pulvertaft, R. G.: Tendon grafts for flexor tendon injuries in the fingers and the thumb. J. Bone Joint Surg., *38B*:175, 1956.

Tubiana, R.: Evaluation des résultats après réparation des tendons longs fléchisseurs des doigts. Ann. Chir., *33*:659, 1979.

Wakefield, A. R.: Hand injuries in children. J. Bone Joint Surg., *46A*:1226, 1964.

Williams, G. S.: Hand injuries in children. Late problems and primary. Clin. Plast. Surg., *4*:503, 1977.

Part Two

SURGERY OF
NERVES

INTRODUCTION

EVOLUTION OF THE CONCEPTS AND TECHNIQUES USED IN THE REPAIR OF PERIPHERAL NERVES

RAOUL TUBIANA

The treatment of traumatic lesions of the peripheral nerves remains one of the most complex and most controversial problems that the hand surgeon has to face. In this chapter we shall not restrict our study to the intrinsic nerves of the hand but will include root and trunk lesions of the upper limb affecting the hand.

Trauma to the peripheral nerves of the upper limb results in a wide range of lesions. Open wounds may vary from partial lacerations to extensive wounds with contusion or loss of substance. Other wounds are closed; these include compressions, injections (which may result in necrosis), and avulsions, particularly of the brachial plexus. The treatment must be adapted to the etiology.

HISTORICAL SURVEY

The work of Augustus Waller (1859) on the distal degeneration of a peripheral nerve after sectioning marked the beginning of our knowledge of this field.

After the earliest attempts at nerve suturing (Arnemann, 1787; Baudens, 1836; Flourens, 1828) and nerve grafting (Albert, 1885; Philipeaux and Vulpian, 1870), the greatest progress in the treatment of such lesions came during wars, when the great number of injuries gave surgeons a wealth of experience. The American Civil War resulted in the work of Hammard (1868) and Weir Mitchell (1872). The First World War provided material for the work of Dejerine (1915), Foerster (1916), Nageotte (1917), and Tinel (1918), and the Second World War brought into prominence the work of Seddon (1948) and Sunderland (1954), who later were to publish important studies (Seddon, 1975; Sunderland, 1972, 1979). The Korean and Vietnam Wars were to be followed by the work of Omer and of Spinner, recently gathered in a common publication (Omer and Spinner, 1980).

For a long time the treatment of peripheral nerve repair had remained virtually unchanged. It was based on the concept that restoration of nerve trunk continuity will allow axon progression and restoration of function.

The study of the internal structure of the nerve trunks revealed their considerable complexity (Sunderland, 1945–1959). Each fascicle contains motor, sensory, and sympathetic (autonomic) fibers in varying proportions. Although there are pure sensory nerves, there are not entirely motor nerves. The different fascicles in the nerve trunk continually branch and divide, forming a complicated plexus surrounded by connective tissue. These structural features exert a profound effect on the final destination of those regenerating axons which enter the distal stumps of a repaired nerve.

AXONAL LOSS

After injury to a nerve trunk, axonal loss at the suture line is considerable. There are four main causes (Sunderland, 1979):

1. Some axons are blocked and others deviated by developing scar tissue.

2. There is constant atrophy in the distal end of the nerve trunk. This involves only the funiculi, not the connective tissue. Nerve trunk atrophy is influenced by the duration of denervation and can involve 60 to 70 per cent of the volume of the funicular part of nerve three months after sectioning. Atrophy is also influenced by the relative amounts of funicular epineural tissue.

3. Some axons become lost in the epineural tissue.

4. Regenerating axons may be sidetracked at the suture line or misdirected as they advance and ultimately fail to reach and establish appropriate connections with functionally related end organs, e.g., a sensory fiber which enters a motor tube.

Axons that overcome these obstacles and reach the periphery and end organs can properly transmit nerve impulses only if a myelin sheath has re-formed along the whole length. Incomplete remyelinization results in slowing of the rate of transmission of motor and sensory impulses; this is usually the case following traumatic lesions.

The quality of functional recovery depends only in part on the number of axons that succeed in reaching the periphery. It is now proved that axon regeneration does not, per se, guarantee good functional recovery.

The restoration of nerve function depends upon two distinct stages: (1) repair and re-generation of nerve structure and (2) establishment of new and functional connections between nerve endings and receptor end organs.

These facts explain the evolution of the treatment of peripheral nerve lesions during the last decades. The surgeons first tried to improve the quality of nerve repair, which no longer could be based on the simple restoration of nerve trunk continuity but on the reduction of the axonal loss by a better coaptation of the nerve ends.

Surgeons are now trying to improve other factors which influence the quality of functional recovery following nerve repair.

SUTURES AND GRAFTS

As pointed out by Moberg (1980), the term nerve repair is not semantically precise. Nerve repair involves many factors other than opposition of the nerve ends, as accurate as it may be. The term "nerve surgery" seems preferable to "nerve repair."

On the basis of careful studies of the numerous repairs performed during World War II, Seddon (1948) showed that secondary suturing is preferable to primary suturing* because the risk of infection is lessened, the extent of the lesion is easier to evaluate, the sutures have a better grip on scar tissue, and elective surgery allows the repair to be performed by an experienced surgeon.

To allow approximation of the nerve ends after resection of neuromas and gliomas, the nerve was widely freed from adjacent tissue and the joints were flexed. Grafts were reserved for cases of extensive tissue loss, for it was believed that they presented even more obstacles than simple suturing. Seddon has commented about his experience with nerve grafts in a personal letter to the author, sections of which are reproduced here.

For these reasons the indications for nerve grafts were reduced to the few cases when extensive nerve loss made direct suturing technically impossible despite such maneuvers as elongation of the nerve, transposition or joint flexion.

Under such conditions it is not surprising that the success rate with grafts was low, with the exception of digital nerve grafts. In such cases Seddon (1963) found that one could be more generous in the distal resection. How-

---

*At that time only epineural suturing was performed.

LAKE HOUSE,
24 GORDON AVENUE,
STANMORE, MIDDX, HA7 3QD

8th January 1977

Professor R Tubiana, M.D.
47 Quai des Grands Augustins
Paris 6
France

Dear Raoul

There are two main snags about nerve grafting to which I have
drawn attention in my book. The first is that the axons have to
cross *two* suture lines, and anyone familiar with the behaviour of
axons at a cut surface of a nerve will know how irresponsibly they
behave. They send out any number of branches whereas, as far as
I can see, surgeons who have no knowledge of neuropathology
imagine in their innocence that the axon behaves just like tooth-
paste or an artist's colour coming out of its tube, one stream which
obligingly enters one Schwann tube. They do nothing of the kind
and this confusing process happens twice over with a nerve graft.
The other serious snag is that the funicular pattern of a nerve is
never constant over more than a centimetre or two, so except in a
very clean cut repaired primarily people are deluding themselves
when they think that they can carry out accurate matching of
funiculi. I have tried, with magnification, though not, I confess,
with the elegant instruments now at your disposal.

My best wishes to you for the New Year.

Yours sincerely,

Herbert J. Seddon

ever, there were also many failures following
suturing (Sakellarides, 1962; Onne, 1962).
Hand surgery was then in active development, and the poor results of nerve surgery
were increasingly troubling. Epineural suturing as practiced up to that time offered little
chance of improvement. Edshage (1964), in
a thesis inspired by Moberg, showed on histological sections that even if an epineural
suture appears satisfactory when viewed from
outside, "internal examination" shows gross
malorientation and poor approximation of
fascicular groups.

At about the same time Smith (1964) described the segmental vascularization of the
peripheral nerves using the mesoneurium. It
appeared that excessive "mobilization" of
nerves was associated with the risk of their
devascularization.

Research was conducted along three principal lines: improving the orientation and

coaptation of the nerve ends, limiting connective tissue proliferation, and filling the
gap between the nerve ends.

IMPROVING THE ORIENTATION AND COAPTATION OF THE NERVE ENDS

Surgeons had long been attempting to improve the approximation of divided nerve
ends. In 1915 Stoffel recommended the use
of magnifying glasses during surgery for nerve
lesions and Marie, Meige, and Gosset (1915)
used "perioperative electrical stimulation to
precisely approximate the peripheral end
with the corresponding lesions of the central
end." However, only in recent years have
optical magnification and perioperative stimulation become generally used.

In 1964 Smith suggested the use of the
microscope to improve approximation of the
nerve ends. Until that time the microscope

had been used for experimental surgery in the laboratory but only rarely in human surgery (for delicate operations involving the eye and ear). Use of the operating microscope was adopted by certain surgeons in the hope of improving fascicular realignment, thereby facilitating axonal regrowth (Michon and Masse, 1964). Hakstian (1968) used electrical stimulation to distinguish between motor and sensory fascicles. Serious objections were soon raised. The operations were lengthened as a result of the new technique. Fascicular identification proved in practice to be very difficult, in particular after resectioning a nerve of any degree of importance. Finally, prolonged manipulation of the nerve extremities and multiplication of intraneural sutures increased connective tissue reactions and risked compromising the aim of the operation. Initial statistics comparing the results of traditional suturing operations and those using a microscope were not in favor of the latter (Braun, 1966).

These technical difficulties have caused many surgeons to continue to use traditional techniques, which they still support vigorously against proponents of the newer microsurgical methods. For this reason, advocates of both techniques have been invited to contribute to this section. We have asked two surgeons with wide experience in peripheral nerve surgery, Donal Brooks and Hanno Millesi, to explain the principles and techniques of their sometimes opposing concepts. It appears to us more and more that, in spite of opposing views, many points of convergence appear between these attitudes, which may at first seem too dogmatic. Indeed everyone now agrees that the use of optical magnification, despite its limitations, allows for more accurate surgical repair, the utilization of finer sutures, better hemostasis, better approximation of nerve endings, and sometimes the possibility of performing fascicular suturing. We believe that a too dogmatic approach should be avoided: epineural and perineural suturing techniques both have their respective places, depending on the nerve involved, the level of the division, and the timing of the repair. Each of these points merits further consideration.

Nerve Suturing Techniques

Many nerve suturing techniques have been described. Since each suture is a foreign body that causes a variable degree of inflammatory reaction, the use of removable sutures with pullout wires has been suggested—or even the elimination of all sutures and replacement by adhesive substances based upon fibrin (Egloff and Narakas, 1982; Matras et al., 1972; Vespasiani and Biancardi, 1980). This technique saves considerable time (see Chapter 55). Attempts have also been made to envelop the nerve extremities with vascular segments or millipore, in the hope of avoiding migration of the axons and preventing scar tissue invasion.

For many years sutures were inserted into the periphery of the nerve, based upon the connective tissue sheath or epineurium. Since the epineurium is very fragile, particularly in fresh lesions, some surgeons employ an additional stay suture using a variety of techniques (Philipeaux and Vulpian, 1870; Seddon, 1972; Snyder et al., 1968). A similar procedure has been reintroduced by Tsuge et al. (1975) in the form of an "anchoring suture."

The desire to improve fascicular realignment, theoretically possible using the microscope, has led to a search for new suturing procedures. In order to distinguish between these various suturing techniques, whose terminology is not always as clearly defined, the intraneural topography must be borne in mind. Each nerve fascicle consists of a group of axons and is surrounded by a highly specialized sheath, the perineurium. The fascicles forming the nerve are surrounded by a connective tissue layer, the epineurium, which infiltrates between the fascicles. Thus, the epineurium is at one and the same time peripheral and intraneural in location. Depending on their position, sutures may be (A) epineural-peripheral, (B) epineural-intraneural or perifascicular, (C) perineural or fascicular, or (D) mixed epiperineural (Fig. 41–1). If precisely carried out, direct perineural suturing (Sunderland's group funicular suture) ensures improved alignment of the fascicles—at the price of additional trauma. The surgeon now has the possibility of choosing the type of suturing technique, weighing its advantages and disadvantages according to the circumstances.

Epineural Suturing. Epineural suturing consists first of the insertion of two diametrically opposed supporting sutures mounted on fine forceps, which facilitate manipulation of the nerve during suturing of one surface and then, after being turned over, that of the opposite surface (Fig. 41–2).

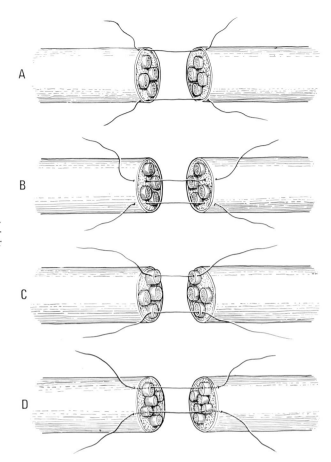

Figure 41–1. Different types of nerve sutures. *A*, Epineural (epineural-peripheral). *B*, Perifascicular (epineural-intraneural). *C*, Fascicular or perineural or group funicular. *D*, Epiperineural.

Fascicular Perineural Suturing. The sutures are tied on the perineurium, bringing together homologous fascicular groups. This theoretically satisfactory technique comes up against great difficulties when the fascicular groups are numerous and small. The isolation of multiple fascicles (Tupper, 1980) results in veritable "spaghettization" of the nerve and the theoretical advantage of greater precision is counterweighed by an increase in surgical trauma. Fascicular suturing is sometimes indicated in partial divisions.

Interfascicular Suturing. Michon (1979) inserts sutures through the epineurium, which also deeply penetrates the interfascicular spaces (Fig. 41–3). This orientates the approximation in axial rotation. In addition some epineural sutures are inserted.

Mixed Epiperineural Suturing. Bora (1976) and Bourrel et al. (1978, 1981) advocate the insertion of sutures through both the epineurium and the external part of the perineurium of the peripheral fascicular groups. The central fascicles are not sutures in order to avoid

leaving suture material within the nerve (Fig. 41–1*D*).

The Nerve Involved

From a theoretical standpoint, fascicular alignment is of value particularly for mixed sensory and motor nerves. This must be precise, since an error in the orientation of a whole fascicular group runs the risk of more complete failure than epineural suturing. The type of fascicular structure of the nerve may guide the choice of suturing technique.

The reconstructed model of the plexiform nature of the musculocutaneous nerve in the arm devised by Sunderland, to which opponents of microsurgery constantly refer, presents an overly pessimistic view of the structure of the peripheral nerves. Perineural suturing is possible in certain nerves at certain sites. Millesi (1980) distinguishes four varieties of nerves on the basis of their fascicular structure:

1. Nerves with a monofascicular structure

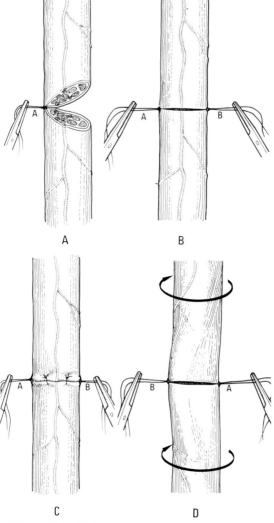

A   B

C   D

Figure 41–2. Early epineural suture. Orientation of the nerve ends is facilitated by the disposition of the superficial vascular system. *A* and *B*, the first two diametrically opposed sutures. *C*, Anterior suture. *D*, Nerve turned for insertion of posterior sutures. A continuous suture may compress the nerve and is inadvisable.

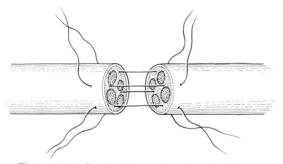

Figure 41–3. Guide suture material passing between fascicular groups.

containing only one fascicle. The epineural suture is adequate.

2. Nerves with an oligofascicular structure. When four or five large fascicles are present, it seems logical to attempt to approximate them using perineural sutures.

3. Nerves with a disorganized polyfascicular structure. This type of structure is seen particularly in the proximal part of a main nerve trunk where the fascicles are intermingled. This is the indication for epineural suturing, with a few sutures sometimes placed between the fascicles to effect alignment.

4. Nerves with organized polyfascicular structure. This type of structure is seen chiefly in the distal part of a nerve trunk before its division.

Site of Sectioning

We have stated that the proximal part of a nerve often has a disorganized polyfascicular structure unsuitable for perineural suturing. By contrast, in the distal part, the structure of the nerve is more organized. The distal extremity of the upper limb is the area most exposed to trauma and where repair is most frequent. The microdissections of Sunderland (1972), Rabischong and Bonnel (1975), and Jabaley et al. (1980) and the operative experience of more and more surgeons have shown that it is possible to identify fascicular groups within the nerves. Such distinct groups sometimes can be identified for a variable, sometimes considerable, length, especially above the levels of origin of the collateral or terminal branches. Interconnections between fascicular groups are also less numerous in the distal part of the nerve.

In addition to study of the macroscopic anatomy of the nerve trunks, one must now be acquainted with the microscopic intraneural fascicular anatomy (see Color Plate III). Even in the distal part of the limbs, accurate approximation of the fascicular patterns of the two divided nerves ends, although theoretically possible, can pose a major problem in practice.

The technical methods described by Millesi permit the "mapping" of both nerve ends, but one must not underestimate the difficulties of identifying the fascicular pattern at each level of section, even though identification is simplified by the use of the microscope. Recent research has been aimed at distinguishing between motor and sensory fibers; so far it has concentrated on histochemical and electrophysiological investigations.

Gruber and Zenker (1973) showed that it is possible to identify motor fibers using an acetylcholinesterase stain. Freilinger et al. (1975) used this histochemical technique to distinguish between motor and sensory fibers in histological specimens. However, this technique requires almost two days and two surgical stages; moreover, its reliability is dubious. Attempts are being made to shorten this period (Engle et al., 1980). Hakstian (1968), Van de Put et al. (1969), and Gaul (1977) have investigated funicular topography using direct intraneural stimulation. Terzis et al. (1976) have applied this electrophysiological information to a perioperative study of lesions in continuity, which are notoriously difficult to treat.* The small magnetic field induced by the passage of a compound action potential along a nerve can now be amplified and may simplify intraoperative nerve recordings (Hentz et al., 1986).

Timing of the Operation

It is easier to orientate the nerve ends properly at the time of primary repair, using the superficial blood vessel distribution and the shape of the nerve as guides. Early peripheral epineural suturing is technically difficult because it is difficult to anchor material in the connective tissue, which is still fragile at this stage. Guide sutures can be inserted, passing between the fascicular groups of the two nerve extremities (Fig. 41–3).

Although technically difficult—and despite a theoretical biological handicap, since connective tissue regrowth precedes axonal regrowth—experience has shown that when the wound is clean and the surgeon is skilled, primary sutures may give very good results with only one operation and only one hospitalization. In addition, primary suture provides the optimum conditions for repair of partial nerve lesions and avoids difficult secondary intraneural neurolyses. Above all, emergency surgery gives the opportunity to repair damaged vessels as well as the nerves. It now seems excessive to advocate only the secondary repair described by Seddon. Such an attitude, reminiscent of the "no man's land" dogma of Bunnell in regard to the flexor tendons of the fingers, is now also no

longer applicable. Seddon's attitude concerning the nerves probably reflected the unfavorable conditions associated with wartime injuries and preantibiotic period when wound infection was the most damaging complication.

The state of the wound will obviously influence the repair of the nerve. When emergency conditions are unfavorable, in particular, where a lesion is contused, the procedure should be limited to approximation of the nerve ends using two sutures in order to limit retraction. Secondary nerve repair follows when local conditions are suitable a few days (delayed, primary) or a few weeks (early secondary) following the injury (one must remember that there will often be a gap to be filled between the nerve ends).

LIMITING CONNECTIVE TISSUE PROLIFERATION

One of the reasons that make the results of nerve repair so unpredictable is that the nerve is composed of tissues of different origins. Axons and connective tissues have different ways of regeneration and their cicatrization has different timing. Epineurium is distinct from the perineurium, which is a clearly differentiated connective tissue structure.

Although the surgeon's attention has long been directed toward axon regrowth, few have taken interest in the connective tissue reactions following nerve injuries. Connective tissue is the major constituent of nerves, surrounding, nourishing, and protecting the nerve fascicles. Since 1967 Millesi has emphasized the need to attempt to limit connective tissue proliferation, which not only is interposed between sectioned nerve ends but may occur even after a closed injury in the peripheral epineurium, in the interfascicular spaces, and in the perineurium. This connective tissue reaction is much more marked after injury with contusion or infection than after a clean section. Because the scar tissue interposed between the nerve ends forms a barrier to the nutrition and passage of the regenerating axons, it must be removed completely before coaptation.

Attempts have been made in animals to decrease fibroblastic activity and stop collagen synthesis (Pleasure et al., 1976) but have not yet led to any human application. According to Millesi, tension on a nerve suture

---

*Terzis describes this technique at greater length in Chapter 45. Bedeschi reports his experience in Chapter 46.

is an essential factor in fibrosis. For this reason he recommends the use of nerve grafts to avoid tension. He has also shown that resection of a collar of epineurium at the suture site decreases connective tissue proliferation.

Surgical trauma represents a further aggression, and less traumatic surgery using microsurgical techniques is a definite contribution in limiting connective tissue proliferation. Use of the microscope has also made possible delicate intraneural neurolyses.

FILLING THE GAP BETWEEN THE NERVE ENDS

The Interfascicular Nerve Graft

As a result of Millesi's work there is currently an interest in "rehabilitating" nerve grafts. Millesi believes that passing a graft through the two suture zones represents less of an obstacle to axonal regrowth than passing through a simple suture under tension (Millesi, 1968; Millesi et al., 1972). He has shown that a nerve graft taken from a subcutaneous sensory nerve in the same subject (most often the sural nerve) offers the best practical possibility of recovery (Millesi, 1977, 1980). It is certain that his technique carried out under microscopic control, using several thin grafts, each of an appropriate length for the different damaged fascicle groups, and "step cutting" the ends has notably improved results in comparison with those with larger traditional grafts (Fig. 41–4).* However, the "routine" graft, which

---
*Described in Chapter 55.

he suggests when the loss of substance exceeds 2 cm., remains controversial.

Secondary suturing still has its partisans when loss of substance is moderate. The amount of substance loss that can be tolerated is difficult to evaluate. It varies according to the site and the judgment of the surgeon. If a graft is decided upon it is essential to avoid grafting under tension and after extensive mobilization of the nerve ends, which can bring all the disadvantages together. Statistics (Gelmacher and Albers, 1981) show that the quality of the result varies inversely with the length of the graft, but the result seems to depend more on the amount of loss of nerve substance than on the length of the graft (Millesi, 1984).

Vascularized Nerve Graft

Recent progress in microsurgery permits free vascular nerve grafts and seems to be valuable particularly when the graft is long and the nerve bed is fibrous and of poor quality (Taylor and Ham, 1976) (see Chapter 57).

Other Procedures Designed to Fill the Gap Between the Divided Nerve Ends

In addition to nerve grafting several procedures have been described to fill the gap between separated nerve ends. Hand surgeons should be familiar with these procedures, as well as their indications and limitations, the latter being related to the site of the lesion and the quality of the blood supply.

Traction on the Nerve Ends. Simple traction on the nerve extremities can be used

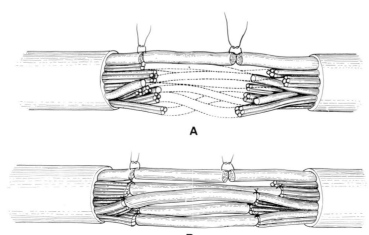

A

B

Figure 41–4. Interfascicular nerve grafts (Millesi). *A*, Microscopic dissection identifies several apparently corresponding fascicular groups on the two nerve ends. *B*, Several fascicular groups are brought together, in order to reduce the number of bridge grafts to four or five or sometimes less, according to the nerve and the level of the repair.

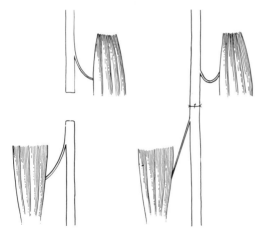

Figure 41–5. If there is a nerve gap to be closed by epineural suture and distal and proximal muscular branches are present, the distal muscular branch will be under tension and the proximal branch will be relaxed.

only to close short gaps of 3 cm. or less, this figure varying from one surgeon to another. The tension at the suture line should be no greater than the breaking point of a 10–0 suture.

Mobilization of the Nerve Ends. Mobilization of the nerve ends by means of careful epineural dissection under microscopic visualization sometimes can achieve a gain of 3 to 4 cm., but care must be taken not to jeopardize the blood supply of the nerve, and the dissection should not be carried beyond 6 to 8 cm. despite the existence of the endoneural microcirculation.*

The presence of collateral branches close to the suture tends to restrict the mobilization, especially if they lie distally. Intraneural dissection of the motor fibers proximal to the suture sometimes can provide extra play (Fig. 41–5).

Flexion of the Joints. When the nerve lies on the flexor side, flexion of the joints also can yield a gain of several centimeters. Thus flexion of the wrist can give an extra 3 cm. and flexion of the elbow, an extra 5 cm., but it must be pointed out that the ulnar nerve can benefit only from elbow flexion if it is first transposed anteriorly. However, extension of the joints after suturing stretches the nerve, and this, if done too rapidly, can produce intraneural fibrosis. For this reason, extension must be progressive during the stage of cicatrization and not exceed 10 degrees a week.

---

*See the chapter by Lundborg in Volume I.

Transposition of the Nerve. At certain sites some gain can be achieved by transposing the nerve. Thus the ulnar nerve can be transposed to the anterior aspect of the elbow (Fig. 41–6), the median nerve in front of the pronator teres, and the terminal motor branch of the ulnar nerve lateral to the hamate in the carpal tunnel (Boyes, 1955).

Shortening the Skeleton. Shortening the skeleton is useful when the nerve division is associated with a fracture or a pseudarthrosis or during replantation after amputation.

Nerve Transfers. Finally, nerve transfers or *neurotizations* are possible when the motor or sensory function to be restored justifies the sacrifice of a healthy nerve. It must contain a significant number of fibers analogous to those to be replaced. Neurotizations, which require one or more intercostal nerves, are now commonly utilized in the treatment of brachial nerve lesions.*

Other transfers are possible at all levels, although they are uncommonly indicated: thus, rami originating from the third and fourth cervical roots, the spinal accessory nerve, or even the proximal stump of C5 can be transferred in brachial nerve lesions. In the arm the musculocutaneous nerve (beyond the point where it supplies the biceps) has been used with success to repair the radial or median nerve. In the forearm the anterior sensory branch of the radial nerve has been transferred onto the medial nerve, and Strange (1947) has described a procedure (which we have used successfully on several occasions for a "pedicled nerve graft") whereby the ulnar nerve is transferred onto

---

*Described in Chapter 62.

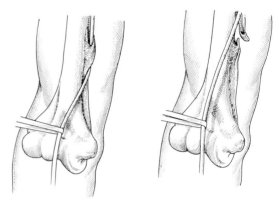

Figure 41–6. Transposition of the ulnar nerve at the elbow. Division of the intermuscular septum may gain additional length.

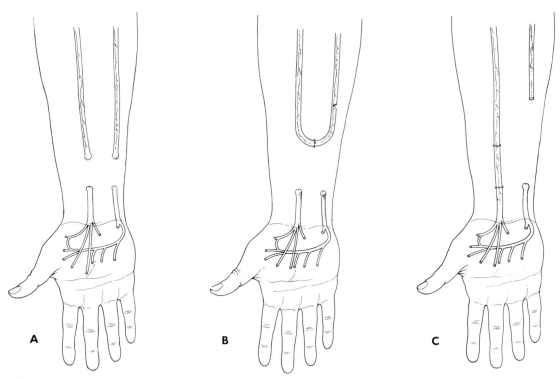

Figure 41–7. Pedicled nerve graft of St. Clair Strange. *A*, Division of the ulnar and median nerves with a significant loss of nerve resulting in a large defect. *B*, The distal end of the proximal stump of the ulnar nerve is sutured to the distal end of the proximal stump of the median nerve. The ulnar nerve is partially divided proximal to the anastomosis, leaving intact a segment of epineurium that carries the longitudinal blood vessels. *C*, Six months later. The distal segment of the ulnar nerve is then separated and used as a graft to bridge the defect in the median nerve.

the median nerve, allowing the bridging of a gap of up to 10 cm. long (Fig. 41–7). In the hand the nerve of the third lumbrical muscle has been transferred to the thenar branch of the median (Fig. 41–8) (Schultz and Aiache, 1972), and the sensory nerve of one digit has been sutured to a functionally more useful collateral nerve.

Evaluation of Results

It is difficult to choose among these methods. Only by comparing the results in equivalent series in terms of age, nature of the lesions, site, timing of surgery, and technique used may help be obtained in selecting one or another method. And this is where we fall into further difficulties inherent in the evaluation of results. This is a long term process, and many surgeons have become fatalistic as a result of their partial or total failures. It is now proved that recovery continues for about four years from the repair (Önne, 1962; Marsh and Barton, 1987). Muscle power can be scored on the M.C.R. (Medical Research

Council, 1954) 0 to 5 scale, but we still lack objective tests to measure sensation (see

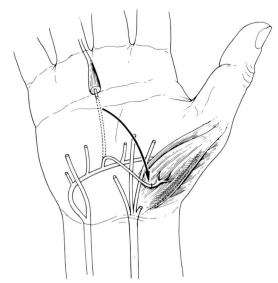

Figure 41–8. The motor branch to the lumbrical of the ring finger is divided as distally as possible and sutured directly to the thenar motor branch of the median nerve.

Chapter 47). Besides, anatomical variations, anastomoses and overlapping of nervous territories may well explain a number of pseudosuccessful "reinnervations." These problems are dealt with in Chapter 51 by Sir Sydney Sunderland.

TRAUMATIC LESIONS OF THE BRACHIAL PLEXUS

Thanks to the courage and tenacity of some pioneers, we now operate directly on brachial plexus lesions, which have increased with the rise in motorcycle accidents. Suturing, nerve grafting, neurolysis, and neurotization now bring hope of partial, if limited, recovery that only a few years ago was inconceivable. Such surgery is highly delicate and time consuming. Alnot, Millesi, Narakas, Morelli, Sedel and Wynn Parry describe their experience in Chapters 59 to 65. These chapters discuss the current art of management of traumatic lesions of the brachial plexus. They demonstrate that nerve surgery should be performed early—if possible no later than three or four months following the injury and preferably during the two first months.

THE EVOLUTION OF NERVE REPAIR MANAGEMENT

One is now able to have an overview of the evolution of the ideas and techniques related to the treatment of peripheral nerves. Many concepts appear contradictory and serve to confuse the surgeon's mind: primary or secondary suture, mandatory nerve grafts, epineural or perineural suture, with or without the use of microscope. However, in the main part, the situation is now clear. Routine secondary suture as recommended by Seddon is no longer the first line treatment and is only performed when primary suture is contraindicated. Routine secondary nerve grafting has not proved superior to primary repair, when this is feasible. However, Millesi has clearly shown that interfascicular cable grafts give better results than either trunk grafts or direct suture under tension. Either epineural or perineural suture can be chosen according to the nerve involved and the level of the repair. Magnification is now used routinely.

It has been the hope of many surgeons that the use of microsurgical techniques would be a turning point in the treatment of peripheral

nerve lesions. The increased use of the microscope has not led to a parallel increase in good results, with occasional disappointment. Expectations were too great and perhaps without sufficient basis. There is no doubt that there is still a high percentage of failures and imperfect results.[*]

Nevertheless the results of nerve repair techniques have progressively improved in recent years as shown by the example of a few surgeons who have had much practice in dealing with such lesions. By contrast, the results remain the same for those who perform such surgery only occasionally. Use of the microscope cannot miraculously improve the technique and results overnight, and it is essential to emphasize the lengthening apprenticeship required. Such opposition as exists is between surgeons with wide experience in nerve repair and others with less experience. Microsurgery is no panacea for all the problems of peripheral nerve surgery, as stressed by Narakas (1979) in a provocative editorial entitled "Why Is My Peripheral Nerve Surgery so Poor?" Although the reestablishment of axonal continuity does not guarantee functional recovery, it is obviously a necessary prerequisite. It is also very important to take note of the *other factors* which influence prognosis.

In a study comparing the results of two series of repairs of the median and ulnar nerves in the forearm by the same surgeon using either standard epineural techniques without the microscope in one group or epi- and perineural microscopic suture in the other, Marsh and Barton (1987) note that the age of the patient and the delay from injury to repair have much more influence on recovery than use of the microscope. All authors note the importance of these two factors (see Chapter 50), but few have evaluated the role of associated lesions.

The nerve lesion constitutes only one part of the wound, the viability of surrounding tissues having a significant influence on prognosis. Merle and Michon have been able (see Chapter 58) to demonstrate clearly the beneficial effect of vascular repair on the results of nerve repair. Thus, there is an imperative need to repair both nerve and vessels as an emergency, rather than delaying surgery until a time convenient to the surgeon.

Other factors also influence the quality of

---

[*]The factors influencing that prognosis are considered in Chapter 47.

the results. Individual factors influence functional recovery. The re-establishment of functional circuits depends essentially but not entirely on the number of regenerated axons that reach maturity. The potential for nerve recovery varies in each patient. "It is clear that it is not so much how nerve tissue is available, but what one does with what is available that decides function" (Wynn Parry, 1984). One observation from Alain Gilbert (1986) is particularly significant. He has found, following ulnar nerve repair in children, that he obtained 80 per cent functional recovery of intrinsic muscles in the dominant limb, but only 30 per cent on the nondominant side. These figures suggest that the connections are re-established more readily on the side that has greater use in children. Although age is a major factor influencing sensory and motor recovery, other factors are also involved. Re-education and motivation of the patient following a nerve injury have an influence on recovery not previously realized. This emphasizes the value of pre- and postoperative care and individual efforts at readaptation. The development of abnormal positions must be avoided at all costs by using postural splints, with every effort made to maintain the mobility of all joints and the power of nonparalyzed muscles. Electrical stimulation of denervated muscles has failed to prove its worth and is little used today. Physiotherapy based upon regular exercise will prevent wasting and maintain the patient's morale and his will to achieve a successful result. Use of the limb must be maximally encouraged; this represents the best means for preventing pain. After repair of mixed nerves, especially the median nerve, sensory rehabilitation, which consists of the learning by the cerebral cortex of a new code of information by the use of repetitive exercises, improves the functional results (Wynn Parry, 1978; Dellon and Curtis, 1971).

BASIC RESEARCH CONTRIBUTION

While the surgeons were looking for more and more sophisticated techniques, much remarkable research was being done on many aspects of peripheral nerve physiology, intraneural microvascularization, histochemistry, molecular biology, electromicroscopy, and reovery of sensation, among others.

Some of these studies have been reported in Volume I (see Chapters 55, 56, and 57 by E. Peacock, M. Jabaley, and G. Lundborg). The following chapters in this volume (Chapters 42, 43, 44, 45, and 46) will illustrate some other aspects of this research activity.

This new information has changed our knowledge of the complex biological systems and mechanisms involved in axon regeneration and functional recovery. Better communication and collaboration between scientists and clinicians interested in peripheral nerves will suggest ways of overcoming persisting difficulties.

What help can the surgeon expect from the therapeutic standpoint? He seeks the answer to a number of questions:

Must the nerve ends be coapted?

Are there neurotrophic factors which facilitate regenerating axons to selectively seek out the proper endoneurial tubes?

How can we minimize the wasteful loss of axons during regeneration?

What is the value of synthetic biodegradable nerve guides?

How can one distinguish sensory and motor nerve fibers at operation?

Can axon growth be improved by effective acceleration?

How can connective tissue proliferation be controlled at the repair site in order to facilitate the passage of regenerating axons and at the same time restore the tensile strength of the nerve?

Is nerve homografting possible with the help of immunosuppressive therapy?

How can one accurately investigate sensory recovery?

"Embryonic" answers already exist. Immense progress remains to be made. This can result only from multidisciplinary cooperation and the refinement of surgical and electrophysiological techniques. All suggest the desirability of grouping the treatment of peripheral nerve lesions in specially equipped centers.

A multicenter study of peripheral nerve injuries is currently being organized. By using a standard protocol, all clinical information will be computer analyzed. It is hoped that the analysis of such data will provide answers to some of the many questions in this field.

The frequent sequelae of such lesions, all the more severe when the lesions are proximal, may be considerably improved by secondary reconstructive surgery, described in Volume IV.

REFERENCES

Albert, E.: Einige Operationen an Nerven. Wien. Med. Presse, 26:1285, 1885.

Alnot, J. Y., Huten, D., Largier, A., and Henin, D.: Réparation primitive des plaies tronculaires des nerfs mixtes. Ann. Chir., 32(9):527–535, 1978.

Arnemann, J.: Versuche über die Regeneration der Nerven. Vandenhoech et Ruprecht, Göttingen, 1787.

Baudens, J. B. L.: Clinique des plaies d'armes à feu. Paris, Baillière, 1836.

Bonnel, F., Mailhe, P., Allieu, Y., and Rabischong, P.: Bases anatomiques de la chirurgie du nerf médian au poignet. Ann. Chir., 34(9):707–710, 1980.

Bora, F W., Pleasure, D. E., and Didizan, N. A.: A study of nerve regeneration and neuroma formation after suture by various techniques. J. Hand Surg., 1:138, 1976.

Bourrel, P.: L'exploration itérative avec neurolyse interfasciculaire après réparation primitive des lésions des nerfs de la main. Méd. Trop., 30(3):672–679, 1970.

Bourrel, P.: Techniques de sutures nerveuses. Médecine et Armées, 6:243–246, 1978.

Bourrel, P., Ferro, R., and Lorthioir, J. M.: Résultats cliniques comparés des sutures nerveuses "mixtes" péri-épineurales et des sutures névrilemmatiques. Ann. Chir., 35(4):286–294, 1981.

Boyes, J. H.: Repair of the motor branch of the ulnar nerve in the palm. J. Bone Joint Surg., 37A:920, 1955.

Braun, . W.: Comparative studies of neurography and sutureless peripheral nerve repair. Surg. Gynecol. Obstet., 122:15–18, 1966.

Brooks, D.: The place of nerve grafting in orthopaedic surgery. J. Bone Joint Surg., 37A:299, 1955.

Buck-Gramcko, D.: Discussion. Symposium: Indication, technique and results of nerve grafting. Vienna, May 22, 1977. Handchirurgie, Sonderheft n° 2.

Bunge, R. P.: Cytological factors influencing nerve growth and regeneration. Proc. 6th Int. Congr. of Electromyography, Stockholm, 1979. A. Persson Ed., 87–92.

Bunnell, S., and Boyes, J. H.: Nerve grafts. Am. J. Surg., 44:64, 1939.

Cabaud, H. E., Rodkey, W. G., McCarroll, R. H., Mutz, S. B., and Niebauer, J. J.: Epineural and peripheral fascicular nerve repairs; a critical comparison. J. Hand Surg., 1:131–137, 1976.

Chanson, L., Michon, J., Merle, M., and Delagoutte, J. P.: Etude des résultats de la réparation de 85 nerfs dont 49 gros nerfs. Rev. Chir. Orthop., 63(Suppl. II):153–160, 1977.

Dardour, J. C., and Hamonet, Cl.: Plaidoyer en faveur de la rééducation des troubles de la sensibilité de la main. Ann. Chir., 29(11):999–1004, 1975.

Déjerine, M., and Mouzon, J.: Les lésions des gros troncs nerveux des membres par projectiles de guerre, les différents syndromes cliniques et les indications opératoires. Presse Méd., 23:153, 1915.

Dellon, A. L., Curtis, R. M., and Edgerton, M. T.: Reeducation of sensation in the hand following nerve injury and repair. Plast. Reconstr. Surg., 53:297–305, 1974.

Dellon, A. L.: Evaluation of Sensibility and Reeducation of Sensation in the Hand. Baltimore, Williams and Wilkins, 1981.

Desbonnet, P.: Réparation des nerfs périphériques du membre supérieur. Analyse informatique de 110 cas. Montpellier, Thèse, 1985.

Edshage, S.: Peripheral nerve suture. A technique for improved intraneural topography. Acta Chir. Scand. (Suppl.), 331:1, 1964.

Egloff, D. V., and Narakas, A.: Rapport préliminaire sur l'emploi de la colle fibrine (Tissucol) dans les greffes nerveuses. Ann. Chir. Main, 2:101–115, 1983.

Engel, J., Ganel, A., Melamed, R., Russon, S., and Farine, I.: Choline acetyl transferase for differentiation between human motor and sensory nerve fibres. Ann. Plast. Surg., 4:376–380, 1980.

Foerster, O.: Lecture: Ausserordentliche Tagung der Deutschen Orthopädischen Gesselshaft, Berlin, Feb. 8–9, Münch. Med. Wschr., 63:283, 1916.

Flourens, P.: Expériences sur la réunion ou cicatrisation des plaies de la moelle épinière et des nerfs. Ann. Sci. Nat., 13:113, 1828.

Freillinger, G., Gruber, H., Holle, J., and Mandl, W.: Zur methodik "sensomotorisch" differenzieter Faszielnaht peripherer Nerven. Handchirurgie, 7:133, 1975.

Gilbert, A., and Kaadan, D. G.: Paralysies des muscles intrinsèques des doigts chez l'infant. Communication XXIe Réunion du G.E.M., Paris, Ann. Chir. Main, 53:218–219, 1986.

Gruber, H., and Zenker, W.: Acetyl cholinesterase: histochemical differentiation between motor and sensory nerve fibers. Brain Res. 51:207, 1973.

Hakstain, H. W.: Funicular orientation by direct stimulation. An aid to perhipheral nerve repair. J. Bone Joint Surg., 50A:1178, 1968.

Hentz, V. R., Wikswo, J., and Abraham, G.: Magnetic measurement of nerve action currents: a new intraoperative recording technique. Peripheral Nerve Repair and Regeneration, 1:27–36, 1986.

Jabaley, M. E.: Current concepts of nerve repair. Clin. Plast. Surg., 8:33–44, 1981.

Jabaley, M. E., Wallace, W. H., and Heckler, F. R.: Internal topography of major nerves of the forearm and hand: a current review. J. Hand Surg., 5:1–18, 1980.

Kater, S., and Letourneau, P.: Biology of the Nerve Growth Cone. New York, Alan Liss, Inc., 1985.

Lundborg, G., and Hansson, H. A.: Studies on the growth pattern of regenerating axons in the gap between the proximal and distal nerve ends. In A. Gorio, H. Millesi, S. Mingrino (Eds): Post-traumatic Peripheral Nerve Regeneration. Experimental Basis and Clinical Implications. New York, Raven Press, 1981, pp. 229–239.

Lundborg, G., Dahlin, L. B., Danielsen, N., Gelbergman, R. H., Longo, F. M., Powel, H. C., and Varon, C.: Nerve regeneration in silicone chambers. Influence of gap length and presence of distal stump components. Expl. Neurol., 76:361–375, 1982.

MacFarlane, R. M.: Commentary on "Experimental studies on the effects of tension intraneural microcirculation in sutured peripheral nerves" by Y. Miyamoto, S. Watari, K. Tsuge. J. Plast. Reconstr. Surg., 63(4):564, 1979.

Marsh, D., and Barton, N.: Does the use of the operating microscope improve the results of peripheral nerve suture? J. Bone Joint Surg., 1987 (in press).

Matras, H., Dinges, H. P., Lassmann, H., Mammoli, B.: Wr. Med. Wschr., 37:517, 1972.

Medical Research Council: Peripheral nerve injuries. Spec. Rep. Ser. Med. Res. Coun. No. 282, London, H.M.S.O., 1954.

Merle, M., Amend, P., Foucher, G., and Michon, J. (Rapport de R. Tubiana): Plaidoyer pour la réparation primaire microchirurgicale des lésions des nerfs périphériques. Etude comparative de 150 lésions du nerf médian et du nerf cubital avec un recul supérieur à 2 ans. Chirurgie, *110*(8–9):761–771, 1984.

Michon, J.: Les techniques modernes de réparation des nerfs périphériques. *In* J. Michon, E. Moberg (eds.): Les Lesions Traumatiques des Nerfs Périphériques. Monographies du G.E.M. Expansion Scientifique Française, Paris, 1979, pp. 115–121.

Michon, J., and Masse, P.: Le moment optimum de la suture nerveuse dans les plaies du membre supérieur. Rev. Chir. Orthop. Répar. App. Moteur, *50*:205, 1964.

Millesi, H.: Zum Probem der überbrückung von Defekten periphen Nerven. Wien. Med. Wschr., *118*:182–187, 1968.

Millesi, H., Meissl, G., and Berger, A.: The interfascicular nerve grafting of the median and ulnar nerves. J. Bone Joint Surg., *54A*:727, 1972.

Millesi, H., Meissl, G., and Berger, A.: Further experience with interfascicular grafting of the median, ulnar and radial nerves. J. Bone Joint Surg., *58A*:209, 1976.

Millesi, H.: Looking back on nerve surgery. Int. J. Microsurg., *2*:143–158, 1980.

Millesi, H.: The current state of peripheral nerve surgery in the upper limb. Ann. Chir. Main, *3*:18–34, 1984.

Millesi, H., and Terzis, J. K.: Problems of terminology in peripheral nerve surgery: Committee report of the International Society of Reconstructive Microsurgery. Microsurgery, *4*:51–56, 1983.

Mitchell, S. W., Morehouse, G. R., and Keen, W. W.: Gunshot Wounds and Other Injuries of Nerves. Philadelphia, J. B. Lippincott Co., 1864.

Mitchell, S. W.: On the diseases of nerves resulting from injuries in contributions relating to the causation and prevention of disease and to camp diseases. *In* A. Flint: United States Sanitary Commission Memoirs, New York, 1867.

Miyamoto, Y., Watari, S., and Tsuge, K.: Experimental studies on the effects of tension in intraneural microcirculation in sutured peripheral nerves. Plast. Reconstr. Surg., *63*:398–403, 1979.

Moberg, E.: Future hopes for the surgical management of peripheral nerve lesions. *In* Michon, J., and Moberg, E.: Traumatic Nerve Lesions of the Upper Limb. Edinburgh, Churchill Livingstone, 1975.

Moberg, E.: Sensibility in reconstructive limb surgery. Symposium on the neurologic aspects of plastic surgery, S. Fredericks, G. Brody (Eds.) chapter 4. St. Louis, C.V. Mosby, 1978.

Moberg, E.: Techniques to determine the clinical result of nerve regeneration. 1st Congress of the Int. Fed. of Societies for Surg. of the Hand, Rotterdam, June 17–21, 1980.

Moberg, E.: Traumatic injuries to the brachial plexus. Surg. Clin. North Am., *61*(2):341–351, 1981.

Nageotte, J.: Sur la greffe des tissus morts et en particulier sur la réparation de perte de substance des nerfs à l'aide de greffons nerveux conservés dans l'alcool. Compte-rendu Séanc. Soc. Biol., *80*:459, 1917.

Narakas, A.: Why is my peripheral nerve surgery so poor? Int. J. Microsurg. *1*(2):50–52, 1979.

Omer, G., and Spinner, M.: Management of Peripheral Nerve Problems. Philadelphia, W. B. Saunders, 1980.

Önne, L.: Recovery of sensibility and sudomotor activities in the hand after nerve suture. Acta Chir. Scand. Suppl., 300, 1962.

Philipeaux, J. M., and Vulpian, E. F. A.: Note sur des essais de greffe d'un tronçon du nerf lingual entre les deux bouts de ce nerf hypoglosse, après excision d'un segment de ce dernier nerf. Arch. Physiol. Norm. Pathol., *3*:618, 1870.

Pleasure, D., Bora, F. W., Lane, J., and Prockop, I. D.: Regeneration after nerve transection of collagene synthesis. Exper. Neurol., *45*:72–78, 1971.

Rabischong, P., and Bonnel, F.: Systématisation endoneurale des nerfs du membre supérieur. Réunion du G.E.M., Montpellier, 1975.

Rushworth, G., Dickson, R. A., O'Hara, J., and Tricker, J.: Nerve gap repair and the quality of regeneration. Proc. 6th Int. Congr. of Electromyography. Symposia. Stockholm, June 17–20, 1979. A. Persson (Ed.), pp. 131–136.

Sakellarides, H.: A follow-up study of 173 peripheral nerve injuries in the upper extremity in civilians. J. Bone Joint Surg., *44A*:140, 1962.

Samii, M.: Klinische Resultäte der autologen Nerventransplantation. Med. Mitt. Melsungen, *46*:197–202, 1972.

Schultz, R. J., and Aiache, A.: An operation to restore opposition of the thumb by nerve transfer. Arch. Surg., *105*:777, 1972.

Seddon, H. J.: War injuries of peripheral nerves. Br. J. Surg., War Surgery (Suppl. 2, Wound of the Extremities), 325, 1948.

Seddon, H. J.: Nerve grafting J. Bone Joint. Surg., *45B*:447, 1963.

Seddon, H.: Surgical Disorders of the Peripheral Nerves. Edinburgh, Churchill Livingstone, 1975.

Seddon, H.: Personal letter, 1977.

Sedel, L.: Résultats des greffes nerveuses. Rev. Chir. Orthop. App. Moteur. *564*(4):284–288, 1978.

Smith, J. W.: Microsurgery of peripheral nerves. Plast. Reconstr. Surg. *33*:317, 1964.

Smith, J. W.: Factors influencing nerve repair. II. Collateral circulation of peripheral nerves. Arch. Surg., *93*:433, 1966.

Snyder, C. C., Webster, H. D., Pickens, J. E., Hines, W. A., and Warden, G. D.: Intraneural neurorraphy: A preliminary clinical and histological evaluation. Ann. Surg., *167*:691, 1968.

Spinner, M.: Injuries to the Major Branches of Peripheral Nerves of the Forearm. 2nd ed. Philadelphia, W. B. Saunders, 1978.

Stoffel, A.: Ueber die Behandlung verletzer Nerven im Kriege. Münch. Med. Wschr., *60*:1365, 1915.

Strange, F. G., St. C.: An operation for nerve pedicle grafting. Preliminary Communication. Br. J. Surg., *34*:423, 1947.

Sunderland, S.: Funicular suture and funicular exclusion in the repair of severed nerves. Br. J. Surg., *40*:580, 1954.

Sunderland, S.: Nerves and Nerve Injuries. 2nd ed. Edinburgh, Churchill Livingstone, 1978.

Sunderland, S.: The pros and cons of funicular nerve repair. J. Hand Surg., *4*:201–211, 1979.

Symposium sur les paralysies traumatiques du plexus brachial de l'adulte. J. Y. Alnot, Y. Allieu, F. Bonnel, N. Cadre, F. Bonnel, B. Frot, D. Huten, M. Mansat, H. Millesi, A. Narakas, L. Sedel. Rev. Chir. Orthop., *63*:17–125, 1977.

Taylor, G. I., and Ham, F. J.: The free vascularized nerve graft. Plast. Reconstr. Surg., *57*:413–426, 1976.

Terzis, J. K., Dykes, R. W., and Hakstian, R. W.:

Electrophysiological recordings in peripheral nerve surgery: a review. J. Hand Surg., *1*:52, 1976.

Tinel, J.: Le signe du "fourmillement" dans les lésions des nerfs périphériques. Presse Med., *47*:378–389, 1915.

Tinel, J.: Nerve Wounds. London, Bailliere, Tindall and Co., 1917.

Tsuge, K., Ikuta, Y., and Sakaue, M.: A new technique for nerve suture. The anchoring funicular suture. Plast. Reconstr. Surg., *56*:496, 1975.

Tupper, J.: Fascicular Nerve Repair and Regeneration. Its Clinical and Experimental Basis. St. Louis, C. V. Mosby, 1980, p. 320.

Van de Put, J., Tanner, J. C., and Huypens, L.: Electrophysiological orientation of the cut ends in primary peripheral nerve repair. Plast. Reconstr. Surg., *44*:378, 1969.

Varon, S., and Williams, L. R.: Peripheral nerve regeneration in a silicone model chamber: cellular and molecular aspects. Peripheral Nerve Repair and Regen., *1*:9–25, 1986.

Vespasiani, A., and Biancardi, G.: La sutura dei nervi periferici in chirurgia della mano mediante usi di colla di fibrina. Rev. Chir. della Mano, *17*:235–238, 1980.

Waller, A.: Experiments on the section of the glossopharyngeal and hypoglossal nerves of the frog and observations of the alteration produced thereby in the structure of their primitive fibrils. Phil. Trans. B., *140*:423, 1850.

Wynn Parry, C. B.: The management of peripheral nerve injuries and traction. Lesions of the brachial plexus. In. Rehabil. Med., *1*:9–20, 1978.

Wynn Parry, C. B.: Rehabilitation of the Hand. 4th ed. London, Butterworths, 1981.

Wynn Parry, C. B.: Recent trends in surgery of peripheral nerves. Int. Rehab. Med., *3*:169–173, 1981.

Wynn Parry, C. B.: Symposium on sensation. J. Hand Surg., *9B*(1):4–6, 1984.

ANATOMY, BIOLOGY, AND EXAMINATION

Chapter 42

THE BIOLOGY OF REGENERATION IN PERIPHERAL NERVES

Jean-Claude Mira

It has been a long time since experiments in merotomy demonstrated the trophic function of the cell nucleus. The latter is now known to be essential to cell life, an enucleated cell fragment being incapable of surviving more than a few days. In this respect the nerve cell behaves essentially like other cells. Thus, the cell body is essential for the growth and maintenance of the axon and for the close relationships that exist between the neuron and the tissues it innervates. These relationships are profoundly disturbed by trauma to the nerve, and separation of a nerve fiber from its cell body triggers a chain of events that affects the whole system, i.e., the cell body, the fiber itself, and related effectors or receptors. The structure and function of this system are severely disturbed, and in the most severe lesions the system as a whole may disintegrate.

The absence of protein synthesis within the axon explains why the latter is unable to survive once it is parted from its trophic center. Under normal circumstances it makes up for this deficiency by importing macro-

molecules from satellite cells (e.g., Schwann cells) and by transporting substances synthesized in the perikaryon.

Axonal transport constitutes an essential source of proteins and organelles, which are essential for the maintenance and survival of the axon. Droz and Leblond (1963) were the first to show that most of the axonal proteins are synthesized in the cell body and transported along the axon. This fact emphasizes the amount of work required of the cell body to maintain permanent metabolic equilibrium and ensure the survival of the axon and its terminals. The nature of this equilibrium to a certain extent has been elucidated in the last few years.

The manufacturing activities of the neuron were suspected as far back as 1838 by Remak, who regarded the nucleated cell body as the source of all substances making up the nerve fiber. Later Waller clearly demonstrated the dependence of the axon on the cell body. In 1906 Scott suggested that a substance elaborated in the perikaryon entered the nerve fiber and passed down to its extremities

383

where it took part in impulse transmission. However, it was Weiss and Hiscoe (1943) who were the first to demonstrate, by means of staged ligatures on the nerve fibers, that materials synthesized in the cell body were continually being transported along the axon. In addition to this slow component (1 to 5 mm. per day), which involves the transport of materials concerned with the maintenance and growth of the axon, there is now known to be a second, faster mechanism (150 to 400 mm. per day) for the transport of substances involved in normal synaptic function. Finally a third transport mechanism has been demonstrated, which functions like the latter but in the opposite direction.*

This notion of "neuronal dynamics" is an important one, because it stresses the significance of the intra-axonal traffic of substances synthesized in the cell body, which takes place simultaneously with impulse conduction along the axon membrane (i.e., the axolemma). It has been shown that blocking this flow by means of alkaloids such as colchicine produces the same signs of distal denervation as a section or a crush injury of the nerve fiber. Yet surgeons are called upon more often to treat compressions (e.g., median or carpal tunnel syndrome) by stopping intra-axonal flow than by anatomical transections.

The diagram in Figure 42–1 defines some of the terms which will frequently recur in the descriptions that follow:

Retrograde degneration involves the changes that occur in the proximal stump of the neuron, including the cell body but excluding a short segment immediately proximal to the lesion. This segment undergoes (to use Cajal's terminology) a *traumatic degeneration* which is in every way identical with that affecting the distal stump. The changes are the same regardless of the site and nature of the lesion and are so constant that they can be said to constitute the only universally accepted law of neuroanatomy. This predictable sequence of events is known as *Wallerian degeneration*, in memory of the physician who first described it in the middle of the nineteenth century. It can be defined as all the histological, biochemical, and physiological changes that reflect the inability of the nerve fiber to maintain its structural and functional integrity once it is separated from its cell body.

These changes are definitive and irreversible. Yet, in the course of the ensuing *regeneration,* the relationships between the nerve cells and the tissues they innervate are at least partly restored. Thus when a nerve is damaged, the part of the fibers that are still connected to the trophic center does not degenerate, even if it undergoes certain changes, and soon sends out new axoplasmic outgrowths to replace the lost parts.

An analysis of the disturbances that follow nerve injuries and their possible reversibility is of enormous importance for clinicians because it enables them to repair, by surgical and therapeutic means, the accidental or congenital lesions that affect the integrity of the nervous system and its dependent end organs. For this purpose, it is imperative that the surgeon should be informed of the changes that damage the nerve cells and their dependent effectors and receptors (e.g., muscle fibers), the degree of reversibility of these changes, and the surgical possibilities of improving the quality of the functional recovery.

DEGENERATION

The histopathological consequences of a peripheral nerve lesion depend on a large number of factors, which include the nature, the severity, and the site of the lesion. Seddon (1943) has defined three degrees of nerve injuries:

Neurapraxia implies a temporary interruption of conduction but with no loss of axon continuity and no recognizable morphological changes. Wallerian degeneration does not set in and function is spontaneously and fully recovered.

In *axonotmesis*, axonal continuity is interrupted, but the connective tissue sheaths are intact. A neuroma does not develop. Although Wallerian degeneration involves all the nerve fibers, regeneration progresses normally within the preserved basal lamina tubes and nerve function usually returns.

In *neurotmesis*, the continuity of the whole nerve is broken and the gap between the stumps becomes filled with a neuroma. Some axons do manage to thread their way through the neuroma and succeed in reaching the

---

*For further details, the reader may wish to consult the publications of Droz (1981), Grafstein (1977), Grafstein and Forman (1980), Lasek and Hoffman (1976), Lubinska (1975), and Ocho and Worth (1978).

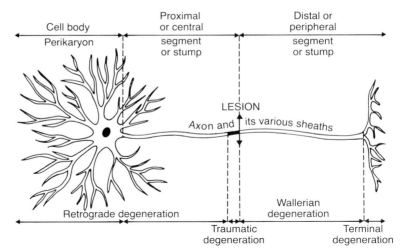

Figure 42–1. Diagrammatic representation of the parts of a nerve cell.

distal stump. The functional recovery is delayed and its quality is profoundly altered because of the absence of a continuous pathway.

Sunderland (1978) has put forward a classification of nerve lesions in order of increasing severity based on the effects rather than the cause of the injury. The first and second degrees correspond to Seddon's neurapraxia and axonotmesis, respectively, and the other three represent subdivisions of neurotmesis according to the site and size of the neuroma.

PRESERVATION OF AXONAL CONTINUITY: CONDUCTION BLOCK

Interruption of nerve conduction, without loss of axonal continuity, can result from compression, from experimental or accidental ischemia, from the action of various therapeutic agents, or from localized cooling. In this type of lesion, the conduction block is restricted to the damaged segment: proximal and distal to that segment, the nerve fiber still responds to electrical stimulation. After a period of inactivity of variable duration, the affected segment recovers full function; there is no Wallerian degeneration and the changes responsible for the nerve block are totally and spontaneously reversible.

INTERRUPTION OF AXONAL CONTINUITY: DEGENERATION

The lesions that interrupt axonal continuity also induce extensive changes within the nerve. These include traumatic and retrograde degeneration proximally to the site of injury, and Wallerian degeneration distally.

Changes in the Proximal Segment

Localized destruction of axons results in the following changes:

Changes in the terminal part of the proximal segment have been described under the names of "ascending degeneration," "indirect Wallerian degeneration," and "traumatic degeneration." We prefer the latter appellation to describe changes that histologically, biochemically, and physiologically are identical to those observed in Wallerian degeneration.

Changes in the cell body of the parental neuron are defined as "chromatolysis" or "axon reaction," a process first described by Nissl at the end of the nineteenth century.

Changes in the nerve cells that bear synaptic relations with the parental neuron are known as "transneuronal degeneration."

Traumatic Degeneration. The region of the nerve immediately proximal to the lesion side undergoes morphological and physiological changes that result directly from the trauma and affect all the nerve fiber components. The severity and extent of these changes vary according to the nature and severity of the lesion and also with the type of fiber involved. If the injury does not rupture the connective tissue sheaths, the changes affect only the first two or three internodal segments (1 to 2 mm.). However, if the continuity of the nerve has been broken, the changes can spread over 4 mm. or more.

These degenerative changes are similar to those observed in the distal segment (Wallerian degeneration), but here they are reversible. Indeed the first manifestations of regeneration are recognizable very soon (they are discussed later on). However, there persists in the affected segment a reduction in the caliber of the nerve fibers and in the conduction velocity (20 to 30 per cent after crash injury; 20 to 40 per cent after sectioning).

Retrograde and Transneuronal Degeneration. After interruption of axonal continuity, the cell body usually undergoes profound structural, metabolic, and physiological changes. These represent the reaction of the parent cell body to sectioning of its axon.*

From the cytological point of view, this "axon reaction," also known as "chromatolysis," is recognizable at a very early stage, usually within a few hours after the lesion is inflicted. The nucleus migrates to the periphery of the cell body; the latter swells at first and then retracts; the Nissl bodies become scattered across the cytoplasm. Outside the cell body, the microglial cells start to proliferate from the second day and there is hypertrophy of the astrocytes. The retraction of the cell body and the glial reaction induce a marked reduction in the number of somatic synapses, which in turn may lead to a deafferentation of the neuron, whose function may be temporarily abolished.

Nevertheless, injury to an axon does not always result in retrograde changes in the parent cell body. In experimental animals, values given for the number of affected neurons vary from 10 to 90 per cent. Accordingly, the range of responses varies considerably: some neurons remained unaffected, others undergo profound changes that often end in cell death or atrophy, and an intermediate group displays responses of varying severity that are partly or fully reversible. The disturbances begin to regress at about the time when the regenerating axons reach their end organs but persist to some degree until axonal maturation is complete (through the third to tenth week or longer). The earliest signs of recovery are the return of the nucleus to the cell center and the reappearance of the compact aggregates of granular endoplasmic reticulum (Nissl bodies). The time elapsing before the onset of recovery

depends on many factors (severity of injury, animal, etc.) but it is usually two to three weeks.

This reactive phase can last several weeks, and its evolution toward reversal to normality or toward neuronal degeneration depends on the reversibility of the axonal injury. If functional regeneration ensues (with re-establishment of appropriate peripheral connections), most of the neurons (85 to 95 per cent) resume a normal appearance, gliosis is reduced, and the synapses reappear. If, however, regeneration is impossible, a large number of neurons degenerate (20 to 75 per cent of the motoneurons in the ventral horns, according to various estimates) and secondary glial proliferation follows. In the most severe lesions, the nerve cells that hold synaptic relations with the cell body of the degenerated neuron can also be affected; this process is known as transneuronal or transsynaptic degeneration (Becker, 1952).

This "axon reaction" probably represents the response of the cell body to information carried from the site of the lesion by "reverse" or "retrograde traumatic" transport (Kristensson, 1984). Indeed within 15 minutes after sectioning there is an accumulation of rapidly transported materials, and one or two hours later some of these materials are carried back to the cell body: this is the "reverse flow," which is different from the normal retrograde flow, whereby intra-axonal materials are transported toward the cell body at a rate of 200 to 300 mm. per day, a rate comparable to that of the rapid anterograde flow.

Changes in the Distal Segment

Despite the more refined techniques now available, the sequence of events that characterizes Wallerian degeneration has not yet been described, let alone elucidated. The results reported in the literature are highly variable and sometimes contradictory. These discrepancies can be partly explained by the fact that the duration of the degenerative process varies with the type of fiber (sensory fibers degenerate faster than motor fibers) and with different types of lesions. The duration also varies with the level of the lesion (the more proximal the lesion, the longer the axon can survive on its metabolic reserves), with the diameter of the fiber (smaller fibers degenerate faster, but the initial diameter of

---

*See the reviews by Lieberman (1974), Grafstein (1975, 1983), and Grafstein and McQuarrie (1978).

a degenerating fiber is difficult to assess), with the structural organization of the level examined (Ranvier's node, myelin or axon), and finally with the distance that separates the segment examined from the actual lesion (the endings degenerate faster than the proximal segments).

It is now universally accepted that Wallerian degeneration advances progressively and centrifugally from the lesion toward the periphery. This is compatible with the hypothesis put forward by Scott at the beginning of the century and taken up and developed more recently by several authors, including Lubinska (1977, 1982): The integrity of the nerve fibers is maintained under the stimulus of a neurotrophic factor, which also inhibits the lytic potentialities of the Schwann cells. This factor is synthesized within the nerve cell body and is carried along the axon by axoplasmic flow. Following nerve injury, this flow is not immediately blocked in the distal stump, but there is a progressive reduction in the amount of the factor arriving from the lesion site; when its concentration falls below a critical level, the Schwann cells become "activated" and induce disruption of both the axon and the myelin sheath. The brief time lag between the injury and the onset of Wallerian degeneration suggests that the trophic factor is transported by rapid anterograde flow.

Wallerian degeneration occurs in two phases. At first there is a conduction block but no recognizable morphological changes, even under electron microscope. This is followed by fragmentation of the axon and myelin.

Axon Degeneration. When the axonal continuity is interrupted, the terminal part of the proximal stump and the whole of the distal stump undergo structural, biochemical, and physiological changes. The earliest manifestation of this degenerative process is the accumulation of various organelles at the extremity of the two stumps, the obvious result of cessation of axonal transports. This is followed by a series of further changes that eventuate in the total disappearance of the axon within 48 to 72 hours and comprise internodal dilation, nodal retraction, accumulation of organelles in the paranodal regions (mitochondria and dense bodies), swelling of the smooth endoplasmic reticulum, disappearance of the neurotubules and neurofilaments, and disintegration of the mito-

chondria. The number of lysosomes increases in parallel with acid phosphatase activity. Finally, disintegration of the axolemma leads to fragmentation of the axon.

Axonal degeneration has important physiological repercussions. Impulse conduction along the axolemma ceases within two to five days in the motor fibers (although it may persist for up to eight days in sensory fibers), resulting in total paralysis of the muscles supplied by the injured fibers.

Myelin Degeneration. The changes in the myelin pass through two successive phases. The first, which lasts about one week, consists essentially of physical fragmentation of the sheath with no significant chemical changes. The second phase, which lasts from the beginning of the second week to the end of the third, is characterized by the chemical breakdown of the myelin with production of cholesterol esters, which are reutilized later in the synthesis of the myelin.

The first physical changes take the form of irregularities within the orderly architecture of the compact myelin; these become noticeable within two hours after a crash injury. The next stages are well known: the terminal swellings of the myelin lamellae retract and coil up, producing a widening of the nodes. The myelin breaks up at the Schmidt-Lanterman incisures, which increase in number. This results in the formation of fragments of various shapes and sizes containing axonal debris and given the name of "digestion chambers." From the third day onward these are found mostly in the cytoplasm of the Schwann cells, which are responsible for the digestion of most of the debris.

The myelin starts to fragment from the second day at the site of the lesion, and this process spreads rapidly toward the periphery. The smallest fibers are affected first, and the degeneration advances at a rate of some 250 mm. a day. When the small fibers have fragmented, the process starts in the larger ones, but here it only progresses at a daily rate of 50 mm. However, three days after sectioning the myelin of some large fibers is still apparently intact (Lubinska, 1977).

The Schwann Cells. The reaction of the Schwann cells is evident within 24 hours after the injury. The nucleoli become clearly visible within the swollen nucleus. The cytoplasm, which is normally scanty except in the perinuclear, nodal, and paranodal regions, increases in volume, becomes vacuolated, and shows a marked increase in inclusions. There is enlargement of the granular endoplasmic reticulum, multiplication of the free ribosomes and polysomes, an increase in the number of mitochondria and lysosomes, the appearance of numerous vacuoles containing axon and myelin debris in different stages of breakdown. The Schwann cells are the site of intense metabolic activity and clearly play an important part in the resorption of the products of nerve fiber degeneration. This very unusual appearance has led to some confusion, because it is difficult to distinguish these "activated" Schwann cells from the macrophages, which also contribute to the scavenging of nervous debris, at least in the vicinity of the lesion.

The Schwann cells multiply actively, and their mitotic activity is greatest when Wallerian degeneration and accumulation of debris are at their peak. This suggests that their proliferation is triggered by a chemical factor released by the breakdown of the axon and/or the myelin, or by physical factors resulting from their fragmentation. The time of maximal mitotic activity of the Schwann cells varies in different species, different nerves, and different fibers within the same nerve (5 to 25 days according to different authors). This activity then drops progressively, and the Schwann cells tend to line up longitudinally within the persisting basal laminae to form the "bands of Büngner," which later act as guidelines for regenerating axons.

The role of Schwann cells in Wallerian degeneration is still not clear and several hypotheses have been put forward. It is reasonable to assume that their contribution is at least twofold:

In the digestion of axon and myelin debris, they behave like true macrophages. Within three days after the injury, the cytoplasm of numerous Schwann cells is seen to contain myelin debris of various shapes and sizes. This suggests that the activated cell is capable of autophagia, because it digests some of its own substance (i.e., myelin) with the help of its own enzymes but cannot phagocytose "alien" myelin. However, it can phagocytose exogenous elements (heterophagia), since axonal debris can be seen among the myelin debris within the so-called "digestion chambers." All this confirms the morphological variability of the Schwann cells during the degeneration of nerve fibers. From the third day onward, apparently two distinct categories of Schwann cells develop—those that help in the digestion of the axon and myelin and that probably were already present within the nerve, and those that are not concerned with the digestive process and are presumably new cells arising from proliferation of the first.

The Schwann cells also aid in the synthesis of the numerous collagen fibrils that invade the scar and endoneural spaces of the distal segment.

The Schwann Cell Basal Laminae. A feature peculiar to the Schwann cell is the basic lamina that covers it and is molded to the cell's shape. In the succession of Schwann cells surrounding each normal myelinated and unmyelinated fiber, the basal lamina forms a narrow tube along the whole fiber and runs uninterrupted from one cell to the next, even at the nodes. The basal lamina together with the adjacent endoneural collagen fibrils are often referred to as "Schwann's tubes" or "endoneural tubes," an extension of the term introduced in 1942 by Holmes and Young to describe the "slough" of the original fiber that persists during degeneration and whose walls are formed by the "neurilemma" and endoneurium.

In the course of Wallerian degeneration, the basal laminae remain intact both in the proximal segment and in the distal segment where they contribute to the formation of the bands of Büngner. For this reason Pease (1960) put forward the concept of the basal lamina as a lasting microskeleton. When the myelin begins to fragment, the fiber takes on a characteristic, moniliform appearance. At the swellings where the debris accumulates, the diameter of the fiber increases manifold, forcing the basal lamina tube to dilate accordingly, even if the latter remains essentially circular in cross section. Between the varicosities, all remains of the initial fiber are the basal lamina and/or some Schwann cells; in such cases, the lumen of the tube is often narrowed and flattened and usually its wall becomes markedly and irregularly folded (Fig. 42–2).

Study of the peripheral nerves and other tissues (skeletal muscles, renal tubules and glomeruli, capillaries, pulmonary tissue, etc.) has demonstrated remarkably similar behavior of the basal lamina under experimental or pathological conditions wherein the trophicity or normal function of the cells it covers is affected. Indeed when the cell (or, in the

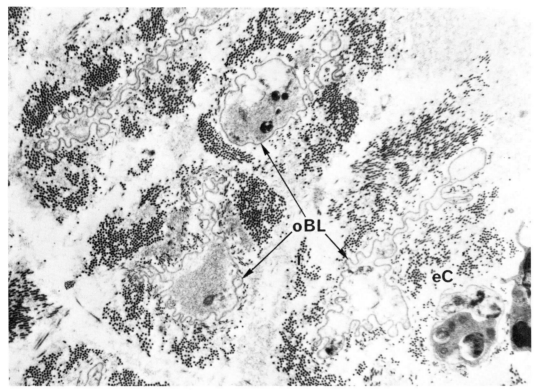

Figure 42–2. Degenerating sciatic nerve of the rat: transverse section through the frozen area (three days after localized freezing). There is some flattening of some segments of the tube formed by the markedly folded old basal lamina. These tubes contain fine granular material and vesicles. The bundles of endoneural collagen fibrils are slightly disorganized while the endoneural spaces are filled with ground substance ($\times$ 9200). eC = endoneural collagen, oBL = old basal lamina.

case of the neuron, part of the cell) must be replaced, the old basal lamina always appears flattened and folded; this is the case with the peripheral nerves (Mira, 1972; Thomas, 1964a), the spinal roots (Nathaniel and Pease, 1963), the muscle fibers and their capillaries (Vracko and Benditt, 1972; Couteaux and Mira, 1984, 1985), and the renal tubules (Cuppage et al., 1967).

The Connective Tissue Sheaths. The perineurium does not appear to undergo major changes except after nerve sectioning, when there is proliferation of the perineural cells attempting to reconstitute the missing part. Some also contribute to the formation of the cicatricial tissue and the neuroma.

The changes in the endoneurium also vary with the nature and severity of the lesion. The conventional light microscope reveals a notable cellular reaction in the necrosed zone. The cell population in a degenerating nerve increases manifold (the number of nuclei can increase up to eightfold), but the

origin of the cells (Schwann cells, fibroblasts, leucocytes, macrophages) has not yet been elucidated. The exact nature of the cells involved in the resorption of axon and myelin debris is still a subject of controversy, but it is probably safe to assume the following:

1. At the site of a traumatic injury where rupture of the basal lamina is observed and a cellular reaction and exudation of leukocytes with edema formation occur, part of the digestion is carried out by exogenous cells (migrating monocytes) and by endogenous cells (macrophages derived from the vascular pericytes, mesenchymatous cells, and histiocytes).

2. In regions of the nerve farther from the lesion, where the basal lamina has preserved its continuity and the vascular reaction is absent or minimal, the scavenging of breakdown products is carried out by endogenous cells (i.e., Schwann cells).

Collagenization of the endoneurium continues for about one year after the injury.

This intense fibrosis results in compression of the bands of Büngner and reduction of the caliber of the fascicles—by 20 to 40 per cent after two months and by 70 per cent after six months. After this time, no significant reduction occurs. The origin of this endoneural collagen is still disputed: it could come from the fibroblasts (Thomas 1964b) or from the Schwann cells themselves (Nathaniel and Pease, 1963). However, it is indisputable that the Schwann cells play a part in the production of collagen (Bunge et al., 1980; Mira, 1972, 1980). This is not surprising if we remember the considerable differences in behavior of the Schwann cells under normal physiological conditions on the one hand and the exceptional circumstances of degeneration and regeneration on the other (intense metabolic activity, mobility, division, autophagia, and heterophagia). However it may be, the laying down of numerous collagen fibrils around the Schwann tubes would appear to constitute one of the main obstacles to the return of normal function after reinnervation.

REGENERATION

All these changes are not permanent, and during regeneration, there is at least partial re-establishment of the relations normally existing between the nerve cells and the tissues they innervate. Within 24 hours after an injury to a peripheral nerve, fine axoplasmic outgrowths issue from the fiber extremity, which has retained its continuity with the cell body. These axonal sprouts penetrate the distal stump and develop along the bands of Büngner. These appear as long strands of Schwann cells, well orientated within the intact basal laminae, which guide them toward the periphery and ensure their myelination. The regenerated axons may ramify in turn, the collaterals always coming off at a node.

Regeneration, however, is never as simple as the foregoing descriptions may suggest. It can be regarded as complete only if the activity of the regenerated nerve is comparable to what it was prior to the injury. Functional recovery results from a combination of complex phenomena depending on central, local, or regional factors. Thus, if regeneration is to succeed, it must restore appropriate connections between the nerve centers and the end organs. For this to occur,

it is essential that each one of the thousands of fibers from the proximal segment cross the scar, return to its original bed, and be guided to the immediate vicinity of its own end organ. Such accurate orientation can be achieved only if the basal laminae remain intact at the lesion site, a situation that obtains after crush injuries but not after nerve sectioning.

For this reason, having studied regeneration in the sciatic nerve of the rat after local crushing and total sectioning we developed a new type of experimental lesion in which the axons were divided without upsetting the organization of the various connective tissue sheaths (Mira, 1972, 1977, 1980). Such a lesion corresponds to axonotmesis (in the classification of Seddon) and to a second degree lesion (Sunderland's classification). The technique, which is readily controlled and perfectly reproducible, consists in localized freezing *in situ*, using a liquid nitrogen cryoprobe at whose tip the temperature is dropped rapidly to about $-180°$ C. The axon and myelin sheath immediately undergo irreversible changes, but the connective tissue sheaths (epineurium, perineurium, endoneurium) and the blood vessels they contain do not appear to be affected by the cold. Moreover, the basal laminae surrounding both the myelinated and unmyelinated fibers run intact through the frozen segment and into the distal stump (Mira, 1971; Basbum, 1973). This technique therefore enables us to study nerve regeneration under extremely favorable conditions.

Regardless of the type of lesion and its severity, the process of regeneration can be divided into four main stages:

1. Return of the nerve cell body to normal from the retrograde effects of the lesion.

2. Axonal regeneration, which involves elongation and sprouting in the proximal segment, crossing of the lesion site, and elongation and sprouting in the distal segment.

3. Restoration of appropriate connections with the end organs.

4. Maturation of the regenerated fibers, i.e., recovery of their anatomical characteristics (number, diameter, distribution) and functional properties.

RECOVERY OF THE NEURON

The onset of regeneration is marked by the resumption of anabolic activities, including protein synthesis, in the damaged neuron. This in turn allows the return of axoplasmic transport and favors axonal elongation, since, as Weiss and Taylor stressed in 1944, the growth of nerve fibers requires a continuous supply of metabolites from the cell body. Any drop in supply results in a slower growth rate, smaller axons, and incomplete myelination. These parameters are only partially controlled by the cell body since experiments on heterologous grafts have shown that the Schwann cells are also involved in the regulation of axon diameter (Aguayo et al., 1977): abnormally small "trembler" mouse axons enlarge and myelinate fully in the presence of normal Schwann cells; by contrast, normal axons regenerating in the presence of "trembler" Schwann cells become thinner and myelin deficient.

Some authors have tried to measure the *latent period*, i.e., the time required for the neuron to recover and enable regeneration to begin. This varies with the site and severity of the injury: the nearer the lesion to the cell body, the more marked the retrograde changes and the longer the recovery time. This is understandable, because the regenerating axons have a greater distance to travel and the end organs go through a longer period of denervation. The relation between the latent period and the severity of the injury, is much more difficult to define. The lesions that do not actually break the continuity of the nerve can be more or less severe, and the degree of severity is almost impossible to quantify. It would appear, however, that the latent period varies in proportion with the severity of the lesion as well as with the type of neuron involved—the sensory neurons, especially those from the spinal ganglia, being affected more rapidly and more severely than the motor neurons. As a rule, the latent period lasts from a few hours to two weeks when the nerve continuity is preserved, but it may be as long as several months after nerve sectioning or avulsion at more proximal levels.

Some modern workers have introduced the notion of "*initial delay*," which is the sum of the latent period and the time required for the regenerating axons to cross the zone of traumatic degeneration. In the sciatic nerve of the rat this initial delay is 1.3 days for adrenergic axons (McQuarrie et al., 1978), 1.6 days for sensory axons (McQuarrie et al., 1977), and 2.2 days for motor axons (Black and Lasek, 1976). These values, however, can vary significantly with the species studied and the type of lesion inflicted.

Retrograde changes consequently can be of great importance and can interfere with the quality of regeneration by limiting the number of available axons, disturbing the function of regenerated fibers and modifying the pattern of activity, thus rendering them less effective. A detailed review of the role of the cell body in regeneration has been published by Cancalon (1984), Forman (1983), Grafstein and McQuarrie (1978), Kristensson (1984), and McQuarrie (1983).

AXONAL REGROWTH TO THE SITE OF LESION

Because the length of the segment affected by traumatic degeneration varies with the lesion and the type of nerve, the extremity of the apparently normal axon inevitably lies at a variable distance from the lesion and from the cell body. Since it is at this level that the first signs of regeneration occur, some axons will have farther to travel toward the lesion site and thence to grow up to the periphery. They all lie within their original basal lamina, which will only have suffered some damage at the site of the lesion.

Within hours of the injury, fine axoplasmic outgrowths appear at the fiber extremity. Microcinematography shows a club shaped axon ending (the "growth cone") alive with short processes capable of ameboid movements. This has been confirmed by scanning electron microscopy. However, it is likely that these first precocious axonal outgrowths degenerate before the onset of the definitive sprouting phase on the second day.

Further development of the axon requires a continuous supply of metabolic material at the growth cone in the same way as the nerve, to preserve its integrity, requires a continuous supply of trophic substances and replacement materials in the axon and its terminals. The rates of protein synthesis and of axonal transport increase in parallel; there is no new mechanism involved but rather an overall adaptation to the needs created by the lesion.

In the proximal stump, regeneration can be detected electrophysiologically within 24 to 36 hours after the lesion and histologically by the second day at the level of the most distal node of Ranvier that remained undamaged (Mira, 1980). It is in fact a heminode since, when the various debris have been

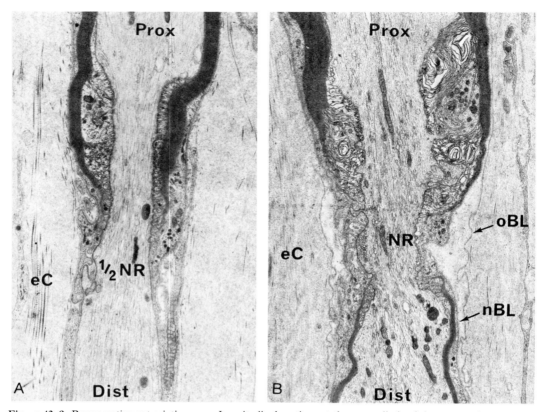

Figure 42–3. Regenerating rat sciatic nerve: Longitudinal sections at the upper limit of the necrosed area.

A, Five days after freezing: When the myelin debris has disappeared, the proximal part of an axon is seen to be ensheathed by normal myelin, while its distal part is not myelinated. This is a hemi-node of Ranvier (× 10,000). Dist = distal segment of nerve fiber, eC = endoneural collagen, ½NR = hemi-node of Ranvier, Prox = proximal part of nerve fiber.

B, Nine days after freezing: Myelination of the regenerating fibers has started by the end of the first week. A reconstituted node of Ranvier can be distinguished, which is made up of two hemi-nodes, a normal complex one proximally and a simpler one distally. The proximal part of the axon is always ensheathed by normal myelin, while the distal part carries only a thin sheath. Note the presence of two distinct basal laminae (× 7800). Dist = distal part of nerve fiber, eC = endoneural collagen, NR = node of Ranvier, nBL = new basal lamina, oBL = old basal lamina, Prox = proximal part of nerve fiber.

resorbed, it is observed that the proximal part of the axon is ensheathed by normal myelin whereas the distal part is not myelinated (Fig. 42–3A). Myelination of the regenerating axons begins toward the end of the first week; it is then noticeable that the proximal segment has a normal myelin sheath whereas distally the sheath is only a few lamellae thick (Fig. 42–3B).

During the first two weeks there is a phase of active axonal sprouting in the necrosed zone and in the distal segment. Although in the normal nerve each myelinated fiber basically consists of a single axon, in the regenerating nerve two myelinated structures are found—"simple" myelinated fibers with a single axon and "compound" fibers made up of

at least two myelinated and several unmyelinated axons (Figs. 42–4 and 42–5). We have continued to use the name *"faisceaux de régénération"* which Nageotte (1922) used to describe the somewhat unusual structures found in the early stages of nerve regeneration (Mira, 1972). Similar structures seen by different authors have been given the names "clusters," "Schwann cell families," and "regenerating units."

In the early stages of regeneration, unusual complex and temporary structures are found consisting of myelinated and umyelinated fibers ensheathed by a common basal lamina. It was generally assumed that these compound fibers result from the sprouting of a single initial fiber, and this has now been

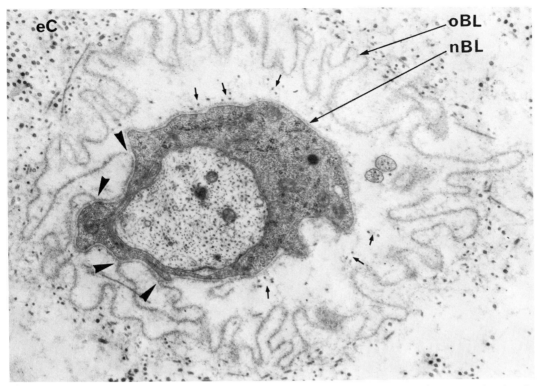

Figure 42–4. Regenerating rat sciatic nerve: Transverse section in the necrosed segment (nine days after freezing). The old basal lamina shows gross foldings, while the new one closely outlines the Schwann cell. Note the junctions between new and old basal laminae (*arrowheads*). A number of collagen fibrils run longitudinally in the extracellular spaces between the laminae (*arrows*) (× 19,800). eC = endoneural collagen, nBL = new basal lamina, oBL = old basal lamina.

confirmed by electron microscopic examination of semiserial sections made after localized freezing (Mira, 1972, 1980).

At the upper border of the necrosed area, some fibers, from the second day onward, begin to ramify actively within the intact basal lamina, which has resisted the freezing. This is the old basal lamina tube that still runs parallel to the fiber axis but now presents numerous folds of varying depth; the Schwann cell plasma membrane is therefore no longer in close apposition to the base of the deepest gutters (Fig. 42–4). The axonal tip gives off one (Figs. 42–3A and B) or more (Fig. 42–6A) terminal outgrowths of various sizes. More distally, in the regenerated segment, collaterals originate always at the level of a node of Ranvier (Fig. 42–6B). All these sprouts develop within the old basal lamina tube and form a *faisceau de régénération*. The bare peripheral axons are progressively wrapped with cytoplasmic expansions from the Schwann cells and thus acquire their own

individual Schwann sheath. By the fifth day short segments of the new basal laminae with free extremities form in close contact with the Schwann cell plasma membrane parts not covered by the old tube. By the sixth day, these new segments link up with the old ones so that the Schwann cell is now ensheathed by a continuous basal lamina closely enveloping its plasma membrane. Longitudinal collagen fibrils then appear within the extracellular spaces created between the two basal laminae (Fig. 42–7). These fibrils are at first scanty and thinner than those of the adjacent endoneurium, but they soon increase in number and in thickness. By now the small cluster of regenerating axons has become a *faisceau de régénération*. Myelination begins around some of the axons by the end of the first week, and the process, although uneven, is essentially similar to that described by Geren (1954) in the course of normal growth. By the fourth week the old basal lamina, which still encloses all the fibers of a *faisceau de*

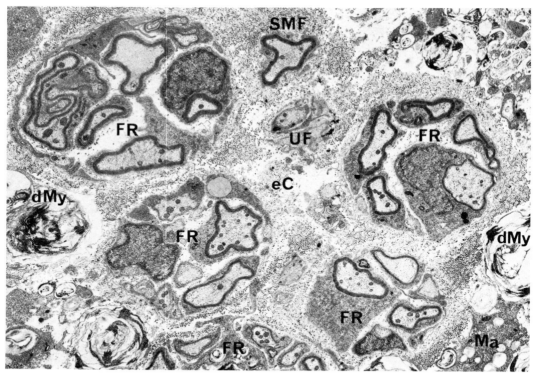

Figure 42–5. Regenerating rat sciatic nerve: Transverse section in the necrotic area (15 days after freezing). Several *"faisceaux de régénération"* are scattered among unmyelinated fibers and "simple" myelinated fibers, some degenerating and others regenerating ($\times$ 4300). dMY = degenerating myelin, eC = endoneural collagen, FR = *faisceau de régénération,* Ma = macrophage, SMF = "simple" myelinated fiber, UF = unmyelinated fiber.

régénération, disintegrates and allows the release of new fibers into the endoneural spaces (Mira, 1980, 1981). These fibers are not all myelinated and the "bare" ones soon degenerate. Thus, although the number of axonal outgrowths is some six to seven times greater than in the normal nerve, the eventual number of regenerated and fully myelinated fibers is only one and one-half to two times the original number (Mira, 1976a, 1977).

The evolution of Schwann cell basal laminae, as observed over time on semiserial ultrathin sections, shows that each *faisceau de régénération* is in fact a morphological entity made up of all the terminal and collateral sprouts originating from a single myelinated fiber and confined for three or four weeks within a common basal lamina; it is the old tube that covers the original healthy myelinated fiber. In addition, the formation and evolution of the *faisceaux de régénération* explain the increase in number of myelinated fibers within regenerating peripheral nerves. They also reveal that the Schwann cell is responsible for its own basal lamina and that it can in fact give rise to new ones under

certain experimental or pathological conditions. Finally, these investigations confirm the important part played by the Schwann cells in the production of endoneural collagen fibrils during regeneration.

Axonal sprouting is not restricted to the regenerating zones. At the beginning of the second week, new fine collaterals can be seen originating in the proximal stump that remained apparently normal, some 3 to 4 mm. proximal to the upper limit of necrosis (Mira, 1976a, 1980, 1981). It is worth stressing that these small sprouts can only be seen during the second postoperative week, whereas sprouting appears in the necrosed area by the second day.

There are at least two possible explanations for this apparent difference between the visualization times of two phenomena whose evolution is similar even though they occur in different zones of the nerve:

1. The whole "machinery" of the neuron is geared at first toward the rapid replacement of damaged parts of the nerve. To this end, the axon must ramify and grow lengthwise toward the necrosed area and the distal seg-

ment of the nerve. It requires some time therefore (i.e., that needed by the outgrowths to reach their end organs) before the cell body can promote the formation and growth of fine collaterals in the apparently normal part of the damaged nerve.

2. The existence of a deliberately "belated" compensatory mechanism to make up for possible faulty regeneration distally. However it may be, the fine collaterals that originate within the basal lamina of the parent fiber develop proximodistally, join the more distal sprouts, and contribute to the formation of a *faisceau de régénération*.

CROSSING OF THE LESION SITE AND GROWTH IN THE DISTAL SEGMENT

Preserving the Continuity of the Connective Tissue Sheaths

When the continuity of the connective tissue sheaths (especially the basal laminae) has not been too severely damaged by the lesion (as is the case after a crash injury), regener-

ating fibers usually cross the injury zone without much ado. Because the axon is usually confined within its original tube throughout the period of regrowth, regeneration tends to occur in a relatively orderly way along the path of the old nerve and in the midst of Schwann cells orientated in longitudinal columns. Despite the relatively severe fibrosis that tends to narrow the bands of Büngner throughout the regenerating zone, restoration proceeds until it is complete because the axons inevitably reach the end organs they innervate prior to the injury. The pattern of innervation is about the same as the original one, and nerve function is restored. Under our own experimental conditions (i.e., crushing of the sciatic nerve shortly after its entry into the sciatic fossa, and controls at standard levels of the nerve to the medial head of the gastrocnemius muscle, the contralateral nerve being used as control), the number of regenerated and fully myelinated fibers average 115 ± 7 per cent and the diameter 80 per cent of the control even two years after the injury (Mira, 1976a).

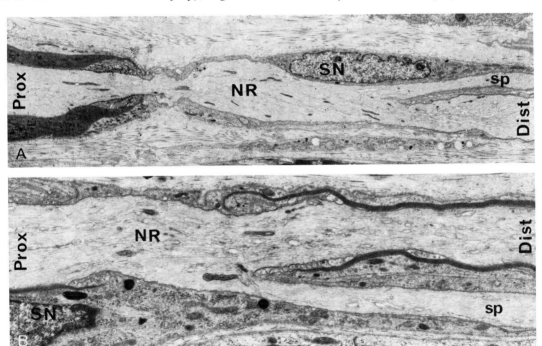

Figure 42–6. *A*, Regenerating rat sciatic nerve: Longitudinal sections passing through nodes of Ranvier and showing collateral sprouting.

A, Five days after freezing: At the upper limit of the necrotic area, a collateral sprout is seen coming off a reconstituted node of Ranvier. It is thinner than the parent axon, unmyelinated, and confined within the Schwann cell cytoplasm of the fiber that gives rise to it. Note that the proximal part of the parent axon has a normal myelin sheath, while the distal part lies within a much thinner sheath (× 4000).

B, Thirteen days after freezing. Another instance of axonal outgrowth at a node in the distal part of the frozen zone (× 9750). Dist = distal segment of the fiber, NR = node of Ranvier, Prox = proximal segment of the fiber, SN = Schwann cell nucleus, sp = axonal outgrowth.

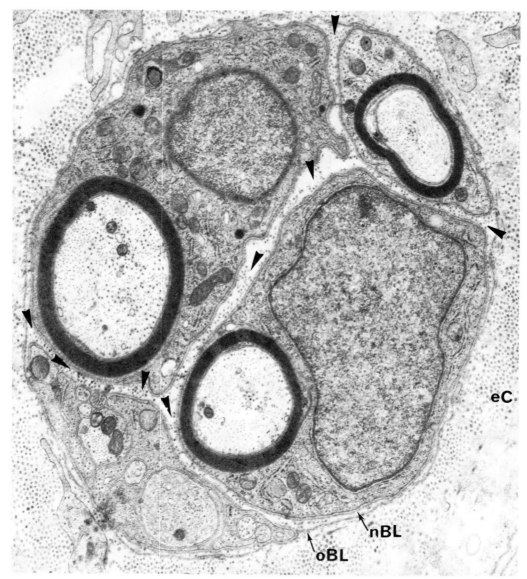

Figure 42–7. Regenerating rat sciatic nerve: Transverse section in the segment frozen 11½ days earlier. A "*faisceau de régénération*" contains 12 axons, only three of which are myelinated. Note that the entire bundle shares a common basal lamina. Each fiber has its own basal lamina sheath formed partly by the old one and partly by the new one. Also note the presence of fine longitudinal collagen fibrils (*arrowheads*) in the extracellular spaces lying between the two basal laminae (× 21,800). eC = endoneural collagen, nBL = new basal lamina, oBL = old basal lamina.

The situation is somewhat different after localized freezing, since the continuity of the basal laminae is fully preserved (Mira, 1971). This facilitates the crossing of the cicatrix for all the regenerating axons that do not have to force their way across a hostile environment. They are guided down to the immediate vicinity of the effectors or receptors of the original nerve. The number of regenerated and myelinated fibers here averaged 125 ± 7 per cent of the control values, and their diameter is almost the same by the beginning of the second year (Mira, 1977). However, although the action potentials show a normal amplitude halfway through the first year (Mira and Pécot-Dechavassine, 1971), the conduction velocity after one year is still 20 per cent below the control value (Mira and Bondoux-Jahan, unpublished study), a possible reason being the shortening of the internodes.

Break in Continuity of the Connective Tissue Sheaths

Sectioning of a nerve implies a break in the continuity of the basal laminae, and this in turn introduces a series of complications that adversely affect the quality of functional recovery and make failure more probable than success.

In the proximal zone undergoing traumatic degeneration and in the distal stump of the severed nerve, there is not only the intense mitotic activity in the Schwann cells mentioned earlier but also active proliferation of the endoneural fibroblasts and perineural cells. There is in addition a vascular reaction resulting in marked edema and swelling of the nerve extremities whose diameters can be two or three times greater than normal.

After sectioning of the nerve, the two stumps come apart, the length of the gap varying with the length of nerve destroyed. Whether or not the distance between the stumps allows suture, the gap becomes invaded by cicatricial tissue of a variable structure, density, and structural organization which has a considerable influence on the future of the nerve. The actively dividing Schwann cells become mobile and migrate toward the gap from both stumps. Also present are perineural cells and numerous endoneural and epineural fibroblasts, which have proliferated at the site of the lesion. There are in addition numerous capillaries (intra-neural and extraneural) emanating from the extremities of the nerve, as well as numerous leukocytes and macrophages, which may be of endogenous or exogenous origin. The latter are the consequence of the inflammatory reaction and the infection resulting from the absence of a continuous perineural barrier. Collagen, which abounds in the bridging tissue, also plays a significant role as the fibrils have a random orientation that interferes with the advance and orientation of the regenerating axons. Several authors have shown that experimental reduction of the amount of scar collagen does assist regeneration (Bora et al., 1972; Lane et al., 1972; Pleasure et al., 1974).

As soon as they leave the proximal stump, where regeneration has progressed under favorable conditions, the axons suddenly find themselves in a new environment constituted by the cicatricial tissue that bridges the gap, yet the axonal outgrowths have to force their way across this hostile environment. It is not surprising therefore that functional recovery is never complete after nerve section regardless of whether surgical repair (grafting or suturing) is attempted. Indeed, the confusion at the scar is such that the ultimate destiny of the axons can be severely affected.

Some fibers escape from the cicatricial tissue but end up in the adjacent tissues. Others fail to clear the barrier, remain confined in the cicatricial tissue, and become involved in a neuroma. Still others succeed in reaching the distal stump where they had more suitable conditions for growth and advance toward the periphery. They do not all develop within a basal lamina appropriate to their function, and many colonize a tube other than the one they occupied prior to the section. These "alien" tubes may or may not guide the axons to an appropriate end organ, and this is, of course, of considerable significance for successful regeneration and functional recovery.

It is not surprising therefore that the original pattern of innervation is never restored after sectioning. In our own experimental studies, when transection was followed by immediate suturing, the number of myelinated regenerated fibers was on average 150 ± 30 per cent of those in the control nerve, and the diameter averaged 50 per cent. When resuturing was not carried out, the number of fibers was 130 ± 32 per cent and the diameter 60 per cent of the control values (Mira, 1976a). Even though the number of regenerated fibers is high as a result of the active ramification of the successful axons, their diameter is markedly reduced, probably as a result of the abundance of collagen deposited in the endoneural spaces.

The Basal Laminae in Regeneration

It is important, finally, to emphasize the essential part played by the basal laminae in the course of regeneration. In 1974 Vracko stated that whatever the tissue studied (peripheral nerve, skeletal muscle, lung, kidney, blood vessel), at least three conditions must be satisfied for anatomical and functional recovery to be complete:

1. The new cells and the extracellular structures must be laid down in such a way that their relations are the same as before the lesion (Vracko, 1974). In peripheral nerves, the basal lamina forms a real frontier between the fiber and the endoneurial spaces filled by connective tissue, keeping the fiber within a suitable microenvironment whose modifications might be detrimental to its function. In addition, the basal lamina seems to possess some degree of polarity; thus, the regenerating axons that succeed in reaching the distal stump of a severed nerve can continue to grow only if they enter a basal lamina tube. Those that fail to find their way into such a tube soon perish.

2. The replacement cells should be of the same type as those present prior to the lesion. The basal lamina seems to have some affinity for certain types of cells. Some authors believe that specific markers are present on its inner face and are identified by a given type of cells as being of that type. This would seem to be confirmed by the fact that proliferating muscle cells do not recognize the basal lamina of renal cells (Vracko, 1974).

In peripheral nerves, it has been suggested that the tissues of the distal stump exert some attraction on regenerating axons, thus reducing the number of axons that become lost or blocked at the suture line. In mammals, however, the growth of proximal fibers and their penetration into the distal tubes are apparently nonselective. There is no evidence of chemotaxis or of a particular affinity of the axons for their original pathways. Thus, the motor and sensory fibers are incapable of selecting the tube that could lead them to an end organ appropriate to their function. For example, the motor fibers supplying a flexor muscle may become scattered at random among alien tubes leading to an extensor muscle or to sensory receptors. These stray fibers continue to grow, but their maturation suffers; such axons never achieve full growth and myelination, but they may still recover useful function (Sunderland, 1978).

3. The number of replacement cells should be roughly the same as the normal state. In this respect, the basal lamina seems to play a part in the initiation and control of cell multiplication. Thus, when the basal lamina of a muscle, lung, or kidney is exposed, the cells proliferate as long as a segment of the tube remains empty. The absence of bared surface would appear to be a negative signal for the arrest of tissue restoration (Vracko, 1974).

In peripheral nerves, however, there is no evidence that the basal lamina is involved in the initiation or arrest of Schwann cell multiplication. But this possibility cannot be excluded, for the basal laminae of the distal stump persist long enough to allow the Büngner's bands formation, and the intense proliferation of Schwann cells ceases only when the tubes have been filled with new cells. However, it remains to be proved that the initiation and arrest of Schwann cell divisions are controlled by basal laminae.

RATE OF REGENERATION

The rate of regeneration can be defined as the rate of growth of the axonal outgrowths. This corresponds roughly to the speed of the slow component of orthograde axonal transport, i.e., 1 to 5 mm. per day. This has been measured using histological, physiological, electrophysiological, and autoradiographical techniques. In mammals this varies between 2 and 5 mm. per day after crushing and 1 to 4 mm. after sectioning (Graftstein and McQuarrie, 1978). After localized freezing the rate is 4.12 ± 0.06 mm. per day.

All fibers, however, do not regenerate at the same rate. Sensory axons grow by 2.0 to 4.8 mm. per day after crush injuries and 1.5 to 3.5 mm. per day after sectioning. For motor axons the daily rates are 2.8 to 4.4 mm. and 1.3 to 2.3 mm, respectively, and for adrenergic fibers 3.9 mm. per day after a crush injury. In man the rate of growth varies between 1.0 and 2.4 mm. for sensory axons and 1.1 to 3.6 mm. for motor axons (Sunderland, 1978).

The rate of regeneration depends on a variety of factors, such as the nature of the lesion (growth is faster if the basal lamina is left intact), the distance between the axonal extremity and the cell body (growth is slower as the distance increases), the type and diameter of fibers involved (sensory fibers regenerate faster), the age, and species, as well as some physical and chemical factors, including the temperature.

MATURATION OF REGENERATED FIBERS AND FUNCTIONAL RECOVERY

The functional effectiveness of the regenerated fibers depends primarily on two complementary, but chronologically distinct, events, namely, the growth in length of the axon and the degree of maturation of the fiber. Both processes occur proximodistally, but maturation involves complex changes that are slower than axonal growth and are still in progress long after the neuron has reestablished contact with its end organs.

The axonal tip, which advances toward the periphery, is always "bare" i.e., without individual Schwann cell or myelin sheaths, and the original architecture of the fiber must be restored in order for normal function to return. After acquiring its Schwann cell sheath, the axon becomes myelinated. Myelination is progressive and always lags behind axon growth as in fetal development. It occurs at a rate of 2 to 4 mm. per day and appears to depend on the diameter of the axon. The myelin sheath of regenerated fibers, however, is thinner than normal, even if the axon ends up with a normal diameter. Moreover, in contrast with the normal nerve in which the internodes increase in length with the axon diameter, in the regenerated nerve the internodal length is curiously the same for all fibers (ca. 300 to 400 mμ) and shorter than in the normal nerve.

Many authors believe that maturation can start only when the regenerated nerve fibers have reestablished their anatomical and functional connections with the end organs. Under the most favorable conditions (i.e., when nerve continuity has been preserved), reinnervation can be theoretically perfect. However, after sectioning, the normal diameter and distribution are never achieved and maturation is much slower than after crush injuries.

Contact of the axons with a functionally related end organ is still not sufficient for the return of function. Additional time must elapse before it is restored. The return of motoricity occurs in several successive stages: the regenerated fibers after a crush injury reach the motor endplates after about 12 days, but a contraction is elicited only by nerve stimulation after 18 days, and the functional reflex returns only after about 23 days (Gutmann and Young, 1944). Functional recovery also depends on the density and pattern of innervation, on anatomical and functional readjustments to make up for deficiencies in the axonal response, and finally on the arrest and reversal of the trophic changes resulting from denervation and inactivity. The exact role of each is still undetermined, because it is not yet possible to study them separately.

MAIN FACTORS INFLUENCING REGENERATION

Unfavorable Factors

Axonal growth and functional recovery are affected by a variety of factors acting at different levels of the nervous pathway, from the neuronal cell body down to the peripheral tissues innervated by the injured axon.

Factors Intervening in the Proximal Segment. Some factors intervene in the proximal segment. Thus the capacity of the neuron to sprout a new axon toward the periphery is of considerable importance because it conditions the anatomical and functional continuity with the end organs. The axon is under the trophic control of the cell body, which may itself have been damaged by the lesion. Retrograde changes can therefore affect the quality of regeneration and restrict the recovery potential by reducing the number of axons available, by disturbing the function of regenerated fibers, and by modifying the patterns of activity that become less effective. However, not all lesions are irreversible and not all lesions lead to cell death. A large proportion of neurons retain their power of regeneration even after repeated lesions (vide infra). There is no doubt, however, that the intensity of the "axon reaction," the time required for the neuron to recuperate, and the extent of the residual disturbances can all affect the capacity of the neuron to regenerate new sprouts, to ensure their growth and maintenance, and therefore to ensure the rate, extent, and quality of the functional recovery.

Factors Intervening at the Site of the Lesion and in the Distal Segment. Other factors intervene at the site of the lesion and in the distal segment. The cicatricial tissue that joins the ends of a severed nerve or develops at the site of a crush injury has a marked effect on regeneration to an extent that varies with its volume, density, nature, and architecture. It can have a constrictive effect as it interferes both with the growth in length and later with the maturation of the regenerating axons. In addition, the large increase in collagen deposited around the Schwann tube within the endoneural spaces of the distal segment results in a reduction of their diameter, and this in turn is bound to affect the completeness of regeneration.

The influence of the caliber of the Schwann tubes has been the subject of numerous studies and the results can be summed up as follows: if the large central fibers can distend a smaller peripheral tube, the latter induces a significant and permanent reduction in regenerated axon diameter and therefore in its physiological properties. By contrast, when the axon enters a tube larger than the one it occupied previously, its diameter will be no greater than normal.

Factors Intervening at the Periphery. A third set of factors intervene at the periphery. A regenerating axon can mature fully only if it can establish appropriate connections with a functionally related end organ; reconnection with an "alien" organ results in incomplete myelination and maturation. Further, Edds (1949, 1950) has shown (and this was confirmed by later workers) that some fibers may become hypertrophied and give off extensive outgrowths when their peripheral connections are increased experimentally. This demonstrates the influence of peripheral tissues on their nerve supply, but it also suggests the presence of possible compensatory mechanisms when reinnervation is incomplete.

Compensatory Mechanisms

The quality of anatomical and functional recovery depends, inter alia, on the number of regenerating axons that succeed in reaching the periphery and on the extent to which the original innervation has been restored. Although regeneration usually has to struggle against unfavorable factors, some mechanisms appear to exist that to some extent can counteract their nefarious influence.

Axonal Sprouting. There is now ample experimental evidence that the neurons preserve for a long time their capacity to give off new outgrowths capable of replacing the missing parts and of restoring the continuity between nerve centers and the periphery. These outgrowths to some extent can improve the quality of recovery as they make up for the loss of some neurons as a result of retrograde degeneration, the inability of severely injured adjacent neurons to give off new axons, the block or misdirection of some axons as they cross the cicatricial tissue, and the failure of other axons to enter appropriate basal lamina tubes.

Conversely, it is conceivable that overabundant axonal ramification could have an unfavorable influence on the quality of regeneration by overloading the neuron with an unduly large number of outgrowths (the nerve cell is then forced to disperse its potentialities withir too great a number of axons so that it is unable to control effectively any one; consequently, maturation will be inadequate and incomplete) and by considerably increasing the risks of block or misdirection of axons at the suture line. Some outgrowths from a common parent fiber can enter different tubes while others from different fibers colonize the same channel. As a result, one central fiber may become connected to several end organs while some end organs may never be reinnervated.

The Influence of Distal Stump Tissues. The influence of the tissues on the distal segment has already been mentioned. It is worth noting, however, that there is experimental evidence suggesting that myelinated axons exert some form of attraction on unmyelinated regenerating axons. Normal gastric function is restored in the rabbit 150 days after crushing of the abdominal vagus nerve. If the cervical vagus nerve is injured, however, gastric function fails to return to normal even after 670 days. Histological examination then shows that the unmyelinated fibers of the regenerating cervical vagus have not grown into the abdominal vagus as one would expect, but along the recurrent laryngeal nerve, which contains far more myelinated fibers than the vagus (Evans and Murray, 1954).

The Influence of Peripheral Tissues. The influence of the peripheral tissues seems even more significant. The nerve terminals are being constantly remolded in the vicinity of the end organ. Exner, as early as 1885, believed that the nerve fibers are part of a dynamic association with the periphery, that they can adapt to changing circumstances and even make up for the destruction of adjacent axons. It was not until 1950 that Edds and others experimentally confirmed Exner's theory. Thus when the motor supply to a muscle is damaged, intensive collateral sprouting can be seen in the course of regeneration. Numerous axonal outgrowths are given off by the surviving fibers or by those reaching a muscular territory first. This was demonstrated experimentally before being described in various forms of human neuropathy. The same is known to occur with the sensory and autonomic nervous systems.

The mechanism of collateral sprouting has now been studied at length. The most generally accepted theory is that the target tissue continually manufactures a substance that stimulates axonal sprouting but whose effects are neutralized by the liberation of a factor carried to the nerve terminals by axonal transport. If its arrival is delayed or obstructed, the adjacent nerves give off collaterals, which colonize the territory of the injured nerve. This has been shown to occur when axoplasmic transport is blocked by colchicine (Aguilar et al., 1973).

Effects of Repeated Injuries

It was pointed out earlier that many neurons retain their capacity to regenerate functionally effective pathways even after repeated injuries.

Holmes and Young (1942) observed that the capacity of the proximal segment to send out new fibers is not diminished after a second lesion, even if it occurs within one week or one year after the first lesion. Gutmann (1948) also observed that repeated lesions of the same nerve do not affect the regenerative potential of axons: repeated crush injuries were followed by functional recovery, and the rate of regeneration was virtually unchanged after eight experimental lesions, successful reinnervation of muscles being the rule. Gutmann and Holubar (1951) even suggested that a "prophylactic" crush of the proximal stump of a severed nerve actually stimulates the nerve cells and intensifies their

metabolic activity, the rate of conduction velocity and the amplitude of the action potentials being greater than in the control side. Ducker et al. (1969) believed that axonal regrowth was faster than a second lesion, provided a gap of 2 to 3 weeks intervened. In the spinal cord, however, the metabolic response of the neurons was not so intense the second time round.

More recent experimental work shows that a "conditioning" lesion inflicted before the "test" lesion could facilitate the response in some neurons. The observations can be summed up as follows:

1. Regeneration of the motor fibers (McQuarrie, 1978; Sébille and Bondoux-Jahan, 1980a) and sensory fibers (McQuarrie et al., 1977) is accelerated, whereas that of adrenergic fibers is slowed considerably (McQuarrie et al., 1978).

2. The "initial delay" (i.e., the time required for the neuron to recover and enable regeneration to begin, and for regenerating axons to cross the zone of traumatic degeneration) is shortened from 1.6 to 0.9 days for sensory fibers (Forman et al., 1980) and from 1.3 to 0.6 days for adrenergic fibers (McQuarrie et al., 1978).

3. The overall number of regenerated fibers is not increased (McQuarrie, 1979) and can even be reduced (McQuarrie et al., 1978). The results are, however, different after repeated localized freezings. Thus one month after one to five cold injuries made three weeks apart, the number of myelinated fibers increased progressively after the first three lesions but remained constant thereafter (ca. 220 per cent of the control). If the counts were made one to 24 months after the third and final freezing, the number of myelinated fibers decreased by some 30 per cent early in the second month and remained at about 190 per cent of the control values (Mira, 1979).

4. Facilitation of the axonal response is noticeable when the "test" lesion is inflicted at least 48 hours after the "conditioning" lesion; it seems to be maximal between 7 and 14 days and regresses after 21 days.

5. Finally, motor function returns earlier but only if the denervated muscle is submitted to daily electrical stimulation (Sébille and Bondoux-Jahan, 1980a). This form of stimulation appears to prevent muscle atrophy resulting from denervation after the "conditioning" lesion.

Recent developments in this field are encouraging and further research might well lead to improvement in the rate and quality of clinical recovery after nerve lesions.

Chemical Factors

In the present state of knowledge, there is no known form of chemical therapy capable of promoting nerve regeneration or protecting the neuron against degeneration of metabolic or toxic origin. The introduction of such a therapy would represent a tremendous advance in the treatment of traumatic and other lesions of the peripheral nerves. Much work has been devoted to this subject but so far with little success. The best known such agent is the *Nerve Growth Factor* (NGF), which under normal conditions or in the course of regeneration does facilitate axon growth. Secreted in small amounts by various target tissues and taken up by the growth cone, nerve growth factor is transported to the cell body via the retrograde axonal flow. Within the perikaryon it enhances the synthesis of proteins—namely that of tubulin, the main constituent of the neurotubules—which are essential in the formation and growth of both axons and dendrites. It must be stressed, however, that this factor influences specifically the growth of unmyelinated sympathetic fibers and exerts no beneficial effect on motor and sensory myelinated fibers.

Apart from nerve growth factor, *thyroid hormone* (T_4) is the only naturally occurring substance known to influence the regeneration of central and peripheral nerves in the healthy animal. As yet it has not been used clinically because the dose required to accelerate peripheral nerve regeneration is only marginally less than that causing thyrotoxicosis. Thyroxine appears to promote functional recovery by acting on the maturation of motor and sensory fibers. Recent work has thrown some light on its mode of action, at least in the fetus where it triggers off the polymerization of tubulin; its absence causes an interruption in the elongation of axons and dendrites. Destruction of the thyroid of a rat fetus results in a marked reduction of interneuronal connections, and after birth the young rat is incapable of learning simple tasks that it would normally be expected to perform with no difficulty.

Among other factors likely to be of thera-peutic use in the not too distant future are *isaxonine,* * *cyclophosphamide*, and *spermine*. Isaxonine is a pyrimidine compound that appears to facilitate or accelerate protein synthesis and to stimulate intraneuronal metabolism and axonal growth, the latter by up to 45 per cent. It can also shorten the time required for functional recovery in sensory fibers (by 50 per cent) and motor fibers (by 35 per cent). Like thyroxine, isaxonine would facilitate nerve fiber regeneration by promoting the synthesis and/or polymerization of tubulin (Hugelin et al., 1979; Legrain, 1977). It also increases the number of muscle fibers with multiple innervation (Pécot-Dechavassine and Mira, 1985).

Cyclophosphamide and spermine act by promoting the growth of medullary and motor neurons. Animal experiments have shown that the recovery of motor function is accelerated 60 per cent by cyclophosphamide and 140 per cent by spermine. Similarly the latent period is reduced by 40 and 50 per cent, respectively. Their mode of action is ill understood, but it is believed that both substances activate the metabolism of motor neurons whose axons have been injured (Sébille and Bondoux-Jahan, 1980b).

---

*While this review was in progress, some cases of human hepatitis related to the treatment were detected. The manufacturer subsequently decided to suspend sales of isaxonine pending more precise information on the mechanism responsible for hepatic toxicity.

REFERENCES

Aguayo, A. J., Attiwell, M., Trecarten, J., Perkins, S., and Bray, G. M.: Abnormal myelination in transplanted trembler mouse Schwann cells. Nature, 265:73–74, 1977.

Aguilar, C. E., Bisby, M. A., Cooper, E., and Diamond, J.: Evidence that axoplasmic transport of trophic factor is involved in the regulation of peripheral nerve fields in salamanders. J. Physiol. (London), 234:449–464, 1973.

Basbum, C. B.: Induced hypothermia in peripheral nerve: electron microscopical and electrophysiological observations. J. Neurocytol., 2:171–187, 1973.

Becker, H.: Retrograde und Transneuronale Degeneration der Neurone. Abh. Akad. Wiss. Lit., No. 10. Weisbaden, Steiner, 1952.

Black, M. N., and Lasek, R. J.: The use of axonal transport to measure axonal regeneration in rat ventral motor neurons. Anat. Rec., 184:360–361, 1976.

Bora, F., Lane, J., and Prockop, D.: Inhibitors of collagen biosynthesis as a mean of controlling scar formation in tendon injury. J. Bone Joint Surg., 54:1501–1508, 1972.

Bunge, M. B., Williams, A. K., Wood, P. M., Uitto, J., and Jeffery, J. J.: Comparison of nerve cell and nerve cell plus Schwann cell cultures, with particular emphasis on basal lamina and collagen formation. J. Cell Biol., *84*:184–202, 1980.

Cancalon, P.: The relationship of slow axonal flow to nerve elongation and regeneration. *In* Elam, J. S., and Cancalon, P. (Eds.): Axonal Transport in Neuronal Growth and Regeneration. New York, Plenum Pub. Co., 1984, pp. 211–241.

Couteaux, R., and Mira, J. C.: Dédifférenciation et remodelage des plaques motrices consécutifs à des lésions expérimentales localisées des fibres musculaires. C. R. Acad. Sci., *3*:299, 1984.

Couteaux, R., and Mira, J. C.: Remodeling of neuromuscular functions during repair of muscle fibers. *In* Changeux, J. P., et al. (Eds.): Molecular Basis of Nerve Activity. Berlin, de Gruyter, 1985, pp. 35–45.

Cuppage, F. E., Neagoy, D. R., and Tate, A.: Repair of the nephron following temporary occlusion of the renal pedicle. Lab. Invest., *17*:600–674, 1967.

Droz, B., and Leblond, C. P.: Axonal migration of proteins in the central nervous system and peripheral nerves as shown by autoradiography. J. Comp. Neurol., *121*:325–346, 1963.

Droz, B.: Axonal transport in peripheral nerves. Intern. J. Microsurg., *3*:93–98, 1981.

Ducker, T. B., Kempe, L. G., and Hayes, G. J.: The metabolic background for peripheral nerve surgery. J. Neurosurgery, *30*:270–280, 1969.

Edds, M. V., Jr.: Experiments on partially deneurotized nerves. II. Hypertrophy of residual fibers. J. Exper. Zool., *112*:29–48, 1949.

Edds, M. V., Jr.: Hypertrophy of nerve fibers to functionally overloaded muscles. J. Comp. Neurol., *93*:259–275, 1950a.

Edds, M. V., Jr.: Collateral regeneration of residual motor axons in partially denervated muscles. J. Exper. Zool., *113*:517–551, 1950b.

Exner, S.: Notz zu der Frage von der Faservertheilung mehrerer nerven in einen Muskel. Pflügers Arch. Ges. Physiol., *36*:572–576, 1885.

Forman, D. S.: Axonal transport and nerve regeneration. A review. *In* Kao, C. C., and Bunge, R. P. (Eds.): Spinal Cord Reconstruction. New York, Raven Press, 1983, pp. 75–86.

Forman, D. S., McQuarrie, I. G., Labore, F. W., Wood, D. K., Stone, L. S., Braddock, C. H., and Fuchs, D. A.: Time course of the conditioning lesion effect on axonal regeneration. Brain Res., *156*:213–225, 1980.

Geren, B. B.: The formation from the Schwann cell surface of myelin in the peripheral nerves of chick embryos. Exper. Cell Res., *7*:558–562, 1954.

Grafstein, B.: The nerve cell body response to axotomy. Exper. Neurol., *48*:32, 1975.

Grafstein, B.: Axonal transport: the intracellular traffic of the neuron. *In* Handbook of Physiology. Bethesda, American Physiological Society, 1977, Vol. 1, pp. 697–717.

Grafstein, B., and Forman, D. S.: Intracellular transport in neurons. Physiol. Rev., *60*:1167–1283, 1980.

Grafstein, B.: Chromatolysis reconsidered. A new view of the reaction of the nerve cell body to axonal injury. *In* Seil, F. J. (Ed.): Nerve, Organ and Tissue Regeneration: Research Perspectives. New York, Academic Press, 1983.

Grafstein, B., and McQuarrie, I. G.: Role of the nerve cell in axonal regeneration. *In* Cotman, C. W. (Editor): Neuronal Plasticity. 155–195, New York, Raven Press, 1978.

Gutmann, E.: Effect of delay of innervation on recovery of muscle after nerve lesions. J. Neurophysiol., *11*:279–294, 1948.

Gutmann, E., and Holubar, J.: Atrophy of fibers in the central stump following nerve section and the possibilities of its prevention. Arch. Intern. Stud. Neurol., *1*:314–324, 1951.

Gutmann, E., and Young, J. Z.: The reinnervation of muscle after various periods of atrophy. J. Anat., *78*:15–43, 1944.

Holmes, W., and Young, J. Z.: Nerve regeneration after immediate and delayed sutures. J. Anat., *77*:63–97, 1942.

Hugelin, A., Legrain, Y., and Bondoux-Jahan, M.: Nerve growth promoting action of isaxonine in rat. Experientia, *35*:626, 1979.

Kristensson, K.: Retrograde signaling after nerve injury. *In* Elam, J. S., and Cancalon, P. (Eds.): Axonal Transport in Neuronal Growth and Regeneration. New York, Plenum Publishing Co., 1984, pp. 31–43.

Lane, J., Bora, F., Prockop, D., Heppenstall, R., and Black, J.: Inhibition of scar formation by the proline analog cis-hydroxyproline. J. Surg. Res., *3*:135–137, 1972.

Lasek, R. J., and Hoffman, P. N.: The neuronal cytoskeleton, axonal transport and axonal growth. *In* Cell Mobility: Microtubules and Related Proteins. Cold Spring Harbor, New York, Cold Spring Harbor Laboratory, 1976, pp. 1021–1051.

Legrain, Y.: Méthode de comparaison de la vitesse de régénération des fibres du nerf sciatique de rat. J. Physiol. (Paris), *73*:13–22, 1977.

Lieberman, A. R.: Some factors affecting retrograde neuronal responses to axonal lesions. *In* Bellairs, R., and Gray, E. G. (Editors): Essays on the Nervous System, Oxford, Clarendon Press, 1974, pp. 71–105.

Lubinska, L.: On axoplasmic flow. Intern. Rev. Cytol., *17*:241–296, 1975.

Lubinska, L.: Early course of Wallerian degeneration in myelinated fibers of the rat phrenic nerve. Brain Res., *130*:47–64, 1977.

Lubinska, L.: Patterns of Wallerian degeneration of myelinated fibers in short and long peripheral stumps and in isolated segments of rat phrenic nerves. Interpretation of the role of the axoplasmic flow of the trophic factor. Brain Res., *233*:227–240, 1982.

McQuarrie, I. G.: The effect of a conditioning lesion on the regeneration of motor axons. Brain Res., *152*:597–602, 1978.

McQuarrie, I. G.: Accelerated axonal sprouting after nerve transection. Brain Res., *167*:185–188, 1979.

McQuarrie, I. G.: Role of the axonal cytoskeleton in the regenerating nervous system. *In* Seil, F. J. (Ed.): Nerve, Organ and Tissue Regeneration: Research Perspectives. New York, Academic Press, 1983, pp. 51–88.

McQuarrie, I. G., Grafstein, B., Dreyfus, C. F., and Gershon, M. D.: Regeneration of adrenergic axons in rat sciatic nerve: effect of a conditioning lesion. Brain Res., *141*:21–34, 1978.

McQuarrie, I. G., Grafstein, B., and Gershon, M. D.: Axonal regeneration in the rat sciatic nerve: effect of a conditioning lesion and of dbc-AMP. Brain Res., *132*:443–453, 1977.

Mira, J. C.: Maintien de la continuité de la lame basale des fibres nerveuses périphériques après "section" des axones par congélation localisée. C. R. Acad. Sci. D., *273*:1836–1839, 1971.

Mira, J. C.: Effets d'une congélation localisée sur la structure des fibres nerveuses myélinisées et leur régénération. J. Micr. (Paris), *14*:155–168, 1972.

Mira, J. C.: Etudes quantitatives sur la régénération des fibres nerveuses myélinisées. II. Variations du nombre et du calibre des fibres régénérées après un écrasement localisé ou une section totale. Arch. Anat. Micr. Morphol. Exper., *65*:255–284, 1976a.

Mira, J. C.: Observations histophysiologiques sur la dégénérescence et la régénération des fibres nerveuses périphériques à la suite d'une congélation localisée. *In* Guiraud, B., and Mansat, M. (Editors): Pathologie du Nerf Périphérique. Paris, Editions Médicales Pierre Fabre, 1976b, pp. 9–23.

Mira, J. C.: Etudes quantitatives sur la régénération des fibres nerveuses myélinisées. III. Variations du nombre et du calibre des fibres régénérées après une congélation localisée. Arch. Anat. Micr. Morphol. Exper., *66*:1–16, 1977.

Mira, J. C.: Quantitative studies of the regeneration of rat myelinated fibres: variations in the number and size of regenerating nerve fibers after repeated localized freezings. J. Anat., *129*:77–93, 1979.

Mira, J. C.: Contribution à l'Etude de la Régénération du Nerf Périphérique et des Changements du Muscle Squelettique Strié au cours de sa Réinnervation. Thèse de Doctorat d'Etat. Paris, Université Pierre-et-Marie Curie, 1980.

Mira, J. C.: Degeneration and regeneration of peripheral nerves: ultrastructural and electrophysiological observations, quantitative aspects and muscular effects. Intern. J. Microsurg., *3*:102–132, 1981.

Mira, J. C., and Pécot-Dechavassine, M.: Effets d'une congélation localisée d'un nerf périphérique sur la conduction de l'influx nerveux, au cours de la dégénérescence et de la régénération. Pflügers Arch., *330*:5–14, 1971.

Nageotte, J.: L'organisation de la Matière Vivante dans ses Rapports avec la Vie. Etudes d'Anatomie Générale et de Morphologie Expérimentale sur le Tissu Conjonctif et le Nerf. Paris, Alcan, 1922.

Nathaniel, E. J. H., and Pease, D. C.: Collagen and basement membrane formation by Schwann cells during nerve regeneration. J. Ultrastruct. Res., *9*:550–560, 1963.

Ochs, S., and Worth, R. M.: Axoplasmic transport in normal and pathological systems. *In* Waxman, S. G.

(Editor): Physiology and pathobiology of Axons. New York, Raven Press, 1978.

Pease, D. C.: The basement membrane: substratum of histological order and complexity. *In* Proceedings of the 4th International Congress on Electron Microscopy. Berlin, Springer Verlag, 1960, pp. 139–155.

Pécot-Dechavassine, M., and Mira, J. C.: Effect of isaxonine on skeletal muscle reinnervation in the rat. An electrophysiological evaluation. Muscle and Nerve, *8*:105–114, 1985.

Pleasure, D., Bora, F. W., Jr., Lane, J., and Prockop, D.: Regeneration after nerve transection: effect of inhibition of collagen synthesis. Exper. Neurol., *45*:72–78, 1974.

Scott, F. H.: On the relation of nerve cells to fatigue of their nerve fibers. J. Physiol. (London), *34*:145–162, 1906.

Sebille, A., and Bondoux-Jahan, M.: Effects of electric stimulation and previous nerve injury on motor function recovery in rats. Brain Res., *193*:562–565, 1980a.

Sébille, A., and Bondoux-Jahan, M.: Motor function recovery after axotomy: enhancement by cyclophosphamide and spermine in rat. Exper. Neurol., *70*:507–515, 1980b.

Seddon, H. J.: Three types of nerve injury. Brain, *66*:237–288, 1943.

Sunderland, S.: Nerves and Nerve Injury. Edinburgh, E. & S. Livingstone, 1978.

Thomas, P. K.: Changes in the endoneurial sheaths of peripheral myelinated nerve fibres during Wallerian degeneration. J. Anat., *98*:175–182, 1964a.

Thomas, P. K.: The deposition of collagen in relation to Schwann cell basement membrane during peripheral nerve regeneration. J. Cell. Biol., *23*:375–382, 1964b.

Vracko, R.: Basal lamina scaffold. Anatomy and significance for maintenance of orderly tissue structure. A review. Am. J. Pathol., *77*:314–346, 1974.

Vracko, R., and Benditt, E. P.: Basal lamina: the scaffold for orderly cell replacement. Observations on regeneration of injured skeletal muscle fibres and capillaries. J. Cell Biol., *55*:406–419, 1972.

Weiss, P. A., and Hiscoe, H. B.: Experiments on the mechanisms of nerve growth. J. Exper. Zool., *107*:315–395, 1943.

Weiss, P. A., and Taylor, A. C.: Impairment of growth and myelination in regenerating nerve fibers subjected to constriction. Proc. Soc. Exper. Biol., *55*:77–80, 1944.

Chapter 43

SURGICAL ANATOMY OF THE PERIPHERAL NERVES

Yves Allieu

and François Bonnel

Without claiming to be comprehensive, we wish to include here a number of notions that ought to be familiar to every surgeon working on peripheral nerves. Some have been known for a long time; others represent recently acquired knowledge. Since the introduction of magnifying aids in this type of surgery, a more detailed knowledge of the structure of the nerve trunk has become essential.

STRUCTURE OF THE PERIPHERAL NERVE TRUNK

THE FASCICLE: THE BASIC UNIT OF THE PERIPHERAL NERVE TRUNK

The fascicular concept of nerves is the basis of most modern neurosurgical techniques. The fascicle consists of a group of nerve fibers within a specialized sheath of connective tissues known as the perineurium. This sheath, which has a well differentiated ultrastructure, must be regarded as a boundary between two environments: the endoneural space, which communicates with cerebrospinal fluid, and the connective tissue (Figs. 43–1 and 43–2). The perineurium consists of collagen fibers arranged longitudinally and sometimes circumferentially. Their diameter varies between 400 and 800 Å, and together their total thickness is 5 microns. By electron microscopy these perineural cells are seen to bear a close morphological resemblance to Schwann cells. Under the optical microscope the perineurium appears as a distinct membrane separating the fascicles. On the larger peripheral nerve trunks it is visible to the naked eye, but it is visualized more clearly with the operating microscope. It appears as a smooth, finely ringed sheath under slight tension with razor-sharp edges when cut. When the nerve is cut, its fascicular contents (nerve fibers and connective tissue) jut out like a snail's horn. The infrafascicular tissue is gelatinous and oozes out, as if under pressure, from the perineural sheath, surface tension being responsible for the characteristic translucent club shaped appearance of the fascicular contents jutting out of the perineurium (Fig. 43–3). In surgical procedures the perineurium should always be preserved; Spencer has shown that damage to it results in an axonic explosion. It is a fragile structure and must be handled with utmost care.

At low magnification ($\times$ 10) the fascicles sometimes seem less numerous than they are found to be on histological examination. This is the result of insufficient optical resolution. Some fascicles may be stuck together, forming a bundle, of which the surgeon can see only the outside. As the magnification is increased, better visualization allows separation of the fascicles by careful microdissection. The fascicles now appear more numerous and can be differentiated through their readily identifiable perineural sheaths. Inadequate visualization at operation is responsible for the difference between the histological fascicle and the surgical fascicle, the latter often consisting of a bundle (Fig. 43–4) (Rabischong and Bonnel, 1975). For this reason we cannot talk in terms of fascicular grafts: as a rule, using Millesi's technique (Millesi et al., 1972) one would transplant three or four fascicles for an ulnar nerve and five or six for a median nerve. In practice, therefore, the nerve graft must be regarded not as individual

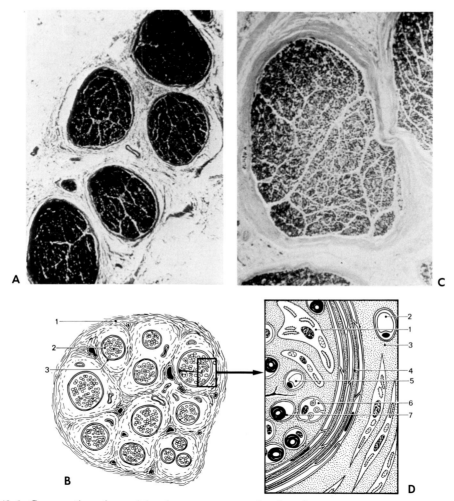

Figure 43–1. Cross section of a peripheral nerve as seen under the microscope. *A,* Low power view. Note the fascicular composition, with epineurium that is loose and not well defined. *B,* Schematic representation. 1 = Epineurium, 2 = fascicle, and 3 = perineurium. *C,* High power microscopic view. *D,* Ultrastructure of the nerve as seen under the electron microscope, showing part of the fascicle. 1 = Fibroblast, 2 = vasa nervorum, 3 = epineurium, 4 = perineurium, 5 = capillary, 6 = unmyelinated nerve fiber, and 7 = myelinated nerve fiber.

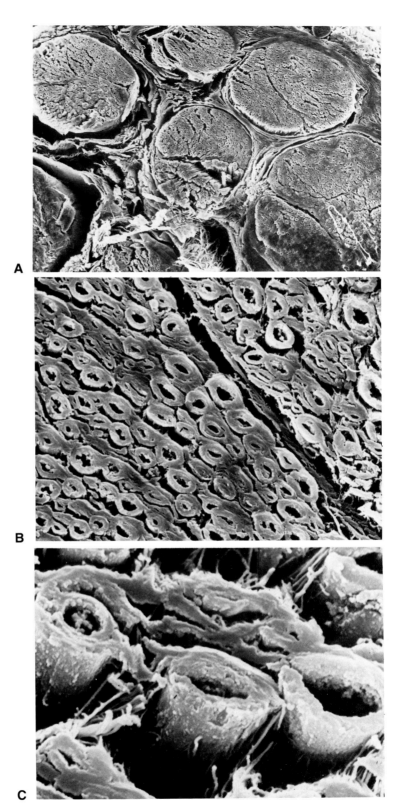

Figure 43–2. Cross section of a peripheral nerve by scanning electron microscopy. *A*, Cross section of human sural nerve ($\times$ 240). *B*, Two fascicles juxtaposed, showing their junction with myelinated fibers ($\times$ 1600). *C*, Detail of myelinated fibers ($\times$ 2000). (Courtesy of V. Meyer and J. Smahel.)

fascicles but as bundles free of perifascicular connective tissue (Fig. 43–5).

CONNECTIVE TISSUE

The fascicles are loosely clothed by connective tissue. It is composed of collagen fibers varying in diameter from 600 to 1100 Å. The latter, which run between the fascicles, condense at the surface of the nerve to form the epineurium. Regardless of the arrangement of the connective tissue, however, the fascicle remains the anatomical unit of the nerve. The epineurium is related to the surrounding connective tissue, especially the tissue associated with blood vessels, and it itself carries small vessels. The epineurium is therefore distinct from the perineurium or perifascicular sheath, which is the only clearly differentiated connective tissue structure. It is a much looser entity, lying between the fascicles and in close association with the

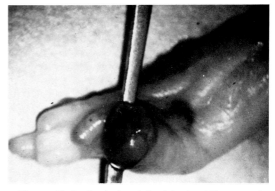

Figure 43–3. An isolated fascicle (× 20). Note the well-defined perineurium. The axoplasm bulges from the cut end of the fascicle.

connective tissue separating the nerve from the surrounding structures. This explains the changes of orientation of the fascicles, which do not occupy a fixed position within a rigid system.

This fascicular conception of the nerve

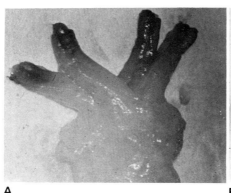

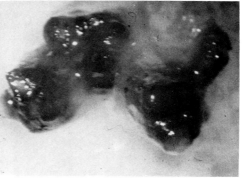

A   B

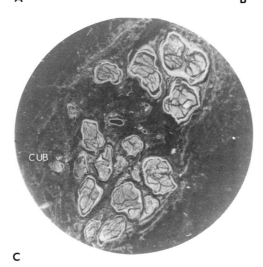

C

Figure 43–4. A, Surgical dissection of ulnar nerve at the wrist. The sensory and motor groups of fascicles have been separated into two groups (the "surgical fascicles") (× 10). B, Examination of the surgical fascicles under magnification (× 20) shows their multifascicular structure. C, Ulnar nerve at the wrist. The division into the motor and sensory groups of fascicles is particularly well shown. Each division is able to be artificially separated into two or three groups of fascicles (the surgical fascicles). Note the poorly defined epineurium between the fascicles (Weigert-Landau stain).

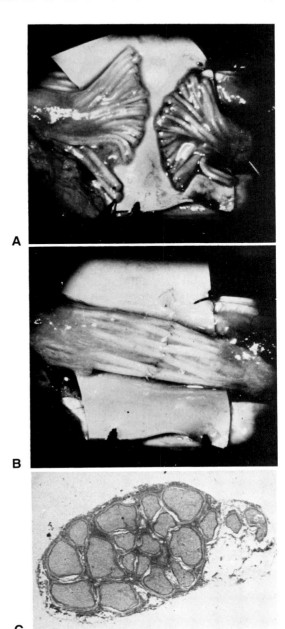

Figure 43–5. *A* and *B,* Interfascicular suture of the median nerve at the wrist, as seen preoperatively. (Courtesy of J. W. Tupper). The fascicular dissection is surgically possible but the advisability of this procedure is questioned. *C,* Section of the median nerve at the wrist. The division into "surgical fascicles" (which may contain four or five fascicles) is shown. The fine dissection allows for the identification of each fascicle (total 20 to 30). The multifascicular structure makes the identification of the thenar motor branch difficult (Weigert-Landau stain). (Courtesy of F. Bonnel and P. Rabischong.)

trunk explains the shortcomings of the classic neurolysis, in which only the nerve trunk is freed, as compared with intraneural perifascicular neurolysis, which frees every fascicle from strangling connective tissue.

The proportion of connective tissue within individual nerves is variable (between 10 and 82 per cent) but always quite high (Table 43–1). The smaller and the more numerous the fascicles, the greater the connective tissue content (Fig. 43–6). The notion of the percentage of connective tissue, which has been studied by Sunderland, appears to be extremely relevant in the light of recent physiological work on nerve repair. As we know, cicatrization in connective tissue constitutes the chief obstacle to nerve regeneration. This partly explains the good results obtained in

Table 43–1. PERCENTAGE OF CONNECTIVE TISSUE AND NERVE TISSUE IN NERVES OF THE UPPER EXTREMITY (after Sunderland) AS SEEN ON CROSS SECTION

Nerves	Perineural Connective Tissue	Epineural and Interfascicular Connective Tisue	Neural Tissue
Radial	11	67	22
Circumflex	13	77	10
Median	10	63	27
Ulnar	4	82	14
Musculocutaneous	30		70

certain zones where the connective tissue element is least, e.g., the radial nerve within its canal. Proliferation of the epineurium can block regeneration of the nerve fibers, and Millesi et al. (1972) advocate its resection.

In addition to the connective tissue (the epineurium and perineurium) there is also abundant connective tissue in the endoneural tubes (Fig. 43–7). These longitudinally disposed collagen fibers have a diameter between 300 and 650 Å. In man it has not been possible to show the Plenk-Laidlow and Key-Retzius layers described by Thomas (1963) in the rabbit and by Gamble and Eames (1964) in rats.

Around the unmyelinated fibers are invaginations of Schwann cells, which surround groups of collagen fibers, forming "collagen pockets." These collagen fibers seem to increase mechanical resistance to traction on the axons.

In summary, therefore, a nerve is made up of a number of fascicles grouped within a perifascicular sheath (the perineurium),

which itself separates the fascicles from the surrounding connective tissue. The perineurium or fascicular sheath thus is in effect a barrier between two environments—one intrafascicular, which communicates with the subarachnoid space, and the other extrafascicular, consisting of the epineurium, itself a differentiated component of the surrounding connective tissue.

The fascicular sheath is a structure that must be respected at all costs, for damage to it results in endoneural hemorrhage. The epineurium is a nonspecific connective tissue that can be subjected to surgical dissection but when sclerosed can hinder neural regeneration.

THE FASCICULAR ARRANGEMENT

Sunderland (1975), whose work in this field forms the basis of our knowledge, has shown clearly that the nerve is not organized like a cable, with well individualized, parallel fascicles, but is in fact plexiform. This is important to the surgeon because it indicates a somewhat restricted scope for repair.

The fascicles, which vary in number at different points, divide and converge to form an intricate plexus. In addition, their position within the nerve trunk is variable. The positional and directional variations are such that in a resection of 15 mm., for example, it may be impossible to reapproximate and realign the severed fasciculi accurately (Sunderland, 1945).

The inextricable plexus is somewhat simplified in the distal regions and at the points where collaterals emerge (Fig. 43–8). At these levels fiber exchanges are fewer, and it is often possible to identify individual fibers by perifascicular intraneural dissection. The process of fasciculation is progressive, being more marked distally as the connective tissue

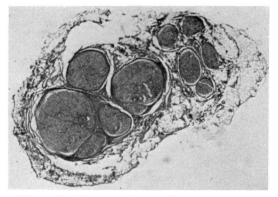

Figure 43–6. Section of the radial nerve at the level of the radial groove of the humerus. Note the few fascicles and the small amount of perineurium. This explains the good results from surgical repair obtained at this level.

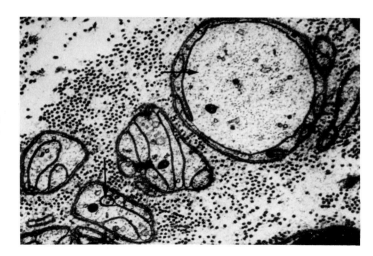

Figure 43–7. Electron microscopic study showing an unmyelinated axon surrounded by collagen fibers.

becomes more differentiated. This was well shown by Allieu and Rabischong, 1970. The fasciculation becomes also more selective distally, differentiation occurring before the actual emergence of the collaterals from the trunk. The fascicles at that stage are much simpler, containing only those fibers that share the same destination. In the more proximal areas of the nerve, by contrast, the fascicles (i.e., those not concerned with the upper branches) are composite, carrying within the same sheath motor, sensory, and autonomic fibers (Fig. 43–9). The mixed arrangement in the proximal parts of the nerve (Fig. 43–10) explains why a high partial sectioning may not have a significant effect on function (Sherren, 1907). It is also responsible for the late recovery of nerve function seen after surgical repair even when accurate fascicular approximation has not been achieved at operation.

In the more distal zones of the nerve where

selective fasciculation has occurred, accurate approximation is obligatory. A fascicular repair therefore requires precise orientation of the nerve extremities: thus, in repair of the median nerve, the most important step is the identification of the thenar branch. Thus, to some extent the selective fasciculation at the terminal zones facilitates reorientation after an intraneural perifascicular neurolysis (Fig. 43–11). This is often possible with the ulnar nerve at the wrist, where by perifascicular dissection one may be able to distinguish the fascicular groups belonging to the motor branch from those belonging to the sensory branch. Separate repairs of the motor and sensory components may then be feasible. However, in the median nerve, which at this level is plurifascicular and whose fascicles are similar in size and shape, identification of the thenar branch is possible only when the loss of nerve tissue is minimal.

As for the collaterals, they can usually be

Figure 43–8. Fascicular structure of a nerve (after Carayon). A = proximal plexiform zone, B = site of origin of collateral branches, C = terminal zone.

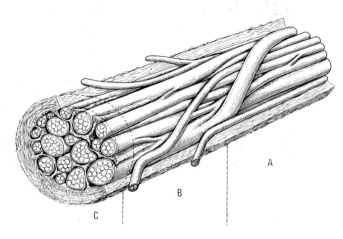

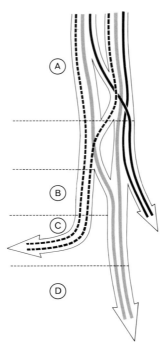

Figure 43–9. Fascicular organization. A = the proximal composition of a fascicle. The fascicle contains fibers for different destinations. B = Simple fascicle with a collateral. At this level, retrograde endoneurolysis is possible. C = Collateral. D = Simple fascicle ending in a terminal branch. Retrograde endoneurolysis is possible.

individualized by proximal dissection well beyond their "apparent" origin from the nerve trunk. Sunderland (1945) has studied the distance over which individual fascicles can be traced within the nerve. The surgical pos-

sibilities of selective fasciculation have been described and exploited by Carayon (1962), who showed that in the course of suturing nerve in certain well defined regions, some fascicles, such as the less important sensory collateral branches, could be safely excluded. Thus, in the radial nerve on the posterior aspect of the arm, the lateral cutaneous branch, whose fascicles make up 11 to 22 per cent of that section of the nerve (Sunderland, (1945), can be separated from the main part of the nerve trunk. Similarly, it is possible to isolate above the elbow those fascicles that form the anterior sensory branch.

The same applies to repair of the ulnar nerve in the middle third of the forearm. Here again, according to Sunderland (1978), one can exclude from suturing the dorsal cutaneous branch, which makes up 20 per cent of the fascicles and lies posteromedially.

Intraneural neurolysis of the collaterals may have other surgical applications. Thus, when the ulnar nerve is freed at the elbow, it is relatively easy to trace the articular fibers and motor fibers of the flexor carpi ulnaris proximally in order to facilitate its transposition anteriorly, a maneuver that is not feasible unless the collaterals are divided or the nerve is submitted to intraneural dissection, the latter being preferable (Fig. 43–12).

Not only do the fascicles exchange fibers, they do not occupy a fixed position within the nerve trunk. They change their relative position within the nerve, and the nerve is subject to variations in position. Within its connective tissue framework its shape de-

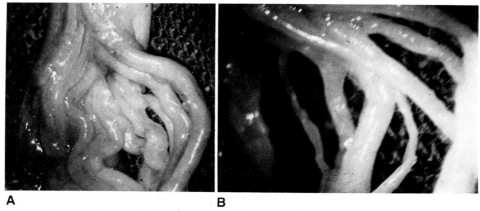

A   **B**

Figure 43–10. Intraneural perifascicular neurolysis of the proximal plexiform zone of the sciatic nerve. A, The beginning of the neurolysis, isolating the fascicular groups (× 10). B, A later stage of the dissection in which some individual fascicles have been isolated (× 25). Note the plexiform structure and the interfascicular connections.

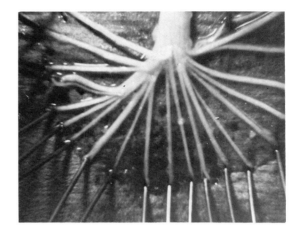

Figure 43–11. Dissection of the "terminal zone" of the median nerve at the wrist showing the fasciculi. Note the absence of the interfascicular connections.

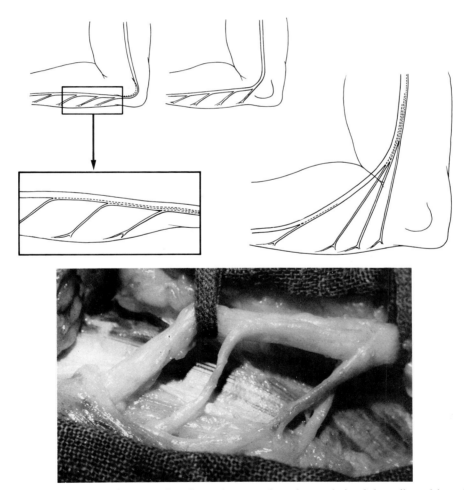

Figure 43–12. Diagrammatic and operative views of retrograde endoneurolysis of the collateral branches of the ulnar nerve during its transposition at the elbow (after Carayon).

pends on the adjacent peripheral anatomical
structures and varies along its course with the
position of the limb. Thus, in pronation or
supination it may rotate on its axis. All these
factors make accurate fascicular orientation
and realignment difficult even when tissue
loss is minimal (Figs. 43–13 and 43–14). Histological sections taken 1 cm away from the
C5 root of the brachial plexus have shown
different fascicular arrangements at different
levels. With the same protocol an analysis of
3 cm. of the median nerve in the forearm
showed an incongruous fascicular pattern

with regard to topography and diameter.
Only the appearance of the fascicles can assist
in nerve reorientation, and then only if they
can be distinguished one from another, which
is not always the case.

The difficulties involved in fascicular mapping of a nerve will now be obvious (Sunderland, 1978), for any attempt at such mapping
can be made only on nerve segments that
have been taken out of their context, and
that are often frayed, twisted, and inevitably
distorted by the sectioning itself. An accurate
mapping of fascicular topography is obviously

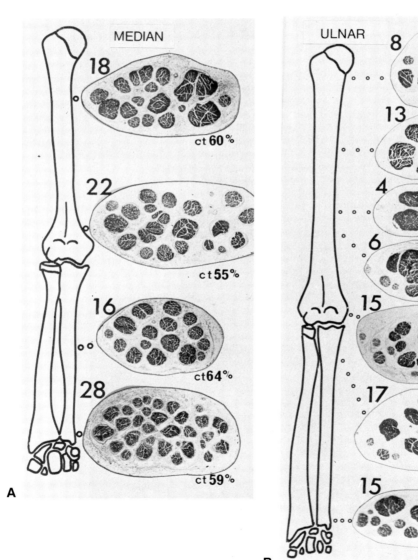

Figure 43–13. *A* and *B*, Histological section of the median and ulnar nerves at different levels of the limb. The qualitative and quantitative variations of the fascicles are precise. There is a high percentage of both perifascicular and interfascicular connective tissue.

Illustration continued on opposite page

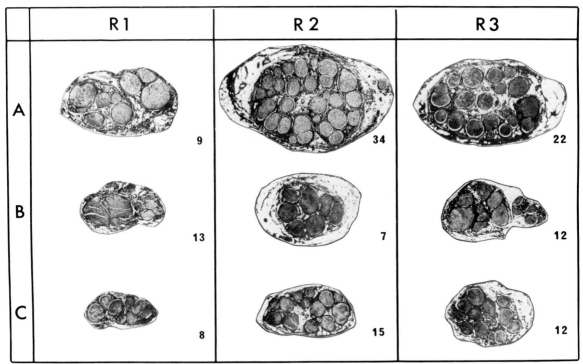

C

Figure 43–13 *Continued C*, Histological sections of the radial nerve in three patients at three levels. A = proximal to the radial groove, B = at the level of the radial groove, C = distal to the radial groove. There is an important variation in the number and topography of the fascicles in different specimens. *D*, Histological sections of the radial nerve in seven specimens.

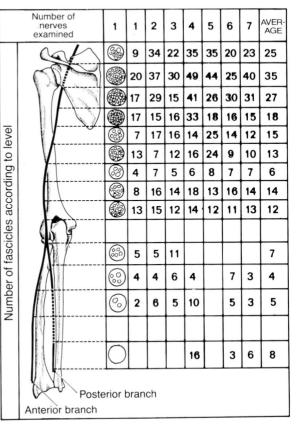

Number of nerves examined		1	1	2	3	4	5	6	7	AVERAGE
			9	34	22	35	35	20	23	25
			20	37	30	49	44	25	40	35
			17	29	15	41	26	30	31	27
			17	15	16	33	18	16	15	18
			7	17	16	14	25	14	12	15
			13	7	12	16	24	9	10	13
			4	7	5	6	8	7	7	6
			8	16	14	18	13	16	14	14
			13	15	12	14	12	11	13	12
			5	5	11					7
			4	4	6	4		7	3	4
			2	6	5	10		5	3	5
						16		3	6	8

Posterior branch
Anterior branch

D

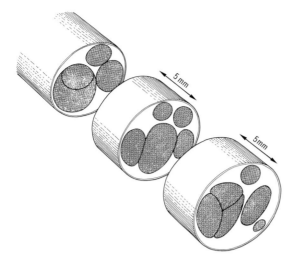

Figure 43–14. Serial histological sections of the C5 root of the brachial plexus over a 1 cm. distance.

illusory; at best such mapping can provide only general guidelines.

Serial histological studies on the roots of 10 brachial plexuses and seven radial nerves in humans showed numerous variations in the topography and diameter of the fascicles from one subject to another. A precise systematization as proposed by Sunderland does not seem possible to us (Fig. 43–15).

Our observations, however, do permit us to make some general observations about organization. Thus, for the roots of the brachial plexus, we found in the T1 root a small number of fascicles whose diameters varied between 2.4 and 2.6 mm. The roots of C5, C6, and C8 have a larger number of fascicles whose diameters are between 700 microns and 2.60 mm. The C7 root has a large number of fascicles with diameters from 15 microns to 1.29 mm.—much too small for fascicular repair to be possible.

In our analysis of the radial nerve we could distinguish three segments: the first segment proximal to the radial groove of the humerus has many fascicles (average, 35). The second segment in the radial groove has an average of six fascicles. The third distal segment has an average of 14 fascicles.

We have not been able to confirm at surgery the topography described by Sunder-

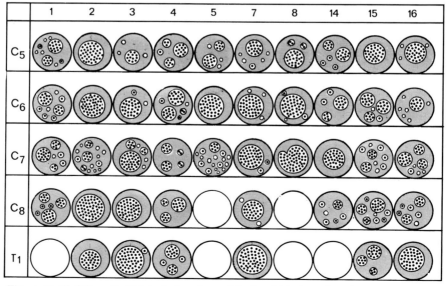

Figure 43–15. Schematic histological sections of the brachial plexus based on ten specimens.

land. More recent studies of numerous specimens have shown that the fascicular arrangement varies from one subject to another and even from one side to another. It would appear, therefore, that we cannot rely on research involving systematic fascicular mapping to help us solve our surgical problems. Only by carefully comparing the numbers, position, shape, and volume of the fascicles in the section can one hope to achieve some sort of match. It is sometimes possible, if tissue loss is minimal, to improve the chances of a good "fit" by close examination and making drawings of the two cross sections (Millesi, 1977).

Millesi and Terzis (1983) presented to the committee of the International Society of Reconstructive Surgery a classification distinguishing four types of intraneural structure: (1) a cross section consisting of one big fascicle, (2) a cross section consisting of a few large fascicles, (3) a cross section consisting of many fascicles of different sizes arranged in groups, and (4) a cross section consisting of many fascicles of different sizes without any group arrangement. Surgical techniques will be adapted to each type and differ for each nerve (Fig. 43–16).

THE FASCICULAR CONTENT

Two important factors must always be kept in mind—the existence of an intrafascicular connective tissue between the nerve fibers (the endoneurium), and the absence of segregation of the fibers within the fascicles.

In addition to the nerve fibers, the fascicles contain connective tissue—the endoneurium—made up of cells and an extracellular matrix. Thus, even at the fascicular level, approximation of nerve tissue may be hindered by a connective tissue barrier.

All the fascicles contain motor, sensory, and autonomic fibers. In a "mixed" fascicle the fibers will have different destinations. Thus, as far as the "simple" fascicles are concerned, it is possible to talk of a pure sensory nerve, but we must now substitute the term "muscular nerve" for motor nerve. Indeed, Rabischong has shown that even the terminal muscular branches include, in addition to the motor fibers, sensory fibers that mediate proprioceptive regulation; hence, the danger of malorientation at the intrafascicular level.

To the technical impossibility of accurately aligning each individual axon, must be added the very large and variable number of nerve fibers contained within the fascicles that make up the nerves. We have been able to determine their number in the nerves of the upper limb in seven specimens (Table 43–2).

These observations help to explain the difficulties of nerve regeneration, now well documented by ultrastructural studies. Nerve regeneration results from displacement of the cone of elongation of the axon as a result of traction. Elongation stops as soon as the axon comes into contact with connective tissue. Axonal growth succeeds as long as it encounters Schwann cells, i.e., as long as the fiber finds its way within the endoneurium. Accurate matching of motor and sensory fasciculi is also vital. As soon as contact is established between a nerve fiber and a muscle fiber, a motor endplate develops, the original territory of the nerve fiber. However, recovery of motor function depends on central orientation of the nerve. Sensory nerves, by contrast, are thus unable to initiate muscular activity, and malorientation means that this "neurotization" is doomed to failure. The problem of nerve regeneration therefore is a dual one—that of control of cicatrization, itself an obstacle to regeneration, and the no less complex problem of orientation, which, as anatomical studies have shown, goes well beyond the simplistic concept of fascicular approximation.

Table 43–2. NUMBER OF NERVE FIBERS (AXONS) WITHIN NERVES OF THE UPPER LIMB IN SEVEN SUBJECTS

Nerve	1	2	3	4	5	6	7	Mean
Median	7,457	14,606		21,899	27,190		20,296	18,288
Musculocutaneous					7,203	3,063	7,917	6,061
Ulnar	13,537		22,690	14,836	22,690	11,950	12,773	16,412
Radial	13,806	10,029	20,067	32,210		15,291	27,750	19,858
Circumflex	8,437	4,967						6,702

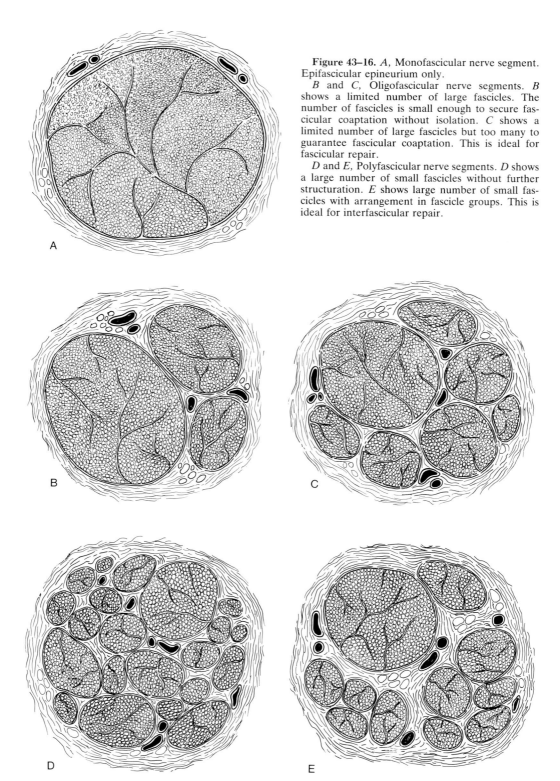

Figure 43–16. *A*, Monofascicular nerve segment. Epifascicular epineurium only.

B and *C*, Oligofascicular nerve segments. *B* shows a limited number of large fascicles. The number of fascicles is small enough to secure fascicular coaptation without isolation. *C* shows a limited number of large fascicles but too many to guarantee fascicular coaptation. This is ideal for fascicular repair.

D and *E*, Polyfascicular nerve segments. *D* shows a large number of small fascicles without further structuration. *E* shows large number of small fascicles with arrangement in fascicle groups. This is ideal for interfascicular repair.

THE VASCULAR SUPPLY OF PERIPHERAL NERVES

The blood supply to nerve trunks has been the subject of countless anatomical and physiological studies. Contrary to earlier belief, these studies have shown that the arterial supply is no less important to the maintenance of neural transmission than is anatomical continuity between the body of the neuron and its axon. We shall distinguish between the conventional macroscopic anatomical studies with which we associate the names of Quenu and Lejars (1892), Adams (1941), Sunderland and Smith (1966), and the more recent studies of microvascularization by Lundborg and Branemark (1968). This microvascularization at the fascicular level is one that conditions surgical dissection.

MACROSCOPIC VASCULARIZATION

The peripheral nerve receives its blood supply at regular intervals through vessels originating from larger limb arteries or their collaterals. The patterns of supply vary among individuals and between the two limbs in the same individual. The blood flow shows regional variations and appears to be more abundant near the joints. The feeder artery can approach the nerve directly or run for some distance along the surface of the nerve in a variety of ways (Sunderland). It may be terminal and penetrate the nerve directly or run for some distance along the surface of the nerve before entering its sheath, in which case it constitutes a useful operative landmark when a severed nerve is resutured. It may leave the nerve after supplying it, it may penetrate the nerve and run in its core, and it may even perforate the nerve without giving off any nerve branch.

According to Smith (1966), all vessels approach the nerve through the mesoneurium, a fine sheet of connective tissue that connects the epineurium to the neighboring connective tissue.* The width of the mesoneurium varies; it tends to be greater in the vicinity of joints where the nerve is more mobile. This enables the nerve to move without jeopard-

izing its blood supply. A mesoneurium accompanies the nerve trunk throughout its course as it does the collaterals and terminals. The term "mesoneurium," suggesting a specific entity comparable to the mesentery, may not be justified (Rabischong, 1975). It consists in fact of a thin sheet of undifferentiated connective tissue, such as is found around all vascular axes, which merges into the epineurium–connective tissue complex. But as Smith (1966) has shown—and this is important surgically—the vessels form a system of arcades overlapping at their extremities and lying within the mesoneurial sheet, which is itself inserted on the nerve along a straight line. Although in semantic terms we should not talk of a mesoneurium, the fact remains that surgically this structure is comparable to the mesotendon and mesentery.

The vascularization of the nerve is a well defined entity, and the mesoneurium must always be treated with the utmost care during surgical dissections. One cannot avoid dividing it during a neurolysis, but the arcade arrangement enables one to use certain technical maneuvers by which the blood supply of the nerve is spared as much as possible in the course of extensive dissection (Fig. 43–17).

The mesoneurium allows the surgeon to take the nerve and its blood supply together in free vascularized nerve grafts (Taylor, 1926).

Breidenbach and Terzis (1986) distinguished three types of nerve vascularization in view of their utilization for free vascularized nerve grafts: type 1, no dominant pedicle; type 2, one dominant pedicle; type 3, multiple dominant pedicles. Type 1 cannot be utilized for a vascularized graft. Only type 2 (superficial radial nerve, superficial peroneal nerve) or type 3 (saphenous nerve, ulnar nerve) can be used (Fig. 43–18).

MICROVASCULARIZATION OF THE PERIPHERAL NERVES

Lundborg and Branemark (1968) have reported their findings in regard to microvascularization of the peripheral nerves. They demonstrated that the nerve has a dual vascular system—an extrinsic (perifascicular) system and an intrinsic (intrafascicular) system, which communicate freely (Fig. 43–19).

*See Chapter 35 in Volume I.

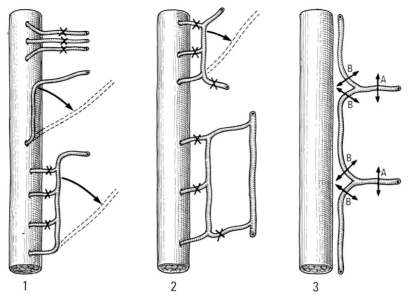

Figure 43–17. Macroscopic vasculature of a peripheral nerve. Technique for preserving the vascularization of a nerve in extended neurolyses (after Sunderland). Different types of ligature are used, based on the vascular anatomy.

The Extrinsic System

As they reach the nerve, accompanied by venules and variable numbers of capillaries, the feeding arteries run longitudinally in the epineurium in both directions. These longitudinal vessels give off collaterals, which are distributed around the various fascicles within the perineurium. There are extensive anastomoses between the epineural vessels that form an extrafascicular plexus. This extrafascicular extrinsic system communicates with the intrafascicular system.

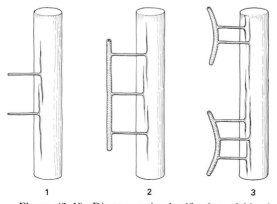

Figure 43–18. Diagrammatic classification of blood supply to nerves. 1 = no dominant pedicle, 2 = one dominant pedicle, 3 = multiple dominant pedicles.

The Intrinsic System

The intrafascicular vascular bed lies within the endoneurium. Continuous throughout the length of the nerve, it consists of capillaries that are mostly longitudinal, although some run transversely and obliquely.

Thus, vascularization of the nerve trunks provides further support for the conception of the fascicle as an anatomical unit. The two systems, extrinsic and intrinsic, complement each other to a large extent; hence, the absence of serious functional consequences when a feeding artery is deficient. This had been amply demonstrated experimentally even by early workers, such as Adams (1941). Stripping a nerve over a short distance does not produce significant ischemia, because the intrafascicular network is able to supply the nerve fibers. Similarly, a cut nerve will bleed at both ends even after an extensive mobilization, which means that a nerve can be mobilized after a dissection of several centimeters. Safe surgical limits cannot yet be set because of a lack of accurate transposable data regarding the variability of the arterial pattern; until such information is available, preservation of the blood supply, i.e., of the mesoneurium, remains the golden rule. Thus, a nerve can be freed by dissection over a limited distance provided the intraneural vessels are intact. The presence of a rich longi-

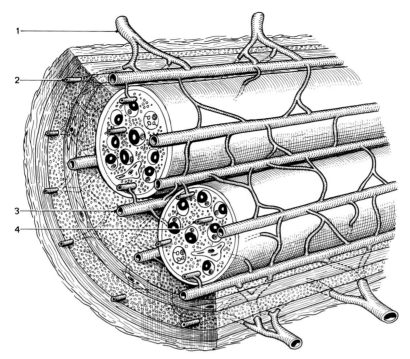

Figure 43–19. Intraneural microvascular structure of a peripheral nerve. 1 = vessels of the nutrient artery, 2 = epineural system, 3 = interfascicular system, 4 = intrafascicular system.

tudinal intrafascicular network permits some intraneural dissection. This damages the extrinsic system, as it is difficult to avoid the interfascicular epineural vessels. In such cases every effort should be made to spare the mesoneurium on the posterior aspect of the nerve. This is usually possible in decompression of the median nerve at the wrist.

Although the vascular arrangement is, to a certain extent, favorable to neurolysis, it also renders the nerve vulnerable to compression and traction forces. This was demonstrated in the rabbit by Lundborg and Rydevick (1973), who blamed the tortuous helicoidal arrangement of the intrafascicular microvascular architecture. The same factor could explain the damaging effect of tension developing during nerve repair.

The venous system closely parallels the arterial system, but the lymphatic channels follow a different pattern. They can be found in the epineurium but not in the perineurium or endoneurium. Here again the perineurium acts as a barrier between two different "environments." This may explain the resistance of the nerve, or more specifically the fascicles, to infection.

The nervi nervorum carry sympathetic vasomotor fibers to the vessels of the nerve trunk and sensory fibers from the epineurium (Kuczynski, 1974).

GENERAL OBSERVATIONS REGARDING THE ANATOMY OF THE NERVE TRUNKS

ANOMALOUS DISTRIBUTION

Anomalies are relatively common, especially in the hand; hence, the difficulties in evaluating results unless a precise clinical examination has been made preoperatively. The classic motor and sensory territories are subject to variation, and we cannot consider here all the known variations. However, their frequent occurrence should always be kept in mind. The anomalies may be secondary to variations in the distribution of the collaterals or terminals, and to anastomoses between the nerve trunks.

Variations in the Distribution of Collaterals and Terminals

Such variations can be found in the same nerve. Thus, the extensor carpi radialis and brevis can be innervated entirely not by the radial nerve itself but by its posterior motor branch. The same muscle may be innervated by two different adjacent nerves. The flexor profundus may be supplied by the collaterals of either the median or the ulnar nerve.

Anomalous distribution of the sensory collateral branches of the digital nerves is also common. Thus, sensation of the fourth and even the third finger may be mediated by either the ulnar or the median nerve. As for the pulp of the thumb, its lateral side is supplied to a variable extent by the radial nerve.

Anastomoses

The functional significance of nerve anastomoses is not obvious, but they explain the overlaps observed. Anastomoses and fiber exchanges are common between the musculocutaneous and median nerves in the upper half of the forearm. Medioulnar anastomoses are the best known, and explain the variability in the innervation of the thenar muscles in particular (anastomosis of Martin Gruber in the forearm and anastomosis of Riche and Cannien in the hand). Another anastomosis worth knowing about is that of Froment Rauber, between the deep branch of the ulnar nerve and the posterior interosseous nerves at the level of the dorsal interosseous muscles. This interesting communication, which produces overlap of the flexion and extension territories, could explain the sparing of the intrinsic muscles in some cases of ulnar palsy.

The "Exposed Zones" Concept

The peripheral nerves have to pass through inextensible osteoligamentomuscular tunnels, where they are exposed to mechanical damage, especially compression, which can affect their blood supplies. Sunderland (1978) believes that the epineurium constitutes the best protection against compression, and that nerves, which have many small fascicles and a high percentage of epineural connective tissue, are less vulnerable to compression than are those with fewer fascicles, such as the ulnar nerve at the elbow. This theory is not borne out by clinical experience, which shows the vulnerability of the multifascicular median nerve in the carpal tunnel. However, the apparent lack of fascicles in a nerve is

often due to the tight packing of the fascicles, as a result of mechanically induced sclerosis of the epineurium. The notion of exposed zones could explain some apparently spontaneous neurological syndromes of the upper limb. There are in fact two particularly narrow channels—the carpal tunnel for the median nerve and the osteofibrous canal under the arch of the flexor carpi ulnaris for the ulnar nerve.

Other fibromuscular tunnels are found less commonly. They include the epitrochlear ring at the humeral canal for the median nerve, the muscular buttonhole of the pronator teres, and the arch of the flexor superficialis communis, also for the median nerve. Similarly the radial nerve may be compressed at the arch of Fröhse. As for the classic canal of Guyon, in which the ulnar nerve may undergo compression, it is a topographical reality but not an inextensible tunnel. Compression of the nerve at that level is due to secondary causes.

The zones of true fibromuscular compression are rare and somewhat variable. Thus, certain anomalies may give rise to nerve compression—Ganzer's muscle in the forearm, and anomalous insertions of supernumerary muscles in the hand.

The syndromes resulting from nerve compression in the forearm and hand have been well described by Spinner (1980).* The real causes of the neural lesions, however, are still not known, and may include compression, microtrauma, friction, or vascular disturbances (Lundborg, 1970; Ochoa et al., 1972). This illustrates the chief difficulty in all studies of the peripheral nervous system, i.e., that of extrapolating to human clinical practice observations made during animal experimentation.

---

*See chapter on Nerve Compression in the Forearm, Elbow, and Arm in Volume IV.

REFERENCES

Adams W. E.: The blood supply of nerves. J. Anat., 76:323–341, 1941.
Allieu, Y.: La chirurgie nerveuse périphérique: conceptions actuelles et perspectives d'avenir. Cahiers Réed. Réadapt. 10:237–243, 1975.
Allieu, Y.: Exploration et traitement direct des lésions nerveuses dans les paralysies traumatiques par élongation du plexus brachial chez l'adulte. Rev. Chir. Orthop., 63:107–122, 1977.
Allieu, Y., and Rabischong, P.: Systématisation endo-

neurale des nerfs du membre supérieur. Presentation at meeting of H Groupe d'Etude de la Main, Marseille, 1975.

Allieu, Y., and Alnot, J. Y.: Résultat des sutures nerveuses sous microscope. Rev. Chir. Orthop., 64:276–283, 1978.

Bonnel, F.: Configuration interne histo-physiologique du plexus brachial. Rev. Chir. Orthop., 63:35–38, 1977.

Bonnel, F.: Structure fasciculaire des nerfs périphériques—membre supérieur. Neurochirurgie, 28:71–76, 1982.

Bonnel, F., Allieu, Y., Bruner, P., Gilbert, A., and Rabischong, P.: Anatomical and surgical principles of the brachial plexus in the newborn children. Int. J. Microsurg., 2:12–15, 1980.

Bonnel, F.: Histologic structure of the ulnar nerve in the hand. J. Hand Surg., 10A(2):264–269, 1985.

Bonnel, F., Allieu, Y., Sugata, Y., and Rabischong, P.: Anatomico-surgical bases of neurotization for root avulsion of the brachial plexus. Anat. Clin., 1:291–296, 1979.

Bonnel, F., Mailhe, D., Allieu, Y., and Rabischong, P.: The general anatomy and endoneural fascicular arrangement of the median nerve at the wrist. Anat. Clin., 2:201–207, 1981.

Bonnel, F., and Rabischong, P.: Anatomy and systematization of the brachial plexus in the adult. Anat. Clin., 2:289–298, 1981.

Breidenbach, W. C., and Terzis, J. K.: The blood supply of vascularized nerve grafts. J. Reconstr. Microsurg., 3:43–55, 1986.

Carayon, A.: La neurolyse fasciculaire. J. Chir., 83:435–472, 1962.

Curtis, R. M., and Eyersman, W. W.: Internal neurolysis as an adjunct to the treatment of the carpal tunnel syndrome. J. Bone Joint Surg., 55A:733, 1973.

Gamble, M. J., and Eames, R. A.: An electron microscope study of the connective tissues of human peripheral nerve. J Anat. (Lond.) 88:655–683, 1964.

Jabaley, M. E., Wallace, W. H., and Heckler, F. R.: Internal topography of major nerves of the forearm and hand: a current view. J. Hand Surg., 5:1–18, 1980.

Kakstian, R. W.: Funicular orientation by direct stimulation: an aid to peripheral nerve repair. J. Bone Joint Surg., 50A:1178–1186, 1968.

Kuczynski, K.: Functional micro-anatomy of the peripheral nerve trunks. Hand, 6:1–10, 1974.

Lundborg, G.: Ischemic nerve injury. Experimental studies on intraneural microvascular pathophysiology and nerve function in a limb subjected to temporary circulatory arrest. Scand. J. Plast. Reconstr. Surg., Suppl. 6, 1970.

Lundborg, G., and Branemark, P. I.: Microvascular structure and function of peripheral nerves. Vital microscopic studies of the tibial nerve in the rabbit. Acta Microcirc., 1:66–88, 1968.

Lundborg, G., and Devick, B.: Effects of stretching the tibial nerve of the rabbit. A preliminary study of the intraneural circulation and the barrier function of the perineurium. J. Bone Joint Surg., 55B:390–401, 1973.

Millesi, H.: Surgical management of brachial plexus injuries. J. Hand Surg., 2:367–379, 1977.

Millesi, H., Meissl, G., and Berger, A.: The interfascicular nerve grafting of the median and ulnar nerve. J. Bone Joint Surg., 54A:727–750, 1972.

Millesi, H., and Terzis, J. K.: Problems of terminology in peripheral nerve surgery: committee report of the International Society of Reconstructive Microsurgery. Microsurgery, 4:51–56, 1983.

Ochoa, J., Fowler, T. J., and Gilliatt, R. W.: Anatomical changes in peripheral nerves compressed by a pneumatic tourniquet. J. Anat., 113:433–455, 1972.

Poirier, J.: L'ultrastructure des nerfs périphériques. Presse Méd., 20:23–26, 1968.

Quenu, J., and Lejars, F.: Etude anatomique sur les vaisseaux sanguins des nerfs. Arch. Neurol., 23:1–15, 1892.

Rabischong, P., and Bonnel, F.: Systématisation endoneurale des nerfs du membre supérieur. Presentation at meeting of H Groupe d'Etude de la Main, Montpellier, 1975.

Seddon, H. J.: Surgical Disorders of the Peripheral Nerves. London, Churchill Livingstone, 1975.

Sherren, J.: Injuries of the nerves. New York, William Wood, 1907.

Smith, J. W.: Factors influencing nerve repair collateral circulation of peripheral nerves. Arch. Surg., 93:433–437, 1966.

Spinner, M.: Management of Peripheral Nerve Problems. Philadelphia, W. B. Saunders Company, 1980, pp. 569–592.

Sunderland, S.: The intraneural topography of the radial median, and ulnar nerves. Brain, 68:243–298, 1945.

Sunderland, S.: Nerves and Nerve Injuries. Ed. 2. London, Churchill-Livingstone, 1978.

Taylor, I. G., and Ham, F. J.: The free vascularized nerve graft. Plast. Reconstr. Surg., 57:413–425, 1976.

Terzis, J. K.: Principles, practices, and techniques of peripheral nerve surgery. In Daniel, R. K., and Terzis, J. K. (editors). Reconstructive Microsurgery. Boston, Little Brown, 1977.

Thomas, P. K.: The connective tissue of peripheral nerve: an electron miscroscope study. J. Anat., 97:35–44, 1963.

Chapter 44

RECENT ADVANCES IN PERIPHERAL NERVE SURGERY: BASIC RESEARCH AND CLINICAL APPLICATION

Joel Engel

Abraham Ganel

Batia Yaffe

Sarah Pri-Chen

Sarah Rimon

and Yeheskell Shemesh

Multiple factors influence the final outcome in patients with severed nerves. Some factors can be dealt with, but others are still enigmas attracting intense research efforts. Refinement of surgical techniques, microsurgical anastomosis, nerve grafting, and the development of modern suture materials have contributed significantly in improving the results of treatment. Increasing the rate of nerve regeneration, prevention of wallerian degeneration, inhibition of scar formation within and outside nerve fibers, and maintenance of functional denervated "target organs" are topics currently being investigated all over the world.

In this chapter biochemical and electrophysiological methods that are currently used or are potentially effective in improving the results of nerve anastomosis will be described.

Biochemical Compounds Affecting Nerve Anastomosis and Nerve Degeneration

Batia Yaffe

Recovery of motor and sensory function following neurorrhaphy is inhibited by excessive scarring and neuroma formation at the anastomosis site and by wallerian degeneration of the distal neural stump and denervation atrophy of the muscles.

SCAR AND NEUROMA FORMATION

Scar formation is essential for normal wound healing. However, excessive proliferation of scar tissue and collagen at the neurorrhaphy site forms an obstacle to the budding of axons (Sunderland, 1978). Subsequent maturation of collagen and shrinkage of the scar may have an additional constricting effect on nerve tissue, creating a chronic entrapment syndrome at the suture site. Several methods and different substances have been tried experimentally to reduce the amount of scar formation.

Graham and coworkers (1973) demonstrated decreased scarring and histological evidence of nerve regeneration after neurorrhaphy following treatment with triamcinolone. In a primate model triamcinolone acetonide instilled locally around the nerve anastomosis site immediately after the repair was shown to have a beneficial effect on the regeneration of nerves (Graham et al., 1982). The results of treatment were measured 12 months after repair by study of the conduction velocity of the repaired nerve, the amplitude of the evoked response, and histological examination of the distal stump. The systemic administration of steroids failed to prevent scar formation at the anastomosis site (Kline et al., 1971; Lundborg et al., 1981).

Cis-hydroxyproline, an analogue of proline, acts as a specific inhibitor of collagen biosynthesis by preventing the formation of a normal collagen triple helix. Bora and associates (1983) showed that the formation of a nerve scar after injury is significantly reduced by the local administration of Alzamer, a cis-hydroxyproline in a bioerodable vehicle.

By slowly disolving the Alzamer at a predetermined rate, small amounts of cis-hydroxyproline are released locally, favorably affecting the nerve anastomosis. The same investigators had reported previously that if given subcutaneously four to 21 days after transection and reanastomosis of the sciatic nerves in rats, cis-hydroxyproline diminishes collagen formation and neuroma formation at the suture line and increases the myelin content of the distal segment (Pleasure et al., 1974). Lundborg (1981), in a preliminary study comparing the effects of systemic administration of steroids and cis-hydroxyproline, reported increased conduction velocity in the repaired nerves of cis-hydroxyproline treated rats.

Hastings and Peacock (1973) succeeded in reducing collagen accumulation after neurorrhaphy by creating vitamin C deficiency in guinea pigs.

NERVE AND MUSCLE DEGENERATION

Progressive wallerian degeneration in the distal stump of a transected or crushed nerve, leaving a narrowed and distorted distal tubular structure, is another obstacle for budding axons (Gutmann and Young, 1944; Richter et al., 1979; Sunderland and Bradley, 1950). Some investigators believe that wallerian degeneration can be minimized by the use of more precise microsurgical techniques of primary nerve repair (Brunelli, 1981). Triiodothyronine (T_3) and dibutyryl-3':5' cyclic adenosine monophosphate (AMP) have been reported to accelerate recovery from wallerian degeneration and to enhance axonal sprouting (Cockett and Kierman, 1973; Pichichero et al., 1973; Roisen et al., 1972).

Wallerian degeneration and muscular denervation atrophy are mediated by proteolytic enzymes. Specific enzymatic inhibitors might slow these degradation processes and thereby facilitate functional recovery following neurorrhaphy.

425

Hurst et al. (1983) treated rats with leupeptin (a thiol protease inhibitor) after transecting and suturing the sciatic nerve. Nerve and muscle degeneration in the treated group was delayed as compared with that in the control animals. Nerve degeneration was measured after six months by determining wet muscle weight and by histological, histochemical, and electron microscopic analyses. Another in vivo study demonstrated that the administration of leupeptin, pepstatin, and aprotinins partly prevented the early (24 hours) denervation induced decrease in muscle weight and protein content, in addition to reducing the decrease in acetylcholine esterase activity in denervated muscle (Fernandez and Dnell, 1980).

As yet there is little clinical proof of the beneficial effects of any of these methods in human patients.

Nerve Growth Acceleration: In Vivo and In Vitro Studies

SARAH PRI-CHEN

SARAH RIMON

The capacity for nerve regeneration involves recapitulation of the neonatal state of a neuron (Pate-Skene and Willard, 1981). Most mammalian central nervous system neurons fail to express the genes for growth associated proteins. This may explain their limited capacity to regenerate after axonal injury. By contrast, neurons in the peripheral nervous system are capable of expressing growth associated protein genes, a necessary but insufficient condition for regeneration.

In peripheral nerve lesions, protective (e.g., perineurium) barriers are broken and the axons have to grow in the environment of a healing wound. Restoration of the proper microenvironment is essential for optimal regeneration. One approach to improving the microenvironment is to use a cuff to insure precise anastomosis with minimal adhesions, isolate the anastomosis from ingrowing fibrous tissue, guide the sprouting axons to the end organ, preventing sprouting sideways, and create longitudinal alignment of components at the junctional tissue. Because it is imperative to provide the nerve with a blood supply from its vicinity, a compromise between complete isolation and external ingrowth must be achieved. Cuffing methods described in the past include the use of filter tubes of millipore, porous stainless steel, micropore, decalcified bone, arteries, veins, fascia lata, tantalum, gelatine, rubber, and various metals (Campbell et al., 1961; Freeman, 1964; Kuhn and Hall, 1974; Maw and Loizean, 1971; Rosen et al., 1980). All these cuffing materials failed, some because of a foreign body reaction, whereas others were sealed too perfectly, depriving the nerve of its environmental supplies. The desire for an inert implant led to experimentation with silicon tubes (Midgley and Woolhouse, 1968), and other studies led to the search for biological materials for cuffing.

Finsterbush et al. (1982) showed that isolation of a nerve involved in a soft tissue injury by use of a split silicone cuff greatly reduces the damaging effect of the surrounding scar tissue on the nerve. The protected nerve is able to glide freely during mobilization of the limb. The blood supply to the nerve is maintained through the split in the Silastic cuff by the formation of a new mesoneurium.

Lundborg and his collaborators introduced a pseudosynovial tube as an experimental model for studying peripheral nerve regeneration (Lundborg, 1981; Lundborg et al., 1982a,b). They used a mesothelial tube to bridge a 12 mm. gap in the rat sciatic nerve. Their studies demonstrated the restoration of normal morphology of the nerve and a good electromyographic recording from the reinervated muscles. Good results were achieved only when both the proximal and distal stumps were inserted into the tube. When the interstump gap was left unbridged, negligible functional regeneration occurred. These results are similar to those obtained with nerve grafts.

For neuronal survival and regeneration a continuous supply of neurotropic factors is essential (Varon and Adler, 1980, 1981). The best known neurotropic factor is nerve growth factor (Levi-Montalcini, 1966; Varon, 1975). It supports survival and elicits neurite outgrowth of sympathetic or sensory neurons in tissue cultures. Other neurotropic factors from Schwann cells and skeletal muscle extracts have been less well characterized (Smith and Appel, 1983; Varon et al., 1981), but have been shown to exert neurotropic effects on ganglionic and spinal cord cells and motor neurons in vitro.

Lundborg et al. (1982b) claim that neurotropic factors accumulate in vivo in mesothelial or silicone chambers containing both proximal and distal stumps. Thus Lundborg's model constitutes a sort of "tissue culture" in situ. The fluid that accumulates contains considerable neurotropic activity for sensory, motor, and sympathetic neurons. Neurotropic factor directed to sensory neurons appears several hours after transection, whereas neurotropic factor directed to motor and sympathetic neurons appears after several days. These different dynamics indicate that these tropic activities are due to different factors. Neurotropic growth factor cannot account for the increased survival of the cells, because antibodies to neurotropic growth factor do not eliminate the observed tropic effect.

In similar experiments Politis et al. (1982) showed that the cells in the distal stump of a transected nerve exert a tropic effect on the regeneration of proximal stump. This effect is mediated over distances of several millimeters via diffusible factors.

Glial cells grown in tissue culture release a macromolecule that promotes neurite extension (Monard and Gunther, 1983). It has been shown that nonendocrinic active fragments of ACTH have neurotropic effects on the sciatic nerve in the rat (Schotman et al., 1983).

Gangliosides are cell membrane associated molecules present in high concentrations in the nervous system (Leeden, 1978). Local application of gangliosides to the site of a crush injury in the sciatic nerve increases the number of regenerating axons (Sparrow and Grafstein, 1982). Daily intraperitoneal injection of gangliosides also enhances sprouting of transected rat sciatic nerve (Gonio et al., 1983).

Adhesion to a substratum appears to be a prerequisite for the survival, differentiation, and proliferation of normal cells. The substratum on which peripheral axons elongate is provided by cell surface and intracellular matrices of connective tissue, or by surfaces of Schwann cells in the distal nerve segment during regeneration (Adler et al., 1981). In vitro coating of dishes with cationic polymers such as polylysine and polyornithine has been proved to support the attachment and survival of dissociated peripheral and central neurons, but the attached neurons exhibited limited neurite regeneration (Manthorpe et al., 1983). The conditioning media of various cells contain a factor called polyornithine attachable neurite promoting factor, which produces dramatic increases in neurite production in peripheral neurons but has no effect on central nervous system neurons (Adler et al., 1981).

During peripheral nervous system development, longitudinal axonal growth may be influenced by basement membrane components, e.g., glycoproteins, such as fibronectin and laminine (Baron-Van Evercooren et al., 1982), that provide "directional" information in the form of longitudinal gradients. Experiments have shown that the addition of purified fibronectin mediates the attachment of dissociated cells to collagen. Laminine has recently been localized in the basement membrane at the neuromuscular junction and around Schwann cells in peripheral nerves. Its stimulative effect on neurite growth was found to be more pronounced than that with fibronectin (Baron-Van Evercooren et al., 1982).

Studies have shown that microcarriers coated with cationic groups, such as diethylaminoethane, have positive effects on the adherence and spreading of growth cells (Reuveny et al., 1983). On the basis of these observations, we used nylon thread to which diethylaminoethane groups were covalently bound to test their capacity to bind neurite promoting factors (NPF).

The nylon threads were treated with diethylaminoethane for varying lengths of time—0, 1.5 hours, 3.5 hours, and 5.5 hours. The number of diethylaminoethane groups bound to the thread was found to be proportional to the reaction time. Three animals were used for each reaction time determination. The thread was wound around a polyethylene tube seven times. The tube length was 13 to 15 mm. and its internal diameter, 2.5 mm. (This length is sufficient to bridge a 7 mm. gap in the sciatic nerve of the rat.) Both stumps of the cut nerve were introduced into the tube, resting on the charged nylon threads. The tube was secured to the surrounding tissue (muscle) with four sutures. The tubes were rejected by the rats (as foreign bodies); hence the positive charge effect could not be evaluated.

In order to overcome the chemical inertness of commercially available silicone tubes, we are currently using a Silastic 382 medical grade elastomer (Dow Corning) into which various substances are incorporated. We have incorporated hemoglobin and dextran blue, and the tubes that were formed were either red or blue, respectively. These polymers remained entrapped in the Silastic tubes even after long soaking in buffers.

To test the activity of the entrapped protein we incorporated catalase into the polymerized tubes. The catalase entrapped in these tubes decomposed hydrogen peroxide efficiently, proving that the catalase did not lose its enzymatic activity. These results encouraged us to incorporate into Silastic tubes or chambers cationic synthetic substances like polyornithine or natural substances available from human sources, such as fibronectin or laminine. These tubes are being used to bridge 10 to 12 mm. gaps in transected sciatic nerves of rats, and their effect on the "in vitro" system is being tested.

Nerve Fascicle Identification

ABRAHAM GANEL

JOEL ENGEL

In cases of complete transection of mixed peripheral motor and sensory nerves, the matching of the cut ends of a nerve is a complicated but most significant problem. Inappropriate matching of a proximal motor nerve stump with a distal sensory nerve stump and vice versa will result in failure of motor or sensory recovery. Precise differentiation between these two kinds of nerve fascicles is essential for successful surgical treatment. There are few purely sensory or purely motor nerve fascicles. Unless motor to motor and sensory to sensory axon anastomosis is achieved, some mismatching is inevitable. It is therefore imperative to know which fascicle is the most motor and which is the most sensory so as to permit a "logical" matching between nerve fascicles. Even in regard to the current "group fascicular" suture technique, this information is extremely important in order to restore function.

Over the years various methods have been developed to improve fascicle matching in cases of mixed peripheral nerve transections.

ANATOMICAL ORIENTATION

Sunderland (1978) focused his studies on the anatomical division and fusion of the funiculi along nerve trunks. The change within the funicular plexus over short distances requires a thorough knowledge of the various cross sections of each nerve along its course in the extremity. Funicular atrophy of the distal nerve stump causes discrepancies in the sizes of the funiculi at the nerve ends and prejudices the entry of regenerating axons into the funiculi of the distal stump.

Sunderland (1981) recommends the restoration of nerve trunk continuity on a funicular basis, using a group funicular technique. He advocates the use of blood vessel location to obtain correct alignment of the nerve ends during repair and study of specific morphology of the funicular groups at the nerve end as another guide.

Sunderland's method, as well as other similar methods of intraoperative sketching of the fascicular pattern of intraneural topography (Millesi, 1969; Walton and Finseth, 1977), requires a fundamental knowledge of the fascicular pattern at different levels of various nerves, and all are time consuming. Even with these methods the precise function of each fascicle is still unknown; thus errors in matching are inevitable.

NERVE STIMULATION

Hakstian (1968) developed a technique of intraoperative direct nerve stimulation to differentiate between motor and sensory nerve fascicles. This method requires full intraoperative cooperation by the patient and thus is done under local anesthesia with no tourniquet. These inconveniences limit the extent of surgery and are associated with marked discomfort to the patient and disadvantages for the surgeon. This electrophysiological method, which has been used by various investigators (Grabb et al., 1970; Vandeput et al., 1969), is restricted to use with freshly lacerated nerves, since severed nerve fibers no longer conduct after 72 hours.

Nakatsuchi et al. (1980) reported good results using an electrophysiological method to obtain funicular orientation of the proximal stump in old nerve lacerations. Because the distal stump in old lacerations was not responsive to electrical stimulation, its dissection was essential.

Gaul (1983) has modified the electrophysiological general anesthesia "wake-up" technique currently used to monitor spinal cord function during corrective spinal surgery. He uses general anesthesia, in which the patient is not intubated, to permit intraoperative conversation after the patient is awakened with pure oxygen by mask. It is essential that the proper balance of medication be maintained to maximize the patient's response and to minimize his apprehension and pain. The

430

patient is requested to name the digit in which he feels the stimulus, and in this way the proximal stump is searched for major sensory fascicles. The distal stump is searched by observation of the twitching in the appropriate intrinsic muscles of the hand. Gaul's results reconfirm the applicability of this method in recent nerve injuries; in late cases distal nerve dissection is often required for motor nerve identification.

HISTOCHEMICAL METHODS

A histochemical method for nerve fascicle differentiation was developed by Gruber and his associates (1976). They demonstrated a difference in the distribution of acetylcholinesterase in motor and sensory funiculi, using a specific staining technique. The essential difference appears in the myelinated fibers: In motor funiculi about half the myelinated fibers are stained, whereas nearly all the myelinated fibers in sensory funiculi are unstained. The major handicap of this technique is the slow biochemical reaction, which requires 25 to 30 hours of incubation, and the consequent need for two operations—an initial operation to obtain nerve slices and mark the nerve cut ends, and a second one two to three days later for definitive repair.

ADDITIONAL BIOCHEMICAL ASSAYS

Extensive work in the use of biochemical methods to differentiate between motor and sensory nerve fascicles has been performed by our group (Engel et al., 1980; Ganel et al., 1982). We have tried to estimate acetylcholinesterase activity by a rapid radiobiochemical assay. However, the acetylcholin-esterase activity in motor fibers was only about two times higher than that in sensory fibers, and therefore unsuitable for precise identification because many fascicles contain a mixture of motor and sensory fibers. Another enzyme was therefore investigated.

We studied the activity of choline acetyltransferase, also called choline acetylase or chAC, in different nerve fibers. Choline acetyltransferase promotes the synthesis of acetylcholine from choline and acetylcoenzyme-A (Fig. 44–1). By using nerve slices and nerve homogenates obtained from fresh human cadavers it was possible to demonstrate choline acetyltransferase activity eight times greater in motor nerve fascicles than in sensory nerve fascicles (Engel et al., 1980). The relatively fast biochemical method—taking about 60 minutes from the time a nerve fascicle specimen is obtained—and its precise identification as a motor fascicle, a sensory fascicle, or a combined fascicle with the predominance of one of these two—suggested the clinical applicability of this method.

In another study, in an attempt to estimate the effect of time on this method (the duration of the method's applicability), we measured choline acetyltransferase activity after complete transection of the sciatic nerve in rats (Ganel et al., 1981). There was a steady increase in choline acetyltransferase activity in the proximal nerve stump and a rapid drop in the distal nerve stump (Fig. 44–2). Ninety-six hours following transection no appreciable activity could be detected in the distal segment. The increase in the proximal segment was followed by a slight decline and leveling off at about twice the normal level. This study suggested that by using the enzymatic nerve differentiation technique, an end to end nerve anastomosis could be performed within the first 96 hours. In late nerve injuries the different fasciculi in the proximal nerve

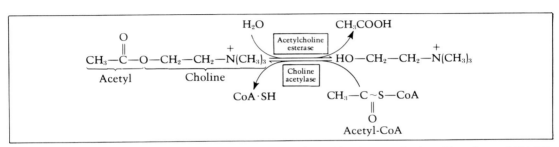

Figure 44–1. Enzymatic activity of choline acetyltransferase. (From Engel, J., et al.: Ann. Plast. Surg., *4*:376–380, 1980.)

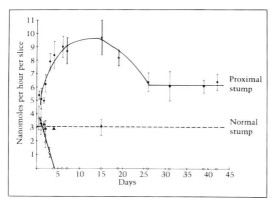

Figure 44–2. Choline acetyltransferase activity changes measured up to the forty-fifth day following transection of the sciatic nerve in rats. (From Engel, J.: Ann. Plast. Surg., 6:228–230, 1981.)

stump could be identified for up to 45 days. Neurolysis and anatomical tracing of the different fascicles in the distal nerve stump would permit precise matching.

Our study was expanded to include clinical use of this biochemical nerve identification technique. In a preliminary review the intra-operative use of this nerve differentiation technique was reported (Ganel et al., 1982). Three patients with late nerve injuries (two to five months) underwent operation. Two required end to end nerve anastomosis and one, cable grafts. Precise identification of the various fascicles in the proximal stump was achieved in all these patients. In the distal stump the nerve fascicles were anatomically identified by following them to their "target organs." In contrast to animal studies, we detected choline acetyltransferase activity in the distal segment that was different for the various fascicles five months after transection.

Biochemical nerve identification is applicable for intraoperative use, requiring only 60 to 80 minutes from resection of nerve samples to the obtaining of final results. It is our routine in all late and fresh nerve injuries to base the anastomosis on the results of this nerve identification technique. Although long term follow-up data on the clinical use of this technique are lacking, such information is gradually being accumulated.

Cortical Monitoring—Somatosensory Evoked Potentials

YEHESKELL SHEMESH

Conventional nerve conduction studies can be used to detect pathological processes in the distal segment of peripheral nerves; the proximal segments are technically not easily accessible to stimulating electrodes. Monitoring of somatosensory evoked potentials recorded on the scalp permits assessment of the entire length of the somatosensory pathway.

The somatosensory evoked potential was first recorded by Dawson in 1947 in a patient suffering from myoclonic epilepsy, a disease characterized electrophysiologically by enhancement of the amplitude of the evoked response; therefore no sophisticated equipment was required for its monitoring (Dawson, 1947; Kelly et al., 1981). Subsequently Dawson developed his averager, a small computer clearing all background noise, which averages the evoked response and gives a clear and simple average potential (Dawson, 1951, 1954). This development initiated the present explosive increase in studies of evoked potentials.

The somatosensory evoked potential has been used to evaluate peripheral nerve lesions, brachial plexus disorders, radiculopathy, silent lesions in multiple sclerosis, spinal cord injury, and brain stem and cerebral lesions (Assmus, 1981; Dorfman et al., 1980; Eisen and Elleker, 1980; Hume and Cant, 1981; Jones, 1979; McDonald, 1980; Van Beek et al., 1986; Zverina et al., 1977).

The somatosensory evoked potential is mediated mainly via peripheral sensory fibers (type IA; Lloyd, 1943) and centrally through the dorsal column medial lemniscal system. Smaller fibers (types II, III, and C) may also contribute to the potential after passing in the anterolateral column (Alpsan, 1981; Yamada et al., 1978).

Peripheral stimuli, such as finger tapping, muscle stretching, and electrical stimulation of peripheral sensory nerves, elicit a response that travels along the sensory fibers to the dorsal root ganglia and then in a cephalad direction in the ipsilateral posterior columns to the dorsal column nuclei. (Chappa and

Allan 1982; Pratt et al., 1979; Starr et al., 1981). The evoked response then crosses to the opposite side and travels to the thalamus in the medial lemniscus. The transmission of information from the thalamus continues to the frontoparietal sensory motor cortex (Fig. 44–3). Surface electrodes placed on the intact human scalp can be used to detect the somatosensory evoked potential. By amplifying 10^4 to 10^5 times and averaging these electroencephalographic data, a clear and reproducible graph of the somatosensory evoked potentials can be obtained (Fig. 44–4).

Such graphs reflect components of varying latencies, each of which is evaluated in relation to its latency and amplitude. The components can be compared to the complex evoked by stimulating the opposite hand or opposite leg. Differences in amplitude of 50 per cent or more between both sides have been found to be significant (Desmedt and Noel, 1973).

Recent studies tend to emphasize peak latency and interpeak latency as the most

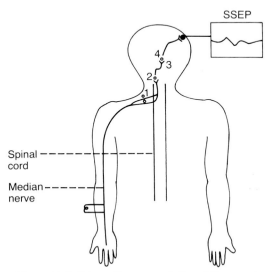

Figure 44–3. Schematic representation of the somatosensory pathway following right median nerve stimulation. 1 = dorsal root ganglia, 2 = dorsal column nuclei, 3 = medial lemniscus, 4 = thalamus. The somatosensory evoked potential (SSEP) is recorded over the sensory parietal cortex.

433

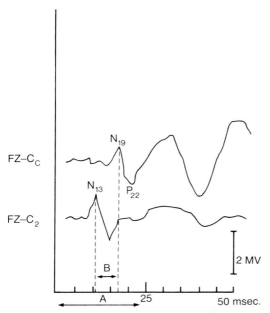

Figure 44-4. Schematic drawing of the short latency somatosensory evoked potential resulting from stimulation of the median nerve at the wrist. Each tracing is the average response to several stimuli delivered at a rate of five per second. FZ-C_c = the recorded tracing over the sensory parietal cortex contralateral to the stimulated limb. FZ-C_2 = the recorded tracing over the C2 vertebra. A = "short latency" components of the response, B = interpeak latency between C_2 and C_c, P = positive, and N = negative.

clinically relevant somatosensory evoked potential parameter, especially the latencies of the earliest components of the somatosensory evoked potential complex (Dorfman and Bosley, 1979; Sances et al., 1978). Latencies less than 25 ms. when stimulating an arm and less than 45 ms. when stimulating a leg are considered as the "short latency components." These short latency components are remarkably stable within the normal milieu of a recording laboratory. They are not affected by drowsiness, sleep, or light anesthesia (Abrahamian et al., 1983). However, barbiturates, halothane, and other medications affect somatosensory evoked potential monitoring enough to make the technique unreliable (Bunch et al., 1983). Moreover, short latency components are the first to disappear in tourniquet induced ischemia. It has been found that the largest myelinated fibers are the first to fail following use of a tourniquet (Yamada et al., 1981). Since the tourniquet is used in most surgical interventions on the extremities, this technique can not be used in such cases unless the tourni-

quet is released for at least 12 minutes (Yamada et al., 1981).

Spinal cord monitoring has been introduced recently during intraoperative correction of spinal curves. This technique includes the monitoring of both cortical and cervical spine somatosensory evoked potentials. The latter is performed by adding recording electrodes over the cervical spine.

It has been found experimentally that a combination of cortical and cervical spine monitoring of the somatosensory evoked potential enables us to differentiate between ischemia induced and mechanically induced intraoperative neurological complications (Larson et al., 1980; Yamada et al., 1981).

Landi et al. (1980) used such monitoring intraoperatively in cases of brachial plexus injury. They recorded the somatosensory evoked potential after direct root stimulation. They grafted the root distally only in roots where the somatosensory evoked potential was recorded (indicating nerve continuity from the root lesion site cephalad). Because preganglionic nerve lesions are irreparable, the somatosensory evoked potential provides important prognostic information regarding the involved root.

We have used the somatosensory evoked potential technique in peripheral nerve lesions. These studies were based on the theoretical assumption that if a somatosensory evoked potential is recorded following proximal nerve stump stimulation, the stimulated fascicle is a sensory one. Stimulation of a motor nerve fascicle elicits retrograde conduction only to the lower motor neuron, and the impulse will not pass in a cephalad direction. Therefore, stimulation of a motor nerve fascicle will not record a somatosensory evoked potential. This promising method can be used to differentiate between motor and sensory nerve fascicles on the proximal side of a severed peripheral nerve.

This method, involving an immediate nerve differentiation technique, is simple to use and shorter than any other known method and obviates the need for the Hakstian wake-up technique currently used (Hakstian, 1968).

In animal experiments that we performed, fascicular nerve stimulation of the proximal stump of the sciatic nerve in rats with bipolar electrodes elicited a good somatosensory evoked potential response. Recordings were made with silver–silver chloride disc electrodes, and potentials were displayed on an oscilloscope (Midelec, MS-91 type).

Encouraging results were obtained using this technique clinically. During an operation on a 36 year old male who had sustained complete transection of the median nerve in the forearm seven months previously, both the choline acetyltransferase enzymatic nerve differentiation technique and the somatosensory evoked potential technique were used (Engel et al., 1980). Three cable grafts were performed following nerve fascicle identification based on both methods. A good correlation was found between these methods, making possible the identification of two proximal stumps as almost purely sensory and one as almost purely motor. No halothane was given as anesthesia, and the tourniquet was released for 10 minutes prior to stimulating the nerves.

Another patient, 55 years old, suffered incomplete amputation of the right forearm with laceration of the ulnar and median nerves. Nerve repair was undertaken three weeks following injury, and again both methods of nerve fascicle identification were compared. For the median nerve there was complete correlation between both methods, identifying two sensory and one motor fascicle in the proximal stump. For the ulnar nerve we were unable to get a reproducible somatosensory evoked potential after stimulating the proximal side. We attribute this difficulty to technical problems resulting from the different sizes of the stimulating electrodes and the small size of the sensory nerve fascicles. The biochemical method was used successfully to identify two predominantly sensory and two predominantly motor fascicles.

In a third, 23 year old patient a neuroma of the ulnar nerve was found. Direct stimulation of the nerve fascicles distal to the neuroma elicited a reproducible somatosensory evoked potential. Thus we were dealing with neuroma in continuity. Intraneural neurolysis was performed.

Presently we have more problems in using the technique with ulnar nerve sensory fibers than with median nerve sensory fibers. Refinement of various technical aspects is still in process. We are evaluating the best stimulation methods, recording electrodes, technical ways to avoid spread of a stimulus to neighboring fascicles, and anesthetic drugs. We believe that the somatosensory evoked potential technique holds great promise in nerve fascicle identification in cases of peripheral nerve injury.

REFERENCES

Abrahamian, H. A., et al.: Effects of thiopental on human cerebral somatic evoked responses. Anesthesiology, 24:650–657, 1963.

Adler, R., et al.: Polyornithine-attached neurite-promoting factors (PNPF); culture sources and responsive neurons. Brain Res., 206:129–144, 1981.

Alpsan, D.: The effect of the selective activation of different peripheral nerve fiber groups on the somatosensory evoked potentials in the cat. Electroencephalogr. Clin. Neurophysiol., 51:589–598, 1981.

Assmus, H.: Somatosensory evoked cortical potentials in peripheral nerve lesions. In Barber, C. (Editor): Evoked Potentials. Baltimore, University Park Press, 1980, pp. 437–442.

Baron-Van Evercooren, A., et al.: Nerve growth factor, laminin and fibronectin promote neurite growth in human fetal sensory ganglia cultures. J. Neurosci. Res., 8:179–193, 1982.

Bora, F. W., Unger, A. S., and Osterman, A. L.: The local inhibition of nerve scar by the bioerodable vehicle, Alzamer, carrying cis-hydroxyproline. Presented at the Thirty-eighth Annual Meeting, American Society for Surgery of the Hand, Anaheim, California, March 7 to 9, 1983.

Brunelli, G.: Is it possible to avoid wallerian degeneration? Experimental study and practical consequences. In Gorio, A., et al. (Editors): Post-traumatic Peripheral Nerve Regeneration. Experimental Basis and Clinical Implications. New York, Raven Press, 1981.

Bunch, W. H., Scarff T. B., and Trimble, J.: Spinal cord monitoring. J. Bone Joint Surg., 65A:707–709, 1983.

Campbell, J., et al. Microfilter sheath in peripheral nerve surgery. J. Trauma, 1:1939:1961.

Chappa, K. H., and Allan, H. R.: Evoked potentials in clinical medicine. N. Engl. J. Med., 20:1205–1209, 1982.

Cockett, S., and Kierman, J.: Acceleration of peripheral nervous regeneration in the rat by exogenous triiodothyronine. Exp. Neurol., 39:389–394, 1973.

Dawson, G. D.: Investigations in a patient subject to myoclonic seizures after sensory stimulation. J. Neurol. Neurosurg. Psychiatry, 10:141–162, 1947.

Dawson, G. D.: A summation technique for detecting small signals in a large irregular background. J. Physiol., 115:2–3, 1951.

Dawson, G. D.: A summation technique for the detection of small evoked potentials. Electroencephalogr. Clin. Neurophysiol., 6:65–84, 1954.

Desmedt, J. E., and Noel, P.: Averaged cerebral evoked potentials in the evaluation of lesions of the central somatosensory pathway. In Desmedt, J. E. (Editor): New Developments in Electromyography and Clinical Neurophysiology. Basel, S. Karger, AG, 1973, Vol. 2, pp. 352–371.

Dorfman, L. J., and Bosley, T. M.: Age-related changes in peripheral and central nerve conduction in man. Neurology, 29:38–44, 1979.

Dorfman, L. J., et al.: Use of cerebral evoked potentials to evaluate spinal somatosensory function in patients with traumatic and surgical myelopathies. J. Neurosurg., 52:654–660, 1980.

Eisen, A., and Elleker, G.: Sensory nerve stimulation and evoked cerebral potentials. Neurology, 30:1097–1105, 1980.

Engel, J., et al.: Choline acetyltransferase for differentiation between human motor and sensory nerve fibers. Ann. Plast. Surg., 4:376–380, 1980.

Fernandez, H., and Dnell, M. J.: Protease inhibitors reduce effects of denervation on muscle end plate acetylcholinesterase. J. Neurochem., 35:1166–1171, 1980.

Finsterbush, A., et al.: Prevention of peripheral nerve entrapment following extensive soft tissue injury using silicone cuffing. Clin. Orthop., 162:276–281, 1982.

Freeman, B. S.: Adhesive anastomosis techniques for fine nerves: experimental and clinical techniques. Am. J. Surg., 108:529–532, 1964.

Ganel, A., et al.: Choline acetyltransferase nerve identification method in early and late nerve repair. Ann. Plast. Surg., 6:228–230, 1981.

Ganel, A., et al.: Intraoperative nerve fascicle identification using choline acetyltransferase—a preliminary report. Clin. Orthop., 165:228–232, 1982.

Gaul, J. S.: Electrical fascicle identification as an adjunct to nerve repair. J. Hand Surg., 8:289–296, 1983.

Gonio, O., Marini, R., and Zanoni, R.: Muscle reinnervation. III. Motoneuron sprouting capacity; enhancement by exogenous gangliosides. Neuroscience, 8:417–429, 1983.

Grabb, W. C., et al.: Comparison of methods of peripheral nerve suturing in monkeys. Plast. Reconst. Surg., 46:31–38, 1970.

Graham, W. P., et al.: Enhancement of peripheral regeneration with triamcinolone after neurorrhaphy. Surg. Forum, 24:457, 1973.

Graham, W. P., et al.: Efficacy of triamcinolone acetanide following neurorrhaphy—an electroneuromyographic evaluation. Ann. Plast. Surg., 9:230–237, 1982.

Gruber, H., et al.: Identification of motor and sensory funiculi in cut nerves and their selective reunion. Br. J. Plast. Surg., 29:70–73, 1976.

Gutmann, E., and Young, J. Z.: Reinnervation of muscle after various periods of atrophy. J. Anat., 78:15–43, 1944.

Hakstian, R. W.: Funicular orientation by direct stimulation. An aid to peripheral nerve repair. J. Bone Joint Surg., 50A:1178–1186, 1968.

Hastings, J. C., and Peacock, E. E.: Effect of injury, repair and ascorbic acid deficiency on collagen accumulation in peripheral nerves. Surg. Forum, 24:516, 1973.

Hume, A. L., and Cant, B. R.: Central somatosensory conduction after head injury. Ann. Neurol., 10:411–419, 1981.

Hurst, L. C., et al.: Inhibition of neural and muscle degeneration after epineural neurorrhaphy. Presented at the Thirty-eighth Annual Meeting, American Society for Surgery of the Hand, Anaheim, California, March 7 to 9, 1983.

Jones, S. J.: Investigation of brachial plexus traction lesions by peripheral and spinal somatosensory evoked potentials. J. Neurol. Neurosurg. Psychiatry, 43:107–116, 1979.

Kelly, J. J., Sharbrough, F. W., and Daube, J. R.: A clinical and electrophysiological evaluation of myoclonus. Neurology, 31:581–589, 1981.

Kline, D. G., and Hapes, G. J.: The use of an erodable wrapper for peripheral nerve repair. J. Neurosurg., 21:737, 1964.

Kline, D. G., et al.: Dexamethasone treatment of partially injured nerves. Curr. Top. Surg. Res., 3:173, 1971.

Kuhn, W. E., and Hall, J. L.: A nerve implant prosthesis for facilitating peripheral nerve regeneration. In Horwitz, J., and Targressen, O.: Biomaterials. Washington, D.C., National Bureau of Standards, 1975, pp. 91–98.

Landi, A., et al.: The role of somatosensory evoked potentials and nerve conduction studies in the surgical management of brachial plexus injuries. J. Bone Joint Surg., 62B:492–496, 1980.

Larson, S. J., et al.: Evoked potentials in experimental myelopathy. Spine, 5:299–302, 1980.

Leeden, R. W.: Ganglioside structures and distribution: are they localized at the nerve ending? J. Supramol. Struct., 8:1–17, 1978.

Levi-Montalcini, R.: The nerve growth factor. Its mode of action on sensory and sympathetic nerve cells. Harvey Lect., 60:217–259, 1966.

Lloyd, O. P. C.: Neuron patterns controlling transmission of ipsilateral hind limb reflexes in cat. J. Neurophysiol., 6:293–326, 1943.

Lundborg, G.: In Gorio, A. (Editor): Posttraumatic Peripheral Nerve Regeneration; Experimental Basis and Clinical Implications. New York, Raven Press, 1981.

Lundborg, G., et al.: Reorganization and orientation of regenerating nerve fibers, perineurium and epineurium in preformed mesothelial tubes—an experimental study on the sciatic nerve in rats. J. Neurol Sci. Res., 6:265–280, 1981.

Lundborg, G., et al.: Nerve regeneration across an extended gap: a neurobiological view of nerve repair and the possible involvement of neurotrophic factors. J. Hand Surg., 7:580–587, 1982a.

Lundborg, G., Longo, F. M., and Varon, S.: Nerve regeneration model and trophic factors in vivo. Brain Res., 232:157–161, 1982b.

Manthorpe, M., et al.: Laminin is a polyornithine-binding neurite promoting factor. J. Neurochem., 41:S43C, 1983.

Maw, R. B., and Loizean, A. D.: Functional regeneration of nerves in dogs when filter tubes are used. J. Oral Surg., 29:848–852, 1971.

McDonald, W. I.: The role of evoked potentials in the diagnosis of multiple sclerosis. In Bauer, H. J., Poser, S., and Ritter, G. (Editors): Progress in Multiple Sclerosis Research. New York, Springer-Verlag, 1980, pp. 564–568.

Midgley, R. D., and Woolhouse, R. M.: Silicone rubber sheathing as an adjunct to neural anastomosis. Surg. Clin. N. Am., 48:1149, 1968.

Millesi, H.: Wiederherstellung durchtrennter peripherer nerven und nerventransplantation. Munch. Med. Wschr., 111:2669–2674, 1969.

Monard, D., and Gunther, J.: A glia derived protease inhibitor which modulates neurite outgrowth. J. Neurochem., 41:S89A, 1983.

Nakatsuchi, Y., Matsui, T., and Honda, Y.: Funicular orientation by electrical stimulation and internal neurolysis in peripheral nerve sutures. Hand, 12:65–74, 1980.

Pate-Skene, J. H., and Willard, M.: Axonally transported proteins associated with axon growth in rabbit central and peripheral nervous systems. J. Cell Biol., 89:96–103, 1981.

Pichichero, M., Beer, B., and Clody, D.: Effects of dibutyryl cyclic AMP on restoration of function of damaged sciatic nerve in rats. Science, 182:724–725, 1973.

Pleasure, D., et al.: Regeneration after nerve transection: effect of inhibition of collagen synthesis. Exp. Neurol., *45*:72–78, 1974.

Politis, M. J., Ederle, K., and Spencer, P. S.: Tropism in nerve regeneration in vivo. Attraction of regenerating axons by diffusible factors derived from cells in distal nerve stumps of transected peripheral nerves. Brain Res., *253*:1–12, 1982.

Pratt, H., et al.: Mechanically and electrically evoked somatosensory potentials in humans. Neurology, *29*:1236–1244, 1979.

Reuveny, S., et al.: Factors affecting cell attachment, spreading and growth on derivatized microcarriers. I. Establishment of working system and effect on the type of the amino-charged groups. Biotechnol. Bioengin. Symp., *25*:469–480, 1983.

Richter, H. P., Frosch, D., and Ketelsen U. P.: Functional and morphological motor regeneration after different periods of denervation and following microsurgical suture of the peroneal nerve. Experimental study in the rabbit. Acta Neuroclin. (Wein) (Suppl.), *28*:605–607, 1979.

Roisen, F., et al.: Cyclic adenosine monophosphate stimulation of axonal elongation. Science, *175*:73–74, 1972.

Rosen, J. M., Kaplan, E. N., and Jewett, D. C.: Suture and sutureless methods of repairing experimental nerve injuries. *In* Jewett, D. L., and McCarrol, H. A., Jr.: Nerve Repair and Regeneration. Its Clinical and Experimental Basis. St. Louis, The C. V. Mosby Company, 1980, pp. 235–243.

Sances, A., Jr., et al.: Early somatosensory evoked potentials. Electroencephalogr. Clin. Neurophysiol., *45*:505–514, 1978.

Schotman, W. A., et al.: Neurotrophic action of ACTH on nerve regeneration. J. Neurochem., *41*:S 30 D, 1983.

Smith, R. G., and Appel, S. H.: Extracts of skeletal muscle increase neurite outgrowth and cholinergic activity of fetal rat spinal motor neurons. Science, *219*:1079–1080, 1983.

Sparrow, J. R., and Grafstein, B.: Sciatic nerve regeneration in ganglioside treated rats. Exp. Neurol., *77*:230–235, 1982.

Starr, A., et al.: Cerebral potentials evoked by muscle stretch in man. Brain, *104*:149–166, 1981.

Sunderland, S.: Nerve and Nerve Injuries. Ed. 2. Edinburgh, Churchill Livingstone, 1978.

Sunderland, S.: The anatomic foundation of peripheral nerve repair technique. Orthop. Clin. N. Am., *12*:245–266, 1981.

Sunderland, S., and Bradley, K. C.: Denervation atrophy of distal stump of severed nerve. J. Comp. Neurol., *93*:401–409, 1950.

Van Beek, A. L., Massac, E., Jr., and Smith, D. O.: The use of signal averaging computer for evaluation of peripheral nerve problems. Clin. Plast. Surg., *13*:407–418, 1986.

Vandeput, J., Tanner, J. C., and Huypens, L.: Electrophysiological orientation of the cut ends in primary peripheral nerve repair. Plast. Reconstr. Surg., *44*:378–382, 1969.

Varon, S.: Nerve growth factor and its mode of action. Exp. Neurol., *48*:75–92, 1975.

Varon, S., and Adler, R.: Nerve growth factors and control of nerve growth. Curr. Top. Dev. Biol., *16*:207–252, 1980.

Varon, S., and Adler, R.: Trophic and specifying factors directed to neuronal cells. Adv. Cell Neurobiol., *2*:115–163, 1981.

Varon, S., Skaper, S. D., and Manthorpe, M.: Trophic activities for dorsal root and sympathetic ganglionic neurons in media conditioned by Schwann and other peripheral cells. Dev. Brain Res., *1*:73–78, 1981.

Walton, R., and Finseth, F.: Nerve grafting in the repair of complicated peripheral nerve trauma. J. Trauma, *17*:793–796, 1977.

Yamada, T., et al.: Somatosensory evoked potentials elicited by bilateral stimulation of the median nerve and its clinical application. Neurology (Minneap.) *28*:218–223, 1978.

Yamada, T., Muroga, T., and Kimura, J.: Tourniquet-induced ischemia and somatosensory evoked potentials. Neurology (N.Y.), *31*:1524–1529, 1981.

Zverina, E., et al.: Somatosensory cerebral evoked potentials in diagnosing brachial plexus injury. Scand. J. Rehabil. Med., *9*:47–51, 1977.

Chapter 45

ELECTROPHYSIOLOGICAL TECHNIQUES IN SURGERY OF PERIPHERAL NERVES SERVING THE HAND

JULIA K. TERZIS

The dramatic difference between true recovery of function in a repaired peripheral nerve and the more common partial return of gross sensibility is a strong incentive to continue to develop our understanding of the processes involved in regeneration of peripheral nerves and to continue to improve the techniques used in their repair. This chapter presents the historical perspective of the complexities of the problem of repair and a description of recent attempts to improve functional recovery in denervated structures with the use of electrophysiological techniques.

HISTORICAL PERSPECTIVE

In 1850 Waller described degeneration of the distal stump secondary to proximal transection. He observed the progression of events leading to complete degeneration of the distal parts of the hypoglossal and glossopharyngeal nerves in the frog, while to his fascination the proximal parts remained intact. He concluded that the nerve cells were responsible for the nourishment of the peripheral fibers.

Distal stump degeneration was a critical finding and formed the basis for the unique problems associated with peripheral nerve injuries. Surgeons since that time have attempted to put the two nerve ends together to take advantage of the regenerative capacity of the central neurons. Failures in repair could not be blamed on a lack of growth potential, since the formation of neuromas

from the proximal nerve stump was proof of attempts of the neuron to repair itself.

Despite major achievements over the last century in the field of peripheral nerve surgery, the overall outcomes of nerve repairs to date can claim only a modest improvement over initial results. Part of the problem resides with the lack of properly conducted studies to quantitate the various factors that influence regeneration following a nerve repair procedure. This scarcity of information reflects a lack of objective means in assessing modalities associated with nerve injury and repair; unreliability of clinical studies, since most are based on subjective data; a lack of universally accepted methods of assessing returning sensibility; justified hesitation in extrapolating controlled experimental findings to human patients because of variations among species (Kline et al., 1964a,b); and gaps in our understanding of the basic pathophysiology of the peripheral nerve.

The functional complexity of the peripheral nervous system has not always been appreciated anatomically. Motor and sensory fibers look deceptively alike under the highest resolution of the electron microscope, and anatomical landmarks indicating the presence or absence of a myelin sheath are not always accompanied by functional correlates.

Only by applying functional criteria in assessing peripheral nerve lesions can intraneural topography be appreciated in vivo and proper identification of proximal and distal fascicles be achieved.

Electrophysiological techniques can provide the objective tool needed for the func-

438

tional assessment of lesions associated with injuries to peripheral nerves. The study of neural excitability was rapidly advanced when the nerve action potential could be easily and reliably recorded. That a wave of electrical disturbance passes outward from the stimulating site along the nerve fibers was known from the work of Helmholtz (cf. Brazier, 1959). In 1850 Helmholtz measured the speed of conduction of nerve impulses by means of a special galvanometer that he constructed. Duchenne (1806–1875) was responsible for developing clinical electrophysiology. He applied the principle of the induction coil discovered by Faraday in 1831 to the investigation of nervous system diseases. However, the foremost neurophysiologist at the turn of the nineteenth century was Sherrington (1857–1952). His work, *The Integrative Action of the Nervous System,* published in 1906, laid the foundations for all modern concepts of central nervous system function (Sherrington, 1906). He introduced the term "synapse" to account for the interactions between nerve cells. In 1922 electrophysiology took a major step forward in the work of Erlanger and Gasser (Erlanger and Gasser, 1937). They studied the compound nerve action potential and demonstrated the range of nerve fiber conduction and other features of the evoked response and the refractory period of nerve. Later the work of Adrian, Hodgkin, and Huxley on the functional aspects of excitable resting membranes, myelin sheath, and nodes of Ranvier (Cansey, 1960; McHenry, 1969) led to the application of nerve conduction studies to clinical practice by Hodes et al. (1948).

RECORDING OF AN ACTION POTENTIAL

The basic apparatus needed for such a recording is illustrated in Figures 45–1 and 45–2. A brief stimulating pulse is delivered to the nerve through the stimulating electrodes. The nerve action potential propagates along the nerve to the recording electrodes. The voltage change developed by the nerve during an action potential is quite small and needs to be amplified more than 1000 times for oscilloscopic display. If both legs of the recording electrode are allowed to pick up the impulse, a diphasic action potential results (Fig. 45–3A). This happens because of the reversal of the potential difference be-

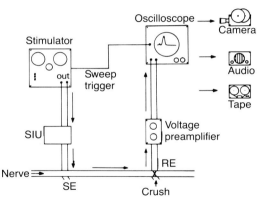

Figure 45–1. Diagrammatic illustration of the basic recording apparatus needed for recording a compound action potential (CAP). SIU = stimulus isolation unit, SE = stimulating electrodes, and RE = recording electrodes.

tween the two recording electrodes as the action potential moves from the first to the second. If conduction to the second electrode is blocked, for example by crushing the

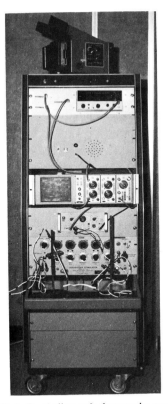

Figure 45–2. Recording unit that can be used for both experimental and clinical work. Starting from above: camera, electronic counter, audio, oscilloscope, preamplifier, and stimulator. Note the recording electrodes (*left*) and stimulating electrodes (*right*) on the base.

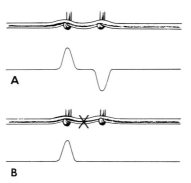

Figure 45–3. *A*, Diphasic action potential when both recording electrodes are allowed to pick up the signal. *B*, Block instituted between recording electrodes resulting in a monophasic action potential.

nerve, a monophasic action potential results (Fig. 45–3*B*). This is a more convenient form in which to study nerve impulses and is the one used widely today.

A diagrammatic illustration of an action potential is shown in Figure 45–4. The first deflection corresponds to the time that the stimulating pulse is applied to the nerve and is called the stimulus artifact. The period of time elapsing between the stimulus artifact and the onset of the response is known as the latency and represents the time required for the action potential to travel a distance from the stimulating to the recording sites. If this distance is known, the speed or conduction velocity of the propagated action potential can be determined by the equation $V = D/T$, where V is the conduction velocity, D is the distance in meters between the stimulating cathode and the first recording electrode, and T is the time in seconds elapsing between the stimulus artifact and the beginning of the action potential (latency).

The conduction velocity is the most precise and the most easily measured property of a nerve fiber and can be correlated reliably

with other properties of nerve fibers, such as the fiber diameter and internodal length.

Erlanger and Gasser (1937) considered the relationship between conduction velocity and fiber diameter in connection with the reconstruction of the compound action potential. When a single fiber is stimulated, a single spike is generated, which is referred to as an all or none response (Hill, 1932). Because of the practical difficulty in isolating single mammalian fibers and recording single fiber activity, multifiber preparations have been utilized to gain much of our knowledge of the physiological properties of nerve trunks. Such simultaneous activation of multifiber preparations results in a compound action potential, which is merely the algebraic sum of individual fiber action potentials. Although the individual fibers in a nerve trunk each obey the all or none law, the compound action potential is a continuously graded response whose amplitude and shape are affected by increments in the stimulus strength. This is because its contributing fibers have different fiber diameters, different thresholds of excitation, and different conduction velocities. The larger myelinated A-α fibers with the lowest thresholds to stimulation and the fastest conduction velocities appear first following application of a threshold stimulus to the nerve. Following a further increase in stimulus strength, other nerve groups successively add their responses to the total (Gasser and Grundfest, 1939). These later-appearing groups are subgroups of the A group of myelinated fibers, namely, α, β, δ, the α group having the lowest threshold and the δ group the highest. A-δ fibers, being the very finely myelinated fibers, add their action potential at the end (Fig. 45–5). At still higher stimulus strengths, a much later-appearing and smaller potential is added by the unmyelinated C group of fibers. An intermediate B group of myelinated fibers is present only in autonomic nerves (Ochs, 1965).

Hursh (1939) correlated the fastest conduction velocities (CV) in different nerves with the largest fiber diameters (FD) and showed that the proportionality factor was 6, e.g., CV/FD = 6. More recently Boyd (1964, 1965) and Boyd and Davey (1968) have found a smaller ratio (4.5) for smaller fibers. In addition, it has been shown that this ratio varies from species to species, by Sanders and Whitteridge (1946), Cragg and Thomas (1957, 1964), McLeod and Wray (1967), Tasaki (1953), and Kiraly and Krnjević (1959).

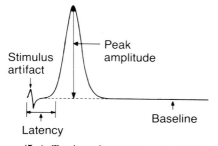

Figure 45–4. Tracing of an action potential, demonstrating stimulus artifact, latency, and peak amplitude.

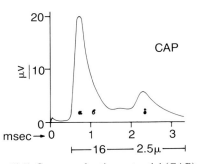

Figure 45–5. Compound action potential (CAP), demonstrating subgroups of the A group in sequence based on fiber diameters and conduction velocities.

Although the electrical signals obtained from single-fiber preparations are at present of little use to the clinician, the compound action potential elicited upon stimulation of multifiber preparations—whether it is the whole nerve trunk, a group of fascicles, or even a single fascicle—can yield a remarkable amount of information about the functional status of the nerve. The examiner, however, must be able to appreciate the meaning of the observed responses and correlate them with his clinical findings. Only then can accurate decisions be made about how to manage a particular nerve lesion.

An understanding of the presence or absence of the evoked response, the conduction velocity of the signal, and the amplitude and shape of the wave form is needed before one can meaningfully apply electrophysiological recordings in the clinical situation.

Absence of Compound Action Potential

The absence of a compound action potential is an indication of total conduction block across the tested nerve segment. It can occur early in a neuropraxic lesion, in which there is localized interruption of nerve conduction without distal degeneration of the nerve axon. In such a lesion, proximal and distal conduction is preserved. In addition, total absence of the compound action potential occurs across axonotmetic and neurotmetic lesions. The former carries a better prognosis and implies a certain degree of reversibility, for the continuity of the endoneurial tubes and connective tissue framework of the nerve is retained, the injury mainly being restricted to the axons. A crush injury of a nerve may represent such a lesion, with eventual return of the compound action potential upon regeneration. The latter, neurotmesis, reflects a severe injury with disruption of all supportive tissues and axoplasm. Recovery is usually poor, and return of the compound action potential is never complete.

Presence of Compound Action Potential

This is an indication of functioning neural tissue. Stepwise recordings of the compound action potential along an injured nerve can be of great assistance in delineating the actual site and extent of the lesion, thus focusing surgical treatment in a region of proven conduction failure. Extensive neurolysis procedures can be avoided, thus preventing further trauma to the nerve.

The Conduction Velocity of the Compound Action Potential

The speed of impulse transmission along a nerve is a very precise property of peripheral nerves and reflects the sizes of the contributing fibers, degrees of myelination, and their internodal lengths. There is a linear relationship between internodal length of a nerve fiber and its conduction velocity (Fullerton and Barnes, 1966; Lascelles and Thomas, 1966; Vizoso and Young, 1948). If the distance between the stimulating and recording sites is known along with the time interval from the stimulus artifact to the onset of the action potential (latency), the conduction velocity can be calculated. Since this parameter reflects axonal diameters and degrees of myelination, disease states, compression phenomena, and regeneration attempts following injury may be identified by alterations in the speed of impulse transmission.

Amplitude of the Compound Action Potential

The size of the compound action potential can be used only in relative terms; that is, meaningful information can be obtained only by comparison with a recording from a similar normal nerve or fascicle. Only then can one assess the significance of a decrease in amplitude and make the decision to preserve a damaged fascicle instead of carrying out resection and repair. In a normal nerve the amplitude of the compound action potential is an indication of the number and size of the contributing nerve fibers (Jacobson and Guth, 1965). The amplitude of the signal in a regenerating nerve is an index of the number and size of functioning regenerating fibers and can be used clinically to assess the degree of functional return.

In a regenerating nerve, following a neurotmetic lesion, it has been shown that the full normal fiber diameters and the normal distribution of fiber sizes are never reconstituted (Cragg and Thomas, 1964; Gutmann and Sanders, 1943). Thus, the amplitude of the compound action potential never returns to preinjury levels. In neuropraxic lesions, fiber diameters and their respective distribution are fully reconstituted with time, and the conduction block and decrease in amplitude of response are completely reversible. In axonotmetic lesions, full wallerian degeneration develops distally, and recovery may be partial or complete, depending on the level and degree of injury and the functional status of the end organs upon reinnervation. Thus, the eventual amplitude that the compound action potential attains varies with all these factors.

Shape of the Compound Action Potential

The normal bimodal distribution of the compound action potential may be disrupted by injury (Fig. 45–5). A qualitative impression of the functional status of the nerve can be obtained from its wave form and can assist in ascertaining the degree of functional loss. Depending on the temporal dispersion and the number and size of regenerating fibers, the compound action potential obtained from an injured nerve may be broader in shape and may have irregular contours. Multiple peaks may be present, reflecting underlying fiber activity. Resumption of the preinjury wave form with time indicates maturation of the constituent nerve fibers.

CLINICAL USES OF ELECTROPHYSIOLOGICAL TECHNIQUES

This section does not include a discussion of the conventional uses of electrophysiological techniques, since such information is readily available (Licht, 1961). Instead, recent clinical contributions are discussed with a view toward future applications of these procedures in peripheral nerve surgery.

The assessment of neural function for control of muscles has been widely studied in conjunction with electromyography (Howard, 1970; Licht, 1961). Attempts to measure

muscle function by Hodes et al. (1948) led to the first report on the motor conduction velocities of peripheral nerves in man.

In 1949 Dawson and Scott introduced a method of examining sensory impulses in human peripheral nerves by applying electrical stimulation to the median or ulnar nerve at the wrist. The afferent volley was recorded proximally by surface electrodes placed over the nerve trunks. Later this method was modified to eliminate the contribution of motor fibers as the digital nerves were stimulated by ring electrodes (Dawson, 1956). These techniques have been used extensively in the investigation of patients with sensory and motor disorders (Ballantyne and Campbell, 1973; Buchthal and Rosenfalck, 1966, 1971; Gilliatt and Sears, 1958; Veale et al., 1973).

In 1968 electrophysiological techniques were used by Kline in the intraoperative assessment of peripheral nerve injuries (Kline, 1968; Kline and DeJonge, 1968; Kline et al., 1969; Kline and Hackett, 1975; Kline and Nulsen, 1972; Vanderark et al., 1970). Compound action potentials were measured from exposed peripheral nerves, and a better indication of function along with a more accurate definition of the extent of the lesion was provided.

Hakstian in 1968 also utilized electrophysiological techniques clinically not to deduce the degree of function but instead to depict the intraneural topography of severed nerves. Electrical stimuli were applied intraoperatively to units smaller than the whole nerve in both the proximal and distal stumps, thus achieving sensory and motor fascicular differentiation. Similar identification procedures were tested by Vandeput in 1969 in an experimental series (Vandeput et al., 1969). In both studies the outcomes of nerve repairs were superior when these orienting techniques were employed.

After extensive experimental work in which electrophysiological recordings were used to determine the effects of tension in a nerve anastomosis and the effects of surgical technique in the outcome of a nerve repair (Terzis et al., 1975; Terzis and Williams, 1976), these procedures were utilized in the intraoperative setup to determine axonal carry-through at a fascicular level in lesions in continuity (Williams and Terzis, 1976).

Lesions in continuity are challenging and difficult to treat. There are discrepancies between the gross appearance of the lesion and the functional integrity of the nerve, making

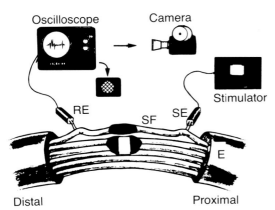

Figure 45–6. Technique of single fascicular recordings for nerve lesions in continuity. E = resected epineurium, SE = stimulating electrode, RE = recording electrode, N = neuroma, and SF = single fascicle tested.

decisions favoring resection over neurolysis especially difficult. Converting a partial lesion to a complete one by sacrificing remaining intact axons can cause a great loss to the patient, especially since the outcome of nerve repairs is so unpredictable. At the same time, wasting valuable time waiting for end organ reinnervation and hoping for return of function may permanently jeopardize the chances of functional restoration.

Single fascicular recordings applied to lesions in continuity have greatly assisted the surgeon in determining the precise site of the lesion, the extent of involvement, and the severity of axonal loss (Fig. 45–6). The functional status of individual fascicles can be determined intraoperatively with this technique, and can provide a guide for surgical treatment. Careful analysis of the compound action potential leads to maximal preservation of intact neural tissue by a careful intraneural neurolysis, while resection and primary repair can be limited to fascicles that have no axonal carry-through.

More recently the use of applied electrophysiology has been expanded in a new, exciting direction (Terzis, 1976a). A technique has been developed that allows the precise mapping of the neural distribution of single fascicles of cutaneous nerves on the skin surface (Terzis, 1976b). The principles guiding the uses of this technique involve the multifiber recording of the receptive fields of afferent fibers that are mechanically stimulated. Furthermore, altering the conditions of the mechanical stimulus allows single sensory fibers to be studied in isolation and their response characteristics to be measured (Terzis and Williams, 1974).

Sensory mapping techniques for the first time have been applied clinically to solve crucial problems in reconstructive surgery (Fig. 45–7). These procedures allow the design of donor neurovascular flaps to provide immediate sensory skin coverage to demanding anesthetic areas; sensory depleted hands can gain tactile gnosis, and vulnerable areas in paraplegics can be transformed into pressure sensors. The design of neurovascular flaps entails the identification of the overlapping territory of an anatomically proven vascular supply and an electrophysiologically determined sensory nerve distribution. Such areas of vascular and neural autonomy, when raised as free flaps in the experimental model, always lead to complete survival (Daniel et al., 1975).

Following experimental success, the effectiveness of this technique was tested clinically. The first successful neurovascular free flap, designed on the dorsum of the foot, provided immediate coverage and, at the end of a year, functional sensibility in the previously anesthetic hand of a laborer (Daniel et al., 1976b). In addition, awareness of pressure sensibility was obtained to various extents in three cases in which intercostal neurovascular island flaps were used to cover pressure sores in paraplegic patients (Daniel et al., 1976a).

These more recent uses of electrophysiological techniques in peripheral nerve surgery have made it possible to speculate about future applications. Recent advances in elec-

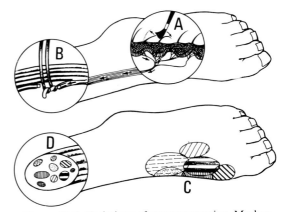

Figure 45–7. Technique of sensory mapping. Mechanical stimulation applied on the skin surface (*A*) elicits an afferent volley of impulses that travel orthodromically and are picked up by the recording electrode (*B*). Sensory mappings depicting the neural distribution of each fascicle can be precisely outlined on the potential donor skin area (*C*) and corresponding individual fascicles (*D*).

tronics with integrated circuitry will soon lead to the development of highly automated, miniaturized recording equipment that can be easily used by the surgeon in the intraoperative situation to facilitate nerve repair procedures. Furthermore, it is conceivable that finer diagnostic resolution will be mandated in the future in the management of peripheral nerve lesions; the "fascicular" era will be followed by an intrafascicular level of assessment at which function of multifiber groups within a fascicle will be determined. Finally, the management of peripheral nerve lesions may require functional assessment at the level of individual fibers.

Single fiber activity has been recorded from peripheral nerves in man for almost 15 years (Hensel and Boman, 1960; Konietzny and Hensel, 1975; Torebjörk, 1974; Torebjörk and Hallin, 1970; Vallbo and Hagbarth, 1968; Van Hees and Gybels, 1972). Both sensory and motor units have been studied in human subjects by inserting tungsten microelectrodes through the skin into peripheral nerves (Fig. 45–8). One important finding has been that the response characteristics in man are comparable to those obtained from corresponding mechanoreceptors in primates.

Clinical usage of percutaneous microelectrode recordings can be anticipated in diagnosing peripheral nerve lesions, assessing neural regeneration at any level following injury to a peripheral nerve, determining the timing of re-exploration after a nerve repair procedure, studying the response characteristics of mechanoreceptive units following reinnervation, assessing returning motor function at the level of the motor unit, depicting intrafascicular topography prior to nerve repair, and determining the axonal transmission through the two anastomoses in nerve graft procedures.

Applications of electrophysiological techniques in peripheral nerve surgery may lead to significant advances in conquering the problems associated with neural lesions, and may improve dramatically our results with nerve repairs. The future promises to be exciting.

REFERENCES

Ballantyne, J. P., and Campbell, M. J.: Electrophysiological study after surgical repair of sectioned human peripheral nerves. J. Neurol. Neurosurg. Psychiatr., 36:797, 1973.

Boyd, I. A.: The relation between conduction velocity and diameter for the three groups of efferent fibres in nerves to mammalian skeletal muscle. J. Physiol. (Lond.), 175:33, 1964.

Boyd, I. A., and Davey, M. R.: Composition of Peripheral Nerves. Edinburgh, E. P. S. Livingstone, 1968, pp. 1–57.

Brazier, M. A. B.: The historical development of neurophysiology. In Field, J. (Ed.): Handbook of Physiology. Vol. 1. Neurophysiology. Washington, D. C., American Physiological Society, 1959, pp. 1–58.

Buchthal, F., and Rosenfalck, A.: Evoked action potentials and conduction velocity in human sensory nerves. Brain Res., 3:1, 1966.

Buchthal, F., and Rosenfalck, A.: Sensory potentials in polyneuropathy. Brain, 94:241, 1971.

Cansey, G.: The Cell of Schwann. Edinburgh, E. & S. Livingstone, 1960.

Cragg, B. G., and Thomas, P. K.: The relationships between conduction velocity and the diameter and internodal length of peripheral nerve fibres. J. Physiol. (Lond.), 136:606, 1957.

Cragg, B. G., and Thomas, P. K.: The conduction velocity of regenerated peripheral nerve fibres. J. Physiol., 171:164, 1964.

Daniel, R. K., Terzis, J., and Cunningham, D.: Sensory skin flaps for pressure sore in paraplegic patients. Plast. Reconstr. Surg., 1976a.

Daniel, R. K., Terzis, J., and Midgley, R.: Restoration of sensation to an anesthetic hand by a free neurovascular flap from the foot. Plast. Reconstr. Surg., March, 1976b.

Daniel, R. K., Terzis, J., and Schwarz, G.: Neurovascular free flaps. A preliminary report. Plast. Reconstr. Surg., 56:B-20, 1975.

Dawson, G. D.: The relative excitability and conduction velocity of sensory and motor nerve fibres in man. J. Physiol., 131:436, 1956.

Dawson, G. D., and Scott, J. W.: The recording of nerve action potentials through skin in man. J. Neurol. Neurosurg. Psychiatr., 12:259, 1949.

Erlanger, J., and Gasser, H. S.: Electrical Signs of Nervous Activity. Philadelphia, University of Pennsylvania Press, 1937.

Fullerton, P. M., and Barnes, J. M.: Peripheral neuropathy in rats produced by acrylamide. Br. J. Industr. Med., 23:210, 1966.

Gasser, H. S., and Grundfest, H.: Axon diameters in

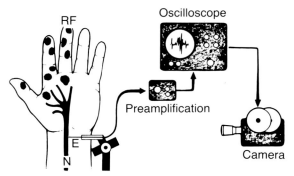

Figure 45–8. Percutaneous microelectrode recordings. A fine tungsten microelectrode (E) is inserted through the skin into a peripheral nerve (N). Mechanical stimulation on the hand demarcates the receptive field (RF) of a single afferent fiber. Altering parameters of penetration allows recordings from multiple units.

relation to the spike dimensions and the conduction velocity in mammalian A fibres. Am. J. Physiol., *127*:393, 1939.

Gilliatt, R. W., and Sears, T. A.: Sensory nerve action potentials in patients with peripheral nerve lesions. J. Neurol. Neurosurg. Psychiatr., *21*:109, 1958.

Gutmann, E., and Sanders, F. K.: Recovery of fiber numbers and diameters in the regeneration of peripheral nerves. J. Physiol., *101*:489, 1943.

Hakstian, R. W.: Funicular orientation by direct stimulation. An aid to peripheral nerve repair. J. Bone Joint Surg., *50A*:1178, 1968.

Hensel, H., and Boman, K. A.: Afferent impulses in cutaneous sensory nerves in human subjects. J. Neurophysiol., *23*:564, 1960.

Hill, A. V.: Chemical Wave Transmission in Nerve. New York, The Macmillan Company, 1932.

Hodes, R., Larrabee, M. C., and German, W.: The human electromyogram in response to nerve stimulation and the conduction velocity of motor axons. Arch. Neurol. Psychiatr., *60*:340, 1948.

Howard, F. M.: The electromyogram and conduction velocity studies in peripheral nerve trauma. *In* Clinical Neurology. Proceedings of Congress of Neurological Surgeons. Baltimore, The Williams & Wilkins Company, 1970, ch. 5.

Hursh, J. B.: Conduction velocity and diameter of nerve fibres. Am. J. Physiol., *127*:131, 1939.

Jacobson, S., and Guth, L.: An electrophysiological study of the early stages of peripheral nerve regeneration. Exp. Neurol., *11*:48, 1965.

Kiraly, J. K., and Krnjević, K.: Some retrograde changes in function of nerves after peripheral section. Quart. J. Exp. Physiol., *44*:244, 1959.

Kline, D. G.: Early evaluation of peripheral nerve lesions in continuity with a note on nerve recording. *34*:77, 1968.

Kline, D. G., and DeJonge, B. R.: Evoked potentials to evaluate peripheral nerve injuries. Surg. Gynecol. Obstet., *127*:1239, 1968.

Kline, D. G., and Hackett, E. R.: Reappraisal of timing for exploration of civilian peripheral nerve injuries. Surgery, *79*:54, 1975.

Kline, D. G., Hackett, E. R., and May, P. R.: Evaluation of nerve injuries by evoked potentials and electromyography. J. Neurosurg., *31*:128, 1969.

Kline, D. G., Hayes, G. J., and Morse, A. S.: A comparative study of response of species to peripheral-nerve injury. I. Severance. J. Neurosurg., *21*:968, 1964a.

Kline, D. G., Hayes, G. J., and Morse, A. S.: A comparative study of response of species to peripheral nerve injury. II. Crush and severance with primary suture. J. Neurosurg., *21*:980, 1964b.

Kline, D. G., and Nulsen, F. E.: The neuroma in continuity: its preoperative and operative management. Surg. Clin. N. Am., *52*:1189, 1972.

Konietzny, F., and Hensel, H.: Warm fiber activity in human skin nerves. Pflügers Arch. Europ. J. Physiol., *359*:265, 1975.

Lascelles, R. G., and Thomas, P. K.: Changes due to age in internodal length in the sural nerve in man. J. Neurol. Neurosurg. Psychiatr., *29*:40, 1966.

Licht, S.: History of electrodiagnosis. *In* Electrodiagnosis and Electrotherapy. Ed. 2. New Haven, LS. Licht, 1961, ch. 1., E.

McHenry, L. C., Jr.: Garrison's History of Neurology. Springfield, Illinois, Charles C Thomas, 1969.

McLeod, J. G., and Wray, S. H.: Conduction velocity and fibre diameter of the median and ulnar nerves of the baboon. J. Neurol. Neurosurg. Psychiatr., *30*:240, 1967.

Ochs, S.: Elements of Neurophysiology. New York, John Wiley & Sons, Inc., 1965.

Sanders, F. K., and Whitteridge, D.: Conduction velocity and myelin thickness in regenerating nerve fibers. J. Phsyiol. (Lond.), *105*:152, 1946.

Sherrington, C. S.: The Integrative Action of the Nervous System. New Haven, Yale University Press, 1906.

Tasaki, I.: Nervous Transmission. Springfield, Illinois, Charles C Thomas, 1953, pp. 81–85.

Terzis, J.: Functional aspects of reinnervation of free skin grafts. Plast. Reconstr. Surg., 1976a. (Submitted for publication.)

Terzis, J.: Sensory mapping. *In* Entin, M. (Editor.): Clinics in Plastic Surgery. Philadelphia, W. B. Saunders Company, January 1976b.

Terzis, J., Faibisoff, B., and Williams, H. B.: The nerve gap: suture under tension vs. graft. Plast. Reconstr. Surg., *56*:166, 1975.

Terzis, J., and Williams, H. B.: Functional aspects of reinnervation of skin grafts. Surg. Forum, *25*:518, 1974.

Torebjörk, H. E.: Afferent C units responding to mechanical, thermal and chemical stimuli in human nonglabrous skin. Acta Physiol. Scand., *92*:374, 1974.

Torebjörk, H. E., and Hallin, R. G.: C-fibre units recorded from human sensory nerve fascicles in situ— a preliminary report. Acta Soc. Med. Upsal., *75*:81, 1970.

Vallbo, A. B., and Hagbarth, K. E.: Activity from skin mechanoreceptors recorded percutaneously in awake human subjects. Exp. Neurol., *21*:270, 1968.

Vandeput, J., Tanner, J. C., and Huypens, L.: Electrophysiological orientation of the cut ends in primary peripheral nerve repair. Plast. Reconstr. Surg., *44*:378, 1969.

Vanderark, G. D., Meyer, G. A., Kline, D. G., and Kempe, L. G.: Peripheral nerve injuries studied by evoked potential recordings. Milit. Med., *135*:90, 1970.

Van Hees, J., and Gybels, J. M.: Pain related to single afferent C fibers from human skin. Brain Res., *48*:397, 1972.

Veale, J. L., Mark, R. F., and Rees, S.: Differential sensitivity of motor and sensory fibres in human ulnar nerve. J. Neurol. Neurosurg. Psychiatr., *36*:75, 1973.

Vizoso, A. D., and Young, J. Z.: Internode length and fibre diameter in developing and regenerating nerves. J. Anat., *82*:110, 1948.

Williams, H. B., and Terzis, J.: Single fascicular recordings: an intraoperative diagnostic tool in the management of peripheral nerve lesions. Plast. Reconstr. Surg., 1976.

Chapter 46

INTRAOPERATIVE ELECTRONEURO-MYOGRAPHIC INVESTIGATION OF PERIPHERAL NERVE LESIONS IN CONTINUITY

Paolo Bedeschi

During the last few years several authors have proposed the utilization of electroneuromyography for the intraoperative study of peripheral nerve lesions (Bedeschi et al., 1979; Bedeschi and Rovesta, 1980; Celli et al., 1979; Kline, 1980; Kline and Nulsen, 1972; Terzis et al., 1980; Williams and Terzis, 1976). This chapter presents the results obtained in the intraoperative use of electroneuromyography in patients with peripheral nerve lesions in continuity.

METHOD

A modular portable model MS 7 Medelec electroneuromyograph with an averager was used. The bipolar electrodes are manufactured at our Institute with beveled points of stainless steel or silver chloride separated by a distance of 3 to 6 mm. They can be sterilized. In special cases (recording small sized nerves, single fascicular groups, and nerves situated at a depth), we use electrodes that are partially coated with insulating material (resin or acrylic cement; Fig. 46–1). The electrodes are sterilized by ethyl chloride gas and are kept ready for use in a double walled plastic casing.

During the operation several centimeters of nerve are first isolated above and below the lesion in continuity. This dissection is carefully carried out by use of a microsurgical technique. After this, the altered nerve section is carefully examined under an operating microscope after hemostasis is effected with a bipolar coagulator, both as regards ischemia and after removal of tourniquet.

Finally, the two electrodes are placed in contact with the epineurium, where they delicately lift the nerve from the surrounding tissues in order to prevent interference phenomena. The stimulator electrode is systematically applied in a proximal position to the lesion with the recording electrode in a distal position. In most cases, when the isolated nerve section exceeds 7 to 8 cm., the test is repeated by stimulating below the lesion and recording above. In this way, the sensory fibers are recorded via the prodrome and the motor fibers are recorded via the antidrome. This avoids the risk of registering potentials from the muscle and not the nerve.

The distance between the two electrodes is generally 5 to 15 cm. The electrical stimulus on the nerve must be very brief (0.1 msec.), with a power difference varying from 0 to 100 volts.

After obtaining a reading at rest without interference, stimulation is begun by gradually increasing the intensity until (when possible) a nerve action potential is recorded, which appears on the oscilloscope. The potential difference is then increased by one-third and the sensitivity of the equipment is regulated according to wave amplitude. The nerve action potential image is blocked with the averager and can be photographed with a Polaroid camera.

For correct clinical application of these

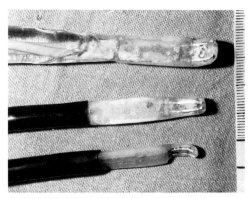

Figure 46–1. Bipolar electrodes are partially coated with insulating material to avoid contact with the surrounding tissues.

intraoperative findings, it is necessary to understand the significance of the presence or absence of the evoked potential, the conduction velocity of the potential itself, and its amplitude and form (see Chapter 45).

CLINICAL APPLICATION

COMPRESSION LESIONS

It is worth remembering that if the peripheral nerve compression lesion is due to a slow, gradual compression, the anatomical and functional nerve damage is essentially correlated with localized ischemia caused by the compression (Sunderland, 1978). During the initial compression phase the more peripheral fibers of the nerve trunk are subjected to earlier functional damage, and this

is particularly true of the larger nerve fibers (Spinner, 1978).

Functional failure of large sized nerve fibers, which are characterized by a greater conduction velocity, explains the resulting slowing of the maximal conduction velocity at the level of the compression. With continuing nerve compression, there is an increase in the pressure of the epineural veins, with edema and consequent fibrosis of the epineurium. Only after prolonged compression is there destruction of the fascicular vascular system, with successive fibrosis of the fascicle itself (Lundborg, 1979).

An exact evaluation of the anatomical and functional damage to a nerve affected by a compression lesion is fundamental in order to carry out efficient microsurgical treatment. The anatomopathological aspects have come to be more widely understood as a result of use of the operating microscope. These can be summarized as follows, in ascending order of seriousness (Bedeschi and Landi, 1976): perineural scarring, fibrotic thickening of the epinevirium, perifascicular fibrosis while the fascicles remain unchanged, perifascicular fibrosis with partial fascicular fibrosis, and massive fascicular fibrosis.

Our intraoperative electroneuromyographic investigations were carried out in 70 patients with peripheral nerve compression lesions of varying seriousness and in various sites. We noted a marked slowing of the maximal conduction velocity at the level of the lesion in the majority of cases (Fig. 46–2). It is evident that the variations in this

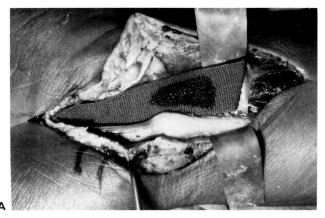

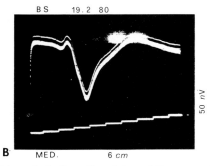

Figure 46–2. Compression lesion of the median nerve in the left carpal tunnel. *A*, Operative picture. After removal of the tourniquet, the distal part of the nerve is already revascularized, while the proximal bulbous portion appears ischemic. Because we found slight fibrosis of the epineurium, we carried out an epineurotomy with an operating microscope to avoid injuring the epineural vessels. *B*, The intraoperative electroneuromyographic examination shows a remarkable delay in the maximum conduction velocity of 50 per cent.

parameter can be correlated with the patient's age, as well as the type and section of the nerve examined. In 13 per cent of the cases we noted the absence of an evoked potential (Fig. 46–3).

We generally encountered a parallel between anatomical damage as shown by the operating microscope and functional damage as shown by intraoperative electroneuromyography. In some cases, however, we observed a dissociation between the two findings, the functional damage being more serious than the anatomical findings might suggest.

I believe that it is important to emphasize that intraoperative electroneuromyographic investigation has been more sensitive than the pre-operative investigation, in that the former often made it possible to record minimal intensity potentials that had been impossible to register before the operation. The overall critical evaluation of the anatomical damage (shown by the operating microscope) and the functional damage (shown by the intraoperative electroneuromyographic examination) enables more precise indications to be given in regard to the type of microsurgical treatment of peripheral nerve compression lesions. In our experience the following indications were found:

External Neurolysis

External neurolysis was used in the absence of epineural fibrosis and in cases showing a slowing of the maximal conduction velocity not exceeding 10 to 20 per cent.

Epineurotomy

Epineurotomy was carried out after removal of the tourniquet in order not to injure the epineural vessels in the presence of modest epineural fibrosis and in cases showing a slowing of the maximal conduction velocity of up to 50 to 60 per cent.

Intraneural Neurolysis

Intraneural neurolysis was used when there was modest perifascicular fibrosis with undamaged fascicles (or very slight fibrosis) and in cases showing marked slowing of the maximal conduction velocity but with the evoked potential still present. Intraneural neurolysis with added epineurectomy appears to be inadvisable, because it damages the vascularization of the nerve, causing further fibrosis (Rydevic et al., 1976).

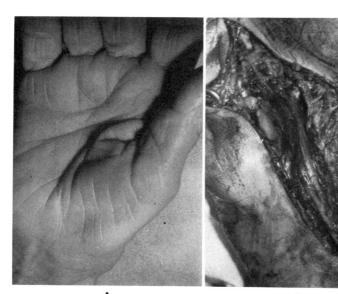
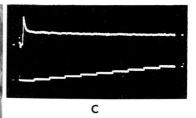

Figure 46–3. Severe compression lesion of the median nerve in the right carpal tunnel of more than two years' duration. *A,* The preoperative picture showed severe atrophy of the external thenar muscles. *B,* Operative picture after the removal of the tourniquet. The operating microscope shows a thickening of the epineurium with perifascicular and fascicular fibrosis. *C,* The intraoperative electroneuromyographic investigation records a complete absence of evoked nerve action potentials. The resection of the fibrotic tract and nerve graft was not carried out because of the age of the patient (69 years old) and the time that had elapsed since the motor paralysis (two years).

Resection of the Fibrotic Section and Nerve Grafting

Resection and nerve grafting were carried out when there was complete fascicular fibrosis and in cases showing complete absence of evoked potentials. (The nerve graft, however, could be ineffective in old lesions, in which irreversible lesions of the effector muscles exist.)

CONTUSIONS

In two cases the examination was carried out a few days after trauma to a radial nerve occurring during internal fixation of a humeral fracture. Although evoked potentials across the injured zone were not recorded in these patients, who presented with complete paralysis, a muscular response was evident upon stimulating the nerve distal to the lesion. Clinical recovery from the paralysis occurred within three months following the trauma and confirmed the lesion as being neurapraxia.

In the other cases the investigation was carried out at least two months after the trauma.

In eight cases an evoked action potential was recorded across the lesion, with a maximal conduction velocity delay of varying degrees and with no (or modest) epineural fibrosis (Fig. 46–4). External neurolysis was carried out with or without epineurotomy, according to the criteria already mentioned in the previous paragraph, and with good long term results.

Resection and nerve grafting were carried out in two cases in which the injured zone showed evidence of diffuse fascicular fibrosis and in which no evoked potential was recorded.

TRACTION LESIONS

The investigation was carried out on damaged nerve trunks in continuity in 27 patients operated on for lesions of the brachial plexus, at least three months after the trauma. The intraoperative electroneuromyographic examination enabled functional continuity of the single nerve trunks to be demonstrated and, furthermore, enabled the proximal level of the lesion to be established exactly. This is difficult to ascertain purely on the basis of anatomical damage seen at operation. In brachial plexus surgery, particularly sophisticated electrophysiological techniques make it possible to evaluate either the integrity of the intraforaminal part of the roots by recording the evoked muscular potentials in the paravertebral muscles and the evoked sensory cerebral potentials (Celli et al., 1979).

PARTIAL DIVISIONS OF NERVES

In three patients operated upon more than two months following the injury, the intra-

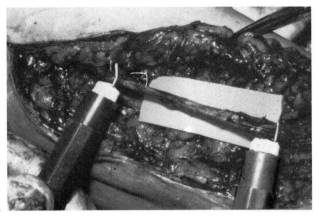
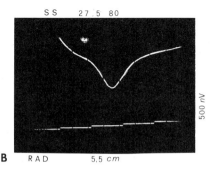

Figure 46–4. Neurolysis of the radial nerve of the right arm. Three months previously a fracture of the humerus occurred, resulting in a contusion injury to the nerve. *A*, Operative picture showing the isolated nerve and the two electrodes proximal and distal to the lesion in continuity. *B*, The recording of the evoked nerve action potential shows a remarkable delay of the maximum conduction velocity. Epineurotomy was carried out with a good follow-up result.

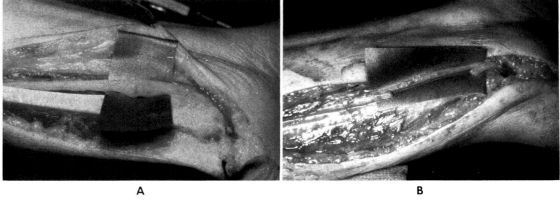

Figure 46–5. Partial division of the ulnar nerve at the left wrist occurring four months previously. *A* and *B*, Operative pictures before and after the resection of the fibrotic segment of the nerve. *C*, After the resection of the partial neuroma, the evoked nerve action potential was unchanged. We carried out a nerve graft to restore the continuity of the resected fascicles.

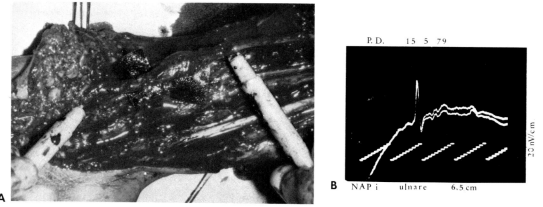

Figure 46–6. Wound of the left wrist treated as an emergency in our clinic three months previously. Originally there were lesions of the ulnar nerve and artery, of the flexor carpi ulnaris, and of most flexors of the fingers. *A*, Operative picture at the reintervention carried out for tenolysis of the flexors of the fingers. At this time we also carried out a neurolysis of the previously sutured ulnar nerve. Examination using the operating microscope showed only slight fibrosis of the epineurium. *B*, At the intraoperative electroneuromyographic examination a polyphasic evoked nerve action potential was demonstrated with a remarkable delay of the maximum conduction velocity, which is typical of regenerating fibers. The follow-up result was very good.

operative electroneuromyographic investigation showed functional nerve continuity that had remained unchanged after resection (and grafting) of the fibrotic zone (Fig. 46–5).

In cases of a partial neuroma, the size of the nerve resection is determined largely by the anatomical findings as seen under the operating microscope. Although extremely interesting and suggestive, the "monofascicular" recordings described by Williams and Terzis (1976) require an extremely deep internal neurolysis, which could be dangerous for nerve vascularization, encouraging perifascicular and fascicular fibrosis (Rydevic et al., 1976).

LESIONS CAUSED BY RADIOTHERAPY

In two patients with lesions of the brachial plexus caused by radiotherapy who were operated upon many years after the mastectomy for mammary carcinoma and radiotherapy, the intraoperative electroneuromyographic investigation revealed much more extensive nerve damage than that which could be discerned by mere observation under the operating microscope.

LESIONS CAUSED BY ISCHEMIA

An intraoperative electroneuromyographic investigation was carried out in four cases of Volkmann's ischemic contracture. In three cases the lesion was two to three months old; in the other case it was over six months old.

In no case was it possible to record evoked potentials in the median nerve, but this was possible in the ulnar nerve in all cases.

A follow-up examination carried out after some time showed good sensory and muscular recovery in the cases in which the median nerve had been decompressed early (together with the ulnar nerve), and an unsatisfactory result occurred in the patient operated upon after six months.

On the basis of experience acquired during the surgical treatment of Volkmann's ischemic contracture, we believe that ischemic damage and the prognosis for nerve recovery (above all for the median nerve) depend on extra- and intraneural fibrosis, which is itself related to the time interval between the trauma and the moment of neurolysis (Bedeschi and Landi, 1976).

RESULTS OF NEURORRAPHY

In six patients who were operated upon in another hospital by neurorraphy without the aid of a microscope, the intraoperative electroneuromyographic examination, carried out at least three months after the first operation showed the complete absence of evoked nerve potentials across the lesion, which involved diffuse fascicular fibrosis when seen under the operating microscope.

In these cases the fibrotic nerve segment was resected and replaced with interfascicular grafts.

In a further operation carried out after several months and for other reasons (tenolysis) in two patients previously operated upon in our Neurorraphy Clinic employing microsurgical technique, the intraoperative electroneuromyographic examination demonstrated evoked polyphasic nerve action potentials across the area of nerve repair with notable conduction velocity delay—a typical expression of fiber regeneration (Fig. 46–6). In special cases in which the intraoperative electroneuromyographic examination is carried out several months after neurorraphy, and when it is possible to record evoked action potentials, but the nerve under the operating microscope shows areas of interfascicular and fascicular fibrosis, it may be advisable to separate the nerve carefully and precisely into two or three fascicular groups and carry out the electrophysiological examination for each fascicular group. It is then possible to resect and replace with grafts the fascicular group across which it has been impossible to record evoked potentials (Kline, 1980; Williams and Terzis, 1976).

The indications for this microsurgical technique must be carefully evaluated in order to avoid causing ischemic damage to the fascicles in which there has been functional postoperative recovery as shown by the recording of evoked nerve potentials.

Together with research in the clinical field, we are carrying out experimental electrophysiological research on rabbits in our Institute with two objectives in view: To identify and eliminate possible causes of electrical interference, which often changes the recorded electrical signals, and to find a more precise quantitative and qualitative relationship between the characteristics of the recorded nerve action potential and the number and type of functioning fibers.

REFERENCES

Bedeschi, P., Canedi, L., and Rovesta, C.: Indagine elettroneuromiografica intraoperatoria nel trattamento delle lesioni compressive dei nervi periferici. Chir. Organi. Mov., 65:253–259, 1979.

Bedeschi, P., and Landi, A.: Aspetti fisio-patologici e possibilità chirurgiche nelle lesioni in continuità dei nervi periferici. Policlin. Sez. Chir., 83:605–610, 1976.

Bedeschi, P., and Rovesta, C.: Utilità dell' elettromiografia intraoperatoria nelle lesioni in continuità dei nervi periferici. Riv. Chir. (In press.)

Celli, L., Canedi, L., and Rovesta, C.: I potenziali muscolari evocati intraoperatori nel trattamento delle lesioni traumatiche del plesso brachiale. Chir. Organi. Mov. 65:399–403, 1979.

Kline, D. G.: Evaluation of the neuroma in continuity. In Omer, G. E., and Spinner, M. (Editors): Management of Peripheral Nerve Problems. Philadelphia, W. B. Saunders Company, 1980, pp. 450–461.

Kline, D. G., and Nulsen, F. E.: The neuroma in continuity its preoperative and operative management. Surg. Clin. N. Am., 52:1189, 1972.

Lundborg, G.: The intrinsic vascularization of human peripheral nerves: structural and functional aspects. J. Hand Surg., 4:34, 1979.

Rydevic, B., Lundborg, G., and Nordborg, C.: Intraneural tissue reactions induced by internal neurolysis. Scand. J. Plast. Reconstr. Surg., 10:3, 1976.

Spinner, M.: Injuries to the Major Branches of Peripheral Nerves of the Forearm. Philadelphia, W. B. Saunders Company, 1978, p. 26.

Sunderland, S.: Nerves and Nerve Injuries. Edinburgh, Churchill Livingstone, 1978.

Terzis, J. K., Daniel, R. K., and Williams, H. B.: Intraoperative assessment of nerve lesions with fascicular dissection and electrophysiological recording. In Omer, G. E., and Spinner, M. (Editors): Management of Peripheral Nerve Problems. Philadelphia, W. B. Saunders Company, 1980, pp. 462–472.

Williams, H. B., and Terzis, J. K.: Single fascicular recordings: an intraoperative diagnostic tool for the management of peripheral nerve lesions. Plast. Reconstr. Surg., 57:562, 1976.

CLINICAL EXAMINATION AND FUNCTIONAL ASSESSMENT OF THE UPPER LIMB AFTER PERIPHERAL NERVE LESIONS

RAOUL TUBIANA

CLINICAL EXAMINATION

A nerve lesion must be sought or suspected in the presence of any open or closed lesion in a region through which one or more nerves pass. A careful and orderly clinical examination is essential.

Repeated examination will be necessary to confirm the diagnosis and observe the evolution of the lesion. Each response obtained on examination, *whether positive or negative,* must be recorded using a standardized protocol. This examination will not be described in detail but its different stages are as follows: history, visual assessment of the limb as a whole, seeking deformities, examination of motor function, examination of sensation, and special investigations.

History involves the circumstances of the lesion, its nature and the chronology of events. Was there loss of consciousness or application of a tourniquet after an injury? Did the motor deficit appear immediately? Later? After reduction of a fracture or dislocation? After an injection? After application of a cast? Did abnormalities of sensation develop simultaneously with the motor deficit or was there a time interval?

Types of pain must be recorded: stabbing, constrictive, "electric shock," burning; constant or paroxysmal; with or without proximal or distal radiation; occurring spontaneously or during movement or pressure; permanent or relieved by rest or analgesics?

General examination is essential. Paralysis of central origin may be erroneously attributed to an injury, or the accident may be due to a central neurological lesion with a fall or loss of consciousness.

Examination of the limb: If an open wound is present, the nerve lesion can be evaluated by careful exploration. Several nerves may be involved. Multiple damage may cause lesions at different points along the same nerve. Concomitant lesions must always be sought: fractures, dislocations, vascular lesions, and so on. When there is no open wound, a contusion must be sought along the course of the nerve.

ANALYTICAL EXAMINATION OF THE MUSCLES

We shall deal here with tests that are used to demonstrate clinically the motor activity of each of the muscles of the upper limb. These tests do not necessarily make use of the normal activity of each individual muscle but aim at dissociating the muscle from its synergists. Most of the maneuvers described are used to produce active mobilization of a more distal segment; it is not so much the actual contraction of a muscle as its efficiency that is tested.

Weakening or disappearance of voluntary movement may be due to one of several causes. Paralysis of the afferent nerve, destruction of muscle tissue (often as a result of ischemia of the fleshy part of the muscle), rupture of the tendon, and tendon block because of adhesions are the more obvious causes. However, one should remember that alteration at its point of angulation will re-

453

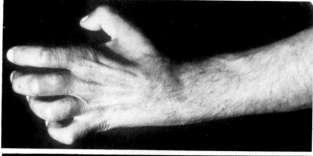

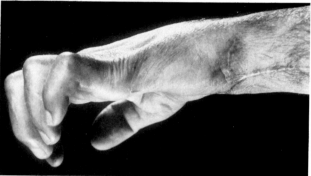

Figure 47–1. Ulnar claw hand.

duce or annul the efficiency of a muscle. This is the case when the pulleys of the flexors are damaged or when the extensor tendons are dislocated into the intermetacarpal spaces. It is also obvious that these tests are valid only if the joint has a normal range of movement.

An abnormal hand posture may be characteristic and establish the diagnosis, as with a typical ulnar claw, or as with wrist drop and flexion of the wrist and metacarpophalangeal joints, pathognomonic of radial nerve palsy (Figs. 47–1, 47–2).

Somewhat less typical is the dissociated radial palsy simulating an ulnar claw in which extension of the thumb and index and middle fingers is preserved (Marie et al., 1917).

Dissociated median nerve forearm palsy resulting from compression or sectioning of the anterior interosseous nerve supplying the flexor pollicis longus, the radial half of the flexor digitorum profundus, and the pronator quadratus also produces a characteristic deformity known as the "anterior interosseous nerve syndrome" (Kiloh and Nevin, 1952; Tinel, 1918) (Fig. 47–3). During pinch the distal phalanges of the thumb and index finger cannot flex and stay in extension.

Clawing of the two ulnar digits, caused by paralysis of the interosseous muscle, is variable. It is usually absent in proximal lesions of the ulnar nerve, because the deep flexors of the ulnar fingers are also paralyzed. The

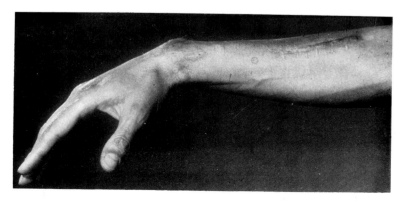

Figure 47–2. The characteristic wrist drop in radial nerve palsy.

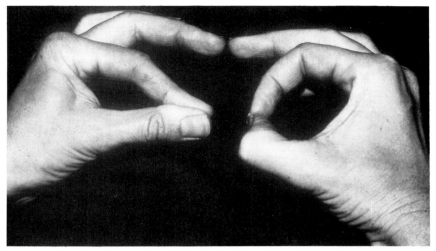

Figure 47–3. Typical pinch attitude in an anterior interosseous nerve palsy.

deformity does not usually involve the index and middle fingers, for paralysis of the interosseous muscles is compensated for by the lumbrical muscles, which are supplied by the median nerve. There is a wide variation in the motor and sensory territories of the median and ulnar nerves.

EXAMINATION OF MOTOR FUNCTION

This examination can be performed in its entirety only after a certain period of time.

The main features of a motor palsy are muscle atrophy and the absence of voluntary contraction.

Demonstration of voluntary contraction is not always easy. Not all muscles are palpable. The nerve supply can be anomalous, and a contraction of a normally innervated muscle can be transmitted to the fibers of an adjacent paralyzed muscle. The reflexes must be tested and compared with those on the healthy contralateral side.

The key of this part of the examination is *The Study of Voluntary Movements*. Accurate assessment of the individual muscles is essential. Muscle power is graded by using the Highet scale adopted by the British Medical Research Council (MRC) (1941) or one of its variations.

M0—no contraction.
M1—flicker (no joint motion).

M2—contraction with mobility with gravity eliminated.
M3—contraction against gravity.
M4—contraction with active movement of normal amplitude against gravity and some resistance.
M5—normal power.

There is a gap between M3 and M4 and many clinicians use an extra grade: M3 +—contraction against resistance.

Examinations are repeated periodically and the results are noted on an appropriate form, such as that shown in Figure 47–4.

We will stress here the importance of testing for movements originating in the arm, forearm, and shoulder. These examinations are mandatory in high trunk lesions and injuries of the brachial plexus (Fig. 47–5).

TESTING THE VOLUNTARY MOVEMENTS OF THE SCAPULAR MUSCLES

SERRATUS ANTERIOR

Nerve supply: Long thoracic nerve ("respiratory" nerve of Bell; C5, C6, C7).

Action: Pulls the scapula forward against the ribs.

Test of muscle function: Using the upper limbs, the patient pushes his body away from a fixed plane. The medial border of the scapula is held against the thoracic plane by

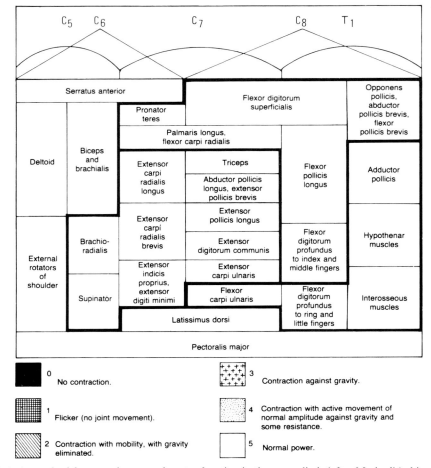

Figure 47–4. A standard form used to record motor function in the upper limb (after Merle d'Aubigne). The areas outlined in heavy black lines enclose those muscles usually supplied by the median, radial, and ulnar nerves. The area on the form for each muscle should be cross hatched or stippled according to its power (scale 0–5): M0, no contraction. M1, flicker of activity (no joint motion). M2, contraction + joint motion (gravity eliminated). M3, contraction + joint motion (against gravity). M4, contraction against gravity + some resistance. M5, normal power.

the serratus anterior unless the latter is paralyzed (Fig. 47–6).

RHOMBOID

Nerve supply: Nerve to the rhomboid (dorsal scapular nerve; C4, C5).

Action: Pulls the lower half of the scapula medially.

Test of muscle function: The patient attempts to push his shoulder backward against resistance. Contraction of the muscle can be felt and sometimes seen (Fig. 47–7).

ANALYSIS OF ARM AND SHOULDER MOVEMENTS

Abduction. Abduction of the arm at the shoulder joint is brought about by the middle part of the deltoid and the supraspinatus (Fig. 47–8).

Flexion. Flexion is produced by the anterior part of the deltoid, the clavicular head of the pectoralis major, the coracobrachialis, and the short head of the biceps (Fig. 47–9).

Extension. Extension results from the action of the posterior part of the deltoid, the latissimus dorsi, the teres major, and the long head of the triceps (Fig. 47–10).

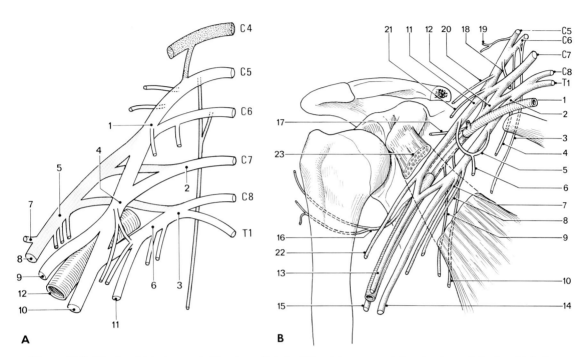

Figure 47–5. The brachial plexus. *A*, Structure. It is traditional to represent the structure of the brachial plexus schematically in the following manner: The fifth anterior cervical root (C5), after receiving the branch from the fourth root (C4), unites with the sixth root (C6) to form the superior trunk. The first thoracic root, after receiving a branch from the second thoracic root, unites with the eighth cervical root (C8) to form the inferior trunk. The seventh cervical root (C7) continues as the middle trunk. Each of these trunks divides into two divisions, one anterior and one posterior. The three posterior divisions unite to form the posterior cord from which the circumflex nerve and radial nerve arise. The anterior division of the superior trunk receives the anterior division of the middle trunk. They unite to form the lateral cord from which the musculocutaneous nerve and the lateral root of the median nerve arise. Finally, the anterior division of the inferior trunk remains independent and forms the medial cord from which the medial root of the median nerve, the ulnar nerve, and the medial brachial cutaneous nerve of the arm and forearm arise. 1, Superior trunk. 2, Middle trunk. 3, Inferior trunk. 4, Lateral cord. 5, Posterior cord. 6, Medial cord. 7, Axillary nerve. 8, Radial nerve. 9, Musculocutaneous nerve. 10, Median nerve. 11, Ulnar nerve. 12, Axillary artery. *B*, Branches of the brachial plexus. 1, Axillary artery. 2, Medial cord. 3, Nerve to serratus anterior. 4, Upper subscapular nerve. 5, Medial anterior thoracic nerve. 6, Anterior thoracic nerve. 7, Medial brachial cutaneous nerve. 8, Medial antebrachial cutaneous nerve. 9, Nerve to latissimus dorsi. 10, Nerve to teres major. 11, Lateral cord. 12, Posterior cord. 13, Median nerve. 14, Ulnar nerve. 15, Radial nerve. 16, Axillary nerve. 17, Inferior subscapular nerve. 18, Dorsal scapular nerve. 19, Nerve to subclavius. 20, Suprascapular nerve. 21, Lateral anterior thoracic nerve. 22, Musculocutaneous nerve. 23, Pectoralis minor muscle.

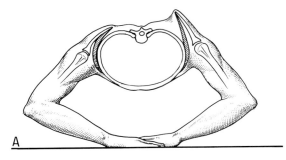

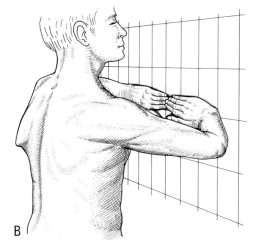

Figure 47–6. Serratus anterior palsy. *A,* Winging of scapula on the left side as seen in this cross section of the trunk. *B,* Clinical test to demonstrate winging of the left scapula.

Adduction. Adduction is due to the combined action of anterior and posterior muscles—anteriorly, the pectoralis major and coracobrachialis and, posteriorly, the posterior part of the deltoid, the long head of the triceps, the teres major, and the latissimus dorsi (Figs. 47–11, 47–12).

Medial Rotation. Medial rotation of the arm is brought about by the subscapularis, the teres major, the pectoralis major, and the latissimus dorsi (Fig. 47–13).

Lateral Rotation. Lateral rotation is achieved by the infraspinatus, the teres minor, and the posterior part of the deltoid.

PECTORALIS MAJOR

Nerve supply: Lateral (C6, C7, C8) and medial (T1) pectoral nerves.

Action: Adducts, lowers, and medially rotates the arm.

Test of muscle function: The patient pulls his arm toward his chest against resistance (Fig. 47–14).

PECTORALIS MINOR

Nerve supply: Branches to the pectoralis minor (C8).

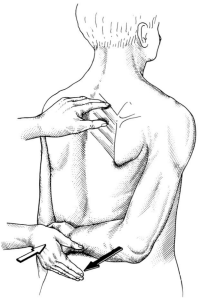

Figure 47–7. Paralysis of the rhomboids. With his arm behind his back, the patient presses his hand backward against resistance. The rhomboid muscle can be seen to contract.

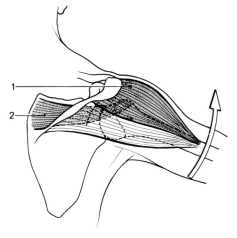

Figure 47–8. The abductors of the shoulder. 1, Middle part of deltoid. 2, Supraspinatus.

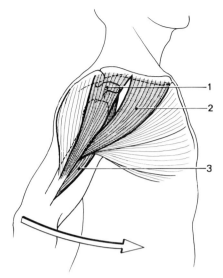

Figure 47–9. The flexors of the shoulder. 1, Anterior part of deltoid. 2, Clavicular head of pectoralis major. 3, Coracobrachialis.

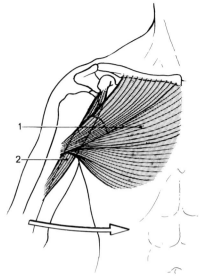

Figure 47–11. The adductors of the shoulder, anterior muscles. 1, Pectoralis major. 2, Coracobrachialis.

Action: Lowers the shoulder.

Test of muscle function: Lowering the shoulder against resistance, the tendon can be felt on the coracoid process (Fig. 47–15).

LATISSIMUS DORSI

Nerve supply: Thoracodorsal nerve from the posterior cord of C6, C7, and C8.

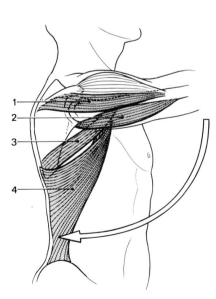

Figure 47–10. The extensors of the shoulder. 1, Posterior part of deltoid. 2, Long head of triceps. 3, Teres major. 4, Latissimus dorsi.

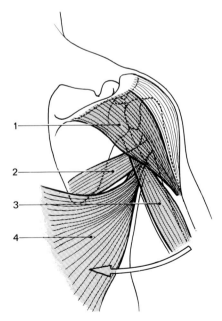

Figure 47–12. The adductors of the shoulder, posterior muscles. 1, Posterior part of deltoid. 2, Teres major. 3, Long head of triceps. 4, Latissimus dorsi.

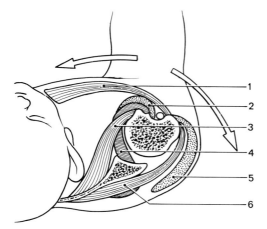

Figure 47–13. Medial and lateral rotators of the shoulder. Medial rotators: 1, Pectoralis major. 2, Latissimus dorsi. 3, Subscapularis. 4, Teres major. Lateral rotators: 5, Posterior part of deltoid. 6, Infraspinatus.

Action: Adductor, extensor, and medial rotator of the arm.

Test of muscle function: Adduction of the arm against resistance demonstrates the lateral border of the latissimus dorsi. The teres

major contracts at the same time (Figs. 47–16, 47–17). Active adduction can be tested with the limb raised or lowered. Moberg (1978), remembering the name given to the muscle by ancient anatomists (musculus scapultor ani: "muscle used to scratch one's bottom"), asks the patient to carry his hand to his buttock against resistance applied by the examiner.

DELTOID

Nerve supply: Axillary nerve (C5, C6).

Action: Abductor of the arm. In addition, the anterior fibers carry the arm forward and the posterior fibers carry it backward (Fig. 47–18A to C).

Test of muscle function:

1. Middle fibers: The patient is asked to abduct his arm against resistance, in the range of 15 to 90 degrees of abduction (Fig. 47–18A, B).

2. Anterior fibers: Elevation of the arm anteriorly against resistance (Fig. 47–18C).

3. Posterior fibers: Elevation of the arm posteriorly against resistance (Fig. 47–18D).

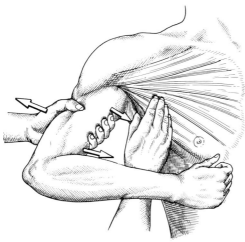

Figure 47–14. Pectoralis major. When the patient adducts his arm against resistance, the muscle belly can be seen and felt.

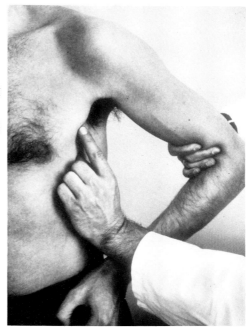

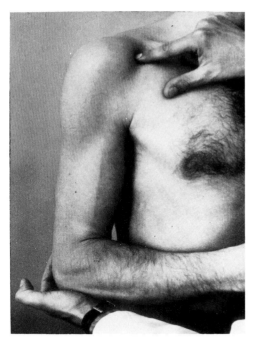

Figure 47–15. Pectoralis minor. The patient depresses his shoulder against resistance. The tendon can be felt at the coracoid process.

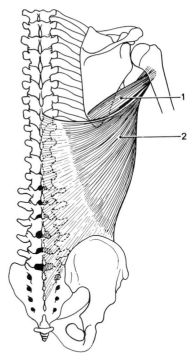

Figure 47–16. Anatomy of the teres major (1) and latissimus dorsi (2).

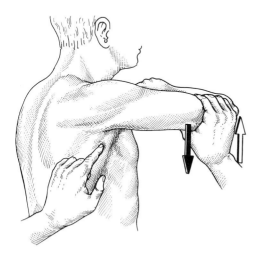

Figure 47–17. Clinical demonstration of the latissimus dorsi. The muscle can be seen when the patient adducts his arm against resistance.

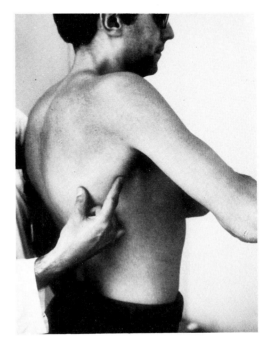

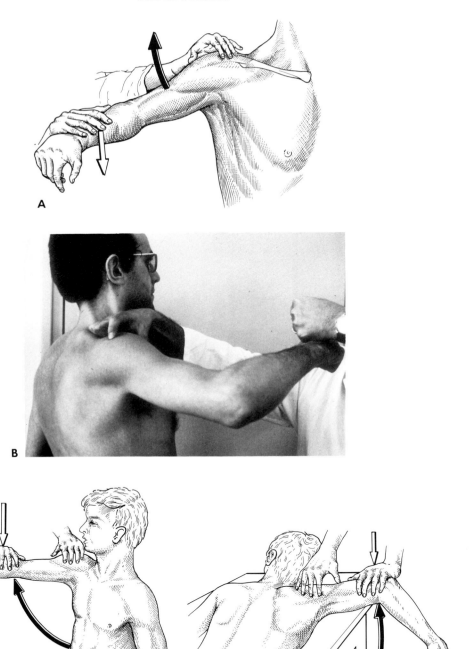

Figure 47–18. Clinical demonstration of the deltoid. *A* and *B*, The middle part of the deltoid is palpated between the thumb and index finger of the examiner when the arm is abducted against resistance and flexed anteriorly 15 to 90 degrees. *C*, Clinical demonstration of the anterior part of the deltoid. The patient is asked to elevate his arm anteriorly against resistance. *D*, Clinical demonstration of the posterior part of the deltoid. The patient is asked to extend the arm posteriorly at the shoulder against resistance.

SUPRASPINATUS

Nerve supply: Suprascapular nerve (C5).
Action: Initiates abduction.
Test of muscle function: With the arm resting alongside the body, the patient attempts to abduct it against resistance. The muscle contraction normally can be felt under the upper part of the trapezius (Fig. 47–19).

INFRASPINATUS

Nerve supply: Suprascapular nerve (C5).
Action: Rotates the arm laterally (Fig. 47–20).
Test of muscle function: Standing up with his arm against his chest and the elbow in 90 degrees of flexion, the patient tries to carry his forearm laterally against resistance (Fig. 47–21*A*). Or, lying prone with his arm in 90 degrees of abduction and his forearm hanging down from the table, the patient tries to externally rotate his arm against resistance (Fig. 47–21*B*).

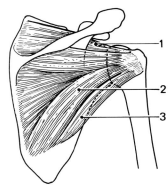

Figure 47–20. Anatomy of the supraspinatus (1), infraspinatus (2), and teres minor (3).

SUBSCAPULARIS (Fig. 47–22)

Nerve supply: Upper and lower branches of the subscapular nerve, arising from the posterior division (C6, C7, C8).
Action: Medial rotation of the arm, adduction.
Test of muscle function: The patient in the prone position (as for infraspinatus testing) tries to internally rotate his arm against resistance (Fig. 47–23).

ANALYSIS OF MOVEMENTS OF THE ELBOW AND FOREARM

Elbow Flexion. Elbow flexion is brought about by the biceps, the brachialis, the brachioradialis, and the pronator teres (Fig. 47–24).

Elbow Extension. Elbow extension is effected by the triceps and the anconeus (Fig. 47–25).

Forearm Pronation. Forearm pronation is effected by the pronator teres and the pronator quadratus (Fig. 47–26).

Forearm Supination. Forearm supination is effected by the biceps and the supinator (Fig. 47–27).

BICEPS BRACHII

Nerve supply: Musculocutaneous nerve (C5, C6).
Action: Flexes the elbow and supinates the forearm.

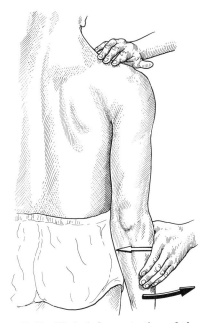

Figure 47–19. Clinical demonstration of the supraspinatus. As the patient abducts his arm against resistance, the muscle contraction can be felt.

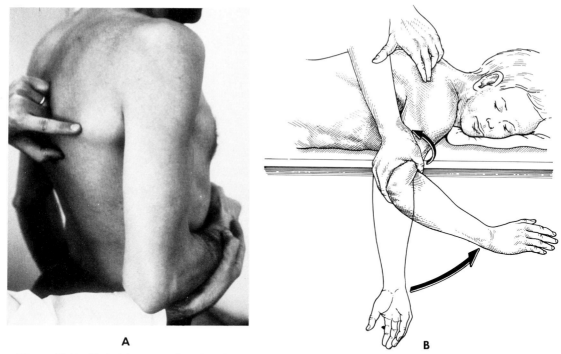

A   **B**

Figure 47–21. Clinical demonstration of the infraspinatus. *A*, The muscle can be palpated when the patient attempts to rotate the arm externally from the position of internal rotation. *B*, The patient lies prone with his shoulder abducted to 90 degrees, the elbow flexed to 90 degrees, and the forearm hanging down. The muscle can be palpated when he externally rotates the arm against resistance.

Test of muscle function: Flexion of the elbow against resistance with the forearm supinated (Figs. 47–28, 47–29).

TRICEPS

Nerve supply: Radial nerve (C5, C6, C7, C8).

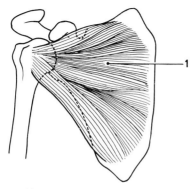

Figure 47–22. Anatomy of the subscapularis.

Action: Extends the elbow; the long head also adducts the arm.

Test of muscle function: With the arm in 90 degrees of abduction (to eliminate the action of gravity) and the forearm hanging down, the patient tries to extend the elbow (Figs. 47–30, 47–31).

BRACHIORADIALIS

Nerve supply: Radial nerve (C5, C6, C7).

Action: Flexes the elbow; also acts as a pronator in full supination and as a supinator in full pronation.

Test of muscle function: Flexion against resistance with the elbow in 90 degrees of flexion and the forearm halfway between pronation and supination (Fig. 47–32).

SUPINATOR

Nerve supply: Radial nerve (C5, C6).
Action: Supinates the forearm.

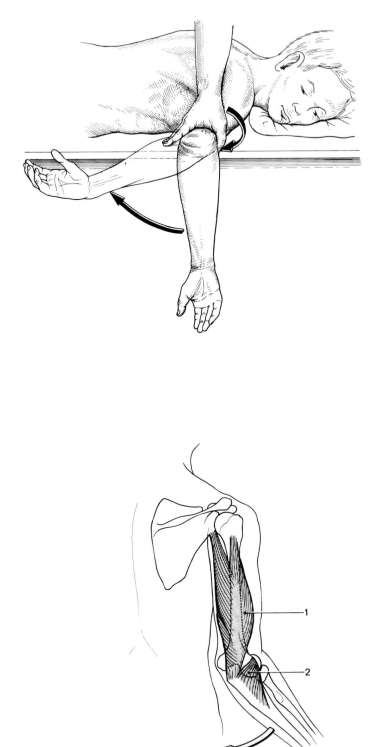

Figure 47–23. Clinical demonstration of the subscapularis. With the patient prone, the reverse procedure for testing the infraspinatus is performed.

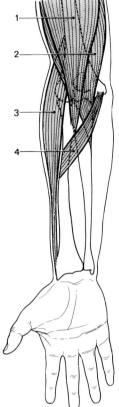

Figure 47–24. Flexors of the elbow. 1, Biceps. 2, Brachialis. 3, Brachioradialis. 4, Pronator teres.

Figure 47–25. Extensors of the elbow. 1, Triceps. 2, Anconeus.

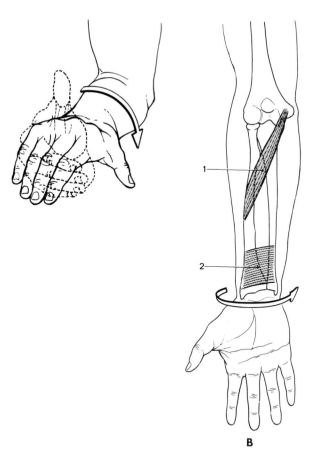

Figure 47–26. Pronation of the forearm. *A*, Movement of pronation. *B*, Muscles of pronation: 1, Pronator teres. 2, Pronator quadratus.

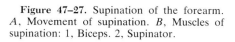

Figure 47–27. Supination of the forearm. *A*, Movement of supination. *B*, Muscles of supination: 1, Biceps. 2, Supinator.

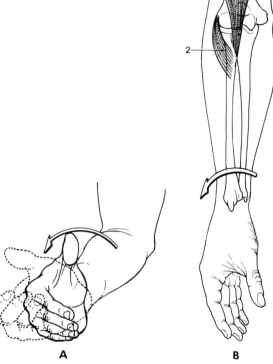

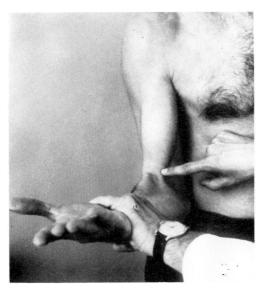

Figure 47–28. Clinical demonstration of the biceps brachii by flexion of the elbow against resistance.

Test of muscle function: With the arm hanging and the elbow extended, the patient attempts to supinate the forearm against resistance (Fig. 47–33).

PRONATOR TERES

Nerve supply: Median nerve (C6, C7).

Action: Pronates the forearm, flexes the elbow.

Test of muscle function: With the elbow flexed, the patient pronates the forearm against resistance. Contraction of the muscle usually can be felt and seen (Fig. 47–34).

ANALYSIS OF MOVEMENTS OF THE WRIST

Wrist Flexion. Wrist flexion is brought about by the flexor carpi radialis, palmaris longus, and flexor carpi ulnaris.

Wrist Extension. Wrist extension is brought about by the extensor carpi radialis longus, extensor carpi radialis brevis, and extensor carpi ulnaris.

Radial Deviation. Radial deviation is brought about by the abductor pollicis longus, extensor carpi radialis longus and brevis, and flexor carpi radialis.

Ulnar Deviation. Ulnar deviation is brought about by the flexor carpi ulnaris and extensor carpi ulnaris.

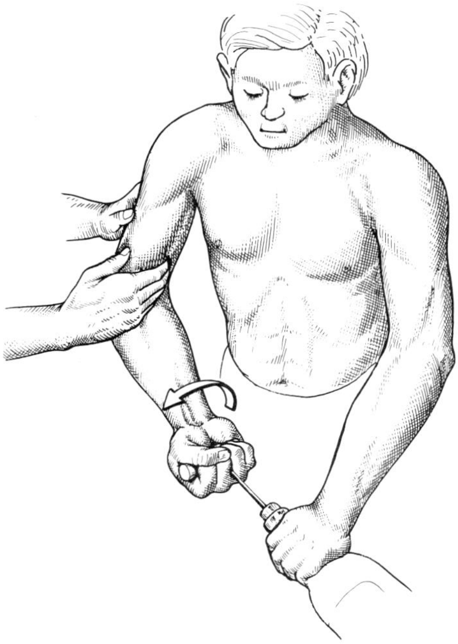

Figure 47–29. Clinical demonstration of the biceps brachii. Flexion of the elbow and supination, as in using a corkscrew, demonstrate the muscle.

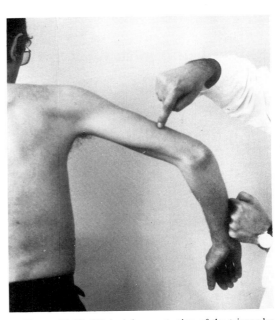

Figure 47–30. Clinical demonstration of the triceps by use of resisted elbow extension.

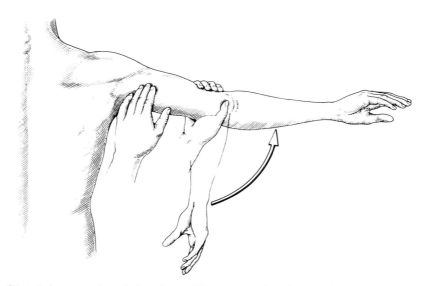

Figure 47–31. Clinical demonstration of the triceps. When testing the triceps, it is important to prevent trick movements that can extend the elbow by using gravity. The arm therefore should be placed horizontally to eliminate the effect of gravity.

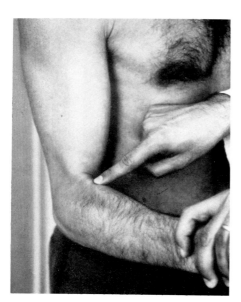

Figure 47–32. Clinical demonstration of the brachioradialis. Resisted elbow flexion is effected with the forearm in 90 degrees of flexion and neutral pronation and supination.

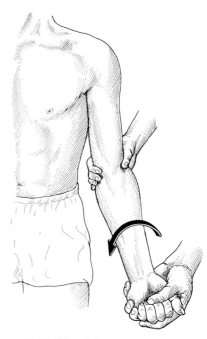

Figure 47–33. Clinical demonstration of the supinator. With the arm hanging by the side and the elbow extended to eliminate the action of biceps, the patient attempts to supinate the forearm against resistance.

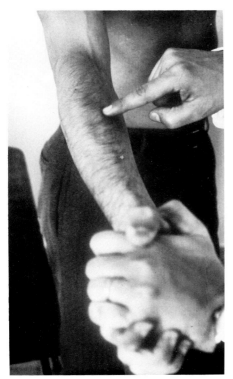

Figure 47–34. Clinical demonstration of the pronator teres. With the elbow and fingers flexed, the patient attempts to pronate the forearm against resistance.

FLEXOR CARPI RADIALIS

Nerve supply: Median nerve (C6).
Action: Flexes the wrist.
Test of muscle function: Flexion of the wrist against resistance (Fig. 47–35).

PALMARIS LONGUS

Nerve supply: Median nerve (C6).
Action: Flexes the wrist.
Test of muscle function: Flexion of the wrist against resistance (Fig. 47–35).

FLEXOR CARPI ULNARIS

Nerve supply: Ulnar nerve (C8, T1).
Action: Flexes the wrist with ulnar deviation.
Test of muscle function: Flexion and ulnar deviation of the wrist against resistance (Fig. 47–36).

EXTENSOR CARPI RADIALIS LONGUS

Nerve supply: Radial nerve (C6, C7).
Action: Radial deviation and extension of the wrist.
Test of muscle function: Extends and deviates the wrist against resistance. The tendon is palpable over the base of the second metacarpal (Fig. 47–37).

EXTENSOR CARPI RADIALIS BREVIS

Nerve supply: Radial nerve (C6, C7).
Action: Extension of the wrist.
Test of muscle function: Extends the wrist against resistance. The tendon is palpable over the base of the third metacarpal (Fig. 47–38). It is difficult clinically to differentiate

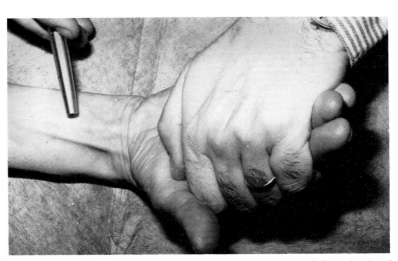

Figure 47–35. Counterflexion of the wrist allows one to test the flexor carpi radialis and palmaris longus, for the tendons are accessible to direct examination.

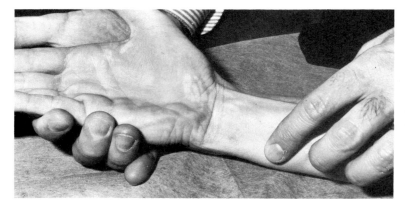

Figure 47–36. The flexor carpi ulnaris is evaluated by a movement counter to ulnar deviation and wrist flexion. Its tendon can be palpated at its insertion into the pisiform.

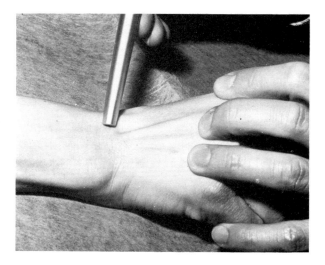

Figure 47–37. Isolated contraction of the extensor carpi radialis longus effects radial deviation of the hand when the wrist is extended. Its tendon is palpable over the base of the second metacarpal.

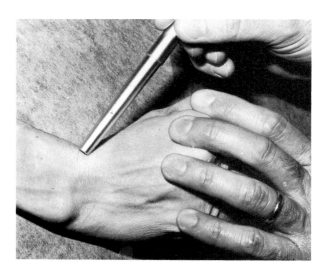

Figure 47–38. Only the extensor carpi radialis brevis is able by itself to effect direct extension of the wrist. Its tendon is palpable over the base of the third metacarpal.

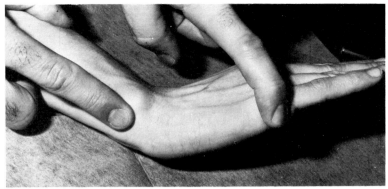

Figure 47–39. The extensor carpi ulnaris is evaluated by counterextension and ulnar deviation of the wrist. Its tendon can be felt at its insertion on the fifth metacarpal.

between the contraction of the extensor carpi radialis brevis and extensor carpi radialis longus. This can have serious consequences in treatment, particularly that of tetraplegia. It is not possible to determine the strength of the extensor carpi radialis brevis without surgical exposure.

EXTENSOR CARPI ULNARIS

Nerve supply: Radial nerve (C7).
Action: Extensor of the wrist in supination, ulnar deviation in pronation.
Test of muscle function: Ulnar deviation of the wrist against resistance in pronation. The tendon is palpable over the base of the fifth metacarpal (Fig. 47–39). The extensor carpi ulnaris is an antagonist of the abductor pollicis longus; their contractions are synchronous. When the thumb is in radial abduction, the contraction of the extensor carpi ulnaris can be palpated.

ANALYSIS OF THE MOVEMENTS OF THE FINGERS

Finger Flexion. Finger flexion is brought about by the flexor digitorum superficialis, flexor digitorum profundus, and the interosseous muscles.
Finger Extension. Finger extension is brought about by the extensor digitorum communis, extensor indicis proprius, extensor digiti quinti proprius, and the interosseous and lumbrical muscles.
Finger Abduction. Finger abduction is brought about by the dorsal interosseous muscles and the abductor digiti quinti.

Finger Adduction. Finger adduction is brought about by the palmar interosseous muscles.

FLEXOR DIGITORUM SUPERFICIALIS

Nerve supply: Median nerve (C7, C8, T1).
Action: Flexion of the proximal interphalangeal joint.
Test of muscle function: Active flexion of the proximal interphalangeal joint of one finger while all the other fingers are held in full extension (Figs. 47–40, 47–41).

FLEXOR DIGITORUM PROFUNDUS

Nerve supply: Median nerve (volar interosseous branch; C8, T1) for the index and long fingers; ulnar nerve (C8, T1) for the ring and little fingers.
Action: Flexion of the distal interphalangeal joint.
Test of muscle function: Flexion of the distal phalanx; the two proximal phalanges are held in extension (Figs. 47–42, 47–43).

EXTENSOR DIGITORUM COMMUNIS

Nerve supply: Radial nerve (C7).
Action: Active extension of the metacarpophalangeal joints of the fingers.
Test of muscle function: Extension of the proximal phalanx against resistance (Fig. 47–44). It is preferable to test the extension of either the middle or ring finger.

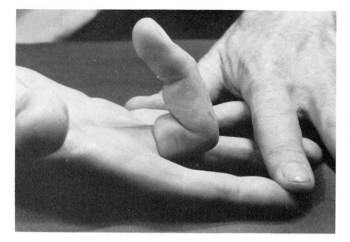

Figure 47–40. Testing the flexor digitorum superficialis. The patient is asked to flex actively one finger, while all the other fingers are held in full extension.

Figure 47–41. By putting all the fingers except the finger to be examined into passive extension, the flexor superficialis overrides the action of its deep flexor. The flaccidity of the distal phalanx, which is put into hyperextension, verifies this absence of contracture of the profundus flexor.

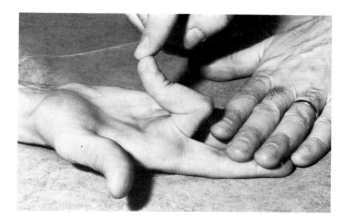

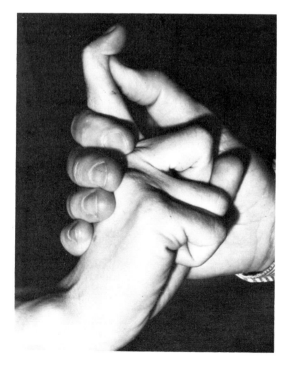

Figure 47–42. The flexor profundus flexes the distal phalanx. If the wrist and the two proximal joints of a finger are put into extension, and the muscle body is kept on tension, contractions of small amplitude can be detected.

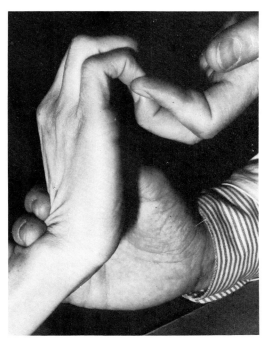

Figure 47–43. The strength of the flexor profundus is evaluated by applying counterpressure to the pulp on the flexed fingers.

EXTENSOR INDICIS PROPRIUS

Nerve supply: Radial nerve (C7).

Action: Extension of the metacarpophalangeal joint of the index finger.

Test of muscle function: With the metacarpophalangeal joints of the long and ring fingers completely flexed to eliminate the action of the extensor communis, the proximal phalanx of the index finger is extended against resistance (Fig. 47–45).

EXTENSOR DIGITI QUINTI PROPRIUS

Nerve supply: Radial nerve (C7).

Action: Extension of the metacarpophalangeal joint of the little finger.

Test of muscle function: With the metacarpophalangeal joints of the long and ring fingers completely flexed, the proximal phalanx of the little finger is extended against resistance (Fig. 47–45).

INTEROSSEOUS MUSCLES

Nerve supply: Ulnar nerve (C8).

Action: The interosseous muscles as a group flex the metacarpophalangeal joints and extend the proximal and distal interphalangeal joints. The dorsal interosseous muscles abduct the index, ring, and little fingers away from the long finger. The palmar interosseous muscles are adductors.

Test of muscle function: The flexion of the metacarpophalangeal joints is tested with the interphalangeal joints in extension (Figs. 47–46, 47–47). Side to side movements of the fingers are partly dependent on the action of the extrinsic muscles. Each finger is tested separately with the metacarpophalangeal joint extended (Figs. 47–48, 47–49).

ABDUCTOR DIGITI MINIMI

Nerve supply: Ulnar nerve (C8).

Action: Abducts the little finger and flexes the metacarpophalangeal joint.

Test of muscle function: Abduction of the little finger against resistance (Fig. 47–50).

Figure 47–44. Evaluation of the extensor digitorum muscle. Passive dorsiflexion of the wrist excludes automatic metacarpophalangeal extension by a tenodesis effect; resistance is applied to the dorsal aspect of the proximal phalanx.

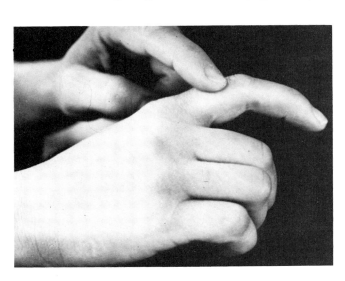

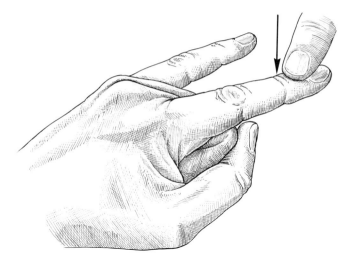

Figure 47–45. Testing the extensor indicis proprius. The metacarpophalangeal joints of the long and ring fingers are flexed to eliminate the action of the extension communis.

Figure 47–46. The interosseous muscles alone are capable of flexing the metacarpophalangeal joints simultaneously with extension of the interphalangeal joints. This is the intrinsic-plus position.

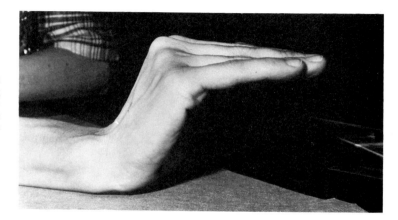

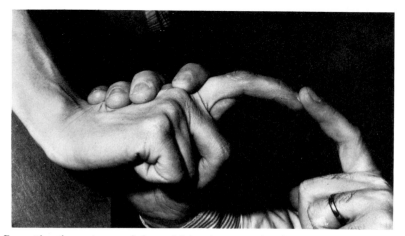

Figure 47–47. By putting the metacarpophalangeal joints into extension first, one can demonstrate a contracture of the interosseous muscles of the corresponding finger, which keeps the interphalangeal joints extended.

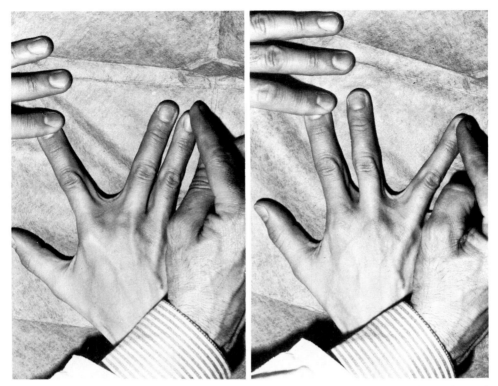

Figure 47–48. The amplitude and precision of voluntary movements of radial deviation of each finger show the quality of innervation of the corresponding interosseous muscles.

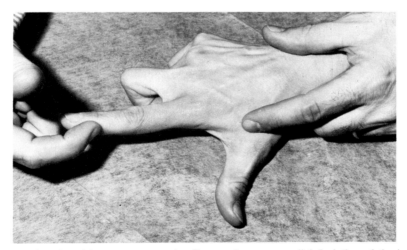

Figure 47–49. The first dorsal interosseous muscle effects active strong radial deviation of the index finger. The muscle belly is palpable; its strength is evaluated by applying counterpressure to the radial side of the finger.

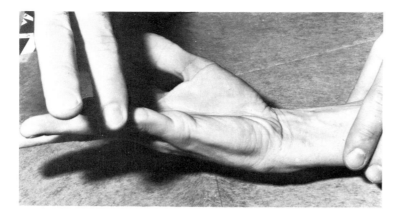

Figure 47–50. The abductor digiti minimi effects strong ulnar deviation of the finger. The contraction of its muscle belly is visible, and its strength can be evaluated by applying counterpressure on the ulnar border of the proximal phalanx.

OPPONENS DIGITI MINIMI

Nerve supply: Ulnar nerve (C8).
Action: Flexion of the fifth metacarpal.
Test of muscle function: Flexion of the fifth metacarpal against resistance (Fig. 47–51).

FLEXOR DIGITI MINIMI

Nerve supply: Ulnar nerve (C8).
Action: Abduction of the little finger.
Test of muscle function: Cannot be tested specifically.

ANALYSIS OF THE MOVEMENTS OF THE THUMB

Flexion. Flexion is produced by the flexor pollicis longus and the flexor pollicis brevis.

Extension. Extension is produced by the extensor pollicis longus and extensor pollicis brevis.

Pronation. Pronation is produced by the abductor pollicis brevis and flexor pollicis brevis.

Supination. Supination is produced by the adductor pollicis and extensor pollicis longus.

ANALYSIS OF THE MOVEMENTS OF THE FIRST METACARPAL

Anteposition. Anteposition is produced by the abductor pollicis brevis and opponens pollicis.

Retroposition. Retroposition is produced by the extensor pollicis longus.

Flexion-Adduction. Flexion-adduction is produced by the adductor pollicis and flexor pollicis brevis.

Extension-Abduction. Extension-abduction is produced by the abductor pollicis longus.

Opposition. Opposition is a combined movement involving all three segments of the thumb column: the first metacarpal moves in anteposition and then in flexion-adduction. This movement is accompanied by an "automatic" longitudinal rotation into pronation. The proximal phalanx flexes, pronates, and radially deviates. The distal phalanx flexes and slightly pronates.

FLEXOR POLLICIS LONGUS

Nerve supply: Median nerve (C8, T1).
Action: Flexion of the interphalangeal joint of the thumb.
Test of muscle function: Flexion of the distal phalanx of the thumb against resistance (Fig. 47–52).

EXTENSOR POLLICIS LONGUS

Nerve supply: Radial nerve (C7).
Action: Extension of the interphalangeal joint and of the metacarpophalangeal joint of the thumb as well as retroposition, adduction, and supination of the thumb column.
Test of muscle function: Retroposition of the thumb column (Fig. 47–53).

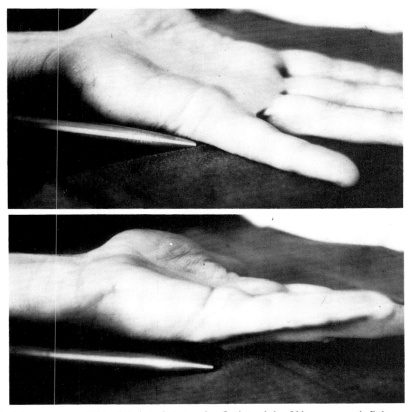

Figure 47–51. The opponens digiti minimi performs active flexion of the fifth metacarpal. Palmar counterpressure on its head can be used to evaluate its strength.

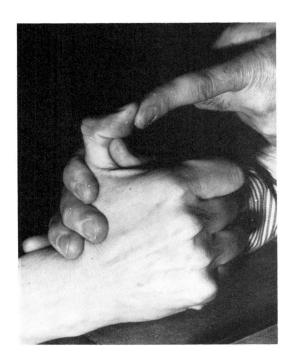

Figure 47–52. Flexion of the interphalangeal joint of the thumb against resistance applied to the pulp makes it possible to evaluate the strength of the flexor pollicis longus.

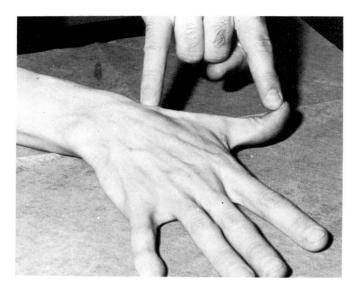

Figure 47–53. Only the extensor pollicis longus is capable of effecting active retropulsion of the column of the thumb and active interphalangeal hyperextension of the thumb.

EXTENSOR POLLICIS BREVIS

Nerve supply: Radial nerve (C7).
Action: Extension of the metacarpophalangeal joint of the thumb.
Test of muscle function: Extension of the proximal phalanx with the distal phalanx semiflexed (Fig. 47–54).

ABDUCTOR POLLICIS LONGUS

Nerve supply: Radial nerve (C7).
Action: Radial abduction of the thumb column. The abductor pollicis longus is a radial abductor of the wrist and is an antagonist of the extensor carpi ulnaris when the wrist is pronated.

Test of muscle function: The patient is asked to move his thumb in radial abduction; the tension of the tendon is felt on the extensor border of the anatomical snuffbox (Fig. 47–55).

ABDUCTOR POLLICIS BREVIS

Nerve supply: Median nerve (C6, C7).
Action: Anteposition of the first metacarpal in the plane perpendicular to the palm as well as lateral deviation and pronation of the proximal phalanx.
Test of muscle function: Anteposition of the thumb against resistance (Fig. 47–56).

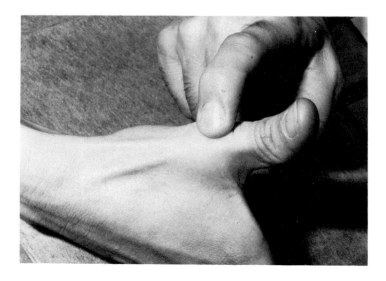

Figure 47–54. Extension of the metacarpophalangeal joint of the thumb simultaneously brings into play the short and long extensors. Evaluation of the short extensor by counterpressure on the dorsal aspect of the proximal phalanx is not as reliable as when the interphalangeal joint is semiflexed.

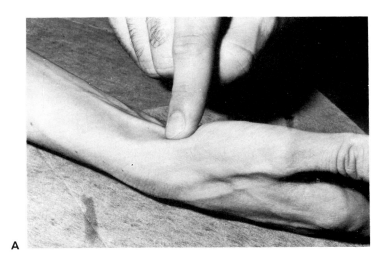

A

Figure 47–55. *A*, Tension in the abductor pollicis longus palpable at the anterior border of the snuffbox is perceptible at the beginning of anteposition, before the abductor pollicis brevis comes into play. *B*, Separation of the thumb in the plane of the palm is effected by the abductor pollicis longus and extensor pollicis brevis.

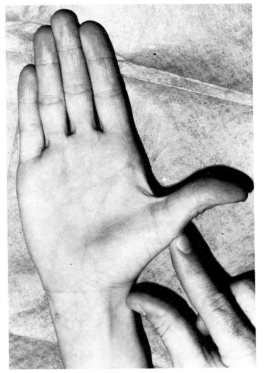

B

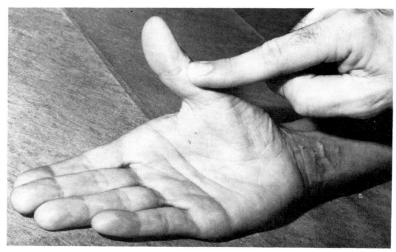

Figure 47–56. The abductor pollicis brevis performs antepulsion of the column of the thumb accompanied by pronation and lateral deviation. Its strength can be evaluated by applying resistance to the radial aspect of the proximal phalanx.

OPPONENS POLLICIS

Nerve supply: Median nerve (C6, C7).
Action: Anteposition of the first metacarpal.
Test of muscle function: Direct palpation of the muscle during anteposition of the thumb against resistance (Fig. 47–57).

FLEXOR POLLICIS BREVIS

Nerve supply: Median nerve (C6, C7) for the superficial portion; ulnar nerve (C8) for the deep portion.
Action: Limited anteposition and flexion-adduction of the first metacarpal and flexion with pronation of the proximal phalanx of the thumb.

Test of muscle function: Difficult to demonstrate unless the other thenar muscles are paralyzed.

ADDUCTOR POLLICIS

Nerve supply: Ulnar nerve (C8).
Action: Approximation of the first to the second metacarpal, flexion-adduction and supination of the thumb column, and extension of the distal phalanx.
Test of muscle function: Approximation of the first and second metacarpals, without flexing the thumb (to eliminate the flexor pollicis longus action) and the wrist extended (to relax the extensor pollicis longus) (Figs. 47–58, 47–59).

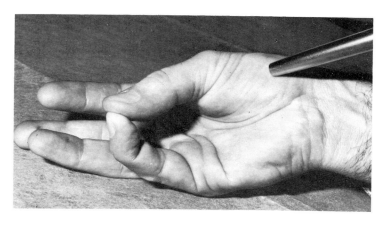

Figure 47–57. The contraction of the muscle belly of the opponens is perceptible in the pulp-to-pulp opposition of the thumb against the little finger.

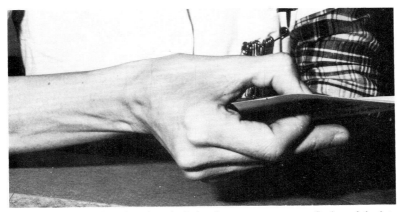

Figure 47–58. When the thumb is forced against the index finger, compensatory flexion of the interphalangeal joint is a sign of weakness of the adductor muscle of the thumb (Froment's sign).

DIFFICULTIES IN TESTING VOLUNTARY MOVEMENTS

Errors of interpretation can have serious consequences. They are due to associated lesions, compensatory movements, and trick movements.

Associated Lesions. Associated traumatic or post-traumatic lesions not involving

nerves, such as tendon divisions, bone and joint injuries, adhesions, and stiffness, can interfere with muscle movements.

Compensatory Movements. One must always remember that no muscle functions in isolation and that the simplest movements require the participation of several muscles (which may well be supplied by different nerve roots). The prime movers, which initi-

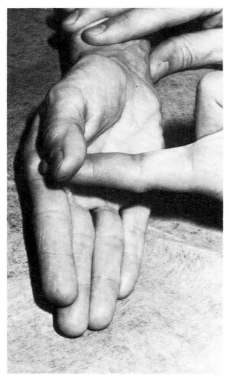

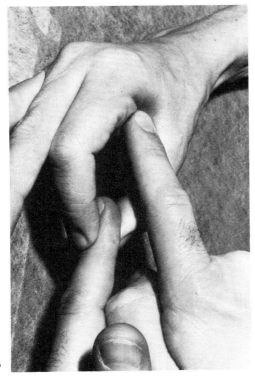

A   B

Figure 47–59. The strength of active closure of the first commissure (*A*) is evaluated by trying to separate the first and second metacarpals, held voluntarily closed. However, the extrinsic muscles of the thumb participate in this adduction. *B*, Participation of the adductor pollicis in closure of the commissure can be verified by direct palpation of the transverse fibers during thumb-index finger pinch.

ate the movement, are assisted by synergists and checked by antagonists and stabilizers. The final movement results from the modulation of these various forces.

The examiner should always take into account possible muscle "compensation." A muscle may have a secondary action, which is usually masked and becomes evident only when the adjacent muscles are paralyzed. Thus, the brachioradialis by itself can flex the elbow when the biceps and brachialis are paralyzed; the extensor digitorum communis can extend the interphalangeal joints if the interosseous muscles are paralyzed, provided the metacarpophalangeal joints are stabilized and hyperextension is prevented (Fig. 47–60). The dorsal expansions of the thenar muscles can extend the distal phalanx of the thumb in paralysis of the extensor pollicis longus, and the abductor pollicis longus can flex the wrist when the flexors are paralyzed.

Deceptive or Trick Movements. Trick movements have a number of causes, one of which is the effect of gravity (Jones, 1919). For example, when one is testing the function of the triceps muscle, the shoulder should be abducted to 90 degrees and internally rotated; thus the muscle can be tested with gravity eliminated. Gravity itself will cause extension of the elbow, even when the triceps is paralyzed, in certain positions of the arm.

Moreover, sudden relaxation of a contracting muscle whose antagonist is paralyzed can stimulate movement in the latter; this is seen in paralysis of the long flexors of the fingers when sudden relaxation of the extensors triggers passive flexion of the metacarpophalangeal joint. In a multiarticular kinetic chain, such as the hand, the extrinsic tendons of the fingers cross several joints. Movements of the proximal joint, e.g., the wrist, can have a tenodesis effect and produce movements of the phalanges. Conversely, in radial palsy, flexion of the fingers can extend the wrist.

The most common sources of error, however, are anomalous innervations and variations in the territories of nerve supply. Such variations are seen most often with the flexor digitorum profundus communis and with the thenar muscles. The territories can be differentiated only by means of selective trunk anesthesia (Highet, 1942). In extensive paralyses, specific peripheral nerve blocks are useful in preoperative evaluation; for example, a peripheral nerve block of the musculocutaneous nerve temporarily eliminates the biceps influence on supination of the forearm. The study of the strength of different varieties of grip (e.g., grasp, thumb-index pinch, lateral and pulp-to-pulp) with a dynamometer is useful to follow the evolution but has no selective value.

TESTING SENSORY FUNCTION

Testing sensation is an essential part of the examination of the hand. The normal cutaneous sensory distribution of the nerve roots and the individual peripheral nerves are

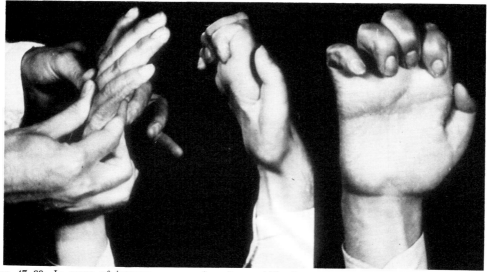

Figure 47–60. In cases of interosseous muscle palsy, stabilization and prevention of hyperextension of the metacarpophalangeal joints allow the extensor digitorum to extend the interphalangeal joints.

shown in Figures 47–61 and 47–62. Sensory skin territories have ill-defined boundaries, and adjacent territories overlap extensively. Thus, sectioning of the radial nerve may produce little to no clinically detectable anesthesia on the dorsum of the hand. The so-called "autonomous" zone of skin supply is much smaller than its potential sensory territory.

The methods of examination of sensibility are discussed in the following chapter. The various techniques in current use can be grouped into three categories: subjective, objective, and functional.

Subjective Tests. Subjective tests requiring full cooperation of the patient test for touch, pain, and temperature (pin prick, cotton wool, von Frey's hairs).

After each examination one should draw on a chart the area of sensory loss. The persistence of complete anesthesia is one of the major signs indicating complete nerve division. By contrast, in the early stages of nerve compression, the area of altered cutaneous sensation may vary from day to day (Dejerine, 1915). During nerve recovery there is a concentric diminution in the area of sensory loss.

Objective Tests. Objective tests requiring no active participation of the patient include the sweat tests, such as the starch and iodine method modernized by Önne (1962), the quinizarine method of Guttmann (1940), and the Ninhydrin test of Moberg (1958). In the wrinkled finger test of O'Riain (1973) the hand is immersed in hot water at 40° C. for 20 to 30 minutes; normal finger pulps wrinkle, whereas denervated pulps remain smooth.

These examination techniques outline the affected territory objectively. However, they give no information about the functional value of the hand as a sensory organ.

Functional Tests (Figs. 47–63 to 47–68). Moberg has carried out extensive studies of the functional sensibility of the hand. He attaches great value to Weber's two point discrimination test for sensibility and added that it appeared to be a good test of proprioception, since most proprioception is from cutaneous afferents rather than from tendons or ligaments. This test, although it requires the patient's cooperation, provides objective data that can be quantified. These measurements are certainly useful, provided the technique is very precise. Because the different areas of the skin of the hand normally present

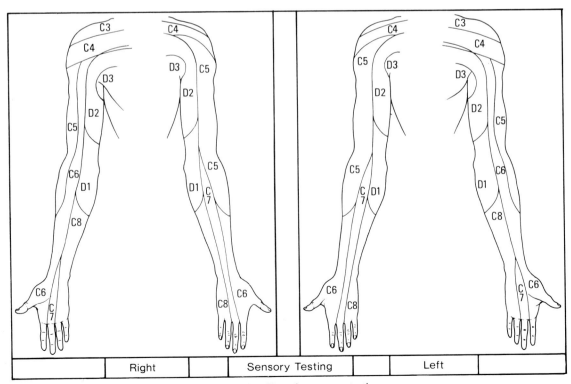

Figure 47–61. Chart for sensory testing.

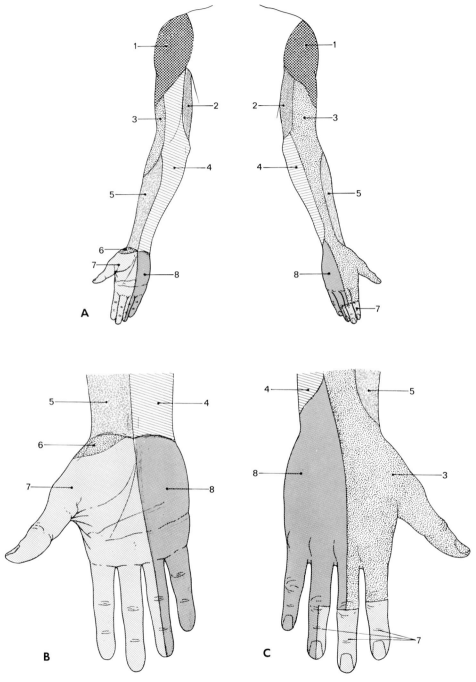

Figure 47–62. *A*, Cutaneous sensory distribution of the peripheral nerves of the upper limb. *B*, Volar aspect of the hand. *C*, Dorsal aspect of the hand. 1, Axillary nerve. 2, Intercostobrachial nerve. 3, Radial nerve. 4, Medial cutaneous nerve of forearm and arm. 5, Lateral cutaneous nerve of forearm (musculocutaneous nerve). 6, Palmar cutaneous branch of radial nerve. 7, Median nerve. 8, Ulnar nerve. There is a considerable variation in the cutaneous areas supplied by each nerve.

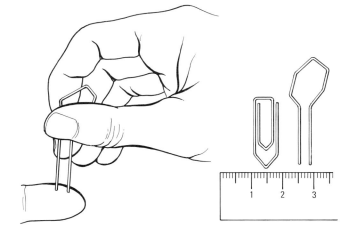

Figure 47–63. Technique of the Weber two point discrimination test. (After Moberg, 1958.)

regional variations in sensibility, it is recommended that the corresponding areas of both hands be compared (Fig. 47–63).

However, a number of reports have indicated that many individuals can acquire good discriminative sensitivity despite the persistence of two point discrimination of more than 20 mm. (Onne, 1962).

A better knowledge of the neurophysiology of cutaneous sensibility explains this fact (see Vol. I). The sensory nerve fibers may terminate free or in a specific structure, such as a Meissner corpuscle, Merkel disk, or Pacinian corpuscle. The sensory endings possess a threshold; that is, there exists a physically definable stimulus of appropriate quality to which they respond with the discharge of a nerve impulse (Mountcastle et al., 1972). The large myelinated fibers (group A-beta fibers)

mediate the perception of touch and are divided into two populations, based on the way in which they respond to a constant touch stimulus (Mountcastle): the quickly adapting fibers (the most numerous) and the slowly adapting fibers. The quickly adapting fibers are further divided into two groups: (1) one responds maximally to a vibratory frequency in the range of 2 to 40 Hz and corresponds to a moving-touch perception, and (2) the other group responds best in the range of 60 to 300 Hz.

The Weber two point discrimination test measures essentially the reinnervation of slowly adapting receptors, whereas the rapidly adapting receptors, essentially the Meissner corpuscles, are the first to be reinnervated (Dellon, 1976; Wynn Parry, 1981).

Dellon (1978) has described a test to eval-

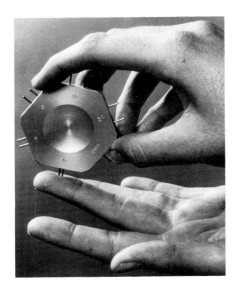

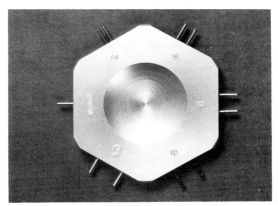

Figure 47–64. The Mannerfelt-Ulrich "sensitometer."

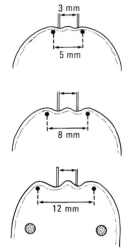

Figure 47–65. Increased pressure on the skin applied by the examiner in testing two point discrimination depresses a larger area of skin and the test will become unreliable. With light pressure, the two point discrimination will be 5 mm., but if the pressure is increased, a 3 mm. distance will be appreciated as if it were a 12 mm. distance.

.uate the mechanical receptors, which are rapidly adapting. The moving two point discrimination test can be considered as a dynamic Weber test. The sensorimeter, the spread of which can be increased from a value of 2 mm., is moved longitudinally on

the surface of the skin along the axis of the digit, with the pressure just sufficient to be perceived by the patient.

The validity of the test has been proved by the capacity to identify those patients who had a 20 mm. two point discrimination according to Weber but a normal Dellon test (3 mm.). It appears that the use of the Weber and Dellon tests allows a better evaluation to the functional sensibility.

Tests of integrated function: It is necessary in addition to add timed functional tests which allow the real evaluation of the practical use of sensation by the patient, e.g., the identification of the shape and texture of objects in a set time. The pick-up test of Moberg (Fig. 47–68), which necessitates the perceptive gnosis of several mobile digits, allows a repeatable numerical evaluation that depicts the area of pinch that is really used and is an excellent dynamic test, giving information on the discrimination and proprioceptive function.

In reality, the evaluation of sensibility in which so many nerve circuits are involved is so complex that it seems necessary to use many different types of examination—a battery of tests—to give a true perception. (See Chapter 51.)

Scales for the assessment of sensibility, more or less similar to the motor scales, are

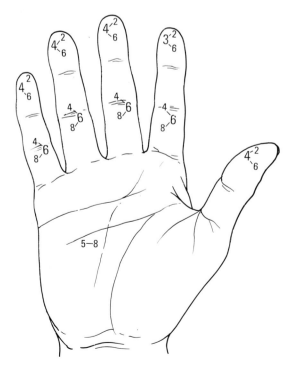

Figure 47–66. Values of discrimination in the Weber test in millimeters in the different zones of the palm. The largest figure indicates the average values and the two others, the minimal and maximal values. (After Moberg, 1958.)

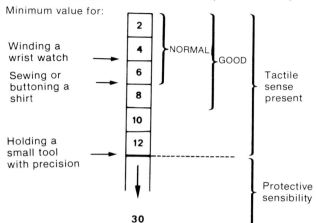

Figure 47–67. Recovery of the capacity for discrimination.

based mainly on the British Medical Research Council scale (Seddon, 1975).

SENSORY RECOVERY

S0—Absence of sensibility in the autonomous area.

S1—Recovery of deep cutaneous pain sensibility within the autonomous area of the nerve.

S2—Return of some degree of superficial cutaneous pain and tactile sensibility within the autonomous area of the nerve.

S3—Return of superficial cutaneous pain and tactile sensibility throughout the autonomous area, with disappearance of any previous overresponse.

S3+—Return of sensibility as in stage 3, with some recovery of two point discrimination within the autonomous area.

S4—Complete recovery.

Moberg believes that this sensibility scale is inadequate. He believes that there should be additional ratings between S3 and S4, and that all lower ratings are useless to the reconstructive surgeon. Moberg estimates that

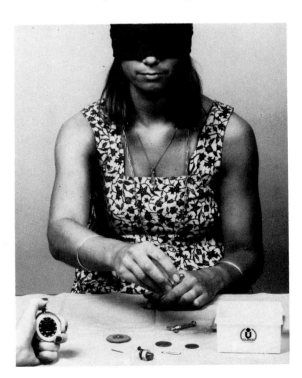

Figure 47–68. The Moberg "pick-up" test.

when pulpar two point discrimination is greater than 10 mm., meaning inadequate cutaneous sensibility, vision is necessary to control manual dexterity. In severe paralysis, particularly tetraplegia, it is indispensable to evaluate both visual (O) and cutaneous (Cu) input.

Pain can interfere with all functional tests, as well as disturbing patient activities. An objective assessment of pain is very difficult, if not impossible.

ASSESSING SYMPATHETIC FUNCTION

It is customary to group arbitrarily under the heading "sympathetic" the various trophic disorders that follow peripheral nerve lesions. Lesions of the sympathetic fibers have a direct action on sweating and circulation. Other so-called "trophic disorders" depend on both sensory and sympathetic fibers.

After sectioning of a peripheral nerve, one often sees changes in the texture of the skin, which becomes dry, loses its elasticity, and develops a thinner epithelium. The nails become striated and brittle; their growth is slowed. The hairs may be longer and bushier, and elsewhere they atrophy and disappear, especially in patients with causalgia. In such patients the skin is often cyanosed, an indication of reduced blood flow. As a rule, the temperature of the skin is lower in the paralyzed zone, and even after reinnervation the part remains sensitive to cold. The consistency of the subcutaneous tissues also changes: The fat pads of the pulps and palm atrophy; this is most evident in the index

finger after median nerve palsy. Atrophy of the skin, changes in blood flow, loss of sensation, and impairment of protective reflexes all increase the risk of injury and predispose to ulceration. These appear readily as a result of repeated minor trauma, pressure, or burns. Healing is slow to occur. The exposed anesthetic zones must be protected by wearing gloves, and the patient should be warned against injuries, which may lead to mutilation.

ELECTRICAL TESTS IN LESIONS OF THE PERIPHERAL NERVES

Electrodiagnostic tests are particularly useful for the detection, localization, and prognosis of lesions of the peripheral nerves. They include electromyography, nerve conduction speed measurements distal to the lesion, and the study of action potentials. (See Chapter 62, Vol. I, by Wynn Parry).

Early electrodiagnosis is of limited interest. The process of wallerian degeneration can be recorded only four to five weeks after nerve division. Apart from helping in the detection of denervation, these tests can record spontaneous changes or changes after a nerve repair. However, it is always necessary to compare the clinical and electromyographic data.

REFERENCES

The references for this chapter will be found at the end of Chapter 50.

Chapter 48

SENSIBILITY EVALUATION

Evelyn J. Mackin

Although sensibility evaluation of the hands has been studied for centuries, it is still by no means completely understood. Much of the literature and widely practiced techniques of sensibility evaluation remain in need of further scientific investigation.

Moberg (1960) has long emphasized that the important factor in sensory function is one of quality and not merely the presence or absence of sensibility. He observes, "Why should the mere perception of touch or pain by the hand be accepted as a sign of normal sensation, when the perception of light is never identified with the normal capacity to see?" We must therefore question whether hand sensibility as it pertains to function can be discussed merely on the basis of known modalities for touch, pain, cold, and warmth. Testing the skin with a safety pin for pain, with cotton wool for touch, and with test tube contact for warmth or cold is inadequate for estimating functional loss. It is often impossible to duplicate these tests periodically and obtain comparable quantitative results (Omer and Spinner, 1975).

The development of microsurgical techniques has increased the need to improve the validity of our clinical methods of sensibility evaluation. We need to know whether one type of surgical repair is better than another. Since sensory and motor function is never completely recovered, it is of the utmost importance that we establish as the point of comparison the patient's condition immediately following the injury rather than his or her normal condition prior to the injury. Moberg (1978) defined the problem by stating that only the pooled results from many centers can provide us with answers, but to be meaningful these data must result from measurements on an identical scale with identical devices.

Consistent with these principles, sensibility testing at the Hand Rehabilitation Center in Philadelphia, Pennsylvania, does not depend upon gross methods such as cotton wool, pin pricks, or any single test. Rather we use several complementary quantitative tests repeated at regular intervals to answer three questions: Is protective sensation present? Is light touch present? And if light touch is present, what is the level of discriminative sensation (Callahan, 1983)? Our battery of tests for the assessment of sensibility may be divided into three groups—the modality test (Semmes-Weinstein monofilaments), functional tests (two-point discrimination, moving two-point discrimination, localization, and the Moberg pick-up test), and nerve conduction studies. We believe that this test battery most closely approximates the Moberg ideal of "quality" by broadening the range of hand function tested.

Modality tests evaluate the perception of the four modalities—warmth, cold, pain, and light touch–deep pressure. Von Frey first described the use of graded stimuli to evaluate cutaneous sensibility in the late 1800's. In an attempt to standardize the technique, he found that horsehairs of varying thicknesses bend at specific milligrams of axial loading pressure. By pressing on the skin with a thorn glued to the end of a hair until the hair started to bow, von Frey obtained a measure of the pressure sensibility of nerve fibers in the skin. He calibrated the hairs on a balance, varying stiffness by changing length and by using hairs of different densities. He recorded pressure sensibility by noting whether a given hair touched to the skin produced any sensation.

In 1960 Semmes and Weinstein and their colleagues made the testing procedure more exact when they reintroduced von Frey's method, using nylon monofilaments mounted in Lucite rods. The monofilaments, known as the Semmes-Weinstein pressure aesthesiometer,* are calibrated to exert specific pressures. Twenty graduated filaments, differing in pressure, are included in the testing kit (Fig. 48–1). The filaments are marked with numbers ranging from 1.65 to 6.65. The filament number represents the logarithm of 10 multiplied by the force in milligrams required to bow the filament. Except for the very largest, all filaments buckle as the examiner presses them against the skin (Fig. 48–2). As long as first-order buckling is maintained, the pressure exerted on the skin varies only with the length and diameter of the calibrated filament, not with the force applied by different examiners. First-order buckling is the bowing produced in a properly applied

Semmes-Weinstein filament, in which the lower end of the mounted filament is "pinned." This position is achieved when the examiner applies only those lateral forces necessary to keep the top end directly over the lower end when the filament is in contact with the skin (Levin et al., 1978).

Hand-held instruments used as a stimulus carry with them the vibration of the examiner's hand and the variable application amplitude of the examiner. Bell and Tomancik (1986) reported that the design of the Semmes-Weinstein filaments provides a relatively more controlled testing stimulus than other hand-held instruments. The design of the filaments provides constant length but increasing diameters that buckle when a specific value is reached. This provides unique control and an objective, reproducible stimulus to use in the testing of peripheral nerve function.

In 1967 von Prince and Butler used the

*Research Designs, Inc., Suite 103, 7320 Ashcroft Street, Houston, Texas 77081.

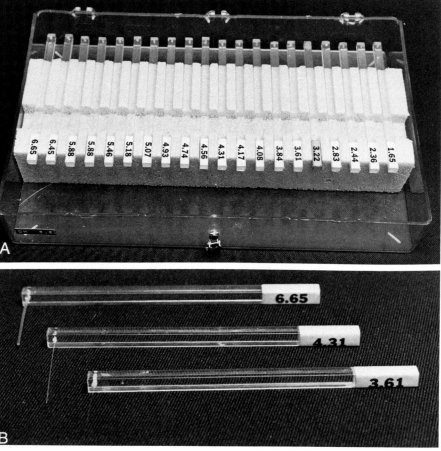

Figure 48–1. *A,* Twenty calibrated filaments, varying in pressure, are included in the testing kit. *B,* Close-up view of filaments.

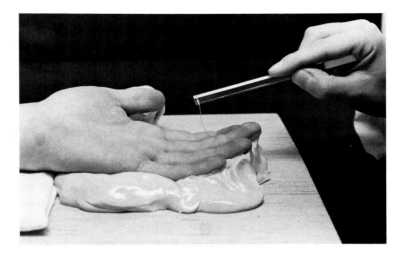

Figure 48–2. First order buckling. The monofilament is applied perpendicular to the hand or digit surface. Pressure is increased until the monofilament bends. The patient's hand is supported in putty because motion misleadingly improves test results.

Semmes-Weinstein monofilaments clinically to test light touch–deep pressure in patients with peripheral nerve injuries from war wounds. They required perception of touch by a given filament and localization of the area of touch for an accurate response. They correlated two-point discrimination and perception of light touch as measured by the monofilaments to develop an interpretive scale that divides the patient's performance into graduated levels of sensibility. These levels are designated as normal, diminished light touch, diminished protective sensation, and loss of protective sensation.

FUNCTIONAL TESTS

TWO-POINT DISCRIMINATION

Light touch two-point discrimination establishes the presence of functional sensation or the fine sensibility required to manipulate small objects. It involves touching the skin with one or two blunt points of an eye caliper or Boley gauge (Fig. 48–3). Both instruments are calibrated in millimeters. The points of an eye caliper must be ground flat to eliminate sharpness. The distance between the points is varied, and the patient is required

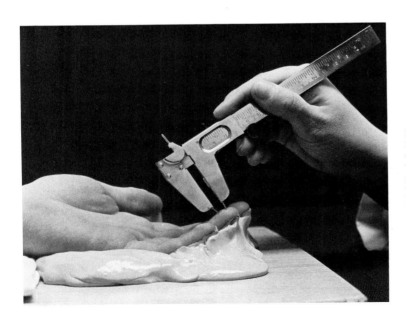

Figure 48–3. Light touch two-point discrimination test to determine whether the patient can discriminate between being touched with one or two points and the minimal distance at which the two points are recognized. The testing instrument is a Boley gauge.

to recognize whether he has been touched with one or two points. The points are applied along a longitudinal axis in the center of the finger tip. Investigators have differed in regard to the proper threshold value for this test. McDougall (1903) placed it at eight correct answers out of 10 for two-point stimuli. Pontin (1960), Mannerfelt (1962), and Moberg (1962) each required seven. Pontin also required that the patient give at least seven correct answers out of 10 for one point stimuli (Onne, 1962). The American Society for Surgery of the Hand recommends seven correct answers out of 10 for two-point discrimination. The value of this test has been variously assessed. Moberg (1960, 1962) stated that there is no better test for evaluating tactile gnosis, although he conceded that the test is not ideal because it requires the patient's cooperation.

Werner and Omer (1970) found in the administration of 4000 tests in 787 patients that the presence of light touch does not necessarily indicate that light touch two-point discrimination is present. Therefore, light touch two-point discrimination is an essential part of the sensibility evaluation for demonstrating the presence of functional sensation.

Moving Two-Point Discrimination

Although the classic Weber (1835) "static sensory" two-point discrimination test does correlate with the hand's ability to perform static grips, critical investigators found that it did not always parallel active hand function (Mannerfelt, 1962; Seddon, 1972). Parry and Salter (1976) observed that active movement is fundamental in hand function and that a "static test" such as two-point discrimination is "irrelevant to function."

The sensation that something is moving across the surface of the fingertips is mediated by the quickly adapting fiber-receptor system. The Weber test evaluates only the slowly adapting fiber-receptor system. In 1978 Dellon introduced the moving two-point discrimination test in which the stimulus is moved along the finger. He further demonstrated that moving two-point discrimination can be evaluated prior to the classic two-point discrimination because both the quickly and slowly adapting fibers are being stimulated. Since the sensation of moving touch is recovered distally sooner than that of constant touch, the moving two-point discrimination

test can give information concerning the results of nerve repair sooner than the static two-point discrimination test (Dellon, 1978).

The test involves moving the Boley gauge along the surface of the fingertips. Dellon recommends orienting the patient to the test as follows. Just one of the two points of the Boley gauge is moved along the fingertips, and the patient is asked what he perceives to have occurred. He is reinforced by being told that only one moving point of the gauge was used. Next, both ends of the gauge, separated by 5 to 8 mm., are moved along the surface of the fingertips. The patient is questioned again and is reinforced as before by being told that both points were used.

Dellon recommends beginning the test with a greater separation of the points of the Boley gauge, 5 to 8 mm., and working down to 2 mm. in order to further orient the patient to the testing procedure. The Boley gauge is randomly alternated between one and two points, and 7 out of 10 patient responses must be correct at any separation of the points before the examiner proceeds to a smaller separation. Testing is stopped at 2 mm., which represents normal two-point discrimination.

LOCALIZATION

Localization has been tested by various investigators using different instruments. Werner and Omer (1970) used the Semmes-Weinstein monofilaments to classify the patient's response according to point localization instead of area localization, as in the von Prince study. Area localization is the ability to recognize the stimulus but not at the exact point, whereas point localization is the identification of the exact point. The patient closes his eyes while the examiner touches the skin with a given filament. If the patient perceives the stimulation, he opens his eyes and identifies the touch point. A $3/8$ inch diameter wooden dowel is used to localize the stimulus. A correct response is one in which the point stimulated must be covered by the wooden dowel or be in contact with a point on the circumference of the dowel. Correct or incorrect responses are recorded in the appropriate area on a worksheet. Werner and Omer recommend that point localization be required in sensibility evaluation of the hand because it reveals more precise sensibility (Omer and Spinner, 1975; Werner and Omer, 1970). Slowness of response and unsure localization are signs of depressed sensibility.

MOBERG PICK-UP TEST

The Moberg pick-up test is a test of function (Fig. 48–4). A box of approximately nine small everyday objects is placed on the table in front of the patient. The objects might include such items as a nut and a bolt, a paper clip, coins, a safety pin, and a screw. The patient is asked to pick up the objects one at a time from the table top and put them into a box, first with his injured hand and then with the uninvolved hand. He does this first with eyes open and then with eyes closed. The examiner times the patient with a stopwatch and observes the manner of prehension.

TEST BATTERY

Sensation is the perception through the senses, or the subjective appreciation of a physical stimulus. Sensibility is the capacity for sensation, that is, the ability to perceive a physical stimulus.

Sensibility testing begins by gathering background information, including an accurate history of the injury, a subjective description of his symptoms by the patient, assessment of trophic changes, joint range-of-motion measurements, muscle evaluation, and quantitative tests of motor function, in-

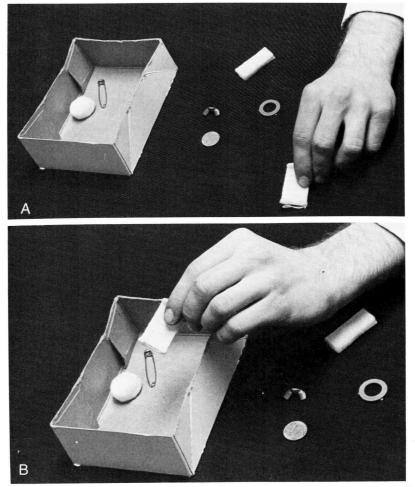

Figure 48–4. *A,* The Moberg pick-up test. *B,* The test assesses the patient's functional aptitude in picking up objects one at a time and placing them in a container, first with the eyes open and then with the eyes closed.

cluding grasp and pinch. After this information has been gathered, the sensibility tests are administered. A detailed evaluation is mandatory if accurate data are to be available for comparison studies. Without such careful evaluation it is impossible to determine whether a patient's recovery following a nerve injury is progressing on schedule or is slower than anticipated.

Testing should be done in a sound-resistant or quiet room with only the therapist and patient present. A quiet, distraction-free environment is of the utmost importance, since nothing (a child crying, people talking, typing) should interfere with the patient's or examiner's concentration. The room temperature should be comfortable and free of excess humidity.

BACKGROUND INFORMATION

History. One records the age, sex, occupation, hand dominance, date of the injury, location of the injury, mechanism of injury, diagnosis, date and type of surgical procedure, and other pertinent information. The date of the injury and the type of surgical procedure are essential data because each defines a predictable time course for recovery. Each characteristically influences recommendations for treatment, sensory re-education, and return to work. Notation of the mechanism of injury aids the examiner in understanding differences in individual recovery. If, for example, the patient sustained a severe crushing injury with massive tissue damage, scarring and pain may affect grip strength and loss of muscle power. In contrast, nerve lacerations with little other tissue damage present a better prognosis (Wilgus, 1982).

Subjective Description of Symptoms by the Patient. One should include the patient's description of his symptoms and of his ability to use his hand: numbness, pins and needles, tingling, pain, burning, improvement noted with rest, and ability to carry out activities of daily living. Activities and hand positions that make the condition worse should be noted. Not all patients are good historians. A patient who states that his hand "feels fine" may show a measurable loss of sensibility. Another patient who says that he "feels nothing" in the median nerve distribution may be amazed at how much he does "feel" after the surgeon uses a local anesthetic to block the ulnar nerve.

Sympathetic Function. The absence of perspiration in an area supplied by a peripheral nerve, most readily demonstrated on the palmar surface, is indicative of a peripheral nerve lesion. Sympathetic nerves travel in company with sensory nerves to the hand. Perspiration ceases instantly when a sensory nerve is severed, causing the skin in the anesthetic area to have a very dry appearance. Although perspiration is an indication of sudomotor activity, there is no relationship between the return of sweat production and the quality of sensibility recovery. The Ninhydrin sweat test developed by Aschan and Moberg (1962) has been used as an objective test in uncooperative patients to obtain information about the function of a nerve. O'Rian in 1973 recorded that the skin of denervated fingers does not wrinkle when exposed to water (104° F) for a prolonged period (30 minutes) as does normal skin. This test is useful in children. A wrinkled fingertip indicates nerve activity.

Trophic changes occur when there is an interruption of the normal nerve supply. Decreased nutrition will be evident in the texture and condition of the skin, finger pulps, nails, and hair, as well as in an increased susceptibility to injury and in slowed healing. Dryness and eventual loss of the normal papillary ridges of the palmar skin are noted after a few weeks of denervation. Early on, the skin is thin and smooth. In long-term cases the skin becomes shiny and inelastic. Nail changes may include striations, ridges, slowed growth, and hardness. In response to the atrophy of the soft tissue of the finger, the nail may conform to the shape of the atrophied pulp. Hair may become longer and finer in the denervated area or may fall out. Atrophy of the epidermis and underlying tissue causes the skin to become more delicate and more susceptible to injury. Burns, blisters, cuts, and bruises on the fingers are often indicative of an insensitive hand. Healing takes longer than in normal skin because of decreased vascularity and nutrition.

Vasomotor changes are noted: temperature, color, and edema. Is the patient's skin warm to the examiner's touch? Does the patient complain of cold intolerance? After complete denervation, and in some incomplete lesions, the skin will feel warm to the touch because of vasodilation secondary to paralysis of the vasoconstrictors. This warm phase, lasting two to three weeks or longer, is gradually superceded by a phase in which the skin feels cool to the touch. The skin appears flushed or rosy during the warm phase and mottled during the cool phase. Assessing color by comparing the injured hand to the uninjured hand is helpful. Edema may occur as the result of circulatory changes. The presence of edema or infection may affect the true validity of the evaluation (Callahan, 1983).

Joint Range of Motion. Active and passive range-of-motion measurements are evaluated with a goniometer (Fig. 48–5). Since active motion of a joint cannot exceed its passive motion, both must be assessed. Limitations in active motion may be caused by adhesions between the tendons, such as flexor digitorum superficialis and flexor digitorum profundus, or between the tendons and the surrounding tissues. Limitations in passive range of motion are indicative of a problem within the joint.

The American Society for Surgery of the Hand recommends that in addition to recording individual joint motion, digital motion be computed as total active motion (TAM) and total passive motion (TPM). TAM equals the total of active flexion measurements of the metacarpophalangeal, proximal interphalangeal, and distal interphalangeal joints of a digit, minus the active extension deficits of the same three joints. TPM is computed in the same manner with passive flexion and extension measurements being used. TAM and TPM can then be expressed as a single numerical value reflecting both the extension and flexion capacities of a single digit.

Muscle Evaluation. A voluntary muscle test will establish the level of function and provide an estimate of the strength of the active muscles. Manual grading of weak muscles and the identification of normal muscles must be accurately recorded. Motor functions are evaluated by observing and testing muscle actions. Trick movements must be detected. Asking a patient to duplicate a movement demonstrated by the therapist avoids confusion. Comparison of the patient's injured hand with his uninjured hand can help detect subtle losses or variations in the patient's innervation patterns.

Grasp and Prehension. Prehension and grasp measurements are checked and compared with those of the uninvolved extremity. The grip of the nondominant hand is generally slightly less than that of the dominant hand. Grip strength is measured on the adjustable Jamar dynamometer (Fig. 48–6). The combined efforts of the intrinsic and extrinsic muscles are evaluated on levels 1, 2, and 3. Primarily extrinsic muscle function is evaluated on levels 4 and 5. The patient's cooperation will be demonstrated during the Jamar dynamometer test. Normal adult grip measurements for the five consecutive handle positions create a bell curve. The first position is the least favorable for strong grip, followed by the fourth and fifth positions. The strongest grip measurement occurs at the second and third handles. Knowledge of this normal grip curve can assist in identifying malingerers.

Pinch can be quantitated on the pinch meter. Pulp as well as key pinch should be evaluated and recorded (Fig. 48–7). Three-way chuck pinch may also be assessed (pulp of thumb to pulp of index and long fingers) as well as grasp measurements; comparisons are made with the opposite hand.

Proprioception. With normal sensation the patient with vision blocked can identify the positional and directional change in a finger

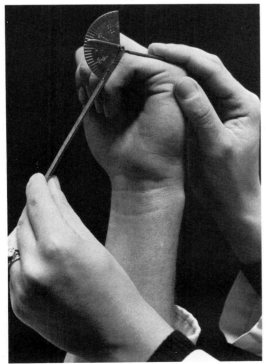

Figure 48–5. Active and passive ranges of motion are measured with a goniometer.

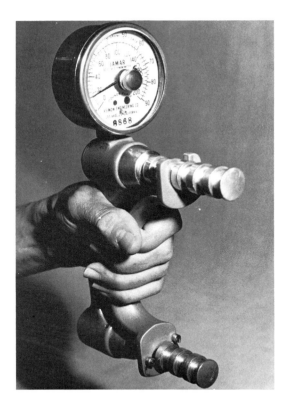

Figure 48–6. Grip strength is measured on the five levels of the adjustable Jamar dynamometer.

when performing passive movements of the interphalangeal joints (Omer, 1981). To test proprioception, the examiner supports the patient's finger laterally and moves it 0.5 to 1.0 cm. in any direction. The patient must identify the angle through which the joint is moved.

THE MODALITY TEST (SEMMES-WEINSTEIN MONOFILAMENTS)

When testing is begun, the area of sensory dysfunction is mapped out. The examiner draws a probe lightly across the patient's hand, beginning with an area of normal sensibility and progressing slowly to an area of suspected abnormal sensibility. A pen or any instrument that is not sharp or too wide may be used. The patient with his vision blocked is asked to indicate immediately when and whether he perceives a change in feeling. The examiner marks the skin with a felt tip pen where the sensory change occurs. The process is repeated until the proximal, distal, and lateral borders of sensory dysfunction have been determined (Fig. 48–8). The examiner then tests for light touch within this area.

Mapping makes the testing quicker and more effective, because follow-up evaluations require only that the area of dysfunction in the initial examination be re-evaluated. The process may be repeated during successive evaluations. It gives the patient and the examiner the opportunity to note whether the area mapped out diminishes in size or remains the same over a period of time. An alternate method is to have the patient himself outline the area of dysfunction in his hand. The results of the mapping can be recorded on an outline of a hand for serial comparison (Callahan, 1983).

Documentation is assessed by the use of a worksheet that has a grid superimposed on an outline of the hand (Fig. 48–9). The grid, devised by von Prince and Butler (1967), is divided into squares or zones. Transverse lines correspond to the flexion creases of the digits and palm. Longitudinal lines are parallel with the rays of the hand. The examiner visualizes the grid on the patient's hand, applies the filament to a given zone in random sequence, and asks the patient to respond. Correct or incorrect responses can be recorded in the appropriate area on the worksheet.

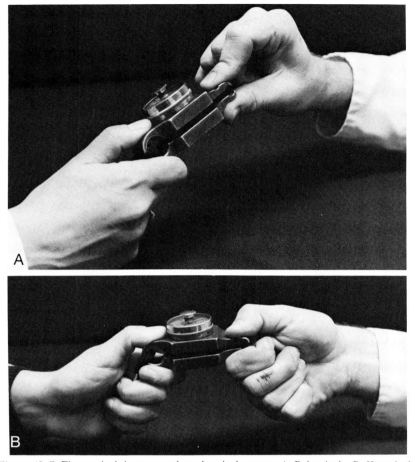

Figure 48–7. Finger pinch is measured on the pinch meter. *A*, Pulp pinch. *B*, Key pinch.

Figure 48–8. The examiner draws a probe across the skin to determine the proximal distal and lateral borders of sensory dysfunction. Vision is blocked by having the patient close his eyes or by the use of a wooden screen.

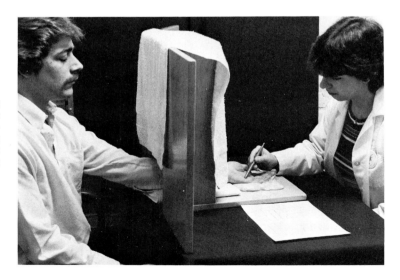

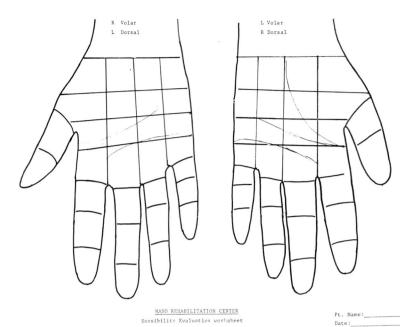

R Volar
L Dorsal

L Volar
R Dorsal

Figure 48–9. Documentation is more accurate with the use of a worksheet that has a grid superimposed on an outline of the hand. The grid is divided into seven palmar zones. The transverse lines correspond to the flexion creases, and the longitudinal lines correspond to the rays of the hand.

HAND REHABILITATION CENTER
Sensibility Evaluation worksheet

Pt. Name:_____
Date:_____

The patient's hand must be fully supported on the table. At the Hand Center we prefer to support the hand in putty (Brand, 1980; Fig. 48–2). Vision is blocked by asking the patient to close his eyes or by the use of a wooden screen (Fig. 48–8). The patient must also be in a position that does not cause discomfort in the arm.

Clinical testing techniques using the Semmes-Weinstein monofilaments have been developed by von Prince and Butler (1967), Werner and Omer (1978, 1981), and Bell (1978, 1983). Testing should begin with the uninvolved extremity. This allows the patient to become familiar with the testing procedure, and the examiner can establish the patient's normal level of sensibility. Higher values may be considered normal when the measurements of the uninvolved extremity are higher than established normal values.

The initial test following a nerve laceration or crush includes both surfaces of the involved hand, with special emphasis on the area of dysfunction as determined by mapping. The examiner visualizes the "grid" on the patient's hand and applies the monofilament at the center of any given zone (Fig. 48–10). Should a more detailed evaluation be needed (e.g., following digital nerve repair), the zones can be subdivided. Some examiners may prefer to mark the responses with a felt pen directly on the patient's hand for easier reference.

The monofilament is applied perpendicular to the skin until the monofilament bends (Fig. 48–2). The top end of the filament must be applied directly over the lower end when the filament is in contact with the skin. Testing is begun with filament 2.83, which tests for normal light touch sensibility. With patients who have severe dysfunction, the examiner may choose to begin testing with a higher numbered filament. Skin that is callused will have a higher sensory threshold than uncallused skin. These areas should be noted and considered in the interpretation of the results.

When monofilaments 1.65 through 4.08 are used, the filament is applied three times in a chosen zone. The filament is applied to the skin for 1 to 1.5 seconds, held in place for 1 to 1.5 seconds, lifted for 1 to 1.5 seconds, and then applied two more times in the same manner. The filament must not slip on the skin when it is being applied, for this will give an additional stimulus clue to the patient. When filaments 4.17 through 6.65 are used, only one stimulation is applied in a chosen zone. With the patient's hand supported in putty and his vision blocked, the examiner touches the skin with a filament. As soon as the patient perceives the pressure of the stimulus, he responds by saying the word "touch." He must respond accurately to the specific filament on two nonsuccessive trials before testing in a zone is considered complete. If the first response is accurate and

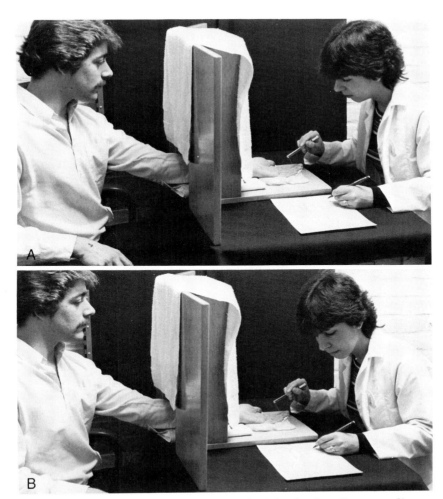

Figure 48–10. The examiner visualizes the "grid" on the patient's hand and applies a monofilament to the center of any given zone. *B,* The response is recorded on a grid superimposed on an outline of the hand.

the second inaccurate, a third trial is used to make a final assessment of that zone. When the responses are inaccurate for two trials with a given filament in a particular zone, the examiner returns to that zone at varying intervals with thicker filaments until a correct response is elicited. If a response is not obtained with the thickest filament marked 6.65 in a particular zone, a pin-prick test is used as a final test of sensibility in that zone.

Callahan (1983) emphasizes the importance of accurate recording of responses, because it is easy to forget where the stimulus has been applied previously and how the patient responded. Careful recording makes the test shorter, more accurate, and more valid in serial comparison tests. It also documents inconsistencies in the responses of a suspected malingerer. She suggests a code for the worksheet as follows: +2.83 (first posi-

tive response to 2.83 monofilament), + +2.83 (second positive response; testing complete in that zone), −2.83 (first negative response to 2.83), − −2.83 (second negative response to 2.83; test at random intervals with thicker filaments until accurate responses are obtained), +3.22 (first positive response to 3.22), and so on. Detailed documentation of this nature requires a worksheet with a life sized outline of the hand to provide space for notations. The examiner may prefer to devise his own code.

The scale of interpretation shown in Table 48–1 enables the examiner to make a meaningful interpretation of the sensibility test results. The norms in the scale, although not standardized, are based on clinical testing of hundreds of nerve-injured hands (Werner and Omer, 1970). The numerical values of the filaments recorded on the worksheet are

Table 48–1. LIGHT TOUCH–DEEP
PRESSURE: SCALE OF INTERPRETATION

Code		Filament
Green	Normal light touch	2.36–2.83
Blue	Diminished light touch	3.22–3.61
Purple	Diminished protective sensation	3.84–4.31
Red	Loss of protective sensation	4.56–6.65
Red lined	Unresponsive to 6.65	

transferred to a color coded outline of a hand
for easy reference and serial comparison
(Bell, 1978, 1983; Fig. 48–11). The colors
correspond to the sensibility levels in the
scale of interpretation. For example, the
color green indicates normal light touch
(2.83) perceived, blue indicates diminished
light touch (3.22–3.61) perceived, purple indicates diminished protective sensation
(3.84–4.31) perceived, and red (4.56–6.65)
indicates loss of protective sensation. A red
lined area indicates that no filament was
perceived.

According to a study conducted by Levin
et al. (1978), an advantage of the Semmes-
Weinstein filaments in measuring threshold
sensitivity is their ease of application. However, correct interpretation of the results requires an understanding of the factors that

can affect those results. According to their
engineering analysis, the principal factors
that can lead to variations in the stress required to buckle or bend a filament are the
method of application by the examiner, variations in the elastic modulus due to elevated
temperatures or high humidity, differences in
the ends of the filaments, and variations in
the attachment of the filaments to the handles. Extreme humidity affects the stiffness
of the lighter Semmes-Weinstein monofilaments and therefore changes the pressure
that they exert on the skin. The filaments
should be stored where they will not be
affected by humidity. With continued use or
mistreatment, the filaments become bent.
These should not be used until they are
straightened. Time seems to correct the bend
(Werner and Omer, 1970). Filaments that
cannot be manually realigned should be replaced.

FUNCTIONAL TESTS

Static Two-point Discrimination. The Weber two-point discrimination test is used to
further quantify the level of sensibility (Bell,

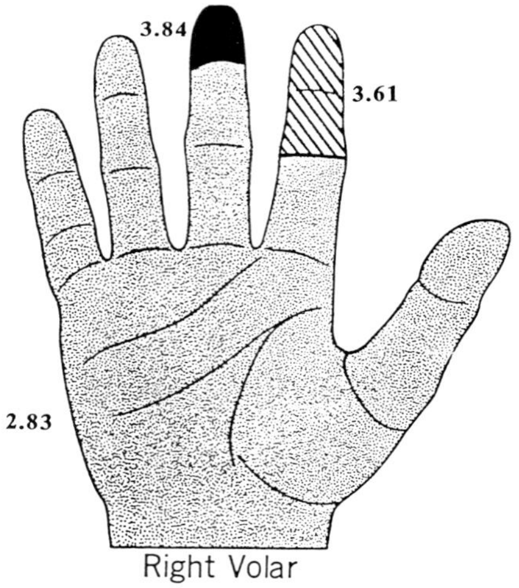

Right Volar

Light Touch-Deep Pressure (Von Frey)

		Filament Log No
	Normal	2.36—2.83
	Diminished light touch	3.22—3.61
	Diminished protective touch	3.84—4.31
	Loss of protective sensation	4.56—6.65
	Unresponsive to 6.65	

Figure 48–11. A coded outline of the hand is an
easy reference for serial comparison.

1983). The test determines the minimal distance at which a patient can discriminate between being touched with one or two points. Moberg (1958) prefers to use an ordinary paper clip with a wire diameter of about 0.9 mm. as the testing instrument. Paper clips are not used by many examiners because the manufacturing process results in a sharp barb on one end of the clip, which stimulates pain receptors. A Boley gauge* (or other caliper with blunt ends) is recommended (Fig. 48–3). In addition the Boley gauge measures the exact distance between the points in millimeters and can be adjusted in 1 mm. increments.

The test procedure should be explained and demonstrated first while the patient observes. His hand should be fully supported on putty (Fig. 48–2) or the examiner's hand. During testing, the patient's vision is blocked with the use of a screen, or the patient is asked either to close his eyes or look in another direction when the stimulus is applied. The gauge is set at a 5 mm. distance between the two points. One point is touched or two points are touched in random sequence along a longitudinal axis in the center of the finger tip. In applying two points, both points should contact the skin simultaneously. The instrument is applied lightly to the point of blanching of the skin (Omer and Spinner, 1975). The patient must respond each time he feels the stimulus. Ten separate stimuli are given. Seven out of 10 responses must be correctly identified. If the patient cannot distinguish seven out of the 10 stimulations correctly, the distance between the two points is increased and the stimulation is repeated until the patient gives the required accurate responses. Testing is stopped at 15 mm. if the response is nondiscriminatory.

The interpretation of scores is based on the American Society for Surgery of the Hand Clinical Assessment Recommendations:

1. Normal—less than 6 mm.
2. Fair—6 to 10 mm.
3. Poor—11 to 15 mm.
4. Protective—one point perceived
5. Anesthetic—no point perceived

Moberg states that 6 mm. of two point discrimination is necessary on both sides of the pinch to wind a watch or to put a 5 mm.

*Research Designs, Inc., Suite 103, 7320 Ashcroft Street, Houston, Texas 77081.

nut on a screw; 6 to 8 mm. for sewing with an ordinary needle or buttoning a small button; and 12 to 15 mm. for handling small precision tools. Above 15 mm. two-point discrimination, gross tool handling may be possible but only with decreased speed and skill. The test values are recorded on a serial test form.

Point Localization. Point localization using the Semmes-Weinstein monofilaments is treated as a separate functional test at our Hand Rehabilitation Center. It is considered to reflect a higher level of perception than simple recognition of a stimulus. Considered to be a test of functional sensation, localization is particularly useful in evaluating the functional capacity of the hand after nerve repair. Poor localization can limit function.

With the patient's hand fully supported on putty and his vision blocked, the examiner applies a filament to the center of a particular zone. The examiner begins with the lowest numbered filament that resulted in a positive response during light touch testing. As soon as the patient perceives the stimulus, he opens his eyes and localizes the touch point by pointing to it (Fig. 48–12). The filament is applied only once to each zone. The speed of the response is related to the level of sensibility. If the patient correctly localizes the stimulus, a dot is marked in the corresponding zone on a worksheet. A worksheet with the grid superimposed on the outline of a hand is again more useful for documentation of the testing results. If the stimulus is incorrectly localized, an arrow is drawn on the worksheet from the point of the stimulation to the point, area, or finger where the touch is referred (Fig. 48–13). This mapping of the patient's responses gives the patient and the examiner a picture of the patient's level of localization. Serial testing should show fewer and shorter arrows (Callahan, 1983).

Moberg Pick-up Test. Tactile gnosis is the fine sensibility of the finger pulps that permits recognition of what is being touched without the aid of sight. Moberg (1978) has stated that a hand without tactile gnosis is "blind" and is useless without the aid of vision. Every evaluation of sensibility in the hand should include a test of tactile gnosis.

The pick-up test introduced by Moberg (1958) assesses general sensibility and tactile gnosis. The advantage of the pick-up test is that it combines sensibility with motion re-

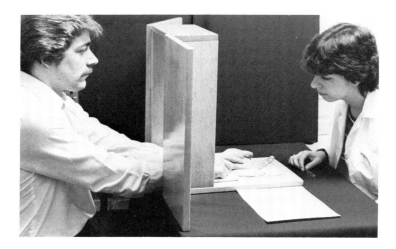

Figure 48–12. The patient localizes the touch point by pointing to it.

quiring active manipulation and recognition of an object. The patient is required to pick up nine objects of different shapes and sizes, one at a time, as quickly as he can and place them in a container (Fig. 48–4). The objects can include such items as a safety pin, a paper clip, a screw, a key, a marble, coins, and a nut and bolt. The test is first done with the involved hand and then with the uninvolved hand. The patient is then asked to close his eyes and the test is repeated. The patient is timed with a stopwatch each time he performs the test. The rapidity and the manner of prehension are recorded, and a comparison is made between the involved and uninvolved hands. When picking up objects with his vision blocked, the patient will not use regions of poor sensibility. If sensibility in the median nerve is impaired, the patient will pick up the object with his thumb and ring and little fingers instead of normally using the thumb and index finger.

The test can be made more difficult by asking the patient to name or describe the objects as he picks them up with his eyes closed (Moberg, 1958). Omer (1981) suggests that on occasion a piece of chalk be used as an object so that the chalk residue remains to show the functional surfaces of the hand.

Periodic tests will indicate the changing status of coordination. Omer (1981) found that the normal time for picking up nine objects is less than 10 seconds. However, the importance of this test is that the examiner can observe the patient's functional aptitude for picking up the objects.

NERVE COMPRESSION LESIONS

Recent studies by Dellon (1981) and Gelberman (1981) indicate that vibration testing is useful in patients with suspected nerve compression because the quickly adapting fibers that mediate vibration are affected early.

Testing is done with the vibrometer. At the Hand Rehabilitation Center we use the Biothesiometer, an amplitude-variable fixed

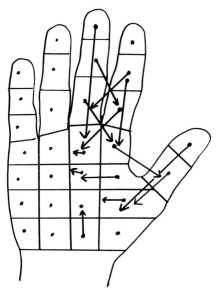

Figure 48–13. Arrows drawn from the point of stimulation to the point where the touch is referred give the examiner and the patient a picture of the patient's level of localization.

frequency (120 cps) instrument. The end of the vibrometer is held in contact with the volar pad of the index and little fingertips while the stimulus intensity is gradually increased. The threshold is read as the voltage required to deliver the perceived stimulus. By measuring the threshold of vibration perception in volts, the Vibrometer allows a more objective test than would a tuning fork.

NERVE CONDUCTION STUDIES

Nerve conduction/velocity testing measures the speed at which impulses travel over the course of a peripheral nerve. Helpful in determining the state of regeneration and documenting advances in the regenerating nerve, it is an important tool to complete the clinical evaluation.

STRESS TESTING

Nerve compression syndromes often occur as a result of repetitive trauma to the hands. Objective documentation can sometimes be difficult or elusive, particularly if the symptoms are subacute or intermittent at the time of testing, or both, and the onset of such symptoms is positional or activity induced. An extensive sensory/motor examination is essential for appropriate documentation. The complexity of this problem is such that the battery of tests employed should be performed under resting conditions and following provocative or stressful activities. This latter element allows for documentation of marginal early developing or intermittent compartment syndromes based on position or activity.

ASSH NERVE FUNCTION EVALUATION

The American Society for Surgery of the Hand Clinical Assessment Committee (1984) reviewed the merits of the various clinical tests for evaluating nerve function and recommended that four areas of evaluation be considered essential when following the progress of patients in cases of peripheral nerve injury and repair: (1) sensibility testing, (2) motor testing, (3) subjective evaluation, and (4) sudomotor function.

Basic sensory testing should include tests of stationary three-point discrimination and moving two-point discrimination. In addition, it is strongly suggested that the von Frey filaments (Semmes-Weinstein) be used, as well as a timed performance test (three coins: 5¢, 10¢, and 25¢).

Basic motor testing should include use of the Jamar grip tester (all five positions) and the pinch meter (key pinch and three-jaw pinch).

The physician's record of the patient's subjective evaluation of his own status (e.g., pain, dysesthesias, cold intolerance, functional limitations) and a statement relative to sudomotor function should also be included in the evaluation.

SUMMARY

No single method of sensibility evaluation may be appropriate for every patient or the choice of every examiner. Different clinicians use different tests. However, the complexity of sensibility is such that no single test or category of tests in clinical use today can provide the full picture of sensibility. Therefore the most complete picture will result from a carefully chosen battery of tests selected to answer three questions: Is protective sensation present? Is light touch present? And if light touch is present, what is the level of discriminative sensation? With this in mind, the battery of tests used at the Hand Rehabilitation Center in Philadelphia, Pennsylvania, includes the Semmes-Weinstein pressure aesthesiometer, two-point discrimination, (status as well as moving) point localization, the Moberg pick-up test, and nerve conduction studies. We have found that this battery of tests provides the desired information in the majority of patients referred for sensibility evaluation.

Isolated tests of nerve loss and recovery are of little value. Postoperative results must be compared with the preoperative status to indicate whether and how much improvement has been obtained. An appropriate battery of tests should be repeated at intervals of approximately 12 weeks to chart the changing status of the injured nerve (Fig. 48–14). Since they are quantitative tests, they have meaning for other examiners and the patient.

Cutaneous sensibility has been studied since the time of Aristotle (350 B.C.). Von Frey's classic study in 1895 merits him special

Text continued on page 508

HAND REHABILITATION CENTER
901 Walnut Street
Philadelphia, PA 19107

SENSIBILITY EVALUATION SUMMARY
(Nerve Laceration Study)

Name _____   Eval # _____

Chart # _____   Date _____

Dominance _____   Ex _____

History

Patient Subjective Description

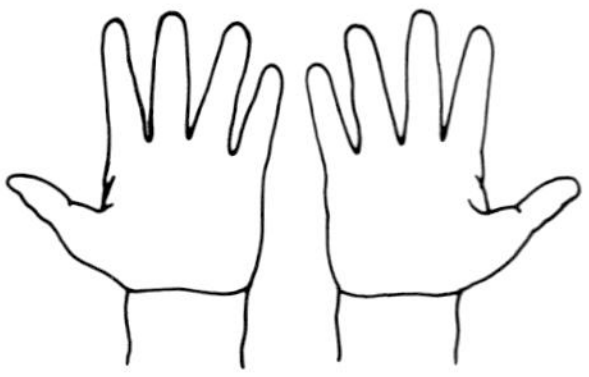

Anesthesia
Hypesthesia
Paresthesia

Muscle Function   Sympathetic Function

Grip (lbs.)   (Jamar# ____)   Pinch (lbs.)
        R   L
1.   ____   ____   Lateral R) ____ L) ____
2.   ____   ____   Pulp   R) ____ L) ____
3.   ____   ____   3 Point R) ____ L) ____
4.   ____   ____
5.   ____   ____

A

Figure 48–14. A detailed and careful documentation is required if accurate evaluation is to be available for comparison studies.

HAND REHABILITATION CENTER
(Nerve Laceration Study)

Chart # _____

TACTILE GNOSIS: Moberg Pick-up Test   Comments
            #Objects _____
                R   L
Eyes Open   __sec.   __sec.
Eyes Closed __sec.   __sec.

_____

Static 2PD *(Normal: 5 mm)   Moving 2PD (Normal: 2 mm)
      I II III IV V   I II III IV V
R)   /   R)
L)   /   L)

_____

Light Touch-Deep Pressure**   Localization
                                    (Stimulus: _____)

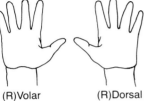
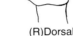

(R)Volar   (R)Dorsal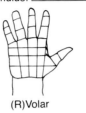

                                    (R)Volar

_____

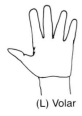

(L) Volar

_____

	**Light Touch–Deep Pressure Scale		*AASH 2 PD
Green	—Normal	1.65–2.83	2 mm– 6 mm Normal
Blue	—Diminished Light touch	3.22–3.61	6 mm–10 mm Fair
Purple	—Diminished protective sens.	3.84–4.31	11 mm–15 mm Poor
Red	—Loss of protective sens.	4.56–6.65	1 Point only Protective
Red Lined	—Unresponsive to 6.65		No Points Anesthetic

B

Figure 48–14 *Continued*

Illustration continued on following page

HAND REHABILITATION CENTER
901 Walnut Street
Philadelphia, PA 19107

SENSIBILITY EVALUATION SUMMARY
(Nerve Compression Study)

Name _____   Eval # _____

Chart # _____   Date _____

Dominance _____   Ex _____

History:

Patient Subjective Description

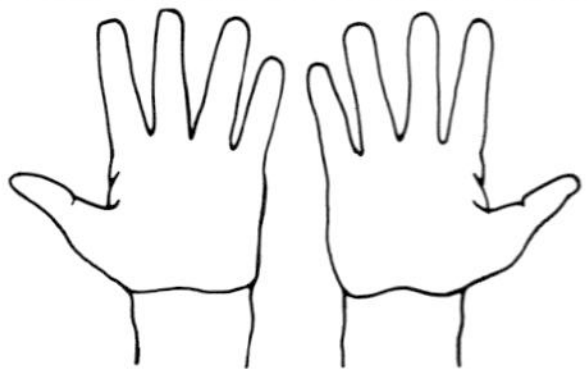

Anesthesia
Hypesthesia
Paresthesia

	R	L			R	L
Tinel's	___	___	day		___	___
Phalen's	___	___	Paresthesia			
EMG	___	___	night		___	___
M-NC	___	___	Pain		___	___
S-NC	___	___	Weakness		___	___
S-NC Stress	___	___	Stress Activities		___	___
					___	___
					___	___

Muscle Function

Grip (lbs)	(Jamar#)		Pinch (lbs)
	R	L	
1	___	___	Lateral R) ___ L) ___
2	___	___	Pulp R) ___ L) ___
3	___	___	3 Point R) ___ L) ___
4	___	___	
5	___	___	

C

Figure 48–14 *Continued*

HAND REHABILITATION CENTER
(Nerve Compression Study)

Chart # _____

TACTILE GNOSIS: Moberg Pick-up Test

	# Objects _____

VIBRATION (Vibrometer)

	II (P$_3$)	V(P$_3$)

	R	L
Eyes Open	sec.	sec.
Eyes Closed	sec.	sec.

R) _____ Volts _____ Volts

L) _____ Volts _____ Volts

Comments:

Static 2PD *(Normal: 5 mm)
    I II III IV V
R)   /
L)   /

Moving 2PD (Normal: 2 mm)
    I II III IV V
R)
L)

Light Touch—Deep Pressure**   stress: _____   stress: _____

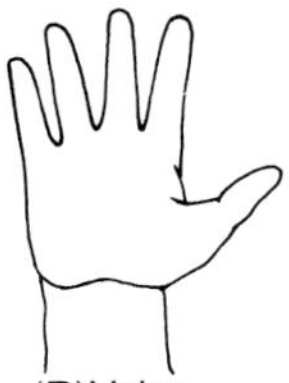

(R)Volar 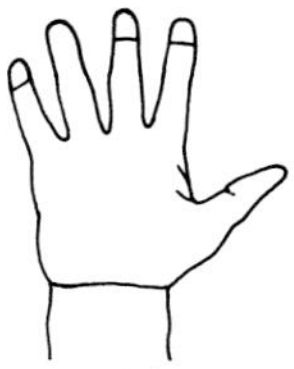   (R)Volar 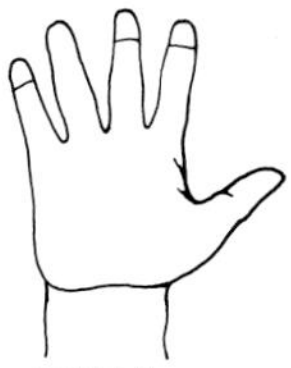   (R)Volar

rest

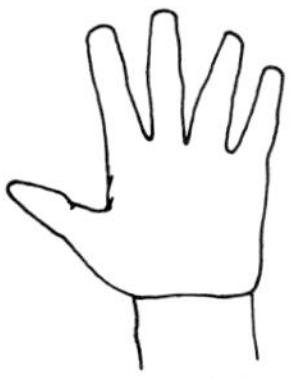

(L) Volar

	**Light Touch-Deep Pressure Scale	
Green	—Normal	1.65–2.83
Blue	—Diminished light touch	3.22–3.61
Purple	—Diminished protective sens.	3.84–4.31
Red	—Loss of protective sens.	4.56–6.65
Red Lined	—Unresponsive to 6.65	

*ASSH   2 PD

2 mm– 6 mm	Normal
6 mm–10 mm	Fair
11 mm–15 mm	Poor
1 Point only	Protective
No Points	Anesthetic

D

Figure 48–14 *Continued*

praise. In the process of learning, new techniques and new ideas have emerged through the clinical studies of Moberg, von Prince, Werner, Omer, Dellon, and Bell. Much is yet to be learned, as indicated by the differing opinions and testing techniques. Critical scientific investigations by these examiners and others have provided us with the basis from which to draw upon and further develop our methods of assessing the quality of sensibility remaining in the hand following a nerve injury.

REFERENCES

American Society for Surgery of the Hand: A report of the Clinical Assessment Committee. Am. Soc. Surg. Hand News, Suppl. B, *3,* January 1984.

Aschan, W., and Moberg, E.: The Ninhydrin finger printing test used to map out partial lesions to hand nerves. Acta Chir. Scand., *123:*365, 1962.

Bell, J.: Sensibility evaluation. *In* Hunter, J. M., Schneider, L. H., Mackin, E. J., and Bell, J. (Editors): Rehabilitation of the Hand. St. Louis, The C. V. Mosby Company, 1978.

Bell, J.: Light touch-deep pressure testing using Semmes-Weinstein monofilaments. *In* Hunter, J. M., Schneider, L. H., Mackin, E. J., and Callahan, A. D. (Editors): Rehabilitation of the Hand. Ed. 2. St. Louis, The C. V. Mosby Company, 1983.

Bell, J. A.: Sensibility testing: state of the art. In Hunter, J. M., Schneider, L. H., Mackin, E. J., and Callahan, A. D. (Editors): Rehabilitation of the Hand, Ed. 2. St. Louis, The C.V. Mosby Company, 1983.

Bell, J., and Tomancik, L.: Repeatability of the Semmes-Weinstein Monofilament. Presented at the ninth annual meeting of the American Society of Hand Therapists, New Orleans, 1986.

Brand, P. W.: Functional manifestations of sensory loss. Presented at Symposium on Assessment of Levels of Cutaneous Sensibility, USPHS Hospital, Carville, Louisiana, September 1980.

Callahan, A.: Sensibility testing: clinical methods. *In* Hunter, J. M., Schneider, L. H., Mackin, E. J., and Callahan, A. D. (Editors): Rehabilitation of the Hand. Ed. 2. St. Louis, The C. V. Mosby Company, 1983.

Dellon, A. L.: Moving two-point discrimination test. *In* Evaluation of Sensibility and Re-education of Sensation in the Hand. Baltimore, The Williams & Wilkins Company, 1981, Ch. 8, pp. 124–125.

Levin, S., Pearsall, G., and Ruderman, R.: Von Frey's method of measuring pressure sensibility in the hand: an engineering analysis of the Weinstein-Semmes pressure aesthesiometer. J. Hand Surg., *3:*211–216, 1978.

Mannerfelt, L.: Evaluation of functional sensation of skin grafts in the hand area. Br. J. Plast. Surg., *15:*136–154, 1962.

Moberg, E.: Objective methods for determining the functional value of sensibility in the hand. J. Bone Joint Surg., *40B:*454–476, 1958.

Moberg, E.: Evaluation of sensibility of the hand. Surg. Clin. N. Am., *40:*375, 1960.

Moberg, E.: Criticism and study of methods for examining sensibility of the hands. Neurology, *12:*8–9, 1962.

Moberg, E.: Sensibility in reconstructive limb surgery. *In* Fredericks, S., and Brody, G. S. (Editors): Neurophysiology and Sensation. Symposium on the Neurologic Aspects of Plastic Surgery. St. Louis, The C. V. Mosby Company, 1978, Vol. 17, Ch. 4, pp. 30–35.

Omer, G.: Physical diagnosis of peripheral nerve injuries. Orthop. Clin. N. Am., *12:*207–228, 1981.

Omer, G. E., and Spinner, M.: Peripheral Nerve Testing and Suture Techniques. A.A.O.S. Instructional Course. St. Louis, The C. V. Mosby Company, 1975, Vol. 24, pp. 122–143.

Onne, L.: Recovery of sensibility and sudomotor activity in the hand after nerve suture. Acta Chir. Scand. (Suppl. 300), 1962.

O'Rian, S.: New and simple test of nerve function in the hand. Br. Med. J., *22:*615, 1973.

Parry, C. B. W., and Salter, M.: Sensory re-education after median nerve lesion. Hand, *8:*250–257, 1976.

Seddon, H. G.: Surgical disorders of the peripheral nerves. Baltimore, Williams & Wilkins, 1972, p. 43.

Semmes, J., Weinstein, S., Ghent, L., and Teaber, H. L.: Somatosensory Changes After Penetrating Brain Wounds in Man. Cambridge, Harvard University Press, 1960.

Von Frey, M., and Kiesow, F.: Ueber die Function der Tastorperchen. Ztschr. Psychol. Physiol. Sinnesory. Leipz., *20:*126–163, 1899.

Von Prince, K., and Butler, B.: Measuring sensory function of the hand in peripheral nerve injuries. Am. J. Occup. Ther., *21:*385–396, 1967.

Weber, E. H.: Veber den Tastinn. Arch. Anat. Physiol. Wissensch. Med., 152–160, 1835.

Werner, J. L., and Omer, G. E.: Evaluating cutaneous pressure sensitivity of the hand. Am. J. Occup. Ther., *24:*5, 1970.

Wilgus, E. F., and Wilgus, E. F. S.: Techniques for diagnosis of peripheral nerve loss. Clin. Orthop., *163:*8–14, 1982.

Chapter 49

PARALYSIS OF THE PERIPHERAL NERVES

RAOUL TUBIANA

Here we consider the course, relations, and distribution of the main nerves of the upper limb. The topographic anatomy of these nerves, dealt with in Volume I, is completed here by a short description of their endoneural anatomy. Since the classic studies of Sunderland (1972), this work has been continued and completed by Bonnel et al. (1978, 1980) and by Jabaley (1980). It is well known by surgeons using an operating microscope. The clinical features of nerve paralyses of the upper limb are dealt with in detail in Volume IV, where several chapters are devoted to the reconstructive treatment of nerve lesions and nerve compression syndromes.

AXILLARY NERVE PALSY

The axillary or circumflex nerve (C5 and C6) is the lateral terminal branch of the posterior cord. It runs alongside the posterior circumflex artery at the lower border of subscapularis. Together they form a neurovascular pedicle that winds around the surgical neck of the humerus from medial to lateral and from anterior to posterior, under cover of the deltoid muscle (Fig. 49–1).

The fascicular pattern of the axillary nerve is variable. Sunderland (1968) found that the fascicles ranged in number from one to 15. In the axilla there is usually a single large motor nerve fascicle accompanied by fine satellites.

The axillary nerve supplies the teres minor and the deltoid (Coene, 1985). Paralysis of the nerve leads to loss of abduction of the arm. Its sensory fibers supply the skin on the posterolateral aspect of the shoulder.

The axillary nerve can be injured in dislo-

cation of the glenohumeral joint, by fractures of the surgical neck, or when compressed in the axilla, e.g., by crutches. It is at risk during surgical operations when the shoulder joint is approached from the posterior or lateral aspect.

RADIAL NERVE PALSY

The radial nerve continues the posterior cord (C5, C6, C7, C8, and T1). Lying at first behind the axillary artery, it runs distally in the arm by winding around the posterior aspect of the humerus from medial to lateral (Fig. 49–2). It continues in the lateral bicipital groove. As it reaches the humeroradial joint line, the radial nerve divides into two terminal branches (Fig. 49–3), the *anterior sensory* branch, which runs down the forearm under the brachioradialis, lateral to the radial artery, and a *posterior motor* branch, the posterior interosseous nerve, which penetrates the supinator muscle by passing under the arcade of Frohse (1908) (Fig. 49–4). This is fibrous in about one-third of cases and may cause compression. The nerve winds around the neck of the radius between the two heads of the supinator. In 25 per cent of all cases it lies flush against the periosteum for about 3 cm. (bare area) when the forearm is supinated, and it is more vulnerable at this level (Spinner, 1978). The nerve then emerges from the supinator in the posterior compartment of the forearm. After giving off branches to all the muscles in this compartment, it runs along the posterior aspect of the interosseous membrane and sends sensory branches to the wrist and carpometacarpal joints.

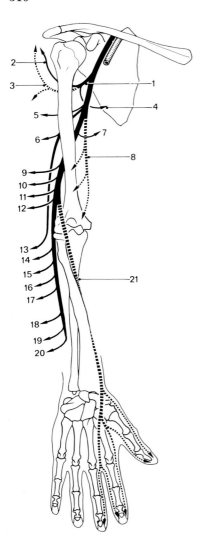

Figure 49–1. The radial and axillary nerves; muscles supplied and cutaneous distribution. The forearm is pronated. 1, Axillary nerve. 2, Deltoid. 3, Cutaneous branch to shoulder. 4, Teres minor. 5, Triceps (long). 6, Triceps (lateral). 7, Triceps (medial). 8, Medial cutaneous branch. 9, Brachioradialis. 10, Extensor carpi radialis longus. 11, Extensor carpi radialis brevis. 12, Supinator. 13, Anconeus. 14, Extensor digitorum communis. 15, Extensor digitorum to fifth digit. 16, Extensor carpi ulnaris. 17, Abductor pollicis longus. 18, Extensor pollicis brevis. 19, Extensor pollicis longus. 20, Extensor indicis proprius. 21, Anterior sensory branch. The sensory branches are shown as dotted lines.

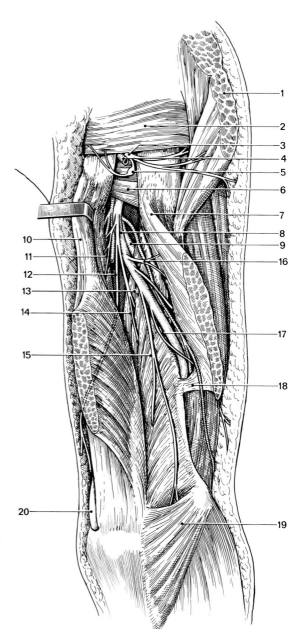

Figure 49–2. Dissection of the posterior arm to show the axillary and radial nerves (right arm). 1, Deltoid muscle (posterior part reflected anteriorly). 2, Teres minor. 3, Axillary nerve emerging with posterior humeral circumflex artery (4) through the quadrilateral space. 5, Branch to teres minor, showing a ganglion. 6, Teres major. 7, Lateral head of triceps. 8, Radial nerve with the profunda brachii artery (9). 10, Long head of triceps. 11, Nerve to long head triceps. 12, Medial cutaneous nerve of arm. 13, Short head of triceps. 14, Superior nerve to short head of triceps. 15, Inferior nerve to short head of triceps and anconeus. 16, Superior nerve to lateral head of triceps. 17, Inferior nerve to lateral head of triceps. 18, Lateral intermuscular septum. 19, Anconeus. 20, Ulnar nerve.

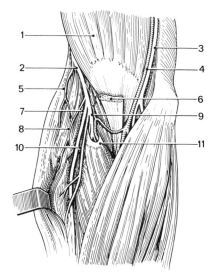
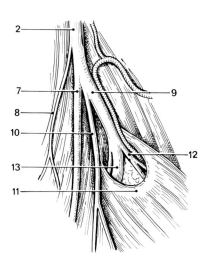

Figure 49–3. The radial nerve at the level of the elbow. 1, Brachialis. 2, Radial nerve. 3, Median nerve. 4, Brachial artery. 5, Branch to brachioradialis. 6, Cut end of biceps tendon. 7, Anterior branch of radial nerve. 8, Branch to extensor carpi radialis longus. 9, Posterior motor branch of radial nerve. 10, Branch to extensor carpi radialis brevis. 11, Arcade of Frohse. 12, Branches to supinator. 13, Posterior interosseous nerve.

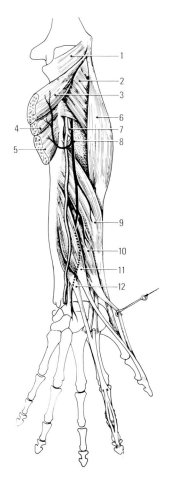

Figure 49–4. The posterior compartments of the forearm showing the posterior interosseous nerve and its branches (deep planes only). 1, Anconeus. 2, Supinator. 3, Extensor digitorum. 4, Extensor digiti minimi. 5, Extensor carpi ulnaris. 6, Brachioradialis. 7, Posterior interosseous artery. 8, Motor branch of radial nerve (posterior interosseous). 9, Abductor pollicis longus. 10, Extensor pollicis brevis. 11, Extensor pollicis longus. 12, Extensor indicis.

The radial nerve supplies all the extensors of the elbow, the wrist, and the fingers. The two distal phalanges of the fingers can also be extended by the interosseous muscles.

By contrast, its sensory territory is relatively limited (the lateral half of the dorsum of the hand), and the autonomous zone is restricted to the dorsal aspect of the first interosseous space, so that sensory nerve palsy is functionally insignificant. However, sectioning of the small sensory branches of the radial nerve at the wrist can give rise to painful neuromas.

In the arm the anterior (superficial) and posterior (interosseous) divisions of the radial nerve can be traced as fascicles for 7.2 to 9 cm. above their point of division (Color Plate III). The single fascicle of the posterior interosseous nerve branches 35 mm. distal to its origin, giving off a division for the supinator.

On the motor side, radial nerve palsy results in:

1. Paralysis of the triceps. This rarely results from radial nerve injury, because the fibers supplying this muscle arise high in the axilla.

2. Paralysis of the supinator. This is partially compensated by the biceps and by shoulder movements.

3. Loss of three movements essential to hand function, which, unlike the paralysis of the triceps and supinator, cannot be compensated for: extension of the wrist (all three wrist extensors are supplied by the radial nerve); extension and retroposition of the thumb, which are brought about by the extensor pollicis longus, abductor pollicis longus, and extensor pollicis brevis; and extension of the proximal phalanges of the fingers.

The close anatomical relationship of the radial nerve with the humeral shaft accounts for the high incidence of radial nerve injuries associated with fractures of the humerus. As the radial nerve crosses the spiral groove on the posterior aspect of the humerus, it is not in contact with the bone. They are kept apart by thin sheets of muscle. They come into direct contact only at the lateral supracondylar border of the bone. At this level the nerve crosses the inextensible fascia to enter the lateral bicipital groove. It is somewhat stretched at this point, and lack of mobility accounts for its vulnerability in humeral fractures (Holstein and Lewis, 1963).

Primary radial nerve palsies are commonly associated with fractures of the middle and distal thirds of the humeral shaft. These fractures are usually characterized by lateral angulation and overriding of the distal fragment. Seddon (1947) demonstrated that actual division of the nerve was rare and emphasized that emergency treatment should be directed at proper closed management of the fracture, with frequent evaluation of the status of the nerve injury before any operative intervention is undertaken.

This conservative approach is now being reconsidered. Vichard (1982) found that in more than 25 per cent of his cases of radial nerve palsy associated with a humeral fracture, there was either complete disruption or significant entrapment of the nerve. The advantage of early operative intervention in these cases is obvious. It is possible that this increase in the severity of the radial nerve lesions is a result of the frequent association today of severe multisystem trauma with this injury. Iatrogenic radial nerve palsy is a separate problem. It results from the technique of closed reduction or surgical exposure and is unrelated to the type of fracture.

PARALYSIS OF THE MUSCULOCUTANEOUS NERVE

The musculocutaneous nerve arises from the lateral cord of the brachial plexus, lateral to the axillary artery. It enters the arm by piercing the coracobrachialis from medial to lateral and runs between the biceps anteriorly and the brachialis posteriorly to the lateral bicipital groove of the cubital fossa (Fig. 49–5). It then becomes superficial on the lateral side of the biceps tendon and the medial cephalic vein and, as the lateral cutaneous nerve of the forearm, divides into its two terminal branches, an anterior branch for the anterolateral aspect of the forearm and a posterior branch that supplies the posterolateral aspect of the skin.

The collateral motor branches supply the coracobrachialis, biceps, and brachialis. Lesions of these branches result in considerable impairment of elbow flexion. Loss of the adductor action of the coracobrachialis can be compensated for by the pectoralis major.

Fascicular Anatomy

In the segment of the nerve traversing the coracobrachialis muscle, the fascicular bun-

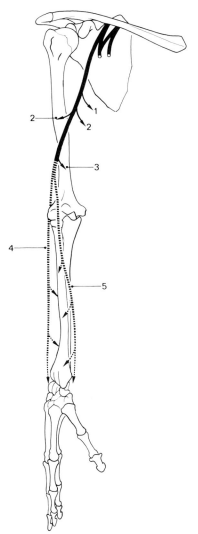

Figure 49–5. The musculocutaneous nerve; muscles supplied and cutaneous distribution. 1, Coracobrachial branch. 2, Biceps brachii. 3, Anterior brachial branch. 4, Posterior branch (sensory). 5, Anterior branch (sensory). The sensory branches are shown as dotted lines.

dles form a complex plexus, so that they are impossible to dissect. The terminal branch, the lateral cutaneous nerve of the forearm, has a similar pattern.

MEDIAN NERVE PALSY

The median nerve arises from two roots, one from the lateral cord of the plexus (C6 and C7) and the other from the medial cord (C8 and T1). The two roots arch around the

axillary artery and join anterior to it (Fig. 49–6). Thus formed, the median nerve runs distally in the anteromedial compartment of the arm. In the cubital fossa the nerve lies medial to the artery, covered by the bicipital aponeurosis, and passes between the two heads of the pronator teres and under the fibrous arch joining the two heads of the flexor digitorum superficialis. It crosses an-

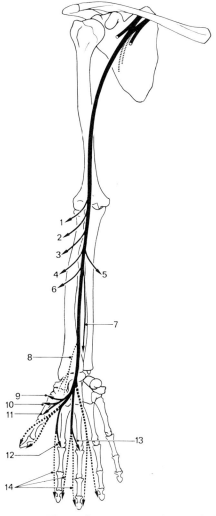

Figure 49–6. The median nerve; muscles supplied and cutaneous distribution. 1, Pronator teres. 2, Palmaris longus. 3, Palmaris brevis. 4, Flexor digitorum superficialis. 5, Flexor digitorum profundus to second and third digits. 6, Flexor pollicis longus. 7, Pronator quadratus. 8, Palmar cutaneous branch. 9, Abductor pollicis brevis. 10, Superficial branch to flexor pollicis brevis. 11, Opponens pollicis. 12, First lumbrical. 13, Second lumbrical. 14, Digital nerves (sensory). The sensory branches are shown as dotted lines.

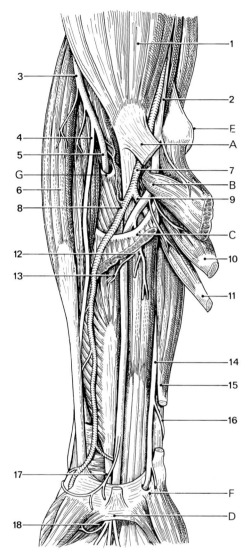

Figure 49–7. Dissection of the anterior aspect of the forearm to show the median nerve, radial nerve, and ulnar nerve. The common sites of compression of the three nerves are shown. 1, Biceps brachii. 2, Median nerve. 3, Radial nerve. 4, Sensory terminal branch of radial nerve. 5, Motor terminal branch of radial nerve. 6, Brachioradialis. 7, Brachial artery. 8, Radial artery. 9, Ulnar artery. 10, Flexor carpi radialis. 11, Palmaris longus. 12, Branch of anterior interosseous nerve to flexor digitorum profundus to index and middle fingers. 13, Branch of anterior interosseous nerve to flexor pollicis longus. 14, Ulnar nerve. 15, Flexor carpi ulnaris. 16, Dorsal cutaneous branch of ulnar nerve. 17. Palmar cutaneous branch of the median nerve. 18, Thenar branch of median nerve.

Common sites of nerve compression in the forearm. Median nerve: A, Expansion of biceps. B, Two heads of pronator teres. C, Flexor digitorum superficialis. D, Carpal tunnel. Ulnar nerve: E, Medial epicondylar groove. F, Guyon's canal. Radial nerve: G, Arcade of Frohse.

terior to the ulnar artery and enters the anterior compartment of the forearm, closely bound to the deep surface of the flexor digitorum superficialis, within the muscle sheath (Fig. 49–7). As the muscle changes to tendon in the lower half of the forearm, the median nerve runs first lateral to the index tendon and then anterior to it and lateral to the tendon of the medial finger. It runs under the flexor retinaculum, and as it emerges from the carpal tunnel, it divides into its terminal branches to the lateral thenar muscles, to the radial two lumbricals, to the skin of the lateral half of the palm and the palmar skin of three and one-half digits, and to the skin covering the dorsum of the distal and medial phalanges of the radial three and one-half digits.

The median nerve gives off numerous motor branches to the anterior forearm muscles. Above the elbow the medial epicondylar branch to the pronator teres arises. It accompanies the anterior interosseous artery in the gap between the flexor pollicis longus and the flexor digitorum profundus and sends fibers to both muscles (but to only the lateral heads of the flexor digitorum profundus) and to the pronator quadratus.

The median nerve can be compressed at several points along its course—between the heads of the pronator teres, in the fibrous bridge between the heads of the flexor digitorum superficialis, and, of course, within the carpal tunnel.

Fascicular Anatomy

The *fascicular anatomy* of the median nerve is relatively constant in the forearm, where the fascicles are arranged in clearly defined bundles. The recurrent thenar branch is composed of two fascicles. It joins the nerve on its volar and radial side and can be traced proximally for about 70 mm. The palmar cutaneous branch is also arranged in two separate fascicular bundles, which can be traced proximally for about 190 mm. The flexor digitorum superficialis branches are variable. The anterior interosseous nerve can be traced for about 150 mm. It gives off in its intraneural course the motor branch to the flexor carpi radialis. The pronator teres branch has been dissected within the nerve for a distance of 100 mm. without encountering any bundle exchange.

During its superficial course through the

wrist the median nerve is particularly exposed to trauma; hence, the high incidence of low median nerve palsy. Such trauma results in loss of the most essential function of the nerve, sensibility of the prehensile zone, which includes the pulp skin of the all important thumb and index and middle fingers.

It is easier to compensate for paralysis of the lateral thenar muscles, because the flexor pollicis brevis is partly or wholly supplied by the ulnar nerve and therefore is frequently spared.

Sectioning of the median nerve above the elbow produces, in addition to the intrinsic lesions of the hand already described, paralysis of the flexor pollicis longus, flexor digitorum superficialis, and lateral half of the flexor digitorum profundus, resulting in loss of flexion of the distal phalanges of the thumb, the index finger, and sometimes the middle finger. Pronation of the forearm is usually preserved, because the high branches to the pronator teres are given off above the elbow. More proximal lesions of the median nerve severely impair pronation.

ULNAR NERVE PALSY

The ulnar nerve arises from the medial cord of the brachial plexus and lies at this point medial to the medial cord contribution to the median nerve. Its fibers come from the C7, C8, and T1 roots. It runs medial to the humeral artery, goes through the medial intermuscular septum, and passes between the medial epicondyle of the humerus and the olecranon (Fig. 49–8). It enters the forearm between the humeral and ulnar origins of the flexor carpi ulnaris and descends within the anteromedial compartment of the forearm under cover of the flexor carpi ulnaris. At the wrist, lying on the medial side of the ulnar artery, it runs with the latter in the so-called Guyon osteofibrous canal (distinct from the carpal tunnel). Just distal to the pisiform it divides into its two terminal branches—the superficial sensory branch, which supplies the medial skin of the hand, and the deep motor branch, which winds around the hook of the hamate, crosses the sharp lower border of the opponens digiti minimi muscle, and, under cover of the deep flexor tendons, reaches the adductor pollicis and flexor pollicis brevis muscles on the lateral side of the hand (Fig. 49–9).

The ulnar nerve supplies the flexor carpi ulnaris and the two ulnar heads of the flexor digitorum profundus. In the lower third of the forearm, it gives off the dorsal cutaneous branch that supplies the skin on the ulnar half of the dorsum of the hand. Between them, the median and ulnar nerves supply all the intrinsic muscles of the hand: the deep

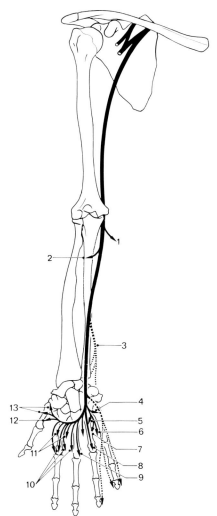

Figure 49–8. The ulnar nerve; muscles supplied and cutaneous distribution. 1, Branch to flexor carpi ulnaris. 2, Branch to flexor digitorum profundus supplying fourth and fifth digits. 3, Dorsal cutaneous branch. 4, Palmar cutaneous branch. 5, Branch to abductor digiti minimi. 6, Branch to opponens digiti minimi. 7, Branch to flexor digiti minimi. 8, Fourth lumbrical branch. 9, Third lumbrical branch. 10, Branch to palmar interosseous muscles. 11, Branch to dorsal interosseous muscles. 12, Deep branch to flexor pollicis brevis. 13, Branch to adductor pollicis. The sensory branches are shown as dotted lines.

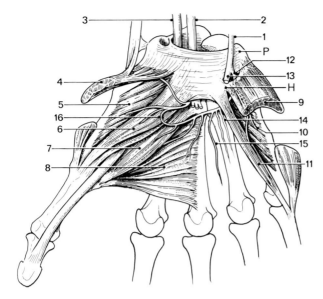

Figure 49–9. Dissection of the palm to show the deep branch of the ulnar nerve. 1, Ulnar nerve. 2, Median nerve. 3, Flexor pollicis longus. 4, Abductor pollicis brevis. 5, Opponens pollicis. 6, Flexor pollicis brevis. 7, Adductor pollicis, oblique fibers. 8, Adductor pollicis, transverse fibers. 9, Abductor digiti minimi. 10, Opponens digiti minimi. 11, Flexor digiti minimi. 12, Motor branch of ulnar nerve. 13, Sensory branch of ulnar nerve. 14, Branches to ulnar two lumbrical muscles. 15, Branches to interosseous muscles (only one shown). 16, Anastomosis between thenar branch of median nerve and deep motor branch of ulnar nerve (anastomosis of Riche and Cannieu). P, Pisiform. H, Hamate.

terminal branch of the ulnar nerve sends fibers to all the intrinsic muscles of the fingers (except the two lateral lumbricals), to the adductor pollicis, and to the deep head of the flexor pollicis brevis. In fact, the respective territories of the median and ulnar nerves are poorly defined, and anastomoses occur in the forearm* (in 15 per cent of cases, according to Mannerfelt [1966]) and in the palm (anastomoses of Riche and Cannieu [1897]), which explains the frequent anomalies of distribution (Fig. 49–10).

The ulnar nerve can be compressed at various points:

1. In the lower third of the arm the nerve enters the posterior compartment by passing through an osteofibrous foramen (Fig. 49–11). This is formed laterally by the medial intermuscular septum (which is attached to the humerus), above by a fibrous expansion of the coracobrachialis, and laterally by the medial head of the triceps. Distally the foramen may be narrowed by inconstant insertions of the triceps that form Struthers' arcade (1854).

2. At the elbow the nerve passes through a narrow channel between the medial epicondyle and the olecranon, where it may be compressed (Fig. 49–12). Then the nerve runs between the humeral and ulnar heads of the flexor carpi ulnaris under a fibrous arcade, which must be divided to relieve compression at that level (Osborne, 1970).

_____
*Martin-Gruber anastomosis.

3. The nerve can also be compressed in the wrist as it courses through Guyon's canal, whose floor is formed by the flexor retinaculum (inserted on the pisiform) and whose

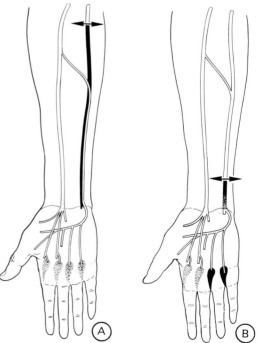

Figure 49–10. Diagram to shown the Martin-Gruber anastomosis between the median and ulnar nerves in the forearm. In high lesions of the ulnar nerve (A), the anastomosis from the median nerve can result in prevention of paralysis of the ulnar innervated intrinsic muscles. In lesions of the ulnar nerve distal to the anastomosis (B), this will not occur.

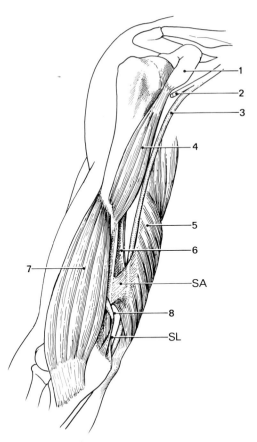

Figure 49–11. Dissection to show the ulnar nerve in the arm and its common sites of compression. 1, Coracoid process. 2, Musculocutaneous nerve. 3, Ulnar nerve. 4, Coracobrachialis. 5, Medial head of triceps. 6, Medial intermuscular septum. 7, Brachialis. 8, Supracondylar spur. SA, Struther's arcade. SL, Struther's ligament.

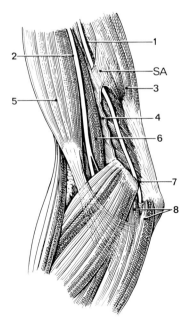

Figure 49–12. The ulnar nerve at the elbow. 1, Ulnar nerve. 2, Median nerve. 3, Triceps. 4, Medial intermuscular septum. 5, Biceps. 6, Brachialis. 7, Medial epicondylar groove. 8, Two heads of flexor carpi ulnaris. SA, Struther's arcade.

roof is formed by an expansion of the flexor carpi ulnaris (Fig. 49–13).

The deep terminal branch courses under the fibrous band that stretches from the pisiform to the hook of the hamate, giving origin to the abductor and flexor digiti minimi brevis.

The ulnar nerve is most vulnerable at the elbow and at the wrist.

Fascicular Anatomy

The distal part of the ulnar nerve can be easily microdissected. The dorsal cutaneous branch forms an independent fascicle that can be traced proximally well above the epicondyle. Jabaley et al. (1980) suggest the use of this branch as a graft in cases in which it may be considered expendable.

Sensory ulnar palsy affects both the palmar and dorsal aspects of the ulnar half of the hand. The autonomous zone of the ulnar nerve is limited to the skin of the distal two phalanges of the little finger.

Motor ulnar palsy, by contrast, has far more serious functional consequences (Table 49–1). Distal ulnar nerve lesions produce the classic claw deformity of the fingers. There is

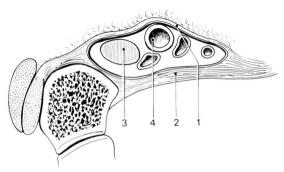

Figure 49–13. The space of Guyon (transverse section). 1, Volar ligament of wrist. 2, Flexor retinaculum. 3, Ulnar nerve. 4, Ulnar artery.

Table 49–1.   SYMPTOMS AND SIGNS IN ULNAR NERVE PARALYSIS*

Original Description By	Year	Symptoms and Signs
Duchenne	1867	Clawing of the ring and little fingers.
		The little finger cannot be adducted to the ring finger.
		Inability to play high notes on the violin because the flexor carpi ulnaris and opponens digiti quinti are paralyzed, and there is loss of sensibility of the little finger.
Jeanne	1915	Hyperextension of the metacarpophalangeal joint of the thumb in pinch grip; Jeanne's sign.
Froment	1915	Pronounced flexion of the interphalangeal joint of the thumb during adduction toward the index finger; Froment's sign.
Masse	1916	Flattening of the metacarpal arch.
André-Thomas	1917	The wrist tends to fall into volar flexion during action of the extensors of the middle finger.
Pollock	1919	Inability to flex the distal phalanx of the fifth finger.
Pitres-Testut	1925	The transverse diameter of the hand is decreased.
		Radial-ulnar abduction of the metacarpophalangeal joint of the middle finger is impossible.
		Inability to shape the hand to a cone.
Wartenberg	1939	Inability to adduct the extended little finger to the extended ring finger; Wartenberg's sign.
Sunderland	1944	Inability to rotate, oppose, or supinate the little finger toward the thumb; Sunderland's sign.
Fay	1954	Inability of the thumb to reach the little finger in true opposition (probably a misinterpretation of the author because the little finger cannot always reach the thumb in cases of paralysis of the opponens of the little finger).
Bunnell	1956	The thumb no longer pinches against the index finger to make a full circle.
Egawa	1959	Inability of the flexed middle finger to abduct radially and ulnarly and to rotate at the metacarpophalangeal joint.
Mumenthaler	1961	On abduction of the little finger against resistance, no normal dimple in the hypothenar region because of paresis of the palmaris brevis musculature.
Mannerfelt	1966	With increasing force in the collapsed pinching grip, a flexion position, often more than 90 degrees of the proximal interphalangeal joint, is to be seen. The distal interphalangeal joint is hyperextended and the radial part of the pulp slides in a proximal direction along the ulnar part of the thumb.

*Adapted from Mannerfelt, L.: Studies on the hand in ulnar nerve paralysis. A clinical-experimental investigation in normal and anomalous innervation. Acta Orthop. Scand., Suppl. 87, 1966.

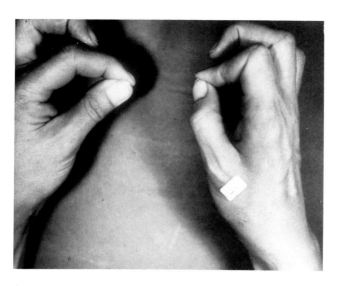

Figure 49–14. Ulnar palsy (on the right), showing Froment's sign in the thumb and hyperflexion of the proximal interphalangeal joint of the index finger. The distal interphalangeal joint is hyperextended and the radial part of the pulp slides in a proximal direction along the ulnar part of the thumb. (Courtesy Dr. L. Mannerfelt.)

wasting of the interosseous muscles and the thenar and hypothenar eminences. There is hyperextension of the metacarpophalangeal joints and flexion of the interphalangeal joints. This posture is less obvious in the index and middle fingers because the lateral lumbricals, supplied by the median nerve, remain functional. The claw is more marked when the deep flexor retains its tonicity. In the thumb, paralysis of the adductor causes a significant loss of pinch strength. Furthermore, in pinch, the distal phalanx of the thumb assumes a position of flexion (Froment's sign [1915]) and the proximal phalanx hyperextends when the flexor pollicis brevis is also paralyzed (Jeanne, 1915). In terminal thumb-index pinch, the patient cannot make an "O" with the two digits (Bunnell, 1956),

the metacarpophalangeal joints have a tendency to hyperextend, and the proximal interphalangeal joint of the index finger tends to hyperflex (Mannerfelt, 1966; Fig. 49–14). The deformity is less marked in proximal lesions because the flexor profundus is also paralyzed. In ulnar nerve lesions at the elbow, the flexor carpi ulnaris is usually spared, in part or in toto.

The clinical features are different in partial lesions and in combined lesions.

REFERENCES

References for this chapter will be found following Chapter 50.

Chapter 50

NERVE REGENERATION AND PROGNOSIS FOLLOWING PERIPHERAL NERVE INJURY

Raoul Tubiana

THE SIGNS OF NEURAL REGENERATION

Two general principles must be kept in mind: Recovery occurs from proximal to distal, and the signs of sensory recovery precedes those of voluntary motor activity.

Tinel's Sign

The first detectable clinical sign of recovery is Tinel's sign. Percutaneous percussion of the nerve trunk distal to the lesion (as far as the level of axonal regeneration) produces a "pins and needles" sensation distally in the territory of distribution of the cutaneous nerve. This sign was described in the same year (1915) by Hoffmann and by Tinel. In an article that has become a classic, Tinel distinguished between peripheral paresthesia, a sign of axonal regeneration, and local pain, which indicates irritation of the nerve. He emphasized the significance of this test in monitoring regeneration of the nerve, but stressed that the sign is neither constant nor easy to interpret.

Technique

Percussion must be gentle, done with the tip of the finger or, more accurately, with the blunt tip of a felt pen or a rubber eraser. One should avoid inaccurate mechanical stimulation with a large object and restrict percussion to the course of the nerve. Most clinicians percuss from a distal point upward along the course of the nerve trunk until they reach the site at which percussion triggers paresthesia. Others work in reverse from the site of the lesion downward until the induced paresthesia disappears. The reaction can be compared to that produced by a weak electric current, unpleasant but not painful. It is important to remember that the sensation is felt peripherally, in the area of the cutaneous distribution of the nerve, and differs from the sometimes painful sensation felt at the point of direct pressure on the nerve caused by neuroma formation or by irritation of pain fibers. A similar peripheral reaction can be obtained by electric stimulation using a cathode 1 cm. in diameter applied to a point over the course of a nerve, and a broader anode at some other point on the body (Moldaver, 1978). Even when a continuous stimulus is applied, the sensation is felt as an intermittent vibration.

Clinical Significance of Tinel's Sign

The "pins and needles" sensation resulting from percussion is caused by regeneration of the sensory axons, which are very sensitive to pressure. The sign thus signifies a favorable prognosis and enables one to follow the progress of the regenerating nerve. Only percussion of the tactile fibers (not those transmitting pain, heat, and cold) triggers the pins and needles sensation.

Changes in the results of Tinel's test reflect the progress of axonal regrowth, which varies from person to person and is faster in the proximal part of the limb than at the extremities. It is faster after spontaneous healing than after nerve suturing. In the latter situation axonal regrowth usually occurs at a rate of 1 to 2 mm. per day (Jung, 1941; Sunderland and Bradley, 1952). A positive response over a long segment of nerve suggests unequal rates of growth of various tactile fibers.

Tinel's sign has fallen occasionally into disrepute, because it sometimes has been absent when a nerve was in fact regenerating and at other times has been positive when exploration showed an absence of continuity between the nerve ends (Woodhall and Beebe, 1956). Some authors, however, have attached great significance to the test (Henderson, 1948).

Tinel himself pointed out that the sign is absent in certain circumstances:

1. It is absent in the early stages following injury or nerve suturing. According to Tinel, the sign appears only four to six weeks after the injury. In fact, this is very variable because axonal growth depends on a number of factors, but it can be said that the time is roughly proportional to the severity of the lesion.

2. The sign may be difficult to elicit if the nerve lies deep to a large mass of muscle.

3. Tinel's sign cannot be demonstrated when the lesion is proximal to the posterior root ganglion.

The prognostic value of this sign is not absolute, for not all the regenerating tactile fibers necessarily recover. Some lose their way; others just stop growing. Even if they continue growing within the nerve sheath, they may follow the wrong route. Thus, a false positive result is elicited when sensory fibers grow into motor sheaths.

Finally the test has no quantitative value; it can be positive with only a few fibers regenerating—hence its limited functional significance.

In spite of all these limitations, the sign is clinically useful when, within a few weeks after the injury or suturing, light percussion distal to the lesion triggers the pins and needles sensation peripherally, and when, in the course of the following weeks, percussion at the same level produces a weak response, which increases in strength if tapping is done more distally. This appears to confirm axonal growth. Interrupted progress must be regarded as alarming, and when this persists, and the absence of other signs of regeneration (to be discussed) confirms it, surgical exploration is indicated. Steady distal progression of the sign, unless contradicted by other factors, suggests a good prognosis, even though the sign gives little information concerning the functional quality of reinnervation.

Too much should not be expected of Tinel's sign, which must be interpreted only in conjunction with other clinical findings.

SENSORY RECOVERY

Sensory recovery progresses in time and space according to the following successive stages:

1. First perception of pain and temperature (small caliber pain fibers regenerate more rapidly). Protective sensation is thus established.

2. Perception of low frequency vibratory stimuli (30 Hz) as well as moving tact sense.

3. Per static tact sense, at the same time as perception of high frequency vibratory stimuli (256 Hz).

4. Two point discrimination (Weber test) is the last form of sensation to develop.

This recovery pattern is used by Dellon as a guide in his sensory rehabilitation program.

MOTOR RECOVERY

Motor recovery is always slower than sensory recovery. The first sign of motor recovery is regression of the atrophy in the territory normally supplied by the injured nerve. Later a weak contraction can be detected in the first muscle supplied by the nerve distal to the lesion. The contraction, however, is not powerful enough to produce movement or to overcome gravity.

Precise electromyographic studies can show signs of motor recovery before any clinical evidence of activity can be demonstrated, provided the electrodes are placed close to the point where the nerve penetrates the muscle.

It should be pointed out that these early signs of neural regeneration, both clinical and electromyographic, are of limited prognostic value: they suggest a favorable outcome but offer no guarantee of functional recovery.

Although it is necessary to detect the early signs of neural regeneration, it is equally essential to follow its progress. Regeneration can be halted at any stage, and there is frequently a marked difference between motor recovery and sensory recovery. As far as the latter is concerned, pain usually appears before tactile sensation returns. Sensation returns first to the proximal margin of the anesthetic zone. It is important to record the interval between the reappearance of contraction in the first muscle supplied distal to the nerve suture and that in the next. Regeneration can slow down or even cease before reaching the extremity of the limb. All these variations make difficult the decision to undertake and the timing of secondary repairs.

FACTORS AFFECTING PROGNOSIS

The prognosis after a traumatic lesion of a peripheral nerve depends on a large number of factors not enumerated here. Countless neurophysiological studies have been devoted to axonal regeneration and to the reinnervation of muscle fibers and sensory receptors in the skin, yet many questions remain unanswered. However, the surgeon should evaluate the available facts, including results of the clinical examination and electrophysiological studies, and operative findings.

We distinguish here between local factors, general factors, and factors related to treatment.

LOCAL FACTORS

The nature and severity of the nerve injury, its site, and the associated lesions are important determinants of prognosis.

Nature of the Lesion

Traumatic lesions of the peripheral nerves can be classified into two categories—open lacerations and compressions.

From the prognostic point of view, it is probably fair to say that open injuries are more ominous than closed injuries because of the risk of infection and of cicatricial tissue formation. This, however, is a very rough distinction. Partial sectioning may be less damaging than compression caused by a plaster cast or a displaced fracture.

As a general rule, a slowly progressive lesion carries a better prognosis than does one that produces sudden paralysis, and a partial lesion carries a better prognosis than does a total lesion.

Other more accurate methods of classification take into account the histological lesions of the nerve trunk. Thus, Seddon (1943) recognized three groups of lesions:

1. Neurapraxia implies interruption of nerve conduction with preservation of anatomical continuity of all neural structures. Its main clinical feature is a dissociated and transitory paralysis that affects primarily large-diameter fibers. It is thus predominantly motor, but also gives rise to sensory changes: the proprioceptive fibers are affected more than the touch fibers, and the latter more than the pain fibers. Recovery occurs in the reverse order.

These transitory paralyses were described as long ago as 1864 by Mitchell, who observed them following bullet injuries in which the bullet passed close to the nerve without hitting it. This type of paralysis can also be triggered by momentary traction or by compression, such as that resulting from the use of crutches.

Electrical tests show no sign of degeneration, conduction is preserved, and fibrillations may be present. This type of paralysis is typically transitory.

Studies have been designed to elucidate these transitory paralyses, which were thought at first to be due to ischemia resulting from transitory compression (Denny-Brown and Brenner, 1944). More recently Lundborg (1970) postulated anoxia in the fascicular microcirculation caused by venous obstruction in the epineurium.* Kuczynski (1974) suggested an electrolytic imbalance at the nodes of Ranvier. In the same year Gilliat et al. and Ochoa demonstrated microscopic mechanical lesions resulting in demyelination at the nodes. The latter lesions are the slowest to recover; the process of remyelination takes about 60 days.

In cases of incomplete paralysis caused by compression with no axonal degeneration, the prognosis must be good. However, because such neurapraxic lesions are due to a variety of causes, some may take months to recover. If after three months there is no sign of recovery, neurolysis to relieve the compression must be considerred (Spinner, 1978). Recovery then occurs in a few days unless demyelination has occurred, in which case reinnervation of the muscles takes two to three months.

---

*See Chapter 57 in Volume I.

2. Axonotmesis is a term coined by Seddon (1943) to describe loss of continuity of axons and of their myelin sheath, while the rest of the nerve trunk is intact: Schwann cells, endoneurium, perineurium, and epineurium. The motor, sensory, and sympathetic paralysis is total, and electrical tests show signs of neural degeneration. Reinnervation can occur spontaneously; its duration depends on the site of the lesion.

3. Finally, there is neurotmesis, which implies either a physical division of the nerve trunk or complete destruction of the intraneural architecture when spontaneous recovery is impossible, despite apparent continuity. Such lesions occur after traction injuries, toxic injections, and prolonged ischemia. Clinically it is impossible to differentiate between axonotmesis and neurotmesis without allowing the lesion to follow its course. Waiting too long for spontaneous recovery, however, is not without danger. Exploration may be necessary to establish the prognosis and attempt surgical repair.

Sunderland's classification distinguishes five degrees of lesions (Table 50–1). The first degree corresponds to neurapraxia, and the second is not unlike axonotmesis. The third degree implies, in addition to axonal destruction and wallerian degeneration, destruction of the internal fascicular structure by edema, stasis, ischemia, segmental hemorrhage, or other factors. This gives rise to intrafascicular fibrosis, which in turn impedes regeneration. The period of denervation of the peripheral tissues is more prolonged than that occurring after a second degree lesion; in the course of regeneration there may be an exchange of fibers, and the quality of functional recovery suffers.

The fourth degree is characterized by complete disruption of the fascicular organization. The perineurium is destroyed, and although the continuity of the nerve trunk is preserved, it is reduced to a cord of connective tissue. This type of lesion necessitates partial resection of the cicatricial tissues.

A fifth degree lesion implies a break in continuity of the nerve.

When the nerve has been severed, the prognosis depends to some extent on the amount of nerve tissue lost. Other local factors are also relevant—the type of nerve and whether it is sensory, motor, or mixed. The extent of contusion and subsequent fibrosis also has a considerable influence on the nerve repair.

Site of the Lesion

The site of the lesion can influence the prognosis in a number of ways. The more proximal the lesion, the farther the axons have to travel to reinnervate the extremity of the limb. In addition to the distance, there are the dangers inherent in the delay in reinnervation. The obstacles include exhaustion of the nerve cell, interstitial fibrosis, progressive atrophy, and degeneration of the muscle fibers.

Recovery of the intrinsic muscles of the hand following a high nerve lesion is exceptional.

Another factor that worsens the prognosis in proximal lesions is the extent of retrograde axonal degeneration, which is always greater in lesions close to the cell body. This phenomenon can lead to the death of nerve cells, or at best may reduce the regenerating capacity of the axon, which may be unable to reach the extremity of the limb. Retrograde degeneration is also influenced by the severity of the trauma, the site of nerve division, and the nature of the injury. It is more marked after avulsions and after injuries by high velocity missiles.

The Nerve Involved

From a prognostic standpoint, risks of directional errors concerning the axons seem greater when the nerve is "mixed." All motor nerves contain sensory fibers. Repair of predominantly motor nerves (e.g., the radial nerve) carries a better prognosis than that of "mixed" nerves containing a high percentage of sensory fibers (e.g., the ulnar and above all the median nerve).

Associated Lesions

Associated traumatic lesions of muscle, bone, and blood vessels increase the scarring

Table 50–1. CORRELATION BETWEEN SEDDON'S AND SUNDERLAND'S CLASSIFICATIONS

Seddon	Sunderland
Neurapraxia	First degree
Axonotmesis	{ Second degree { Third degree
Neurotmesis	{ Fourth degree { Fifth degree

around and ischemia of the damaged nerve. The state of the "nerve bed" also influences the quality of the repair.

Emergency repair of the vessels, as is increasingly widely practiced, probably has a beneficial effect on the state of the muscle fibers, avoiding or delaying their degeneration and thus permitting late reinnervation.

GENERAL FACTORS

The age of the patient is of such importance that any analysis of results must be made by age groups if it is to be valid. Every series published so far confirms that the best results are obtained in young subjects (Hallin et al., 1981). After the age of 30 the chances of success are reduced. It has been suggested that in children the axons have a shorter distance to travel because the limbs are shorter, the capacity for regeneration is greater, and there is probably the possibility of participation by a still adaptable nervous system (Almquist and Olofsson, 1973).

The effect of age on conduction velocity has been studied by several investigators. Thomas and Lambert (1960) reported that in children five years old or less, conduction velocity is slower than that in the adult. This is readily explained by the fact that the rate of conduction is directly proportional to the diameter of the fibers, and this changes little after the age of five. At the other end of the scale, conduction velocity decreases with age, by about 10 per cent at the age of 60 years, owing to local ischemia and reduced permeability of the cell membrane (Wagman and Lesse, 1952).

The Effect of Delay on the Prognosis

This problem is far from simple, and one must differentiate between delays in spontaneous regeneration compatible with functional recovery and delays between the injury and the repair compatible with functional recovery.

Delays Prior to Spontaneous Recovery. These include (1) the initial latent period (Sunderland, 1968), which corresponds to the time needed by the axon to cover the distance of the retrograde degeneration in addition to that needed for it to cross the injured zone of the nerve; (2) the period taken by the axons to cover the distance between the site

of injury and the peripheral connections; and (3) the time required for the regrown axons and their reinnervated terminal corpuscles to be converted into functional units.

These delays are inevitably longer after proximal lesions, because retrograde degeneration is more marked, the axons have farther to travel, and the peripheral tissues remain denervated longer.

It appears that, in practice, the latent period is proportional to the severity of the lesion. In the majority of cases the first signs suggesting regeneration appear after six months, although in some proximal lesions the latent period may be even longer.

Delays Prior to Nerve Repair. It has now been virtually established that the limiting factor is not so much the regeneration capacity of the nerve cell as the degeneration of the denervated muscles (Sunderland, 1950). Some nerve cells probably retain for years the capacity to grow new axons. By contrast, the period during which a denervated muscle can recover useful function is shorter. This delay in muscle recovery depends on the number of useful axons reaching the muscle and the number of surviving muscle fibers capable of reinnervation. Each of these must be considered in more detail.

The number of functional axons reaching the denervated muscles is necessarily smaller than normal by an amount that varies with the number of neurons surviving retrograde degeneration, the number of axons whose growth is stopped by fibrosis at the level of the injury, the number of axons misdirected outside the fascicles, and the number of axons misdirected within the fascicles.

The number of muscle fibers capable of reinnervation depends on the degree of destruction at the time of injury, the secondary degenerative changes in the muscles leading to atrophy and sclerosis, and the capacity for connection between the extremities of the nerve fibers reaching the motor end plates, and the restoration of sufficient neuromuscular units to achieve useful motor function.

Gutmann and Young (1944) believed that the longer the delay in reinnervation, the less the chances of return of motor function, because the proportion of reinnervated motor end plates is rapidly reduced when atrophy sets in. Also, the formation of new end plates slows because they are probably less efficient than the old. The number of fibers destined not to be reinnervated increases with time. It follows, therefore, that the earlier reinnervation occurs, the better are the chances for functional recovery.

It has been shown that the delay prior to a nerve repair affects the quality of the results. Figures published by the U.S. Army Medical Services concerning nerve suturing performed during World War II showed that every delay of six days before the repair reduced the quality of the result by 1 per cent (Woodhall and Beebe, 1956).* Analyzing their results in microsurgical repair of nerve injuries, Zilch and Buck-Gramcko (1975) found that 85 per cent of their failures occurred when the repair was performed more than four months after the injury.

Delay between injury and nerve repair has much stronger effects on the functional scores than on the electrophysiological measures (Marsh and Barton, 1987). For these authors there is particular deterioration after a delay of about two months.

Delays Compatible with Reinnervation After Nerve Repair. The delay usually noted as being compatible with good recovery of muscle function ranges from 12 to 18 months. It seems unlikely that muscles that have been denervated for 18 months will regain useful function (Zachary and Roaf, 1954). However, Bowden and Gutmann (1944) have shown in muscle biopsy studies that reinnervation remains possible for up to three years. Now that repairs after brachial plexus lesions are more frequent, reinnervation has been seen to occur after more than two years. It should be pointed out, however, that the late reinnervations occurred in young patients and in muscles relatively free of atrophy and sclerosis as a result of regular physiotherapy. It is important to point out that function continues to improve for at least four years (Nicholson and Seddon, 1957; Önne, 1962; Marsh and Barton, 1987). This notion is perhaps not widely appreciated by surgeons. Assessments of final results of nerve repair therefore require follow-up times in excess of four years.

From a practical viewpoint, it is worth stressing that:

1. Nerve repair should be carried out as soon as local conditions are favorable.

2. As soon as paralysis has been diagnosed, a course of physiotherapy should be prescribed to keep the joints supple and to prevent muscle fibrosis.

3. The more proximal a lesion, the earlier the repair should be performed.

4. When assessing the theoretical chances for recovery, the surgeon should add the preoperative delay to the time needed for the growing axon to reach the paralyzed muscle (on the basis of an average of 1 mm. a day). If the total is greater than 18 months, it is often wiser, especially if the patient is not young, to combine a nerve repair with palliative surgery to correct the motor deficit resulting from lack of function of the paralyzed muscles, provided this does not produce a further deficit.

5. By contrast, sensation (or at least protective sensation) can return after much longer delays—seven years or more in some of our cases. Protective sensation, however, should not be confused with the return of "stereognosis," which is difficult to obtain even with early repair.

PROGNOSTIC FACTORS PERTAINING TO TREATMENT

The prognostic factors pertaining to treatment are extremely important. It is now agreed that the surgical procedure should be delicate and nontraumatic, that the "nerve bed" (at the site of the repair) should be cleared of scar tissue, and that excessive dissection and suturing under tension should be avoided. The use of operating microscopes, bipolar coagulation, microinstruments, and microsutures has now become commonplace. Accurate realignment of the nerve ends is always desirable but difficult to achieve. Some of the chapters that follow are concerned with microsurgical techniques in nerve repairs. The controversy concerning primary and secondary repairs by suturing and grafting is also considered in detail.

Emphasis should be placed on the influence on prognosis of the experience and careful technique of the surgeon.

PROGNOSTIC FACTORS RELATING TO OTHER ASPECTS OF TREATMENT AND THE PATIENT

The functional prognosis is in great part dependent upon the state of the paralyzed

---

*See Chapter 82 on "War Injuries of the Hand."

limb, e.g., the remaining muscles and the suppleness of the joints. Hence, the fundamental importance of physiotherapy, which as soon as paralysis is present must be undertaken to overcome abnormal positions and stiffness, maintain the strength of the remaining muscles, and enforce maximal use of the limb by the patient. This treatment is continued throughout the course of nerve regeneration.

A will to recover on the part of the patient and his ability to play a role was long unrecognized. This explains why certain individuals are capable of discriminative use of the hands in spite of severely disturbed sensitivity test results. Rehabilitation of sensitivity is also based upon the possibility of improving use of the regenerated nerve potential. After motor paralysis, the efforts of the patient to use his limb and obtain best use of the reinnervated muscles help considerably in his adaptation to the new circumstances.

REFERENCES

Almquist, E. E., and Olofsson, E.: Bilan électrique et clinique des sutures nerveuses en fonction de l'âge. *In* Lésions traumatiques des Nerfs Périphériques, 1972.

Bonnel, F., Durand, Y., Blotman, F., and Godebout, Y.: Anatomie et Systematisation Fasciculaire du Nerf Médian. Paris, Masson, 1978.

Bonnel, F., Mailhe, P., Allieu, Y., and Rabischong, P.: Bases anatomiques de la chirurgie fasciculaire du nerf médian. Ann. Chir., *34*:707–710, 1980.

Bowden, R. E. M., and Gutmann, E.: Denervation and re-innervation of human voluntary muscle. Brain, *67*:273, 1944.

Cannieu, J. M. A.: Recherches sur une anastomose entre la branche profonde du cubital et le médian. Bull. Soc. Anat. Physiol. (Bordeaux), *18*:339–340, 1897.

Coene, L. N. J. E. M.: Axillary nerve lesions and associated injuries. Printed in Holland by De Kempenaer Oegstgeest, 1985.

Dellon, A. L.: The moving two-point discrimination test: Clinical evaluation of the quickly adapting fiber receptor system. J. Hand Surg., *3*:474–481, 1978.

Denny-Brown, D., and Brenner, C.: Paralysis of nerve induced by direct pressure and by tourniquet. Arch. Neurol. Psychiat., *51*:1–26, 1944.

Frohse, F., and Frankel, M.: Die Muskeln des Menschlichen Armes. *In* Bardeleben's Handbuch der Anatomie des Menschlichen. Jena, Fisher, 1908.

Gilliatt, R. W., Ochoa, J., Rudge, P., and Neary, D.: The cause of nerve damage in acute compression. Trans. Am. Neurol. Assoc., *99*:71–74, 1974.

Gruber, W.: Ueber die Verbindung des Nervus medianus mit dem Nervus ulnaris am Unterarme des Menschen und der Sängethiere. Arch. Anat. Physiol., *37*:501–522, 1870.

Gutmann, E., and Young, J. Z.: The re-innervation of muscle after various periods of atrophy. J. Anat., *78*:15, 1966.

Guyon, F.: Note sur une disposition anatomique propre à la face antérieure de la région du poignet et non encore décrite. Bull. Soc. Anat. Paris (2nd Series), *6*:184–186, 1861.

Hallin, R. G., Wiesenfeld, I., and Lungnegard, H.: Neurophysiological studies of peripheral nerve function after neural regeneration following nerve suture in man. Int. Rehab. Med., *3*:187–192, 1981.

Henderson, W. R.: Clinical assessment of peripheral nerve injuries. Tinel's test. Lancet, *2*:801, 1948.

Highet, W. B.: Procaine nerve block in investigation of peripheral nerve injuries. J. Neurol. Psychiat. (London), *5*:101, 1942.

Hoffmann, P.: Ueber eine Methode den Erflog einer Nervennaht zu beurteilen. Med. Klin., *11*:359–350, 1915.

Holstein, A., and Lewis, G. B.: Fractures of the humerus with radial nerve paralysis. J. Bone Joint Surg., *45A*:1382, 1963.

Jabaley, M. E., Wallace, W. H., and Keckler, F. R.: Internal topography of major nerves of the forearm and hand: a current view. J. Hand Surg., *5*:7–18, 1980.

Jones, F. W.: Voluntary muscular movements in cases of nerve lesions. J. Anat., *54*:41, 1919.

Jung, R.: Die allgemeine Symptomatologie der Nervenverletzungen und ihre physiologischen Grundlagen. Nervenarzt, *11*:494, 1941.

Kiloh, L. G., and Nevin, S.: Isolated neuritis of the anterior interosseous nerve. Br. Med. J., *1*:850–851, 1952.

Kuczynski, K.: Functional micro-anatomy of the peripheral nerve trunks. Hand, *6*:1–10, 1974.

Lundborg, G.: Ischemic nerve injury. Experimental studies on intraneural microvascular pathophysiology and nerve function in a limb subjected to temporary circulatory arrest. Scand. J. Plast. Reconstr. Surg., Suppl. 6, 1–113, 1970.

Mannerfelt, L.: Studies on the hand in ulnar nerve paralysis. A clinical-experimental investigation in normal and anomalous innervation. Acta Orthop. Scand., Suppl. 87, 1966.

Marie, P., Meige, H., and Patrikios: Paralysie radiale dissociée simulant une griffe cubitale. Rev. Neurol., *24*:123–124, 1917.

Marsh, D., and Barton, N.: Does the use of the operating microscope improve the results of peripheral nerve suture? J. Bone Joint Surg., (*B.*), 1987.

Martin, R.: Tal om Nervus allmanna Egenskaper i Mannsikans Kropp. Stockholm, Lars Salvius, 1763.

Mitchell, S. W., Morehouse, G. R., and Keen, W. W.: Gunshot wounds and other injuries of nerves. Philadelphia, J. B. Lippincott Company, 1864.

Moberg, E.: Objective methods for determining the functional value of sensibility in the hand. J. Bone Joint Surg., *40B*:454–476, 1958.

Moberg, E.: The Upper Limb in Tetraplegia. Stuttgart, Georg Thieme Verlag, 1978.

Moldaver, J.: Tinel's sign. Its characteristics and significance. J. Bone Joint Surg., *60A*:412–413, 1978.

Nicholson, O. R., and Seddon, N. J.: Nerve repair in civil practice: results of treatment of median and ulnar nerve lesions. Brit. Med. J., *2*:1065, 1957.

Ochoa, J.: Schwann cell and myelin changes caused by some toxic agents and trauma. Proc. Roy. Soc. Med., *67*:3–4, 1974.

Omer, G. E., and Spinner, M.: Management of Peripheral Nerve Problems. Philadelphia, W. B. Saunders Company, 1980.

Önne, L.: Recovery of sensibility and sudomotor function in the hand after nerve suture. Acta Chir. Scand. (suppl.), *100*:1, 1962.

Osborne, G.: Compression neuritis of the ulnar nerve at the elbow. Hand, *2*:10–13, 1970.

Riche, P.: Le nerf cubital et les muscles de l'éminence thénar. Bull. Mem. Soc. Anat. (Paris). *5*:251–252, 1897.

Seddon, H. J.: Three types of nerve injury. Brain, *66*:237, 1943.

Seddon, H. J.: Nerve lesions complicating certain closed bone injuries. J. Am. Med. Ass., *135*:691, 1947.

Seddon, H. J.: Surgical Disorders of the Peripheral Nerves. Ed. 2. Edinburgh, Churchill Livingstone, 1975.

Spinner, M.: Injuries to the Major Branches of Peripheral Nerves of the Forearm. Ed. 2. Philadelphia, W. B. Saunders Company, 1978.

Struthers, J.: On some points in the abnormal anatomy of the arm. Br. Foreign Med. Chir. Rev., *14*:170, 1854.

Sunderland, S.: Capacity of reinnervated muscles to function efficiently after prolonged denervation. Archs Neurol. Psychiat. (Chicago), *64*:755, 1950.

Sunderland, S.: Nerves and Nerve Injuries. Baltimore, The Williams & Wilkins Co., 1968.

Sunderland, S., and Bradley, K. C.: Rate of advance of Hohhmann-Tinel sign in regenerating nerves. Arch. Neurol. Psychiatr. (Chicago), *67*:650, 1952.

Thomas, J. E., and Lambert, E. H.: Ulnar nerve conduction velocity and H-reflex in infants and children. J. Appl. Physiol., *15*:1, 1960.

Tinel, J.: Le signe du "Fourmillement" dans les lésions des nerfs périphériques. Press. Med., *47*:388–389, 1915.

Vichard, P., Tropet, Y., Landecy, G., and Briot, J. F.: Paralysies radiales contemporaines des fractures de la diaphyse humérale. Chirurgie, *108*:791–795, 1982.

Wagman, I. H., and Lesse, H.: Maximum conduction velocities of motor fibers of ulnar nerve in human subjects of various ages and sizes. J. Neurophysiol., *15*:235, 1952.

Woodhall, B., and Beebe, G. W.: Peripheral Nerve Regeneration. Washington, D.C., United States Government Printing Office, 1956.

Wynn Parry, C. B.: Recent trends in surgery of peripheral nerves. Int. Rehab. Med., 3:169–173, 1981.

Zachary, R. B., and Roaf, R.: Lesions in continuity. *In* Seddon, H. J. (Editor): Peripheral Nerve Injuries. London, H. M. Stationery Office, 1954, ch. 2, p. 57.

Zilch, H., and Buck-Gramcko, D.: Ergebnisse der Nervenwiederherstellungen an der oberen Extremität durch Mikrochirurgie, Handchirurgie, 7:21–31, 1975.

Chapter 51

END RESULT ASSESSMENT FOLLOWING NERVE REPAIR AND ITS IMPLICATIONS

SYDNEY SUNDERLAND

Assessment of the end result is an essential element in the saga of nerve repair, with implications relating to the determination of disability ratings, to monitoring of the effectiveness of surgical practices and procedures, thereby ensuring the preservation of surgical standards, and to the evaluation of innovations introduced with a view to improving the generally disappointing record of nerve repair. However, before consideration of these and other issues, background information germane to the subject of end result assessment is discussed.

GENERALIZATIONS RELATING TO END RESULT ASSESSMENT

The objective of nerve repair, regardless of the particular form it takes, is to restore those connections that existed between neurons and their peripheral endings prior to the injury, so that the pattern of innervation is precisely the same as the original. Although this is an ideal that can never be realized (Sunderland, 1978), the objective remains one of at least maximizing the restoration of functionally useful pathways.

To achieve this, nerve repair must be designed not only to assist axon regeneration but, and even more important, also to ensure that regenerating axons will grow into the endoneurial tubes of the distal stump of the severed nerve in a manner that will favor the restoration of functionally useful connections with the periphery. Nerve repair, then, is concerned with much more than axon regeneration, its ultimate objective being function-

ally useful regeneration. This is the prerequisite for functionally useful recovery, and it is in the attempt to achieve this that nerve repair faces its greatest challenge.

FACTORS COMPLICATING EVALUATION OF RECOVERY ATTRIBUTABLE TO NERVE REPAIR

It is important to appreciate that the improvement following nerve repair is not due solely to nerve regeneration and tissue reinnervation. Other factors are involved whose roles and significance should be understood lest they confuse evaluation of the benefits conferred by the repair.

An all too common source of error in end result assessment studies is the failure to recognize the significance of anomalous motor and sensory innervations and the use of supplementary muscle actions to compensate for the continued paralysis or paresis of some muscles, for example, the capacity of the flexor pollicis longus to compensate for the loss of the adductor pollicis in ulnar nerve paralysis.

Non-neural factors, in the form of loss of muscle substance, the division of tendons, the formation of restrictive scar tissue and adhesions, and joint and periarticular abnormalities, should also be identified, lest their contribution to a residual disability be misinterpreted.

Finally, some of the improvements in motor performance following nerve repair could be due to the hypertrophy of reinnervated muscle fibers to compensate for those that

528

are never reinnervated. The possible role of the sensory overlap from neighboring intact cutaneous nerves, and the ingrowth of sensory terminals from the same source, in reducing the area of cutaneous sensory loss should also be constantly kept in mind.

That function can be further improved by remedial training after nerve regeneration has ceased has interesting implications. It means, inter alia, that of two patients, one may benefit still further from remedial training, whereas the other will fail to do so, despite the fact that reinnervation has suffered to the same extent in both. Expressed in another way, it means that differences in the quality of recovery do not necessarily reflect differences in reinnervation following regeneration. Account should be taken of this factor when assigning a rating to a new method of repair on the basis of the quality of the recovery. In such studies some value, no matter how subjective, must be placed on one patient's capacity to benefit from remedial training as opposed to another's inability or unwillingness to do so.

The relevance of these points to end result evaluation is illustrated by reference to an inquiry into the merits of homografting in West Germany in the early 1970's. At that time some sensational claims in favor of homografting were being made by Jacoby and his associates (1970). These impressive claims, which were in striking contrast to the experience of other surgeons, were subsequently referred to the German Society of Neurosurgeons for an opinion on the merits of the method. The society, mindful of the necessity for investigating operative successes that differed radically from those of other surgeons, set up a neutral commission to undertake a critical evaluation of Jacoby's results. He accepted a request to submit for examination by the commission the data relating to the eight patients operated on 12 to 18 months previously that he regarded as having obtained the best results. The Commission's inquiries revealed that the allegedly good results were not the result of axonal regeneration and the return of function in the repaired nerves, but were based on a misinterpretation of neurological findings (Kuhlendahl et al., 1972). This incident serves to stress the decisive importance in taking account of all possible factors in assessing the end result in order to confirm or disprove the claim that a particular innovation has been responsible for improving the quality of recovery.

THE TIME FACTOR IN END RESULT ASSESSMENT

Recovery following nerve repair is a continuing process until an end point is reached beyond which no further improvement occurs. It is not possible to determine the end point in advance of the event, because the time taken to reach it is influenced by many complex factors and so is subject to considerable individual variation.

Nerve regeneration and the functional maturation of restored pathways are usually completed within three years after the repair. Further improvement then depends on the patient's ability to exploit, by remedial training, the new but changed pattern of innervation prevailing after regeneration has ceased. This final phase of recovery in most cases continues steadily into the fifth year, but in exceptional cases it may not be completed until the tenth year, or even later. It is for this reason that some end result assessments are undertaken prematurely. With the foregoing proviso in mind, a five year end point may be regarded as a reasonable compromise for purposes of comparison. Alternatively a condition that remains unchanged for two years is unlikely to show further improvement later.

END RESULT ASSESSMENT AND EVALUATION OF INNOVATIVE PROCEDURES INTRODUCED TO IMPROVE THE RESULTS OF NERVE REPAIR

The results of nerve repair continue to be disturbingly uncertain and too often, decidedly bad, the number of unsatisfactory recoveries increasing as more critical standards for testing and evaluating function are applied. This disappointing scenario explains the ceaseless search for new ways of removing the uncertainty from surgical repair and converting it into a more consistent and rewarding undertaking. In this search for improvement it is clear that any new method, procedure, technique, or management policy directed to improving the results of nerve repair should survive only if it can be conclusively shown that it, and it alone, is responsible for the improved results. In this respect accurate end result assessments of recovery provide the only acceptable yardstick by which to judge the effectiveness of any new method or procedure. In pursuing this theme, reference should be made to the difficulty in transferring experimental physiological data to the human clinical situation and to the limited role of animal experimentation in problem solving.

In the first place, though axon counting and the detection of regenerating axons by histological and electrophysiological methods may provide information about the numbers of axons regenerating below the suture line, the outcome, particularly in mixed nerves, remains in doubt. This is because the destination of the axons is not known. Thus, motor axons could be advancing down "sensory" endoneurial tubes to the skin, and regenerating cutaneous sensory processes could be in "motor" endoneurial tubes that will take them into muscles.

Second, experimental conditions are rarely comparable to those commonly characterizing civilian accidents and battle casualties, and end result assessments in the experimental animal bear little relation to the human situation. Motor and sensory functions in the forepaws of the rat, rabbit, cat, and dog are in no way comparable to the manipulative skills and the stereognostic sense of the human hand, which are peculiarly human attributes.

One should not, therefore, lean too heavily upon experiments, which, although they may tell us much about regeneration, tell us little about the functional value of that regeneration to a patient. The use of primates in experimental studies has much to commend it, although it still falls short of the ideal.

Functionally useful motor and sensory recovery depends not only on the numbers of axons reinnervating skin and muscles, and the extent to which their structural features and physiological properties are restored but, more important, on the restoration of patterns of innervation that are the basis for the coordinated activity of groups of muscles and discriminative sensory functions. In this respect the clinic alone can provide the data on which to base decisions regarding conflicting claims.

Returning to the clinical situation, experience reveals that assigning a value to a particular method or procedure on the basis of the end result is more difficult than might at first appear. This is because establishing such a cause and effect relationship is subject to several possible sources of error.

One difficulty is that all too often references to recovery are expressed in the most general terms and lack the detail essential for a valid comparative study.

Another important source of error concerns the difficulty in excluding the influences of other variables that are coincidental contributors to the end result. It is now known that many factors combine in an exceedingly intricate manner to influence the outcome after nerve repair, and that each of these factors is, in turn, subject to a wide range of variation. As a consequence, a study to determine the relative merits of different methods or procedures should, in order to offset the influences of coexisting variables, be undertaken in patients of about the same age and with a standard type of lesion, as this relates to the nerve injured, the nature, severity, and level of the injury, the retrograde neuronal reaction to the injury, the internal structure of the nerve at the site of injury, and so on. Unfortunately this prerequisite is difficult to satisfy in clinical practice, for in no two patients are the conditions associated with the injury identical in every respect. This, however, does not deter some investigators from concentrating exclusively on a particular feature of the repair and, in doing so, overlooking the coexistence of other variables that are contributing to the end result.

END RESULT ASSESSMENT AND THE PRESERVATION OF SURGICAL STANDARDS

The outcome of any surgical procedure should always be subjected to a detailed and critical examination in order to determine in what respect the end result meets, exceeds, or falls short of expectations. In the absence of this type of scrutiny, surgery inevitably degenerates into a thoughtless mechanical exercise devoid of any hope of improvement.

END RESULT ASSESSMENT AND ITS MEDICOLEGAL IMPLICATIONS

The automobile, industry, and iatrogenic injuries from surgery, along with Workmen's Compensation and other measures for compensating the victims of accidents, have combined to create a demand for medical assessment of injuries for legal purposes, particularly when litigation is involved. In this context accurate end result assessments of nerve injury and nerve repair are essential for establishing disability ratings of patients.

END RESULT ASSESSMENT AND THE COLLECTION OF CLINICAL DATA

In civilian practice it is unusual to find clinics especially created for the exclusive study and treatment of patients with peripheral nerve injuries. On the contrary, not only are such patients dispersed geographically, but in any one area they are also treated in a variety of specialist surgical departments: orthopedic, neurological, hand, plastic, and so on. All this means that patients with nerve injuries are unlikely to accumulate in sufficient numbers in any one clinic or consulting room to satisfy the investigational instincts of the surgeon. Furthermore, when so many variables are interlocked in complex ways to influence the course of regeneration and the quality of the final recovery, it is difficult, when only a limited number of patients is available for study, to decide with certainty whether some selected variation in the repair is or is not responsible for an improved recovery.

One way of overcoming limitations imposed in this way would be to pool clinical data from several sources, in order to create a series large enough to permit meaningful comparisons and correlations. An essential prerequisite for this sort of exercise, however, is the need for standardized, precise, accurate clinical documentation relating not only to the details of the injury and the repair but also to the quality of the final recovery.

THE END RESULT ASSESSMENT

Following nerve repair, recovery proceeds somewhat irregularly, some parts of the peripheral field served by the repaired nerve recovering in advance of, and to a greater extent than, others. In general the progression is from proximal to distal, but in the final state, recovery is not uniform but presents a patchy distribution in which some muscles or cutaneous areas either fail to

recover or show residual disabilities of varying severities.

It is assumed that the reader is familiar with testing methods and the conditions under which testing is performed (Sunderland, 1978).

Regarding sensory testing, two points deserve special mention. Conventional testing for pain sensibility (pinprick) and tactile sensibility (Frey hair or its equivalent) involves the repeated application of a point stimulus over the affected cutaneous area. Even though these stimuli can be graded, this is a somewhat artificial way of testing for a sensory response because larger cutaneous areas are normally stimulated so that afferent receptors are activated not singly but in large numbers, the acuity of sensory perception being greatly increased when larger areas are stimulated. Thus, pin scratch (Denny Brown and Yanagisawa, 1973; Kirk and Denny Brown, 1970) or the use of a device that permits several needle points to be applied simultaneously to a test area (Sunderland, 1978) constitutes a more effective stimulus than do single pinpricks; light stroking with a fine wisp of cotton wool is also more effective in eliciting a response than is the application of a Frey hair. Sensory testing in these ways often elicits a response when a single sharply localized stimulus fails to do so. Moreover the results of Frey testing do not correlate well with functional sensibility.

The second point is that movement is an essential component of texture discrimination and object identification, which depend on the repetitive stimulation of a succession of quickly and slowly adapting touch receptors as the object and the skin are moved or rubbed in relation to one another between the thumb and fingers.

A study of the recovery process reveals that it proceeds in several phases, in which, as already mentioned, it is important to distinguish between axonal regeneration and functional recovery.

Phase 1

During this phase, which involves axonal regeneration, the presence and advance of growing axon tips can be detected by electrophysiological methods, or by following the progression of Hoffmann-Tinel sign. These methods give no clue to the destination of regenerating axons and so are not reliable indicators of useful regeneration.

PHASE 2

During this phase, end organ connections are re-established. Reinnervation potentials can now be detected in muscles by electromyography, and muscles respond to stimulation of the nerve trunk but not to voluntary effort. Although repeated electromyographic examinations and strength duration curve testing reveal whether reinnervation is continuing or has been arrested, the methods give no clue to the ultimate outcome, for this is expressed in terms of useful functional recovery.

The presence of fine regenerating sensory terminals in the muscles is heralded by the appearance of tenderness when the muscle is squeezed. This sign usually precedes the return of voluntary contractions and in this respect assumes prognostic significance.

The presence of regenerating sensory terminals in the skin is revealed by the appearance of the crude protective elements of cutaneous sensation, which collectively represent what is generally referred to as protopathic sensation. The skin is still insensitive to light touch, but pinprick gives rise to an extremely unpleasant, stinging, widely radiating sensation, which is difficult to localize.

PHASE 3

This phase of recovery depends on the progressive maturation of regenerated axons. It is marked by the appearance of feeble palpable muscle contractions and perhaps a flicker of movement in response to voluntary effort. Regarding sensory recovery, the unpleasant features of the protopathic response to pinprick and extremes of temperature are less pronounced, but the affected cutaneous territory remains insensitive to light touch.

Testing during this phase reveals that the conduction velocity in regenerating nerve fibers gradually improves. However, it is never fully regained. Furthermore, the conduction velocity recordings for regenerated nerve fibers do not correlate with the clinical result, and such electrical testing lacks prognostic value.

PHASE 4

This phase of recovery is dependent on increasing numbers of "axons" reaching muscles, joints, and skin and their further development into mature nerve fibers.

Motor recovery is marked by a gradual increase in the range and power of individual affected movements. This recovery is often expressed in terms of an accepted scale:

M1. Feeble contractions too weak to produce movement.

M2. Feeble movement but not against resistance or gravity. In this state the muscle may maintain a part in a position into which it has been passively moved.

M3. Movement against gravity and some resistance; easily fatigued.

M4. Movement against gravity and strong resistance; improved endurance.

M5. Normal in every respect.

A more precise assessment of motor function can be expressed in terms of the range and power of individual movements measured and compared as a percentage of the corresponding recordings on the sound side. In making such an evaluation, care should be taken to exclude the influences of uninvolved muscles.

When other muscles normally combine with the recovering muscle to produce a movement (for example, the flexor carpi radialis and the flexor carpi ulnaris combining to produce wrist flexion), the function of the affected muscle is then described as strong, weak, or feeble, depending on the state of the muscle and its tendon in response to voluntary effort as ascertained by inspection and palpation; the power, efficiency, and fatigability of the movement it is assisting to produce; and the extent to which other muscles are called upon to assist the movement (for example, the flexor pollicis longus compensating for a paresed adductor pollicis).

Assessment of motor recovery should also include a reference to any reduction in muscle wasting, as this is provided by measurements of the circumference of the limbs at standard levels. This, however, is not practicable when the parts are affected by soft tissue injury or edema. Normal lateral differences between the two limbs and the development of a use hypertrophy of uninvolved muscles on the affected or opposite side may also complicate assessments of residual wasting.

Sensory recovery during this phase is marked by the gradual reappearance of the

Table 51–1. SENSIBILITY RATINGS

Pinprick (P)	Light Touch (T)	Two Point Discrimination (D)	Ridge Test (R)	Temperature (T°)
P1 Pinprick interpreted as an ill defined change of state. This is presumably due to the deformation of deep tissues.	T1 Awareness of a change of state at high thresholds.	D1 Defective two point discrimination.	R1 Recognition only at high elevations of the ridge.	T°1 Insensitive to cold and heat except at very low (0° C.) and high (55° C.) temperatures, respectively, when the delayed effect is unpleasant.
	T2 Radiating tingling sensation. Not localized.	D2 Normal.	R2 Recognition toward the lower elevations of the ridge.	
P2 Can now distinguish between the head and point of the pin. The latter gives rise to an unpleasant stinging sensation with considerable radiation and false reference. Not localized.	T3 Light touch just perceived as such. Crude localization.		R3 Normal.	T°2 Temperatures below 15° C. and above 50° C. are readily identified as cold and hot, respectively. No appreciation of temperatures between 15 and 50° C.
	T4 Light touch readily recognized as such but with reduced acuity. Localization to within 2 cm.			
	T5 Normal.			
P3 Sharp tingling or stinging sensation with some radiation and false reference. Poor localization.				T°3 Temperatures below 25° C. and above 40° C. are correctly identified as cold and hot, respectively. No appreciation of temperatures between 25 and 40° C.
P4 A localized sensation of sharpness with no or little radiation.				
P5 Normal.				
				T°4 Normal.

discriminative aspects of sensation, such as the perception of joint movement; weight and pressure perception; the identification of degrees of sharpness; tactile, texture, and temperature discrimination; and tactile localization, all of which constitute the building blocks of the stereognostic sense.

Regarding the different cutaneous sensory modalities, a value can be assigned to each by suitably designed testing methods. All testing relates to the autonomous field served by the nerve compared with the corresponding area on the contralateral side. A suggested simplified formula for sensory recovery is shown in Table 51–1, but this could be

further simplified for rapid clinical use in the manner shown in Table 51–2.

Two point discrimination is tested in the conventional way by compass points and for the hand is regarded as the only reliable index to the functional value of sensory recovery (Hubbard, 1972; Moberg, 1958, 1960, 1962, 1975; Omer, 1974; Önne, 1962). The normal threshold for two point discrimination varies from individual to individual and from area to area over the surface of the body. Thus, normal values range from 2 to 5 mm. for the digital pads, 5 to 10 mm. for the palm, and 30 to 50 mm. for the forearm and leg. Tactile discrimination remains grossly defective with

Table 51–2. SIMPLIFIED SENSORY RECOVERY RATINGS

Sensibility	Absent	Markedly Impaired	Slightly Impaired	Normal
Protective	P0	P1	P2	P3
Tactile	T0	T1	T2	T3
Temperature	T°0	T°1	T°2	T°3
Tactile discrimination	D0	D1	D2	D3
Object identification	O0	O1	O2	O3

two point discrimination thresholds between 8 and 12 mm. and is absent with thresholds exceeding 12 mm. However, what is of more importance is the magnitude of the difference between the corresponding readings on the two sides.

Clinical tests for tactile discrimination provide the closest correlation with functional recovery. These tests reveal the patient's ability to recognize differences in the textures of fabrics of varying grades of smoothness and roughness and sandpaper of different grades of coarseness as these are rubbed across the finger tips or examined between the terminal pads of the thumb and fingers.

A useful method of testing tactile discrimination, appropriately called the ridge method, was first described by Renfrew (1960, 1969) and subsequently developed by Poppen et al. (1979). The value of the ridge test lies in the fact that it relies on movement between the skin and the surface of the object, thereby generating an array of sensory receptor activity. The device consists of a thin, smooth, rectangular block of plastic, 10 by 1.5 cm. One surface of the block carries a narrow linear ridge, which gradually increases in prominence from zero elevation at one end of the block to a height of 1.5 mm. at the other. For the purpose of rating tactile sensibility the ridge is suitably calibrated by dividing the block by transverse lines into eight 1 cm. segments, the height of the ridge in each segment exceeding that in the preceding segment. The patient is instructed to inform the examiner when, with eyes closed, he first feels an irregularity as the digit is firmly moved over the surface of the device and along the ridge, thereby bringing increasing heights of the ridge into contact with the skin. Normally the elevation is perceived within the first 1 cm. segment of the ridge. However, the greater the residual sensory defect, the higher the ridge before an irregularity is first detected; sensation may be so defective that the patient is unable to detect the ridge.

For the lower limb Clawson and Seddon (1960) have advocated a useful recovery assessment based on the daily activities of the individual. The following recovery ratings are based on their scale:

Grade 1. The limb is normal in every respect.

Grade 2. Slight generalized or localized residual disability, which appears only after long periods of walking or standing. There is no pain, and special footwear is not needed.

Grade 3. There is an obvious residual motor and sensory disability, which is maximal below the knee. Special shoes and some mechanical aid are necessary to support the arches of the foot and to assist ambulation. There is no disabling hypersensitivity of the sole and no pain, but the leg and foot ache after prolonged use of the limb.

Grade 4. Walking is greatly restricted. There is troublesome hypersensitivity of the sole and moderate to severe pain. Despite attention to foot toilet, pressure sores develop, but they can be controlled. The disability is sufficiently marked to limit the choice of an occupation.

Grade 5. Motor and sensory functions are grossly impaired, and there are marked troublesome trophic changes and severe incapacitating pain, which is often causalgic. These are the cases that raise the question of amputation.

PHASE 5

This phase of recovery involves the restoration of the motor and sensory mechanisms by which the various sensory modalities and individual muscles are integrated to permit the efficient performance of a wide range of normal daily activities. It is dependent on the re-establishment of correct end organ relationships so that the new pattern of innervation is precisely the same as the original. This is essential for the complete recovery of complex movements and, in the case of the hand, manipulative skills and the return of the refinements of sensory perception and acuity that are essential for object identification and the normal use of the hand in the efficient performance of daily tasks.

However, following surgical repair, the loss of some axons at the suture line and the entry of others into foreign endoneurial tubes mean that the restored pattern of innervation is both defective and incomplete in comparison with the original. Structural imperfections originating in this way impair function and, in the case of the hand, limit its efficient use in the performance of normal daily tasks.

In this respect it is important to remember that motor and sensory functions are interdependent. Thus, much of a residual motor disability may be due to a sensory defect rather than to muscle weakness. At the same time, objects must be handled as well as felt in order to give full scope to sensory discrimination and object identification.

Clinical tests to evaluate this final phase of recovery should be directed to the patient's ability to cope with a wide range of daily activities. Such tests are limited only by the ingenuity of the clinician and the time at his disposal. How rapidly and efficiently can the patient pick up and handle dexterously a series of objects of varying sizes and shapes, both with and without visual supervision? How accurately can he recognize objects solely by feeling and handling them? Does the patient know whether he is holding an object when the act cannot be checked visually? Is he constantly dropping objects and injuring affected skin and joints? Does the hand become useless in the dark or when he is unable to see what he is attempting to do with it? Are movements clumsily performed because of a lack of sensory information and persisting muscle weakness and incoordination, when carrying out such daily tasks as shaving, dressing and undressing, writing, sewing, cooking and handling cutlery, tools and utensils? The list could easily be extended. Admittedly it is often difficult to put a value, other than one expressed in subjective terms, on these refinements of functional recovery, but unless end result assessments include a reference to them, the evaluations will have limited value as a basis for comparing the relative merits of different procedures and techniques.

Finally, it is a matter of common observation in everyday life that motor performance and sensory acuity can be greatly improved by practice and experience. It should not, therefore, be surprising that in well motivated patients, intensive remedial training with, and later without, visual guidance can be effective in improving the quality of the recovery after nerve repair (Bowden, 1954; Davis, 1949; Dellon et al., 1974; Omer, 1973; Sunderland, 1978). In evaluating the end result it is therefore important not to overlook the fact that the residual motor and sensory disability consequent on incomplete and imperfect axonal regeneration can be improved by retraining directed to increasing the patient's ability to use, to greater advantage, new and altered patterns of motor and sensory innervation.

In this respect the very young are known to have a decided advantage. Almquist and Eeg-Olofsson (1970) attributed the better results in children after nerve repair to the adaptability of the young patient's sensory cortex rather than to peripheral factors such as the maturation of regenerated nerve fibers. They also reported that good two point discrimination was never restored in patients more than 10 years old. In the author's experience the younger teenager also enjoys some advantages in this respect, and it is always well worth exploiting the regeneration that has occurred in the adult by intensive remedial retraining.

The basis for this continued improvement in function is, presumably, the adaptive readjustment of flexible patterns of activity at central levels. The readjustments permit the more effective use of reinnervated muscles while sensory mechanisms are no longer unresponsive to the altered signal patterns reaching them from the periphery, so that the patient learns to recognize and identify an altered profile of sensory impulses and to relate the new sensations to a past event. With the passage of time the dedicated patient has a remarkable capacity for improving the quality of the recovery and for adjusting to his residual disability.

It is difficult to put a time limit on this last phase of recovery, depending as it does on a further set of factors such as the general attitude, intelligence, patience, perseverance, and motivation of the patient. It is a slow process, and certainly extends into the fifth year; in some patients it can extend well beyond this time. Therefore, although it is true that the effects of some "methods on trial" may be immediately apparent, it may not be possible to assess others until many years after the repair. From this it is clear that many end result assessments have been and continue to be made prematurely.

MISCELLANEOUS FACTORS AFFECTING THE END RESULT

While attention is concentrated on the restoration of motor and sensory functions after nerve repair, it is important not to overlook the adverse effects that persistent pain and residual trophic changes can have on the final outcome.

INCOMPLETE OR FAILED SYMPATHETIC REINNERVATION

Sympathetic nerve fiber regeneration and reinnervation generally follow the same pattern as that recorded for somatic nerves; sympathetic responses gradually improve although secretion of sweat remains depressed in most patients. Önne (1962) was unable to detect any correlation between the functional value of restored sensation and secretion of sweat.

Observations in patients with sympathectomized limbs indicate that the loss of sympathetic innervation does not adversely affect somatic motor or sensory function. However, troublesome trophic disturbances are more likely to develop and persist when sympathetic denervation is associated with a residual sensory defect.

RESIDUAL TROPHIC CHANGES

The trophic regulatory control that the nervous system exercises over the skin and subcutaneous tissues is served by sensory and sympathetic fibers, which combine to control the complex nutritional requirements of these tissues.

Following denervation, the general appearance, color, and texture of the skin change, the terminal digital pads atrophy, and the skin becomes dry and unduly susceptible to injury and ulceration from even minor trauma. With reinnervation these trophic disturbances regress, but in the absence of satisfactory reinnervation they persist and may severely restrict the usefulness of the part. The end result assessment should carry a reference to the adverse effect that any such trophic disturbance may have on function.

PERSISTENT PAIN AND TROUBLESOME DYSESTHESIAS

Pain and discomfort often make an appearance during regeneration when a sensitive neuroma develops at the site of the repair, the cutaneous field previously insensitive becomes hyperalgesic, and there are tenderness and aching in recovering muscles. These sensory disturbances normally regress with advancing recovery. However, the development of an exquisitely sensitive and painful neuroma at the suture line or the development and persistence of hyperalgesia and hyperpathia in the cutaneous field of the recovering nerve may severely restrict the usefulness of the hand or foot. The end result assessment should detail this information. Thus, the distressing hyperesthesias of the sole that often follow repair of the tibial nerve below the origin of the branches innervating the calf muscles may leave the patient worse off than before.

Causalgia is a special case: when it is present, spontaneous pain may be so severe and compelling that it incapacitates the patient and makes him a nervous wreck, despite the state of motor and sensory function.

CONCLUDING COMMENT

It should never be forgotten that many factors combine in complex ways to influence regeneration and the quality of the recovery. Concentration on one factor to the exclusion of others involves its abstraction from the total reality under investigation. Unless consideration is given to what is being left out of immediate account, the results of such studies are capable of grave misinterpretation. A worthwhile innovation may be inadvertently judged valueless and a worthless one incorrectly claimed to be of value.

REFERENCES

Almquist, E., and Eeg-Olofsson, O.: Sensory-nerve conduction velocity and two-point discrimination in sutured nerves. J. Bone Joint Surg. *52A:*791, 1970.

Bowden, R. E. M.: Factors influencing functional recovery. *In* Seddon, H. J. (Ed.): Peripheral Nerve Injuries. Medical Research Council Special Report Series No. 282. London, H. M. Stationary Office, 1954, p. 298.

Clawson, D. K., and Seddon, H. J.: The late consequences of sciatic nerve injury. J. Bone Joint Surg., *42B:*213, 1960.

Davis, D. R.: Some factors affecting the results of treatment of peripheral nerve injuries. Lancet, *1:*877, 1949.

Dellon, A. L., Curtis, R. M., and Edgerton, M. T.: Reeducation of sensation in the hand after nerve injury and repair. Plast. Reconstr. Surg., *53:*297, 1974.

Denny-Brown, D., and Yanagisawa, N.: The function of the descending root of the fifth nerve. Brain, *96:*783, 1973.

Hubbard, J. H.: The quality of nerve regeneration. Factors independent of the most skillful repair. Surg. Clin. North Am., *52:*1099, 1972.

Jacoby, W., Fahlbusch, R., Mackert, B., Braun, B., Rolle, J., and Schnell, J.: Überbrückung peripherer

Nervendefekte mit lyophilisierten und desantigenisierten homologen Transplantaten. Münch. Med Wochenschr., *112*:586, 1970.

Kirk, E. J., and Denny-Brown, D.: Functional variation in dermatomes in the macaque monkey following dorsal root lesions. J. Comp. Neurol., *139*:307, 1970.

Kuhlendahl, H., Mumenthaler, M., Penzholz, H., Röttgen, P., Schliack, H., and Struppler, A.: The treatment of peripheral nerve injuries with homologous nerve grafts. Acta Neurochir., *26*:339, 1972.

Moberg, E.: Objective methods for determining the functional value of sensibility in the hand. J. Bone Joint Surg., *40B*:454, 1958.

Moberg, E.: Evaluation of sensibility in the hand. Surg. Clin. North Am., *40*:357, 1960.

Moberg, E.: Criticism and study of methods of examining sensibility in the hand. Neurology (Minneap.), *12*:8, 1962.

Moberg, E.: Method of examining sensibility of the hand. *In* Flynn, J. E. (Ed.): Hand Surgery. Ed. 2. Baltimore, The Williams & Wilkins Company, 1975.

Omer, G. E.: Sensibilité et sensations au niveau de la main. Ann. Chir., *27*:479, 1973.

Omer, G. E.: Injuries to nerves of the upper extremity. J. Bone Joint Surg., *56A*:1615, 1974.

Önne, L.: Recovery of sensibility and sudomotor activity in the hand after nerve suture. Acta Chir. Scand., Suppl. 300, 1962.

Poppen, N. K.: Clinical evaluation of the von Frey and two point discrimination tests and correlation with a dynamic test of sensibility. *In* Jewett, D. L., and McCarroll, H. R. (Eds.): Symposium on Nerve Repair: Its Clinical and Experimental Basis. St. Louis, The C. V. Mosby Company, 1979.

Poppen, N. K., McCarroll, H. R., Doyle, J. R., and Niebauer, J. J.: Recovery of sensibility after suture of digital nerves. J. Hand Surg., *4*:212, 1979.

Renfrew, S.: Aesthiometers. Lancet, *1*:1011, 1960.

Renfrew, S.: Fingertip sensation. A routine neurological test. Lancet, *1*:396, 1969.

Sunderland, S.: Nerves and Nerve Injuries. Ed. 2. Edinburgh, Churchill Livingstone, 1978.

PERIPHERAL NERVE REPAIR

Chapter 52

SURGICAL APPROACHES TO THE NERVES OF THE UPPER LIMB

Marius Fahrer

Of the many and varied surgical approaches to the nerves of the upper limb, the ones selected for inclusion in this chapter are the simplest, and few alternatives are given. This chapter is intended as a practical guide. Exposure of the brachial plexus from neck to axilla is treated elsewhere in this volume.*

EXPOSURE OF THE AXILLARY NERVE

The frame of the quadrangular space and the two divisions of the axillary nerve running around the posterior aspect of the surgical neck of the humerus can be well exposed from the posterior aspect.

POSTERIOR SHOULDER APPROACH (KOCHER MODIFICATION)

The skin is incised from the tip of the acromion along the acromion and the spine

---

*See Chapter 49.

of the scapula to the base of the spine (Fig. 52–1). After retraction of the skin and superficial fascia, the origins of the posterior head of the deltoid are exposed and detached from the bone by subperiosteal dissection (to minimize bleeding). The muscle is then reflected laterally and separated from the underlying infraspinatus muscle. (Often muscular fibers and a common fascia connect these muscles, complicating the dissection.) The teres minor muscle is then identified; the origin of the deltoid should not extend beyond the lateral border of the latter.

The axillary nerve is exposed in the quadrangular space (limited above by the teres minor, below by the teres major, medially by the long head of the triceps, and laterally by the humerus). It runs proximally to the posterior circumflex artery and to the venae commitantes as it follows its circumflex course around the surgical neck of the humerus. At this level the nerve is not in direct contact with the bone (it is maintained against the deep surface of the deltoid by a strong fascia) and divides into its two branches—posterior and anterior. The posterior branch

539

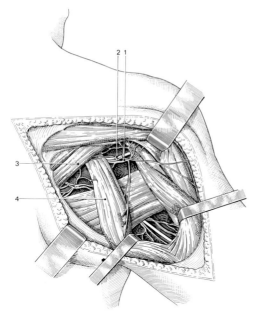

Figure 52–1. Exposure of the axillary nerve by the posterior shoulder approach (modified Kocher approach). The nerve is found in the humeral-tricipital space (quadrilateral space of Velpeau) constituted by the teres minor at the top, the teres major below, the humerus laterally, and the long head of the triceps medially. Below the teres major, visible when the long portion of the triceps is retracted, may be seen the radial nerve with the deep muscular branch of the brachial artery. 1 = posterior circumflex artery, 2 = axillary nerve, 3 = teres minor, and 4 = long head of triceps.

gives off a cutaneous branch for the shoulder, winding around the posterior border of the deltoid before piercing the investing fascia and becoming superficial. A branch for the teres minor, originating from a common trunk with the cutaneous branch, was found in 26 of 36 cases—a ganglion-like swelling before the nerve reaches the muscle but there are no ganglionic nerve cells in this swelling (Gitlin, 1957). The branch for the spinous (posterior) head of the deltoid penetrates the muscle through its deep aspect after a short horizontal course.

The anterior branch supplies the acromial (middle) and clavicular (anterior) heads of the deltoid muscle. The separate innervation of the posterior head of the deltoid opens the possibility of an alternative approach, the posterior "inverted U."

ABBOT AND LUCAS INVERTED U APPROACH (BOYD, 1961)

The skin incision starts at the level of the ascending branch 5 cm. distal to the spine of the scapula, in its medial third (Fig. 52–2). The horizontal part of the inverted U runs over the spine. The descending branch starts at the angle of the acromion and runs 7.5 to 8 cm. over the space between the posterior and lateral heads of the deltoid. After dissection of the skin and fascia, the posterior head of the deltoid is detached subperiostally from

the spine. The posterior and lateral heads are separated by dissection along the muscular fibers; the splitting of the muscle will coincide with the gap between the anterior and posterior branches of the axillary nerve and posterior circumflex artery. Separation of the muscular heads permits minimal dissection of the skin. The large flap of skin and muscle that results can be turned down to expose the infraspinatus and teres minor muscles and the quadrangular space.

SUPRASCAPULAR NERVE

The lower part of the suprascapular nerve, behind the neck of the scapula and in the

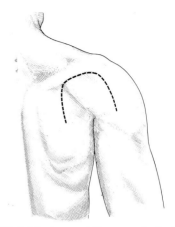

Figure 52–2. The inverted U approach. Incision line.

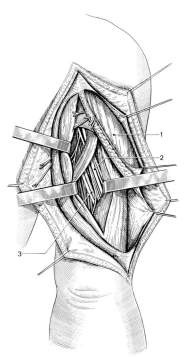

Figure 52–3. Radial nerve. The posterior brachial approach (after Henry). 1 = deltoid, 2 = radial nerve, and 3 = profunda brachii artery.

infraspinous fossa, can be approached via the same posterior exposures, after reflecting downward or dividing the infraspinatus.

RADIAL NERVE

POSTERIOR BRACHIAL APPROACH

Henry (1957) exposes the radial nerve as it leaves the axilla and winds behind the humerus (Fig. 52–3). At this level the nerve is liable to be involved in the complications of fractures of the humeral shaft. The skin is incised from the middle of the posterior border of the deltoid downward to the olecranon. After dissection of the skin and superficial fascia, the deep fascia is divided between the long and lateral heads of the triceps and the space is opened by blunt dissection. The radial nerve and profunda brachii artery and veins run between the origins of the medial and lateral heads of the triceps, crossing the spiral groove at acute angles. The exposure can be completed distally by dividing the lateral head of the triceps.

ANTEROLATERAL BRACHIAL APPROACH

The posterior brachial approach can be modified and combined with Henry's anterolateral approach to the elbow in order to expose the radial nerve in the lower third of the arm and its division into the anterior superficial and posterior interosseous nerves. The skin is incised vertically between the brachialis and the brachioradialis muscles. The incision can be extended dorsally toward the lateral epicondyle and then forward and distally over the extensor carpi radialis longus and the brachioradialis. The fascia between the brachialis and brachioradialis is incised and the interval is exposed by blunt dissection. The radial nerve runs in the intermuscular space filled with fat and can be traced from the lateral intermuscular septum proximally to its bifurcation inside the radial tunnel (Lister et al., 1979; Roles and Maudsley, 1972; Fig. 52–4).

For a more extensive exposure of the posterior interosseous nerve, the skin incision is prolonged distally on the anterior border of the brachioradialis and then extended backward below the lateral epicondyle and down-

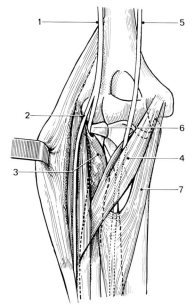

Figure 52–4. The radial and median nerves at the elbow. Note the division of the radial nerve inside the radial tunnel and the relationship of the median nerve to the pronator teres. 1 = radial nerve, 2 = superficial branch, 3 = supinator, 4 = pronator teres (humeral head), 5 = median nerve descending between the two heads of the pronator teres, 6 = posterior interosseous nerve entering arcade of Frohse, and 7 = arcade of flexor digitorum superficialis.

ward behind the extensor carpi radialis brevis (Littler, 1964; Fig. 52–5). The space between the latter and the lateral border of the extensor digitorum (communis) is defined, after which the strong investing fascia of the upper third of the forearm can be incised proximally, in continuation with the natural plane of cleavage. The supinator muscle forms the floor of the exposed area. The posterior interosseous nerve divides either inside the supinator or, more commonly, below the supinator into five to seven branches (Hovelacque, 1927). The superficial branches have a recurrent course, running between the supinator and the extensor digitorum; a blunt dissection of the space between the two muscles may endanger these superficial branches (Spinner, 1972). As the posterior interosseous nerve courses under the supinator, the nerve is crossed by transverse fibers of this muscle. In 30 per cent of the adults examined, Spinner (1968) found this arcade of Frohse to be fibrous and therefore capable of compressing the nerve.

POSTERIOR INTEROSSEOUS NERVE

The posterior interosseous nerve can be approached in the distal half of the forearm for resection as part of a partial or total denervation of the painful wrist joint (Wilhelm, 1966). We follow the technique developed by Buck-Gramcko (1977).

A transverse skin incision is made on the dorsum of the forearm about 7 cm. above the radiocarpal joint line. Dissection of skin and fascia is carried out. The tendons or muscle bellies of the extensor digitorum (communis) and extensor pollicis longus are retracted ulnarward and the extensors carpi radiales longus and brevis and the abductor pollicis longus are retracted radially. The nerve is exposed on the dorsum of the interosseous membrane.

MEDIAN NERVE

As it leaves the axilla, the median nerve runs in front and lateral to the brachial artery. In the middle third of the arm the nerve crosses in front of the artery and courses medial to it. In the arm the nerve can be exposed in the medial bicipital sulcus.

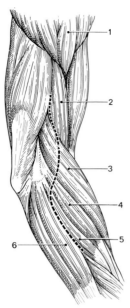

Figure 52–5. Henry's anterolateral approach (modified by Littler) exposes the radial nerve in the lower third of the arm and its division into the anterior and posterior (interosseous) branches. 1 = deltoid, 2 = brachialis, 3 = brachioradialis, 4 = extensor carpi radialis longus, 5 = extensor carpi radialis brevis, and 6 = extensor (communis) digitorum.

MEDIAL NEUROVASCULAR APPROACH IN THE ARM

The site of the incision is given by a line connecting the apex of the axilla to the middle of the cubital fossa (medial side of the biceps tendon; Fig. 52–6). The ulnar nerve also can be exposed on this incision line in the upper and middle thirds of the arm. The relations of the median nerve and brachial artery have already been mentioned.

In the cubital fossa the median nerve lies between the brachial artery and the biceps tendon under the biceps aponeurotic expansion. In the forearm the course of the median nerve can be projected as a line joining the medial aspect of the biceps tendon to the medial aspect of the tendon of the flexor carpi radialis above the wrist. Because of the variable relations of the median nerve (83.3 per cent of the cases between the two heads of the muscle [Fig. 52–4], in 8.7 per cent deep to the muscle [the ulnar head being absent], in 6 per cent deep to the ulnar head, and in 2 per cent through the humeral head; Jamieson and Anson, 1952), Spinner recommends Littler's exposure.

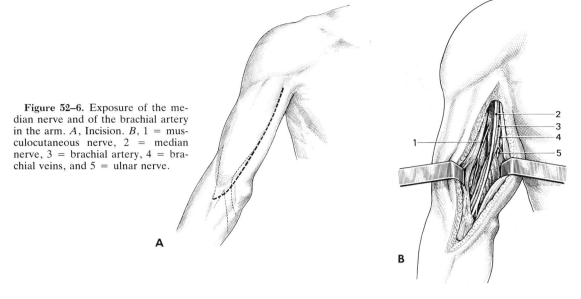

Figure 52–6. Exposure of the median nerve and of the brachial artery in the arm. *A*, Incision. *B*, 1 = musculocutaneous nerve, 2 = median nerve, 3 = brachial artery, 4 = brachial veins, and 5 = ulnar nerve.

LITTLER APPROACH FOR THE MEDIAN NERVE IN THE FOREARM (1964)

The skin is incised along the medial border of the pronator teres, and then along a sinuous course down the anterior forearm it parallels the wrist flexion crease and follows the medial border of the thenar crease in the hand (Fig. 52–7). After division of the fascia, the nerve is exposed above the biceps aponeurotic expansion and traced distally, through the heads of the pronator teres and the flexor digitorum superficialis. At this level the branches of the median nerve arise from its medial and posterior aspects. The anterior interosseous nerve (the main branch originating from the posterior surface of the nerve) can be compressed by the deep (ulnar) head of the pronator teres (Fig. 52–8).

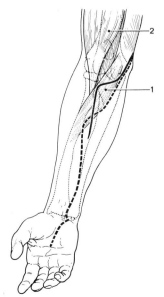

Figure 52–7. Exposure of the median nerve in the elbow and forearm (after Littler). 1 = pronator teres, and 2 = biceps.

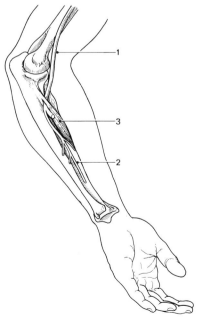

Figure 52–8. Potential compression: fibrous arch of the deep head of the pronator teres. 1 = median nerve, 2 = anterior interosseous nerve, and 3 = deep head of pronator teres.

In the lower end of the palm the palmar cutaneous branch of the median nerve arises from the lateral aspect of the nerve. It runs parallel to the nerve on its lateral side, lateral to the tendon of the palmaris longus. As this tendon divides into its thenar and palmar slips, the palmar cutaneous branch becomes superficial, running through a buttonhole in the tendinous bifurcation. In exposing the nerve in the palm, it is safe to dissect the end of the palmaris longus tendon in order to expose and spare this palmar branch.

In the carpal canal the median nerve runs anterior to the tendons. When opening the flexor retinaculum to expose the nerve, the following points should be remembered:

1. The flexor retinaculum must be divided completely; it is much deeper than expected.

2. The retinaculum should be divided near its ulnar border in order to protect the nerve.

3. Two variations of the median nerve can complicate this rather simple procedure—the exceptionally rare duplication of the median nerve, in which the anterior division runs anterior to the flexor retinaculum, and the much more common one, in which the recurrent thenar branch runs through an orifice or canal through the flexor retinaculum.

The thenar branch can be approached

through the incision used for the opening of the carpal canal.

The digital nerves can be exposed in the distal part of the palm and proximal part of the finger by digitopalmar incisions. If the normal relations are distorted by Dupuytren's bands, the nerves should be exposed in the lumbrical canals and safely traced from there proximally and distally.

ULNAR NERVE

In the upper two-thirds of the arm the ulnar nerve can be exposed by the medial neurovascular approach described for the median nerve (Fig. 52–6). At the level of the humeral midshaft the ulnar nerve pierces the medial intermuscular septum and becomes posterior. In the lower third of the arm and the elbow area, the ulnar nerve can be exposed from behind, in the groove between the medial epicondyle and the olecranon (Fig. 52–9).

Posterior Approach at the Elbow

The skin is incised by a medial longitudinal incision, 10 cm. long, centered behind the medial epicondyle (Fig. 52–10). The deep fascia is divided and the nerve, identified as it passes behind the medial epicondyle, can then be freed upward and downward. This exposure can be used for anterior transpositions of the nerve as well as for exploring the cubital tunnel in cases of entrapment of the nerve, because of the fibrous arch joining the two heads of the flexor carpi ulnaris or an anomalous anconeus epitrochlearis muscle.

In the lower two-thirds of the forearm the ulnar nerve runs under the flexor carpi ulnaris muscle, with the ulnar artery and its venae comitantes lateral to it. It can be exposed through a longitudinal anteromedial incision on the lateral border of the muscle.

In the wrist and hand the nerve can be compressed at three different levels in a course of less than 2 cm. (Fahrer and Millroy, 1981):

1. In the ulnar nerve canal, between the volar carpal ligament and the flexor retinaculum (Fig. 52–11).

2. In Guyon's "loge," located distal to the canal, in the basal area of the thenar eminence.

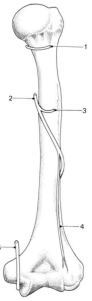

Figure 52–9. The nerves related to the posterior aspect of the humerus. 1 = axillary nerve, 2 = radial nerve, 3 = branch to lateral head of triceps, 4 = branch to lower part of medial head of triceps and anconeus, and 5 = ulnar nerve.

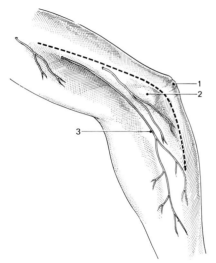

Figure 52–10. Posterior approach at the elbow for exploring the cubital tunnel. The ulnar nerve can be transposed anteriorly by the same approach. 1 = olecranon, 2 = medial epicondyle, and 3 = branches of the medial cutaneous nerve of the forearm.

3. The motor branch can be compressed under the fibrous arch of origin of the abductor digiti minimi and flexor digiti minimi brevis. A few millimeters distally, it can be compressed from behind by the fibrous arch of origin of the opponens digiti minimi muscle.

EXPOSURE OF THE DISTAL ULNAR NERVE

The skin is incised along a sinuous line, starting 5 cm. above the wrist, curving along

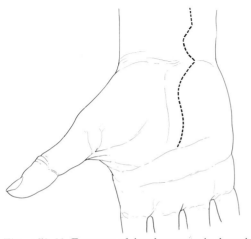

Figure 52–11. Exposure of the ulnar nerve in the wrist and palm. The incision is shown.

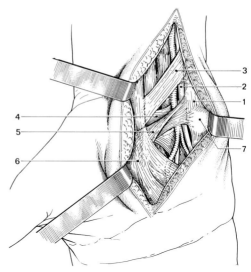

Figure 52–12. Exposure of the ulnar nerve in the palm. Superficial plane. 1 = tendon of flexor carpi ulnaris, 2 = ulnar nerve, 3 = volar carpal ligament forming the roof of the tunnel, 4 = flexor retinaculum, 5 = superficial tendon fibers of flexor carpi ulnaris running into the palmar aponeurosis, 6 = palmar aponeurosis, and 7 = pisiform bone.

the distal wrist crease and running in the palm over the hook of the hamate (Fig. 52–12). After dissection of the skin and fascia, the volar carpal ligament is divided to expose the ulnar nerve and artery in the ulnar nerve canal (Fig. 52–13). The thick retinaculum is

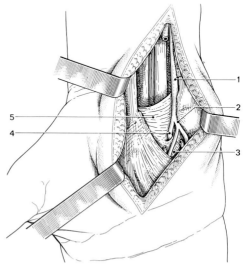

Figure 52–13. Exposure of the ulnar nerve in the palm. The volar carpal ligament is excised. 1 = ulnar nerve proximal to its division, 2 = superficial branch of the ulnar nerve, 3 = abductor digiti minimi, 4 = deep branch of the ulnar nerve running under the fibrous arch of the origin of the abductor and short flexor of the little finger, and 5 = flexor retinaculum.

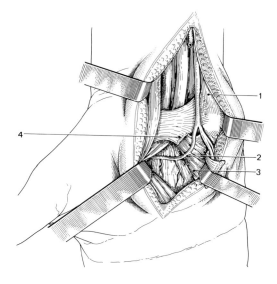

Figure 52–14. Exposure of the ulnar nerve in the palm. The apex of the hook of the hamate bone is resected. The fibrous arch of origin of the abductor and flexor brevis digiti minimi is retracted medially. The flexor tendons are retracted laterally. The deep branch of the ulnar nerve is now fully exposed. 1 = tendon of the flexor carpi ulnaris, 2 = deep branch of the ulnar nerve, 3 = opponens digiti minimi, and 4 = flexor retinaculum on the resected hook of the hamate.

incised with the skin over Guyon's canal, and the palmaris brevis muscle is then divided to expose the division of the ulnar nerve into its motor and digital branches. The lateral part of the fibrous arch of the abductor and flexor brevis is detached from the hook of the hamate and carefully retracted medially, avoiding damage to the branches innervating the hypothenar muscles (Fig. 52–14). The deep motor branch is then exposed at its origin. It can be explored further in the palm, together with the deep palmar arch, by laterally retracting the flexor tendons with the lumbricals (Fig. 52–15).

EXPOSURE OF THE DORSAL CUTANEOUS BRANCH

The skin is incised on a longitudinal line along the medial border of flexor carpi ulnaris, starting about 10 cm. above the ulnar head. The skin is dissected and the dorsal cutaneous branch exposed, piercing the deep fascia about 2 cm. proximal to the ulnar head. If the branch pierces the fascia below the level of the ulnar head, the fascia is incised on the border of the flexor carpi ulnaris, the muscle is retracted laterally, and the dorsal

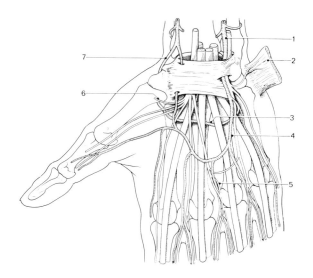

Figure 52–15. Relationship between the arteries and the terminal branches of the median and ulnar nerves in the palm. 1 = ulnar artery, 2 = palmaris brevis, 3 = deep palmar arch, 4 = superficial palmar arch, 5 = Hartmann's loop around a digital artery, 6 = recurrent branch of the median nerve, and 7 = radial artery.

branch is exposed as it runs parallel to the ulnar nerve.

EXPOSURE OF THE MEDIAL COLLATERAL DIGITAL BRANCH AT THE BASE OF THE LITTLE FINGER

If retracted fibrous bands alter the relations of the digital nerves in Dupuytren's contracture, the medial collateral digital nerve of the little finger can be found in the fibrous angle formed by the band of the superficial transverse metacarpal (natatory) ligament laterally and the lateral cutaneous tendon of the abductor digiti minimi medially (Tubiana, 1975).

REFERENCES

Buck-Gramcko, D.: Denervation of the wrist joint. J. Hand Surg., 2:54–61, 1977.

Boyd, H. B.: In Campbell's Operative Orthopaedics. Ed. 4. St. Louis, The C. V. Mosby Company, 1963.

Fahrer, M., and Millroy, P. J.: Ulnar compression neuropathy due to an anomalous abductor digiti min-imi. Clinical and anatomical study. J. Hand Surg., 6, 1981.

Gitlin, G.: Concerning the gangliform enlargement (pseudoganglion) on the nerve to the teres minor muscle. J. Anat., 91:466–470, 1957.

Henry, A. K.: Extensile exposure. Ed. 2. Edinburgh, E. & S. Livingstone, 1957.

Hovelacque, A.: Anatomie des nerfs craniens et rachidiens et du systeme grand sympathique. Paris, G. Doin, 1927.

Jamieson, R. W., and Anson, B. J.: The relation of the median nerve to the heads of origin of the pronator teres muscle. A study of 300 specimens. Quart. Bull. Northwest. Univ. Med. School, 26:34–35, 1952.

Lister, G. D., Belsole, R. B., and Kleinert, H. E.: The radial tunnel syndrome. J. Hand Surg., 4:52–59, 1979.

Littler, J. W.: Principles of reconstructive surgery of the hand. In Converse, J. M. (Editor): Reconstructive Plastic Surgery. Philadelphia, W. B. Saunders Company, 1964.

Roles, N. C., and Maudsley, R. H.: Radial tunnel syndrome: resistant tennis elbow as a nerve entrapment. J. Bone Joint Surg., 54B:499–508, 1972.

Spinner, M.: The arcade of Frohse and its relationship to posterior interosseous nerve paralysis. J. Bone Joint Surg., 50B:809–812, 1968.

Spinner, M.: Injuries to the Major Branches of Peripheral Nerves of the Forearm. Philadelphia, W. B. Saunders Company, 1972.

Tubiana, R.: Personal communication, 1975.

Wilhelm, A.: Die Gelenkdenervation und ihre anatomihschen Grundalagen. Hefte Unfallheilk., 86:1–109, 1966.

Chapter 53

GENERAL PRINCIPLES OF NERVE REPAIR

Donal M. Brooks

In 1872, just over 100 years ago, Silas Weir Mitchell published his book, *Injuries of Nerves*. His observations were based on experience gained in the American Civil War. The impetus of two World Wars has done much to increase our knowledge of these injuries and to stimulate the formulation of principles of nerve repair, but the technical problem of reuniting a severed nerve has not been solved in a satisfactory manner.

When it is considered that a severe nerve comprises tens of thousands of axons on one end, destined for an equal number of empty Schwann sheaths on the other, it is remarkable how successful our crude surgical endeavors can be.

It was thought by some that the advent of the operating microscope would go a long way toward solving at least the problem of accurate apposition of nerve ends. It soon became apparent, however, that such a technique involving the suturing of funicular nerves could be applied only when the topographical arrangements of the nerve bundles were identical. Because nerves are often crushed at the time of injury, unless divided in the source of an operation, some resection of the damaged stumps is inevitable. With trimming, the topographical arrangement changes rapidly. Thus, when it comes to the practical task of uniting the nerve ends under a microscope, funicular apposition made possible by the increased magnification becomes even less tidy than a well executed epineural repair. Millesi (1967) has to a certain extent overcome this problem. He inserts strands of cutaneous nerve between the nerve ends and matches the bundle arrangements as best he can.

FACTORS INFLUENCING RECOVERY AFTER NERVE REPAIR

TIME AFTER INJURY

In theory a nerve should be repaired as soon as possible after it has been divided. In practice this is not always desirable. For example, injuries involving tendon, bone, and nerve require, first, stabilization of the fracture, second, repair of the tendon, and last, suturing of the nerve. Our experience in the Second World War showed that the quality of recovery after nerve repair began to deteriorate when more than six months had elapsed after the injury (Medical Research Council, 1954). Perhaps even more important from the surgeon's point of view is the fact that within this period time, the results do not differ significantly.

PRIMARY AND SECONDARY NERVE SUTURING

The controversy between the supporters of primary and secondary nerve repairs will never be settled by argument; fortunately, the outcome is unimportant. When local conditions at the primary operation are not favorable for formal nerve repair, the nerve ends should be simply tacked together to prevent retraction and to preserve their correct orientation. There are those who advocate the use of Silastic nerve cuffs to facilitate secondary nerve repair. One thing is certain: when tendons and nerves are simultaneously damaged at the level of the wrist, secondary nerve repair should not be undertaken until tendon function is virtually normal. This may mean a delay of six to eight weeks. Premature surgery can cause gross adhesions.

EFFECT OF DELAY IN MUSCLE

Denervation of muscle leads to wasting and loss of its normal electrical excitability in response to a short-diuration stimulus. After prolonged denervation certain changes take place within the muscle, giving rise to fibro-fatty infiltration of contractile tissue. These changes take 18 months to two years to develop fully. They are accelerated if in addition to nerve damage there is an element of muscle ischemia. In cases of severe injury, denervated muscle histologically resembles tendon.

The practical significance of this effect is such that it imposes a time limit for nerve repair, after which motor recovery cannot be expected to occur. This time limit is about 18 months and clearly is related to the distance between the site of injury and the motor point of the nearest muscle.

EFFECT OF DELAY ON SENSORY FUNCTION

No such time limit exists for the return of sensory function. We have, in fact, repaired nerves 25 years after injury to restore protective sensitibility in the hand. Sensory end organs are capable of regeneration irrespective of the delay in nerve repair. Naturally the quality of sensibility regained is affected by the time that has elapsed since injury.

In a late nerve repair the practical problem of uniting a normal sized proximal stump to a grossly shrunken distal stump arises. This can be overcome to a certain extent by a surgical technique, but the suture line is never very satisfactory.

SITE OF THE LESION

PROXIMAL LESIONS

The site of the lesion has an important bearing on the prospects for recovery after nerve repair. The more proximal the lesion, the less chance there is of a functional recov-

ery in the distal muscles. The rate of nerve regeneration is approximately 2 mm. a day. In high lesions, therefore, by the time the axons have reached the extremity of the limb, the adverse changes in muscle referred to earlier have occurred.

Although regular stimulation of the denervated muscle by application of long-duration electrical current can delay the onset of these muscle changes (Jackson, 1945), evidence has been accumulated to confirm that it cannot prevent them. Our present state of knowledge does not justify the regular use of electrotherapy or confirm the hope of earlier investigators that it would improve the quality of motor recovery after nerve repair.

It seems probable that there are other factors responsible for the poor recovery after repair of high lesions. It may be that changes in the anterior horn cells that can be demonstrated in proximal neural lesions determine the capacity of the cell to support a long column of axoplasm (Platt, 1920). There is no doubt that as regeneration progresses distally, the rate becomes progressively slower, as shown in Peacock (1963).

From a surgical standpoint, this means that in open wounds of the brachial plexus, the only part of the plexus worth repairing is the upper trunk because of the relatively short distance required for axonal regeneration (Brooks, 1949). In the lower limb, repair of the sciatic nerve above the lower third of the thigh will not enable the patient to discard a toe-raising apparatus, but will give useful recovery in the calf muscle and may confer some sensibility on the sole of the foot (Clawson, 1960).

DISTAL LESIONS

Distal lesions have their own special problems. When a nerve is damaged at the point where it breaks up into its terminal branches, such as the ulnar nerve at the level of the pisiform, or the median nerve in the distal half of the carpal tunnel, the surgeon is faced with the difficulty of uniting three or four distal branches to a single proximal stump. While this can be achieved by direct suturing, a case can be made for nerve grafting in such circumstances. Furthermore, an operating microscope is very helpful. Unfortunately, in the situations cited, the surroundings for the graft are not favorable for revascularization and the proximity of tendons poses difficulties in immobilization.

PARTIAL LESIONS

Partial lesions at this level require careful consideration. For example, a partial lesion of the median nerve at the level of the wrist in which normal sensibility for the most part is retained in association with a motor paralysis is best left alone. It is wisest to deal with the motor paralysis by tendon transplantation rather than attempt a partial repair and run the risk of damaging the intact sensory fibers.

By the same token, sensibility in the ulnar area is relatively unimportant compared with motor function. When motor function is largely retained, it is wisest not to operate.

DIGITAL NERVE LESIONS

When digital nerves are damaged the digital vessels are frequently also involved. This may well be an important factor in considering the results of digital nerve repair. Damage to the vessels can cause ischemic changes in the distal stump of the nerve, with marked collagen formation.

When a single digital nerve is injured in a finger, sensory overlap from the other, in time, usually confers protective sensibility in the previously anesthetized area. For this reason it is difficult to assess accurately the results of digital nerve repair. Perhaps the most important indication for late repair of a divided digital nerve is the presence of a tender neuroma.

It is generally accepted that restoration of sensibility on the sole of the foot is desirable. Furthermore, it is widely held that loss of sensibility on the sole of the foot inevitably leads to trophic disturbances, perforating ulcers, and the like. Our experience is otherwise.

An anesthetic sole becomes vulnerable only if and when a fixed deformity develops. Thus, anesthesia on the sole is not in itself an indication for repair of the posterior tibial nerve in lesions above the ankle.

Perhaps even more important, the hypersensitivity that develops in a previously anesthetized area after late nerve repair may be a positive disadvantage, and has led on

some occasions to the subsequent sectioning of a previously repaired nerve.

This phenomenon can occur in the hand after repair of a single digital nerve. Each digital nerve injury must be considered on its own merits if the question of late repair arises. Primary repair of a digital nerve is always desirable.

FINDINGS AT OPERATION

NEUROMA IN CONTINUITY

Not infrequently, when a nerve is exposed at operation, a neuroma in continuity is found. Should it be resected? Palpation of the nerve between the finger and thumb is a useful guide to the amount of scar tissue present. A large soft fusiform neuroma in continuity is compatible with useful recovery and should be left. Alternatively, a hard neuroma implies marked intraneural fibrosis and a poor outlook. When one is in doubt, it is much better to do a "trial section" than to be unrealistically optimistic.

By "trial section" is meant making a transverse cut slowly through the nerve at the point of maximal firmness. If nerve bundles are not seen, the section is continued until the nerve is severed. Inspection of the stumps will then show a smooth homogeneous surface consistent with marked collagenization. Therefore, formal resection and suturing are executed. If, however, discrete bundles are encountered, the sectioning is discontinued and the epineurium closed by one or two sutures. One always resects a doubtful lesion.

THE DIVIDED NERVE

In 80 per cent of open wounds associated with a degenerative nerve lesion, the nerve at operation is found to be divided, with a well developed proximal neuroma and a small distal glioma. The nerve ends are resected until good pouting bundles are seen. This is commonly carried out by use of a razor blade. Over the years more sophisticated techniques have been developed to ensure that the nerve ends are divided squarely. Some have surrounded the nerve ends with wax or plastic cuffs, and Tarlov and Epstein (1945), among others, devised a neurotome for this purpose.

GAP AFTER RESECTION-METHODS OF CLOSURE

The resulting gap after resection is closed by flexing the appropriate joint. Whereas it may be possible to close a gap of 2.5 or 3.0 cm. in the median nerve by flexing the wrist to 60 or 70 degrees, it is better to obtain length by flexing the elbow joint to a right angle. This means that in subsequent extension of the elbow, the stretch is taken over a longer segment of nerve than if the wrist were extended.

In the case of the ulnar nerve, if wrist flexion is not sufficient, full mobilization of the nerve with anterior transposition at the elbow becomes necessary. For closure of large gaps if may be necessary to expose the median nerve as far as the elbow and to strip the motor branches. There is no doubt that extensive mobilization of a main nerve is harmful.

Formerly it was believed that the blood supply of a nerve was derived mainly from longitudinal vessels that ran in the epineurium and within the nerve. The work of Smith (1966) and others has provided ample evidence that much of a nerve's blood supply reaches it through a fine mesentery extending throughout its course. This is inevitably destroyed during mobilization by open operation.

If closure of a gap is achieved by acute joint flexion, then inevitably when postoperative extension of the joint is begun three weeks later, a severe traction lesion will be imposed on the nerve (Highet and Sanders, 1943). There is therefore a biological rather than an anatomical limit to the closure of gaps by this method.

A set of "critical resection lengths" has been worked out for each nerve (Medical Research Council, 1954). The exact figures are unimportant. As a good working rule, if the wrist joint has to be flexed more than 40 degrees, or the elbow joint more than 90 degrees, an alternative method of nerve repair should be used.

TENSION AT THE SUTURE LINE

Undue tension at the suture line is harmful in several respects. In the first instance, separation of the nerve ends may occur. It necessarily implies poor apposition of nerve bundles. Furthermore, if there is any oozing from the nerve ends, a hematoma can develop, with subsequent scar formation.

Because hemorrhage occurring at the suture line is so harmful, it is customary to release the tourniquet before repair.

For some years it was our custom to apply gold markers to each side of the suture line and then by serial radiographs to ensure that separation had not occurred. Interestingly enough, in the rare event of separation of the suture, it always occurred within the first three weeks, while the limb was immobilized in plaster of Paris, and not when the joint was being extended. It seems, therefore, that the nerve ends are more likely to be blown apart by a hematoma than to separate during joint extension.

ABNORMAL METHODS FOR CLOSURE OF LARGE GAPS

Bone Shortening

Even in peacetime, shotgun injuries are not uncommon. Not only is part of the nerve (or nerves) blown away at the time of injury, but frequently bones may be shattered.

In such circumstances, when there is a large gap in the nerve, bone shortening is justifiable. By the same token, if a nonunited fracture is present at the time of secondary nerve repair, bone shortening can be considered.

Bulb Suturing

This is a method by which a large gap can be closed by stretching the nerve in two stages. At the first operation, full mobilization of the nerve is carried out by open dissection and flexion of the appropriate joint. At that session the unresected neuroma and glioma are united by a silk suture. Thereafter the joint is gradually extended by means of serial plaster casts. At the second operation a formal resection is carried out and the gap is again closed by flexing the joint. After a further period of three weeks in plaster, the joint is gradually extended for the second time. There is no doubt that this does inflict a traction lesion on the nerve, and it should be regarded as a maneuver to be used only in extenuating circumstances.

AUTOGENOUS NERVE GRAFTING

THE USE OF CUTANEOUS NERVES

Cutaneous nerves can be used as grafting material to restore continuity in a nerve. Because of their small diameter, they are quickly revascularized and provide a nearly normal pathway for regenerating axons. The donor nerves most frequently used in peripheral nerve surgery are the medial cutaneous nerve of the forearm, taken from the upper arm, and the sural nerve of the lower limb. Either provides a graft with an average length of 22 cm. The resultant sensory deficit in either instance is well tolerated. They are commonly used in any of four ways: interfascicular nerve repair, cable grafting, inlay grafting, and digital nerve grafting.

For some years Millesi (1967), using an operating microscope, has sought to improve the results of nerve repair by matching, as far as possible, the bundle patterns in the two stumps and restoring fascicular continuity by means of cutaneous nerve grafts. With this method there is no tension at the suture line such as may occur after epineural nerve repair. The technique is time consuming, and it requires the use of an operating microscope by a surgeon who has had special experience with it.

The inlay graft is particularly suitable for partial lesions of nerves when there is a lateral neuroma. After excision of the damaged segment, the resulting gap can be neatly bridged with a strand or strands of a cutaneous nerve. Similarly, in the repair of digital nerves in the palm of the hand, single strands of a cutaneous nerve can be useful.

Closure of large gaps in a main nerve, such as the median nerve in the forearm, can be achieved by constructing a cable of several strands of cutaneous nerve whose total diameter is equal to the cross sectional area of the nerve to be repaired.

Millesi sutures has interfascicular grafts at either end. When using cutaneous nerves it is often simpler to "glue" the nerve ends with a plasma clot formed by the interaction of thrombin and fibrinogen (Seddon and Medawar, 1942). Care must be taken to confine the "glue" to the site of repair, for otherwise it could cinterfere with revascularization of the graft.

MAIN TRUNK GRAFTS

When two main nerves are damaged such that neither can be repaired by direct suturing, a free graft of the less important nerve can be used to bridge the gap in the other. For example, in the forearm the ulnar neve is used to restore continuity in the median nerve. There is evidence to suggest that in such circumstances it is wisest to use the distal segment for grafting material. The metabolic requirements for a predegenerate graft are rather less than if the proximal segment is used. Since it is a free graft, its surival is precarious. It will be obvious that whenever a free graft is used, the vascularity of its surroundings becomes important for its survival. In the forearm it is nearly always possible to bypass scar tissue and arrange a suitable bed, whereas in the hand, local conditions are unfavorable, and this is reflected in the results of digital nerve grafting.

THE PEDICLE NERVE GRAFT

When severe Volkmann's ischemia of the forearm is present in addition to muscle damage, the median and ulnar nerves may also be affected (Holmes et al., 1944). After resection of ischemic neural tissue, direct suturing is never possible. A free graft cannot survive in an ischemic environment. In such circumstances the pedicle nerve graft operation devised by Strange (1947) is partularly applicable.

At the first stage of this two stage procedure the proximal neuromas of both nerves are resected and the ends united. The gap to be closed is estimated. The ulnar nerve is then exposed in the upper arm, and all but its epineural vessels is divided or encircled with a stout silk suture at the point that will allow sufficient nerve to close the gap in the forearm.

Not less than six weeks later, at the second stage, the ulnar nerve is swung down as a pedicle and united to the distal stump of the median nerve at the level of the rist joint.

The results of this procedure are spectacular. Protective sensibility is restored in the median area of the hand and functional opposition of the thumb is regained. Results to date have shown that of all methods of nerve grafting, the pedicle nerve graft is the most reliable.

HOMOGRAFTS

Despite extravagant claims by some authors regarding the use of specially prepared homografts, it can be stated that as in other areas of tissue transplantation, the problem of the immune reaction that they provoke remains unsolved. They are useless.

REFERENCES

Adams, W. E.: The blood supply of nerves. 2. The effects of exclusion of its regional sources of supply on the sciatic nerve of the rabbit. J. Anat., 77:243, 1943.

Barnes, R., Bacsich, P., and Wyburn, G. M.: A histological study of a pre-degenerated nerve graft. Br. J. Surg., 33:130, 1945.

Barnes, R., Bacsich, P., Wyburn, G. M., and Kerr, A. S.: A study of the fate of nerve homografts in man. Br. J. Surg., 34:34, 1946.

Bentley, F H., and Schlapp, W.: Experiments on the blood supply of nerves. J. Physiol. (Lond.), 102:62, 1943.

Brooks, D. M.: Open wounds of the brachial plexus. J. Bone Joint Surg., 31B:17, 1949.

Brooks, D. M.: The place of nerve grafting in orthopaedic surgery. J. Bone Joint Surg., 37A:299, 1955.

Campbell, J. B., Bassett, C. A. L., and Bohler, J.: Frozen, irradiated homografts shielded with microfilter sheaths in peripheral nerve surgery. J. Trauma, 3:302, 1963.

Campbell, J. B., Bassett, C. A. F., Giraldo, J. M., Seymour, R. J., and Rossi, J. P.: Application of monomolecular filter tubes in bridging gaps in peripheral nerves and for prevention of neuroma formation. J. Neurosurg., 13:635, 1956.

Clawson, D. K., and Seddon, H. J.: The results of repair of the sciatic nerve. J. Bone Joint Surg., 42B:205–212, 1960.

Doupe, J., Barnes, R., and Kerr, A. S.: Studies in denervation: effect of electrical stimulation on circulation and recovery of denervated muscle. J. Neurol. Psychiat. (Lond.) 6:136, 1943.

Edshage, S.: Peripheral nerve suture. A technique for improved intraneural topography evaluation of some materials. Acta Chir. Scand., Suppl. 331, 1964.

Gutmann, E., and Guttmann, L.: Effect of galvanic exercise on denervated and reinnervated muscles in rabbit. J. Neurol. Neurosurg. Psychiatr., 7:7, 1944.

Gutmann, E., and Young, J. S.: The reinnervation of muscle after various periods of atrophy. J. Anat. 78:15, 1944.

Highet, W. B., and Sanders, F. K.: The effects of stretching nerves after suture. Br. J. Surg., 30:355, 1943.

Holmes, W.: Histological observations on the repair of nerves by autografts. Br. J. Surg., 35:167, 1947.

Holmes, W., Highet, W. B., and Seddon, H. J.: Ischaemic nerve lesions occurring in Volkmann's contracture. Br. J. Surg., 32:259, 1944.

Jackson, E. S. C.: The role of galvanism in the treatment of denervated voluntary muscle in man. Brain, 68:300, 1945.

Marmor, L.: Regeneration of peripheral nerves by irradiated homografts. J. Bone Joint Surg., 46A:383, 1964.

Medical Research Council: Peripheral Nerve Injuries. Special Report Series, Medical Research Council, No. 282, London, Her Majesty's Stationery Office, 1954.

Michon, J., and Masse, P.: Le moment optimum de la suture nerveuse dans les plaies du membre supérieur. Rev. Chir. Orthop. Repar. Appar. Moteur., 50:205, 1964.

Millesi, H., Ganglberger, J., and Berger, A.: Paper presented at the 83rd Congress of the german Surgical Society in Munich, 14th April, 1966. Chir. Plast. Reconstr., 3:1967.

Mitchell, S. W.: Injuries of Nerves. Philadelphia, J. B. Lippincott Company, 1872.

Ognev, B.: Metal Prostheses for Nerves, 1966.

Peacock, E. E., Jr.: Restoration of sensation in hands with extensive median nerve defects. Surgery, 54:576–586, 1963.

Platt, H.: Results of bridging gaps in injured nerve trunks by autogenous fascial tubulization and autogenous nerve grafts. Br. J. Surg., 7:384, 1920.

Pollock, L. J., and Davis, L.: Peripheral Nerve Injuries. New York, Hoeber, 1933.

Sanders, F. K.: The repair of large gaps in the peripheral nerve. Brain, 65:281, 1942.

Sanders, F. K., and Young, J. S.: The degeneration and reinnervation of grafted nerves. J. Anat., 76:143, 1942.

Seddon, H. J.: The use of autogenous grafts for the repair of large gaps in peripherl nerves. Br. J. Surg., 35:151, 1947.

Seddon, H. J.: Nerve grafting. J. Bone Joint Surg., 45B:447, 1963.

Seddon, H. J.: Nerve suture and nerve grafts in the upper limb. Tenth International Congress: Société Internationale de Chirurgie Orthopaedique et de Traumatologie. Brussels. Acta Medica Belgica, 1967, p. 739.

Seddon, H. J., and Holmes, W.: Late condition of nerve homografts in man. Surg. Gynecol. Obstet., 79:342, 1944.

Seddon, H. J., and Medawar, P. B.: Fibrin suture of human nerves. Lancet, 2:87, 1942.

Smith, J. W.: Microsurgery of peripheral nerves. Plast. Reconstr. Surg., 33:317, 1962.

Smith, J. W.: Factors influencing 'nerve' repair. 1. Blood supply of peripheral nerves. Arch. Surg., 3:335, 1966.

Spurling, R. G., Lyons, W. R., Whitcomb, B. B., and Woodhall, B.: Failure of whole fresh homogeneous nerve grafts in man. J. Neurosurg., 2:79, 1945.

Strange, F. G. St. C.: An operation for nerve pedicle grafting: preliminary communication. Br. J. Surg., 34:423, 1947.

Sunderland, S.: Blood supply of peripheral neves: practical considerations. Arch. Neurol. Psychiatr., 54:283, 1945d.

Tarlov, I. M., and Epstein, J. A.: Nerve grafts: importance of adequate blood supply. J. Neurosurg., 2:49, 1945.

Zachary, R. B., and Holmes, W.: Primary suture of nerves. Surg. Gynecol. Obstet., 82:632, 1946.

Chapter 54

NERVE ANASTOMOSIS AND GRAFT WITH FIBRIN GLUE

Alain Gilbert

The idea for using the adhesive properties of fibrin was first described in 1909 by Bergels (1909), who suggested using a blood clot. Applying fibrin glue to peripheral nerves was proposed in 1940 by Seddon and Medawar (1942), who used a plasma glue enriched with fibrinogen and thrombin. The problem presented by these glues was not so much with their adhesive properties as with the risk of the anastomosis rupturing, caused by too rapid dissolution of the clot. Only in the 1970s did the use of fractionation permit the formation of stable and homogeneous glues offering greater durability.

These glues have been used for a variety of applications, but nerve anastomosis is one of the most interesting. Following the work of Matras et al. (1973) and Kuderna (1979), an important clinical trial by Egloff and Narakas (1983) has recently demonstrated the clinical usefulness of these glues in human beings.

PRINCIPLES AND METHODS OF ACTION

Fibrin glue is a biological adhesive, with a human fibrinogen and calcified thrombin base which is completely reabsorbed within a few days during the healing process. The fibrinogen is concentrated and fortified with Factor XIII and fibronectin. The components are lyophilized to ensure their conservation and must be reconstituted in an aqueous solution at 37°C. at the moment of application. Thrombin, when mixed with fibrinogen, transforms into a soluble fibrin monomer. Factor XIII and calcium trigger the polymerization of fibrin.

The rapidity of the reaction is regulated by the concentration of thrombin, and can vary from seconds to minutes. The addition of aprotenin protects the fibrin clot for 12 to 15 days (Figs. 54–1 and 54–2).

TECHNIQUE FOR USE

The technique differs according to whether an immediate anastomosis or a graft is glued.

IMMEDIATE ANASTOMOSIS

Retraction of a freshly divided nerve results in a certain amount of tension and thus hinders using only the glue as an adhesive. A few 9-0 or 10-0 epiperineurial sutures to

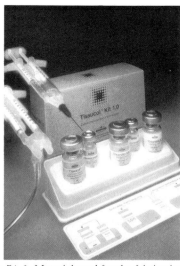

Figure 54–1. Material used for the fabrication of fibrin glue.

554

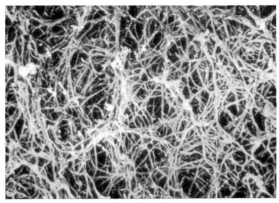

Figure 54–2. The fibrin clot.

orient the nerve and relieve this tension are necessary. The glue, which should be prepared ahead of time (around 10 min.), is applied around the sutures, while excessive penetration between the extremities is avoided.

Note: once prepared, the glue keeps for several hours.

NERVE GRAFT (Figs. 54–3 and 54–4)

Contrary to Egloff and Narakas (1983), who use sutures for approximation before applying the glue to nerve grafts, we use only

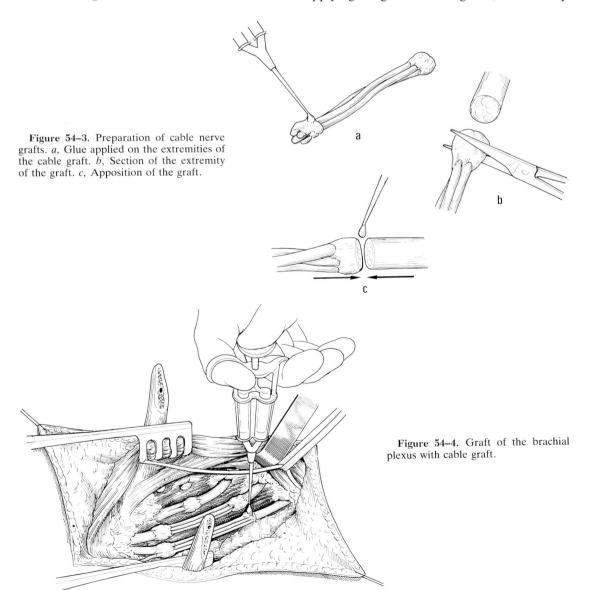

Figure 54–3. Preparation of cable nerve grafts. *a*, Glue applied on the extremities of the cable graft. *b*, Section of the extremity of the graft. *c*, Apposition of the graft.

Figure 54–4. Graft of the brachial plexus with cable graft.

the glue when there is no tension. The extremities of the grafts are placed within the anastomotic zone with forceps, and the glue is applied around this zone. Within a few seconds, there is sufficient adherence.

This technique saves considerable time, especially in brachial plexus surgery. In this particular instance, a review of 60 brachial plexus operations, with a following for up to two years, has shown comparable and sometimes astonishingly good results with this method when compared to suturing. In particular, grafts of roots ruptured near their truncal division have become easier to repair while they remain difficult to suture. These clinical results have been confirmed by those of Egloff and Narakas.

CONCLUSION

Fibrin glue, as it has been used in Europe for several years, seems to provide clinical results at least equal to those techniques using conventional sutures. It has a certain advantage, in that it saves time, and another lesser known advantage, that is, the temporary formation of a regeneration chamber that favors axonal growth by protecting it from the external environment.

The main risk with glue fabricated from human serum is the transmission of diseases such as hepatitis or AIDS, but the laboratory examinations (Scheele et al., 1981) used to detect these and prevent their transmission make this unlikely.

REFERENCES

Becker, C., Gueuning, C., and Graff, G.: Réparation de nerf périphérique: Intérêt des colles biologiques et de la suture épipérineurale dans les interventions tardives. Ann. Chir. Main, 4(3):259–262, 1985.

Bergels, S.: Uber Wirkungen des Fibrins. Dtschr. Med. Wochenschr., 35:633–665, 1909.

Egloff, D., and Narakas, A.: Anastomoses Nerveuses par fibrino-collage. Ann. Chir. Main, 2:101–115, 1983.

Kuderna, H.: Fibrin Kleber System Nervenklebung. Dtsch. Zahn.-Mund-Kerer-u-Gesishts Chirg., 3:32S–35S, 1979.

Matras, H., Dinges, H. W., Mamoli, B., and Lassmann, H.: Non-sutured nerve transplantation. J. Max. Fac. Surg., 1:37–40, 1973.

Panis, R., and Scheele, J.: Hepatitisrisiko bei der Fibrinklebung in der HNO-Chirurgie. Laryng.-Rhinol., 60:367–368, 1981.

Redl, H., Schlag, G., Stanek, G., Hirschl, A., and Seelich, T.: In vitro properties of mixtures of fibrin seal and antibiotics. Biomat, 4:29–32, 1983.

Scheele, J., Schricker, K. Th., Goy, R. D., Lampe, I., and Panis, R.: In Schattauer, F. K. (Ed.): Hepatitisrisiko der Fibrinklebung in der Allgemein chirurgie. Vol. 32. New York, Springer Verlag, 1981, pp. 783–788.

Seddon, H. J., and Medawar, P. B.: Fibrin suture of human nerves. Lancet, 2:87–92, 1942.

Tarlov, I. M., Denslow, C., Swarz, S., and Pineles, D.: Plasma clot suture of nerves. Arch. Surg., 47:44, 1943.

Chapter 55

TECHNIQUE OF PERIPHERAL NERVE REPAIR

Hanno Millesi

a. Selection of Technique in Surgery of Peripheral Nerves

Advances in peripheral nerve surgery have been achieved by the development of microsurgical techniques and the use of physiological approaches. At the SICOT Meeting (Societé International de Chirurgie Traumatologique et Orthopaedique) in Tel Aviv in 1972, the value of microsurgical techniques in the repair of injured peripheral nerves was confirmed. However, some still hold the view that conventional techniques can yield equally satisfactory results, and that the technical efforts connected with microsurgery are not worthwhile. Furthermore, sophisticated equipment and trained surgeons are not uniformly available. Therefore, at the moment neither method of repair is universally accepted, and the surgeon has to make up his mind by selecting the optimal technique for each case. The following pages contain advice that I hope will aid in making this choice, based on an analysis of the literature and on personal experience. Consequently this material may be controversial.

PRIMARY VERSUS SECONDARY REPAIR

The arguments in favor of primary repair are that time is saved and that no further surgery is required. Moreover, the proximal and the distal nerve stumps are still elastic and not retracted. Finally, no scarring is present at the time of surgery. On the other hand, there are disadvantages: The amount of damage to the nerve stumps cannot be estimated, and the danger of infection is greater. Depending on the size and condition of the original wound, complications are more likely. The circumstances are not always favorable for repair. Finally, when secondary repair is selected, another operation must be performed, and thus some time is lost.

One advantage of secondary repair is that the timing can be selected so that the secondary operation is done when conditions are ideal. The operation is scheduled when the patient's general state is satisfactory for a major operation and optimal conditions in regard to personnel and technical equipment are fulfilled. From a biological point of view, there are two opinions about the optimal time for repair:

1. In the third or fourth week after the injury Schwann cell activity reaches its peak, the epineurium has thickened somewhat to make epineurial suture easier, and healing of the original wound has progressed (Holmes and Young, 1942; Seddon, 1944).

2. Starting at day 4 after the injury, the enzymatic activity of the ganglion cells increases (Kreutzberg, 1963). The ganglion cells remain enlarged for 10 to 20 days (Ducker et al., 1969). The axons of the proximal stumps are thickened as a result of an increase in axoplasmic flow, which reaches its maximum at days 3 to 4 (Weiss and Hiscoe, 1948). At this time also, the first axon sprouts are formed. These considerations suggest that the earliest date for the secondary repair is about the fifth or sixth day.

Independent of biological considerations, the date for the secondary repair is selected as early after the accident as the general state of the patient, the amount of edema, and the state of the wound allow. The amount of damage to the two nerve stumps can be estimated more accurately because of the early fibrotic changes that can be seen in the damaged area. The operation can be focused on the nerve repair because other problems, such as fractures and skin loss, have been managed at the primary operation.

In conclusion, primary repair should be done when there is a clean skin wound without skin defect; when there is a clean laceration of the nerve without damage to the stumps, and without defect; when the nerve stumps are easily found in the wound; and when there is no additional damage to other structures such as bone and tendons. In all other circumstances, secondary repair is more advisable. It should be performed as early as general and local conditions allow.

PRIMARY REPAIR

If the conditions for primary repair exist, an epineurial nerve repair is an excellent technique. In the majority of these uncomplicated cases, a satisfactory result will be achieved. If after five to six months no sign of regeneration is present (Tinel's sign progression, electromyographic evidence), the suture site should be re-explored. An external neurolysis is performed first. The thickened epineurium is then incised and is resected except for a small strip on the opposite side of the nerve. Then intraneural neurolysis is carried out. In some cases this might be sufficient to induce regeneration, but if the suture site is scarred, it is resected and interfascicular nerve grafting is performed. The preserved strip of epineurium maintains continuity.

If microsurgical equipment is available, either of two techniques can be used:

1. Epineurial nerve repair with guide sutures (Michon and Masse, 1964). This technique is useful for nerves consisting of many small fascicles (proximal levels), which makes fascicular realignment impossible.

2. Fascicular or interfascicular nerve repair after resection of the epineurium. This technique is superior for nerves that have a limited number of fascicles, already arranged according to their function (distal levels).

Nerves of the caliber of the digital nerves are united by two loose sutures after the epineurium has been peeled back. In nerves with one, two, or three large fascicles, good fascicular alignment can be achieved by either technique.

EARLY SECONDARY REPAIR

CASES WITHOUT DEFECT

Nerve repair can be performed according to the principles already outlined for primary repair.

CASES WITH MAJOR DEFECTS

The prognosis for nerve repair becomes poor if end to end suturing is performed under tension. A nerve graft offers a better chance. The axon sprouts grow more easily across two good suture lines than across one poor, scarred suture line. The methods used to overcome a nerve defect are described in detail with the discussion of nerve grafts.

Autologous Free Trunk Graft

This technique can be used only when a trunk graft is available as a donor. There is danger of central fibrosis if the diameter of the graft is too great. Seddon (1972) reported 17 good and seven fair results and ten failures from trunk grafting.

Autologous Pedicled Trunk Graft

Autologous trunk grafts survive well if transplanted, with microvascular anastomosis, and blood circulation is restored immediately (Strange, 1947). Neurotization occurs more rapidly than in free grafts. This could be of great advantage under favorable conditions, e.g., in brachial plexus surgery.

Preserved Homografts (Allografts)

Early optimistic reports on the successful use of lyophilized homografts such as that by Jacoby et al. (1970) could not be substantiated (Kuhlendahl et al., 1972). The results with preserved homografts are inferior to the results with neurotization autografts (Schröder and Seiffert, 1970). Therefore, a preserved homograft should be used only when there is no possibility of autografting.

Cable Grafts

The successful use of this type of graft has been reported by Seddon (1947, 1972) and Brooks (1955). The majority of operations utilizing cable grafts were done in the years after World War II. Since then, this technique has been used only occasionally. Nomura et al. (1970) were not pleased with the results of cable grafting.

Interfascicular Grafting

By use of the "interfascicular" grafting technique, satisfactory results can be achieved even in patients with longstanding defects (Millesi, 1968; Millesi et al., 1967, 1972). These results have been confirmed by the experiences of other centers (Anderl, 1973; Bedeschi, 1972; Buck-Gramcko, 1971; Furlan et al., 1973; Narakas and Verdan, 1969; Palazzi et al, 1971; Salvi, 1973; Samii and Willebrand, 1970; Samii and Kahl, 1972). Interfascicular nerve grafts yield good results only when the technique is performed in a very exact way. Tension must be avoided. The graft must be longer than the defect when the limb is in full extension.

According to our present knowledge, the best results in the repair of nerves with long defects can be achieved by the interfascicular nerve grafting technique.

CASES WITH MINOR DEFECTS

There is still controversy about the definitions of minor and major defects, as well as the defects that can be repaired by end to end suturing and those that should be grafted. Opinions of individual surgeons give evidence of their confidence in the value of nerve grafts. It seems logical to assume that end to end suturing with one suture line is superior to a graft with two suture lines, and as a result many surgeons have difficulties in familiarizing themselves with nerve grafting.

Of course one must consider all other possible techniques to overcome a defect (e.g., anterior transposition of the ulnar nerve in the elbow area) before grafting is considered.

Flexion of the adjacent joints can help to overcome a defect, but it should be used with caution because the suture line will be stretched when mobilization is begun, and this can damage the axon sprouts. Flexion to reduce a defect should never be used when grafting is performed.

By mobilization of the nerve stumps, length can be gained, and this can help to close the gap.

My point of view is that if by mobilization of the nerve stumps, by transposition, or by bone shortening the nerve stumps can be united without tension in the neutral position of the extremity, end to end suturing should be performed. In all other cases grafting is indicated.

In the case of the median or the ulnar nerve in the distal half of the forearm, the distance that can be filled by mobilization under favorable conditions is about 2.5 cm. I am sure that good results can be achieved by end to end suturing in cases of longer defects, but the average result in a great number of cases will be inferior. Nicholson and Seddon (1957) and Sakellarides (1962) reported a marked deterioration in the average result in cases in which the defects were longer than 2.5 cm.

LATE SECONDARY REPAIR

When late secondary repair is done, the retracted nerve stumps have contracted so much that the resulting distance between the two nerve stumps is equivalent to a defect caused by loss of neural tissue or by resection of the neuroma. Under these circumstances end to end suturing can be performed only with considerable tension, and therefore nerve grafting is indicated much more frequently than in early secondary repairs. There is a good chance of motor recovery as long as 18 months after the neural lesion is sustained. In young patients some motor recovery can be observed after an even longer time interval. Return of sensibility (at least protective sensibility) has been seen after an interval of several years. Therefore, repair of important nerves, such as the median nerve, is indicated even if a long time has elapsed following the injury.

b. Secondary Repair of Peripheral Nerves by Grafts

Without doubt, end to end suturing of a transected peripheral nerve is the method of choice to re-establish continuity if one wants the nerve stumps to heal without a gap and with minimal scar tissue formation. In a clean laceration of the nerve without loss of neural substance, this can be accomplished by primary or early secondary repair. In late secondary repairs, even under favorable conditions, much tension is necessary to unite the two stumps, because of retraction. If there is a real defect, it is much more difficult to achieve good union, and alternative methods of closing the defect must be considered.

ORIGIN OF NERVE DEFECTS

ELASTIC RETRACTION

Owing to the elasticity of peripheral nerve tissue, the two nerve stumps retract after transection. Some force is necessary to stretch the segments of nerve proximal and distal to the site of division to reunite the two stumps. In the sciatic nerve of the rabbit, this force is between 6 and 10 gm. (Millesi, Berger, and Meissl, 1972). When the tissue loses its elasticity, much more force is needed to overcome the gap that forms as a result of retraction even without loss of neural tissue (Fig. 55–1). To avoid tension, it is much better to use a nerve graft to bridge the gap than to stretch the nerve. Because there is no real defect, the fascicular patterns of the two cross sections correspond very well, and corresponding fascicles can be easily identified.

LOSS OF SUBSTANCE

When the initial trauma destroys nerve substance, a real defect is formed. It may be increased by elastic retraction or by fibrotic changes. In this situation the fascicular patterns of the cross sections do not correspond exactly. This difference increases with the length of the defect.

The loss of substance can be caused by trauma, operation (excision of a tumor), ischemic necrosis, and other factors.

FIBROSIS

After severe damage, fibrotic changes occur in the area. Such damage develops in the two stumps of a transected nerve when the laceration was not clean. It occurs in a blunt injury, by ischemia, or by compression.

Fibrosis increases the gap between the two stumps of a transected nerve by contraction. The fibrotic parts have to be resected before continuity is re-established. Thus, a real defect may be formed, or, when there is already a loss of substance, the defect may be increased. The fascicular patterns of the cross sections do not correspond exactly, and the

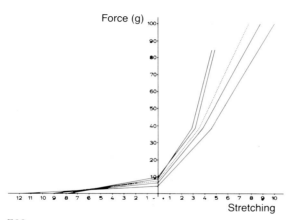

Figure 55–1. Relationship between force (vertical, in g) and stretching (in percentage of free length) of the extrapelvic sciatic nerve of the rabbit. After transection, the two stumps are retracted, forcing a gap between 8 and 12 per cent of the free length of the nerve between its exit from the pelvis and its division (left side). A force between 6 and 10 g was necessary to reunite the two stumps. With an increasing amount of resection, the two stumps had to be stretched to be brought into contact again, as an increasing amount of force had to be applied to achieve this. With a resection of more than 3 to 5 per cent the force rose rapidly.

difference increases with the length of the gap.

EFFECTS OF TENSION ON NERVE REGENERATION

It is generally accepted that the result of a nerve repair is influenced by the tension at the suture line. Careful follow-up studies have revealed a marked deterioration of the functional results in median and ulnar nerve repairs when defects are longer than 1 inch (2.5 cm.) (Nicholson and Seddon, 1957; Sakellarides, 1962). Therefore, avoidance of tension is recommended.

EFFECTS AT OPERATION

Good union is more difficult to achieve when tension is increased. The nerve stumps are traumatized because it is difficult to place the sutures, and more sutures are needed. Some of the stitches may not hold. If the adjacent joints are flexed to reduce the tension, the exposure is compromised and the operation is more difficult to perform. More attention is paid to technical details to achieve and secure union than to the accuracy of the fascicular alignment. There is always the danger of lateral gap formation if the distance between two stitches is too great. There is the danger of rupture if the flexed position is not maintained carefully during wound closure and dressing. This risk is further increased by increases in the amount of tension and the length of the defect.

When the sciatic nerve of the rabbit is stretched, the actual force required increases slowly when the stretching amounts to less than 2 or 3 per cent of its extrapelvic length. However, there is a steep increase in the force needed when the nerve is stretched more than 3 per cent (Millesi, Berger, and Meissl, 1972).

EFFECTS DURING THE EARLY HEALING PERIOD

Even with special instruments it is difficult to create a very smooth surface on the two cross sections. The tissue within the perineural tubes, being under higher pressure, tends to protrude. Therefore, when epineurial suturing is carried out tightly, the fascicles

buckle (Edshage, 1964). When the suturing is done loosely, a gap may occur between the two cross sections. This gap increases if the suture is under tension. It is filled by connective tissue. As the gap increases, more distance and more obstacles have to be overcome by the outgrowing axon sprouts.

If there is a lateral gap between two stitches at the circumference, connective tissue can grow in from the surrounding areas. The amount of connective tissue formation is directly related to the amount of tension at the suture line.

By immobilization of the affected part in a flexed position, the amount of tension can be reduced and its consequences postponed. When the period of immobilization ends and the patient starts to extend his joints again, the suture line and the nerve are gradually stretched. Healing at this time is so far advanced that rupture is avoided, but hypertrophy and stretching of scar tissue occur even after long periods of immobilization. In controlled experiments we demonstrated all these consequences of nerve suturing, even when tension had been moderate (Millesi et al., 1967, 1970, 1972). Our results were confirmed by the experimental study of Samii et al. (1972).

An interesting experiment by Ventimiglia (1973) showed a significantly better tensile strength during the first seven days when tension was avoided.

EFFECTS DURING THE LATE HEALING PERIOD

There is a widespread opinion that the axon sprouts are bound to grow toward the end organs if they succeed in crossing the suture line. Therefore, it would seem to be sufficient to maintain immobilization until the axons have passed into the distal stump. Actually, the process is not that simple. In the later phases of healing, when the scars are maturing, scar shrinkage occurs. Axons that have already reached the distal stump can suffer fatal damage as a result of constricting scar tissue contracture. We have observed this both in animal experiments and in histological studies of human specimens.

In nine patients who had recently been injured, nerve suturing was done under moderate tension using classic techniques. There was no regeneration. Therefore, in each patient, the suture line was exposed again and resected and the gap bridged by nerve grafts. Histological investigation showed degenerating axons in three of the nine cases, even though the initial nerve suturing had been done several months previously (Seitelberger et al., 1969). This proves that many of the axons that reached the distal stump have suffered damage, probably by constriction at the suture site. There is strong evidence that the amount of scar shrinkage is related to the amount of tension. The effects of stretching are seen not only at the suture line but also proximal to the site of injury, in the form of a disseminated degeneration, as described by Highet and Holmes (1943).

TECHNIQUES OF MANAGEMENT OF NERVE DEFECTS

STRETCHING THE NERVE

Under the circumstances of secondary repair, much force is needed to approximate the nerve ends even when there is no actual defect but merely the gap produced by elastic recoil.

The question of the amount of stretching a nerve can bear without damage has been discussed at length. The argument is put forward that when a femur is lengthened by osteotomy, the sciatic nerve can tolerate a great deal of stretching. This, however, is an intact nerve, and the force is distributed along its entire length. When the nerve is transected, the tensile force focuses at the suture line.

By mobilizing the two nerve stumps, the gain in length by stretching can be increased. Wide mobilization deprives the nerve of its segmental blood supply and may preclude optimal circulation (Smith, 1966). The consequences of stretching the nerve can be postponed by flexing the adjacent joints to achieve a tensionless union, but these consequences will reappear when mobilization starts. Therefore, the average results under these conditions remain rather poor.

The amount of stretching can be reduced by dividing the reconstructive procedure into two steps. At the first operation the neuroma and the glioma are not resected, but united by suturing (Bulb suturing). At the second stage, when the nerve is already stretched, the fibrotic part is resected and the end to end suturing is carried out.

REROUTING THE NERVE

Certain anatomical conditions offer the opportunity to gain an advantage by rerouting the transected nerve. This advantage can be twofold: a real gain in length, because the new course of the nerve is significantly shorter; and better use in shortening the distance by flexion of the adjacent joints.

The removal of the hook of the hamate offers a real gain in length for the deep branch of the ulnar nerve because the new course is shorter (Boyes, 1955).

Anterior transposition of the ulnar nerve at the elbow level offers a real gain of 2 to 3 cm. in length as a result of the new shorter course. By flexing the elbow joint, the distance between two stumps can be shortened another 4 to 5 cm., but in this situation all the disadvantages of stretching the nerve have to be considered.

Transposition of the transected radial nerve around the medial aspect of the upper arm and the transected median nerve superficial to the superficial head of the pronator teres gives adequate relief only when the elbow joint is flexed (Finochietto, 1961). Therefore, there is no real gain.

BONE SHORTENING

Shortening the bone to reduce the distance between two nerve stumps is advocated by some. In pseudarthrosis of the involved bone, when an osteotomy is indicated, one can make good use of this technique. An osteotomy of a normal bone is not justified, because the real gain is limited and nerve grafts give excellent results without the risks.

NERVE GRAFTING

The use of nerve grafting is the logical way to bridge a nerve defect. Nerve grafts have been used for 100 years (Albert, 1885). They were initially used as a last resort when all other methods to achieve a direct union had been exhausted. The view was held (and still is) that a graft must always yield inferior results compared with direct nerve suturing. When a graft is used, the regenerating axons must cross two suture lines. Logically this should be more difficult than crossing one. This is true under experimental conditions, when there is no defect. In clinical practice this situation is rare. Usually there is a defect, especially when the two stumps are resected, until normal nerve tissue is encountered. Then a real tension-free union is not possible. Experiments and clinical experience have taught us that a nerve graft that avoids tension and provides two ideal suture lines gives better results than one scarred suture line achieved under tension (Millesi et al., 1970, 1972).

The length of the graft does not influence the result. Therefore, the graft can be long enough to cover the whole defect in the extended position of the limb, and no attempt to reduce this distance is necessary.

BASIC TECHNIQUES OF NERVE GRAFTING

AUTOGRAFTS

When the donor nerve is derived from the same individual, immunological problems are not encountered.

Free Trunk Grafts

Free grafting of a main nerve trunk has two serious drawbacks. The function of the donor nerve is sacrificed, and the surface area of the nerve trunk graft is rather small in relation to its tissue volume. After free grafting, the graft can survive only if the circulation is re-established in a reasonably short time. For the tissue in the center of a trunk graft, the ischemic period is longer than for a tissue in the periphery. It may be so long that the neural tissue is damaged and only the connective tissue survives. The neurotization of the graft is then impaired.

Pedicled Trunk Grafts

Poor results with free trunk grafts led to the technique of pedicled nerve grafting. By this technique the graft always has a very good blood supply, and there is no danger of damage (Strange, 1947). The donor nerve must be sacrificed. Therefore, this technique has been used when two parallel nerves, e.g., the median and the ulnar, have been destroyed for long distances. In a case of bilateral involvement, a cross arm nerve graft was tried. Good results with regard to return of sensibility were reported.

Vascularized Trunk Graft

To avoid ischemic damage when performing a free transplantation of a nerve trunk, Taylor and Ham (1975) developed a technique that permitted the re-establishment of circulation within the nerve by microvascular anastomosis. Considerable success has been reported with this technique. In regard to cell survival, these grafts are as good as pedicled trunk grafts, but they also share the disadvantage of being trunk grafts. It has not yet been well established whether the regeneration along such a graft occurs significantly faster than along a free graft.

Cable Grafts

The use of unimportant cutaneous nerves as donors for autografting was described by Bielschowsky and Unger in 1917. Such cutaneous nerves have a much better surface area–tissue volume relationship than others, and thus the risk of central damage is minimal. Bunnell and Boyes (1939) and Seddon (1943) formed cable grafts to achieve the same caliber as the nerve to be repaired by uniting several cutaneous nerves. The cable graft was used in the same way as trunk graft and sutured to the proximal and distal stump by epineurial stitches.

Interfascicular Nerve Grafts

With this technique, instead of uniting cutaneous nerves to form a cable, the distal and proximal stumps are divided into smaller units, each with about the same diameter as the donor nerve (Fig. 55–2).

The dissection starts in the normal portions of the proximal and distal stumps. The epineurium is incised and reflected. By blunt dissection in the interfascicular tissue, several groups of fascicles are separated. The dissection then proceeds toward the stump ends. The level where the neural tissue loses its normal appearance and fibrosis starts is defined exactly. Each group of fascicles is transected exactly at this level. Then the epineurium is resected. This offers an additional advantage because the epineurium is one of the main sources of connective tissue proliferation, and its removal at the level of the suture line reduces the formation of connective tissue.

The nerve grafts are then inserted between the corresponding groups of fascicles of the

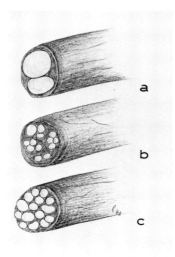

Figure 55–2. Basic types of fascicular patterns: Monofascicular pattern (not shown), oligofascicular pattern (*a*) with two to eight fascicles, polyfascicular pattern with group arrangement (*b*), and polyfascicular pattern without group arrangement (*c*).

proximal and distal stumps (Figs. 55–3 to 55–5). The grafts are laid into the defect individually, and no attempt to form a cable is undertaken.

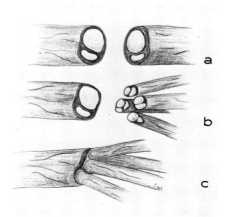

Figure 55–3. Oligofascicular pattern with two large fascicles. There is only a small amount of nonfascicular tissue in the cross section. Exact coaptation of the fascicles can be achieved by handling the epifascicular epineurium. Resection of the epineurium does not provide any advantage (*a*). With nerve grafting, the large fascicle can be covered easily with three cutaneous nerve grafts (fascicular grafting 1:3) and the small fascicle with one graft (fascicular grafting 1:1). The coaptation can be secured by a few epineural stitches (*b, c*). If the stumps consist of five to eight or ten fascicles, the coaptation of the central fascicles cannot be guaranteed by epifascicular stitches. Isolating each of the several large fascicles and performing a fascicular coaptation or fascicular grafting would be the better solution.

The nerve grafts must be long enough to avoid tension. Without tension, one 10-0 or finer stitch at the end of each graft is sufficient to achieve a good union. The suture helps to bring the cross section of the graft and the cross section of the fascicle group into good contact without traumatization by touching, and it secures the union for a short time. After 20 minutes the two ends stick together by natural clotting (Millesi, Berger, and Meissl, 1972). Experiments in rabbits have shown that the tensile strength of such a union after 24 hours is already between 15 and 30 gm.

After the nerve grafting the skin wound is closed carefully to avoid separation by improper handling. The elbow is extended, and the wrist joint is in the neutral position during the entire operation. Then a plaster cast is applied with the elbow and wrist in exactly the same positions to avoid tension. Ten days after the operation the cast is removed, and the patient begins active exercise. At this time the union is strong enough to withstand motion. This operation should be carried out under the microscope, using very fine instruments and minimizing surgical trauma (Fig. 55–6).

The exposure is done under tourniquet control. When all anatomical landmarks have been defined, the tourniquet is removed and the wound is compressed for 20 minutes. This time can be used to take the graft. The grafting procedure is carried out without a tourniquet. Suction drainage is not used.

Fascicular Nerve Grafting

This term means that each fascicle of the proximal stump is united by one graft with the corresponding fascicle of the distal stump. For a median nerve 20 or more grafts would be needed. The grafts must be thinner than the usual donor nerve. The sural nerve, for instance, must be divided into subunits. For these reasons this technique can be used only with nerves having a few large fascicles, for example, the sciatic nerve of the rabbit. In surgical practice use of this technique is associated with increased tissue damage.

FRESH HOMOGRAFTS (ALLOGRAFTS)

Fresh homografts provoke an immunological response. At present such grafts are not used. Careful selection of the donor and

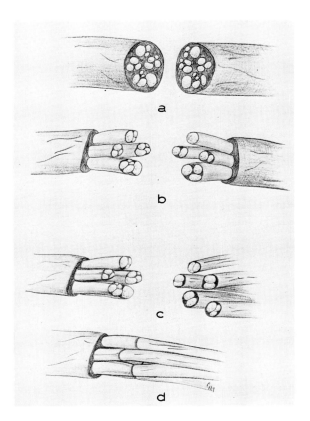

Figure 55–4. Polyfascicular nerve segment. Fifteen fascicles of different sizes are arranged in four groups (*a*). After partial resection of the epineurium and isolation of the groups, a coaptation of the two stumps of each group can be achieved, reducing the amount of epineural connective tissue as a source of connective tissue proliferation and diminishing the chance of malalignment, i.e., fascicular to nonfascicular tissue (*b*). When grafting is used, each fascicle group is connected with one cutaneous nerve (interfascicular grafting) (*c*). Interdentation of the individual coaptation increases stability (*d*).

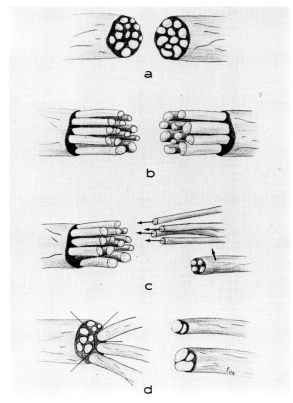

Figure 55–5. Polyfascicular nerve segment with 13 fascicles and 11 fascicles in the other stump, as a result of a small nerve defect and rapid changing of the fascicular pattern along the course. If a surgeon attempts to perform a fascicular coaptation after isolation of the individual fascicles and much dissection, he would face the problem of having to deal with the different number of fascicles in each stump. An error in the identification of corresponding fascicles would have more severe consequences, e.g., in stump-to-stump coaptation, which in this case still remains the optimal solution. The alignment of the fascicles can be improved by interfascicular stitches (not shown). If fascicular grafting is attempted, cutaneous nerves, such as the sural nerves, have to be split into their individual fascicles (*c*), which again increases the surgical trauma. In such a case we try to connect corresponding sectors of the stumps by individual nerve grafts (*d*) (sectoral grafting).

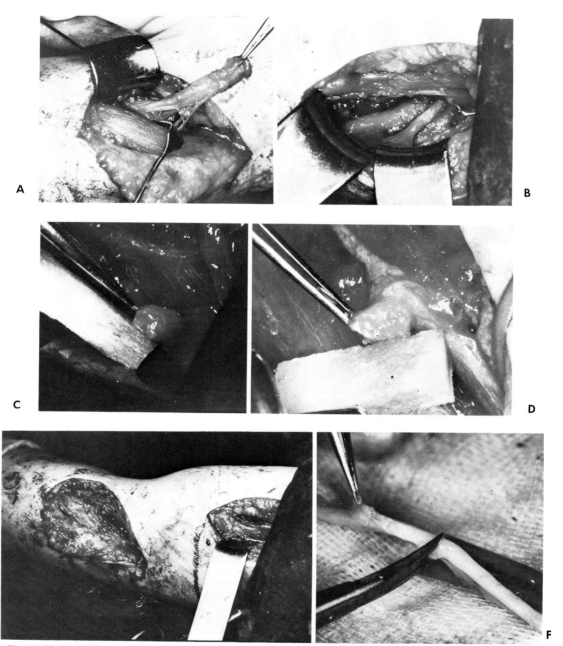

Figure 55–6. *A*, Distal stump near the elbow joint. Note the branches to the brachioradialis and extensor carpi radialis longus muscle. *B*, Proximal stump in the middle of the upper arm. *C*, Proximal stump after preparation. *D*, Distal stump after preparation. *E*, A tunnel is created connecting the two sites of coaptation. *F*, Sural grafts are provided and trimmed to proper length.

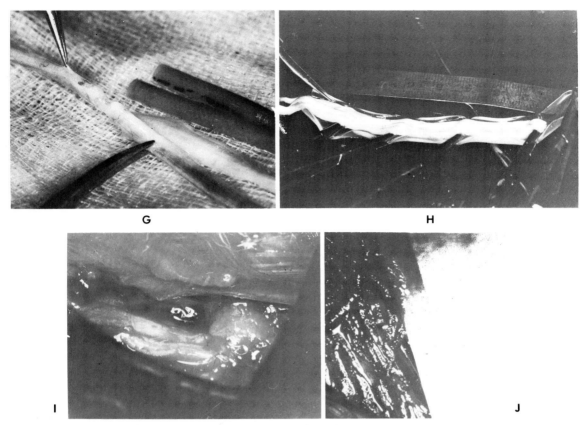

G

H

I

J

Figure 55–6 *Continued. G*, The epineurium of the graft ends and is shifted away to avoid covering the cross section. *H*, The grafts are placed in an open rubber tube. *I*, The proximal ends of the grafts are coapted to the proximal stump by one or two stitches per graft. *J*, The same is done at the distal end of the grafts.

immunosuppressive treatment would be necessary. Because the latter treatment is not without danger to the patient, it is questionable whether it can be justified for a nerve graft.

PRESERVED HOMOGRAFTS (ALLOGRAFTS) AND HETEROGRAFTS (XENOGRAFTS)

Preserved grafts are less immunogenic than heterografts. They are not real grafts but collagen frameworks without living cells. At present, the following methods to preserve such grafts are advocated:

Irradiation

Irradiation was proposed by Marmor (1963). This technique is still in the experimental stage.

Preservation in Cialit Solution

Successful use of nerve preserved in cialit solution (sodium 2-ethylmercurithiobenz oxazole-5-carboxylate) to bridge defects has been reported by Afanasieff (1971) and Motta (1971).

Preservation by Lyophilization

This technique has been used by Weiss (Weiss 1942; Weiss and Taylor, 1943). Lyons and Woodhall (1949) reported one success in 26 uses. Later, Jacoby claimed successful use of this method in 85 per cent of their cases (Jacoby, 1972; Jacoby et al., 1970). Some of the patients of Jacoby et al. who had good results were examined by other surgeons and neurologists. In all these cases the grafts were found to be nonconductive (Kuhlendahl et al., 1972). These experiences remind us of the need for caution in evaluating results.

PROBLEMS CONNECTED WITH NERVE GRAFTING

PROVIDING THE GRAFT

The use of a nerve trunk as a graft without loss of function is possible in the case of an amputee or when two nerves are involved and only one is to be repaired. The disadvantages of trunk grafts have been mentioned. Suitable donor nerves for cable and interfascicular nerve grafts are described in Chapters 57 and 58.

The Sural Nerve

The sural nerve usually originates from the tibial nerve in the lower part of the popliteal fossa. It can be identified and dissected out easily within the tibial and sciatic nerves up to the distal third of the thigh.

The sural nerve in the average adult is 30 to 40 cm. long. An additional 8 to 10 cm. can be gained by following the course of the nerve within the tibial and sciatic nerves.

The sural nerve has a diameter approximately equal to that of a common digital nerve. The sural nerve can be divided if the defect involves two collateral nerves and one common digital nerve. The diameter of the sural nerve matches well the diameters of the musculocutaneous, axillary, and accessory nerves. For the ulnar nerve, three or four, and for the median nerve, five or six, pieces of sural nerve are needed.

As a consequence of resection of the sural nerve, a small area of hypoesthesia develops at the lateral side of the heel and the foot. None of the hundreds of patients whose sural nerves we have resected has complained about this functional loss.

There have also been no complaints of a neuroma problem in our cases. I always resect such a long portion of the nerve that the proximal stump disappears under the fascia, even when I do not need that long a segment.

Medial Cutaneous Nerve of the Forearm

The medial cutaneous nerve of the forearm is excised by three transverse incisions. It provides a good nerve graft 20 cm. long, somewhat thicker than the sural nerve. The distal parts after the division are rather thin and difficult to use. The effect of excising this nerve is hypoesthesia along the medial part of the forearm. The zone supplied by this nerve can extend into the area usually supplied by the ulnar nerve. Therefore, we do not use this nerve as a graft when the ulnar nerve is involved.

Medial Cutaneous Nerve of the Arm

The medial cutaneous nerve of the arm originates from the medial cord too (C8, T1). It follows the course of the medial cutaneous nerve of the forearm and becomes subcutaneous in the proximal third of the arm. It provides a rather thin, short graft.

Lateral Cutaneous Nerve of the Thigh

The lateral cutaneous nerve of the thigh originates from L2. It enters the thigh just medial to the anterior superior iliac spine, turns laterally and supplies the lateral aspect of the thigh. It is found near the anterior superior iliac spine. One must bear in mind that at this level the nerve is still deep to the fascia. It is the only structure that turns in a laterodistal direction. The nerve provides a graft 15 to 20 cm. long. In its distal part the nerve has several branches. Sometimes it is difficult to find, and occasionally it is absent.

Saphenous Nerve

The saphenous nerve is a branch of the femoral nerve. It follows the neurovascular bundle and emerges superficial to the adductor muscles going to the medial aspect of the leg. It supplies the skin of the lower medial part of the leg, ankle, and foot proximal to the metatarsophalangeal joint. One can obtain a long graft. To preserve a sufficient nerve supply to the foot, one should avoid using this nerve together with the sural nerve.

Intercostal Nerves

The intercostal nerves are rather thin and have many branches. They are found between the layers of the external and internal intercostal muscles just below the inferior margins of the corresponding ribs. I have had no personal experience in using them as grafts, but have used them on several occasions for nerve transfers in cases of brachial plexus lesions.

Repair of Long Defects

In the majority of cases it is not difficult to obtain sufficient nerve material for repair of even long defects. There are two special situations in which the amount of grafting material may not be sufficient. These are long defects of the sciatic nerve and brachial plexus lesions. In these cases preserved homologous material could be used if it were more reliable.

With a long defect of the sciatic nerve, a part of the proximal stump can be used as a nerve graft to bridge the defect of the remaining cross section (Seddon, 1948).

NEUROTIZATION OF THE GRAFT

AUTOGRAFTS

After excision of the graft, its axons and myelin sheaths undergo wallerian degeneration. If the circulation within the graft is reestablished soon, the connective tissue cells and the Schwann cells survive. The Schwann cells proliferate and form Büngner's bands within the endoneurial tubes. Axon sprouts from the proximal stump have simply to cross the proximal suture line. Within the graft they meet ideal conditions. They can proceed along the Schwann cells of Büngner's band to the distal end of the graft. There is no need for structural changes, because the fascicular pattern of the graft is preserved. As already mentioned, when a trunk graft is used, the ischemic period may be prolonged in the central parts of the graft owing to the unfavorable relationship between surface area and tissue volume. The original fascicular pattern is destroyed, and fibrosis occurs. Under these conditions the neurotization is more complicated, and a new fascicular pattern must be established (Schröder and Seiffert, 1970).

Thin cutaneous nerve grafts have a much better surface area–tissue volume relationship, especially when the grafts have circumferential contact with the graft bed. When they are packed together to form a cable, parts of their surfaces come into contact with other grafts and not with the graft bed. Therefore, the chance of survival is optimal with the interfascicular technique, which employs individual nerve segments.

PRESERVED HOMOGRAFTS

Preserved homografts are not real grafts, but merely a nonvital collagen framework. After grafting, fibroblasts grow in, the original collagen framework is removed, and new collagen fibers are produced. When axons from the proximal stump enter the graft, they meet unfavorable conditions. It is not possible for them to proceed along the graft. The only way to achieve neurotization is by the formation at the proximal stump of a neuroma that includes Schwann cells, connective tissue, vessels, and axons. This neuroma grows along the graft (neuromatous neurotization according to Schröder and Seiffert, 1970). This explains the unreliability of results in using preserved grafts.

Within certain limits the length of the graft is not related to the functional result. It does not play a role when the graft is 3 or 5 or 7 cm. long. It is therefore a mistake to try to shorten the distance between the two stumps by mobilization or flexion of the adjacent joint just to be able to use a shorter graft.

Increased tension jeopardizes the functional result.

Because wallerian degeneration occurs within the graft, it is not important whether the graft is inserted in an orthodromic or antidromic direction.

Motor axons usually have larger diameters than do sensory axons. When cutaneous nerves are used as grafts, only sensory endoneurial tubes are available. This may be an unfavorable factor, but there is no alternative.

IDENTIFICATION OF CORRESPONDING FASCICLES

The fascicular patterns differ considerably along the course of a single nerve (Sunderland, 1968). Several authors believe that it is impossible to identify corresponding fascicles when there is an intervening defect between the nerve ends. This is true at a proximal level. There, the nerve fibers for specific functions are distributed diffusely over the cross section, so that a third of the cross section of a nerve can be incised without visible loss of function (Sherren, 1907). It is because of this diffuse distribution that there is a good chance that the axons will find the correct connections when the fascicles are united by grafts.

More distally the nerve fibers are well arranged according to their functions, and here it is essential to unite the corresponding fascicular ends. We try to achieve this in the following way.

For a lesion of the median nerve in the distal forearm, the median nerve is exposed up to its division in the proximal palm. The motor thenar branch is identified and followed proximally to the level of the lesion. An exact sketch is made of the distal cross section. In this sketch we can define very well the motor thenar branch and the fascicles going to the thumb, the index finger, and other regions. A sketch is made of the proximal cross section too. The two sketches are carefully studied, and the corresponding fascicles identified. Identification is easy in cases of short defects, but it becomes more difficult with longer defects. It is clear that the probability of achieving a good result decreases with the length of the defect. It is the amount of loss of neural substance that influences the result, not the length of the graft.

Freilinger et al. (1975) use a staining technique to differentiate motor and sensory axons. Unfortunately this technique takes two days for staining, which reduces its practical value.

COMPLICATIONS

Any complication, such as hematoma, infection, or wound rupture, will jeopardize the chances of a satisfactory result. The complications that are especially related to grafting procedure are the following:

THE GRAFT DOES NOT TAKE

This may happen when the graft bed was very fibrotic and the situation was not rectified by previous plastic surgical procedures. The graft transforms into a fibrotic band. Tinel's and Hoffmann's signs are not obtained along the course of the graft. If after two to three months Tinel's and Hoffmann's signs are still positive at the proximal end of the graft, it should be exposed and eventually the grafting should be repeated.

BLOCK AT THE PROXIMAL SUTURE LINE

The proximal suture line may be blocked by scar tissue in spite of a good take of the graft. The symptoms are the same as those described in the preceding paragraph. If Tinel's and Hoffmann's signs have not progressed within two to three months, the graft should be exposed.

BLOCK AT THE DISTAL SUTURE LINE

Because of the ingrowth of scar tissue, the distal suture line may be blocked when the axon sprouts reach this level.

When trunk grafts with classic epineurial suturing have been used, the distal suture lines have often been blocked when the grafts were longer than 3 cm. In such cases Tinel's and Hoffmann's signs progress to the level of the distal end of the graft and stop. When no further progression occurs after two to three months, the graft should be exposed, the distal suture line resected, and end to end suturing performed (Bsteh and Millesi, 1960; Davis and Cleveland, 1934; Lewis, 1923). Since the advent of the interfascicular technique, this complication has occurred only rarely.

MANAGEMENT OF SPECIFIC SITUATIONS

SEVERE SCARRING

When the original trauma has produced severe scarring, it is essential to correct this cicatrization by plastic surgery to provide a good bed for the graft. This may require use of a pedicled skin flap to cover the area of the future graft.

There are exceptional cases in which plastic surgical repair would require several steps and much time would be lost. In such cases it is possible to create a new graft bed, bypassing the area of the original injury.

ASSOCIATED BONE AND TENDON INJURIES

Usually the skeleton should be stabilized prior to the nerve repair. When there is a pseudarthrosis and bone shortening is indicated, one can gain as much as 3 to 4 cm. to achieve union of the nerve by end to end suturing.

When there is an associated tendon injury, the nerve is repaired in the first stage at the same time that Silastic rods are introduced for the tendons. In a second operation the Silastic rods are replaced by tendon grafts without exposure of the site of the neural lesion.

COMPLETE TRANSECTION OF THE NERVE NOT REPAIRED PRIMARILY

In this situation the indication for surgery is clear (Fig. 55–7). The two nerve stumps are exposed. Two approaches are possible.

1. The nerve is exposed by a longitudinal zigzag incision, including the site of the original injury. This is done when the length of the nerve defect is not known or when there are doubts that the lesion is complete.

2. The nerve stumps are exposed by two transverse incisions proximal and distal to the site of injury, leaving the injured area alone. After the two stumps are prepared, the grafts are introduced into tissue tunnels uniting the proximal and distal incisions. This maneuver is indicated in long defects with much scar tissue at the site of the original injury when complete transection has been confirmed during the primary wound closure.

The two nerve stumps can be prepared in two ways.

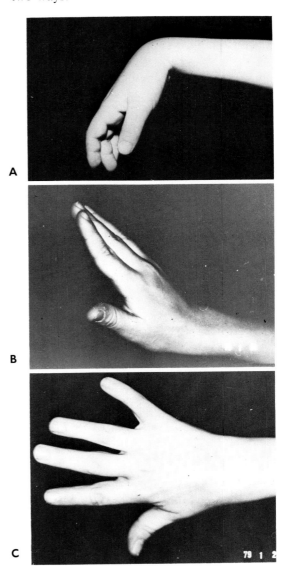

Figure 55–7. *A*, Right humerus fracture with complete high radial nerve palsy. Exploration was carried out 10 months after the accident. The distance between the two stumps of the radial nerve was 3.5 cm. Both stumps were severely fibrotic. After proper resection the final distance to be bridged was 9 cm. Four cutaneous nerve segments of 8 cm. in length were used (one sural, one cutaneous antebrachii medialis). Four months later muscle contraction can be detected in the extensor carpi radialis longus, eight months later satisfactory motor function was noted (average M 3,75). *B* and *C*, After two years, motor function is 4,5 but the patient cannot fully extend the digits in dorsiflexion of the wrist. This function returned at the end of the fourth year.

1. Serial transverse sections are made, starting within the neuroma or glioma until a cross section with a normal appearance is encountered. For this maneuver different apparatuses can be used (Edshage, 1964; Gosset, 1969; Stellbrink, 1969; Wilhelm, 1965).

2. Microsurgical dissection is performed, starting with an incision of the epineurium in the normal parts of the nerve and proceeding toward the neuroma. At the junction of normal and abnormal nerve tissue blunt dissection in the interfascicular tissue becomes more difficult. For each fascicle group the exact level of loss of normal appearances is defined, and the fascicle group is transected at this level. With this technique the resection of the stumps is rather generous, but this is important for the final result.

COMPLETE TRANSECTION OF THE NERVE WITH PRIMARY OR EARLY SECONDARY REPAIR WITHOUT RETURN OF FUNCTION

The problem in these cases is to determine the time when further delay would be futile. Electromyographic findings are often interpreted too optimistically because they may show that some axons have crossed the suture line. When after four to six months Tinel's and Hoffmann's signs are still obtained at the neural suture line and there is no sign of regeneration, the original suture should be exposed.

When Tinel's and Hoffmann's signs have progressed along the nerve, one can wait, so long as there is evidence of progressive regeneration.

After exposure, the site of the original suture could be resected and the two stumps freshened by transverse segmental resection. I prefer to incise and reflect the epineurium by use of a longitudinal incision, starting in the normal parts proximally and reaching the normal parts distally. The epineurium is resected, leaving intact a narrow strip on the deep side to prevent retraction of the stumps. The fascicles are then isolated by microsurgical interfascicular dissection.

COMPLETE TRANSECTION OF THE NERVE WITH PRIMARY OR EARLY SECONDARY REPAIR WITH PARTIAL BUT NOT SATISFACTORY RETURN OF FUNCTION

In these cases it is much more difficult to define the indications for reintervention.

Clinical observations, such as electromyographic evidence showing no progress for several months, and individual considerations such as the age of the patient may indicate the final decision.

After exposure, the suture line should not be resected, because regenerated nerve fibers might be sacrificed. By use of longitudinal microsurgical dissection, regenerated fascicles can be isolated and spared. Only the fascicles or groups of fascicles showing fibrotic changes are resected and replaced by grafts.

PARTIAL LESION OF THE NERVE

The site of the lesion is exposed, the damaged part of the nerve is defined by microsurgical dissection, and the interrupted fascicles are replaced by grafts.

OLD LESIONS

In young individuals, return of motor function has been achieved as long as three years after injury. When the patient is young and does not have complete muscular atrophy, repair of motor nerves should be attempted within this period.

Regeneration of sensory function in the form of useful protective sensibility can occur even after many years. Therefore, repair of a nerve with an important sensory function (e.g., the median nerve) should be undertaken even many years after injury. In a second stage, motor function can be improved by a tendon or muscle transfer.

Nerve grafting is sometimes indicated even when long periods have elapsed since injury to prevent the recurrence of painful neuromas. The best means of avoiding neuroma formation is to allow the axon to grow into the distal stump.

SUGGESTIONS FOR IMPROVING RESULTS

WRAPPING THE SUTURE LINE OR THE WHOLE GRAFT

By wrapping, the ingrowth of connective tissue and the aberration of axon sprouts should be prevented.

Early results obtained with the use of micropore membranes for wrapping led to optimistic reports (Böhler, 1962; Campbell et al., 1961). It was believed that the micropore membrane would allow nutrition by plasmatic circulation but prevent the ingrowth of cells and so prevent cellular homograft reactions. The long term results were disappointing (Böhler, 1966).

The use of resorbable material such as collagen sheets was suggested (Braun, 1964, 1966).

Silastic nerve cuffs to protect the suture line were designed (Campbell, 1966; Ducker and Hayes, 1967; Lehmann and Hayes, 1967).

Animal experiments have demonstrated that in spite of a satisfactory macroscopic appearance, significant connective tissue proliferation derived from the epineurium remains inside the wrapping. Without wrapping there was no ingrowth of connective tissue from the surroundings provided good apposition was achieved (Millesi, Berger, and Meissl, 1972).

Jacoby et al. (1970) wrapped their lyophilized homografts with lyophilized dura. Metz and Seeger (1969) used collagen to wrap lyophilized homografts.

"Sutureless" Nerve Suturing

The thesis was put forward that results of nerve repair could be improved if sutures were avoided and the union of the two ends was achieved by use of tissue glues (Heiss and Faul, 1965). Cyanoacrylate derivatives were used. The tissue glue causes considerable connective tissue proliferation. Even when contact between the glue and the cross section of the nerve is carefully avoided, the experimental results are inferior to those obtained with other methods (Berger et al., 1967; Berger and Millesi, 1969).

To avoid sutures and the foreign body reaction they cause, it would be ideal to rely on the natural clotting of the normal wound fibrin. The tensile strength of this union, however, is not great. Attempts have therefore been made to improve the tensile strength by use of homologous and heterologous fibrin (Tarlov and Benjamin, 1943; Young and Medawar, 1940). However, Lyons and Woodhall (1949) described tissue reactions to these fibrin deposits. Matras and Kuderna (1975) increased the tensile strength after interfascicular nerve grafting by putting a fibrinogen concentrate with thrombin and calcium on the coaptation.

When tension at the suture site can be avoided completely, the tensile strength of the normal wound fibrin is sufficient to maintain the union (Millesi, Berger, and Meissl, 1972). As a matter of fact, the interfascicular grafting technique relies on the natural clotting mechanisms. The single 10-0 or 11-0 suture that is used at each end of the graft serves more to orientate graft and corresponding fascicle group with minimal trauma than to contribute to the tensile strength.

Further improvement in the results of nerve repair could be expected if connective tissue proliferation could be reduced by the use of drugs. There are several possible ways to interfere with collagen production. Research work in this direction is under way in several centers.

RESULTS

It is extremely difficult to evaluate the results of nerve repair, and it is even more difficult to compare results reported by different investigators.

Objective criteria for evaluation are still lacking. More and more we appreciate how common are anomalies of innervation, which, when present, may simulate a good functional result. In the average case, the result depends on the age of the patient, the time elapsed since the injury, the level of the injury, the length of the defect (loss of neural substance)—with a secondary repair there is usually a defect, surgical technique, which plays an important role (maximal accuracy and sense for meticulous details are a sine qua non), and the method used.

With the greatest caution, the following problems should be considered:

Grafting Versus Suturing

Earlier in the chapter, in discussing nerve grafting, I mentioned experiments demonstrating that under ideal conditions a graft gives much better results than does suturing the nerve under moderate tension. This was confirmed in an exacting study carried out by Samii et al. (1972).

Ashworth et al. (1971) reported the management of long median nerve defects in 15 patients by maximal mobilization of the nerve

Table 55–1. RESULTS OF RADIAL NERVE REPAIR BY NERVE GRAFTING

M5			M4			M3			M2		
Age (years)	Interval (months)	Defect (cm.)	Age (years)	Interval (months)	Defect (cm.)	Age (years)	Interval (months)	Defect (cm.)	Age (years)	Interval (months)	Defect (cm.)
19	18	4.0	8	3	8.5	8	12	12.5	62	3	10.0
30	1	3.0	22	8	6.0	42	29	9.0			
21	11	10.0	53	4	4.0	26	7	6.0			
42	3	3.0	25	5	8.0	16	3	14.0			
25	8	15.0	34	3	12.0						
16	3	6.0	26	18	8.0						
11	2	9.0	63	0	10.0						
22	5	6.0	9	10	7.0						
33	4	8.0	10	29	10.0						
62	6	4.0	18	6	8.0						
25	6	8.0	49	5	12.0						
32	6	11.0	24	7	10.0						
64	1	2.0									

and maximal flexion of the joints. In all the cases some protective sensibility returned. In four cases some activity of the thenar muscles was even achieved.

In a series of cases of median nerve injury in which the defects were longer than 5 cm., seven of 11 patients treated by interfascicular nerve grafting achieved motor function of M4 to M5, and eight of the 11 had useful two point discrimination.

AUTOGRAFTS VERSUS HOMOGRAFTS

The excellent results that Jacoby et al. (1970, 1972) claimed to have achieved with

Table 55–2.   RESULTS OF MEDIAN NERVE REPAIR BY NERVE GRAFTING ACCORDING TO HIGHET'S SCHEME (M0–M5, S0–S4)*

	Mixed Innervation of Thenar Muscles — Age-Interval-Defect (months; cm.)			M4–M5 — Age-Interval-Defect (months; cm.)			M3 — Age-Interval-Defect (months; cm.)			M2 — Age-Interval-Defect (months; cm.)			M1 — Age-Interval-Defect (months; cm.)			M0 — Age-Interval-Defect (months; cm.)		
	21	4	5.0	19	6	2.5				23	4	7.0						
	20	1	2.0	22	8	8.0												
	25	2	3.5	18	7	7.0												
	40	2	2.0	21	2	6.0												
S3 + −4	27	2	3.5	10	9	5.0												
	49	1	6.5	9	2	5.0												
	44	8	5.0	20	3	5.0												
	7	2	2.0	46	5	3.5												
	13	4	4.0	50	2	2.0												
				10	4	4.0												
	21	4	4.5	35	6	2.0	43	8	5.0	41	28	15.0						
	21	2	6.0	19	2	4.0	44	36	12.0									
	46	4	2.0	50	2	3.0	48	18	7.0									
S3	24	4	5.0				25	2	5.0									
	27	2	4.0				6	5	4.0									
	52	12	4.5															
	30	9	10.0															
	23	5	4.0															
S2	61	3	4.0															
	26	11	16.0															
S1																		
S0																		

*Thirty-nine cases, there is a high percentage of mixed innervation of the thenar muscle.

Table 55–3. RESULTS OF ULNAR NERVE REPAIR BY NERVE GRAFTING ACCORDING TO HIGHET'S SCHEME (M0–M5, S0–S4)

Mixed Innervation	M4–M5	M3	M2+	M2	M1	M0
AGE-INTERVAL-DEFECT (months; cm.)	AGE-INTERVAL-DEFECT (months; cm.)	AGE-INTERVAL-DEFECT (months; cm.)*	AGE-INTERVAL-DEFECT (months; cm.)*	AGE-INTERVAL-DEFECT (months; cm.)*	AGE-INTERVAL-DEFECT (months; cm.)*	AGE-INTERVAL-DEFECT (months; cm.)*
4 5 2.0						
18 10 6.0						
	11 2 5.0	13 6 5.0				
	11 3 6.0*	55 4 2.0				
	12 2 5.0					
	12 3 3.0*					
S3+ − 4	7 4 4.5					
	20 36 7.0					
	23 2 5.0					
	28 9 5.0					
	40 6 3.0					
	11 12 5.0	18 3 2.0	25 7 10.0*	31 48 20.0*		
	12 3 10.0*	34 31 20.0*	18 7 13.0*	17 6 6.0*		
	17 5 7.0	39 11 18.0*	37 6 3.0			
	16 6 4.0	40 8 5.0				
	21 4 6.0	48 3 6.0*				
	22 7 2.0*	49 4 4.0				
S3	19 1 3.0*	45 5 4.0				
	49 2 4.0*	54 8 3.0				
	63 13 3.0*	56 2 3.0				
	64 1 2.0					
	67 13 3.0*					
	25 2 3.0*					
	27 10 4.0					
S2			25 8 6.0*			28 5 15.0*
						16 4 6.0*
S1			64 2 16.0*			
S0				44 7 11.0		33 6 19.0*

*Defect = proximal lesion.

lyophilized homografts were not supported by the results of a critical examination by a commission of the German Society for Neurosurgery (Kuhlendahl et al., 1972). In none of the eight cases examined could any sign of recovery be demonstrated.

Afanasieff (1971) reported 44 nerve repairs using Cialit preserved homografts. In less than half the cases protective sensibility returned. The return of motor function was poor. Motta (1971) compared autografts with Cialit preserved homografts and confirmed the superiority of the autografts. Doi, et al. (1971) re-examined six patients who had nerve repairs using Cialit preserved homografts. In none of these cases was there any definite sign of regeneration. At the present time the results achieved by use of preserved homografts are so unreliable that they should be considered for use only after all possibilities for autografting are exhausted.

DIFFERENT TECHNIQUES OF AUTOGRAFTING

Seddon (1972) reported 17 good results in 25 cases after trunk grafts in the upper extremity. In 1948 Seddon had described the danger of central necrosis in trunk grafts. This is an additional reason to appreciate his results. During the same period, 13 pedicled nerve grafts were carried out, with eight good results. Of 22 cable grafts, nine patients achieved good results, four achieved fair results, and nine were failures.

The results in using interfascicular nerve grafts are presented in Tables 55–1 to 55–4. Excellent results have been achieved by Samii and Kahl (1972) using the interfascicular grafting technique. Some of these cases were controlled by the commission of the German Society for Neurosurgery, and the results confirmed. Palazzi and Marrero (1971), Be-

Table 55–4. RESULTS OF COMBINED MEDIAN AND ULNAR NERVE REPAIR*†

	M4–M5		M3		M2+		M2		M1		M0	
	Age·Interval·Defect (months; cm.)		Age·Interval·Defect (months; cm.)		Age·Interval·Defect (months; cm.)		Age·Interval·Defect (months; cm.)		Age·Interval·Defect (months; cm.)		Age·Interval·Defect (months; cm.)	
S3+	M19 4 5.0	U19 4 5.0	M15 5 20.0				M23 6 7.0				M12 48 19.0	
	M10 4 12.0	U10 4 6.0	M39 18 13.0				M10 18 3.0				M12 49 12.0	
–4	M13 2 5.0		U55 10 3.0									
	M19 2 4.0											
	M51 0 2.0	U51 0 2.0	M15 5 6.0	U15 5 7.0	U15 5 20.0		M69 9 5.0		M38 8 6.5	U38 8 4.0		
	M10 29 NN†	U10 29 8.5	M11 2 4.0	U11 2 4.0	U39 9 7.0		M18 9 7.0		M49 11 13.0			
	M18 6 7.0	U18 6 7.0	M62 4 3.0		U18 6 9.0		M10 3 1.5	U49 11 4.0			U18 9 15.0	
	M39 9 5.5		M46 3 4.0		U26 3 9.0							
					U1 16 8.0							
					U19 3 4.0							
S3		U46 3 4.0	M55 10 16.0									
		U13 2 5.0	M36 3 13.0									
		U23 6 11.0	M59 3 6.0									
		U19 2 4.0	U39 18 11.0									
		U10 3 9.0	U69 9 5.5									
			U39 9 3.0									
			U10 18 NN†									
S2			U62 4 7.0				M47 13 7.0				M61 16 NL†	
			U47 13 5.0				M39 9 8.0					
							M18 6 18.0					

*Twenty-nine patients with 30 extremities involved. In two extremities after tissue loss resulting from a severe electrical burn, only the continuity of the median nerve was repaired. Fifty-five grafting procedures, two end to end nerve repairs, and one neurolysis were performed (Median—28 grafts, one end to end repair, one neurolysis; ulnar—27 grafts, one end to end repair).

†NN = end to end repair, NL = neurolysis.

deschi (1971), and Salvi (1973) have also reported good results by use of this technique.

REFERENCES

Albert, E.: Einige Operationen an Nerven. Wien. Med. Presse, *26*:1285, 1885.

Afanasieff, A.: Les homogreffes des nerfs conserves pa le Cialit. Chir. Main (Toulouse), *31*:19–26, 1971.

Anderl, H.: Rekonstruktive Eingriffe am peripheren Nerven mittels mikrochirurgischer Operationstechniken. Actuelle Chir., *8*:285–292, 1973.

Ashworth, C. A., Boyes, J. H., and Stark, H. H.: N. med. etwas Schutzsensibilität 4 von 15 gewisse Thenaraktivität. 26th Annual Meeting, American Society for Surgery of the Hand, March 5–6, 1971, San Francisco, Cal.

Bedeschi, P.: Reparation micro-chirurgicale des lesions traumatique des nerfs peripheriques du membre superieur par autogreffes nerveuses. SICOT 12 Abstr. Israel, October 9–13, 1972, p. 522.

Bedeschi, P.: Lesioni traumatiche dei nervi periferici. LVI Congresso della Societa Italiana di Ortopedia e Traumatologia, Rome, Nov. 10, 1971.

Berger, A., Ganglberger, J., and Millesi, H.: Experimentelle Untersuchungen zur Nervennaht mit Klebstoffen. I. Intern. Kongress Klebstoffe Wien, Sept. 1967.

Berger, A., and Millesi, H.: Verwendung von Klebstoffen zum Verschluß von Hautwunden und zur Vereinigung durchtrennter peripherer Nerven. Kunststoffe in der Chirurgie, Symposium, Innsbruck, Feb. 16, 1969, Vol. 13, pp. 173–178.

Bielschowsky, M., and Unger, E.: Überbrückung großer Nervenlücken.. Beiträge zur Kenntnis der Degeneration und Regeneration peripherer Nerven. J. Physiol. Neurol., *22*:267, 1916–1918.

Böhler, J.: Nervennaht und homoioplastische Nerventransplantation mit Milleporeumscheidung. Referat gehalten am 28.4.1962 bei der Tagung der Deutschen Gesellschaft Chir., München.

Böhler, J.: Vortrag am X. Kongress der SICOT, Paris, Sept. 9, 1966.

Boyes, H. J.: Repair of the motor branch of the ulnar nerve in the palm. J. Bone Joint Surg., *37A*:920, 1955.

Braun, R. M.: Comparative studies of neurorrhaphy and sutureless peripheral nerve repair. Surg. Gynecol. Obstet., *122*:15, 1966.

Braun, R. M.: Experimental peripheral nerve repair. Surg. Forum, *15*:452, 1964.

Brooks, D.: The place of nerve grafting in orthopaedic surgery. J. Bone Joint Surg., *37A*:299, 1955.

Bsteh, F. X., and Millesi, H.: Zur Kenntnis der zweizeitigen Nerveninterplantation an ausgedehnten peripheren Nervendefekten. Klin. Med., *12*:571, 1960.

Buck-Gramcko, D.: Wiederherstellung durchtrennter peripherer Nerven. Handchir. Praxis, *15*:55–63, 1971.

Bunnell, S., and Boyes, H. J.: Nerve grafts. Am. J. Surg., *45*:64, 1939.

Campbell, J. B.: Kongress der SICOT, Paris, Sept. 9, 1966.

Campbell, J. B., Basset, C. A. L., Husby, J., Thulin, C. A., and Fingera, E. R.: Microfilter sheaths in peripheral nerve surgery. A laboratory report and preliminary clinical study. J. Trauma, *1*:139–157, 1961.

Davis, L., and Cleveland, D. A.: Experimental study in nerve transplants. Ann. Surg., *99*:271–283, 1934.

Doi, T., Egawa, T., and Horiki, A.: Clinical Use of Peripheral Nerve Homografts Preserved in Cialit Solution. Proceedings of the 14th Annual Meeting of the Japanese Society for Surgery of the Hand, Osaka, 1971, p. 36.

Ducker, T. B., and Hayes, G. J.: A comparative study of the technique of nerve repair. Surg. Forum, *28*:443–445, 1967.

Ducker, T. B., Kempe, L. G., and Hayes, G. J.: The metabolic background of peripheral nerve surgery. J. Neurosurg., *30*:270, 1969.

Edshage, S.: Peripheral nerve suture. Acta Chir. Scand., Suppl. 331, 1964.

Finochietto, R.: Translacion de Nervoios cubital radial y mediano. Prinsa Med., *48*:503, 1961.

Freilinger, G., Gruber, H., Holle, J., and Mandl, H.: Zur Methodik der "sensomotorisch" differenzierten Faszikelnaht peripherer Nerven. Handchirurgie, *7*:133–138, 1975.

Furlan, S., Rigotti, G., and Barisoni, D.: Conference at 11th Congress, Nat. Societa Italiana di Chirurgia della Mano, Pavia, Dec. 8–9, 1973.

Gosset, J.: Zit. nach Michon J. Die Nervennaht unter dem Mikroskop. Handchirurgie, *2*:75–76, 1969.

Heiss, W. H., and Faul, P.: Nervennaht mit Klebstoff. Langenbeck's Arch. Klin. Chir., *313*:710, 1965.

Highet, W. B., and Holmes, W.: Traction injuries to the lateral popliteal nerve and traction injuries to peripheral nerves after suture. Br. J. Surg., *30*:212, 1943.

Holmes, W., and Young, J. Z.: Nerve regeneration after immediate and delayed suture. J. Anat., *77*:63, 1942.

Jacoby, W.: Langenbeck's Arch. Klin. Chir., *332* (Kongressbericht), 1972.

Jacoby, W., Fahlbruch, R., Mackert, B., Braun, B., Rolle, J., and Schnell, J.: Überbrückung peripherer Nervendefekte mit Lyophilisierten und desantigenisierten Transplantaten. Münch. Med. Wochenschr., *112*:586–589, 1970.

Kreutzberg, G. W.: Changes of coenzyme (TPN) diaphorase and TPN-linked dehydrogenase during axonal reaction of the nerve cells. Nature (Lond.), *199*:393, 1963.

Kuhlendahl, H., Mumenthaler, M., Penzholz, H., Röttgen, P., Struppler, A., and Schliack, H.: Behandlung peripherer Nervenverletzungen mit homologen Nervenimplantaten. Z. Neurol., *202*:251–256, 1972.

Lehmann, R. A., and Hayes, G. J.: Degeneration und Regeneration in peripheral nerve. Brain, *90*:285–296, 1967.

Lewis, D.: Some peripheral nerve problems. Boston Med. Surg. J., *188*:875, 1923.

Lyons, W. R., and Woodhall, B.: Atlas of Peripheral Nerve Injuries. Philadelphia, W. B. Saunders Company, 1949.

Marmor, L.: Regeneration of peripheral nerves by irradiated homografts. Lancet, *1*:1911, 1963.

Matras, H., and Kuderna, H.: The Principle of Nervous Anastomosis with Clotting Agents. 6th Int. Congr. Plast. Reconstr. Surg., Paris, Aug. 24–29, 1975.

Metz, R., and Seeger, W.: Collagen wrapping of nerve homotransplants in dogs. Europ. Surg. Res., *1*:157, 1969.

Michon, J., and Masse, P.: Le moment optimum de la suture nerveuses dans les paies du membre superieur. Rev. Chir. Orthop., *50*:205–212, 1964.

Millesi, H.: Zum Problem der Überbrückung von De

fekten peripherer Nerven. Wien. Med. Wochenschr., *118*:182–187, 1968.

Millesi, H., Berger, A., and Meissl, G.: Experimentelle Untersuchungen zur Heilung durchtrennter peripherer Nerven. Chir. Plast., *1*:174–206, 1972.

Millesi, H., Ganglberger, J., and Berger, A.: Erfahrungen mit der Mikrochirurgie peripherer Nerven. Chir. Plast. Reconstr., *3*:47–55, 1967.

Millesi, H., Meissl, G., and Berger, A.: Entwicklungstendenzen in der operativen Wiederherstellung durchtrennter peripherer Nerven. Bolesti i Ozljeda Sake Medicinska Naklada, Zagreb, 1970, pp. 161–175.

Millesi, H., Meissl, G., and Berger, A.: The interfascicular nerve grafting of the median and ulnar nerves. J. Bone Joint Surg., *54A*:727–750, 1972.

Motta, A.: La nostra esperienza negli innesti di nervo ell-artro superiore. Chir. Main (Toulouse), *31*:11–17, 1971.

Narakas, A., and Verdan, C.: Les greffes nerveuses. Zeitschr. Unfallmed. Berufskrankheiten, *3*:137–152, 1969.

Nicholson, O. R., and Seddon, H. J.: Nerve repair in civil practice. Results of treatment of median and ulnar nerve lesions. Br. Med. J., *2*:1065, 1957.

Nomura, S., Yamada, H., Toda, N., Yasomoto, S., Kobayashi, S., Shiroishi, H., Honda, M., and Shima, I.: Nerve flap method. Report of 8 cases. Proceedings, 13th Annual Meeting, Japanese Society for Surgery of the Hand, Nagaya, 1970, p. 33.

Palazzi, S. C., and Marrero, R. M.: La microcirurgia en las lesiones de los nervios periféricos. Revista de Ortop. y Traumatol. Vol 15, IB, Fasc. 4, 1971, pp. 499–526.

Sakellarides, H.: A follow up study of 173 peripheral nerve injuries in the upper extremity in civilians. J. Bone Joint Surg., *44A*:140, 1962.

Salvi, V.: Problems connected with the repair of nerve sections. Hand, *5*:25–32, 1973.

Samii, M., and Kahl, R. I.: Klinische Resultate der autologen Nerventransplantation. Melsunger Med. Mitteilungen, 46 (No. 116):197–202, 1972.

Samii, M., and Willebrand, H.: Zur Indikation und mikrochirurgischen Technik von autologen Nerventransplantaten. Vortrag Jahrestagung Deutsche Gesellschaft für Neurochirurgie, 1970.

Samii, M., Wallenborn, R., and Scheinpflug, W.: Experimentelle vergleichende Untersuchungen oder Nerventransplantation mit autologen u. lyophilisierten homologen Nerven. Symposium Kassel Wilhelmshöhe, Feb. 3–4, 1972.

Schröder, J. M., and Seiffert, K. E.: Die Feinstruktur der neuromatösen Neurotisation von Nerventransplantaten. Virchows Arch. Abtlg. B. Zellpathol., *5*:219–235, 1970.

Seddon, H. J.: Three types of nerve injury. Brain, *66*:237, 1943.

Seddon, H. J.: The early management of peripheral nerve injuries. Practitioner, *157*:101, 1944.

Seddon, H. J.: Restoration of function in peripheral nerve injuries. Lancet, *1*:418, 1947.

Seddon, H. J.: The use of autogenous grafts for the repair of large gaps in peripheral nerves. Br. J. Surg., *35*:151, 1948.

Seddon, H. J.: War injuries of peripheral nerves. *In* Wounds of the Extremities. Br. J. Surg., War Surg. Suppl. No. 2, 325, 1948.

Seddon, H. J.: Surgical Disorders of the Peripheral Nerves. Edinburgh and London, Churchill Livingstone, 1972.

Seitelberger, F., Sluga, E., Millesi, H., and Meissl, G.: Vortrag gehalten am 21.11.1969 in der Gesellschaft der Ärzte, Wien.

Sherren, J.: Injuries of Nerves and Their Treatment. New York, William Wood, 1907.

Smith, J. W.: Factors influencing nerve repair. I. Blood supply of peripheral nerves. Arch. Surg., *93*:335, 1966.

Smith, J. W.: Factors influencing nerve repair. II. Collateral circulation of peripheral nerves. Arch. Surg., *93*:433, 1966.

Stellbrink, G.: Modifizierter Stenström'scher Nervenhalter für die Chirurgie der peripheren Nerven. Chirurgie, *40*:424–425, 1969.

Strange, F. G. St. C.: An operation for nerve pedicle grafting. Preliminary communication. Br. J. Surg., *34*:423, 1947.

Sunderland, S.: Nerve and Nerve Injuries. Baltimore, The Williams & Wilkins Company, 1968, pp. 27, 38, 63.

Tarlov, I. M., and Benjamin, B.: Plasma clot and silk sutures of nerves: experimental study of comparative tissue reactivities. Surg. Gynecol. Obstet., *76*:366, 1943.

Ventimiglia, N.: Vortrag am 3. Operationskurs über Mikrochirurgie der peripheren Nerven. Mainz, May 1973.

Weiss, P.: Functional nerve regeneration through frozen-dried nerve grafts in cats and monkeys. Proc. Soc. Exp. Biol. Med., *54*:277, 1942.

Weiss, P., and Taylor, A. C.: Repair of peripheral nerves by grafts of frozen-dried nerves. Proc. Soc. Exp. Biol. Med., *52*:326, 1943.

Weiss, P., and Hiscoe, H. B.: Experiments on the mechanism of nerve growth. J. Exp. Zool., *107*:315, 1948.

Wilheim, A.: Verletzungen peripherer Nerven. *In* Traumatologie in der Chirurgischen Praxis. Berlin, Springer-Verlag, 1965.

Young, J. Z., and Medawar, P. B.: Die Kabeltransplantate mit Fibrin. Lancet, *2*:126, 1940.

Chapter 56

DONOR SITES FOR NERVE GRAFTS

Alain Gilbert,
Wilson de Moura,
Ricardo Salazar-Lopez,
and John A. I. Grossman

The problems produced by the loss of nerve substance have always been the subject of many articles and research projects. Various ingenious methods have been proposed but with only equivocal results. Suturing at a distance, with the interposition of silk or catgut (proposed by Assaky in 1886 and Huber in 1895), has yielded clinically poor results (Stopford, 1920). Tubulization with another material, like silicone, millipore, or vein, has given some good experimental results, but the clinical results have been judged insufficient (Chao et al., 1962; Swan, 1941).

Early in this century nerve heterografts were used—either fresh grafts, preserved grafts, or grafts fixed in alcohol (Duroux, 1911; Gluck, 1880; Nageotte, 1917). Some researchers also utilized spinal cord, essentially that of the cat (Gosset and Bertrand, 1937; Mayo-Robson, 1896). Experimental and clinical results were equivocal and the method was abandoned (Bjorkesten, 1948).

Homografts also failed to yield good results, whether they were fresh or preserved (Forssmann, 1900), but a renewed interest in homografts resulted with the appearance of immunosuppressive drugs like cyclosporine A, which allows the graft to behave like an autograft (Green, 1984; Izquierdo, 1984). This new technique may someday be the single answer to the problems posed by loss of nerve substance. Meanwhile the only practical and efficacious possibility we have is the autograft.

CHARACTERISTICS OF A NERVE GRAFT

As with all instances of autotransplantation, we are limited by the difficulty of finding donor sites where morbidity is low. The characteristics of the ideal graft are determined by several factors, well studied by Sunderland (1972). Revascularization of a graft is difficult if the nerve diameter is large. In the case of a large trunk there is often a central necrotic area. The capacity of a graft to revascularize is inversely proportional to the number of fascicles; i.e., the graft is more fragile if it consists of only one or two fascicles, and it revascularizes less well than a multifascicular nerve. The amount of connective interfascicular tissue is equally important: the more developed this connective tissue is, the more difficult will be the revascularization of the fascicle.

The quality of axonal passage between the extremities of the nerve and the graft is influenced by the morphology of the graft. The ideal graft has several fascicles, pressed tightly against each other, with just a small amount of interstitial tissue. A large quantity of interstitial tissue is the source of axonal loss.

The maturation of axons may be influenced by the diameter of the endoneurial tubes of the graft. It is probable that the utilization of grafts after a long period of denervation, if they have endoneurial tubes of small diameter, can complicate the maturation of axons. Some authors claim that the passage and growth of large motor fibers are complicated by the utilization of sensory nerve grafts because their endoneurial tubes have an unacceptably small diameter (Hammond and Hinsey, 1945). However, Simpson and Young (1945) have shown that the diameter of endoneurial tubes can be dilated by larger axons. Even though experiments have demonstrated that sensory nerve grafts with tubes of small diameter can succeed perfectly with motor nerves, it is undoubtedly preferable to choose grafts that have endoneurial tubes with diameters as large as possible.

Fascicular correspondence at the graft extremities can be important for precise suturing, mainly in the repair of mixed nerves. The graft has a fascicular arrangement that varies along its length, with a variable number of fascicles. These variations in arrangement and fascicle number at the graft extremities are a drawback, but considering that the endoneurial tubes of nerve grafts often have a reduced diameter, this scarcely influences the repair. Only in situations like facial paralysis, digital nerve repair, and neurotizations in which the graft is larger than the nerve to be repaired does absolute concordance of fascicular arrangements at the graft extremities become necessary.

The length of the graft and the ease of harvesting are important factors. Some long grafts like the sural nerve are particularly useful for repair in cases of large losses of nerve substance, as in the brachial plexus or some peripheral nerves. It is wasteful to utilize a large nerve like the sural nerve for a graft involving a small loss of nerve substance, as in a digital nerve. It is preferable in such cases to harvest a small graft near the area to be repaired. The deficit at the donor site must also be considered, because the benefits of repair can only be diminished by a poor result at the donor site.

Having determined the ideal qualities of a nerve graft, we can compare several donor sites where we can find not the ideal graft but a graft that will adapt well to the clinical situation under consideration. According to Seddon (1948), nerve trunks are not useful as free grafts because, as we have mentioned, there is a risk of central necrosis. Strange's procedure and, more recently, microsurgical revascularization of nerve grafts permit reconsideration of this judgment. We will see that sensory nerve grafts are quite useful.

SURAL NERVE

Described a long time ago, the sural nerve was recently the object of a detailed study (de Moura and Gilbert, 1984). The medial cutaneous sural nerve emerges 2.5 cm. proximal to the flexor crease of the popliteal fossa, from the posterior tibial nerve. Soon it is accompanied by its artery and satellite vein (Fig. 56–1), and it courses into a groove between the two heads of the gastrocnemius muscle and the soleus muscle. It courses as far as the musculotendinous junction and leaves the groove, through the superficial aponeurosis, and becomes superficial. This passage through the aponeurosis is remarkably constant and occurs about 16 cm. from the inferior extremity of the malleolus in an adult of medium stature (Fig. 56–2). In general, the nerve is rejoined at this level by the lateral cutaneous sural nerve; the trunk formed by the union of these two nerves should be called the *sural nerve proper.*

This nerve almost always lies next to the lesser saphenous vein. About 6 cm. above the extremity of the malleolus, the nerve gives off the first collateral branch, the lateral calcaneous branch. The nerve divides about 2 cm. above the malleolus into posterior and anterior terminal branches (Fig. 56–3). Its total length varies between 31 and 37 cm., according to the length of the limb; its aver-

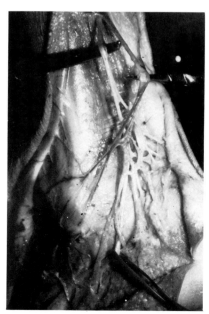

Figure 56–1. The origins of the sural nerve and the lesser saphenous vein.

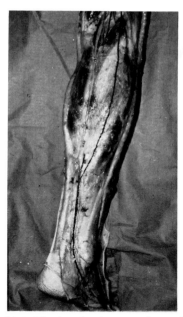

Figure 56–2. The junction between the medial cutaneous sural nerve, which is leaving the aponeurosis, and the lateral cutaneous sural nerve.

age length is 33 cm. The nerve does not have branches in its course through the aponeurosis.

After exiting from the aponeurosis, the nerve receives the lateral cutaneous sural nerve, a huge communication coming from the common peroneal nerve. The superficial cutaneous branch of the common peroneal

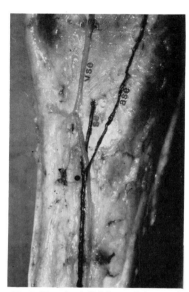

Figure 56–3. Terminal divisions of the sural nerve and lesser saphenous vein. vse = lesser saphenous vein, se = medial sural nerve, and ase = lateral sural nerve.

nerve arises about 3.8 cm. below the popliteal crease and soon gives off an anterior cutaneous branch called the cutaneous peroneal nerve. The lateral cutaneous sural nerve soon becomes superficial and passes over the aponeurosis of the lateral head of the gastrocnemius until it unites with the medial cutaneous sural nerve, about 16 cm. from the extremity of the malleolus. This anatomical configuration is found in 74 per cent of the cases. In 22 per cent of the cases there is no anastomosis and the nerves proceed in a parallel fashion. Finally, in 4 per cent of the cases the anastomosis has another anatomical configuration (Fig. 56–4).

The medial cutaneous sural nerve is a complex composite made up of two nerves that unite into one trunk in the inferior third of the leg. This configuration argues against harvesting the nerve unless it can be directly viewed; otherwise precious grafts may be lost. In 20 per cent of the cases the medial cutaneous sural nerve is smaller than the lateral cutaneous sural nerve, making it necessary to harvest both nerves together. This may be confirmed by the histological structure of this configuration; the medial cutaneous sural nerve at the level of its origin has two large fascicles, and the lateral cutaneous sural has five fascicles. At the level of the sural nerve, the nerve has, on the average, nine fascicles (Fig. 56–5).

Harvesting the nerve must take account of the relatively stable localization of the branches and long portions without any branch. In the child it is preferable to use one longitudinal incision, to avoid destroying the nerve by traction. In the adult it is possible to do the harvesting with several short incisions. A retromalleolar incision allows the nerve to be located and allows the terminal divisions to be sectioned. An oblique or vertical incision 16 cm. from the extremity of the malleolus makes it possible to locate the junction between the medial cutaneous sural nerve and the lateral cutaneous sural nerve. A medial horizontal incision below the popliteal crease allows sectioning of the medial cutaneous sural nerve at its origin. A posterior incision at the level of the peroneal head allows sectioning of the lateral cutaneous sural nerve.

Harvesting proceeds as follows. One locates the terminal branches and then the 16 cm. junction point between the lateral and medial cutaneous sural nerves. With slight traction the precise course of the lateral cu-

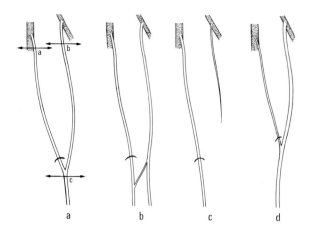

Figure 56–4. Anatomical variations of the sural nerve and its branches. *a*, The most common organization (74 per cent). *b*, Sometimes the two nerves are separated (22 per cent). *c* and *d*, Rare variations.

taneous sural nerve can be found and the nerve is cut at the proximal extremity. With a popliteal incision the medial cutaneous sural nerve can be located and sectioned. By using gentle traction at the level of the junction, the lateral and medial cutaneous sural branches can be harvested, proceeding from the origin on; this makes possible a complete harvesting. In this way the nerve can be harvested with subcutaneous traction in the middle, not high or low, as is often the procedure, to conserve both the nerves. Thus the length of the harvested graft can be doubled (Fig. 56–6).

ANTEBRACHIAL MEDIAL CUTANEOUS NERVE

The antebrachial medial cutaneous nerve is one of the terminal branches of the medial cord. It emerges at the axilla level and follows the vascular nerve complex in the medial aspect of the arm between the short portion of the biceps and the vastus medialis. It becomes subcutaneous, going through the aponeurosis in the median third of the arm and following the basilic vein. Soon it gives

off a cutaneous branch for the region (Fig. 56–7). About 8 cm. above the flexion crease of the elbow, it divides into two branches. A posterior branch goes to the internal or medial aspect of the forearm, crossing the flexion crease of the elbow in front of the epitrochlea. It is a very thin branch, generally formed by two fascicles; this branch is not usable. An anterior branch goes directly to the axis of the ulna and terminates at the

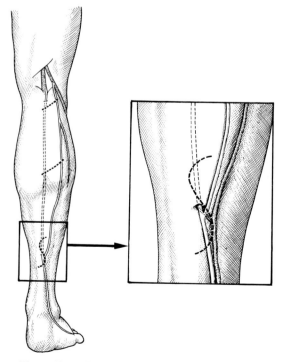

Figure 56–6. Harvesting the sural nerve. The small incisions will allow dissection of the two roots of the sural nerve.

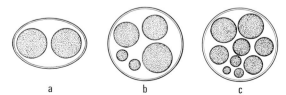

Figure 56–5. Fascicular configurations of the sural nerve. *a*, At its origin; *b*, the lateral cutaneous sural nerve; *c*, at its distal part.

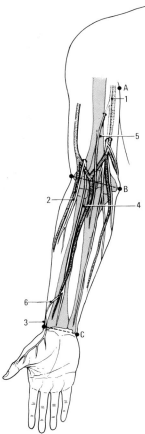

Figure 56–7. Antebrachial medial cutaneous and musculocutaneous nerves. 1 = antebrachial medial cutaneous nerve, 2 = posterior branch of the musculocutaneous nerve, 3 = branch of the superficial radial nerve, 4 = anterior branch of the musculocutaneous nerve, 5 = brachial branch of the antebrachial medial cutaneous nerve, and 6 = anastomosis with the superficial radial nerve. A, B, and C = anatomical levels of the upper extremity.

proximal or medial third of the forearm. This branch is generally formed by three fascicles.

At the level of its emergence, the antebrachial medial cutaneous nerve generally has five fascicles. The usable length of this branch averages 22 cm., from the axilla to its division about 8 cm. above the epitrochlea. With clever technique it is possible to harvest a little more nerve by using the branches at the nerve division at the elbow crease.

Harvesting this nerve is an easy procedure. The nerve can be located through a small incision about 8 to 10 cm. above the epitrochlea. The nerve travels with the basilic vein. With another incision into the axilla region,

the nerve can be found by exerting slight traction near the vascular nerve trunk. The nerve has only a few branches and it can be harvested subcutaneously. The terminal branches, particularly the anterior branch, can be harvested through a small incision at the level of the flexion crease of the elbow; it can be used for grafting digital nerves.

SUPERFICIAL RADIAL NERVE

This branch is formed from the division of the radial nerve about 1 cm. below the flexion crease of the elbow. It travels with the radial artery under the brachioradialis muscle near its anterior border and then under its tendon, becoming superficial between the tendons of the brachioradialis and the extensor carpus radialis longus, about 8 cm. above the radial styloid. About 2 cm. above the styloid the nerve divides into a variable number of terminal branches (Fig. 56–8). On the average there are four branches—two posterior

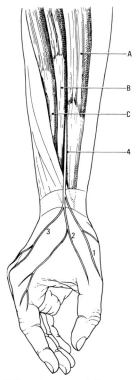

Figure 56–8. Terminations of the superficial branch of the radial nerve. A = brachioradialis, B = extensor carpi radialis longus, C = extensor carpi radialis brevis, and 4 = superficial branch of the radial nerve and its subsequent branches (1, 2, and 3).

branches, one external branch, and one anterior branch. (The superficial branch of the radial nerve has had about 14 fascicles at the level of its origin in our dissections. These findings are somewhat different from those of Sunderland, who found only six fascicles.)

It is possible to harvest up to 22 cm. of graft, depending on the use of a very delicate approach to the division of the nerve at the level of the elbow. Sunderland advised the harvesting of the superficial branch of the radial nerve, but this nerve is not used to a great extent because of the complexity of the approach at the level of the elbow and the substantial risk of neuroma formation at this level. In addition, in some cases the sensory innervation of the thumb depends on the radial nerve, and its harvesting can be cumbersome.

TERMINAL BRANCH OF THE POSTERIOR INTEROSSEOUS NERVE

We are concerned here with the sensory terminal branch of the interosseous posterior nerve. After the nerve gives off several motor branches, the sensory branch travels behind the long and short extensors of the thumb, lying over the posterior surface of the interosseous ligament. The branch courses into the synovial sheath of the common extensor and proceeds to the dorsal face of the carpus. The usable length of this nerve is about 5 to 6 cm. at the level of and proximal to the wrist (Fig. 56–9).

The nerve can be approached through a vertical posterior incision. The posterior annular ligament is opened on its radial side. The extensor communis is retracted, and on its deep face the nerve can be found. More proximally in the forearm this nerve is crossed by the extensor pollicis longus. The nerve lies between the extensor communis and the extensor pollicis longus at the level of the wrist and more lateral to these muscles in the inferior third of the forearm. This is an interesting nerve because it can yield a graft equivalent in diameter to that of a digital nerve. Harvesting is undertaken near the hand, and there is no deficit because the nerve does not provide cutaneous innervation but innervates only the articular capsules of the wrist.

TERMINAL BRANCHES OF THE MUSCULOCUTANEOUS NERVE

After innervating the coracobrachialis, the biceps, and the anterior brachialis muscles, the musculocutaneous nerve becomes sensory. It crosses the muscular mass of the short portion of the biceps diagonally and courses along its lateral border. At the level of the flexion crease of the elbow, the nerve becomes superficial and is called the antebrachial lateral nerve. At a point 1 cm. below the flexion crease it divides into two branches. A thin posterior branch crosses in front of the median cephalic vein and then travels in the direction of the proximal third of the lateral border of the forearm where it

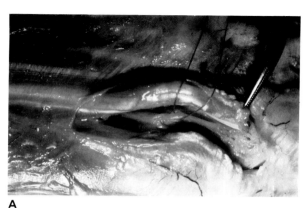

A

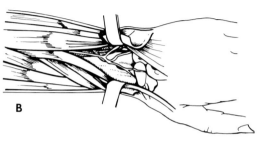

B

Figure 56–9. Terminal branch of the radial nerve. A, Dissection. B, Diagram.

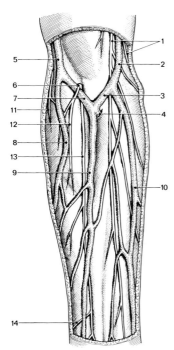

Figure 56–10. Musculocutaneous nerve and its branches. 1 = antebrachial medial cutaneous nerve, 2 = basilic vein, 3 = medial basilic vein, 4 = communicating vein of the elbow, 5 = cephalic vein, 6 = musculocutaneous nerve, 7 = medial cephalic vein, 8 = accessory radial vein, 9 = superficial radial vein, 10 = superficial cubital vein, 11 = external cutaneous branch of the radial nerve, 12 = musculocutaneous nerve (posterior branch), 13 = musculocutaneous nerve (anterior branch), and 14 = anastomosis of the musculocutaneous nerve with the superficial radial nerve.

terminates. An anterior branch crosses behind the median cephalic vein and follows the course of the radial superficial vein up to the middle third of the forearm. The nerve then travels in the direction of the thenar eminence, and about 8 cm. from the radial styloid it divides and anastomoses with a branch of the superficial radial nerve in 60 per cent of the cases (Fig. 56–10).

At its origin the antebrachial lateral nerve has eight fascicles. The anterior branch has four fascicles, and the posterior branch has one fascicle. Only the anterior branch can be used as a graft, and it is difficult to harvest more than 8 cm.

The anterior branch of the musculocutaneous nerve is theoretically a good source of a graft in cases of small losses of nerve substance, but its harvesting often generates a substantial deficit of innervation in the area.

This nerve, then, would be a secondary choice.

OTHER NERVES

Medial Cutaneous Brachial Nerve. This small nerve emerges from the medial cord and soon anastomoses with the lateral perforator branch of the second intercostal nerve. It quickly courses through the aponeurosis at the superior third of the arm and emerges on the medial aspect of the arm as far as the epitrochlea. Sometimes it can be used as a small graft, but it is not dependable and this is not advised.

Peroneal Superficial Nerve. This is the terminal branch of the common peroneal nerve. It courses distally, in front of, and near the lateral aspect of the peroneal area between the insertions of the long peroneal muscles. The nerve travels in front of the peroneal muscles, goes through the aponeurosis, and becomes subcutaneous. In general, at the union of the distal and the medial thirds, the nerve perforates the aponeurosis. Six to 8 cm. above the extremity of the external malleolus, this nerve divides into two terminal branches. One can harvest 22 to 25 cm. of this nerve. However, it innervates the dorsal sole of the foot, and one must think twice before doing this harvesting. The nerve cannot be the first choice as a source of graft, but it may be used if there are no better choices.

CONCLUSION

The choice of donor sites for nerve grafts are multiple because no one nerve has all the specific qualities of the ideal graft. However, we must distinguish situations in which the loss of nerve substance is large or multiple (such as the brachial plexus) from situations in which a smaller digital lesion must be repaired. In the first case the sural nerve is the primary choice, and harvesting it along with the lateral cutaneous sural nerve yields a graft of matchless quality. In the second case, sacrifice of a long large nerve is not necessary, and one must choose a small cutaneous nerve. The interosseous dorsal nerve would seem to answer these demands. In all cases one must consider both residual scarring and sensory deficit in choosing a donor site.

REFERENCES

Assaky, G.: De la suture des nerfs à distance. Arch. Gen. Méd., *17:*529, 1886.

Bjorkesten, G.: Clinical experiences with nerve grafting. J. Neurosurg., *5:*450, 1948.

Chao, Y. C., Tsang, Y. C., and Tsui, C. T.: Nerve regeneration through a gap. An experimental study. Chin. Med. J., *81:*740, 1962.

De Moura, W., and Gilbert, A.: Surgical anatomy of the sural nerve. J. Reconstr. Microsurg., *1:*31–39, 1984.

Duroux, E.: Greffes nerveuses expérimentales. Lyon Chir., *6:*537, 1911.

Forssmann, J.: Zur Kenntnis des Neurotropismus. Weitere Beitrage. Beitr. Path. Anat., *27:*407, 1900.

Gluck, T.: Ueber Neuroplastic auf dem Wege der Transplantation. Arch. Klin. Chir., *25:*606, 1880.

Gosset, A., and Bertrand, I.: Traitement chez l'homme des sections nerveuses périphériques par greffon hétéroplastique médullaire. C. R. Acad. Sci. (Paris), *204:*391, 1937.

Green, C.: Personal communication, 1984.

Hammond, W. S., and Hinsey, J. C.: The diameters of the nerve fibers in normal and regenerating nerves. J. Comp. Neurol., *83:*79, 1945.

Huber, G. C.: A study of the operative treatment for loss of nerve substance in peripheral nerves. J. Morph., *11:*629, 1895.

Izquierdo, P.: Homotransplantation nerveuse avec immunosuppression. Mémoire Diplôme de Microchirurgie, Université Parix, VI, 1984.

Mayo-Robson, A. W.: A case in which the spinal cord of a rabbit was successfully used as a graft in the median nerve of man. Br. Med. J., *2:*1312, 1896.

Mayo-Robson, A. W.: Nerve grafting as a means of restoring function in limbs paralyzed by gunshot or other injuries. Br. Med. J., *1:*117, 1917.

Nageotte, J.: Sur la greffe des tissus morts et en particulier sur la réparation des pertes de substance des nerfs à l'aide de greffons nerveux conservés dans l'alcool. C. R. Soc. Biol. (Paris), *80:*459, 1917a.

Nageotte, J.: Sur la possibilité d'utiliser dans la pratique chirurgicale, les greffons de nerfs fixés par l'alcool et sur la technique à employer. C. R. Soc. Biol. (Paris), *80:*925, 1917b.

Seddon H. J.: The use of autogenous grafts for the repair of large gaps in peripheral nerves. Br. J. Surg., *35:*751, 1948.

Simpson, S. A., and Young, J. Z.: Regeneration of fibre diameter after cross-unions of visceral and somatic nerves. J. Anat., *79:*48, 1945.

Stopford, J. S. B.: The treatment of large defects in peripheral nerve injuries. Lancet, *2:*1296, 1920.

Sunderland, S.: Nerves and Nerve Injuries. Edinburgh, Churchill Livingstone, 1972.

Swan, J.: Discussion on injuries to the peripheral nerves. Proc. R. Soc. Med., *34:*521, 1941.

Chapter 57

VASCULARIZED NERVE GRAFTS

JEAN-JACQUES COMTET

A conventional nerve graft survives within its bed for several days by plasma absorption alone. The first signs of revascularization are discernible only toward the end of the first week. This delay in revascularization explains the different pattern of degenerative changes compared with wallerian degeneration after sectioning of a nerve. The quality of revascularization depends on the graft bed and on the graft itself. In practice, the smaller the diameter of the graft, the quicker and the more complete is the revascularization. Conversely, areas of central necrosis are known to occur within large trunk grafts. Grafts placed in a poorly vascularized bed can suffer to the point of total destruction, as we have observed in the course of secondary repairs.

To encourage revascularization, one is usually well advised to follow the following principles: (1) Use as grafts cutaneous nerves of a small diameter. (2) Spread out the graft to maximize contact with its bed. (3) Carefully prepare the bed in order to avoid secondary sclerosis. (4) If necessary, use a circuitous but healthy route.

Strange's technique of pedicled nerve grafting was the first attempt to graft a nerve along with its blood supply (Strange, 1950). The results, as emphasized by Seddon (1972), have been encouraging. The applications of this technique are limited, however, because one must utilize an adjacent nerve of large caliber whose sacrifice is justified only if it is itself interrupted by a lesion beyond repair.

A nerve graft is also transplanted with its vascularization in two circumstances: a *vascularized graft "in situ,"* as, for example, when the medial cutaneous nerve of the forearm is used without being elevated from its bed to repair part of the median nerve at the level of the arm; and an *island nerve graft,* as, for example, when the peroneal nerve pedicled by a branch of popliteal artery is used to repair the tibial nerve (Oberlin and Alnot, 1985).

The concept of the free vascularized nerve graft (FVNG) with simultaneous microvascular, arterial and venous, reconstruction was introduced by Taylor and Ham (1976). Since then, other donor sites have been described, and Taylor (1984) described composite arterialized neurovenous systems.

EXPERIMENTAL STUDIES

Taylor (1976) demonstrated the possibility of preserving the viability of a nerve after transplantation as an island graft, or after microvascular reconstruction. Restoration of vascular continuity with proximal and distal anastomoses was proved to prevent thrombosis.

According to Lunborg (1975), the sciatic nerve of the rabbit can be distally transected and freed from its extrinsic system along 45 times the nerve width, without any disturbance in intraneural circulation. This could theoretically justify using short cutaneous nerve graft, 50 to 100 mm. long, even if they are vascularized by staggered and nonanastomosed vessels. However, in humans, the additional length of nerve that can be taken beyond the extrinsic vascular system remains debatable.

Jamieson observed experimentally that, unlike the conventional grafts, large free vascularized nerve grafts do not undergo longitudinal and transverse atrophy. Hunt (1983) noted a more even distribution of regular sized axons in vascularized canine nerve graft compared to nonvascularized grafts.

Conversely, according to McCullough (1984), the rate of axon regeneration was not significantly different between vascularized and nonvascularized nerve graft in the rat. Brooke and Seckel (1986) found nonsignificant differences in the number or size of regenerated axons in vascularized and nonvascularized nerve grafts.

According to experiments performed by Wood (Settergren and Wood, 1984; Daly and Wood, 1985), epineurial and endoneurial blood flow at day 4 was found to be significantly better in conventional grafts than in free vascularized nerve grafts taken in healthy tissue.

The effect of the recipient bed quality was studied by Koshima and Harii (1985). After scarifying the bed by means of thermal burns, the number and diameter of regenerating axons in the distal part was significantly greater in free vascularized nerve grafts than in conventional grafts.

DONOR SITES

Peripheral nerves are supplied through a longitudinal epineural and perineural plexus fed by the arteriae nervorum. The latter can arise directly from the main arterial channels or from muscular or cutaneous vessels. They approach the nerve through a mesoneurium. Taylor (1978) classifies nerves into five cate-

gories—A, B, C, D, and E—in descending order of suitability as vascularized nerve grafts (Fig. 57–1). This classification shows that theoretically ideal grafts, if used, would necessitate the sacrifice of an important nerve trunk or arterial trunk. Such sacrifices can be justified only in exceptional circumstances, i.e., amputation of a whole segment or an irreversible lesion of a donor nerve proximal or distal to the potential donor. Sunderland's order of preference for conventional grafts starts with the superficial branch of the radial nerve, followed by the sural nerve and the cutaneous nerve of the forearm (Sunderland, 1968). It happens that these three nerves satisfy all the criteria, including the possession of a nutrient artery of sufficient length and diameter for eventual anastomosis. The anterior branch of the radial nerve falls into Taylor's category A but entails the sacrifice of an important arterial axis.

In Taylor's classification, the sural nerve and the medial cutaneous nerve of the forearm fall into category D by reason of their staggered and multipedicled arterial supply. This, however, does not concur with the anatomical findings, to be discussed. We consider here only the blood supply of the potential donor nerves and refer the reader to Sunderland's work for their other anatomical features such as length, diameter, branches,

Figure 57–1. Classification of the peripheral nerves in terms of their suitability as vascularized transplants. (After Taylor, G. I.: Clin. Orthop. Rel. Res., *133*:56–70, 1978.)

Type A: Ideal case. Long nerve trunk with no collateral supplied through a single segmental parallel arteriovenous system. Examples: anterior branch of the radial nerve, the neurovascular pedicles, ulnar nerve at the forearm, anterior and posterior tibial nerves in the lower leg, median nerve, and brachial artery in the arm.

Type B: Similar arrangement as Type A, but early division of the nerve favors reversal of the graft to avoid the loss of some axons. Examples: intercostal neurovascular pedicle, radial nerve, and deep brachial artery in the arm.

Type C: Rare case. Long nerve trunk with no collateral and a single nutrient feeder artery. Examples: median nerve supplied by an "artery to the median nerve" of good caliber, sciatic nerve supplied primarily by a concomitant artery.

Type D: Same type of nerve trunk as that supplied segmentally through several vessels. Example: sciatic nerve in the thigh. Taylor also includes the medial saphenous nerve and the medial cutaneous nerve of the arm in this group.

Type E: Nerve giving off several collaterals and supplied by several arteries. This is the least suitable type.

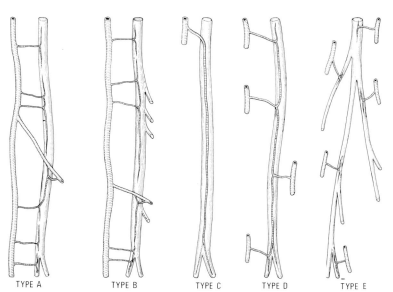

TYPE A   TYPE B   TYPE C   TYPE D   TYPE E

percentage of connective tissue, and fascicular patterns.

CUTANEOUS NERVES AS VASCULARIZED NERVE GRAFT

SUPERFICIAL SENSORY BRANCH OF RADIAL NERVE (Fig. 57–2)

The anatomy of this nerve has been described by Taylor and Ham (1976, 1978). The nerve is as long as the forearm, plus another 3 to 4 cm., which can be dissected microscopically into the proximal trunk or distal to the bifurcation. The mesoneurium can be identified at the middle third of the forearm: it transmits one to four arteriae nervorum, which either come off the radial artery or arise from an arterial arch that crosses the artery anteriorly and supplies the extensors. The radial artery usually can be exposed for 4 to 5 cm. on either side of this arch. Its diameter varies between 1.8 and 4.5 mm. The venous return occurs through the venae comitantes.

The graft is elevated through a longitudinal forearm incision along the course of the radial artery. The dissection is made easier by detaching the brachioradialis tendon. The mesoneurium is carried with the nerve together with some connective tissue, including the muscular branches of the radial artery and the arterial arch feeding the extensors. These branches are all ligated as far as possible from the nerve.

SURAL NERVE

The blood supply to the sural nerve, studied by Fachinelli et al. (1981), comes essentially from the superficial sural artery. The latter arises in 65 per cent of the cases from

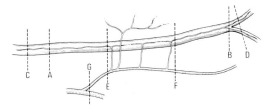

Figure 57–2. Anatomy and blood supply of the superficial branch of the radial nerve. The central segment (AB) can be prolonged proximally by intraneural dissection (CA) and by inclusion of the branches (BD). The middle third is supplied by the radial artery from E to F and the vascular pedicle (EG) can be isolated. (After Taylor, G. I., and Ham, F. J.: Plast. Reconstr. Surg., 57:413–426, 1976.)

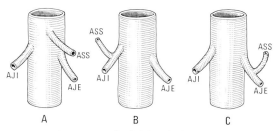

Figure 57–3. A to C, Origin of the superficial sural artery. ASS = superficial sural artery, AJE = lateral sural artery, AJI = medial sural artery. (After Fachinelli, A., et al.: Int. J. Microsurg., 3:57–62, 1981.)

the popliteal artery, in 20 per cent from the medial sural, and in 8 per cent from the lateral sural artery. Its diameter varies between 0.6 and 2 mm. (average, 1.2 mm.). It gives off a cutaneous branch and accompanies the nerve over a distance varying between 4.5 and 33 cm. About seven nutrient branches are given off at intervals of about 4 cm. (Figs. 57–3, 57–4). In 65 per cent of the cases the superficial sural artery supplies the whole length of the sural nerve, while in 35 per cent another vessel provides part of the distal supply.

The sural nerve provides the longest graft of all (40 cm.). It can be folded on itself several times and cut into parallel segments without damaging the mesoneurium.

The nerve graft is taken, with the patient in a prone position, through a long incision along the leg completed by a Z at the popliteal fossa. The first part of the dissection centers on the vascular pedicle, which is ligated at the level of its origin from the popliteal artery. In one of six cases we found the vascular pedicle too narrow to be anastomosed.

MEDIAL CUTANEOUS NERVE OF FOREARM

In 1981 we described a technique for elevating this nerve along with its blood supply (Comtet et al., 1981). In the course of our anatomical studies we found that in the majority of cases the nerve is supplied by the superior ulnar collateral artery, which itself arises from the brachial artery in the upper third of the arm (Fig. 57–5). Its diameter averages 1.2 mm. (range, 1 to 1.5 mm.). Its origin lies about 6.5 cm. distal to the inferior border of pectoralis major with the arm in 90 degrees of abduction. It is usually (but not always) the first medial branch (Lebreton et

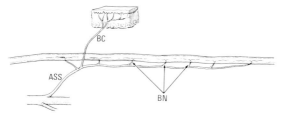

Figure 57–4. Distribution of the superficial sural (ASS). Its cutaneous branch (BC) arises early from the trunk and is supplied by approximately seven feeders (BN). (After Fachinelli, A., et al.: Int. J. Microsurg., 3:57–62, 1981.)

al., 1982). Just before it crosses above and behind the medial intermuscular septum, it gives off a constant anteromedial branch, which has a diameter of 0.8 to 1 mm. There are two known "types" of this arterial branch: In the type I branch (found in 16 of 25 cases) the vessel has a short (10 mm.) trunk after which it gives off its terminal fan of branches to the skin of the medial aspect of the forearm and to the medial cutaneous nerve. In the type II branch (nine of 25 cases) the artery has a long trunk (30 to 40 mm.) that runs vertically behind the basilic vein and gives off four or five staggered horizontal branches to the skin and to the nerve. In some cases it anastomoses with a branch of the inferomedial collateral artery (Fig. 57–5A). In one patient who came to surgery we found that the arterial supply came primarily from the collateral inferomedial artery; in another it came from a muscular branch arising directly from the middle third of the brachial artery.

The composite graft is raised through a longitudinal incision running from the lower border of pectoralis major down to the elbow crease (Fig. 57–5C,D). The loose tissue surrounding the medial cutaneous nerve and the basilic vein is dissected off the superficial fascia. The upper part of the medial intermuscular septum is incised to expose and ligate the superomedial collateral artery distal to the origin of its anteromedial branch. The former is dissected along parts of its course, so that its two ends can be anastomosed, and cut off flush with its origin on the brachial artery. The medial cutaneous nerve and the basilic vein are then divided, and along with the surrounding connective tissue, they are pulled medially to put the superomedial collateral artery under stretch before it is ligated flush with the humeral artery. Occasionally a muscular branch or the inferomedial collateral may have to be used as the chief arterial

pedicle. The graft is usually about 10 cm. long, but its length can be increased if the dissection is carried out proximally into the axillary fossa. It is preferable not to prolong the dissection beyond the bifurcation of the nerve. Usually the brachial cutaneous nerve of the arm is included within the composite graft.

More recently, several donor sites were described: deep peroneal (anterior tibial) nerve in its distal part with the dorsalis pedis artery was used by Rose and Kowalski (1985); saphenous nerve with saphenous artery and superficial peroneal nerve with a branch of the anterior artery were also proposed by Breidenbach and Terzis (1984).

MAJOR NERVES AS VASCULARIZED NERVE GRAFTS

Major nerves may be available in certain circumstances, such as when a limb, or part of a limb, is amputated, paralyzed, or irreparably damaged. They provide group A, B or C type grafts.

The ulnar nerve has been used as a pedicled graft by Strange (1948) and as a free vascularized nerve graft: from the forearm (Bonney et al., 1984; Comtet, 1983) or from the arm (Merle et al., 1984) in brachial plexus injuries when C8 and D1 are avulsed.

Sunderland's studies have shown that the ulnar nerve is supplied by arterial branches from the superior ulnar collateral artery, the posterior ulnar recurrent artery, and the ulnar artery itself.

The upper part of the nerve is also regularly supplied by the axillary artery or one of its branches. Other sources of arterial supply are not constant. It would seem possible therefore to use any of the three portions of the ulnar nerve—brachial, middle (at the elbow), or antebrachial.

In brachial plexus palsies one can utilize the lower antebrachial segment of the nerve (with the ulnar vessels) below the origin of the nerve to the flexor carpi ulnaris and to the flexor digitorum profundus. We now know that in brachial plexus palsies involving the C8 and T1 roots the intrinsic muscles are very unlikely to recover after three months. The nerve is readily accessible at this level but unfortunately contains a much greater percentage of connective tissue than in its proximal third. Bonney et al. have shown that it is possible to prolong the antebrachial

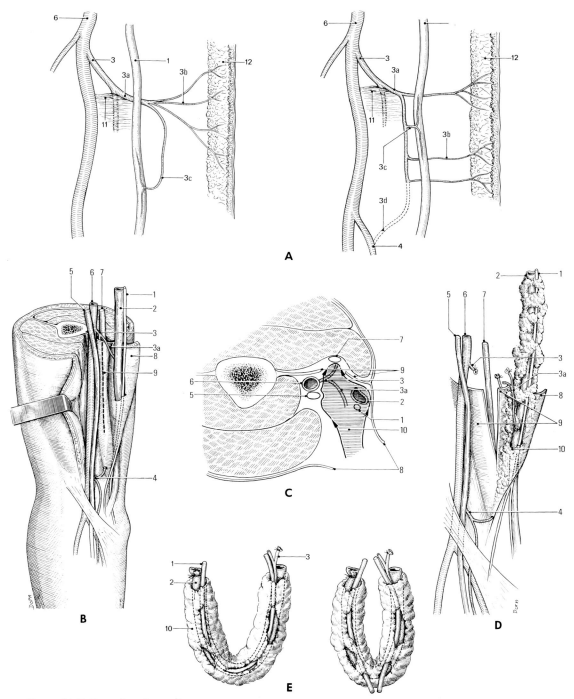

Figure 57–5. Preparing the medial cutaneous nerve of the forearm. *A*, Variations. (After Condamine et al.) *B*, Anterior view after incision of the superficial brachial fascia. *C*, Transverse section showing the tissues that must be included in the transplant. *D*, The transplant is freed from above downward and from medial to lateral. *E*, The graft is folded into a "U." 1 = medial cutaneous nerve of the forearm, 2 = basilic vein, 3 = superior ulnar collateral artery, 3a = anteromedial branch of the superior ulnar collateral artery, 3b = secondary cutaneous branch(es), 3c = secondary branch(es) to the medial cutaneous nerve, 3d = anastomotic branches, 4 = medial collateral that sometimes supplies part of the medial cutaneous nerve, 5 = median nerve, 6 = branchial artery, 7 = ulnar nerve, 8 = superficial brachial fascia incised and retracted, 9 = medial intermuscular septum that must be incised, 10 = adventitial tissue, 11 = inconstant muscular branch that may supply part of the nerve, and 12 = skin.

graft toward the brachial part, although dissection of the posterior ulnar recurrent vessels behind the elbow may prove difficult.

Lebreton et al. (1982) conducted a study of the blood supply of the ulnar nerve in the context of its microsurgical transfer (Fig. 57–6). In 50 dissections they found that in 47 the nerve was supplied by the superior ulnar collateral artery and in two by the inferior ulnar collateral. In one case the nerve was vascularized by several staggered arterioles too small to be anastomosed.

In eight of 10 cases the venous drainage is through a single satellite vein, which reaches the brachial vein 2 to 3 cm. below the origin of the artery and distal to the junction with the basilic vein. In two of 10 cases there are two or more draining veins.

In the arm the ulnar nerve is taken through a straight medial incision. The brachial artery is dissected from above downward and its medial branches identified. The nerve and its arteriovenous pedicle are isolated together with the surrounding tissue behind the medial intermuscular septum. The muscular branches (of which there may be many) are ligated or cauterized. The length of this vascularized graft is at least 13 cm., but injection studies show that the vascularization reaches up to Osborne's arch over a length of 20 cm.

Other major nerves have been used or proposed: median and ulnar nerve with brachial artery in the upper arm (Taylor, 1978) or lateral part of the sciatic nerve in the thigh (Comtet et al., 1985). Possible future free vascularized nerve grafts include radial nerve with the profunda brachii artery, median nerve in the forearm with a large arteria comitans, peroneal nerve with anterior tibial artery, and tibial nerve with posterior tibial artery.

TECHNICAL PROBLEMS

One feature of these grafts is the small area of their capillary bed. For this reason it is important to include in the transplant a sufficient amount of connective tissue to avoid the discrepancy between the ample blood supply and the reduced capillary bed. It is preferable therefore to anastomose the artery at both extremities to produce a lateral rather than terminal circulation. In an experimental series Taylor and Ham reported several cases of thrombosis with a single anastomosis.

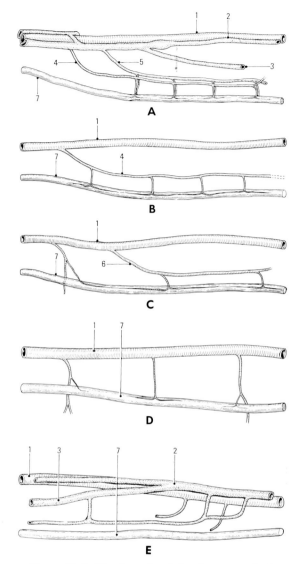

Figure 57–6. Blood supply of the ulnar nerve in the arm. (After Lebreton et al.) A, Normal arrangement of the arteriovenous pedicle. B, Arterial supply, most common type (47 to 50). C, Arterial supply through the distal ulnar collateral (2 of 50). D, Rare Taylor type D (1 of 50). E, Multiple efferent veins (10 of 50). 1 = brachial artery, 2 = brachial vein, 3 = basilic vein, 4 = proximal ulnar collateral artery, 5 = proximal ulnar collateral vein, 6 = distal ulnar collateral artery, 7 = ulnar nerve.

The ideal form of venous drainage is still a subject of debate. We still do not know whether it is better to utilize the larger veins (sural and basilic) with their satellite nerves or whether the venae comitantes are adequate. In the case of the medial cutaneous nerve of the arm, we have seen a flow of venous blood into the basilic vein when the latter was used as drainage route. In some cases, however, the venous flow can be slow enough to give rise to thrombosis. When the grafts are taken from the distal part of the upper limb, the diameter of the larger veins is too wide compared with that of the distal forearm veins. The only solution is then to reroute a dorsal vein; it is in such cases that the venae comitantes may prove useful.

The small diameter of vascularized nerve transplants in itself poses a technical problem. If we exclude the special cases in which a large trunk is available, the diameter of the utilizable nerves is invariably small. Several alternatives have been tried:

1. Place the nerve in a single or multiple U shape in order to double or multiply the overall diameter.

2. Connect the transplant to the more important fascicular group, e.g., the first digital nerves in median nerve repairs.

3. Utilize concomitantly one or more conventional nerve grafts, which are laid on the well vascularized bed of the graft.

RESULTS

It is far too early to express a definitive opinion regarding these transplants, which so far have been attempted mostly in hopeless cases in which spectacular results could hardly be expected. In the pioneer case described by Taylor and Ham (1976), the patient recovered good protective sensibility with fair localization of touch and prick sensation two years after the loss of 22 cm. of the median nerve. Taylor (1978) reported two other cases. In a patient who sustained an electrical burn he utilized the median and ulnar nerves, with accompanying vessels, from the amputated right upper limb to bridge a gap of 20 cm. in the median and ulnar nerves of the left forearm; after nine months protective sensibility had returned. In a second case he utilized the anterior branch of the radial nerve to repair a 20 cm. gap in the median nerve in a complicated forearm injury. At 10 months the first signs of recovery were recorded in the median territory at the palm.

Sural nerve was used by Gilbert in five cases (Fachinelli et al., 1981; Gilbert, 1984). One, a case of Volkmann contracture, was reported in detail. defect of median nerve, 7 cm. long, was repaired with four strands of vascularized sural nerve. Eighteen months later protective sensibility reappeared in the

distribution of the median nerve and the trophic changes disappeared. There was no return of motor function.

Bonney et al. (1984) used vascularized ulnar grafts from the forearm to repair 30 brachial plexus injuries. Results were analyzed for 12 cases with nine favorable results and three failures.

Merle et al. (1984) reported five vascularized unlar nerve grafts from the arm to repair brachial plexus injuries. Although the axonal regeneration seemed to progress more rapidly than in conventional grafts, the final result was not clearly different.

Rose and Kowalski (1985) used free vascularized nerve grafts from the dorsum of the foot after failure of conventional graft in five cases of digital nerve reconstruction. Touch and vibratory sensation was restored in all patients. Average static two point discrimination was 9.5 mm.

Since 1980, we have used free vascularized nerve grafts in 10 cases. Vascularized ulnar nerve was used in four brachial plexus injuries with three favorable results and one failure (neurotization from the spinal accessory). The medial cutaneous nerve of the forearm was used in six cases for particularly unfavorable cases such as long delay, age, long defect, and scarred bed. One technical failure with venous thrombosis was observed. In three cases no return of sensitivity was observed (although trophic ulcers disappeared in one case), while in two cases (median and ulnar defect), an S3 grade of sensitivity was recovered.

CURRENT INDICATIONS

Finally experimental and clinical data have shown that, in normal conditions, free vascularized nerve grafts do not provide better results than conventional grafts. Ideas that vascularization of the graft could compensate for unfavorable factors, such as advanced age and delayed repair, have not been confirmed. However, using free vascularized nerve grafts seems to be justified in two circumstances: along the gap and a scarred bed. Long grafts greater than 150 mm. have proved to give significantly less favorable results than shorter grafts (Sedel, 1978). An explanation for this poorer result could be the delayed revascularization from the recipient bed in the central portion of the conventional graft compared with that of the two ends through the suture line. When the recipient bed is not suitable for an early revascularization of the graft, free vascularized nerve graft is an alternative or a complementary method to other procedures such as resection of scar tissue, rerouting to a healthy area, and utilizing well-vascularized tissues such as cutaneous, muscular flaps, or sliding fascia.

A point in favor of free vascularized nerve graft is the opportunity of using a large trunk from an amputated or irreparably damaged segment (Taylor and Ham, 1976; Taylor, 1978). This is also the cause in brachial plexus injuries with preganglionic avulsion of the lower roots, where the ulnar nerve can be used to repair the territory of C5, C6, or C7.

When necessary, free vascular nerve grafts from Taylor's group A (Taylor, 1978) offer the possibility of repairing a major vessel at the same time as the nerve. When a large trunk is not available, cutaneous nerves can be used: they have the drawback of a small diameter but at least their use entails a minimum sacrifice. Finally, as suggested by Taylor and Ham (1976), we can envisage in the future the vascularized transplantation of larger nerves as allografts from cadavers once the immunological problems have been solved.

REFERENCES

Bonney, G., Birch, R., Jamieson, A. M., and Eames, R. A.: Experience with vascularized nerve grafts. Clin. Plast. Surg., *11*:137–142, 1984.

Breidenbach, W., and Terzis, J. K.: The anatomy of free vascularized nerve graft. Clin. Plast. Surg., *11*:65–72, 1984.

Brooke, R., et al.: Vascularized versus nonvascularized nerve grafts: an experimental structural comparison. Plast. Reconstr. Surg., *78*:211–220, 1986.

Comtet, J. J.: Les greffes nerveuses vascularisées. Acta Chir. Belg., *83*:293–297, 1983.

Comtet, J. J., Bertrand, H. G., Moyen, B., and Condamine, J. L.: Greffe nerveuse vascularisée utilisant le brachial cutané interne avec un pédicule vasculaire. Technique de prélèvement. Lyon Chirurg., *77*:62–63, 1981.

Comtet, J. J., Herzberg, G., and Lemire, J. L.: Utilisation de la portion externe du nerf sciatique comme greffe de nerf vascularisée libre. Group pour l'Avancement de la Chirurgie, Sitges, 1985.

Condamine, J. L., Pheline, Y., and Comtet, J. J.: Etude de la vascularisation du nerf brachial cutané interne. Ses applications à un transfert composite vascularisé. Congres de l'Association des Anatomistes, Limoges, 1982.

Daly, P. J., and Wood, M. B.: Endoneural and epineural

blood flow evaluation with free vascularized and conventional nerve graft in the canine. J. Reconstr. Microsurg., *2*:51–58, 1985.

Fachinelli, A., Masquelet, A., Restrepo, J., and Gilbert, A.: The vascularized sural nerve. Int. J. Microsurg., *3*:57–62, 1981.

Gilbert, A.: Vascularized sural nerve graft. Clin. Plast. Surg., *11*:73–77, 1984.

Hunt, D. M.: A model for the study of free vascularized nerve graft. J. Bone Joint Surg., *65B*:659, 1983.

Jamieson, A. M.: Personal communication.

Koshima, I., and Harii, K.: Experimental study of vascularized nerve grafts: multifactorial analyses of axonal regeneration of nerves transplanted into an acute burn wound. J. Hand. Surg., *10A*:64–72, 1985.

Lebreton, E., Bourgeon, Y., Lascombes, P., Merle, M., and Foucher, G.: Systematisation de la vascularisation de la portion brachiale du nerf ulnaire. Ann. Chir. Main, *3*:211–218, 1983.

Lunborg, G.: Structure and function of the intraneural microvessels as related to trauma, edema formation and nerve function. J. Bone Joint Surg., *57A*:938–948, 1975.

McCarthy, C.: Two stage autograft for repair of extensive damage to sciatic nerve. J. Surg., *8*:319–322, 1951.

McCullough, C. J. et al.: Axon regeneration and revascularization of nerve graft. An experimental study. J. Hand. Surg., *9B*:323–327, 1984.

Merle, M., Lebreton, E., Bouchon, Y., and Foucher, G.: Les greffes nerveuses vascularisées. Premiers résultats. Communication Société Française Chirurgie, Main Rouen, 1984.

Oberlin, C., and Alnot, J. Y.: Utilisation du nerf sciatique poplité externe comme greffe vascularisée. Rev. Chir. Orthop., *71*:(Suppl 2):94–98, 1985.

Rose, E. H., and Kowalski, I. A.: Restoration of sensibility to anesthetic scarred digits with free vascularized nerve grafts from the dorsum of the foot. J. Hand. Surg., *10*:514–521, 1985.

Sedel, L.: Résultats des greffes nerveuses. In Symposium Microchirurgie en Traumatologie. Directors C. Dufourmentel and J. J. Comtet. Rev. Chir. Orthop., *64*:284–289, 1978.

Settergren, C. R., and Wood, M. B.: Comparison of blood flow in free vascularized nerve graft. J. Reconstr. Microsurg., *1*:95–101, 1984.

Smith, J. W.: Factors influencing nerve repairs blood supply of peripheral nerves. Arch. Surg., *93*:335–341, 1966.

Strange, F. G.: The pedicle nerve graft. Br. J. Surg., *35*:331–333, 1948.

Sunderland, S.: Nerves and Nerve Injuries. Edinburgh, Churchill Livingstone, Ltd., 1968.

Taylor, G. I.: Nerve grafting with simultaneous microvascular reconstruction. Clin. Orthop. Rel. Res., *133*:56–70, 1978.

Taylor, G. I., and Ham, F.: The free vascularized nerve graft. Plast. Reconstr. Surg., *57*:413–426, 1976.

Townsend, P. L. G., and Taylor, G. I.: Vascularized nerve grafts using composite arterialised neuro-veinous systems. Br. J. Plast. Surg., *37*:1–17, 1984.

Taylor, G. I.: Nerve grafting with simultaneous microvascular reconstruction. Clin. Orthop. Rel. Res., *133*:56–70, 1978.

Taylor, G. I., and Ham, F. J.: The free vascularized nerve graft. Plast. Reconstr. Surg., *57*:413–426, 1976.

Chapter 58

MICROSURGICAL REPAIR IN 150 PATIENTS WITH LESIONS OF THE MEDIAN AND ULNAR NERVES

Michel Merle,
Philippe Amend,
and Jacques Michon

In assessing the results of peripheral nerve repair, one must consider the background of the patient, the type of injury, and the surgical technique used in order to avoid erroneous conclusions. Since the advent of microsurgical techniques, there has been some discrepancy between the results of primary repair, direct suturing, and secondary nerve grafting. Insufficiently large series involving multiple surgeons, followed by incomplete evaluation of results, may have led a number of readers to the erroneous belief that secondary repair was better than primary repair and that fascicular grafts should always be preferred to direct suturing.

We believe that a statistical study should be based on follow-up data collected for two years or more. The assessor must not be a member of the surgical team involved, and only patients operated upon by senior surgeons familiar with neurovascular microsurgical techniques should be included.

This survey is restricted to lesions of the median and ulnar nerves at the wrist and in the forearm. Our results were subjected to the chi square test and take into account the background of the patient, the type of injury, and the microsurgical techniques employed.

CLINICAL MATERIAL AND METHOD

Between 1977 and 1982, 500 peripheral nerve lesions were repaired in our Hand Assistance Department. In this report we shall review only the 150 median and ulnar nerve lesions at the wrist and forearm, excluding lesions of the radial, sciatic, and femoral nerves, which pose specific problems and are not relevant here.

The 150 lesions occurred in 131 patients, 19 of whom sustained multiple or bilateral injuries. They were all reviewed by one assessor (P.A.), who had not been involved with the surgery, with a follow-up of two to seven years. The ages of our patients ranged between two and 90 years, the majority being between 20 and 30 years of age. Sixty-eight per cent were males and 32 per cent, females.

Type of Nerve Repair. Secondary suturing was performed in 14 cases (9.3 per cent), fascicular grafts were used in 50 cases (33.3 per cent), and primary suturing in 86 cases (57.4 per cent).

The surgical technique used varied according to the nature of the injury. A clean wound repaired as an emergency case was treated by interfascicular suturing (guided suture) combined with epineural stitches, for we believe in achieving a water-tight suture line to protect against invasion by connective tissue and to preserve the epineurium, which has a rich blood supply.

By contrast, a partial nerve lesion was managed by a perineural (or fascicular) suture. This type of lesion is best treated at emergency surgery when fascicular reorientation is still possible.

In the presence of limited fascicular avulsion, we prefer a perineural to an interfascicular suture to avoid catching the fascicles in the suture line.

If the wound is contused, the nerve is repaired primarily with an epineural suture in the knowledge that secondary suturing or grafting will be required six to eight weeks later. The early provisional suture helps to preserve the overall orientation of the nerve and reduces the neurogliomatous reaction. When this is limited to 1.5 cm. or less, direct suturing with little or no tension remains possible.

Fascicular grafting is carried out as described by Millesi, using the sural or medial cutaneous nerve of the arm as a donor. This technique is used when loss of nerve substance makes direct suturing impossible.

Primary suturing of the nerve is performed at the same time as the repair of other lesions of tendons, arteries, and bones, according to the all-in-one-stage principle, with early mobilization. Secondary nerve grafts are best carried out as isolated procedures to avoid the onset of fibrosis, which can affect revascularization of the graft.

EVALUATION OF RESULTS

All patients underwent a clinical and electromyographic examination two to seven years after the nerve repair.

The scoring system used is that of Chanson, which is itself based on that of the Medical Research Council to quantify motoricity and sensibility, but introduces as an additional parameter the patient's "degree of satisfaction."

The three criteria are defined as follows (Table 58–1): G = degree of satisfaction (G4 to G0), M = muscular recovery (M4 to M0), and S = sensory recovery (S4 to S0). The scoring of results is shown in Table 58–2.

ANALYSIS OF RESULTS

The overall results (including all repairs) are included in Table 58–3, which shows that 49.3 per cent of the repairs yielded useful results and 22.7 per cent, average results; 28 per cent resulted in failure.

INFLUENCE OF SEX, AGE, AND TYPE OF INJURY

Sex. As shown in Table 58–4, the sex of the patient is not directly relevant to the result, but it is probably fair to say that the types of injury sustained by the two groups are somewhat different. Contused wounds are more common in industrial injuries sustained mostly by male patients, whereas female patients sustain more clean-cut wounds (from accidents in the home), which carry a better prognosis. Yet the results are less satisfactory in female patients. This may be partly explained by the inclusion of lesions from attempted suicides, which tend to yield poor results owing to lack of cooperation from these patients postoperatively.

Age. By contrast, the patient's age has a marked influence on the result (Table 58–5). The excellent results tend to occur in patients under 30 years of age, the good to average results in the 30 to 60 year age group, and

Table 58–1. CRITERIA FOR EVALUATION OF RESULTS

Patient Satisfaction	Motor Recovery	Sensory Recovery	
G4 No pain or limitation	M4 Contraction possible	S4 Weber test	< 5 mm.
G3 Slight limitation compatible with normal activity	M3 Contraction possible against minimal resistance	S3 Weber test	< 10 mm.
G2 Limitation of activity but no major problem	M2 Contraction possible against gravity	S2 Weber test	< 20 mm.
G1 Constant pain and poor utilization of hand	M1 Contraction possible but not against gravity	S1 Weber test or protective sensibility	> 20 mm.
G0 Severe pain and limitation rendering hand useless	M0 Contraction absent	S0 Anesthesia or nonprotective dysesthesia	

Table 58–2. SCORING OF RESULTS

Results			Score		
			G	M	S
Useful	Excellent	=	4	4	4
	Very good	>	4	3	3
	Good	>	3	2	2
Average	3 2 2	to	2	1	1
Mediocre	2 1 1	to	1	0	0
Failure		<	1	0	0

the failures and mediocre results in those over 60. This militates against a secondary repair when the primary repair yields an acceptable result. Age should always be taken into account when the results in a given series are assessed: a high proportion of children in a series usually improves the overall score significantly.

Type of Injury. If the injuries are broken down into the three main groups (industrial, attempted suicide, and accidents in the home), we find the following (Table 58–6):

1. In 15.6 per cent of industrial injuries there is a good result and in 44.4 per cent an average result.

2. In attempted suicide (usually clean wounds in female patients), 44.4 per cent of the final results are good or very good.

3. After accidents in the home, 67.8 per cent of the results are good, very good, or excellent. This high percentage of successful results can be explained by the fact that this group includes a high proportion of clean cuts in children under 15 years of age.

The nature of the injury, the psychological context (suicide), and the desire for compensation after industrial accidents can lead to great diversity in the results.

INFLUENCE OF FACTORS INHERENT IN THE LESION ITSELF

Level of the Lesion. The level of the lesion of the median and ulnar nerves has a profound effect on the prognosis (Table 58–7). The more proximal the lesion, the poorer the prognosis and the more uncertain is the re-

covery of the intrinsic muscles of the hand. This is due to the length of the regenerating nerve and to the severity of the lesion. For instance, lesions at the level of the wrist have given us 53.5 per cent useful (good, very good, and excellent) results, but lesions at the forearm have given only 36.8 per cent useful results.

Type of Injury. The type of injury also has a bearing on the ultimate functional result (Table 58–8). A useful result (i.e., good, very good, or excellent) was obtained in 52.3 per cent of the patients with a clean cut wound, but the proportion of similar results fell to 40 per cent when the wound was contused. One of the problems is, of course, the difficulty in gauging the extent of the contusion on the nerve. Besides, this type of injury is usually best managed by a secondary fascicular graft.

As for lesions produced by avulsion and crushing, the prognosis is consistently bad.

Type of Nerve Lesion. A partial nerve section repaired at emergency by perineural suturing will yield a useful result in 64.5 per cent of the cases (Table 58–9). If the nerve section is total, only 46.4 per cent of the cases have useful results. The difference lies in the fact that a more accurate reorientation is possible in a partial section. In addition, the intact fascicles can compensate and mask a failure of fiber regeneration.

We have also observed that late repairs of partial sections tend to yield a poor functional result owing to the difficulty in isolating the healthy fascicles once they are embedded in a neuroglioma.

INFLUENCE OF SURGICAL TECHNIQUE ON THE RESULTS

The factors relating to the patient and to the lesion itself are so many and so diverse that the part played by the actual surgical technique is difficult to quantify. In order, therefore, to assess their contribution as well as that of the simultaneous repair of one or more arterial channels, we reviewed 67 total nerve lesions in the wrist and forearm only.

Table 58–3. OVERALL RESULTS IN 150 LESIONS OF THE MEDIAN AND ULNAR NERVES

RESULTS	Failures 28.0%		Average 22.7%	Useful Results 49.3%			
	FAILURE	POOR	AVERAGE	GOOD	VERY GOOD	EXCELLENT	TOTAL
Sutures and grafts	7 (4.7%)	35 (23.3%)	34 (22.7%)	53 (35.3%)	12 (8.0%)	9 (6.0%)	150 (100%)

Table 58–4. RESULTS OF MEDIAN AND ULNAR NERVE REPAIRS ACCORDING TO SEX IN 150 CASES

	Failures			Average Results	Useful Results				TOTAL
	FAILURE	POOR	TOTAL		GOOD	VERY GOOD	EXCELLENT	TOTAL	
Males	4 (3.9%)	24 (23.5%)	28 (27.4%)	22 (21.6%)	41 (40.2%)	6 (5.9%)	5 (4.9%)	52 (51.0%)	102 (100%)
Females	3 (6.3%)	11 (22.9%)	14 (29.2%)	12 (25.0%)	12 (25.0%)	6 (12.5%)	4 (8.3%)	22 (45.0%)	48 (100%)

$\chi^2 = 5.144$. ddl = 5 (nonsignificant).

Table 58–5. RESULTS IN ULNAR AND MEDIAN NERVE LESIONS ACCORDING TO AGE IN 150 CASES

Age (Years)	Failures			Average Results	Useful Results				TOTAL
	FAILURE	POOR	TOTAL		GOOD	VERY GOOD	EXCELLENT	TOTAL	
0 to 9		1 (8.3%)	8.3%		4 (33.3%)	2 (16.6%)	5 (41.7%)	11 (91.6%)	12 (100%)
10 to 19	2 (5.7%)	4 (11.4%)	17.1%	6	18 (51.4%)	3 (8.6%)	2 (5.7%)	23 (65.7%)	35 (100%)
20 to 29	1 (1.8%)	11 (20.0%)	21.8%	13 (23.7%)	22 (40.0%)	7 (12.7%)	1 (1.8%)	30 (54.5%)	55 (100%)
30 to 39	1 (4.7%)	6 (28.6%)	33.0%	8 (38.1%)	6 (28.6%)	0	0	6 (28.6%)	21 (100%)
40 to 49	2 (14.3%)	5 (35.7%)	50.0%	4 (28.6%)	2 (14.3%)	0	1 (7.1%)	3 (21.4%)	14 (100%)
50 to 59	0	2 (40.0%)	40.0%	2 (40.0%)	1 (20.0%)	0	0	1 (20.0%)	5 (100%)
60 to 69	1 (16.7%)	4 (66.6%)	83.3%	1 (16.7%)					6 (100%)
Over 70		2 (100.0%)	100%						2 (100%)

$\chi^2 = 72.31$. ddl = 35. P < 0.001 (very significant). Cramer = 0.31 (strong correlation).

Table 58–6. RESULTS ACCORDING TO TYPE OF INJURY IN 150 CASES

Type of Injury	Failures			Average Results	Useful Results				TOTAL
	FAILURE	POOR	TOTAL		GOOD	VERY GOOD	EXCELLENT	TOTAL	
Industrial injury	3 (6.7%)	15 (33.3%)	18 (40.0%)	20 (44.4%)	7 (15.6%)			7 (15.6%)	45 (100%)
Attempted suicide	2 (11.1%)	3 (16.7%)	5 (27.8%)	5 (27.8%)	5 (27.8%)	3 (16.6%)		8 (44.4%)	18 (100%)
Home and odd job accidents	2 (2.5%)	17 (19.5%)	19 (22.0%)	9 (10.3%)	41 (47.1%)	9 (10.3%)	9 (10.3%)	59 (67.7%)	87 (100%)

$\chi^2 = 42.39$. ddl = 10. P < 0.001 (very significant). Cramer = 0.38 (very strong correlation).

Table 58–7. RESULTS ACCORDING TO LEVEL OF LESION IN 150 CASES

Level of Lesions	Failures			Average Results	Useful Results				Total
	Failure	Poor	Total		Good	Very Good	Excellent	Total	
Wrist	4 (3.6%)	21 (18.7%)	25 (22.3%)	27 (24.1%)	41 (36.6%)	11 (9.8%)	8 (7.1%)	60 (53.5%)	112 (100%)
Forearm	3 (7.9%)	14 (36.8%)	17 (44.7%)	7 (18.5%)	12 (31.6%)	1 (2.6%)	1 (2.6%)	14 (36.8%)	38 (100%)

$\chi^2 = 7.10$. ddl = 2. P <0.025 (significant). Cramer = 0.217 (strong correlation).

Table 58–8. RESULTS ACCORDING TO TYPE OF INJURY IN 139 CASES

Type of Injury	Failures			Average Results	Useful Results				Total
	Failure	Poor	Total		Good	Very Good	Excellent	Total	
Clean cut wounds	1 (0.9%)	24 (22.0%)	25 (22.9%)	27 (24.8%)	41 (37.6%)	10 (9.2%)	6 (5.5%)	57 (52.3%)	109 (100%)
Contused wound	5 (16.7%)	7 (23.3%)	12 (40.0%)	6 (20.0%)	7 (23.3%)	2 (6.7%)	3 (10.0%)	12 (40.0%)	30 (100%)

$\chi^2 = 16.06$. ddl = 5. P <0.01 (significant). Cramer = 0.33 (strong correlation).

Table 58–9. RESULTS ACCORDING TO THE NERVE LESION IN 143 CASES

Type of Nerve Lesion	Failures			Average Results	Useful Results				Total
	Failure	Poor	Total		Good	Very Good	Excellent	Total	
Total sections	5 (4.5%)	32 (28.6%)	37 (33.1%)	23 (20.5%)	39 (34.8%)	6 (5.4%)	7 (6.2%)	52 (46.4%)	112 (100%)
Partial sections	0 (0%)	2 (6.5%)	2 (6.5%)	9 (29.0%)	12 (38.7%)	6 (19.3%)	2 (6.5%)	20 (64.5%)	31 (100%)

$\chi^2 = 12.9$. ddl = 5. P <0.05 (significant). Cramer = 0.30 (strong correlation).

Table 58–10. RESULTS ACCORDING TO TYPE OF MICROSURGICAL REPAIR IN 67 CASES

Type of Repair	Failures		Average Results		Useful Results			
	FAILURE	POOR	TOTAL		GOOD	VERY GOOD	EXCELLENT	TOTAL
Emergency nerve sutures	2 (5.3%)	7 (18.4%)	9 (23.7%)	10 (26.3%)	15 (39.5%)	3 (7.9%)	1 (2.6%)	19 (50.0%)	38 (100%)
Secondary sutures		1 (12.5%)	1 (12.5%)	4 (50.0%)	3 (37.5%)			3 (37.5%)	8 (100%)
Fascicular grafts	2 (9.5%)	10 (47.6%)	12 (57.1%)	4 (19.1%)	5 (23.8%)			5 (23.8%)	21 (100%)

$\chi^2 = 10.15$ ddl = 4. P <0.05 (significant). Cramer = 0.275 (strong correlation).

Table 58–11. INFLUENCE OF ARTERIAL REPAIR ON RESULTS OF EMERGENCY NERVE SUTURES IN 38 CASES

Type of Arterial Lesion	Failures		Average Results		Useful Results			
	FAILURE	POOR	TOTAL		GOOD	VERY GOOD	EXCELLENT	TOTAL
No arterial lesion				3 (23.1%)	7 (53.8%)	2 (15.4%)	1 (7.7%)	10 (76.9%)	13 (100%)
Arterial lesion repaired and functional		2 (14.3%)	2 (14.3%)	3 (21.5%)	8 (57.1%)	1 (7.1%)		9 (64.2%)	14 (100%)
Arterial lesion not repaired or repaired but nonfunctional	2 (18.2%)	5 (45.4%)	7 (63.6%)	4 (36.4%)					11 (100%)

$\chi^2 = 22.25$. ddl = 1. P <0.01 (significant). Cramer = 0.541 (very strong correlation).

To reduce the bias introduced by age, we have concentrated our attention on patients 20 to 49 years of age. This study included 38 primary repairs carried out as emergency procedures, 8 secondary suture repairs, and 21 secondary fascicular grafts.

Table 58–10 shows that primary repair by suturing gives better results than secondary suturing, with the fascicular graft a poor third; the statistical differences are significant.

Several observations can be made in the light of this study:

1. Delayed repairs yielded no very good or excellent results.

2. Primary suturing produced 50 per cent of the useful results.

3. Secondary suturing produced 50 per cent of the average results.

4. Grafting failed in 57.1 per cent of the cases.

5. The percentage of failures in emergency suture repairs was greater than in secondary suturing, but the numbers in the latter group were small. This possibly emphasizes the difficulty in assessing the extent of contusion at emergency operation in a tissue as gelatinous as a nerve.

In addition, total median-ulnar lesions are often complicated by interruption of the radial or ulnar artery. The beneficial influence of arterial repair on the ultimate functional result has been demonstrated in our study and the difference found to be highly significant (Table 58–11).

Thus an isolated nerve lesion with no arterial damage will yield a useful result in 76.9 per cent of the cases. When an artery is repaired and remains patent in the long term, the percentage of useful results is 64.2 per cent. If the artery is not repaired or thromboses after repair, no useful results are recorded.

DISCUSSION

This study concerns 150 lesions of the median and ulnar nerves in which results were scored by a system generally accepted as strict and accurate. Statistical analysis of the results makes it possible to draw some useful conclusions regarding factors related to the patient, the nature of the injury, and the surgical method.

Our results confirm the fact that repairs in children carry an excellent prognosis, whereas the results in aged patients are consistently poor.

The type of injury also influences the prognosis. Industrial accidents can result in the most complex injuries: In this group of patients we found that if the nerve lesion was repaired at emergency surgery, 46 per cent of the patients could resume their occupation within six months, whereas only 30 per cent of those treated by secondary nerve grafts did. Moreover, 70 per cent of the patients treated by nerve suturing returned to their initial occupation; after a nerve graft only 59 per cent did so.

It is tempting, of course, to suggest that the lesions treated by secondary grafting were the most severe. However, in our practice over the last 10 years, the frequency of nerve grafts has been markedly reduced in favor of primary suturing.

This study has also confirmed the impression we had formed in our earlier practice that the result of nerve suturing is significantly improved by early arterial repair. All surgical teams involved in the emergency repair of hand injuries should be aware of this fact. Indeed combined neural and arterial injuries should always be regarded as microsurgical emergencies. This is true for clean wounds as well as for contused ones: vascular repair is essential to preserve the trophicity of tissues that may be called upon to act as a bed for a fascicular graft or to surround a secondary nerve suture. Microscopic examination of the nerve at emergency, the epineural vascularization, and the surrounding tissue may enable the surgeon to restore its overall orientation, a maneuver that is difficult and delicate after secondary resection of the neuroglioma.

This study emphasizes the advantages of primary repair of clean nerve sections and will, we hope, dispel the myth that a secondary repair carries an equal chance of success. Figure 58–1 shows that the results of secondary grafts and sutures have improved but little since 1976.

The only improvements in published results concern lesions in which primary repair was carried out. This concept, however, is not without its drawbacks because it implies the constant availability of fully trained teams of microsurgeons for emergency repairs.

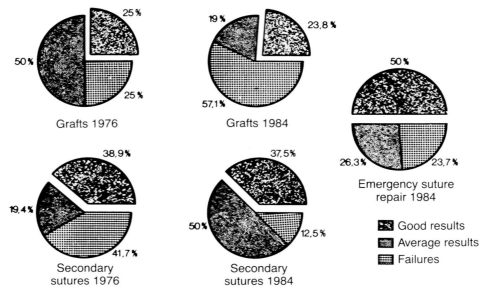

Figure 58–1. Nerve repairs. Comparative statistics.

Every microsurgeon will testify to the technical difficulty of a primary repair when the nerve is gelatinous and its manipulation necessitates the exteriorization of fascicles, which in turn renders apposition difficult.

With the surgeon still ill equipped to differentiate between the sensory and motor fibers traveling within the same mixed nerve trunk, it must be recognized that the only advances in the repair of peripheral nerve lesions in the last 10 years have been the result of improved primary microsurgical techniques of nerve suturing combined with the reconstruction of arterial channels.

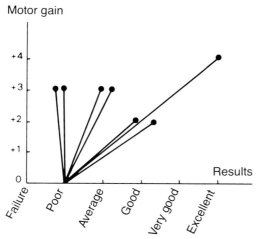

Figure 58–2. Influence of an opposition tendon transfer on the final result.

There is no doubt that the improvements in operating microscopes and in microsurgical equipment, needles, and sutures and the more thorough training of surgeons have heightened the quality and accuracy of epineural, interfascicular, and vascular suturing. But surgery is not the only aspect of the management of peripheral nerve lesions: The development of postoperative dynamic splints to prevent or correct an ulnar claw and the introduction of programs of sensory rehabilitation also make an important contribution to the return of hand function. It is also worth remembering that a simple opposition tendon transfer can convert an average result into a very good one. This is well illustrated by the graph of seven cases in Figure 58–2.

CONCLUSION

A partial or total clean cut of the median or ulnar nerve is best managed by early suturing under microscope control. The frequent association of a vascular lesion means that these injuries must be regarded as emergencies.

Finally, a repair by primary microsutures yields a better result than the best of secondary repairs, whether by direct suturing or by nerve grafting.

THE BRACHIAL PLEXUS

Chapter 59

TRAUMATIC LESIONS OF THE BRACHIAL PLEXUS: RECENT ADVANCES IN MANAGEMENT AND SURGICAL INDICATIONS

RAOUL TUBIANA

Lesions of the brachial plexus have increased in frequency in recent years in parallel with road traffic accidents and the increase in popularity of two wheel motor vehicles. With improved intensive care and better patient survival, the number and severity of brachial plexus lesions have increased. This type of injury is of great social significance in view of the severe residual morbidity, for the majority of patients are in their early twenties. Hence, the effective management of such lesions is of considerable importance. The constitution and distribution of the brachial plexus are shown in Color Plates IV and V.

HISTORICAL ASPECTS

The first clinical description of partial plexus palsy in a newborn was published by Smellie in 1746. Flaubert in 1827 suggested that the paralysis resulting from forcible reduction of long standing shoulder dislocations was due to stretching of the nerve roots. In 1853 Duchenne gave a clinical description of C5-C6 palsies, but it was Erb who in 1874 localized the lesion when he realized that paralysis affecting the deltoid, biceps, brachialis, and brachioradialis did not result from isolated lesions of nerves arising in the plexus but from a lesion of the C5 and C6 roots at the site where they join to form the upper trunk of the plexus. He also suggested that in such cases one should look specifically for a lesion of the suprascapular nerve.

In 1885 Miss A. Klumpke, later to become Dejerine's wife, described lesions of C8-T1, and in a thesis published the same year Secretan summed up contemporary knowledge about lesions of the plexus.

The experimental work of Duval and Guillain (1898) demonstrated the role of stretching when the head and shoulder are pulled apart forcibly. This was later confirmed by Stevens (1934) and by Barnes (1949).

The prognosis remains difficult to establish, depending as it does on the level, extent, and exact nature of the lesion. More accurate localization has been made possible by axon reflex studies (Bonney, 1954), myelography (Murphy et al., 1947), and electromyography, but repeated clinical examinations still form the basis for diagnosis.

As far as treatment is concerned, it would appear that the Englishman Horsley (1899), toward the end of the nineteenth century, was the first to try a surgical approach to plexus lesions in adults, followed in 1903 by his compatriot Kennedy, who dealt with obstetrical lesions. Taylor (1907) in the United States started with obstetrical plexus lesions and in the 1920's operated on adult lesions. In 1903 Harris and Low in England carried out the first nerve transfer, followed by Tuttle (1913) in the United States. Their techniques then were adopted and developed by Foerster (1916–1918) and Vulpius and Stoffel (1920). There followed a period of isolated surgical experiments (Lurje, 1948; Petrov, 1973; Scaglietti, 1942). Seddon and Merle d'Aubigné deserve credit for the first systematic, long-term study of plexus lesions. Like the majority of their surgical contemporaries, in view of the disappointing results of early surgical repairs, they refrained from active intervention and watched for spontaneous recoveries, which fortunately occurred in more than 50 per cent of the cases (Merle d'Aubigné, 1956; Yeoman and Seddon, 1961). They concentrated on late palliative surgery, which they classified (Merle d'Aubigné and Deburge, 1967).

The advent of microsurgical techniques, which without doubt have improved the prognosis in nerve repairs, now justifies a more aggressive attitude. Direct repair of plexus lesions has become routine practice in specialized centers over the last few years, at least in cases in which a clear distinction can be made between lesions in patients who are likely to recover spontaneously and those in which an early surgical repair represents the patient's only hope. Despite the technical problems and doubtful prognosis, the stakes are such that the opportunity for a successful repair must not be missed.

Surgery of the brachial plexus is time consuming and technically difficult, and the results are often disappointing. However, direct suturing, nerve grafts, neurolysis, and neurotization make possible a variable degree of functional recovery. This may be limited when several roots have been totally severed, yet only a few years ago recovery—even minimal recovery—was inconceivable. Alnot, Millesi, Narakas, Morelli, and Sedel, all pioneers in this field, describe their personal experience in other chapters, and in Volume IV Gilbert discusses his results in the repair of obstetrical brachial plexus lesions in children.

Those reports, which sum up the present trends in the management of brachial plexus injuries, show a definite tendency to favor early direct surgical repair; i.e., surgery is now indicated in all cases when no clinical or electromyographic evidence of functional recovery can be elicited three months after the accident. Some authors (e.g., Alnot and Narakas) advocate surgery in certain cases after only a few weeks.

The lesions are so diverse, however, that it is difficult to lay down a definite set of rules. Perhaps they are best summed up on the basis of chronology.

EMERGENCY SURGICAL REPAIR

Emergency surgical repair is indicated in cases of open wounds and when acute compression must be relieved (e.g., drainage of a hematoma, reduction of a fracture, or dislocation of the neighboring bones).

THE FIRST STAGE

During the first stage (i.e., up to two or three months) conservative treatment consists of making an accurate estimate of the level, extent, and severity of the lesions by clinical and other means; physiotherapy, which aims at preserving passive mobility of all the joints of the limb and forestalling the development of stiffness and deformities; and careful watching for every telltale sign of recovery. In certain cases, e.g., after severe accidents leading to total motor and sensory loss in the limb and Horner's syndrome, the diagnosis of root avulsion is so obvious that surgical exploration is indicated within a few weeks after the injury.

THE SECOND MONTH

In the course of the second month, one of two situations may exist.

1. Recovery is evident and progress is rapid. There is no axonal interruption (Sunderland stage 1) and the prognosis is good. Conservative treatment is continued and the progress monitored.

2. There are no signs of recovery. It is now essential to identify preganglionic root lesions as early as possible with the help of all available methods—clinical examination, electromyography, sensory potentials, myelography, and computed tomographic scanning.

If a preganglionic lesion is present, spontaneous recovery is out of the question and surgery represents the only hope. This should take the form of exploration and neurotization. However, although neurotization of the upper roots can restore weak abduction of the shoulder and flexion of the elbow, the same procedure in avulsions of the C8-T1 roots never succeeds in reactivating the intrinsic muscles of the hand. At best one can hope for the return of protective sensibility.

In postganglionic lesions and lesions of the trunks, conservative treatment is continued for another four to eight weeks. During this time it should be possible to differentiate between lesions without axonal interruption (positive results on Tinel testing and electromyography), which correspond to Sunderland stages 2 and 3 lesions (these patients recover spontaneously) and lesions with axonal interruption (absence of Tinel's sign at the plexus) corresponding to Sunderland stages 4 and 5 (spontaneous recovery is impossible). In the latter cases surgical repair must be attempted. Direct suturing is seldom possible and nerve grafts are usually indicated. If the whole plexus cannot be bridged, priority is given to reinnervating the proximal territories.

THREE MONTHS

At the end of three months, if the diagnosis is still in doubt, a full neurological examination is repeated at regular intervals, and the surgical repair is directed at lesions that show no sign of recovery.

If no evidence of recovery is detected, exploration must be attempted. If axonal disruption has occurred, a nerve graft is indicated.

If following initial recovery progress ceases, exploration is indicated with a view to relieving a possible obstruction. The possibility of lesions at different levels must be kept in mind, and neurolysis or a nerve graft is carried out, depending on the findings. The most difficult surgical indications are when it exists as a dyschronological (distal recovery before proximal) or a dissociated recovery (when recovery occurs in only one territory); surgical exploration is again justified after three months.

With modern techniques, surgical exploration produces no serious tissue damage and blood loss is minimal. Even after extensive repairs lasting several hours, the patient can be discharged within a week. There is thus little to lose by early exploration (Narakas, 1985).

AFTER THREE MONTHS

All reconstructive procedures should have been carried out before four months have passed, but this does not imply that direct surgical repair should not be attempted in patients at later stages. Some improvement has been noted after repairs carried out eight to 10 months after the injury, but the prognosis worsens with time.

The most distressing feature in brachial plexus lesions is persistent pain. After root lesions the pain may be relieved by nerve grafts or late neurolysis, and it is now confirmed that pain is far less common in patients who have undergone early surgical repair. After avulsions, pain is more frequent and results of any treatment are unpredictable. Wynn Parry in his chapter (65) studies ways of helping patients with such pain.

Reconstructive surgery as a complement of nerve repairs or in patients in whom these have failed is discussed in detail in Volume IV.

The indications for amputations and for limb appliances have also evolved. As Wynn Parry points out, early amputation of hopelessly paralyzed limbs has been replaced by external dynamic splinting of flaccid limbs whose passive mobility has been preserved by physiotherapy.

The lines of treatment have only been outlined here; they are considered in greater detail in the following chapters. The timing of the repair and the choice of procedure are still debatable in view of the diversity of lesions.

The benefits of these difficult and time consuming repairs, to be analyzed in this section, may appear limited. Their modest objective, after a complete paralysis, is to restore stability of the shoulder, flexion of the elbow, a primitive grip, or protective sensibility, but these "limited" benefits still justify the enormous cost and effort in the opinion of both surgeons and patients.

REFERENCES

Alnot, J. Y., Allieu, Y., Bonnel, F., Cadre, N., Frot, B., Huten, B., Mansat, M., Millesi, H., Narakas, A., and Sedel, L.: Paralysie traumatique du plexus brachial chez l'adulte. Symposium Réunion Annuelle SOFCOT. Rev. Chir. Orthop., 63:17–125, 1977.

Barnes, R.: Traction injuries of the brachial plexus in adults. J. Bone Joint Surg., 31B:10, 1949.

Bonney, G.: The value of axon responses in determining the site of lesion in traction injuries of the brachial plexus. Brain, 77:588, 1954.

Duchenne, G. B.: De l'électrisation localisée. In Diagnostic des Paralysies Cérébrales de l'Enfance, d'avec la Paralysie Atrophique Graisseuse de l'enfance et avec Certaines Paralysies Traumatiques Congénitales. 2nd Ed. Paris, J. B. Bailieres et Fils, 1861, pp. 342–351.

Duval, P., and Guillain, G.: Pathogénie des accidents nerveux consécutifs aux luxations et traumatismes de l'épaule. Arch. Gen Med., 8:5–10, 143–191, 1899.

Erb, N.: Ueber eine eigentliche Lokalisation von Lähmunger im Plexus brachialis. Verhandlungen Heidelberg, Naturhistor. Verein, 1987, pp. 130–136.

Erb, N.: Diseases of the peripheral cerebro-spinal nerves. In Ziemssen, H., (ed.): Cyclopedia of the Practice of Medicine, Vol. XI. London, Searle and Rivington, 1876.

Flaubert, M.: Mémoire sur plusieurs cas de luxation. Rev. Gen. Anat. Physiol. Pathol., 3:55–69, 1827.

Foerster, O.: Die Therapie der Schussverletzungen der peripheren Nerven. In Lewandowski, E. (ed.): Handbuch der Neurologie. Berlin, Erganzungsband, 1929, pp. 1677–1691.

Gilbert, A., Khouri, N., and Carlioz, H.: Exploration chirurgicale du plexus brachial dans la paralysie obstetricale. Rev. Chir. Orthop., 66:33–42, 1980.

Harris, W., and Low, V. W.: On the importance of accurate muscular analysis in lesions of the brachial plexus and the treatment of Erb's palsy and infantile paralysis of the upper extremity by cross-union of nerve roots. Br. Med. J., 2:1035–1038, 1903.

Horsley, V.: On injuries to peripheral nerves. Practitioner 63:131–144, 1899.

Kennedy, R.: Suture on the brachial plexus in birth paralysis of the upper extremity. Br. Med. J., 1:298–301, 1903.

Klumpke, A.: Paralysies radiculaires du plexus brachial. Rev. Med. (Paris), V:591–790, 1885.

Lurje, A.: Concerning surgical treatment of traumatic injury of the upper division of the brachial plexus (Erb's type). Ann. Surg., 127:317–326, 1948.

Medical Research Council: Peripheral nerve injuries.

Spec. Rep. Ser. Med. Res. Coun., No. 282, H.M.S.O., London, 1954.

Merle d'Aubigné, R., and Deburge, A.: Etiologie, évolution et pronostic des paralysies traumatiques du plexus brachial. Rev. Chir. Orthop., 53:23–42, 1967.

Merle d'Aubigné, R., and Deburge, A.: Traitement des paralysies du plexus brachial. Rev. Chir. Orthop., 53:199–215, 1967.

Merle d'Aubigné, R., Benassy, J., and Ramadier, J. O.: Chirurgie Orthopédique des Paralysies. Vol. I. Paris, Masson et Cie, 1956.

Millesi, H.: Résultats tardifs de la greffe nerveuse interfasciculaire. Chirurgie réparatrice du plexus brachial. Rev. Med. Suisse Romande, 9293:511–518, 1973.

Millesi, H.: Brachial plexus injuries. Management and results. Clin. Plast. Surg., 11:115–121, 1984.

Morelli, E., and Pajardi, G.: La microchirurgia nelle lesioni del plesso brachiale. Medico e paziente, 9:1822–1830, 1985.

Murphy, F., Hartung, W., and Kirklin, J. W.: Myelographic demonstration of avulsing injury of the brachial plexus. Am. J. Roentg. Radium Ther., 58:102, 1947.

Narakas, A.: Plexo braquial. Terapeutica chirurgica directa. Tecnica indicacion operatoria, resultados. Cirurgica de los nervios periféricos. Rev. Ortop. Traumatl., 16:856–920, 1972.

Narakas, A.: The treatment of brachial plexus injuries. Internat. Orthop. (SICOT), 9:29–36, 1985.

Petrov, M. A.: Lésions traumatiques du plexus brachial. Traitement chirurgical. Transplantations, résultats éloignés. Mem. Acad. Chir., 99:924–934, 1973.

Scaglietti, O.: Einzelheiten uber Operationstechnik bei Verletzungen der Wurzeln des Plexus Brachialis durch Schusswaffen. Zbl. f. Neurochir., 7:129–144, 1942.

Secretan, H.: Contribution à l'étude des paralysies radiculaires du plexus brachial. Thèse, Paris, Librairie Ollier Henri, 1895.

Seddon, H. J.: Brachial plexus. In Carling, E., and Ross, J. P. (eds.): British Surgical Practice. London, Butterworth, 1948.

Seddon, H. J.: Surgical Disorders of the Peripheral Nerves. Edinburgh, Churchill-Livingstone, 1972.

Smellie, W.: Observations sur les accouchements. Traduction Préville, recueil 30. Cité par Johnson, E. W.: Brachial palsy at birth. Int. Abst. Surg., 3:409, 1950.

Stevens, J. H.: Brachial plexus paralysis. In Codman, E. A. (ed.): The Shoulder. New York, G. Mill, 1934.

Taylor, A.: Results from the surgical treatment of brachial birth palsy. J.A.M.A., 48:96–104, 1907.

Taylor, A.: Brachial birth palsy and injuries of similar type in adults. Surg. Gynecol. Obstet., 30:494–502, 1920.

Tuttle, H.: Exposure of the brachial plexus with nerve transplantation. J.A.M.A., 61:15–17, 1913.

Vulpius, O., and Stoffel, A.: Orthopädische Operationslehre, 2nd Ed. Stuttgart, Enke, 1920.

Yeoman, P. M., and Seddon, H. J.: Brachial plexus injuries: treatment of the flail arm. J. Bone Joint Surg., 43B:493, 1961.

Chapter 60

TRAUMATIC BRACHIAL PLEXUS PALSY IN ADULTS

JEAN-YVES ALNOT

Brachial plexus lesions and their evolution have been the subject of numerous surgical studies that also consider the indications and timing of tendon transfers in view of the resulting palsies. Exploration of the brachial plexus has been advocated with the objective of determining a prognosis rather than undertaking a surgical repair that may seem impossible in the presence of avulsions and massive loss of tissue. The advances in nerve microsurgery and the early results of nerve grafts combined with a better understanding of the pathology of the lesions have shed new light on the problem.

The earliest repairs consisted mostly of neurolyses. Next, a few isolated cases of nerve grafts were reported in the literature, and the Estonian neurosurgeon Pussepp was possibly the first to record a successful result with a nerve graft in 1931. Isolated cases of nerve grafting were reported by Scaglietti (1947), Seddon and Brooks (1949), and Petrov and Solarov (1964). Such repairs have now become possible because of our better understanding of the anatomy of the brachial plexus, our improved surgical approach, and the clearer modern classification of the lesions.

The first part of this chapter will consider the anatomy of the brachial plexus, the clinical features of brachial plexus lesions and their natural history, and finally the indications for surgery. The second part will be concerned with surgical technique and with the indications for direct repairs of brachial plexus lesions. Tendon transfers for consecutive palsies of the shoulder, the elbow, and the hand will be mentioned briefly but not described in detail, as they are considered in Volume IV.

ANATOMY OF THE BRACHIAL PLEXUS

Two points need to be stressed. First, the brachial plexus lies in two planes, anterior and posterior, which are completely independent and do not exchange fibers. Second, it is possible to map out the whole of the brachial plexus, including its cords, its trunks, and even its roots. Based on our own microscopic dissections of the plexus in the fresh cadavers, from its roots to its terminal and collateral branches, and on the histological studies of Bonnel (1977) and Mansat (1977), we have been able to obtain a comprehensive overall picture of the anatomical organization of the brachial plexus.

THE BRACHIAL PLEXUS AND ITS VARIATIONS

The brachial plexus is formed by the anterior branches of the four lowest cervical nerves and by part of the anterior branch of the first thoracic nerve. The roots of the plexus unite to form the three trunks—upper (C5 and C6), middle (C7), and lower (C8 and T1).

Each trunk divides into two branches, anterior and posterior. The anterior branches join to form the two anterior cords, medial and lateral. The medial cord gives rise to the medial root of the median nerve, the ulnar nerve, the medial brachial cutaneous nerve, and the medial antebrachial cutaneous nerve. The lateral cord gives off the lateral root of the median nerve and the musculocutaneous nerve.

607

The posterior divisions unite to form the posterior cord, which gives rise to the radial and axillary nerves. Finally, collateral branches arise from the roots and from the trunks and cords. Therefore, beginning from the division of the trunks, the separation into an anterior and a posterior plane is evident.

Anatomical Features of Clinical Significance

The Posterior Branch of the Spinal Nerve. This branch arises at the vertebral foramen and runs posteriorly, crossing the superior aspect of the posterior part of the transverse process and the neck of the first rib. Clinical or electromyographic involvement of the muscles of the paravertebral gutters is of topographical and prognostic interest, as such involvement serves to differentiate between preganglionic and postganglionic lesions, even though their innervation is metameric and comes from different roots.

The Nerve to the Serratus Anterior Muscle. This nerve arises proximally from the root. It always transmits fibers from C5 and C6, but also frequently transmits fibers from C7, C8, T1, and in particular from C4. This means that involvement of the serratus anterior muscle in the context of brachial plexus palsy is a poor prognostic sign, as it is indicative of a very proximal lesion spread over many root levels.

The Autonomic Fibers. Without discussing the sympathetic ganglia and pathways in detail, it should be noted that the fibers concerned with dilatation of the iris originate in the hypothalamus and travel down the cord to emerge with the first three thoracic roots. From there, they run in the white rami communicantes and cross the stellate ganglion before supplying the dilator muscle of the iris. Horner's syndrome is therefore the result of a lesion involving the ramus communicans of T1 with the stellate ganglion and usually suggests a proximal lesion.

The Phrenic Nerve. Every work-up of a total brachial plexus lesion should include cineradiography of the corresponding hemidiaphragm. Paralysis of the hemidiaphragm signifies a lesion at C4, which not only supplies the phrenic nerve but also is part of the brachial plexus through its connections with C5. Thus, certain collateral nerves of the brachial plexus, notably the nerves to the subscapular muscle and rhomboids (C4-C5),

can be lost. The superficial cervical plexus and the nerve to the trapezius can also be lost, and their area must also be studied.

Anatomical Variations

While this is the classic organization of the plexus, numerous variations exist from one individual to another and even from one side to the other in the same person. Thus, Kerr (1949) reported perfect symmetry in only 39 of 63 bilateral dissections.

We shall now consider variations that can affect the roots as well as the actual structure of the plexus.

Variations in Root Distribution. Classically, consecutive roots contribute to the plexus an anastomotic branch arising from C4 or T2. This contribution has been studied by Kerr (1949), among others, who showed that the participation of C4 is the most common (63 per cent of cases) and that when C4 does not contribute to the plexus, T2 does, and vice versa. When both roots send fibers to the plexus, there is a proportional relationship in the number of fibers contributed.

These differences result in variations in the plexus in relation to the axial skeleton. For this reason a distinction is made between the high or prefixed plexus, which receives an anastomosis from C4, and the low or postfixed plexus, which receives fibers from T2. Seddon (1972) prefers to reserve the terms pre- or postfixed for cases in which all fibers come from C4 or T2, i.e., for plexuses with the arrangement C4 to C8 or C6 to T2, although these are rarely found.

Between the classic and the extreme arrangements is a wide range of variations in the respective contributions to the branches (e.g., large C5 root and small T1 or vice versa) as well as in the mode of origin of the terminal branches, (i.e., in the very structure of the plexus).

Variations in the Structure of the Plexus

VARIATIONS IN CONSTITUTION AND DISTRIBUTION. These have been studied by Turner, Herringham (1866), Wychmann, Schumacher, and Kerr (1918) and concern mostly the trunks. Thus, the upper trunk, which classically arises from C5 and C6, can originate from the union of C5, C6, and C7, or, conversely, it can be absent, with C5 and C6 each dividing into two branches, anterior and posterior, which join in both planes. Similar variations have been reported in the intermediate and lower trunks, but they do not necessarily alter the overall structure of the plexus. Thus, it can be shown that the trunks are only macroscopic entities, resulting from the apposition of two anterior and posterior groups of nerve fibers, and that some of the variations are caused by the more or less proximal approximation or separation of these groups within the same plane.

VARIATIONS IN THE LENGTH OF THE ROOTS, TRUNKS, AND CORDS. Table 60–1 highlights three interesting features:

1. The shortness of C8 and T1, which makes surgical access to this region even more difficult.

2. The great variability of the middle trunk, which is impossible to quantify (it is a transitional element between various types of plexuses, as it is a prolongation of C7 without anatomical differentiation).

3. The variable diameter of the spinal or accessory nerve, C5 being inversely proportional to T1 according to the type of plexus (pre- or postfixed).

THE ANTERIOR AND POSTERIOR COMPONENTS

There is no disagreement whatsoever concerning the division of the trunks into their anterior and posterior branches, which unite to form the anterior and posterior cords. This is amply confirmed by microdissection. Thus, the upper trunk can be split into an anterior and a posterior fiber group, and it appears that these are simply the anterior divisions of the trunk that run together at this level. This separation can sometimes be pursued up to the level of C5 and C6, if necessary by opening the epineurium (Fig. 60–1). Similarly, it can be shown that the middle trunk and C7 actually consist of the apposition of two anterior and posterior fiber bundles.

Finally, at the level of C8-T1 and of the lower trunk the same arrangement is seen, but the dissection also shows that the posterior bundle of T1 makes only a small contribution to the posterior plane of the plexus. Therefore, from the roots down to the terminal and collateral branches, the plexus can be divided into two planes or fiber groups (anterior and posterior) that are quite distinct, do not exchange fibers, and can be studied separately. As a result of microdis-

Table 60–1. MEASUREMENTS OF THE ROOTS AND TRUNKS OF THE BRACHIAL PLEXUS

Length of Spinal Nerves as They Emerge from the Transverse Canal

NERVE	MINIMUM AND MAXIMUM (cm.)	MEAN (cm.)
C5	3.5–4.25	4.07
C6	3.0–4.0	3.14
C7	4.8–6.0	5.80
C8	2.35–3.15	2.53
T1	2.15–3.2	2.46

Length of Primary Trunks

TRUNK	MINIMUM AND MAXIMUM (cm.)	MEAN (cm.)	DIAMETER (mm.)
Upper primary	1.8–3.5	2.7	4–7
Inferior primary	3.5–4.0	3.9	4–7
Middle primary	Extremely variable		

section, one can now trace the nerve fibers from the terminal branches to the root and obtain a "map" of the brachial plexus.

MAPPING OUT THE BRACHIAL PLEXUS

We shall first discuss the posterior plane, which is simple and constant, before discussing the anterior plane, which is complex and variable.

Map of the Posterior Plane

By dissection of the posterior plane of the brachial plexus it is possible to trace every terminal or collateral nerve to its root of origin (Table 60–2). Thus, the axillary nerve originates in C5 and C6 and the radial nerve in C6, C7, C8, and (to a lesser extent) T1. It is also possible to follow the path and determine the position of the fibers in relation to those destined to travel to other nerves, e.g., the axillary fibers always travel above those of the radial fibers (Figs. 60–2, 60–3A). The proportion of fibers within each root and trunk belonging to a given nerve can also be worked out. Thus, we know that the major part of the posterior component of the upper trunk and of the C5 and C6 roots belongs to the axillary nerve, while the radial fibers represent almost all of the posterior component of the middle and lower trunks and of the C7, C8, and T1 roots. A similar map can be worked out for the collateral branches of the posterior component (Fig. 60–3).

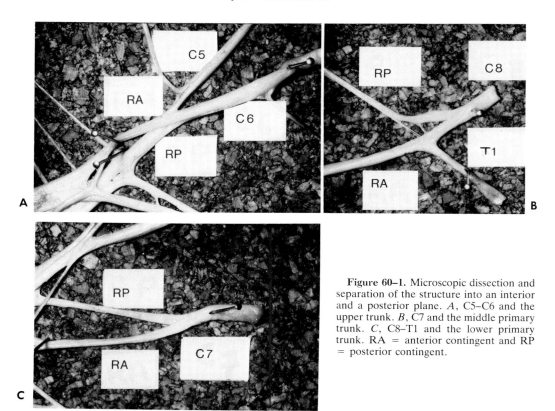

Figure 60–1. Microscopic dissection and separation of the structure into an interior and a posterior plane. *A*, C5–C6 and the upper trunk. *B*, C7 and the middle primary trunk. *C*, C8–T1 and the lower primary trunk. RA = anterior contingent and RP = posterior contingent.

Map of the Anterior Plane

Unlike the posterior plane, the anterior plane is complex and variable (Table 60–3), mostly as a result of the C7 root, whose anterior fibers are shared in variable proportions between the anterior cords. On the basis of these variations, three types of plexus can be distinguished (Fig. 60–3):

1. In type A, the entire anterior component of C7 enters the lateral cord, so that the ulnar nerve contains no C7 fibers.

2. In type B, all the C7 fibers pass into the

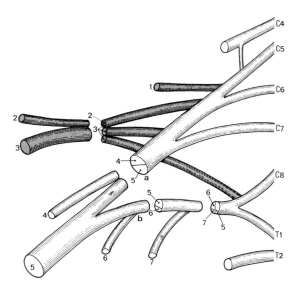

Figure 60–2. Two-plane arrangement of the brachial plexus and simplified mapping.

Table 60–2. ANATOMY OF THE POSTERIOR PLANE

Nerve to subscapularis:	C5-C6
Nerves to levator scapula and to rhomboids	C4-C5
Nerve to serratus anterior:	C4-C5-C6-C7
Nerve to supraspinatus:	C5 or C5-C6
Posterior secondary trunk:	C5-C6-C7-C8-T1
Nerve to teres major: C6	
Nerve to latissimus dorsi: C7	
Radiocircumflex trunk: circumflex: C5-C6	
radial: C6-C7-C8-T1	

medial cord, so that the ulnar nerve is rich in C7 fibers.

3. In type C, the anterior component of the C7 fibers is shared by the lateral and medial cords, producing two subtypes. In subtype C1, the fibers of C7 destined for the medial cord join the cord at or just proximal to the origin of the ulnar nerve, which then contains C7 fibers. In subtype C2, these same fibers join the cord after the origin of the ulnar nerve, which therefore lacks C7 fibers.

This explains why the ulnar nerve will or will not include the fibers from the C7 root. A similar dissection of the posterior fibers will show the following root values for the various nerves (Table 60–3): musculocutaneous nerve—C5, C6, and sometimes C7; median nerve—C6, C7, C8, and T1; ulnar nerve—C7 (sometimes), C8, and T1; and medial cutaneous nerve of the arm and medial cutaneous nerve of the forearm—C8 and especially T1.

Table 60–3. ANATOMY OF THE ANTERIOR PLANE

Anterolateral secondary trunk: C5-C6-C7	
Anteromedial secondary trunk: C8-T1-C7 ±	C7 = shared root

C5: Musculocutaneous
    Pectorals
C6: Lateral root of the median nerve
C7: More common
    Lateral root of the median nerve + + +
    Pectorals
    Musculocutaneous ± ulnar +
    Less common
    Medial root of the median nerve + + +
    Ulnar
C8: Medial root of the median nerve
    Ulnar
    Pectoralis
T1: Medial cutaneous nerve of arm

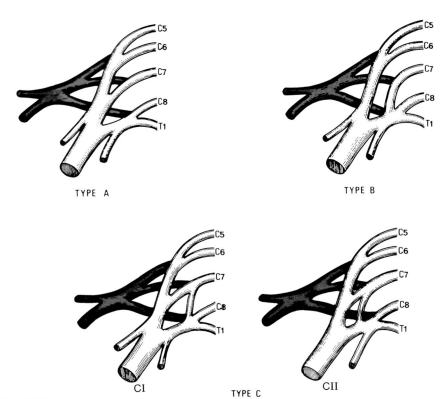

TYPE A   TYPE B

CI   TYPE C   CII

Figure 60–3. Different anatomical types according to the distribution of C7. *Type A*, C7 joins the anterolateral secondary trunk. *Type B*, C7 joins the anteromedial trunk. *Type C*, Intermediate.

This mapping by dissection shows the pathway of the root fibers as well as their position within a given trunk (Figs. 60–2, 60–3). In the lateral cord and superior roots, the fibers of the median nerve run anterior to those of the other terminal branches, i.e., medial cutaneous nerves of the forearm and arm. These fibers then gradually pass under those of the median nerve before arising from the inferior border of the cord. In the two anterior cords, the fibers destined for the pectoral muscles are always anterior to and in the middle of those of the median or the musculocutaneous nerves.

The suprascapular nerve occupies a rather special position in the above arrangement. It consists of a collateral branch of the posterior plane that arises from the terminal of C5 or from the origin of the upper trunk. The nerve receives C5 and sometimes C6 fibers. The fibers run above those of the musculocutaneous nerve, i.e., in the anterior plane. However, if these fibers are traced back to the origin of the C5 and C6 roots, they are found to occupy a position posterior to those of the musculocutaneous nerve. Thus, they join the fibers of the posterior plane, to which the suprascapular nerve belongs, and occupy a position between the radial-axillary fibers behind and the median and musculocutaneous fibers anteriorly.

The proportion of fibers belonging to a nerve in a trunk or root is more difficult to assess in the anterior component. This is especially true for C7, which has a variable distribution, the only constant feature of which is its massive contribution to the median nerve. However, it also makes a variable contribution to the musculocutaneous and ulnar nerves.

CONCLUSIONS DRAWN FROM THE ANATOMICAL STUDY

The two salient points of the above study are the following:

1. The brachial plexus lies in two planes that are independent from the roots to the terminal and collateral branches—a posterior plane, which has a simpler and constant arrangement and supplies the extensors of the upper limb, and an anterior plane, which is complex and variable and supplies the flexors of the upper limb. This variability is due to the unpredictable distribution of the C7 root, hence the three subtypes A, B, C.

2. Using microdissection, it is possible to trace all terminal fibers to their root of origin and to work out the path of these fibers and their relative numerical importance within each trunk, cord, and root of the brachial plexus. A knowledge of the organization of the fibers is of clinical and therapeutic importance. All the muscles of the upper limb are innervated by fibers from two or more spinal roots, and this fact remains the basis of every clinical examination of the limb. However, the numerous anatomical variations explain why it is possible to have different clinical pictures resulting from identical lesions. When performing a nerve graft for loss of nerve substance at the plexus, the surgeon should therefore make every effort to disturb the cortical representation as little as possible (see Fig. 60–5). Knowledge of the plan of the plexus is the best guide for bridge grafting between nerve fibers of the same origin and destined for the same territory. Thus, in repairs of the axillary nerve, the surgeon will use a graft starting from the posterior part of the C5 root. However, it remains extremely difficult to respect the fascicular pattern, and we must distinguish between the histological fascicle and the surgical fascicle, which are actually groups of fascicles.

The histological studies of Bonnel (1977) and Mansat (1977) have not yet revealed the fascicular organization of the nerves, but some useful observations have already emerged. The average number of surgical fascicles for each nerve root is as follows: four in C4, five in C5, six in C7, two in C8, and three in T1. In addition to the fascicular variability, a huge number of fibers are involved in each nerve root. Thus, C5 transmits about 21,000 fibers (14,000 for the posterior radicle and 7000 for the anterior radicle). Finally, the C7 root transmits more fibers than any of the other roots.

ANATOMOPATHOLOGICAL LESIONS

MECHANISM OF INJURY

A lesion can be situated at any level from the origin of the nerve root to the division in the axillary region. The most common lesion results from traction, and Sunderland's classification helps to classify nerve injury as neurapraxia, axonotmesis, or neurotmesis

(Table 60–4). Sunderland (1978) subdivides axonotmesis into a second degree lesion in which recovery is possible, a third degree lesion in which recovery is less probable, and a fourth degree lesion in which it is unlikely. Root avulsion constitutes a special type of brachial plexus lesion to which we shall return later. As Seddon (1972) has pointed out, both the site and the severity of the lesions must be recognized. A proximal lesion can be preganglionic or postganglionic. More distally, lesions are defined as supra- and retroclavicular and later as infraclavicular.

Once we exclude divisions resulting from open wounds, we find that most brachial plexus lesions are caused by traction. One mechanism is peripheral (Fig. 60–4). This results from different types of injuries.

In the first type there is a wrenching of the cervical spine away from the shoulder; 90 per cent of these injuries are secondary to motor cycle accidents involving a fall onto the shoulder. The degree of abduction of the arm at the moment of the fall seems to play a part, while associated antepulsion stretches all the spinal roots, especially the upper ones. Retropulsion with 90 degrees of abduction further increases the tension on the roots and is usually responsible for total paralysis of the upper limb.

The second type of injury, which is less frequent, consists of traction on an upper limb in maximal abduction. This produces a C8-T1 palsy by stretching of the lower roots

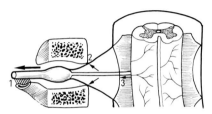

Figure 60–4. Peripheral mechanism of brachial plexus palsy. Lateral traction on the neural complex. The different protective systems include: 1, Fixation to the transverse processes; 2, dural cone and internal orifice of the intervertebral foramen; 3, dentate ligament and indentation of the cord.

and relaxation of the upper roots of the plexus. This type of trauma with its resulting lower root palsy is now seldom seen.

The third type of injury involves a dislocation of the shoulder. It tends to cause lesions of the cords, especially the posterior cord, but there may be concomitant stretching of all the roots. There is, in addition, the injury induced by extreme movements of the cervical column as a result of severe trauma and exaggerated by the added weight of the cranium (Fig. 60–5). This produces tension within the nerve roots followed by stretching and even rupture without actual damage to the dural sheath.

ANATOMOPATHOLOGICAL LESIONS
(Fig. 60–6)

It must be remembered that nerves constitute an elastic system and that section or rupture results in marked retraction of their ends. Lesions of the brachial plexus are usually due to traction and commonly involve a large segment. Repair by direct suturing of the nerve ends is seldom possible. Let us consider the following points:

The lesion can lie anywhere between the spinal origin of the nerve root and the infraclavicular region. Within the nerve itself, the same fascicles can be ruptured at different

Table 60–4. MILLESI'S CLASSIFICATION

Site of the lesion:
    Preganglionic I
    Postganglionic II
    Supra- and retroclavicular III
    Infraclavicular (trunk) (nerves) IV

Transverse extension:
    C5-C6-C7-C8-T1 + C4-T2

Primary trunks:
    Upper = s
    Middle = im
    Lower = i

Secondary trunks:
    Anterolateral second trunk = c
    Anteromedial second trunk = m
    Posterior second trunk = d

Severity of the lesion:
    Sunderland's degrees 1 to 5

Type of the lesion:
    o = open
    r = rupture
    T = traction, first to fifth degree
    K1–K2 = external or internal compression

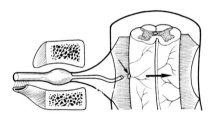

Figure 60–5. Central mechanism of brachial plexus palsy. Rupture of the root at its origin. The dural cone is intact.

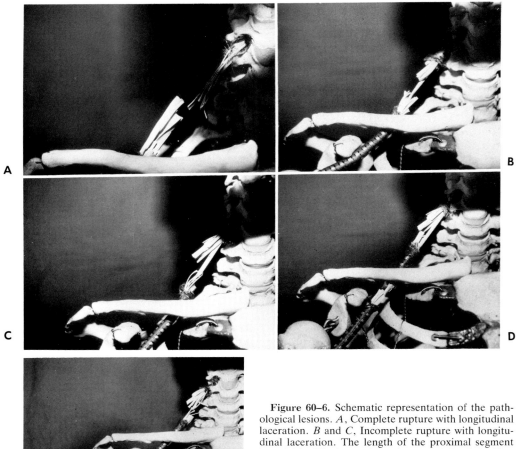

Figure 60–6. Schematic representation of the pathological lesions. *A*, Complete rupture with longitudinal laceration. *B* and *C*, Incomplete rupture with longitudinal laceration. The length of the proximal segment is variable. The longer it is, the more it lends itself to surgical repair. *D* and *E*, Lesions at different levels.

levels, some at their vertebral origin and others in the supraclavicular region, the result being multiple longitudinal lacerations. Only the fibers ruptured distally will regenerate and only some will achieve axonal continuity. Proximal lesions can cause retrograde degeneration that affects anterior horn cells or cells of the posterior ganglia, the latter being equivalent to an avulsion. This explains the failure of some repairs performed on an apparently normal root.

The rupture can be relatively distal, leaving a segment of variable length. The longer the segment, the more feasible will be surgical repair. A rupture may be incomplete, with one or more fascicles in continuity, which would help to explain the long-term partial recoveries that are sometimes seen. These

fascicles, which are often difficult to "identify," must be treated with the utmost care at the time of the surgical exploration.

The lesion can lie at several levels of the plexus, and this can be explained by the presence of two fixed points—one at the transverse process and the other at the coracoid process or at the pectoralis minor, depending on the position of the arm. Thus, one can see supraclavicular lesions associated with infraclavicular lesions at the level of the coracoid or involving the musculocutaneous nerve, which is relatively fixed as it enters the biceps, or the axillary nerve.

In our series of 420 patients operated on from 1974 to 1985, 315 lesions (75 per cent) were supraclavicular and 105 lesions (25 per cent) were infra- or retroclavicular.

Lesions at both supraclavicular and infraclavicular level must be recognized. With forced abduction of the arm the middle part of the plexus is temporarily fixed in the coracoid region. The terminal branches may then be torn with the concomitant production of supraclavicular lesions by sudden bending of the head on the opposite side. Supraclavicular lesions combined with infraclavicular lesions may affect the secondary trunks or be more distal, notably involving the musculocutaneous nerve, the axillary nerve, or the subscapular nerve, each of which has fixed segments along its anatomical course.

The frequency of these two-level lesions (15 per cent of all supraclavicular lesions) thus justifies surgical exploration of the entire plexus.

Finally, there is the root avulsion that is a special lesion. Avulsion of a root as it emerges from the spinal cord results in irreparable lesions. The simultaneous avulsion of the meningeal sheaths and the violence of the force explain the retraction, which occurs in the cervical region, through the transverse foramina. During a cervical exploration it is not uncommon to find all the nerve structures (anterior root, posterior root, and ganglia) bundled up in the interscalene or supraclavicular region.

At the level of the spinal cord, the avulsion can be confirmed by posterior laminectomy, and in the five patients operated on, we found that the root had totally disappeared without any "scarring" of the cord. It is important to stress the significance of root avulsion. The root can have retracted into the cervical region, and the avulsion is recognized at exploration through an anterior approach. It is also possible for the roots to remain in the transverse canal or at the dural orifice, giving an appearance of continuity in the cervical region.

ANATOMOPATHOLOGICAL CLASSIFICATION

The pathological lesions can be classified in order to facilitate the interpretation of results, but all the classifications used are somewhat complicated, as they include a great number of factors.

Millesi's classification* utilizes a formula that tries to express the various possibilities

---

*See Chapter 61.

(Table 60–4). Thus, I (5, 6, 7, 8, 1) 5th d° R signifies a total palsy with avulsion of all the roots at supraganglionic level.

The more clinical classification that we use (Table 60–5) always defines the lesions in terms of the roots injured and the level of injury but also states whether the paralysis is total or partial. The partial lesions associated with the longitudinal tears resulting from stretch injuries can cause very strange clinical pictures, and in cases of spontaneous recovery it is important to make a clear distinction between recovery of the entire territory supplied by a given nerve root or of only one or two muscles in that territory. Direct surgical intervention in partial lesions is hazardous.

Classification is essential for the study of results, especially after surgical repairs. The use of diagrams depicting the various lesions and the nerve repair performed is of great interest for later examinations and should be encouraged (see Fig. 60–5).

CLINICAL EXAMINATION AND ANCILLARY INVESTIGATIONS

A clinical examination complemented by paraclinical investigations aims to give an accurate diagnosis of the lesion.

INITIAL CLINICAL EXAMINATION

The initial examination constitutes an important step, as it serves to localize the damage, to indicate the nature of the lesions, and to make a prognosis concerning their likely evolution. This evaluation involves careful testing of the motor system, sensory system, and trophicity, whether the injury is recent or old.

Table 60–5. CLASSIFICATION OF BRACHIAL PLEXUS LESIONS

C5-C6	Total (complete, massive)
C5-C6-C7-C8	
C7-C8-T1	
C8-T1	*or*
	Partial (incomplete motor or sensory on X roots)
Preganglionic lesions	Roots
Postganglionic lesions	
Supra- and retroclavicular lesions	Trunks
Infraclavicular lesions	Nerves

Motor Examination

While making a careful examination of each individual muscle in turn, the surgeon must be aware of the possibility of trick movements due to contraction of other muscle groups with the same action. The results are recorded on a special form that is kept as a reference for successive examinations. The objective is to detect the roots involved in the injury and to distinguish between root palsies and trunk palsies, keeping in mind the possibility of anatomical variations and the multiradicular innervation of muscles.

The recording of each examination (including findings of amyotrophy, muscle retraction, and joint stiffness) enables the surgeon to follow the evolution of the paralysis. A synopsis of the motor and sensory findings is tabulated and represents a summary of repeated clinical and paraclinical examinations (Fig. 60–7). Muscle function is recorded by the international scoring system (0 to 5), which is useful for comparative purposes but has the disadvantage of being the same for muscles as different as the biceps and hypothenar muscles. Ideally, three more factors should be included in such records: fatigability, muscle reinnervation and "overall shoulder-elbow-hand function."

Sensory Examination

Here both subjective and objective signs must be looked for. The record of objective sensory signs will note hypoesthesia or anesthesia (and sometimes hyperesthesia) and will be transferred to a special sensory chart and expressed in terms of the spinal roots involved. Sensory testing is notoriously difficult to interpret and should be repeated frequently.

Subjective signs (symptoms) such as pain must also be faithfully recorded and can be of two types: the first takes the form of "pins and needles" or "electric shock" sensations provoked by percussion or palpation in the cervical region, the supraclavicular fossa, and the axilla. Such spontaneous symptoms exacerbated by local percussion are significant, as they indicate a distal lesion, usually a neuroma on a root of a trunk. The persistence of a localized electric shock sensation suggests a total rupture. If, however, this sensation is found at successive examinations in the cervical region and then in the supraclavicular and axillary regions (Tinel's sign) it is an indication of axonal growth. The importance of this finding has been stressed by Millesi in the context of the prognosis and indications for surgery.

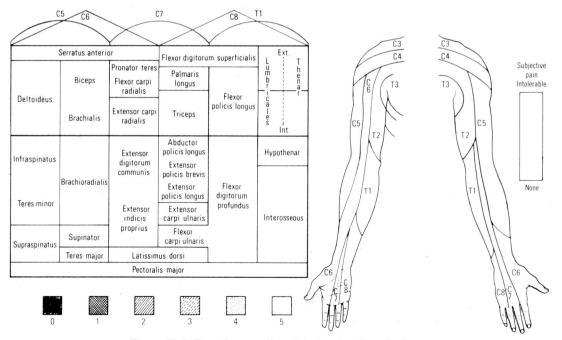

Figure 60–7. Form for recording clinical and ancillary findings.

A second type of pain, which is not localized, is quite distressing and not unlike causalgia. The pathogenesis is hard to define and the treatment is difficult. Participation of the sympathetic nervous system has been suggested. It appears that this causalgia, which is quite rare, occurs mostly after total avulsion of the lower roots of the plexus, which are rich in sympathetic fibers.

Sympathetic Disorders

Examination of the sympathetic nervous system is essential from the start. Sympathetic disorders take the form of vasomotor changes, cyanosis, soft tissue edema, and trophic changes of the skin. Radiologically, they include osteoporosis of the carpus and fingers with secondary stiffness and trophic changes (Fig. 60–8).

The presence of Horner's syndrome

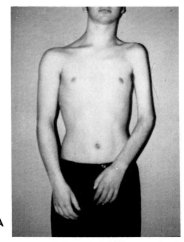

A

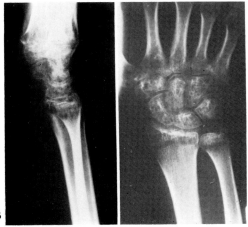

B

Figure 60–8. *A* and *B*, Complete paralysis with distal trophic changes.

(meiosis, ptosis, endophthalmos) must be noted. These signs may regress with time but never completely disappear.

Complete Neurological Examination

This examination aims at detecting signs of cord lesions that might indicate avulsion of a root. These include pyramidal signs in the lower limbs, transitory micturition problems, and blood in the cerebrospinal fluid. Combined lesions finally play a role because they reflect the severity of the initial trauma and also because they worsen the final prognosis, notably in multiple trauma cases. Vascular lesions must be sought and the restoration of continuity after rupture of the subclavian or axillary artery is desirable in all cases because it improves overall trophic status. On the basis of the complete clinical work-up one should then be able to categorize the various lesions as follows:

Supraclavicular Root Lesions. The upper roots (C5-C6-C7) are involved in 20 to 25 per cent of cases in the world literature (22 per cent in our series). Lower root lesions (C8–T1) are rare and are involved in 2 to 3 per cent of cases (3 per cent in our series). A middle root lesion (C7) is never isolated but is always seen in conjunction with an upper or lower root lesion. Total paralysis of all roots (C5-C6-C7-C8-T1) is the most common lesion and was found in 75 per cent in our series. It affects the entire musculature of the upper limb with the frequent exception of the serratus anterior. Sensory loss is variable but disorders of sympathetic origin are marked. The entire limb may be involved equally or upper or lower root involvement may predominate.

Infraclavicular Lesions with Lesions of the Trunks or Terminal Branches of the Plexus. The posterior cord syndrome involves shoulder paralysis, including the deltoid, while preserving some function of the paraspinal muscles. This can also include paralysis of the radial and axillary nerves with occasional involvement of the latissimus dorsi and teres major. The paralysis can be limited to terminal branches, especially the suprascapular and axillary nerves, as well as the musculocutaneous nerve.

One can also observe lesions involving both the suprascapular and the axillary nerves. Lesions of the middle and lateral cords are less common. They can be seen with a fracture of the humerus combined with radial nerve paralysis, which may confuse the picture.

PROGNOSTIC CLINICAL SIGNS

One of the most important aspects of any brachial plexus palsy is the prognosis and the future for the patient. It is obviously difficult to make an accurate forecast in the early stages, but we shall consider the factors that will be taken into account when attempting to formulate a prognosis.

Some clinical features can be regarded as favorable, others as unfavorable. Thus, a patient with a brachial plexus palsy secondary to a dislocation of the shoulder has a 90 per cent chance of recovering completely, which means that the patient can usually be reassured about the prognosis. Similarly, an incomplete paralysis, e.g., one muscle with a score of 1 or 2 in each territory, can be regarded as a good sign.

The following factors, by contrast, are unfavorable:

1. A history of violent trauma involving the plexus as well as the upper limb (Fig. 60–9). In 100 cases we observed 58 long bone lesions and 22 arterial injuries.

2. Involvement of the serratus anterior and the presence of Horner's syndrome, both of which indicate a proximal lesion.

3. The presence of pain and signs suggesting injury to the cord.

ANCILLARY INVESTIGATIONS

Myelography

Our initial experience was based upon metrizamide (Amipaque) myelography only. We

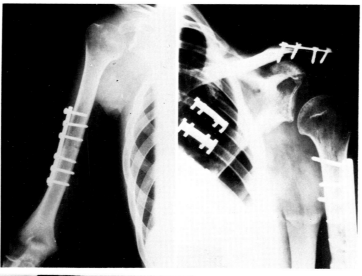

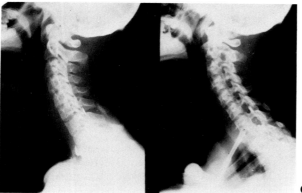

Figure 60–9. *A,* "Medium" trauma. Note the paralyzed shoulder. *B* and *C,* Severe trauma. Crush fracture of the scapula.

defined various radiological abnormalities by comparing radiological appearances with preoperative findings in the cervical region. Study involved the appearance of the meningeal sheaths and that of the roots. In normal myelographs a thin line is clearly seen dividing the root space into two, with juxtaposition of the anterior and posterior rootlets (Fig. 60–10). Radiological lesions can thus be classified and the following appearances are found (Fig. 60–11):

1. Pseudomeningocele, with rupture of the dura mater sheaths, whether large (M) or small (m), corresponds in the majority of cases to root avulsion or to a very proximal lesion at the entrance of the transverse canal, i.e., an irreversible lesion for which surgical repair is impossible. Nerve continuity after tearing off of the dura mater cone seems to be rare, and in any event serious stretch lesions affecting the rootlets is present. Subsequent clinical recovery does not occur in the majority of cases. Exploration by posterior laminectomy has been suggested by certain authors if justified by the clinical situation.

2. Extensive lacunar (L) and filling-defect (d) appearances have the same significance and often coincide with a pseudomeningocele or an adjacent root. In these cases of extended lacunae, laminectomy confirms root avulsion and the presence of adhesions between the cord and the dura mater.

3. Root lesions may occur without obvious sheath involvement (as described above). The two meningeal lips surrounding the root are nevertheless modified. They lose their parallelism and show a tendency to come together ("sulky lips," B). The root itself is the site of diverse lesions, e.g., simple Lipiodol "ball" appearance (G), stretching of a root with disappearance of the central gap (E), or opaque or absent root (O). These abnormalities are suggestive of a root lesion but offer no indication as to its possible severity. In general, partial stretch lesions are present, which can be treated by neurolysis if continuity exists. However, in a certain number of cases there is complete rupture caused by longitudinal splitting. The proximal surgical section passes through a fibrous root containing only 25 to 50 per cent of its potential nerve fibers. It is then difficult to assess the value of the axon capital and subsequent regrowth.

Myelography Combined with Computed Tomography

Since 1980, myelography has been combined with computed tomography (CT). This has led to refinement of our findings.

Large or small meningoceles are more easily seen. Most importantly, it is possible to identify the site of large meningoceles (anterior and especially posterior), which explains why these lesions are rarely found during exploration via a cervical approach. No rootlets are visible in the majority of cases. In some rare cases the visible rootlets are interrupted before penetrating the transverse canal, and lesions may be found at different sites on the anterior and posterior rootlets. Very large meningoceles spreading over two levels can be recognized, thereby avoiding errors of interpretation. Deviation of the cord by localized hematoma due to tearing of the roots can also be better analyzed. Extensive lacunae with adhesions correspond to avulsions after over several levels.

In opaque roots the CT scan often reveals a small meningocele not visible on myelography, which allows better evaluation of the severity of the lesion. Other root abnormalities are also better visualized in association with anterior or posterior rootlet lesions.

Myelography combined with a CT scan gives the most precise information possible of anatomopathological lesions. It forms part of the preoperative assessment, while emphasizing that the appearance of the sheaths and roots must not be interpreted in isolation.

Combined examinations are common. Radiological findings may not be accompanied by typical clinical findings because of anatomical variations. Myelography combined with a CT scan, viewed level by level, will eventually provide essential data via two different approaches:

1. An abnormal appearance indicates a root lesion. Its severity must be assessed according to the features mentioned above. Pseudomeningoceles generally indicate root avulsion and in the majority of cases are located at C7-C8-T1. The CT scan is used to evaluate the state of the rootlets, not only at the level of the meningocele but also at adjacent levels. Rootlets superior to an avulsed root are rarely intact.

2. A normal radiological appearance of the sheaths and roots in the presence of total

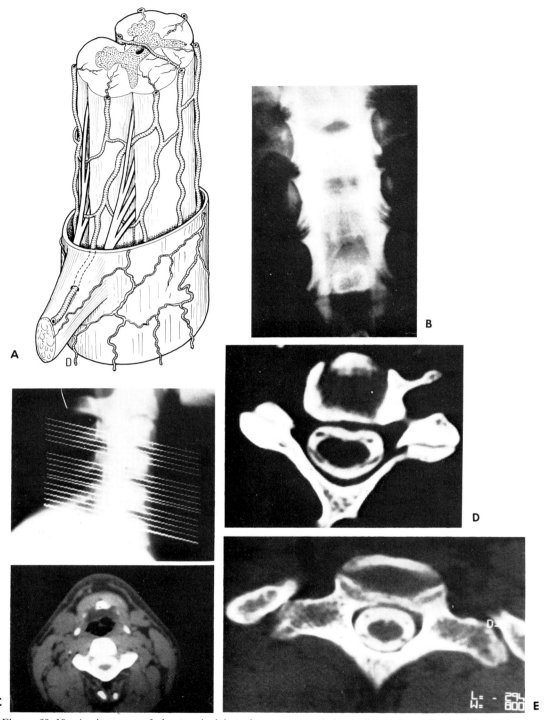

Figure 60–10. *A*, Anatomy of the terminal branches, roots, and dural sheath (from R. Louis). *B*, Normal myelogram. *C*, *D*, and *E*, Scan after injection of Amipaque; normal appearance of the terminal branches.

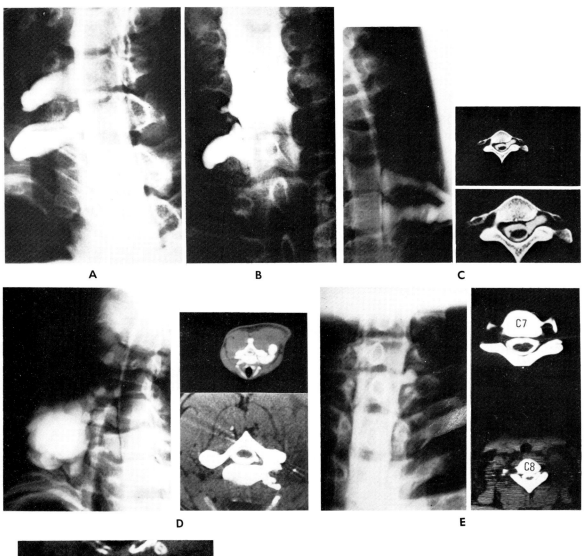

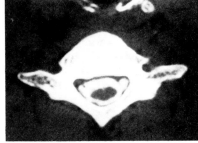

Figure 60–11. *A*, Large meningoceles on C7 and C8. *B*, Meningocele on T1. Opaque root with small meningocele on C8. Opaque root on C7. *C*, Meningoceles shown on the scan with nonvisualization of the terminal branches. *D*, Large posterior meningocele. *E*, Meningocele on C8. Opaque root on the myelogram on C7 and nonvisualization of the terminal branches on the scan. *F*, Small meningocele on the scan with opaque root on the myelogram.

paralysis suggests the possibility of either spontaneous recovery or the discovery of a more distal lesion accessible to direct repair in the cervical region. A normal appearance on myelography alone may correspond to a complete irreversible lesion. In a certain number of cases the CT scan then offers the possibility of confirming this eventuality based on either an equivalent of avulsion by lesions in the transverse canal or rootlet ruptures without any lesion of the connective tissue coverings.

Combined clinical and radiological evaluation gives accurate anatomopathological data essential for preoperative assessment.

Electromyography

The electromyogram forms part of the assessment. Two successive electromyographic examinations should indicate the presence or absence of subclinical reinnervation, reflecting the existence of first-degree lesions. Above all, electromyography is of interest in superior root paralysis.

Study of evoked sensory potentials is felt by certain authors to be of value in assessment based on comparison of the results with radiological and clinical findings.

Psychological Problems

The psychological problems raised by these patients must also be dealt with, attempting to cope with their justifiable anxiety. Is recovery possible? What are you planning to do now? When is operation possible, if necessary? What result can be hoped for?

INITIAL MANAGEMENT

Associated vascular lesions must be repaired immediately. In the absence of vascular lesions, treatment will consist of the prevention of trophic changes and joint stiffness. All traction on the roots must be avoided. The limb is immobilized with a minimum of bracing with the arm in abduction and forward flexion. Active mobilization is started as soon as possible, as is passive mobilization to prevent joint stiffness.

The palsy is assessed by repeated motor and sensory examinations and by progression of Tinel's sign. On the thirtieth day the examination is completed by an electromyogram and in certain cases by a myelogram.

SURGICAL MANAGEMENT

INDICATIONS

The surgical indications depend on how the clinical course evolves. In a certain number of patients (2 of 3) spontaneous recovery occurs in the first month; in other cases the indications for surgery can be decided in light of all the factors discussed above.

Our series of 420 patients operated on between 1974 and 1985 were explored by a cervicoaxillary approach. They were preferably explored early if there was no clinical or electrical recovery at one or several radicular levels.

The delay depends on when the patient was first seen. In our first 100 patients, the exploration was often between the sixth and eighth months, but the tendency now is between the first and second months.

The prognosis depends on the anatomy and type of the lesion and in all cases is dominated by the degree of involvement of the hand. The therapeutic indications also depend on our knowledge of the anatomical lesions which for the first 100 cases are shown in Tables 60–6 and 60–7.

Table 60–6. TRAUMATIC PARALYSES OF THE BRACHIAL PLEXUS: 100 SURGICAL CASES (75 PER CENT TOTAL PARALYSES)

Avulsions or very proximal ruptures: no repair
  C5 2
  C6 8
  C7 7
More distal rupture at emergence from the transverse foramen with extensive lacerations: no repair possible
  C5 1
  C6 1
  C7 1
Rupture with longitudinal lacerations (nerve graft)
  C5 9
  C6 3
  C7 1
  Lateral cord 1
Extensive longitudinal lacerations (neurolyses)
  C5 7
  C6 8
  C7 8
  Lateral cord 1
Anatomic continuity but no response to electric stimulation
  C5 2
  C6 1
  C7 5
Normal appearance—electric stimulation +
  C5 2
  C6 2
  C7 3

Table 60–7. TRAUMATIC PARALYSES OF THE BRACHIAL PLEXUS: 100 SURGICAL CASES (75 PER CENT TOTAL PARALYSES)

Avulsions or very proximal ruptures: no repair
    C5 13
    C7 47
    C6 35
    C8 39
    T1 37
More distal rupture at emergence from the transverse foramen with extensive lacerations: no repair possible
    C5   3
    C6   7
    C7 12
    C8 16
    T1 15
Rupture with longitudinal laceration outside the transverse foramen: grafts to one or more roots possible but assessment of axon capital essential
    C5 43
    C6 16
    C7   4
    C8   4
    T1   3
    Lateral cord   5
Longitudinal elongation with lesions in continuity; neurolyses; assessment of lesion
    C5   6
    C6   6
    C7   5
    C8   4
    T1   6
Anatomic continuity but no response to electric stimulation
    C5   4
    C6   5
    C7   6
    C8 10
    T1 11
Normal appearance—electric stimulation +
    C5   1
    C6   1
    C7   1
    C8   2
    T1   3

In Total Sensory-Motor Paralysis

The decision to operate must be made during the first month (Fig. 60–12). Some patients have a spontaneous recovery after a short delay, but when this does not occur it is not necessary to wait seven or eight months. Several aspects of the clinical course and complementary studies can be described.

1. *Total paralysis without recovery in the first month with avulsions of the lower roots.* Myelography shows myelomeningoceles at C8 and T1, and often on C7; C6 may have an abnormal aspect, and C5 is usually normal. In these total paralyses with avulsions of the lower roots (C7, C8, T1) when there is only one or two remaining normal roots, it

is not possible to graft all the plexus. Our approach now is to look for and obtain reinnervation of the proximal territories.

a. When only one root is to be grafted our choice will be to repair the subscapular nerve and the lateral cord or the anterior division of the upper trunk. The goal is to obtain stabilization of the shoulder, an active pectoralis major to adduct the arm, flexion of the elbow, and some palmar sensibility. The patients must be informed that they will have a complete paralysis of the hand.

b. When there are two roots to be grafted it is possible to also graft some parts of the posterior cord for the radial nerve or axillary nerve function. One must not try to graft everything, and if the roots are small, it is better to place the grafts to the lateral cord and suprascapular nerve.

2. *Total paralysis without recovery in the first month with avulsions of all roots.* With meningoceles on all the roots. At surgery one would find total avulsions of C5 to T1. In these cases neurotizations are indicated using intercostal nerves, the spinal accessory nerve, or superficial cervical plexus. The goal is to have less arm atrophy and elbow flexion by neurotization of the musculocutaneous nerve. The indication for amputation is for us exceptional, and amputation must not be done for pain.

3. *Paralysis which is initially total with spontaneous recovery in the first month.* It is possible to observe a favorable evolution.

a. From proximal to distal. In some cases this evolution can give a more or less complete recovery starting from the shoulder, followed by the elbow and then the hand. In total paralysis after shoulder dislocations this favorable result is frequent (80 to 90 per cent). In other cases the improvement is from proximal to distal, but some facts must be kept in mind: Tinel's sign that does not progress may correspond to a distal rupture or more rarely to fibrosis. Some muscles can be saved in some specific radicular territories and these are usually traction injuries, which may be improved by a neurolysis. The surgical indication will be to explore these cases and perform a neurolysis or repair.

b. Recovery from distal to proximal. In some total paralysis, recovery is rapid at C8 and T1, less at C7, and not at all in C5 and C6. The exploration must be done early because it is a reparable extrascalenic lesion of the proximal roots or upper trunk in most cases.

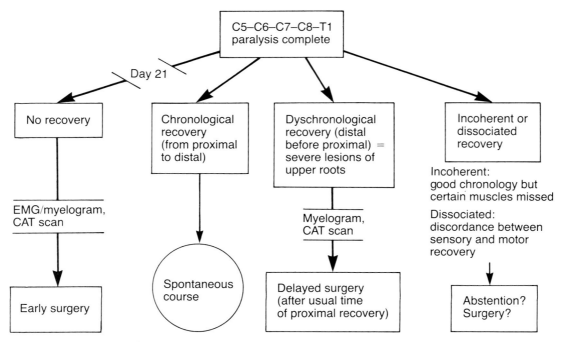

Figure 60–12. Management of supraclavicular total paralyses.

In Paralysis of C5, C6, +/− C7
(Fig. 60–13)

The prognosis is dominated by the fact that the hand is normal or only partially involved but useful. Surgery must be done early because the lesions are often in the scalenic region on the roots or upper trunk, with a good possibility of nerve repair or graft with a satisfactory functional result. The possibility of reconstructive surgery must not prevent the surgeon from performing early nerve repair because the results of direct reinnervation of the muscles are always better than tendon transfers.

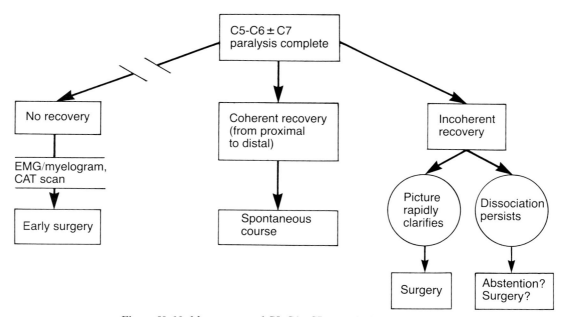

Figure 60–13. Management of C5–C6±C7 supraclavicular paralyses.

In Paralysis of the Lower Roots C7, C8, and T1

The decision for surgery depends on the clinical examination and ancillary studies. Prognosis is dominated by involvement of the hand. If myelography shows the existence of pseudomeningoceles and root avulsion of the lower roots, surgery is not justified. On the contrary, if myelography is normal in the absence of spontaneous recovery, surgery is indicated to explore the lesions and perform necessary nerve repairs. However, it is necessary to keep in mind that even if it is possible to repair, with nerve grafts, lesions of C8 and T1, the distance between the nerve lesion and the hand is such that it is not possible to hope to reinnervate the intrinsic muscles of the hand in adults.

In Infraclavicular Paralysis

Lesions at the level of the shoulder girdle are frequently associated with infraclavicular paralysis. Myelography is normal, and electrical studies are often difficult to interpret. Our tendency now is to operate early. These patients can be divided into two groups:

1. The lesions are distal to the level of the terminal branches of the plexus, such as the suprascapular nerve, axillary nerve, or musculocutaneous nerve, with frequent combined lesions. Clinically, a sensory and motor paralysis implies a complete rupture, and it is necessary to operate before the third month.

2. Lesions at the level of the cords behind and below the clavicle are often associated with muscular lesions. In these cases the diagnosis is most difficult. Fractures of the clavicle or vascular lesions without distal ischemia are surgical indications in the early weeks.

In Old Paralysis

Only pain syndromes are indications for neurolysis. In the current state of surgery of the brachial plexus with early exploration, intolerable painful syndromes are now rare.

THE OPERATIVE EXPOSURE

We use a long zigzag cervicoaxillary incision. The patient is placed on his back with a small cushion under his shoulder and the head turned to the opposite side (Fig. 60–14). The table is placed in the foot-down position in order to achieve orthostatic hypotension. Some surgeons, such as Narakas, operate with the patient sitting up. The upper limb must be included in the surgical field in case traction or pulsion on the scapular region is required. The two lower limbs are prepared for the eventual taking of sural nerve grafts. The surgeon should have at his disposal a bipolar microcoagulator, an adjustable nerve stimulator, and an operating microscope or magnifying loupes.

The incision runs along the posterior border of the sternomastoid and the inferior border of the clavicle toward the coracoid process, ending in the deltopectoral groove. Infiltration of the superficial planes with vasopressin reduces bleeding to a minimum. The flaps are dissected and reflected to expose the operative field, and the exploration proceeds from the cervical to the axillary region. The omohyoid is then identified. Access to the axillary region is made easier by dividing the clavicular head of the pectoralis major to expose the underlying pectoralis minor. The clavipectoroaxillary fascia is resected.

Next the neurovascular structures are iden-

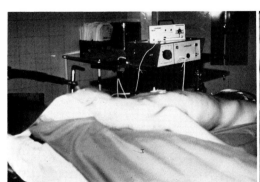
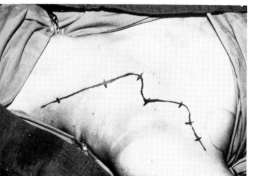

A **B**

Figure 60–14. *A*, Positioning of the patient. *B*, Cervico-axillary approach.

tified and retracted with tapes. Dissection of the nerves can prove extremely difficult in the event of extensive fibrosis. This finding is particularly marked when there has been additional trauma (e.g., scapulothoracic injury, fractured clavicle).

The axillary artery is carefully dissected and the axillary nerve is identified, if necessary with the help of the stimulator. If the dissection is hazardous and the large vessels and pleural dome are at risk, osteotomy of the clavicle may be indicated. Identification of the nerves may be made easier by passing a tape under the clavicle and applying traction or pulsion to the limb.

The exploration extends from the transverse foraminal canal to the axilla and even the upper arm. It will reveal one or more of the following lesions: (1) avulsion of the roots; (2) rupture of a root or primary trunk; (3) partial lesions with persistence of one or two fascicles, which may or may not respond to stimulation; (4) two-tier lesions with ruptures in the supraclavicular region and in the musculocutaneous or the circumflex nerve; and (5) apparent continuity in theoretically avulsed roots (meningocele on myelography) with no response to electrical stimulation. In such cases, one must keep in mind the possibility of a central rupture, which can be confirmed only by posterior laminectomy.

We carried out a posterior laminectomy in five of our early cases, but we now believe that this is no longer indicated, as the combined clinical examination and myelogram should provide enough information about the lesions. The only indication for a posterior laminectomy would be to confirm avulsion of a root in the presence of a normal myelogram and an exploration showing nerve continuity up to the transverse canal. However, it should be possible to come to the right conclusion without the risk of a laminectomy.

Once the damage has been evaluated, the next step is the definitive nerve repair. Osteotomy of the clavicle is necessary only if the dissection is particularly difficult or if one wishes to have access to the C8 and T1 roots when these have been ruptured in the retroclavicular region. At the end of the operation the clavicle is repaired by a plate fixed with screws.

Once the nerve repair is completed, the pectoralis major is reattached and the deltopectoral groove is closed by suturing. The arm is immobilized in a Dujarier dressing and held abducted over a cushion for two weeks, at which point physiotherapy can start.

NERVE REPAIR

This stage is carried out in systematic, stepwise fashion.

Neurolysis

The first step consists of an exoneurolysis, with or without an endoneurolysis. Partial lesions must be treated with the utmost care. It is important to realize that the identification of intact fascicles is extremely arduous and can aggravate existing lesions. Endoneurolysis carries the major risk of interfering with the blood supply.

In 23 of our first 100 cases we performed a neurolysis without grafting or suturing. In two cases of late neurolysis, we noted postoperative deterioration, one of which was followed by recovery after 6 months. We found that late neurolyses were justified only in the presence of persistent pain, as these procedures never resulted in motor or sensory recovery. In all the other 21 cases of "early" neurolysis, some degree of pain relief was obtained, and in five of these we noted some motor and sensory improvement as well. We consider that neurolysis can facilitate recovery in a territory that is already showing signs of recovery.

Nerve Grafting or Repair

Neurolysis is followed by resection of neuromas. The type of repair, whether by direct suturing or grafting, will depend on the extent of tissue loss. Direct suturing is possible in some rare cases, such as avulsion of the C7-C8-T1 roots, when the entire plexus can be lifted to the upper primary trunk or when the C5-C6 roots have been ruptured in the supraclavicular region. Direct suturing is then preferable to a long graft with two "anastomoses"; we were able to do this on two occasions. In the majority of cases, however, a graft will be required to bridge the gap (Fig. 60–15).

There are two important considerations.

1. Appreciation of the proximal nerve stump (Fig. 60–16). Here we must stress the difference between extrascalenic lesions, in which the proximal end is rich in axons, and

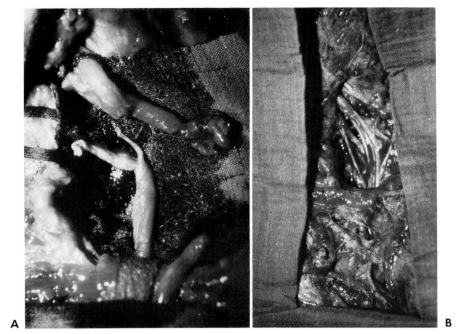

Figure 60–15. *A*, Avulsion of C7 to T1 and rupture of C5 and C6 in the scalene region. *B*, Graft repair of C5 and C6.

intrascalenic lesions, in which the proximal end is flabby and unhealthy looking. In the latter case, regeneration will be hampered by three factors—longitudinal laceration, retrograde degeneration, and fibrosis. This no doubt explains some of our poor results.

2. The length of the graft. This depends on the extent of the lesions and usually varies between 5 and 15 cm. Therefore, a graft sutured in the position of maximal length (i.e., head turned to the other side and slightly extended) should be safe from traction during later movements of the head and neck.

The grafts are taken from the sural nerves and the medial cutaneous nerve of the fore-

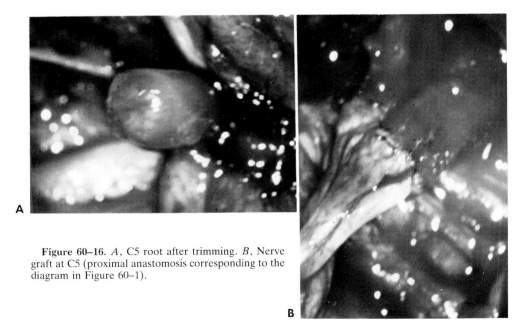

Figure 60–16. *A*, C5 root after trimming. *B*, Nerve graft at C5 (proximal anastomosis corresponding to the diagram in Figure 60–1).

arm. The ulnar nerve can be considered when there has been an avulsion of C7-C8-T1. The graft can be vascularized either by conserving a pedicle or by using it as a free graft and anastomosing the accompanying ulnar artery to the transverse cervical artery.

Postoperative immobilization of the cervical region is not essential if these conditions are satisfied. Again, the upper limb is immobilized in a Dujarier dressing for two weeks.

SPECIFIC PATTERNS OF PLEXUS INJURY
(Figs. 60–17 and 60–18)

On some rare occasions (one of our 61 cases) all the roots are interrupted in the scalene region and it is possible to bridge graft the entire plexus. More commonly, some roots or trunks are interrupted in the supraclavicular region while others show partial or total avulsion. A choice must then be made, as one cannot repair the entire plexus with only one, two, or three roots.

Structures that must be repaired as a priority include the anterolateral secondary trunk, the posterior secondary trunk, and the upper scapular nerve. In our experience, with only one root it is better to bridge the anterolateral secondary trunk plus one posterior element, which can be the upper scapular nerve, the circumflex nerve, or, if the root is large, the posterior secondary trunk. This repair can be complemented by a neurotization using the intercostal nerves.

When the C5-C6 roots have ruptured and C7-C8-T1 have been avulsed, the C5-C6 roots can be repaired using a vascularized ulnar nerve graft. The aim should be to reinnervate the proximal muscles. When the C7-C8-T1 roots are ruptured, their repair is pointless, as the chance for recovery in the intrinsic muscles is virtually nil.

When there is avulsion of all the nerve roots, neurotization through the intercostal nerves can be considered.

A musculocutaneous nerve contains 7900 fibers and the terminal biceps has 2000 fibers, whereas an intercostal nerve contains only 550. Thirty per cent of fibers are necessary to restore some muscle function, but this is the minimum number. About three to four intercostal nerves are therefore needed to repair a musculocutaneous nerve, and even more for an anterolateral secondary nerve trunk. The incision can be a continuation of the initial deltopectoral incision, or another horizontal incision can be made on the mid-axillary line between the insertions of the pectoralis major and latissimus dorsi.

The intercostal nerve lies along the lower

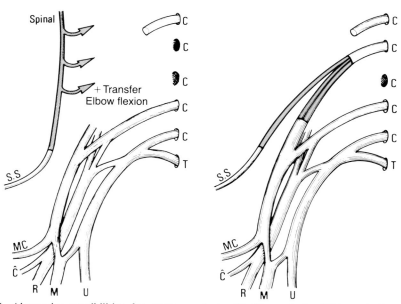

Figure 60–17. Alternative possibilities for nerve repair in C5–C6 paralysis. With a single usable root, the suprascapular nerve and the anterior part of the superior trunk are grafted. If C5 and C6 are avulsed (C7, C8, and T1 intact), direct neurotization of the terminal part of the spinal accessory nerve on the musculocutaneous nerve plus muscle transfer of pectoralis minor or triceps can be done to restore flexion of the elbow.

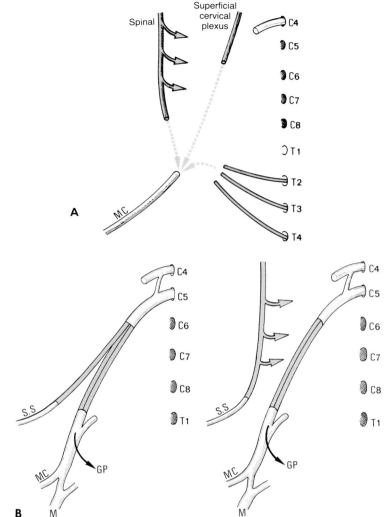

Figure 60–18. Possibilities for nerve repair with total supraclavicular paralysis. *A*, Neurotization in total paralysis with avulsion of all the roots. *B*, Nerve repair with only one usable root, all the others being avulsed. If the root is small, the suprascapular nerve can be neurotized directly by the terminal part of the spinal accessory nerve. Nerve grafts will then be placed on the anterior part of the superior trunk or only on the musculocutaneous nerves.

Illustration continued on following page

border of the rib. It is divided as posteriorly as possible so as to obtain the maximum number of motor fibers. Damage to the pleura with pneumothorax is a theoretical risk, but this did not occur in our series.

Bridging is achieved by an intermediate graft, at least for the fourth, fifth, and sixth intercostal nerves. In a few cases direct suturing is feasible if it has been possible to dissect the musculocutaneous nerve high enough and to take it across to the second and third intercostal nerves.

In our first 100 cases we have performed eight neurotizations of the intercostals, and in five cases we bridged the musculocutaneous on the anterolateral secondary trunk. In one case the median nerve was neurotized, as the musculocutaneous nerve showed irreversible distal lesions. In two cases we per-

formed a bridging of the ulnar nerve or the anterolateral secondary trunk in addition to a graft for the upper roots. The spinal accessory nerve can also be used, provided half its fibers are left to supply the trapezius. In our series this was done twice in two cases of isolated C5 ruptures. Finally, neurotization from the superficial cervical plexus (Brunelli, 1984) is another possible technique.

ASSESSMENT OF RESULTS

Our series includes 420 patients operated on between 1974 and 1985 (315 with supraclavicular lesions and 105 with infraclavicular and retroclavicular lesions). At least two years must elapse before the results can be properly analyzed. This analysis must be crit-

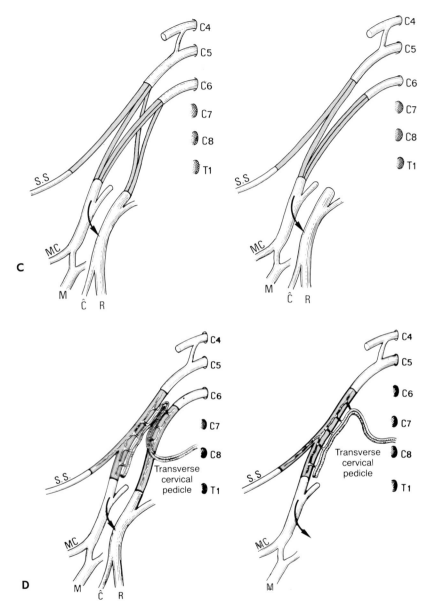

Figure 60–18 *Continued. C*, Nerve repair with two usable roots. If the two roots are small, the nerve grafts are placed on the suprascapular nerve and on the anterior part of the superior trunk. *D*, Utilization of a vascularized ulnar nerve after avulsion of C7, C8, and T1 in cases in which the appearance of the cut nerve is good and when the size of the root corresponds to the size of the ulnar nerve.

ical, and recovery can be attributed to the surgical repair only if there is no other possible way in which it could have occurred.

In cases of avulsion of C7-C8 and T1, if C5 or C5 and C6 are graftable, the problem is simple. Interpretation is more delicate, however, in cases of paralysis with spontaneous recovery of roots or trunks due to second- or third-degree traction lesions or to lacerations sparing some of the fibers. In addition, most muscles receive their nerve supply from more than one root, and anatomical variations are numerous.

Some patients with a C7 avulsion confirmed by myelography and surgical exploration have shown complete recovery in the muscles theoretically innervated by C7, i.e., the triceps and the extensors of the wrist and fingers. This is a typical example of clinical error in which recovery of the C7 root is claimed when in fact the muscles were supplied by C8 and T1. This apparently paradoxical result was explained when the clinical, myelographic, and electromyographic findings were supplemented by surgical exploration with *nerve stimulation*.

Reinnervation after grafting is always a long process. For example, from the motor system point of view, the classic delays of 8 months for the shoulder can be increased to 12 to 15 months if one thinks in terms of useful function.

Some patients recover partial function, which is difficult to quantify. Thus, some patients who had no active movement of the shoulder eventually succeed in actively reducing their previously paralyzed subluxed humeral head. As mentioned earlier, the international 0 to 5 scoring system does not take into account two useful parameters in evaluation of results: the fatigability of the reinnervated muscles and the overall shoulder-elbow-hand function.

Sensory results are also difficult to evaluate, but a successful nerve graft restores a far from negligible protective sensibility as well as an improved trophic state.

SUMMARY OF SURGICAL MANAGEMENT AND RESULTS

Based on the present state of knowledge, the indications for surgery in traumatic brachial plexus palsies can be listed as follows:

1. In total (C5-T1) palsies with avulsion of all the roots, the primary consideration is the patient's future. It is our contention that amputation is very seldom indicated and should not be undertaken because of pain. Functional braces are rarely utilized, and cosmetic prostheses for social use are always less satisfactory than the paralyzed arm.

Neurotization by the intercostal nerves improves the trophicity of the limb and can restore some elbow flexion. However, one should not expect too much of an intercostal neurotization. The patient must learn to live with his paralyzed limb and, if necessary, be redirected toward another occupation.

2. In paralyses of C5-T1 with irreversible lesions of the lower roots, the major problem is the hand lesion. Grafting of the C5-C6-C7 roots can produce reinnervation in the proximal muscles (shoulder and elbow), whereas reinnervation of the long muscles of the hand can be expected in a few cases.

In total C5-C6-C7-C8-T1 paralyses with avulsion of all roots, the problem is to envisage the future with the patient. We feel that amputation is rarely indicated (two cases out of 100: one by crushing of the forearm and one secondarily for personal convenience) and should under no circumstances be considered because of pain.

The functional system is generally unused and aesthetic prostheses for social purposes are always inferior to the paralyzed arm. Neurotization may improve the trophic status of the upper limb and may restore a degree of elbow flexion. No more should be expected of neurotization, and the patient must learn to live with a paralyzed upper limb and be guided in terms of occupational orientation (Fig. 60–19).

In C5-C6-C7-C8-T1 paralyses with irreversible lesions of lower roots, the problem is dominated by involvement of the hand. Repair by nerve graft from the C5-C6 and sometimes C7 roots results in reinnervation of the proximal muscles (shoulder, elbow), and reinnervation of the long muscles of the hand occurs in some cases. The result must be studied in relation to the nerve repair and the therapeutic approach that is to be adopted.

1. When only one root can be used and grafts have been applied to the subscapular nerve and the lateral cord, proximal to the loop of the pectorals, the useful result which can be expected from the repair procedure combines the following.

Active reduction of the paralyzed shoulder but with little or no mobility, particularly in

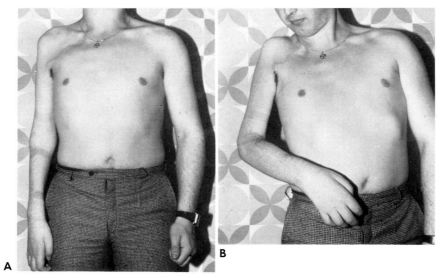

Figure 60–19. Result of neurotization of the intercostal on the musculocutaneous.

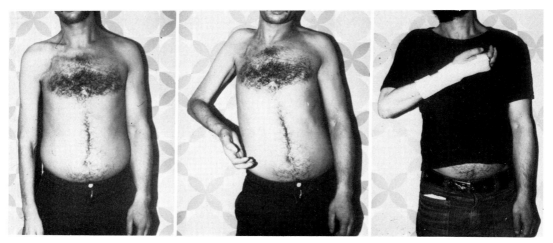

Figure 60–20 *See legend on opposite page*

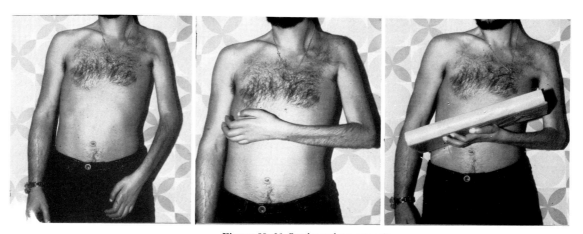

Figure 60–21 *See legend on opposite page*

abduction–external rotation. Stabilization of the shoulder by recovery of the supra- and sometimes infraspinatus muscles, then scored 2, is nevertheless very useful and improves function of the elbow.

A pectoralis major, scored at 3 or 4, is very useful for holding an object against the chest.

Flexion of the elbow, active against gravity and often against resistance, then scored at 4.

A degree of sensation on the palmar surface of the hand.

2. If, in addition to the above, it has been possible to use two roots to bridge part of the posterior cord or place more grafts on the lateral cord, it is reasonable to hope for a degree of extension of the elbow and relative flexion of the wrist and sometimes the digits. The patient must be warned that the hand will remain paralyzed.

In relation to the nerve repair performed, results will be described as useful if recovery is good in all grafted areas. In other cases results will be classified as partial or failure.

In our 107 cases with a follow-up of more than three years (Fig. 60–13) we have had 74 useful recoveries.

a. In these 74 useful recoveries, the result was related to the number of usable roots (Figs. 60–20, 60–21, 60–22).

There was always recovery of elbow flexion

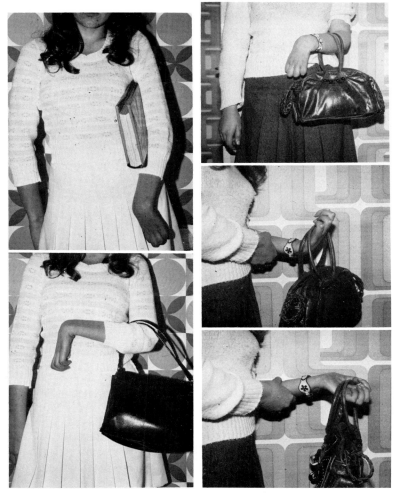

Figures 60–20, 60–21, 60–22. Examples of results after nerve grafts (only C5 and C6 can be grafted; C7–C8 and T1 are avulsed).

and pectoralis major and sensation of the anterior surface of the forearm.

At the shoulder, patients noted stabilization improving elbow function and in six cases reinnervation enabled active abduction to 20 to 30 degrees, but without external rotation.

At the wrist and hand, in the 54 useful recoveries after bridging of two, three, or five roots, 20 patients also recovered wrist flexor muscles.

b. Twenty recoveries were partial, with differences between grafted areas, and there were 11 failures. These 11 failures were related to grafts applied to a fibrous root with midregeneration potential as determined by pathological study of specimens taken from the root resection site and this raises the problem of perioperative assessment of the proximal end of the root.

In paralyses affecting the upper roots, nerve surgery provides the best results (Table 60–8). The frequency of involvement of upper trunk or of the C5-C6 roots in the interscalene region enables repair with maximum success. Reinnervation involves the proximal muscles of the shoulder and elbow, and results obtained at the shoulder are better than those obtained by all possible palliative operations (muscle transfer, shoulder arthrodesis).

Apart from six neurotizations which gave moderate results and 10 neurolyses which resulted in eight improvements, the problem is in fact centered upon grafts from roots or trunks.

We have 52 lesions with a follow-up of more than three years. Results are shown in Table 60–8.

Table 60–8. RESULTS AFTER REPAIR BY GRAFT IN 52 SUPRACLAVICULAR C5-C6-C7 PARTIAL PARALYSES (FOLLOW-UP ≥ THREE YEARS)

Graft	Total Number of Cases	Results
1 root graft	20	1 failure
		4 partial results
		15 useful results
6 cases with C7-C8-T1 intact		
6 cases with C8-T1 intact		
2 root grafts or upper trunk	25	5 partial results
		19 useful results
		1 lost from sight
10 cases with C7-C8-T1 intact		
3 root grafts	7	7 useful results
C8-T1 intact		

Table 60–9. RESULTS AFTER REPAIR BY GRAFT IN LESIONS OF THE TERMINAL BRANCHES OF THE PLEXUS: FOLLOW-UP ≥ ONE YEAR

Lesion	Results
6 isolated lesions of the musculocutaneous nerve	6 good results
22 isolated lesions of the axillary nerve	
3 lesions irreparable by equivalent of muscular avulsion	
1 secondary suture	1 good result
18 nerve grafts	16 good results
	2 moderate results
5 lesions axillary nerve + subscapular nerve	5 moderate results
4 axillary nerve lesions + musculocutaneous nerve	4 good results

Nerve lesions were generally relatively close to effectors, explaining the high proportion of useful results (Fig. 60–23).

In paralyses by infraclavicular lesions (Table 60–9), we have experience with 105 infra- or retroclavicular lesions, explored surgically (neurolysis, nerve graft) among 420 plexus paralyses treated by operation.

From a clinical standpoint, pure syndromes arise from problems and surgery is indicated after three to four months, with the obvious exception of lesions secondary to section by side arm or bullet injuries, which can be operated upon sooner.

Atypical pictures with multiple lesion combination raise the most difficult problems. Sixty per cent of cases recover spontaneously within varying periods of time, which depend upon the distance between nerve lesions and effectors. In the absence of recovery, these relatively distal lesions must be operated upon since they are accessible to nerve surgery (neurolysis or graft) with much better results than in supraclavicular lesions.

We have the following in our statistics:

a. Six isolated lesions of the musculocutaneous (six sutures or grafts) with six good results (elbow flexors at 3 + 4).

b. Sixty-eight infra- or retroclavicular lesions involving secondary trunks: 51 lesions of the posterior cord, treated by neurolysis or by graft—lesion combinations (median nerve, musculocutaneous nerve) were present in 30 per cent of cases; 11 lesions of the lateral cord; 6 lesions of the medial cord.

Follow-up after these operations is too short in the majority of cases, and it is impossible at present to offer any valid sta-

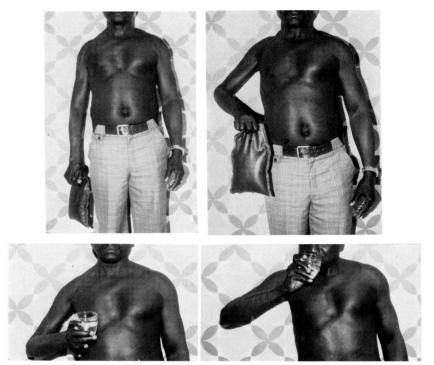

Figure 60–23. Results after graft when C5 and C6 can be grafted and C7, C8, and T1 are intact.

tistics concerning results which, in any case, are very difficult to codify because of lesion combinations and therapeutic combinations (neurolysis or graft in the same patient).

c. Thirty-one lesions of the axillary nerve, isolated (22 cases) or combined with a lesion of the subscapular nerve (five cases) and of the musculocutaneous nerve (four cases). Overall results in these 31 cases were in general favorable (Table 60–9).

In the context of these distal infraclavicular lesions, the distinction must be drawn between the following:

1. Nerve lesions relatively close to their effectors: subscapular nerve, axillary nerve, musculocutaneous nerve, and radial nerve (borderline). Nerve repair by graft is followed by satisfactory recovery in 70 to 80 per cent of cases. However, there are certain difficulties associated with repair, notably of the subscapular nerve, the distal end of which is difficult to find, or the axillary nerve when there is an equivalent of avulsion at muscular level.

2. Nerve lesions distant from their effectors: lateral and medial cords, and median nerve and ulnar nerve. In these cases, even after repair of good quality, results are uncertain, with reinnervation of the flexor mus-

cles of the wrist and digits in 60 per cent of cases but no reinnervation of the intrinsic muscles of the hand. From a sensory standpoint, reinnervation provides very useful protection notably in the territory of the median nerve.

3. The high frequency of lesion combinations must be noted, particularly lesions of the subscapular nerve and lesions of the musculocutaneous nerve, median nerve, or ulnar nerve. Similarly, bone or vascular lesions also influence the overall prognosis.

The treatment of infraclavicular lesions of the brachial plexus requires knowledge of the various possible anatomopathological lesions. The possibilities of nerve grafts or of neurolyses must be understood, and clinical diagnosis, sometimes difficult, must ensure the possibility of early exploration. Knowledge of anatomopathological lesions and progress in microsurgery justify the modern approach to the treatment of brachial plexus lesions.

Precise determination of indications is based upon knowledge of the spontaneous course and the study of long term results (more than two years) after direct repair. In our series of 420 cases treated surgically between 1974 and 1985, results confirm that the direct repair of nerve lesions offers the hope, in an increasingly large number of cases, of obtaining functional results which justify surgery of this type.

Nerve surgery provides the best results in C5-C6 upper root paralyses with reinnervation of the proximal muscles of the shoulder and of the elbow. These functional results should lead to continuing work along these lines with precise and early indications.

Finally, palliative surgery must be discussed in relation to individual cases and the outcome.

PALLIATIVE RECONSTRUCTIVE SURGERY

Palliative surgery can be considered when the limits of maximum recovery, whether spontaneous or following grafting, are reached or passed. The indications and choice of procedure will depend on the site of the residual palsy, the state of the muscles and joints, and the occupation and personality of the patient.

PARALYSIS OF THE SHOULDER

Shoulder paralysis can be palliated in three ways: muscle transplants, ligamentoplasty, and scapulohumeral arthrodesis. Muscle transplants are indicated in isolated C5-C6 palsies and in total palsies with a C5-C6 predominance, when the greatest handicap results from the loss of abduction and of external rotation.

Paralysis of Abduction. The numerous methods put forward include, among others, transplants involving the serratus anterior and the sternomastoid. However, no series has been published as yet. The most commonly used procedures are transplantation of the pectoralis major on the deltoid (Hildebrant) and the trapezius on the humerus (Lange and Mayer; Bateman, 1962). These transplants should be considered only if the rotators of the shoulder (which are essential in abduction) and the fixators of the scapula (serratus anterior, rhomboid major and minor) are intact.

Paralysis of the External Rotators. These muscles are important to the overall function of the upper limb and their reactivation should always be envisaged. The most popular procedures include transplants of the

teres major and latissimus dorsi (L'Episcopo; in Merle d'Aubigné, 1954), but these muscles are frequently involved, at least partially, in C5-C6 palsies.

Ligamentoplasty attempts to provide passive abduction, which is more elastic than in arthrodesis. It is mentioned here only for general interest, as it not performed any longer.

Arthrodesis of the shoulder is a useful procedure in C5-C6 palsies. Its objective is to assist active abduction by the trapezius and to improve the function of a transplant designed to reactivate elbow flexion. The prerequisites for an arthrodesis are: (1) the trapezius and serratus anterior should be normal in order to avoid winging of the scapula, and (2) the position must be accurately adjusted as follows: 60 degrees of abduction, 20 degrees of flexion, 30 degrees of internal rotation. The functional results are satisfactory, especially in manual laborers. An overall abduction of 90 degrees can usually be restored.

The indications for surgery vary according to the type of palsy. In paralysis of abduction and of lateral rotation, many surgeons prefer a transplant, provided the patient is still active and accepts surgery. In combined paralyses of abduction and external rotation, arthrodesis seems preferable, but here again the patient may prefer a "hanging" shoulder to a fixed shoulder.

PARALYSIS OF ELBOW FLEXION

Treatment of this type of paralysis is naturally geared toward restoring elbow flexion, which is so important for placing the hand at the correct height. It is of course desirable to obtain flexion powerful enough to lift a weight, but the gain of flexion against gravity in itself constitutes a substantial surgical achievement. The shoulder is also an important element in upper limb function, and, as we have seen, the elbow may have to be stabilized surgically before some flexion is restored by transplants. The following procedures are most commonly used:

Transplant of the Epitrochlear Muscles (Steindler). This procedure consists of raising the insertion of the epitrochlear muscles by a few centimeters up the humerus so that they can be converted into elbow flexors. It has the advantage of not interfering with the biceps, the partial spontaneous recovery of which, though too weak by itself, can assist the action of the neo-flexors. Provided the flexor carpi ulnaris is intact, this procedure can give the elbow up to 90 or 100 degrees of active flexion.

The undesirable effect of the operation is not so much the extension deficit (which is always observed and constitutes only a minor handicap) as the forearm pronation and flexion of the wrist and fingers, which occur during active flexion of the elbow. The consequent effects on the hand are difficult to avoid, especially in C5-C6-C7 palsies and in partially recovered total palsies.

In such cases, the flexor carpi radialis is not powerful enough, and the work imposed on the epitrochlear head of the flexor superficialis communis is excessive. This useful procedure is therefore indicated mostly in palsies of C5-C6.

Direct Transplants on the Biceps. Several such procedures have been tried. They include the transfer of part or all of the pectoralis major. The latter (Brooks, 1959; Seddon, 1972) is only active with the arm in elevation and anteposition. In the former, only the lower fibers are transplanted (Clark, 1946; Merle d'Aubigné, 1967). This has the advantage of giving the transplant a more direct course but risks necrosis by torsion of the pedicle. These two transplants are seldom indicated.

Second, there is the possibility of transplanting the pectoralis minor (Le Coeur, 1963). This is an interesting approach in paralysis of the upper roots, as the pectoralis minor is supplied by all the roots from C5 to T1. In addition, it has several advantages: function is not interfered with, there are no trick movements, the procedure restores better flexion than the other methods, and arthrodesis of the shoulder is unnecessary. In all the published series, flexion was sufficient to overcome more than gravity, but fatigue set in rapidly. Again, the extension deficit cannot be considered a disadvantage, as it enables the transplant to initiate movement under more favorable conditions.

Anterior Transplant of the Biceps. We consider anterior transplant of the triceps (Bunnell, 1951; and Carroll, 1953) a useful operation that should be reserved for cases of complete paralysis of the biceps and brachialis to avoid the antagonistic effect.

Transplant of the Latissimus Dorsi. Finally, there is the transplant of the latissimus dorsi according to the technique of Hovnanian (1956) or that of Zancolli (1973). This procedure is very appealing, and has become commonly used.

The choice of operation in paralysis of elbow flexion will depend on the type of palsy. Steindler's operation seems the best in isolated C5-C6 lesions. In paralysis of C5-C6-C7 we prefer a pectoralis minor transplant that can be combined with Steindler's procedure. Finally, there is the possibility of a triceps or latissimus dorsi transplant depending on the territorial recovery after nerve grafts.

PARALYSIS OF THE HAND

Paralysis of the hand is the result of a total plexus palsy in which only the upper roots have recovered or, less commonly, of isolated lesions of the lower roots only. After a brachial plexus palsy the paralytic hand does not constitute a characteristic pathological entity as does the ulnar hand or the medioulnar hand. Each case must be evaluated in the overall context of the palsy. The decision to operate and the choice of operation are difficult to make and depend on the motor and sensory conditions prevailing. The following factors must all be taken into account before palliative surgery is undertaken:

1. The state of all transplantable muscles proximal to the paralyzed hand: Only muscles with a score of 4 to 5 should be transplanted if one wants to restore useful function.

2. The overall sensation in the hand: It is well known that motor transplants should not be used if the hand is anesthetic.

The surgical indications can be summarized as follows:

1. Some clinical aspects are not difficult because the paralysis is localized in a specific territory, such as thenar muscles or wrist and finger extensors, and in such cases it is possible to perform classical tendon transfers.

2. Other aspects need discussion because the hand is totally paralyzed with or without sensibility. No indications can be given because arthrodesis, in order to put the wrist and thumb in a functional position, is more cumbersome than useful and can be usefully replaced by orthoses.

3. Others need very detailed discussion, and must be analyzed on a case by case basis. For instance, in cases in which the wrist flexors have recovered either spontaneously

or after a nerve graft, one must not perform a wrist arthrodesis in order to recuperate muscles to be transferred. The hook obtained by wrist flexion can be very useful to lift objects (see Fig. 60–22). Moreover, the muscles that could be transferred never have grade IV strength and could not be useful. Finally, tenodesis of the extensors can be useful for positioning the fingers and obtaining automatic opening of the hand by wrist flexion.

REFERENCES

Adams, R. D.: Disease of Muscles. A Study in Pathology. New York, Harper and Row, 1975, pp. 112–139.

Adelove, A., Kolawove, T., and Odeku, E. L.: Myelography in the diagnosis and prognosis of brachial plexus injuries. West Afr. Med. J., 20:380, 1971.

Adler, J. B., and Patterson, R. L.: Erb's palsy. Long-term results of treatment in 88 cases. J. Bone Joint Surg., 49A:1052, 1967.

Adson, A. W.: The surgical treatment of brachial plexus injuries. Med. Rev., 99:888, 1921.

Adson, A. W.: The gross pathology of brachial plexus injuries. Surg. Gynecol. Obstet., 34:351–357, 1922.

Afanassieff, A.: Les homogreffes des nerfs conservés par le Cialit. Chir. Main, 31:19–25, 1971.

Alexandre, J. H., et al.: Les nerfs du grand dentelé. Arch. Anapathol., 16:185–190, 1969.

Allende, B. T.: Lésions traumatiques du plexus brachial dans la région infra-claviculaire. Rev. Chir. Orthop., 57:131–134, 1971.

Allieu, Y.: Exploration et traitement direct des lésions nerveuses dans les paralysies traumatiques par élongation du plexus brachial chez l'adulte. Rev. Chir. Orthop., 63:107–122, 1977.

Allieu, Y., Privat, J. M., and Bonnel, F.: Paralysis in root avulsion of the brachial plexus: Neurotization by the spinal accessory nerve. Clin. Plast. Surg., 11:133–137, 1984.

Alnot, J. Y.: Paralysie traumatique du plexus brachial chez l'adulte. Symposium, Réunion Annuelle de la SOFCOT. Paris, Nov. 1975.

Alnot, J. Y.: Les lesions et leur mecanisme. Rev. Chir. Orthop., 63:39–43, 1977.

Alnot, J. Y.: Classification anatomopathologique. Rev. Chir. Orthop., 63:55–57, 1977.

Alnot, J. Y.: Examen clinique initial. Rev. Chir. Orthop., 63:58–64, 1977.

Alnot, J. Y.: Technique chirugicale dans les paralysies du plexus brachial. Rev. Chir. Orthop., 63:75–80, 1977.

Alnot, J. Y.: Paralysie Traumatique du Plexus Brachial de l'Adulte. Encycl. Med.-Chir. (Paris), Appareil Locomoteur, 15002, A 10, 9, 1983.

Alnot, J. Y.: Infraclavicular lesions. Clin. Plast. Surg., 11:127–133, 1984.

Alnot, J. Y., and Abols, Y.: Réanimation de la flexion du coude par transferts tendineux dans les paralysies du plexus brachial de l'adulte. Rev. Chir. Orthop., 70:313–323, 1984.

Alnot, J. Y., and Huten, D.: La systématisation du plexus brachial. Rev. Chir. Orthop., 63:27–30, 1977.

Alnot, J. Y., and Jolly, A.: Traitement direct des lésions nerveuses dans les paralysies traumatiques par élongation du plexus brachial chez l'adulte. Intern. Orthop. (S.I.C.O.T.), 5:151–168, 1981.

Ammount, F.: Contribution à l'étude des paralysies du plexus brachial après cancer du sein. These Med., Paris, 1969.

Anderl, H., Ganner, H., and Nowak, H.: Mikrochirurgische transplantationen zür wiederherstellung nach Amplexuslähmungen. Wien. Klin. Wschr., 85:539, 1973.

Apert, A.: Paralysie traumatique radiculaire inferiéure du plexus brachial. Autopsie 33 ans après l'accident. Bull Soc. Med. Hop. Paris, 35:613, 1898.

Babcock, W. W.: A standard technique for operations on peripheral nerves with special reference to closure of large gaps. Surg. Gynecol. Obstet., 45:364, 1927.

Barnes, R.: Traction injuries of the brachial plexus in adults. J. Bone Joint Surg., 31B:10–16, 1949.

Basauri, L., Hudson, H., and Bardales, A.: Diverticuli of the nerve root sheaths. J. Neurosurg., 31:680, 1969.

Bateman, J. E.: An operative approach to supraclavicular plexus injuries. J. Bone Joint Surg., 31B:34–36, 1949.

Bateman, J. E.: Trauma to Nerves in Limbs. Philadelphia, W. B. Saunders Company, 1962.

Bateman, J. E.: Nerve injuries about the shoulder in sports. J. Bone Joint Surg., 49A:785, 1967.

Binns, J. H., and Wynn-Parry, C. B.: Successful repair of a complete brachial plexus lesion. Injury, 2:19, 1970.

Bischoff, A.: Anatomie Chirurgicale des Nerfs Périphériques. Monographie du Groupe d'Etude de la Main (G.E.M.). Paris, Expansion Scientifique Française, 1973, pp. 15–22.

Bjorkesten, G.: Suture of war injuries to peripheral nerves. Clinical studies of results. Acta Chir. Scand. (Suppl. 95), 1:119, 1947.

Bonnel, F.: Configuration interne histophysiologique. Anatomie du plexus brachial. Rev. Chir. Orthop., 63:35–38, 1977.

Bonnel, F., and Rabischong, P.: Le Plexus Brachial. Essai de Systématisation. Paris, G.E.M. Expansion Scientifique Française, 1976.

Bonney, G.: The value of axon responses in determining the site of lesion in traction injuries of the brachial plexus. Brain, 11:588–609, 1954.

Bonney, G.: Prognosis in traction lesions of the brachial plexus. J. Bone Joint Surg., 41B:4–35, 1959.

Bonney, G., Birch, R., Jamieson, A. M., and Eames, R. A.: Experience with vascularized nerve grafts. Clin. Plast. Surg., 11:137–143, 1984.

Boyes, J. H.: Bunnel's Surgery of the Hand. Philadelphia, J. B. Lippincott Company, 1964.

Brand, P. W.: Tendon grafting. Illustrated by a new operation for intrinsic paralysis of the fingers. J. Bone Joint Surg., 43B:444, 1961.

Brewerton, D. A., and Daniel, J. W.: Factors influencing return to work. Br. Med. J., 4:277–281, 1971.

Briston, A. T.: Avulsion of the brachial plexus with a report of 3 cases. Ann. Surg., 36:411, 1902.

Brooks, D. M.: Open wounds of the brachial plexus. J. Bone Joint Surg., 31B:17–33, 1949.

Brooks, D. M.: Open wounds of the brachial plexus in peripheral nerve injuries. Med. Res. Counc. Spec. Rep. Ser., 282:418–429, 1954.

Brooks, D. M., and Seddon, H. J.: Pectoral transplantation for paralysis of the elbow. J. Bone Joint Surg., 41B:36, 1959.

Brown, F. W., and Navigato, W. J.: Rupture of the axillary artery and brachial plexus palsy associated with anterior dislocation of the shoulder. Clin. Orthop. Rel. Res., 60:195, 1968.

Brunelli, G., and Monini, L.: Neurotization of avulsed roots of the brachial plexus by means of anterior nerves of the cervical plexus. Clin. Plast. Surg., 11:149–153, 1984.

Buchthal, F., Rosenfalck, A., and Behse, F.: Sensory potentials of normal and diseased nerves. In Dyck, P. J. et al. (eds): Peripheral Neuropathy. Philadelphia, W. B. Saunders Company, 1975, pp. 442–464.

Buck-Gramcko, D.: Wiederherstellung durchtrennter peripherer Nerven. Chir. Praxis, 15:55–63, 1971.

Buffalini, C., and Pescatori, G.: Posterior cervical electromyography in the diagnosis and prognosis of brachial plexus injuries. J. Bone Joint Surg., 51B:627–631, 1969.

Bunnell, S.: Surgery of nerves of the hand. Surg. Gynecol. Obstet., 44:145, 1927.

Bunnell, S.: Restoring flexion to the paralytic elbow. J. Bone Joint Surg., 33A:566–571, 1951.

Bunnell, S.: Surgery of the Hand, 3rd Ed. London, Pitman Medical, 1956, p. 555.

Cabaud, H. E., Rodkey, W. G., McCarroll, H. R. Jr., Mutz, S. B., and Niebauer, J. J.: Epineural and perineural fascicular nerve repairs. A critical comparison. J. Hand Surg., 1:131–137, 1976.

Cadre, N.: Étude électromyographique des paralysies traumatiques du plexus brachial. Rev. Chir. Orthop., 63:65–66, 1977.

Caldani, cited by Testut, L., and Latarjet, A.: Traité d' Anatomie Humaine. Paris, I. G. Doin et Cie, 1948, p. 562.

Campbell, J. B.: Operation Orthopaedics, 4th Ed. St. Louis, C. V. Mosby Company, 1963, pp. 1464–1471.

Campbell, J. B., and Lusskin, R.: Upper extremity paralysis consequent to brachial plexus injury. Partial alleviation through neurolysis or autograft reconstruction. Surg. Clin. North Am., 52:1235, 1972.

Carayon, A., Cheynet, M., and Blanc, J. F.: Place des arrachements radiculaires dans les élongations du plexus brachial. Rev. Chir. Orthop., 6:855–864, 1959.

Carroll, R. E., and Gartland, J. J.: Flexor plasty to the elbow. An evaluation of a method. J. Bone Joint Surg., 35A:706–710, 1953.

Cashman, M. D.: Monoplegia and Horner's syndrome for pressure palsy. Br. Med. J., 12:1850–1852, 1960.

Celli, L.: Communication lors du Symposium sur les Lesions du Plexus Brachial. Lausanne, August 26, 1976.

Censi, M., et al.: Le lesioni traumatische del plesso brachiale. Riv. Infort. Mal. Prof., 47:925–942, 1960.

Cibert, N.: Des Paralysies Radiculaires Obstétricales du Plexus Brachial. These med., Lyon, 1897 (n 130).

Clark, J.: Reconstruction of biceps brachii by pectoral muscle transplantation. Br. Surg., 34:180–181, 1946.

Clausen, E. G.: Postoperative (anesthetic) paralysis of the brachial plexus. Surgery, 12:933–942, 1942.

Comtet, J. J.: Traitement des Paralysies du Plexus Brachial par Traumatisme Fermé de l'Adulte. These, Lyon, 1962 (n 114, bibliographic).

Comtet, J. J., and Ramet-Girard, R.: Possibilités therapeutiques dans les paralysies du plexus brachial. Les résultats de la reinsertion professionnelle. Arch. Mal. Prof., 29:732–734, 1968.

Comtet, J. J., and Auffray, Y.: Physiologie des muscles

élévateurs de l'épaule. Rev. Chir. Orthop., 56:105–117, 1970.

Cormier, J. M., and Ferry, J.: Paralysie plexique dans les cancers du sein traités. Nouv. Presse Med., 3:1000–1004, 1974.

Creyssel, J., Comtet, J. J., and Fischer, L.: Le pronostic des lésions traumatiques fermées du plexus brachial chez l'adulte. Presse Med., 75:1721–1723, 1967.

Darling, H. C. R.: The surgery of the brachial plexus. Med. J. Aust., 2:335, 1915.

Dautry, P., Apoil, A., Moinet, F., and Koechlin, P.: Paralysie radiculaire supérieure du plexus brachial. Traitement par transpositions musculaires associees (7 cas). Rev. Chir. Orthop., 63:399–407, 1977.

Davies, E. R., Sutton, D., and Bligh, A. S.: Myelography in brachial plexus injury. Br. J. Radiol., 39:362–371, 1966.

Davis, L., Martin, J., and Perret, G.: The treatment of injuries of the brachial plexus. Ann. Surg., 125:647–657, 1947.

Dejerine-Klumpke, A.: Paralysie radiculaire totale du plexus brachial avec phénomènes oculopapillaires: autopsiee 36 jours apres l'accident. Rev. Neurol., 16:637, 1908.

Delanne, A.: Les paralysies du plexus brachial par traumatisme fermé. Tentative de classification. These med., Bordeaux, 1961.

Delbet, P., and Cauchoix, A.: Les paralysies dans les luxations de l'épaule. Rev. Chir. Paris, 41:327–352, 667–687, 1910.

Dellon, L. A.: Reinnervation of denervated Meissner corpuscles. A sequential histologic study in the monkey following fascicular nerve repair. J. Hand Surg., 1:98–109, 1976.

Delmas, A.: Voies et Centres Nerveux. 8th Ed. Paris, Masson, 1969.

Denny-Brown, D., and Doherty, M.: The effects of transient stretching of peripheral nerves. Arch. Neurol. Psychiat., 54:116–129, 1945.

Dhuner, K. G.: Nerve injuries following operations. A survey of cases occurring during a six year period. Anesthesiology, 11:289–293, 1950.

Dolenc, V. V.: Intercostal neurotization of the peripheral nerves in avulsion plexus injuries. Clin. Plast. Surg., 11:143–149, 1984.

Drake, C. G.: Diagnosis and treatment of lesions of the brachial plexus and adjacent structures. Clin. Neurosurg., 11:110, 1963.

Duchenne, G. B.: De l'Électrisation Localisée et son Application a la Pathologie et al Thérapeutique. 3rd Ed. Paris, Bailliere, 1872.

Duval, P., and Guillain, G.: Paralysies Radiculaires traumatiques du plexus brachial. Arch Gen. Med., 2:143–191, 1898.

Duval, P., and Guillain, G.: Paralysies Radiculaires du Plexus Brachial. Steindler Ed. 1905.

Edshage, S.: Acta Chir. Scand., Suppl. 331, 1964.

Erb, W.: Ueber eine eigentumliche Lokalisation von Lähmungen im Plexus brachialis. Verh. Heidelberg Naturhist. Veiren, 130–139, 1874.

Fenart, R.: Développement du plexus brachial chez l'embryon humain. These med., 1956.

Fieux, A.: De la pathogenie des paralysies brachiales chez le nouveau-né. Paralysies obstétricales. Ann. Gynecol. Obstet., 47–52, 1897.

Flaubert, M.: Mémoire sur plusieurs cas de luxation. Rev. Gen. Anat. Physiol. Path., 3:55, 1827.

Flemming, F.: Traitement des lésions fermées du plexus

brachial. Bruns. Beitr. Klin. Chir., *211*:487–503, 1965 (resumé français).

Fletcher, I.: Management of severe tractions of the brachial plexus. J. Bone Joint Surg., *48B*:178, 1966.

Fletcher, I.: Traction lesions of the brachial plexus. Hand, *1*:129–136, 1969.

Foerster, O.: Die Therapie der Schlussverletzungen des peripheren Nerven. Supplement du Handbuch der Neurologie, Chap. 3, pp. 939–941. *In* Lewandowsky, A. (ed.): Hdb. der Neurologie Erganzungsband. Berlin, 1929.

Frazier, C.: Results of peripheral nerve surgery. Med. Opt. of the U.S. Army in the World War. Gov. Printing Office, Washington, II, 1084, 1927.

Frot, B.: La myélographie cervicale opaque dans les paralysies traumatiques du plexus brachial. Rev. Chir. Orthop., *63*:67–72, 1977.

Frot, B., Filippe, G., Olivier, H., Alnot, J. Y., and Duparc, J.: Intérèt de la myélographie cervicale à contraste positif dans l'exploration des lésions traumatiques du plexus brachial chez l'adulte. Ann. Radiol. *16*:715–721, 1973.

Frykholm, R.: The mechanism of cervical radicular lesions resulting from friction or forceful traction. Acta Chir. Scand., *102*:93, 1951.

Galleazzi, R.: Contributo clinico e sperimentale allo studio delle lesioni del plesso brachiale d'origine traumatica. Arch. Orthop. Milano, *20*:1, 1903.

Goldhahn, G.: Plexus-Brachialis-Verletzungen ans neurochirurgischer Sicht. Zentbl. Chir., *92*:225, 1967.

Gournay, J. et al: Un cas de paralysie obstetricale du nerf phrenique gauche associé à une paralysie du plexus brachial du même cote. Bull. Soc. Pediatr. Paris, 523–528, 1936.

Granberry, W. M., and Lipscomb, P. R.: Tendon transfers to the hand in brachial palsy. Am. J. Surg., *108*:840–844, 1964.

Greenfield, A., Sheperd, J. T., and Whelen, R. F.: The part played by the nervous system in the response to cold of the circulation through the finger tip. Clin. Sci., *10*:347–360, 1951.

Grenet, H.: Formes cliniques des paralysies du plexus brachial. Arch. Gynecol. Med., *4*:424, 1900.

Grenet, H., et al.: Paralysie radiculaire du plexus brachial et paralysie diaphragmatique. Bull Soc. Pediat. Paris, *35*:146–150, 1937.

Gros, C., and Cazaban, R.: Kyste extra-dural consécutif à un arrachement radiculaire du plexus brachial. Presse Med., *68*:815, 1948.

Guerbert, M.: Etude pharmacologique du monoiododstearate d'éthyle produit de contraste pour myélographie. Therapie, *21*:1219–1227, 1966.

Gutmann, E., and Gutmann, L.: Effect of electrotherapy on denervated muscles in rabbits. Lancet, *1*:169–170, 1942.

Gutmann, E., and Young, R.: The reinnervation of muscles after various periods of atrophy. J. Anat. *78*:15–43, 1944.

Haftek, J.: Stretch injury of peripheral nerve (acute effects of stretching on rabbit nerve). J. Bone Joint Surg., *52B*:354–365, 1970.

Hakstian, R. W.: Funicular orientation by direct stimulation. An aid to peripheral nerve repair. J. Bone Joint Surg., *50-A*:1178–1186, 1968.

Hamonet, C., and Heuleu, J. N.: Electromyographie. Edit. Med. Univ., Paris.

Heile, B.: Bruns Beitrage, *124*:639, 1921.

Henderson, E. D.: Transfer of wrist extensors to restore opposition of the thumb. J. Bone Joint Surg., *44A*:513–522, 1962.

Hendry, A. M.: The treatment of residual paralysis after brachial plexus injuries. J. Bone Joint Surg., *31*:42–49, 1949.

Heon, M.: Myelogram: a questionable aid in diagnosis and prognosis in avulsion of brachial plexus components by traction injuries. Conn. Med., *29*:260, 1965.

Heon, M., and Strois, J.: La valeur du myélogramme comme aide diagnostique et pronostique dans les lésions traumatiques du plexus brachial. Can. J. Surg., *3*:112, 1960.

Hermingham, W. P.: The minute anatomy of the brachial plexus. Proc. R. Soc. London, *B41*:423–441, 1886.

Hiles, R. W.: Freeze-dried irradiated nerve homograft. A preliminary report. Hand, *4*:79–84, 1972.

Holler, M., and Hopf, H. C.: Pathological associated movements of diaphragm and shoulder muscles following paralysis of the brachial plexus and their significance with regard to peripheral regeneration Electroencephal. Clin. neurophysiol., *26*:438, 1969.

Holmes, W.: Histological observations on the repair of nerves by autografts. Br. J. Surg., *35*:167, 1947.

Holmes, W., and Young, J. Z.: Nerve regeneration after immediate and delayed suture. J. Anat. 77:63–96, 1942.

Holt, S., and Yates, P. O.: Cervical nerve root cysts. Brain. *87*:481, 1964.

Horsley, V.: On injuries to peripheral nerves. Practitioner, *63*:131–144, 1899.

Hovnanian, A. P.: Latissimus dorsi transplantation for loss of flexion or extension at the elbow. A preliminary report on technic. Ann. Surg., *143*:493, 1956.

Howard, F. M., and Schafer, S. J.: Injuries to the clavicle with neurovascular complication. A study of 14 cases. J. Bone Joint Surg., *45A*:1335–1346, 1965.

Howland, W. J., Curry, J. L., and Buttler, A.: Pantopaque arachnoiditis. Experimental study of blood as potentiating agent. Radiology, *43*:489–491, 1963.

Hubert, M. N.: Paralysie traumatique du plexus brachial: approaches du diagnostic topographique et lésionnel. Thèse, Montpellier, 1974.

Hughet, W. B., and Holmes, W.: Traction injuries to the lateral popliteal nerve and traction injuries to peripheral nerves after suture. Br. J. Surg., *30*:212–233, 1943.

Ikeda, K.: Successful peripheral nerve homotransplantation by use of high voltage electron irradiation. Arch. Jap. Chir., *35*:679–705, 1966.

Isch, F.: Electromyographie. Doin Edit., Paris, 1963.

Jabaley, M. E., Burns, J. E., Orcutt, B. S., and Bryant, W. M.: Comparison of histological and functional recovery after peripheral nerve repair. J. Hand Surg., *1*:119–130, 1976.

Jackson, E. C. S.: The role of galvanism in the treatment of denervated voluntary muscles in man. Brain, 68:300, 1945.

Jacoby, W., et al.: Munch. Med. Wschr., *112*:586, 1970.

Jackson, L., and Keats, A. S.: Mechanism of brachial plexus palsy following anesthesia. Anesthesiology, 26:190–194, 1965.

Jaeger, R., and Whitley, W. H.: Avulsion of the brachial plexus—report of 6 cases. J.A.M.A., *153*:633, 1953.

Jelasic, F., and Piepgras, U.: Functional restitution after cervical avulsion with typical myelography findings. Eur. Neurol., *11*:158, 1974.

Jolly, F.: Ueber Infantile Entibindungslahmungen, Neurol. Zb. Lpz., *16:*222, 1897.

Kapandji, I. A.: Physiologie articulaire. Maloine, Paris, 1966.

Kendall, H. O., and Kendall, F. P.: Muscles. Testing and function. Baltimore, Williams and Wilkins, 1949.

Kennedy, R.: Suture of brachial plexus in birth paralysis of the upper extremity. Br. Med. J., *1:*298, 1903.

Kennedy, R.: Further notes on the treatment of birth paralysis of the upper extremity by suture of the 5th and 6th cervical nerves. Br. Med. J., *2:*1065, 1904.

Kerner, Y.: Paralysies traumatiques du plexus brachial. These med., Paris, 1956 (Bibliograph.).

Kerr, A. T.: The brachial plexus of nerves in man. The variations in its formation and branches. Am. J. Anat. *23:*185–395, 1918.

Kerr, A. T.: Cervical plexus injuries as an extension of brachial plexus injuries. J. Bone Joint Surg., *31B:*37–39, 1949.

Kettelkamp, D. B., and Larson, C. B.: Evaluation of the Steindler flexor plasty. J. Bone Joint Surg., *45A:*513–518, 1963.

Klumpke, A.: Contribution a l'étude des paralysies radiculaires du plexus brachial. Rev. Med., *5:*591–615, 739–791, 1885.

Kotani, T., Matsuda, H., and Suzuki, T.: Trial surgical procedures of nerve transfer to avulsion injuries of plexus brachialis. Proc. 12th Congress of the International Society of Orthopaedic Surgery and Traumatology. Tel Aviv. Amsterdam, Excerpta Medica, 1972, p. 348.

Kotani, T., Toyoshima, H., Masuda, H., Suzuki, T., Ishizaki, Y., Iwani, H., Yamano, K., Inque, H., Moriguchi, T., Asaka, K.: The postoperative results of nerve transfer for the brachial plexus injury with root avulsion. Proc. 14th Annual Meeting Japan Society of Surgery of the Hand, Osaka, 1971.

Krenkel, W.: Die Technik der Nervenoperationne unter besonderer Berücksichtigung der Verletzungen des Plexus Brachialis. Heft. Unfallheilk., *81:*267–274, 1965.

Kus, H., and Kedra, H.: Une homogreffe du nerf median avec ses branches de division. Chir. Main, *31:*7–9, 1971.

Lange, M.: Die Behandlung der irreparablen peripheren Nervenletzungen. Wiederherst Chir. Traumat. *1:*240, 1953.

Lange, M.: Die Bedeutung der orthopädischen Erstzoperation für die Behandlung der irreparablen peripheren Nervenlähmungern. Med. Klin., *57:*627, 1962.

Laplane, D.: Les paralysies traumatiques du plexus brachial chez l'adulte. Rev. Praticien, *18:*2733–2745, 1968.

Larsen, E. H.: Injuries to the brachial plexus in adults. J. Bone Joint Surg., *37B:*733, 1955.

Laxorthes, G.: Le Systeme Nerveux Peripherique. Paris, Masson, 1971.

Lecoeur, P.: Procédés de restauration de la flexion du coude paralytique. Rev. Chir. Orthop., *37n:*655–656, 1963.

Leffert, R. D., and Seddon, H. J.: Infraclavicular brachial plexus injuries. J. Bone Joint Surg., *47B:*9–22, 1965.

Leffert, R.: Brachial plexus injuries. Orthop. Clin. North Am., *1:*399–416, 1970.

Leffert, R.: Brachial plexus injuries. New Engl. J. Med., *1:*1059–1067, 1974.

Lester, J.: Pantopaque myelography in avulsion of the brachial plexus. Acta Radiol., *55:*186–192, 1961.

Lewis, T., Harris, K. E., and Grant, R. T.: Observations relating to the influence of the cutaneous nerves on various reactions of the cutaneous vessels. Heart, *14:*1–17, 1927.

Lhermitte, F., and Mamo, H.: Systeme Nerveux et Muscles. Paris, Flammarion, 1973.

Luchey, C. A., and McPherson, S. R.: Tendinous reconstruction of the hand following irreparable injury to the peripheral nerves and brachial plexus. J. Bone Joint Surg., *29A:*560–581, 1947.

Lurge, A.: Le traitement chirugical des traumatismes de la partie supérieure du plexus brachial, du type ERB. Ann. Surg., *127:*317–328, 1948.

Lusskin, R., Campbell, J. B., and Thompson, W. A. L.: Post-traumatic lesions of the brachial plexus: treatment by transclavicular exploration and neurolysis or autograft reconstruction. J. Bone Joint Surg., *55B:*1159–1176, 1973.

McQuillan, W. M.: Nerve isolation techniques: an adjunct to secondary nerve repair. Ass. J. Bone Joint Surg., *49B:*186, 1967.

Mannerfelt, L.: Studies on the hand in ulnar nerve paralysis: a clinical experimental investigation in normal and anomalous innervation. Acta. Orthop. Scand. (Suppl.), *87:*175, 1966.

Mansat, M.: Anatomie topographique chirurgicale du plexus brachial. Rev. Chir. Orthop., *63:*20–26, 1977.

Maroon, J. C., Roberts, E., and Nimoto, M.: Microvascular surgery: simplified instrumentation, technical note. J. Neurosurg., *38:*119–126, 1973.

Masse, P., and Morchoisne, P.: Restauration de la flexion du coude paralytique par transplantation du petit pectoral. Opération de Pol Lecoeur. Rev. Chir. Orthop., *53:*357–372, 1967.

Maurer, G., and Schmidt, H.: Verletzungen der peripheren Nerven. Neurotraumatologie. Munich, Kessel, Gutmann, Maurer, Urban und Schwarzenberg. 1971.

Mayer, L., and Green, W.: Experiences with the Steindler flexor plasty at the elbow. J. Bone Joint Surg., *36A:*775–789, 1954.

Mendelsohn, R. A., Weiner, I. H., and Keegan, J. M.: Myleography demonstration of brachial plexus root avulsion. Arch. Surg., *75:*102, 1957.

Merger, R., and Judet, J.: Paralysie obstetricale du plexus brachial. Prévention et traitement. Nouv. Presse Med., *2:*1935–1938, 1973.

Merle D'Aubigne, R.: Opérations palliatives pour paralysies de la main. V1 Congres de la SICOT, 1954, pp. 262–275.

Merle D'Aubigne, R., Benassy, J., and Ramadier, J. O.: Chirurgie Orthopédique des Paralysies. Paris, Masson, 1956, pp. 122–139.

Merle D'Aubigne, R., and Bombart, M.: Technique de l'arthrodèse de l'épaule par voie postérieure. Rev. Chir. Orthop., *52:*157–163, 1966.

Merle D'Aubigne, R., and Deburge, A.: Etiologie, évolution et pronostic des paralysies traumatiques du plexus brachial. Rev. Chir. Orthop., *53:*23–42, 1967; Traitement des paralysies du plexus brachial, 199–215.

Michon, J., and Masse, P.: Le moment optimum de la suture nerveuse dans les plaies du membre supérieur. Rev. Chir. Orthop., *50:*205–222, 1964.

Miette-Soullier, L.: Traumatismes du Plexus Brachial. These med., Lille, 1962 (bibliographie).

Miller, D. S., and Boswick, J. A.: Lesions of the brachial plexus associated with fractures of the clavicle. Clin. Orthop., *64:*144–149, 1969.

Millesi, H.: Zum Problem der Veberbrückung von Defekten peripherer Nerven. Wien. Med. Wschr., *118:*9, 40, 182–187, 1968.

Millesi, H.: Verletzungen des Plexus brachialis. Munch. Med. Wschr., *3:*26–69, 1969.

Millesi, H.: Verletzungen des Plexus brachialis in allg. und Spezielle chirugische Operationslehre. *In* Wachsmuth, W., Wilhem, A. (eds.): Operationen an der Hand. Berlin, Springer, 1972, pp. 245–249.

Millesi, H.: Indications et résultats des interventions directes: paralysie traumatique du plexus brachial chez l'adulte. Reunion annuelle de la SOFCOT. Paris, Nov. 1975; Rev. Chir. Orthop., *63:*82–87, 1977.

Millesi, H.: Brachial plexus injuries: management and results. Clin. Plast. Surg., *11:*115–121, 1984.

Millesi, H.: Résultats tardifs de la greffe nerveuse interfasciculaire. Chirurgie reparatrice des lésions du plexus brachial. Rev. Med. Suisse Romande, *93:*511, 1973.

Millesi, H.: Ganglberger, J., and Berger, A.: Erfahrungen mit der Mikrochirurgie peripheren Nerven. Chir. Plast. Reconstr., *3:*47, 1967.

Millesi, H., Meissl, G., and Berger, A.: The interfascicular nerve grafting of the median and ulnar nerves. J. Bone Joint Surg., *54B:*727–750, 1972.

Millesi, H., Meissl, G., and Katzer, H.: Zur Behandlung der Verletzung des Plexus brachialis. Vorschlag einer integreirten Therapie. Brun's Beitr. Klin. Chir., *220:*429–446, 1973.

Millesi, H., Meissl, G., and Berger, A.: Further experience with interfascicular grafting on the median ulnar and radial nerves. J. Bone Joint Surg., *58A:*209–218, 1976.

Moberg, E.: Objection methods for determining the functional value of sensibility of the hand. J. Bone Joint Surg., *40B:*454–476, 1958.

Motta, A.: La nostra esperinza negli innesti di nervo all artrosuperior. Chir. Main, *31:*11–17, 1971.

Murphey, F., Hartung, W., and Kirlin, J. W.: Myelographic demonstration of avulsion injuries of the brachial plexus. Am J Roentgenol, *58:*102–105, 1947.

Narakas, A.: La réparation chirurgicale des paralysies du plexus brachial par abord direct des lesions. These, Lausanne.

Narakas, A.: Les résultats des autogreffes fasciculaires au membre superieur. Com. Congrès Franco-Suisse d'Orthop., Berne, 1971.

Narakas, A.: Plexo brachial terapeutica quirurgica directa. Tecnica. Indicacion operatoria. Resultados in cirurgia de los nervos perifericos. Rev. Ortop. Traum. Madrid, 339–401, 1972.

Narakas, A.: Paralysie traumatique du plexus brachial chez l'adulte. Symposium. Reunion Annuelle de la SOFCOT. Paris, Nov. 1975; Les lésions dans les élongations du plexus brachial. Rev. Chir. Orthop., *63:*44–54, 1977.

Narakas, A.: Indications et résultats du traitement chirurgical direct dans les lésions par élongation du plexus brachial de l'adulte. Rev. Chir. Orthop., *63:*88–106, 1977.

Narakas, A.: Paradoxes en chirurgie nerveuse peripherique au niveau du plexus brachial. Med. Hyg., *35:*833–839, 1977.

Narakas, A.: Resultäte der plexus brachialis Rekonstruktion mit autologen Nerventra-splantaten. *In* Buff, H. U., and Glinz, W. (eds.): Urgent Surgery. Straube, Erlangen, 1976, p. 373.

Narakas, A.: The surgical management of brachial plexus injuries. *In* Daniel, R. K., and Terzis, J. K.

(eds.): Reconstructive Microsurgery. Boston, Little and Brown, 1977, Chapter 9.

Narakas, A.: Surgical treatment of traction injuries of the brachial plexus. Clin. Orth. Rel. Res., *133:*71–90, 1978.

Narakas, A.: Thoughts on neurotization or nerve transfers in irreparable nerve lesions. Clin. Plast. Surg., *11:*153–161, 1984.

Narakas, A., and Verdan, C.: Les greffes nerveuses. Z. Unfallmed. Berufsstrankh., *3:*137–152, 1969.

Nelson, K. G., Jolly, P. C., and Thomas, P. A.: Brachial plexus injuries associated with missile wounds of the chest. A report of 9 cases from Vietnam. J. Trauma, *8:*268–275, 1970.

Nulsen, F. E., and Slade, H. W.: Recovery following injury to the brachial plexus. (A follow-up study of 3656 World War II injuries). *In* Woodhall, E., and Beebe, G. W. (eds.): Peripheral Nerve Regeneration. VA Med. Monograph, 1956, p. 389.

Oliveira, J. C. de: Aspects expérimentaux et cliniques de la suture nerveuse peripherique. Rev. Orth. Traum., *21:*161, 1976.

Oostrom, J.: Cervical root avulsion. Arch. Chir. Neerl., *17:*239, 1965.

Paturet, G.: Traite d'Anatomie Humaine, 4. Systeme Nerveux. Paris, Masson, 1964.

Pauly, R., and Cools, M.: Intérêt de la myélographie dans les lesions formées du plexus brachial. J. Radiol. Electrol., *43:*283–287, 1962.

Pecinka, H.: Die operative Behandlung der traumatische Lahmungen des Plexus brachialis. Zbl. Chir., *85:*1678–1682, 1960.

Pecinka, H.: Plexus Verletzungen. 2. Tagung Esterr. ges. f., Unfallchir, 9–11, 9, 1960, pp. 258–260.

Penfield, W.: Late spinal paralysis after avulsion of the brachial plexus. J. Bone Joint Surg., *31B:*40–49, 1949.

Penning, L., and Kerchoffs, P. M.: Recherches expérimentales d'un nouveau moyen de contraste opaque (Duriolopaque). Psychiat. Neurol. Neurochir., *71:*105–108, 1968.

Perricone, G., and Gonzalez-Zerpa, R.: Le paralisi traumatische del plesso brachiale. Chir. Organi. Mov., *52:*1–39, 1963.

Perthes, G.: Ausfuhrung der Nervennaht. *In* Barth, A. (ed.): Erfahrungen im Weltkrieg. Leipzig, 1922, pp. 554–580.

Petrov, M. A., and Solarov, T.: Acad. Chir., *12:*889–892, 1964.

Petrov, M. A.: Transplantation of nerves and roots of the spinal cord. Reconstr. Surg. Traumat. (Karger), *12:*250–262, 1971.

Petrov, M. A.: Lésions traumatiques du plexus brachial. Traitement chirurgical, transplantations, résultats éloignés. Chirurgie, *99:*924–934, 1973.

Puusepp, L.: Die Peripheren Nerven. Chir. Neuropath., *1:*17, 1931.

Rayle, A. A., Gay, B. B., and Meados, J. L.: The myelogram in avulsion of the brachial plexus. Radiology, *65:*65–72, 1955.

Rexed, B., and Wennstrom, K. G.: Arachnoidal proliferation and cystic formation in the spinal nerve-root pouches of man. J. Neurosurg., *16:*73, 1959.

Rigault, P.: Paralysies traumatiques du plexus brachial chez l'enfant. Etude de 7 cas. Rev. Chir. Orthop., *55:*125–130, 1969.

Roaf, R.: Lateral flexion injuries of the cervical spine. J. Bone Joint Surg., *45B:*36–38, 1963.

Robles, J.: Brachial plexus avulsion. A review of diagnostic procedures and report of 6 cases. J. Neurosurg., *28:*434, 1968.

Rohr, H.: Untersuchungen über die Segmentinnervation des Hals-Schulter-Arm-gebietes bei cervikalen Wurzellaesionen. Langenbeck's Arch. Klin. Chir., *301:*873–879, 1962.

Rouviere, H.: Anatomie Humaine. III. Paris, Masson et Cie, 1962.

Roviller, C., et al.: La microscopie électronique et ses applications. Acta Clica 6, 1968; Doc. Geigy, 52–82.

Saha, A. K.: Surgery of the paralyzed and flail shoulder. Acta Orthop. Scand. (Suppl.), 97:1–90, 1967.

Sammi, M.: Aspects modernes de la chirurgie des nerfs peripheriques (Collaboration Lagarrigue, J., et Laxorthes, Y.) Ed Med. P. Fabre, 1977.

Santos Palazzi, R.: La microcirurgia en las lesiones de los nervios perifericos. Rev. Orth. Traum., *15:*499–526, 1971 (Résumé français-anglais).

Sassaroli, S., and Di Giulio, T.: Betrachtungen über das myelographische Bild des sogennantes Ausrissverletzungen des Brachial plexus. Fortsch. Geb. Roentgenstrahl. Nukl. Med., *94:*130–137, 1961.

Scaglietti, O.: Einselheiten über die Operationstechnik bei Verletzungen der Wurzeln des Plexus Brachialis durch Schusswaffen, Zentbl. Neurochir., *7:*129–144, 1947.

Schneck, F.: Subkutane vollständige Zerreissung des Plexus cervicalis. Moratschr. Unfallheilk. Versicherungsmed., *35:*22, 1928.

Schuler, C.: Le traitement des lésions fermées du plexus brachial. Schweiz Med. Wschr., *88:*801–806, 1958.

Seddon, H. J.: Three types of nerve injury. Brain, *66:*237–288, 1943.

Seddon, H. J.: The practical value of peripheral nerve repair. Proc. R. Soc. Med. (Orthop.), *42:*427, 1949.

Seddon, H. J.: Nerve grafting. J. Bone Joint Surg., *45:*447–461, 1963.

Seddon, H. J.: Surgical Disorders of the Peripheral nerves. Edinburgh, Churchill-Livingstone, 1972.

Sedel, L.: Evolution spontanée des paralysies traumatiques du plexus brachial. Rev. Chir. Orthop., *63:*73–74, 1977.

Sedel, L.: Traitement palliatif d'une série de 103 paralysies par élongation du plexus brachial. Evolution spontanée et résultat. Rev. Chir. Orthop., *63:*651–666, 1977.

Sedel, L.: La réparation chirurgicale des lésions traumatiques du plexus brachial. Nouv. Presse Med., 8:691–693, 1979.

Sedel, L.: The management of supraclavicular lesions. Clin. Plast. Surg., *11:*121–127, 1984.

Segal, A.: Contribution à l'étude des differentes techniques de chirurgie réparatrice des paralysies de la flexion du coude. These med., Paris, 1957.

Segal, A., Seddon, H. J., and Brooks, D. M.: Treatment of paralysis of the flexors of the elbow. J. Bone Joint Surg., *41B:*44–50, 1959.

Selig, R.: Die Nervenaht und ihre Erfolge mit besonderer Berücksichtigung der Nervenanatomie und Studien über den Plexus. D. Zeitschr. Chir., *137:*455–465, 1916.

Sharpe, W.: The operative treatment of brachial plexus paralysis. J.A.M.A., *66:*876, 1916.

Smith, J. W.: Microsurgery of peripheral nerves. Plast. Reconstr. Surg., *33:*317–329, 1964.

Smith, J. W.: Factors influencing nerve repair. Arch. Surg., *93:*335–341, 433–437, 1966.

Smith-Petersen, M. N.: A new approach of the wrist joint. J. Bone Joint Surg., *22:*122–124, 1940.

Souttar, H. S., Twinning, R.: Injuries of the Peripheral Nerves. Bristol, John Wright Sons, 1920.

Steindler, A.: Tendon transplantation in the upper extremity. Am J. Surg., *44:*260–271, 1939.

Steindler, A.: Muscle and tendon transplantation at the elbow. American Academy of Orthopaedic Surgeons Instruction Course Lectures. 2nd Vol., Ann Arbor, Mich., J. W. Edwards, 1944.

Steindler, A.: The Traumatic Deformities and Disabilities of the Upper Extremity. Springfield, Ill., Charles C Thomas, 1946.

Stevens, J. H.: Section on brachial plexus paralysis in the shoulder. Monograph by Codmann E. A.: The Shoulder. Privately printed in Boston, 1934.

Sunderland, S.: A classification of peripheral nerve injuries producing loss of function. Brain, *74:*491–516, 1951.

Sunderland, S.: Nerves and Nerve Injuries. 1st ed. Edinburgh, Churchill-Livingstone, 1968, pp. 953–967, 968–980.

Sunderland, S.: Mechanisms of cervical nerve root avulsion in injuries of the neck shoulder. J. Neurosurg., *41:*705, 1974.

Sunderland, S.: Nerves and Nerve Injuries. 2nd Ed., Edinburgh, Churchill-Livingstone, 1978, pp. 854–900.

Sunderland, S., and Bradley, K. L.: Stress-strain phenomena in human spinal nerve roots. Brain, *84:*120–134, 1961.

Tarlov, I. M., and Day, R.: Myelography to help localize traction lesions of the brachial plexus. Am J Surg. 88:266–271, 1954.

Tavernier, L.: Paralysie du plexus brachial: rupture des racines supérieures dans le creux sus-claviculatre. Greffe nerveuse. Lyon. Chir., *29:*90–93, 1932.

Taylor, A. S.: Results from the surgical treatment of brachial birth palsy. J.A.M.A., *48:*96–104, 1907.

Taylor, A. S.: Brachial birth palsy and injuries of similar types in adults. Surg. Gynecol. Obstet., *30:*494–502, 1920.

Taylor, P. E.: Traumatic intradural avulsion of the nerve roots of the brachial plexus. Brain, *85:*579–602, 1962.

Temple, C.: Evaluation of traction injuries to the brachial plexus in adults. South Med. J., *63:*409, 1970.

Terzis, J. K., Dykes, R. W., and Hakstian, R. W.: Electrophysiological recordings in peripheral nerves surgery. A review. J. Hand. Surg., *1:*52–66, 1976.

Testut, L., and Latarjet, A.: Arthrologie. Traite d'Anatomie Humaine. Paris, G. Doin et Cie, 1948, p. 562.

Thomas, C.: Post-radium or metastatic brachial plexus palsy. J.A.M.A., *222:*311, 1972.

Tinel, J.: Le signe du fourmillement dans les lésions des nerfs peripheriques. Presse Med., *47:*388, 1915.

Tinel, J.: Plaie des Nerfs. Paris, Bailliere, 1917.

Tracy, J. F., and Brannon, E. W.: Management of traction plexus injuries (traction types). J. Bone Joint Surg., *40A:*1031–1042, 1958.

Tsuyama, N., Sakaguchi, R., Hara, T., Kondo, T., Kaminuma, S., Ihchi, M., and Ryn, D.: Reconstructive surgery in brachial plexus injuries. Proc. 11th Annual Meeting Japan Society of the Hand. Hiroshima, 1968.

Tsuyama, N., and Hara, T.: Intercostal nerve crossing as a treatment of brachial plexus injury of root avulsion type. SICOT, *12:*521, 1972.

Tubiana, R.: Les dates et les indications des reparations secondaires après lésions des nerfs peripheriques du membre supérieur. Monographies du G.E.M. Expansion Scientifique Francaise, 1973, pp. 87–90.

Tuttle, H. K.: Exposure of the brachial plexus with nerve transplantation. J.A.M.A., *61:*15–17, 1913.

Vincent, F.: Pathogenie et marche de la paralysie dans les luxations de l'épaule. Thèse méd., Paris, 1876.

Warren, J., Gutmann, L., Figueroa, A. F., and Bloor, B. M.: Electromyography changes of brachial plexus root avulsions. J. Neurosurg., *31:*137, 1969.

Weber, E.: Diagnostick und therapie der Plexusverletzungen in Halsberich, Langenbecks Arch. Klin Chir., *301:*881–885, 1962.

White, J. C., and Hanelin, J.: Myelographic signs of brachial plexus avulsion. J. Bone Joint Surg., *36A:*113–118, 1954.

Wiedenmann, O.: Neurologische Stösungen als Forge von Ausrissverletzungen des Plexusbrachialis in Vergleich zu den Befunden des positiven Myelogramms. Z. Orthop., *97:*67–77, 1963.

Wilhelm, K.: Die Veberbrückung von Nervendefekten mit lyophilisierten Nerven. Handchir., *4:*25–29, 1972.

Wilson, A. B. K.: Hendon pneumatic power units and control for prostheses and splints. J. Bone Joint Surg., *47:*435–441, 1949.

Wodley, E. J., and Vandam, L. D.: Neurological sequelae of brachial plexus nerve block. Ann. Surg., *149:*53–60, 1959.

Wright, S.: Applied Physiology. 11th Ed. Revised by Keele, C. A., and Neil, E., London, Oxford University Press, 1966, pp. 211–264.

Wynn-Parry, C. B.: Rehabilitation of the Hand. 3rd Ed. London, Butterworth, 1973, pp. 133–148, 286–294.

Wynn-Parry, C. B.: The management of injuries to the brachial plexus. Proc. R. Soc. Med., *67:*488, 1974.

Yeomann, P. M.: Cervical myelography in traction injuries of the brachial plexus. J. Bone Joint Surg., *36A:*113–118, 1954.

Yeomann, P. M., and Seddon, H. J.: Brachial plexus injuries, treatment of flail arm. J. Bone Joint Surg., *43B:*493–500, 1961.

Yeomann, P. M.: Cervical myelography in traction injuries of the brachial plexus. J. Bone Joint Surg., *50B:*253–260, 1968.

Zancolli, E., and Mitre, H.: Latissimus dorsi transfer to restore elbow flexion. J. Bone Joint Surg., *55A:*1265–1275, 1973.

Zverina, E., and Skorpil, V.: Possibilities of the electromyographic diagnosis of brachial plexus injury. Electroencephal. Clin. Neurophysiol., *26:*233, 1969.

Chapter 61

BRACHIAL PLEXUS LESIONS: CLASSIFICATION AND OPERATIVE TECHNIQUE

Hanno Millesi

Different views have been expressed regarding the indications for operative treatment in brachial plexus lesions. The recommended timing of surgery varies in the literature between immediate intervention and exposure of the plexus after six months.

Pecinka (1960, 1961) suggested splitting the epineurium, but Lange (1961), Rohr (1962), and Weber (1962) found this procedure to be ineffective. Neurolysis was recommended by Bateman (1962), but Seddon (1972) stated in his book, "In Britain there is widespread conviction that operation, although occasionally useful in clarifying the prognosis in infraganglionic lesions, has little to offer in amelioration of the paralysis. We do not share Bateman's attachment to neurolysis."

Nerve grafting is not regarded as a useful technique by Maurer and Schmid (1971) and Sunderland (1968). Seddon (1972) repaired traction lesions in five cases by nerve grafting and obtained useful results in two. In his opinion similar functional results can be achieved by the transfer of the pectoralis major muscle with arthrodesis of the shoulder joint (Clark, 1946), and therefore he has discontinued the use of nerve grafts. The value of nerve grafting is a crucial point in this problem. Because the defects to be overcome are usually so long, end to end nerve suturing is out of the question.

The diagnostic value of exposure was regarded as important (Seddon, 1972), because in cases with a bad prognosis conservative treatment should be limited to prevent the patient from getting used to having only one arm (Yeoman and Seddon, 1963). Once this occurs, the patient has great difficulty in learning to use a prosthesis. Hendry (1949) was opposed to early amputation. He believed that amputation has an unfavorable psychological effect and makes professional rehabilitation more difficult. In the event of an injury or paralysis of the contralateral hand, the patient would be completely helpless.

It seems worthwhile, therefore, to try every possible means to obtain some useful function in the paralyzed arm before considering amputation. Of course, one cannot expect complete recovery, but the severity of the functional loss is so grave for the patient that even a small gain in function means a lot. Amputation can be done if all attempts at other therapy fail. There are several prerequisites for successful therapy.

1. A skillful therapeutic plan from the beginning using all available measures appropriate in the case.

2. Prevention of time loss. Usually too much time is lost with conservative treatment and in establishing the diagnosis.

3. Improvement in surgical technique. By the use of microsurgery the accuracy and effectiveness of neurolysis can be increased. The use of nerve grafts on a larger scale can solve the problems of nerve defects.

We started to pursue an active approach to treatment as just outlined in 1966. In 1969 I presented preliminary results in Lausanne. Since then, 44 patients have been operated upon; the results have been reported in detail elsewhere (Millesi, 1973). Narakas (1972) and Allieu also believed that a more active approach to brachial plexus lesions was indicated and they have produced remarkable results.

Without going into details, in the following

645

pages a simple formula for the classification of brachial plexus lesions is outlined and a plan for the therapeutic and diagnostic steps is given.

A FORMULA FOR THE CLASSIFICATION OF BRACHIAL PLEXUS INJURIES

A formula has to express the following criteria: the level of injury, the longitudinal and transverse extension of the injury, the grade of injury, and the type of injury.

From a functional point of view, four different levels should be distinguished (designated by roman numerals): the supraganglionic part of the root (I), infraganglionic part of the root (II), trunks (supraclavicular; III), and cords (infraclavicular; IV).

If the longitudinal extension of the lesion involves two levels, for instance, supraganglionic and infraganglionic lesions of the same root, this can be expressed as I and II. Involvement of the supraclavicular part (trunks) and the infraclavicular part (cords) would be designated III and IV.

TRANSVERSE EXTENSION

The second part of the formula represents the transverse extent of the injury—the roots, trunks, and cords involved.

The roots are represented by Arabic numerals: 4 = C4, 5 = C5, 6 = C6, 7 = C7, 8 = C8, 1 = T1, and 2 = T2.

Involvement of all roots in a normal case would be expressed as (5, 6, 7, 8, 1). Prefixation of the plexus is expressed as 4, 5, 6, 7, 8.

Postfixation of the plexus is expressed as 6, 7, 8, 1, 2.

At the level of the trunks: s = upper trunk, im = middle trunk, and i = lower trunk.

At the level of the cords: l = lateral cord, m = medial cord, and p = posterior cord.

Grade of Injury

The third component of the formula expresses the grade of injury. The grading system devised by Sunderland (1951) is used:

1. The continuity of the axons is preserved. Electrical reactions remain normal, and if there is no continuous compression, spontaneous recovery occurs in three to eight weeks.

2. The continuity of the axons is destroyed, but the endoneurial tubes are preserved. Wallerian degeneration ensues a few days after injury and the electrical reactions become pathological. If there is no continuous compression, spontaneous recovery can be expected within three to eight months.

3. The continuity of the axons is lost and the endoneurial tubes are destroyed, but the perineurium and fascicular pattern remain intact. Wallerian degeneration follows. A few days after the injury the electrical reactions become pathological. Retrograde degeneration occurs. Spontaneous recovery under favorable conditions is possible, but there is a loss of axons and a new innervation pattern has to be developed

4. The continuity of the axons is lost and the endoneurium and perineurium are destroyed. Wallerian degeneration occurs. A few days after the injury the electrical reactions become pathological. There is more retrograde degeneration than in the grade 3 situation. The fascicular pattern is destroyed and a neuroma in continuity forms. Useful regeneration is unlikely. The epineurium, however, is preserved.

5. There is complete loss of continuity including the epineurium.

TYPES OF LESIONS

The following types should be differentiated:

Open transection: O. Rupture: R. O and R would mean grade 5 damage.

Traction lesion: T. Continuity is preserved. Grade 1 to 4 damage is possible.

Compression: K. The compression can be caused by acute external compression by a bone fragment or hematoma (K1) or by internal compression by nerve tissue edema, intraneural hematoma, fibrosis, or shrinkage of the epineurium (K2).

EXAMPLES OF USE OF THE FORMULA

1. A complete lesion of the brachial plexus with avulsion of all roots from C5 to T1 would be expressed as I (5, 6, 7, 8, 1), 5°, R.

2. A traction lesion of the superior trunk with preserved continuity but a destroyed fascicular pattern would be expressed as III (s), 4°, T.

3. An open transection of the lateral and dorsal cord in the infraclavicular region would be expressed as IV (1, d), 5°, O.

4. If two different levels are involved in different roots, trunks, or cords, they are listed independently separated by a slash mark (/). For example, avulsion of roots C6, C7, C8, and T1 combined with an infraganglionic lesion of C5 would be expressed as II (5), 5°, R/I, (6, 7, 8, 1) 5°, R. The same would be done with other combinations of lesions.

DIAGNOSTIC AND THERAPEUTIC CONSEQUENCES

The aim of surgical treatment in brachial plexus cases is trifold:

1. To prevent further damage by acute compression or infection in open injuries.

2. To achieve neurotization of the peripheral nerves by removing obstacles to spontaneous recovery, re-establishing continuity, and effecting nerve transfer.

3. To improve function by other surgical means, such as muscle transfer, arthrodesis, arthrolysis, tenodesis, or tendon transfer.

Category 1 comprises the surgical treatment of the acute injury, that is, the acute phase. Category 2 comprises the surgical treatment of the brachial plexus, that is, the phase of direct repair. Category 3 comprises the surgical treatment in late or failed cases, that is, the phase of indirect repair.

It is therefore useful to divide the time after a brachial plexus injury into three phases: the acute phase, the phase of direct repair, and the phase of indirect repair. The main difficulty is that brachial plexus lesions can show varying degrees of spontaneous recovery. In the majority of these cases, signs of spontaneous recovery become apparent so late that precious time is lost in cases in which no spontaneous regeneration is going to occur. Early differentiation is therefore essential.

ACUTE PHASE

When the patient is first seen, the presence of a brachial plexus lesion can easily be ascertained by clinical examination. One can differentiate between a complete and a partial lesion and in the latter case between an upper (Duchenne-Erb) and a lower lesion (Klumpke).

There are only two situations that require immediate intervention:

1. If there is an open injury (O), the wound should be treated surgically. The circumstances of the individual case determine whether primary or early secondary repair of the transected parts of the nerves is carried out. The general rules of peripheral nerve repair should be followed in these cases.

2. Immediate intervention is also indicated if there is acute external compression (K1). This can be caused by a bone fragment in a fracture of the clavicle, the first rib, or a transverse process. Removal of small fragments, repositioning, and stabilization of the fracture should be carried out. Another reason for compression is the danger of formation of a hematoma along the scalenus muscles and in the space between the clavicle and the first rib. Such hematomas should be evacuated and the fascial sheaths split.

PHASE OF DIRECT REPAIR

EARLY PHASE I (THREE TO FOUR WEEKS AFTER INJURY)

If neither of the aforementioned indications is present, conservative treatment is followed during this early phase. By neurological examination the level of the injury can be defined approximately. A lesion of the cords (IV) can be assumed if the suprascapular nerve and the thoracodorsal nerve are intact. In lesions of the trunks (III), usually the long thoracic nerve is preserved. If this nerve is also involved, a root lesion (I, II) can be assumed to be present.

Wallerian degeneration along the nerves distal to the lesion will lead to a pathological response to electrical stimulation. If palsy is present and the electrical examination (percutaneous stimulation, strength-duration curve) reveals normal results, the damage is of grade 1. There is a good chance of spontaneous recovery if there is no external compression.

EARLY PHASE II (EIGHT TO TWELVE WEEKS AFTER INJURY)

If there is grade 1 damage, during this period recovery should occur. If recovery is delayed, one has to consider whether external compression is present. Conservative treatment is continued.

In all the other cases there are two possibilities:

Recovery Starts. If a Tinel-Hoffmann sign is obtained and gradually indicates advancement toward the periphery, grade 2 damage is probably present and there is a good chance of spontaneous recovery. Conservative treatment is continued.

No Recovery. If the clinical examination reveals a trunk (III) or cord lesion (IV) at the level of the injury, a Tinel-Hoffmann sign must be present. It then remains to differentiate by further observation between grade 3, 4, or 5 damage. Conservative treatment is continued.

If there is a root lesion, it is necessary to differentiate between supraganglionic and infraganglionic lesions. Although many tests and diagnostic aids have been developed, this differentiation is difficult because combinations of all possible lesions may be present. Table 61–1 lists the results of six common examinations for four typical cases: supraganglionic lesion I, infraganglionic lesion II, an extensive lesion involving both supraganglionic and infraganglionic portions of the roots I and II, and supraganglionic lesions and infraganglionic lesions involving different roots I/II.

From a clinical point of view, the Tinel-Hoffmann sign is very useful. If it is present, one can assume that at least one root is damaged at an infraganglionic level and that axon sprouts have formed. If the sign is not obtained, the lesion is supraganglionic or both supraganglionic and infraganglionic (I and II).

If a lesion of level I or levels I and II is proved, there is no chance of spontaneous recovery nor is direct nerve repair possible. Further waiting is therefore useless. In these cases operation should be performed in this phase before further muscle atrophy develops. The brachial plexus is exposed to confirm the diagnosis. If the diagnosis is confirmed, neurotization of the distal stumps is achieved by nerve transfer using the intercostal nerves as donors.

In cases of infraganglionic damage (II) or combinations (I/II), it is necessary to clarify the degree of the damage before operation is undertaken. Conservative treatment is continued.

EARLY PHASE III (THREE TO SIX MONTHS AFTER INJURY)

In cases of grade 1 damage, recovery should be complete at this time. If not, there is internal compression (K2) and neurolysis is indicated.

In cases of grade 2 damage, recovery will progress. During this phase one should be able to differentiate between grade 3 damage and more severe damage.

In a case of grade 3 damage the Tinel-Hoffmann sign proceeds toward the periphery, and the first signs of recovery should be detectable by clinical or electrophysiological examinations.

In cases of grade 4 damage there also may be a distal movement of the Tinel-Hoffmann sign.

If there is no recovery at all and the Tinel-Hoffmann sign remains at the site of the lesion, one can assume the existence of grade 5 damage or that regeneration is being prevented by external or internal compression (K1, K2).

In all cases without signs of recovery during phase II, operation is indicated (Fig. 61–1). If there is loss of continuity (grade 5 damage, R), the two ends are united by end to end suturing or by nerve grafting after the neuroma and the damaged parts have been resected.

If continuity is preserved (T, K2, K3), external neurolysis is first carried out; that is, the epineurium is split and resected. Then an

Table 61–1. DIFFERENTIAL DIAGNOSIS OF ROOT LESIONS

	I	II	I and II	I/II
Tinel-Hoffmann	Neg.	Pos.	Neg.	Pos.
Electromyography sensory conduction	Normal	Nil	Nil	
Axon reflexes	Pos.	Neg.	Neg.	
Sweat test	Pos.	Neg.	Neg.	Different according to segment
Electromyography of posterior cervical muscles	Neg.	Normal	Neg.	
Myelography	Meningocele or defect	Normal	Pos. or neg.	

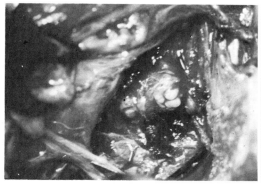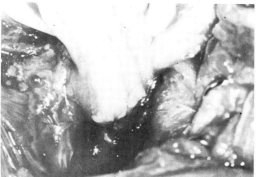

Figure 61–1. Root lesion interruption. *A*, Stumps of the roots C5 and C6 after resection of the neuroma. *B*, The cross sections are covered by sural nerve grafts.

internal neurolysis is performed. In cases of grade 3 damage the operation is then complete. If there is grade 4 damage, resection of the damaged part and re-establishment of continuity by nerve grafting are indicated.

LATE PHASE OF DIRECT REPAIR (AFTER SIX MONTHS)

Patients with grade 1 damage should already have recovered.

In the majority of cases with grade 2 damage, regeneration proceeds during this phase until a useful degree of recovery is reached. If not, or especially if deterioration develops, there is an obstruction, probably as a result of external compression (K1), and neurolysis is indicated.

All other cases showing signs of recovery have had grade 3 damage. This recovery must progress steadily. If there is a prolonged period without signs of recovery, exploration is indicated.

SUMMARY OF THE PHASE OF DIRECT REPAIR

1. Immediate operation is indicated in cases of acute compression or open injury.

2. During early phase I, a rough estimation of the level of injury is possible and cases of grade 1 damage can be differentiated.

3. During early phase II, cases of grade 2 damage can be recognized. The diagnosis of supraganglionic (I) or supraganglionic and infraganglionic (I and II) lesions should be established, and as a consequence, when confirmed by exposure, an intercostal nerve transfer should be performed.

4. During early phase III in all other cases showing no recovery or no satisfactory recovery, neurolysis should be performed or continuity re-established.

5. Direct repair should be accomplished within six months.

6. In the late phase, direct repair is done when after some spontaneous recovery, no further progress is seen.

PHASE OF INDIRECT REPAIR

There are no time limits on this phase of repair.

When the final functional gain following spontaneous recovery or surgery can be evaluated, one should determine the additional functional gain that would be of greatest benefit for the patient. The following procedures are at one's disposal:

1. Arthrodesis of the shoulder joint.

2. Dorsal fixation of the scapula if the clavicle is absent.

3. Transfer of the pectoralis major for partial replacement of the deltoid muscle.

4. Transfer of the pectoralis major to achieve active flexion of the elbow joint (Clark) and transfer of the common head of the forearm flexors to the numeral shaft to achieve active elbow flexion (Steindler).

5. Arthrodesis of the elbow joint.

6. Arthrodesis of the wrist joint.

7. All the other transfers described for irreparable peripheral nerve lesions may be used in cases of partial recovery.

The island flap technique or sensory nerve transfer can be considered if good motor recovery is present with a lack of sensation in important areas.

As more function is achieved by direct

repair, better use can be made of these indirect operations. If motor function by nerve transfer could be achieved in the biceps muscle, the pectoralis major could be used to improve the mobility of the shoulder joint. If not, the pectoralis major muscle must be transferred to the biceps tendon to provide elbow flexion.

The final step in the plan of treatment is amputation at different levels. When all the possibilities of direct and indirect repair have been exhausted, the parts of the arm still without function should be amputated.

In many cases of complete brachial plexus lesions with root involvement (I, II), the level of amputation will be the forearm because the chance for recovery of function in the distal muscles is not good. However, a sensible and workable forearm stump fitted with a good prosthesis is better than a high amputation. This can be considered to have been worthwhile if one has been successful in moving the level of amputation toward the periphery. This was not necessary during the last 10 years.

SURGICAL TECHNIQUE

INCISION

Wide access is necessary and therefore a large incision has to be used. We prefer an incision that starts high in the neck and follows the dorsal border of the sternocleidomastoid muscle. It then continues laterally along the clavicle and in a zigzag fashion down the ventral axillary fold to the arm.

The triangular skin flaps are undermined and reflected. The external jugular vein is ligated. The cervical fascia is split and the scalenus anterior exposed.

ROOT DISSECTION

On the surface of the scalenus muscle, one encounters the phrenic nerve. If one follows this nerve proximally, one usually arrives without difficulty at the C4 root, which is not involved in brachial plexus lesions. Once the layer is defined in normal tissue, it is relatively easy to find the other roots; they emerge between the scalenus anterior and the scalenus medius muscles. Under normal conditions, dissection in the layer between these two muscles is easy, but in brachial

Table 61–2. BRACHIAL PLEXUS LESIONS
1963–1978

Treatment continuing		47
Treatment completed		104
Complete palsy		
Root lesion	44	
Peripheral lesion	20	
Partial palsy		
Root lesion	32	
Peripheral lesion	8	
Total		151

plexus lesions the two muscles, especially the scalenus medius muscle, show fibrotic changes, which make blunt dissection impossible. This muscle fibrosis suggests that an ischemic process may play a role in the pathogenesis of some of the plexus lesions.

The roots lie between the anterior and posterior tubercles of the transverse processes within the sulcus nervi spinalis. The axillary artery is situated in front of the roots. Starting cranially, the roots C5, C6, and C7 are exposed. The lower roots lie between the cupola pleurae and the thoracic wall. Sometimes they can be dissected more easily after distal dissection.

DISTAL DISSECTION

By dissecting between the clavicular part of the deltoid and the pectoralis major muscle, the cephalic vein is exposed and retracted to the lateral side. After the fascia of the infraclavicular fossa has been split, the first major structure encountered is the lateral cord. As the dissection at the lateral side proceeds, the dorsal cord is encountered.

PATHOLOGICAL FEATURES

If root involvement is suspected, the dissection should always start by exposure of the roots. If no proximal stump is encountered, the diagnosis of a supraganglionic lesion is confirmed. A nerve transfer may be carried out (neurotization).

Table 61–3. BRACHIAL PLEXUS LESIONS

Complete Palsy	N	Useful Function
Root lesion	44	28
Peripheral lesion	20	18
Total	64	46

Table 61–4. BRACHIAL PLEXUS LESIONS

Partial Palsy	N	Useful Function
Root lesion	32	26
Peripheral lesion	8	7
Total	40	33

If roots can be defined as short stumps containing nondegenerated nerve tissue, restoration of continuity is indicated.

If there is no loss of continuity, dissection should follow the roots in a peripheral direction into the supraclavicular fossa. Usually the dissection becomes more and more difficult because of scar tissue. Therefore, it is better to start the distal dissection distal to the lesion in healthy tissue.

On a deeper plane and medial to the lateral cord, the posterior cord is exposed near the clavicle. More distally in the infraclavicular fossa, the medial cord, having crossed the subclavian artery, is found medial to the artery. The subclavian vein is more medial still.

After definition of all structures the dissection follows them in a central direction. The clavicle is freed from muscle in this area and elevated. The subclavian muscle is partially split.

Osteotomy of the clavicle gives a better view, but there is some risk to bone healing. Callus formation may cause a narrowing of the space under the clavicle. Therefore, we do not recommend osteotomy. By lifting the clavicle in a cranial or caudal direction, a satisfactory approach can be achieved.

EXTERNAL NEUROLYSIS

In quite a few cases one may find scar tissue with or without disruption of the plexus structures (K2). The scar tissue is carefully removed, and the space under the clavicle is

Table 61–5. BRACHIAL PLEXUS LESIONS: PALLIATIVE SURGERY

Triceps to biceps	10
Pectoralis major	2
Pectoralis minor	1
Latissimus dorsi	5
Trapezius	1
Tendon transfer	
As for radial nerve palsy	4
Arthrodesis, wrist joint, and tenodesis	7
Total	30

widened. The brachial plexus can then be inspected from the roots to the infraclavicular fossa.

If continuity is preserved (T, K2, K3), external neurolysis is completed by excising the fibrotic tissue in the area of the scalenus muscles. The dissection of the roots of C8 and T1 is completed, and the trunks and cords are isolated. The dissection is continued into the axillary groove. Sometimes the pectoralis minor muscle forms a fibrotic constricting band across the cords.

In cases of external compression the operation is finished at this point (K2).

INTERNAL NEUROLYSIS

If the trunks themselves are scarred, the epineurium is split and deflected. It is often thickened and forms a constricting stocking around the nerve tissue (K3). After resection of this part of the epineurium, one sees the nerve tissue expand. In grade 3 and 4 lesions there may be considerable fibrous tissue between the fasciculi or replacing them. The fibrous tissue is excised with the aid of the operating microscope. In grade 3 lesions it is possible to free the remaining structures and give them a chance for spontaneous regeneration. Areas of grade 4 damage should be resected and the defect bridged by nerve grafts. Grade 3 and 4 damage is often present in the same patient and even in the same trunk.

LOSS OF CONTINUITY

If loss of continuity is diagnosed preoperatively and one finds the distal elements of the plexus intact, distal exposure is performed (Fig. 61–2). One starts at the distal healthy parts; the elements of the brachial plexus are followed in a proximal direction until they lose their normal appearance. This point represents the distal end of the lesion. It is not worth performing further dissection, because the fibrotic part is not suitable for neurotization and must be resected.

The trunks and cords consist of many rather small fasciculi, and fibers of different functions are distributed diffusely over the cross section. Therefore, the principles of interfascicular nerve grafting cannot be applied in the same way as in the peripheral nerves (Fig. 61–3).

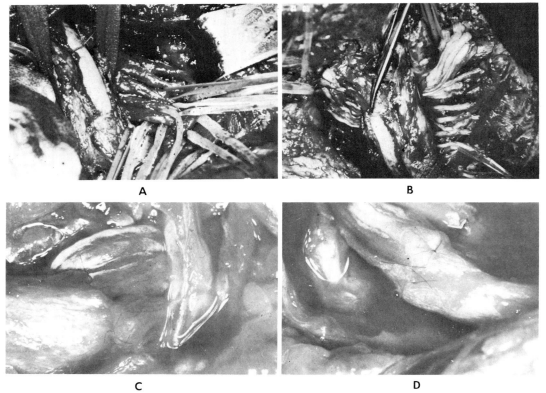

A   B

C   D

Figure 61–2. Peripheral lesions. *A*, The trunks have been explored in the supraclavicular fossa. Shown is the infraclavicular fossa with the vein, the artery, and the medial, lateral, and dorsal cords exposed. *B*, The grafts are in place before performing the coaptation. *C*, A close-up view after coaptation of the stump of a trunk connected with the proximal ends of nerve grafts (right). *D*, View of the distal ends of the grafts connected with the stumps of cords. The operation is performed with minimal exposure and without transection of the clavicle.

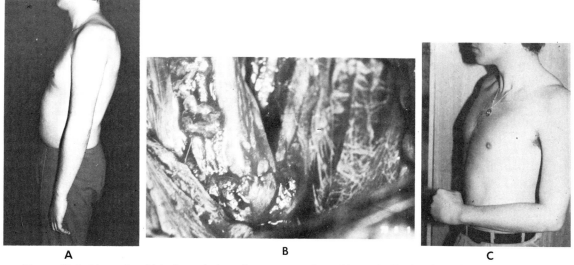

A   B   C

Figure 61–3. Upper brachial plexus lesion after motor cycle accident. *A*, Exploration nine months after the accident. A fourth-degree lesion of roots C5, C6, and the upper trunk was present. Continuity was restored by four cutaneous nerve grafts 6 cm. in length (cutaneous antebrachii medialis). *B*, The distal site of coaptation between grafts (left) and the distal stump (right). *C*, Thirteen months after surgery, good control of shoulder motion and forceful elbow flexion have returned.

Usually there are long defects. If all five roots are ruptured or transected with suitable stumps, it may be difficult to provide enough material to bridge all the defects. In clinical practice these cases seem to be rare.

In all of our cases of complete brachial plexus lesions with root involvement, there was a combination of supraganglionic and infraganglionic lesions. There were three different types:

1. Root C5 interrupted with a suitable stump. Roots C6, C7, C8, and T1 were avulsed (supraganglionic lesion). Formula II, (5), 5°, R/I (6, 7, 8, 1) 5°, R.

In these cases the ulnar nerve is excised and used as a graft. The ulnar nerve was successfully used as a free graft after excision of the epifascicular epineurium and splitting of the nerve in longitudinal direction into smaller units. There is also the possibility of using this nerve as a vascularized nerve graft, following the suggestion of Taylor and Ham (1975). In addition, the two sural nerves and the radial cutaneous nerve of the forearm were applied as grafts.

The root stump of C5 is connected with the distal stump of the dorsal cord, and the accessory nerve is transected distal to its first branches and is connected by a nerve graft with the distal stump of the suprascapular nerve. An intercostal nerve transfer is performed, bringing the axons of C2, C3, and C4 to the median nerve and C5, C6, C7 to the musculocutaneous nerve. In some cases, as a result of the work of Brunnelli (1980), the motor components of the cervical plexus (C3 and C4) were used for neurotization.

2. Root C5 and C6 were interrupted distal to the ganglion with suitable stumps. Roots C7, C8, and T1 were avulsed. Formula II (5, 6) 5°, R°/I (6, 8, 1) 5°, R.

Again the ulnar nerve can be utilized as a graft. The root of C5 is connected with the dorsal cord and the root of C6 with the lateral cord. Intercostal nerve transfers are effected to the thoracodorsal nerve and that portion of the median nerve coming from the medial cord.

3. Roots C5, C6, and C7 were interrupted distal to the ganglion with suitable stumps. Roots C8 and T1 were avulsed. Formula II (5, 6, 7) 5°, R/I (8, 1) 5°, R.

In this case also the ulnar nerve can be used as a donor. C5 is connected with the dorsal cord and C6 and C7 with the lateral cord, including the portion of the median nerve coming from the medial cord.

It should be emphasized that in all cases, avulsion of the roots has to be demonstrated by exploration. It would be wrong to perform a nerve transfer without confirming the avulsion. It is equally dangerous to utilize the ulnar nerve as a donor without demonstrating the avulsion of C8 and T1 (Fig. 61–4).

NERVE TRANSFER (NEUROTIZATION)

Good results using nerve transfer in brachial plexus lesions have been reported by Seddon (1963), Tsuyama et al. (1968), Kotany et al. (1971), and Millesi et al. (1973). The accessory nerve and a different number of intercostal nerves can be used as donors. There are two techniques available:

1. The intercostal nerves can be dissected as far distant as possible to provide sufficient length. The nerves are then rerouted and united directly with the distal stump.

2. The intercostal nerves are exposed below the axilla and transected there. They are united by nerve grafts to the distal recipient stumps. This technique has the advantage that the nerves are thicker at the level of transection and contain many more motor axons than at their extremities. The disadvantage, at least from a theoretical point of view, is that a graft has to be used.

SENSORY TRANSFER

In patients with some function remaining in the hand but with a lack of sensibility in the pulp of the thumb and index finger, the following operation can be done: The site of division of the median nerve in the palm is exposed. The branches to thumb and index finger are defined. The median nerve is dissected in a proximal direction, following the sensory fasciculi for the thumb and index finger. In spite of the changing fascicular pattern, it is possible to continue well up into the forearm. The intercostobrachial nerve is exposed in the axilla and followed as far distal as possible into the arm. The two nerve ends are united by a graft. Useful protective sensibility can be achieved.

CONCLUSION

A brachial plexus lesion is a severe handicap, and any improvement in function will

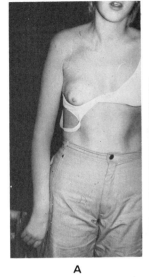

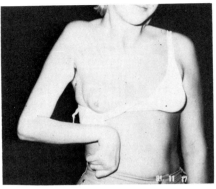

A   B

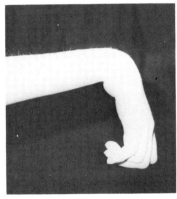

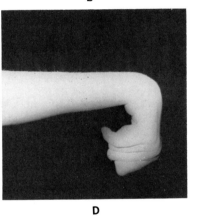

C   D

Figure 61–4. Complete right brachial plexus lesion after traffic accident. Root avulsion of C6, C7, and C8 has been confirmed by computerized tomography. At exploration six months after the accident, root C5 was interrupted and C6, C7, and C8 were avulsed, as anticipated. Root T1 was fibrotic but in continuity. Continuity was restored between C5 and the dorsal root. Neurolysis of T1 was performed, as well as intercostal nerve transfer (intercostal nerves 3, 4, 5, 6, 7) to the lateral source of the median nerve (3, 4) and to the musculocutaneous nerve (5, 6, 7).

At follow-up 22 months after the operation (A), the patient has good control of the shoulder joint (C5) and elbow flexion (intercostal nerve transfer) (B). Strong wrist and finger flexion returned by regeneration along root T1 after neurolysis (C, D). There is no wrist or finger extension. Protective sensibility returned in the median nerve area.

In a second operation, an arthrodesis of the wrist joint was performed and the wrist flexors transferred to provide thumb and finger extension. Although it is often suggested that the ulnar nerve can be used as a graft, it is important to state that this can be done only if complete loss of continuity of C8 and T1 or of the inferior trunk has been proved by direct vision.

be gratefully accepted by the patient. The results are far from satisfactory, and we are still in a phase of development. Successful cases are impressive, but unsuccessful attempts also have to be faced. In the case of failure, amputation can still be done and the patient can be fitted with a prosthesis. The main problem is to speed up the course of reconstructive procedures to prevent muscle atrophy. If we can do this, the loss of time in the failed cases will not be so important. With increasing experience and development we will achieve further improvement in our results.

REFERENCES

Allieu, Y., and Rabischon, S.: Systematisation des nerfs. Presented at Congress of G.E.M., Marseille, 1970.

Bateman, J. E.: Trauma to Nerves in Limbs. Philadelphia, W. B. Saunders Company, 1962.

Brunelli, G.: Neurotisation of avulsed roots of the brachial plexus by means of anterior nerves of the cervical plexus. Intern. J. Microsurg., 2:55–58, 1980.

Clark, J.: Reconstruction of biceps brachii by pectoral muscle transplantation. Br. Surg., 34:180–181, 1946.

Hendry, A. M.: The treatment of residual paralysis after brachial plexus injuries. J. Bone Joint Surg., 31:42–49, 1949.

Kotani, G. T., Toyoshima, Y., Matsuda, H., Suzuki, T., Ishizaki, Y., Iwani, H., Yamano, K., Inoue, H., Moriguchi, T., Ri, S., and Asada, K.: The postoperative results of nerve transfer for the brachial plexus injury with root avulsion. Proceedings, 14th Annual Meeting, Japanese Society for Surgery of the Hand, Osaka, 1971.

Lange, M.: Die Bedeutung der orthopädischen Ersatzoperation für die Behandlung der irreparablen peripheren Nervenlähmungen. Med. Klin., 57:627, 1962.

Maurer, G., and Schmidt, H.: Verletzungen der peripheren Nerven. In Maurer, G., and Schmidt, H. (Editors): Neuro-Traumatologie, Kessel-Guttmann-Maurer, Munich, Urban & Schwarzenberg, 1971.

Millesi, H., Meissl, G., and Katzer, H.: Zur Behandlung der Verletzung des Plexus brachialis Vorschlag einer integrierten Therapie. Bruns' Beitr. Klin. Chir., 220:429–446, 1973.

Narakas, A.: Plexobraquial, terapeutica quirurgica directa, tecnica, indicacion operatoria y resultados. *In* Cirugía de los nervios perifericos. A.S. Palazzi Duarte et coll. Madrid, Tipografia Artistica Alameda, 1972, pp. 339–404.

Pecinka, H.: Plexusverletzungen. 2. Tagung Österr. Ges. Unfallchir., *9*:S258–260, 1960a.

Pecinka, H.: Die operative Behandlung der traumatischen Lähmungen des Plexus brachialis. Zbl. Chir., *85*:1678–1682, 1960b.

Rohr, H.: Untersuchungen über die Segmentinnervation des Hals-Schulter-Armgebietes bei cervikalen Wurzellaesionen. Langenbeck's Arch. Klin. Chir., *301*:873–879, 1962.

Seddon, H. J.: Nerve grafting. J. Bone Joint Surg., *45*:447, 1963.

Seddon, H. J.: Surgical Disorders of the Peripheral Nerves. Churchill Livingstone, 1972.

Steindler, A.: The Traumatic Deformities and Disabilities of the Upper Extremity. Springfield, Illinois, Charles C Thomas, 1946.

Sunderland, S.: A classification of peripheral nerve injuries producing loss of function. Brain, *74*:491, 1951.

Sunderland, S.: Nerve and Nerve Injuries. Baltimore, The Williams & Wilkins Company, 1968.

Taylor, G. I., and Ham, F. Z.: The free vascularized nerve graft. Plast. Reconstr. Surg., *56*:166–170, 1975.

Tsuyama, N., Sakaguchi, R., Hara, T., Kondo, T., Kaminuma, S., Ijichi, M., and Ryn, D.: Reconstructive surgery in brachial plexus injuries. Proceedings, 11th Annual Meeting, Japanese Society of the Hand, Hiroshima, 1968, pp. 39–40.

Weber, E.: Diagnostik und Therapie der Plexusverletzungen im Halsbereich. Langenbecks Arch. Klin. Chir., *301*:881–885, 1962.

Yeoman, P. M., and Seddon, H. J.: Brachial plexus injuries, treatment of the flail arm. J. Bone Joint Surg., *43*:493, 1961.

Chapter 62

NEUROTIZATION OR NERVE TRANSFER IN TRAUMATIC BRACHIAL PLEXUS LESIONS

Algimantas O. Narakas

Neurotization or nerve transfer is used to reinnervate a sensory or motor territory of particular value that has been denervated because of central or peripheral nerve lesions. For this purpose a functional nerve of less value than the one destroyed is used. It must contain a significant number of fibers analogous to those to be replaced and not be essential to the part of the body from which it will be separated.

The healthy donor nerve is cut, and its proximal stump is connected to the postlesional, distal portion of the destroyed nerve or to a denervated muscle or insensitive skin. Union between the donor nerve and the recipient is obtained by direct suturing or implantation, while intermediate nerve grafts are used to bridge a possible gap between the two.

Neurotization implies theoretically five possibilities: cutaneocutaneous neurotization, musculomuscular neurotization, neuromuscular neurotization, neurocutaneous neurotization, and neuroneural (motor or sensory) neurotization. In every variety the donor nerve is meant to provide axonal regrowth sprouts to the recipient.

We will deal only briefly with the first four varieties, emphasizing neuroneural neurotization, particularly when applied to traumatic lesions of the brachial plexus.

CUTANEOCUTANEOUS NEUROTIZATION

Healthy skin eventually spontaneously reinnervates neighboring denervated skin. Skin grafts, skin flaps, or insensitive skin is progressively invaded by collateral sprouting from normally innervated skin in the vicinity. The quality and extension of this colonization remain limited. The progression of sprouts seems to be a matter of chance. Specific receptor organ reinnervation is irregular. In this chapter we will not consider the complex events occurring in this type of neurotization but will discuss the frequently incomplete, patchy, and disharmonious recovery of the different modalities of sensation.

MUSCULOMUSCULAR NEUROTIZATION

Heineke working on the rabbit demonstrated in 1914 that healthy muscle can provide some axonal collateral sprouts to neighboring paralyzed muscle, provided an intimate anatomical contact exists between the two. Erlacher (1914) confirmed this finding, stating, however, that the functional results were poor. Thirty years later Van Harreveld (1945) described the basic mechanisms of this type of neurotization while studying the reinnervation of partially paralyzed muscles.

More recently musculomuscular neurotization has been applied clinically in some specific conditions, as for instance in facial nerve palsy. Thompson (1971) proposed the transfer to the face of the previously denervated extensor brevis of the toes or the palmaris longus. Clinical practice has confirmed the laboratory findings: the reinnervation remains limited and is synchronous with the action of the muscle supplying the axonal sprouts. In addition there is a deficiency in feedback. The sprouts of the efferent motor fibers are able to spread over the surface of the recipient muscle and establish efficient end plates that will allow voluntary contraction of the reinnervated muscle. The afferent fibers, however, have little capacity for the production of new receptors. The muscular fibers and afferent organs remaining in the denervated muscle that are not yet completely degenerated are only by chance reached by axonal sprouts of analogous specificity.

Some of the instances of spontaneous and partial reanimation of muscles in man, particularly of the pectoralis major in cases of Erb's palsy, could be explained by musculomuscular neurotization. In the absence of recovery of the upper trunk, the lower sternal portion of the muscle innervated by the intact medial cord may after a few years effect reinnervation of the upper clavicular portion of the muscle.

NEUROMUSCULAR NEUROTIZATION AND HYPERNEUROTIZATION

According to Steindler (1915), Gersuny (1906) succeeded in 1906 in hyperneurotizing a normally innervated muscle, implanting into it an additional nerve. Later workers did the same, but soon it was apparent that the additional innervation remained very localized, limited to the area of implantation of the supplementing nerve. Aitken studied the phenomenon again in 1950, noting that his predecessors had damaged the muscle fibers during implantation and had denervated them, hyperneurotization being effective only at that level. Actually the so-called hyperneurotization was a reinnervation, a neuromuscular neurotization. As a result of Aitken's work as well as of other researchers, hyperneurotization was discarded; it was admitted that a normally innervated muscle could not accept additional innervation.

Heineke in 1914 succeeded in reinnervating a paralyzed muscle in the rabbit, implanting a functional motor nerve directly into it. Steindler (1916) achieved the same result a year later in the dog. Elsberg in 1917, Weiss in 1930, and Fort in 1940 confirmed these results. Aitken (1950) demonstrated clearly that when a proper technique was used, the implanted nerve established functional motor end plates in the paralyzed muscle.

The research of that period demonstrated the great complexity of the normal innervation of muscles in mammalians, particularly the complexity of reinnervation after paralysis. The direct influence of the denervated muscular fibers on axonal sprouting, the myogenic capabilities of the latter, and the existence of reciprocal tropism were demonstrated even in vitro in the rat by Peterson and Crane (1972) and other researchers.

Sorbie and Porter (1969) quantified the results of neuromuscular neurotization in the dog. After excision of the motor nerve to the flexor carpi radialis (to paralyze it completely), they implanted into it the distal nerve of the flexor carpi ulnaris. The neurotizer produced new motor end plates, while the old ones degenerated in about 40 weeks. Once the plate had regenerated, a muscle fiber became refractory to the establishment of other motor plates. At least half the original strength was recovered. The number of motor axons in the donor nerve proved to be critical for the result. The fate of the spindle efferent and muscle afferent axons in the transferred nerve was not clear. In clinical cases, however, the neurotized muscle was able to function almost normally.

In 1976 Brunelli et al. found evidence not only of efferent motor reinnervation but also of afferent reinnervation, using electron microscopy.

AVULSION OF NERVES FROM MUSCLE

Direct implantation of nerves into denervated muscle is of importance in reconstructive surgery of the upper limb. Industrial, agricultural, construction, and road traffic accidents are responsible for severe mutilations of the upper limb and produce multifocal nerve lesions. In addition to brachial plexus lesions implying root avulsion and trunk or cord ruptures, peripheral nerve lesions are witnessed; a nerve is avulsed at its entry point into the muscle, frequently leaving no distal stump that can be used for repair (Fig. 62–1).

Important nerves, such as the median, radial, and musculocutaneous, may be injured in this way, the other site of injury being

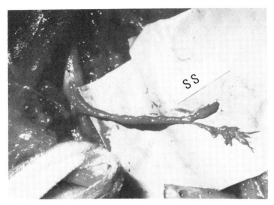

Figure 62–1. Avulsion of the terminal rami of the suprascapular (SS) nerve from the supraspinatus and infraspinatus muscles on the left side of a patient who also had a crush injury to his lateral and posterior cords underneath the clavicle. The latter was divided to explore the injured structures.

found at the plexus (Fig. 62–2). In these cases the muscular rami are avulsed, and the main trunk is ruptured at about the same level but retracted proximally, disconnected from surrounding tissues for long distances, up to 20 cm. Modern surgical procedures can effect the survival of limbs affected by these severe injuries, but serious problems are encountered in rendering them functional. Motor rami can be implanted into muscles, either directly or with the help of intermediate nerve grafts, incising the perimysium. The survival of the main nerve trunk depends mostly on its vascularization and that of the grafts re-establishing its continuity.

Results obtained by the author during the last 10 years, as well as those of Brunelli and Fontana (1982), confirm the validity of neuromuscular neurotization.

NEUROCUTANEOUS NEUROTIZATION

According to Brunelli (1983), it is possible to proceed in the same way for denervated skin. Sensory nerve fascicles or grafts prolonging them are implanted into the deep layers of the skin. Instead of forming neuromas they seemingly provide axonal sprouts that reinnervate the skin. This phenomenon seems to occur in all instances of reinnervation after a superficial wound or surgical incision. This type of neurotization is sometimes associated with pronounced and unpleasant paresthesias, which may persist for months.

NEURONEURAL NEUROTIZATION

In 1873 Letievant proposed the lateral implantation into a healthy nerve of the distal stump of an irreparable nerve. This technique and varieties of it resulted in failures. Direct transfer of a functioning nerve onto an injured nerve, e.g., transfer of the spinal accessory or hypoglossal nerve onto the facial nerve, was used successfully but sometimes with grotesque results.

With regard to brachial plexus injuries, the British neurologist Harris and the surgeon Low were the first to perform a neurotization

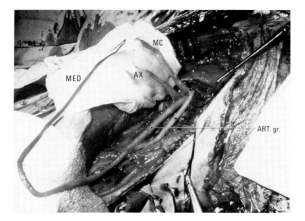

Figure 62–2. Emergency exploration of an infraclavicular lesion of several nerves near their origin and a rupture of the axillary artery, which in this picture is already repaired by a venous graft. There is a rupture of the axillary nerve at the quadrangular space, a low rupture of the musculocutaneous nerve, and a rupture of the ulnar and radial nerves with a very distal avulsion of the median nerve in the forearm, which was fractured. The median nerve was found rolled on itself in the axillary region. This patient was involved in a motorcycle accident and, in addition to fractures of the lower limbs and rupture of the spleen, also had a rupture of the suprascapular nerve at the scapular notch. This latter diagnosis was missed initially and was detected only later when the axillary nerve had recovered but no proper shoulder function could be obtained. Arthrography excluded a rotator cuff rupture. MED = median nerve, AX = axillary nerve, MC = musculocutaneous nerve, and ART gr = grafted axillary artery. The ruptured ulnar and radial nerves cannot be seen in this picture.

in 1903, implanting the distal stump of the ruptured C5 spinal nerve or at least some of its fascicles into the uninjured spinal nerves C6 or C7. They did not report the detailed results in their three cases but stated only that the partial lesion of C6 or C7 did not worsen the condition of their patients.

Tuttle in 1913 considered neurotization of the upper trunk with the spinal accessory nerve, reflecting current practice at that time. Being unable to do so because of the distance between the plexus trunks and the accessory nerve, he used deep motor rami of the cervical plexus. The results in his single case are not known.

Spontaneous neurotization is known to occur after traction injuries to the brachial plexus, particularly in Erb-Duchenne obstetrical palsy. The phrenic nerve or its accessory branches may rupture together with the upper trunk and come into contact with nerve fascicles in the distal part of C5, reinnervating the upper portion of the pectoralis major or the biceps. Muscle contractions synchronous with respiration can be observed in these cases. This has been confirmed more recently by electromyography in both children and adults.

Vulpius and Stoffel (1920), Förster (1929), Steindler (1946), and to a greater extent the Russian surgeon Lurje (1948) (Fig. 62–3) performed different types of neuroneural transfer in irreparable lesions near the plexus or of the plexus itself. Yeomann (1979), working with Seddon (1972), introduced the use of intercostal nerves for neurotization (Figs. 62–4, 62–5), a procedure soon thereafter used by Fantiš et al. (1967). Harris (1921) suggested use of the superficial branch of the radial nerve at the wrist, and Peacock (1963) used the ulnar nerve to neurotize the median nerve. These various techniques are summarized in Table 62–1.

The increase in severe lesions of the brachial plexus in the last 15 years, particularly in patients sustaining multiple trauma who did not survive years ago, as well as the increase in root avulsions, induced Japanese surgeons, such as Kotani and his coworkers (1972) and Tsuyama and Hara (1972), to perform neurotization more often, using the spinal accessory and intercostal nerves (Figs. 62–6, 62–7).

Present-day brachial plexus surgeons are somewhat eclectic in the choice of the type of neurotization they perform. They may use whatever is at their disposal as a source of axons, knowing the value of each and avoiding the aggravation of deficits already present (Allieu et al., 1982; Brunelli, 1980; Celli et al., 1978; Gilbert; Merle, 1980; Millesi, 1983; Morelli, 1983; Narakas, 1982; Sedel, 1982; Sugioka, 1983). Only during the last five years have the techniques of neurotization become more common, and because several years are necessary to evaluate the results, particularly when neurotizing the fibers of the median or ulnar nerve, it is no wonder that world medical literature offers fewer than 10 articles on the subject.

AVULSION OF THE SPINAL ROOTS

In injuries producing an elongation of the brachial plexus between the vertebrae and

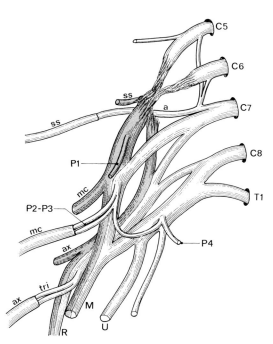

Figure 62–3. Lurje's proposal for nerve transfers in a non-suturable upper trunk C5-C6 lesion (the destroyed and degenerated nerve pathways are shown in gray). The long thoracic nerve of Bell is connected to the suprascapular nerve. Several functional rami of the anterior thoracic nerves for the pectorals coming from an intact C7 are transferred onto the musculocutaneous nerve, and two superior rami for the triceps are connected to the axillary nerve. a = long thoracic nerve of Bell, ss = suprascapular nerve, P1 to P4 = anterior thoracic nerves for the pectorals, ax = axillary nerve, R = radial nerve, U = ulnar nerve, M = median nerve, tri = rami for the triceps, and mc = musculocutaneous nerve.

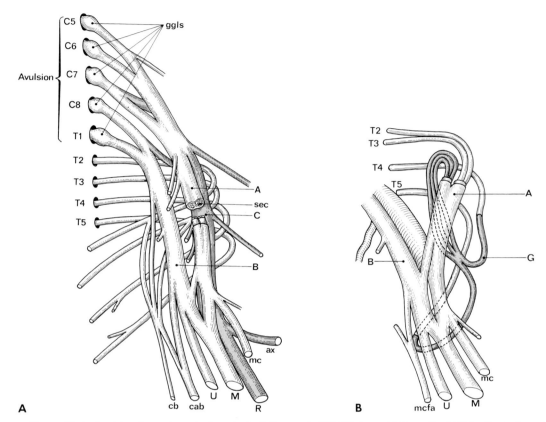

Figure 62–4. Avulsion from the spinal cord of all five roots (C5-T1) in a girl from the Middle East who refused upper arm amputation. Yeoman and Seddon performed a shoulder arthrodesis, amputated the forearm in the middle third for the later fitting of a prosthesis, and transferred intercostal nerves T3 and T4 onto the musculocutaneous nerve, utilizing the useless ulnar nerve as an intermediate graft. They obtained protective sensation of the stump and active flexion of the elbow.

A and *B*, These drawings show a modification of the original salvage procedure, which is an alternative to amputation of the upper arm. All the roots of the plexus are avulsed from the spinal cord; the spinal ganglia protrude at the outer margin of the foraminal canal. At surgery, the lateral cord was transected in its midportion and the distal fascicles were prepared for suture (drawing on right). Using the medial cutaneous nerves for the arm and forearm as an intermediate graft (originating from T1 and T2), the intercostal nerves T2 and T5 are connected to the distal fascicles of the lateral cord in order to neurotize the fibers of the musculocutaneous nerve and some fibers of the median nerve. Utilizing this technique, it is possible to obtain active flexion of the elbow and possibly of the wrist, as well as protective sensation of the thumb and index finger and possibly of the long finger. Because of the frequent anastomosis between the median and musculocutaneous nerves (in about 20 per cent of cases), this procedure has a greater chance for a safe result than the isolated neurotization of the musculocutaneous nerve.

A = lateral cord, B = medial cord, C = posterior cord, G = graft, mc = musculocutaneous nerve, T2 to T5 = intercostal nerves, R = radial nerve, M = median nerve, U = ulnar nerve, cab = medial cutaneous nerve of the arm, ggls = dorsal root ganglia, sec = surgical transection, and ax = axillary nerve.

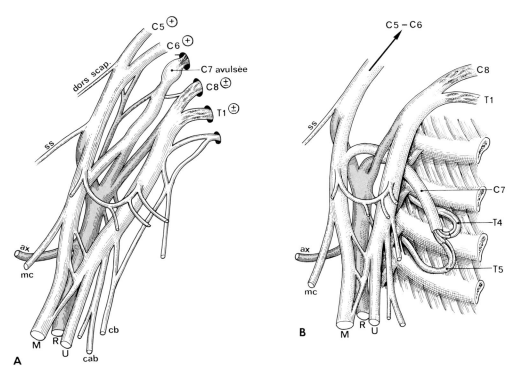

Figure 62–5. *A* and *B*, Isolated avulsion of C7 with integrity of C5 and C6, including the fibers originating from these structures. C8 and T1 are partially damaged but react to perioperative electrical stimulation. The only solution is to neurotize C7 with intercostal nerves T4 and T5, which are unusually well developed in this case. Based on testing, the neurotizing fibers went into the inferior part of the latissimus dorsi and the long head of the triceps. No sensory cross-over was noted. Abbreviations: see preceding illustrations.

Table 62–1. NEURONERVOUS TRANSFERS IN MEDICAL LITERATURE

Letievant, 1873 (France)	Lateral implantation of the stumps of a ruptured nerve into a healthy neighboring nerve.
Harris and Low, 1903 (UK)	Transfer of some healthy proximal fascicles of C6 onto the distal stump of ruptured C5, or of some fascicles of C7 onto ruptured distal C6.
Tuttle, 1913 (USA)	Sensory and motor rami of the cervical plexus deviated onto ruptured upper trunk.
	Accessory spinal nerve transferred onto the upper trunk.
Vulpius and Stoffel, 1920 (Germany)	Transfer of healthy rami for the pectoral muscle onto the ruptured musculo-cutaneous or axillary nerves.
Harris, 1929 (USA)	Sensory superficial branch of the radial nerve deviated onto the damaged median nerve.
Foerster 1929 (Germany)	Transfer of the thoracodorsal nerve (for the latissimus dorsi) onto the axil-lary nerve:
	—of the subscapular nerve onto the axillary nerve
	—of the long thoracic nerve onto the upper trunk
	—of nerves for the pectorals onto the musculocutaneous nerve
Steindler, 1946 (USA)	Transfer of the subscapular nerve onto the long thoracic nerve.
Lurje, 1948 (USSR)	Long thoracic nerve deviated onto the suprascapular nerve.
	Pectoral nerves onto the musculocutaneous nerve.
	One or two rami for the triceps onto the axillary nerve.
Peacock, 1963 (USA)	Ulnar nerve deviated onto the median nerve.
Seddon and Yeoman, 1963 (UK)	Transfer of intercostal nerves onto the musculocutaneous nerve.
Kotani et al., 1964–1972* (Japan)	Spinal accessory nerve deviated onto the upper trunk, the posterior cord, the musculocutaneous nerve.
	Intercostal nerves onto C8, the medial cord, the ulnar, the median, radial, and musculocutaneous nerves.
Tsuyama et al., 1965–1972* (Japan)	Intercostal nerves deviated onto the musculocutaneous nerve.
Fantiš, 1967 (Czechoslovakia)	Intercostal nerves deviated onto different parts of the avulsed plexus.
Narakas, 1972 (Switzerland)	Intraplexal transfers, i.e., some proximal fascicles of a ruptured spinal nerve onto an avulsed root, other parts of destroyed plexus, and use of the above-mentioned methods.
Gilbert, 1983 (France)	Transfer of the healthy pectoral nerves from the contralateral side onto the
Fossati and Iriguaray, (Uruguay)	musculocutaneous nerve in the affected side in two stages with a long intermediate graft.

*Date of publication

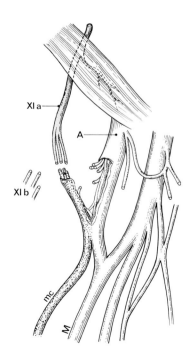

Figure 62–6. The use of the terminal rami of the spinal accessory nerve in a case of C5-C6 avulsion as neurotizers for the fascicles of the muscu-locutaneous nerve. It should be noted that the partial denervation of the upper trapezius thereby produced diminishes the usual exaggerated eleva-tion of the shoulder. An intermediate nerve graft is used if the dissection of the fascicles of the musculocutaneous nerve in the lateral cord does not provide enough length for direct suture. A shoulder arthrodesis must be considered if the control of the scapula is satisfactory. XIa = proximal stump of the spinal accessory nerve, XIb = distal stumps of the terminal rami of the spinal accessory nerve, A = lateral cord, M = median cord, and mc = musculocutaneous nerve.

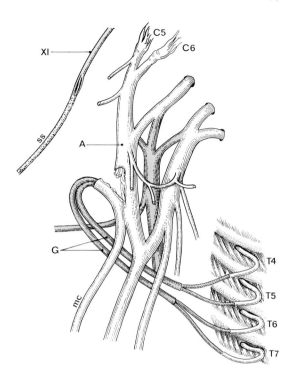

Figure 62–7. Use of the spinal accessory nerve connected to the suprascapular nerve and possibly use of the superior rami of the triceps, which would be connected to the axillary nerve, to restore at least partial function of the shoulder in a case of C5-C6 avulsion. Four intercostal nerves (T4 to T7) are used as neurotizers for the musculocutaneous nerve, utilizing intermediate grafts to restore elbow flexion. XI = spinal accessory nerve, A = lateral cord, T4 to T7 = intercostal nerves, G = sural nerve graft, ss = suprascapular nerve, and mc = musculocutaneous nerve.

clavicle, avulsion of one or more roots from the spinal cord is extremely common. It is found in 75 per cent of the patients with extensive and persisting palsy (Table 62–2). In the majority of these cases the injury happened during use of a two wheeled vehicle, particularly a motorcycle. This has been the experience of all surgeons dealing with this type of injury.

Experimenting on cadavers, Duval and Guillain concluded in 1898 that for anatomical reasons associated with vectors of forces, the upper roots of the plexus (i.e., C5 and C6) were most vulnerable to stretch injuries, such as those occurring during sudden lowering and retropulsion of the shoulder with contralateral inclination of the head. This mechanism would produce an Erb-Duchenne type of lesion—actually a more severe one because instead of rupture of the upper trunk, the lesion would lie more proximally, involving the roots.

The observations of these researchers in studying head injuries induced in cadavers have not been confirmed by clinical and operative findings in more than 1000 cases of surgical exploration by European brachial plexus surgeons. Tables 62–2 and 62–3, corroborated by the anatomical studies of Bonnel et al. (1979, 1980), Celli (1978), Narakas

(1977), and Sunderland (1974), show that upper root avulsion is less common than lower root avulsion. Isolated avulsion of C5 is extremely rare; Birch (1983) has seen it only twice. In more than 300 patients with traumatic brachial plexus lesions who underwent surgical exploration by the author, it has never been observed. We cannot consider in detail here the factors that protect C5 and act to the disadvantage of C6 and particularly of the three lower roots. For this purpose the reader may wish to consult the work of Fritsch (1983), Narakas (1977), and Sunderland (1978).

Avulsions from the spinal cord of C7, C8, and T1 or of C8 and T1 dominate the clinical and surgical picture in brachial plexus lesions. They are associated with elongation of C5-C6, and sometimes of C7, resulting after several months in a Klumpke (1885) type of palsy or a rupture of the upper spinal nerves at the interscalene level with persistent total palsy. An initial isolated Klumpke type of palsy is uncommon. In our series of about 700 cases of traction injuries of the brachial plexus in adults we found only 13 cases, i.e., less than 2 per cent.

In summary, in three quarters of the patients with avulsion of the roots, the brachial plexus surgeon encounters avulsion of the

Table 62–2. RADICULAR AVULSIONS

A. Localization of Plexal Lesions Seen at Operation in 380 Patients

supraclavicular	234
supraclavicular and more distal	26
retroclavicular	41
infraclavicular	77
infraclavicular and more distal	2
Total	380

In 260 cases with supraclavicular lesions, 199 had radicular avulsions (76.5%).

B. Number of Roots Completely Avulsed in 199 Patients

C5	39
C6	95
C7	136
C8	145
T1	137
Total	553

N.B.: Note the low incidence of C5 avulsion (7%) and the frequency of lower root avulsions (76%).

C. Association of Avulsion Lesions in 199 Patients

	NUMBER OF PATIENTS WITH AVULSIONS		
	Certainly complete	Partial	Probably but uncertain
UPPER ROOTS			
C5 alone	1		
C6 alone (C5 ruptured)	11		
C7 alone*	17		
C5 and C6 (C7 either stretched or ruptured)	4	2 for C5	
C6 and C7 (C5 ruptured)	8	3 for C7	1 for C7
C5, C6, C7	7		1 for C5 1 for C7
LOWER ROOTS			
T1 alone (C8 stretched or ruptured	4		1
C8 alone	4	(1 in a postfixed plexus, C8 = C7)	
C7-C8	6	(1 in a postfixed plexus, C7-C8 = C6-C7) (1 in a postfixed plexus, C7 = C6)	
C8-T1, C5-C6-C7 ruptured	28	1 for C8 1 for T1	
C8-T1† C5-C6 stretched, C7 ruptured	2		
C7-C8-T1 C5-C6 ruptured	35	2 for C7	1 for C7
C7-C8-T1† C5-C6 incontinuity	5		
UPPER AND LOWER ROOTS			
C5-C6-C7-C8	2	1 for C5	
C5-C6-C7-C8-T1	19		
C5-C6-C8, T1, C7 ruptured	3		
C5-C7-C8-T1, C6 ruptured	2		
C6-C7-C8-T1, C5 ruptured	34	2 for C6	1 for C5 1 for C6
C6-C7-C8, C5 ruptured, T1 stretched	2		
C6-C7 and T1, C5 and C8 ruptured	1		
C6-C8 and T1, C5 and C7 ruptured	4		

*C5-C6 either ruptured or stretched outside the foramina.
†Note the rarity of isolated type Klumpke palsy (2, 5%).

Table 62–3. NEUROTIZATIONS WITH
ACCESSORY NERVE (XI)

	Number of Patients	Good	Fair	Poor or Nil
A. Transfer onto the musculocutaneous nerve				
Allieu	15	3	7	5
Kotani	5	4	1	0
Merle	7	3	1	3
Morelli	3	2	0	1
B. Transfer onto the suprascapular nerve				
Allieu	2	0	0	2
Narakas	20	8	7	5
C. Transfer onto the upper trunk				
Allieu	3	0	1	2
Kotani	1	1	0	0
Merle	1	0	0	1
D. Transfer onto the posterior cord, the axillary nerve, the radial nerve				
Allieu	5	0	3	2
Kotani	1	0	1	0
Merle	1	0	0	1
Narakas	5	2	2	1
Sedel	3	1	0	2

Note: H. Anderl (Innsbruck, Austria) reports many failures.

four lower roots with extraforaminal rupture of C5 or rupture of C5 and C6 with avulsion of C8 and T1. C7 plays an intermediate role: it is either avulsed or ruptured outside the foramen. Avulsions of two or three upper roots, sometimes of C6 only, occur while the neighboring ones are ruptured or elongated. This situation will result in a more or less useful hand, the upper portion of the limb being paralyzed.

In the majority of these cases the sensorimotor loss is beyond hope, for there are no reconstructive methods to restore even a nearly normal limb. When the paralysis is complete, the choice lies among the omission of surgical treatment, a high level amputation, or a reconstructive procedure (Fig. 62–8), including neurotization even if the results will be very modest or without practical usefulness.

In partial palsy affecting the upper roots—C5 and C6, or C5, C6, and C7, with integrity of C8 and T1—the hand is still useful, but the elbow and the shoulder are paralyzed and scapulothoracic function is sometimes defective. In such cases the repair should combine all available techniques, ranging from arthrodesis to neurotization, with the aim of providing the patient with a utilizable hand. The reverse is equally true: when the lower roots are avulsed without injury to the upper spinal

nerves, the aim should be to reconstruct primitive prehension and some sensation in the hand, the shoulder and elbow being nearly normal. Various types of neurotization can be used for that purpose in combination with more conventional musculotendinous transfers.

Another depressing aspect of root avulsion has to be taken into account, at least when the lower roots are involved—the frequency of permanent and severely painful syndromes, which by themselves and independent of the paralysis ruin all efforts of rehabilitation. Wynn-Parry (1980) found in 108 patients with clinical signs of root avulsion that 98 (90.7 per cent) presented with a pain syndrome. In 42 (38.8 per cent) it was severe and of more than three years' duration. In 14 patients (13 per cent) it persisted for more than 10 years.

In our series of 199 patients with avulsions documented by clinical examination and surgical exploration done more than three weeks after injury (the onset of pain is not always

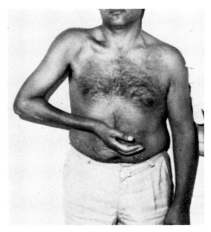

Figure 62–8. Rupture of C5 and avulsion of C6 to T1. Direct neurotization of the suprascapular nerve with two terminal rami of the spinal accessory nerve was performed. Autologous nerve grafts were used between C5 and the lateral cord and the lateral part of the posterior cord, which carries most of the fibers for the axillary nerve. There is synergism between abduction in the shoulder and elbow flexion. The shoulder is elevated at rest; paradoxically it will be depressed when abduction is carried out. This is probably due to contraction of the costosternal portion of the pectoral muscle (a function difficult to explain, as it depends normally on roots C8 and T1, which are avulsed in this patient). It is not clear whether the costosternal portion of the pectoralis major muscle receives an accessory innervation from intercostal nerves or whether it receives a ramus from the lateral cord, which was reinnervated by C5.

immediate), 123 (82 per cent) suffered from pain. More than one third suffered considerably and were using pain killing drugs or narcotics.

There is a striking difference between these patients and those with infraganglionic lesions. Wynn-Parry (1980) found no persisting painful syndromes in patients with distal lesions. In our series of 181 patients with infraganglionic ruptures, only 6 per cent suffered from pain until the surgery was performed. Half of our patients with avulsion who could benefit from reconstructive surgical procedures, including neurotization, were improved or healed with regard to their pain.

At present we cannot explain the positive outcome in this respect of reconstructive neurosurgery in cases implying deafferentation at the spinal cord level (Narakas, 1981). Nevertheless, experience shows that neurotization, when successful, produces favorable results in half the painful conditions. Even if the motor or sensory results are modest, as we will see later, the positive effect on pain justifies use of these procedures.

ANATOMICAL AND NEUROPHYSIOLOGICAL CONSIDERATIONS

Avulsion of a spinal nerve as it emerges from the cord is at present beyond the possibility of direct surgical repair. Admittedly the work of Windle and Chambers in 1950, Clemente and Windle in 1954, Sjöstrand et al. in 1969, Nathaniel in 1973, and Sanjuanbenito et al. in 1976 has shown that some degree of regeneration can occur at the posterior and anterior horns in some vertebrates. Aguayo (1982) has demonstrated that a graft taken from a peripheral nerve and implanted into the spinal cord fills with axonal sprouts although the growth of the axons centripetally is blocked by the neuroglial reaction. The attempt of Jamieson and Eames (1980) to reimplant avulsed roots in five dogs ended in failure. One of the dogs became quadriplegic. It was shown, nevertheless, that the axons grow from the spinal ganglion toward the medulla, but they are stopped at the entry of the spinal cord or curl back as if the medullary tissues had repelled the intruders and resisted any attempt at reorganization, even if local. Jamieson and Bonney (1983) replanted the posterior roots of two spinal

nerves 48 hours after injury but with no positive result after five years.

Thus neuroneural or neuromuscular transfers are among the few present, day techniques that can be used to treat medullary avulsions of brachial plexus roots. When rerouting the proximal axonal end of a healthy nerve onto the distal portion of another one we want to revive, the number of fibers available in the donor ought to be matched with that in the recipient. The density of innervation in muscles is uneven. The trapezius and the latissimus dorsi, of considerable size, are innervated by 1000 to 1700 nerve fibers. At least half of the biceps, a less bulky muscle probably with one half or one third the number of muscular fibers, is innervated by the 6000 afferent or efferent myelinated fibers of the musculocutaneous nerve, the remaining fibers being devoted to the skin. This proportion is even more striking in the intrinsic muscles of the hand. The ratio between the number of innervating fibers and the number of muscle fibers receiving them certainly plays a fundamental role in function; unfortunately it has not been defined.

However, some donor nerves, such as the intercostal nerves, contain a considerable number of sensory fibers for the skin. In most instances only perioperative stimulation or the topographical situation will allow one to distinguish between sensory and motor rami or fasciculi. Histochemical or enzymatic reactions are presently of little use in the operative field. Thus, the mixed nerve may contain a number of fibers irrelevant to motor function.

Finally the discrepancy between what has been lost in an avulsive brachial plexus injury and what is available to compensate for the loss has to be considered.

Bonnel and Rabischong (1980) counted the myelinated fibers in a circumscribed area of known surface in sections of spinal nerves forming the brachial plexus (10 cases). They inferred from the count the total number of myelinated fibers in the whole section. Their results were as follows:

C5: 8,738 to 33,027
C6: 14,227 to 39,036
C7: 18,095 to 40,576
C8: 14,636 to 41,246
T1: 12,102 to 35,600

The total number of myelinated fibers in the whole plexus ranged from 101,864 to 166,214, with an average of 130,000 fibers.

These high numbers have been challenged by other researchers in as yet unpublished works. They found an average of 80,000 to 85,000 fibers when counting in whole sections of spinal nerves. The article by Bonnel and Rabischong (1980) gives the following data for the major nerves arising from the plexus:

Musculocutaneous: 6,061
Median: 18,288
Ulnar: 16,412
Radial: 19,858
Axillary: 6,702
Suprascapular: 3,500

By contrast, the commonly used donor nerves present the following counts:

One intercostal nerve: approximately 1300
Spinal accessory nerve: approximately 1700
Long thoracic nerve: approximately 1600
One ramus going to the pectoral muscles: approximately 400–600

Thus theoretically at least five intercostal nerves would be necessary to effect sufficient neurotization of a musculocutaneous nerve, taking into account the erroneous pathways taken by some axonal sprouts, those blocked at the suture site in cases of direct transfer and at both sutures if an intermediate graft is used. However, we know that a compensating mechanism does exist for these losses: every fiber produces several sprouts, and if Mira's experimental work can be applied to the human (Mira, 1982), an excess of about 30 per cent is to be expected at the proximal stump.

The first lesson to be drawn from these figures is that at exploration of a brachial plexus injury, one should not neglect the axonal end of a spinal nerve ruptured at or just distal to the vertebral foramen. Even in massive avulsions, C5 is often ruptured outside the foramen, between the scalenus muscles, and this stump may contain 8,000 to 33,000 myelinated fibers. Admittedly retrograde degeneration may considerably damage the contents of the proximal stump. Histological examinations of the last slice of the spinal nerve stump, taken when trimming it, have demonstrated destruction of 15 to 80 per cent. Perioperative electrophysiological methods using evoked potentials, as proposed by Sugioka et al. (1982), Landi (1980), and others, to a certain extent permits an evaluation of this retrograde degeneration reaching the cells in the spinal cord.

However, the number of surviving axons remains, even in severe injuries, equivalent to or greater than the number of fibers available in several intercostal nerves, and certainly more than the number of axons in a spinal accessory nerve. Therefore it is important to explore the plexus in search of proximal stumps, particularly at the C5-C6 level and to use them if they are available and a valid choice. It must be stressed again that in severe injuries of the three upper roots, it is important to obtain elbow flexion in order to position a functional hand, that a Steindler procedure in these conditions will have only a limited result, and that, according to Clark, Merle d'Aubigné, and Brooks, a transfer of the inferior part of the pectoralis major will deprive the shoulder of the important residual function of adduction. Under these conditions there is no substitute for some kind of nerve repair reanimating the flexors of the elbow.

When evaluating nerve transfers, we must consider some neurophysiological factors. The nerve fibers participating in the brachial plexus are connected to medullary, thalamic, cortical, and cerebral centers directly concerned with motor and sensory function of the upper limb. They help set the definitive somatic pattern during development. The intercostal nerves, by contrast, have no such wealth of central connections; the cortical representation of the entire thorax is appreciably less than that of the thumb alone. The cortical area of the shoulder is not even one tenth that of the hand alone. A long thoracic nerve or a spinal accessory nerve cannot be compared with the musculocutaneous nerve, not to speak of the median or ulnar nerve. The density of innervation increases as we proceed to the periphery of the upper limb.

Function of the shoulder, including the humeroscapular and scapulothoracic joints, requires about 25,000 to 30,000 fibers originating from the brachial plexus to innervate a muscular volume measured in kilograms and a surface of approximately 10 sq. dm. (Bonnel and Rabischong, 1980; Narakas, 1981). Function of the hand, by comparison, requires about 50,000 myelinated fibers for a muscular volume and a cutaneous surface that are half those of the shoulder.

We have already discussed the discrepancy between the number of fibers transferred onto a damaged nerve and the number it contained originally. In addition there is the impressive difference between the millions of central cells devoted to the multiple functions of the upper limb and the paucity of cells specific for voluntary motion or tactile gnosis in the nerves we may use as neurotizers.

The plasticity of the central nervous system is such that to a certain extent it can adapt to the transfer of function from one soma-tome to another and compensate for the erroneous direction taken by regenerating sprouts. This is most obvious in young indi-viduals, although experience gained with ob-stetrical palsy and their repair is not convinc-ing in this respect. In spite of an ample reinnervation as demonstrated by electro-myography, function may remain poor and faulty; instances of synkinesia are numerous. Paradoxically this happens at a time when the conditions are ideal for compensatory mechanisms to take over and when the so-matic model is not yet fully established. In adults, therefore, central compensation will be less successful.

If such problems are met in repairing nerve trunks, it must be expected that they will be even greater in neurotizations. Centers in the spinal cord and brain related to upper limb function are left deafferentated. By contrast, some of the nerves controlling motor and sensory function of the limb are connected to centers of much less value, which were hitherto not in direct relationship with the upper extremity. This is particularly true in using intercostal nerves for neurotization. One wonders that such a unit can function at all.

From these facts the following deductions can be made when considering neurotization in brachial plexus lesions:

1. Preoperative clinical and instrumental analysis must ascertain whether the plexus rupture is extraforaminal, i.e., whether there are proximal stumps, particularly at the level of C5 and C6 and even C7. Tinel's sign will give some information in this respect, more precise data being obtained by muscle testing, electromyography of deep paraspinal mus-cles, and myelography, searching for nerve action potentials in the periphery and evoked sensory potentials recorded on the brain. The results will aid in the selection of operative measures (Sugioka et al., 1982, 1983).

2. A thorough exploration of the whole plexus must be carried out in every case in the hope of finding a proximal stump as a potential source of axons and not missing a multifocal lesion. Experience has shown that incomplete explorations can fail to demon-strate complete avulsion of C5 to T1, while in these cases our reexplorations have shown C5 alone or C5 and C6 stumps adequate for repair.

Because extraforaminal approach after ET scan and myelography with preoperative and perioperative recordings of evoked potentials cannot absolutely guarantee the absence of rootlet avulsion from the spinal cord, it may be useful to proceed to an exploratory hemi-laminectomy in order to establish the integ-rity of the radiculomedullary junction and to detect partial root avulsions (Privat et al., 1982).

3. The aim of motor neurotization should be the restoration of relatively simple move-ments, such as flexion or extension of the elbow, some abduction in the shoulder, and flexion or extension of the wrist or even of the fingers.

4. Extensive neurotization should be car-ried out on a given nerve at the periphery of the plexus; e.g., three to four intercostal nerves should be rerouted onto the muscu-locutaneous nerve. If two intercostal nerves are used for the musculocutaneous nerve and two others for the radial nerve, synkinesis of the antagonists will be encountered, counter-acting the function sought. In practice, how-ever, differentiated function of antagonists has been obtained and proved by electro-myography (Celli, 1983). Millesi (1977) ob-served active flexion of the elbow by neuro-tizing the musculocutaneous nerve with T2 and extension of the wrist and digits by rerouting T3 and T4 onto the radial nerve. Sedel (1982) has obtained similar results. Such paradoxical facts should be submitted to critical neurophysiological testing and analysis because they imply voluntary control of neuromuscular units that usually do not operate individually. In this respect it must be mentioned that fakirs and acrobats can demonstrate individual function of isolated muscles of the trunk and can contract in succession segments of the rectus abdominis.

5. The neurotization has to be effected in the periphery of the plexus. It would be wasteful in an extraplexus nerve transfer to scatter the available axons over too wide a territory. As is to be discussed, direct neu-rotization of nerve trunks at the interscalene level or of avulsed roots, with donor nerves containing a limited number of axons, leads to an insufficient neurotization unable to ef-fect a valid muscular contraction and also causes synkinesis between antagonists.

6. Unless all roots of the plexus are

avulsed, neurotization must be part of a planned therapeutic program of direct repair and palliative measures.

These principles are not always easy to put into practice for anatomical as well as physiological reasons. Neurotization of the musculocutaneous nerve is a good example. Originating mostly from C5 and C6, the fibers of this nerve leave the plexus in the distal part of the lateral cord to form the nerve that crosses the coracobrachialis muscle. In about one case in six there are crossovers between the median and musculocutaneous nerves and even a common trunk for both of them down to the middle third of the forearm. This situation complicates neurotization of the musculocutaneous nerve, particularly when median function is intact. Long intermediate grafts become necessary.

The situation becomes even worse if C6 is avulsed from the spinal cord while C5 is either ruptured extraforaminally or presents a lesion in continuity. We encountered this situation in about 10 cases in 380 surgical patients. What can be done in such a case?

Repair of only the C5 tracts will not ensure the recovery of active flexion of the elbow if the C6 tracts are left denervated. By using intercostal nerves or the accessory nerve, neurotization of these tracts can be undertaken at a site proximal to the point at which they join C5 to form the upper trunk. Such a proximal neurotization carries the risk of dispersing the axonal end of the donor nerve (Fig. 62–9), leading to hyponeurotization. Because at that level it is difficult to identify with certainty the fascicles that will eventually constitute the lateral cord and to differentiate them from those going into the posterior cord, a proximal neurotization may produce handicapping synkinesis. In addition, the axons coming from the neurotizer will compete at the muscular level with the sprouts from C5 and will probably be eliminated. To avoid this, one can interrupt the musculocutaneous nerve more distally and undertake a neurotization at that level. By doing this one interrupts the fibers regenerating from C5 whose number and functional value are far more important than those of the donor. One may therefore perform a plexoplexus neurotization, as proposed by Harris and Low (1903), connecting the avulsed motor root of C6 to one of the anterior fascicles in the proximal stump of C5. This technique will yield a beneficial result, but flexion of the elbow will be linked to the function of the shoulder (Fig.

62–10). To a large extent the choice of the procedure depends on the condition of the root and the distal tracts. One can omit direct repair of C6 and, if the three lower roots and their pathways are intact, use the lower part of the pectoralis major, as proposed by Clark (1946) and Merle d'Aubigné (1967), or the latissimus dorsi (Zancolli and Mitre, 1973). One also may use a Steindler flexorplasty (Steindler, 1940) or transfer the triceps onto the biceps to restore active flexion of the elbow. If the lower roots are avulsed, which occurs frequently, a judicious decision will be difficult.

SCAPULOTHORACIC AND SCAPULOHUMERAL FUNCTION

When comparing patients with upper palsy (C5-C6 and C5-C6-C7) with patients suffering from a Klumpke type of palsy with paralysis of C8-T1 alone, it is striking to find that in spite of the considerable functional value of the hand, the patients with the lower type of palsy have much greater use of the limb. Hand function is lost, but because the shoulder is functional and allows orientation of the extremity, they can take advantage of it in their private and professional life. This fact underlines the paramount importance of scapulothoracic and scapulohumeral function. All muscles controlling the scapula except the trapezius are innervated by branches originating from the brachial plexus. To a large extent, control of the scapula affects the scapulohumeral joint and if this control is not ensured, there is little hope of reviving shoulder function.

At present there are no surgical means to stabilize a scapula that is out of balance because of an avulsive lesion of C5, C6, and C7. In isolated palsies of the serratus anterior or the trapezius, even if scapulohumeral function is normal, the deficit in range of motion of the shoulder is important. Deterioration of the residual range of motion will result if the scapula is fixed to the thorax; the only positive result will be pain reduction.

Another fact has to be noted. In lesions of C5, C6, and C7 that are not repaired or cannot be repaired, there is always a progressive fixed elevation of the shoulder, because the upward pull of the trapezius, the levator scapulae, and the rhomboids is not balanced by antagonists. In these cases scapulothoracic mobility is considerably reduced

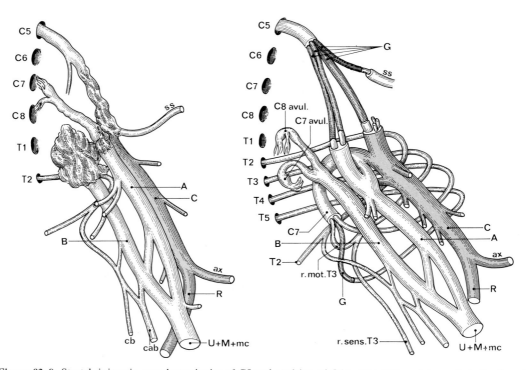

Figure 62–9. Stretch injury in pseudocontinuity of C5 and avulsion of C6 to T1. Although imperfect, the function of the scapulothoracic joint was good in this case. A shoulder arthrodesis could therefore be considered using the axonic capital in C5 to reanimate the pectoralis major, with the elbow flexors directly connecting C5 with the pectoral and musculocutaneous nerves. Unfortunately, the latter forms a common trunk with the ulnar and median nerves. It left the median nerve only in the lower part of the arm, its motor branch being recurrent. The drawing shows the solution chosen in 1974 when the patient was operated upon. An alternative would have been a spinal accessory nerve transfer onto the suprascapular nerve, C5 being grafted onto the upper divisions of the lateral and posterior cords. Five years after the operation this patient had recovered abduction of 60 degrees in the shoulder, combining scapulothoracic and scapulohumeral joint motion. He could rotate his forearm away from the thorax about 20 to 30 degrees, simultaneously performing elbow flexion of more than 90 degrees with a force evaluated at M3+. Active elbow extension as a result of intercostals connected to one distal part of C7 is performed only as an isolated movement when the patient leans on his hand. The hand has no active function but provides protective sensibility in the thumb and the two first long fingers. A = lateral cord, B = medial cord, C = posterior cord, U + M + mc = common trunk of the ulnar, median, and musculocutaneous nerves, cab and cb = medial cutaneous nerves of forearm and arm, ax = axillary nerve, R = radial nerve, G = grafts, ss = suprascapular nerve, r. mot. T3 = motor ramus of third intercostal nerve, and r. sens. T3 = sensory ramus of third intercostal nerve.

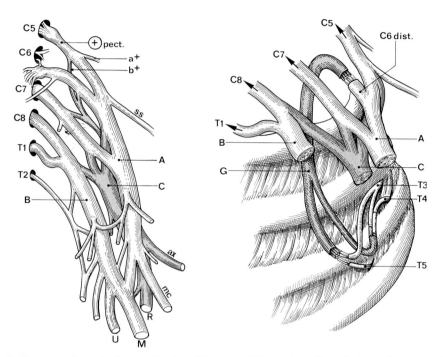

Figure 62–10. Example of proximal neurotization. C5 was partially avulsed, the spinal ganglion protruding at the foramen, but a positive response is obtained when directly stimulating the ramus for Bell's nerve (a⁺) and the dorsal scapular nerve (b⁺), both originating from C5. Direct stimulation of C5 moreover elicits a response in the upper part of the pectoral muscle, and evoked sensory potentials can be recorded at the spinal cord and contralateral cortex. Therefore, C5 should be left alone, as it is impossible to separate the functional fascicles within that spinal nerve from the degenerated ones to neurotize the latter without taking great risks. C6, on the other hand, is completely avulsed. The fascicles can be neurotized as *distally* as possible, i.e., at the level where they merge with those coming from C5 to form the upper trunk. Utilizing an intermediate graft (G), intercostal nerves T3, T4, and T5 are connected to distal C6. The regenerating axons coming from the intercostals will go down the distal pathways in the lateral cord (A) and will be distributed in the original neurotome of C6. But they will also enter the posterior cord (C) and probably innervate muscles with opposite functions. Moreover, these muscles are already partially innervated by C5 and C7. Therefore, the result will be nil or only of academic interest. On the drawing, the cords are interrupted to show the intercostal nerves. B = medial cord, mc = musculocutaneous nerve, M = median nerve, ax = axillary nerve, R = radial nerve, and U = ulnar nerve.

and can be exploited to the advantage of humeroscapular function even if the gain is limited. An arthrodesis of the shoulder should be avoided in such cases at all costs, the acceptability and the functional result of such an operation depending on adequacy of the thoracoscapular joint.

One also must remember that some nerve transfers imply the use of the spinal accessory nerve and rami of the long thoracic nerve. When one uses the distal portion of the spinal accessory nerve, only the upper trapezius will be paralyzed, and this may contribute to bringing the shoulder down. When the lower rami of the nerve to the serratus anterior are used as donors in a nerve transfer, the scapula may tilt forward and a scapula alata will result if the muscles inserting on the coracoid regain their function.

The choice of the procedures therefore implies important functional sacrifices that are added to existing deficits. For this reason the advantages and disadvantages of each procedure have to be evaluated, and the type of neurotization chosen has to form a whole with orthopedic and reconstructive measures.

AVAILABLE TECHNIQUES

Let us consider the nerves available as donors—first those in the vicinity of the plexus and then those farther away.

Among the cranial nerves at our disposal are the eleventh and twelfth. Only the accessory nerve has been used as a neurotizer, by Kotani, Allieu, Merle, the author, and others. Among the cervical nerves, the posterior ramus of the second cervical (Arnold's) nerve, which has numerous muscular branches, can be used as a neurotizer. To the best of our knowledge this has never been done for brachial plexus injuries, but Umashev (1983) has transferred it onto some of the cervical roots in a few cases of post-traumatic quadriplegia. Tuttle (1913), Brunelli (1980), and the author have used rami originating from the third and fourth cervical nerves together with the spinal accessory nerve to neurotize plexus trunks originating from avulsed upper roots. Some Chinese surgeons have used the phrenic nerve as a neurotizer, apparently with success. Lurje (1948) mentioned the possibility also without having

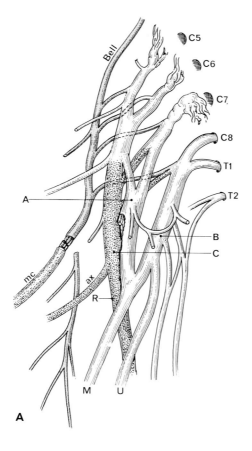

A

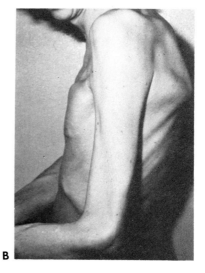

B

Figure 62–11. *A* and *B*, Neurotization of the lateral cord by the distal rami of the long thoracic nerve. When the elbow is flexed simultaneously, a partial scapula alata appears because the lower digitations of the serratus anterior are not paralyzed, whereas the short head of the biceps, coracobrachialis, and pectoralis minor depress the coracoid. Abbreviations: see preceding illustrations.

Figure 62–12. Complex neurotization in avulsion of C5-C6. Restoration of shoulder function and elbow flexion is needed. In this case the long thoracic nerve (of Bell) is partially functional, as it receives a contribution from C4 and C7. The latter nerve is usually at least partially damaged in this type of avulsion injury. Bell's nerve is directly related to the suprascapular nerve (ss). The spinal accessory nerve (XI) is transferred onto the musculocutaneous nerve (mc) utilizing an intermediate graft (G). Two upper rami of the triceps (r. tri) are isolated in the distal part of the posterior cord (C) and connected to two fascicular groups of the axillary nerve (ax). Palliative operations may restore extension of the wrist if needed. A latissimus dorsi transfer (if strong enough) may supplement the flexion of the elbow if the result of the neurotization is poor. The serratus anterior palsy resulting from this technique is a serious handicap for shoulder function. Additional abbreviations: see earlier drawings.

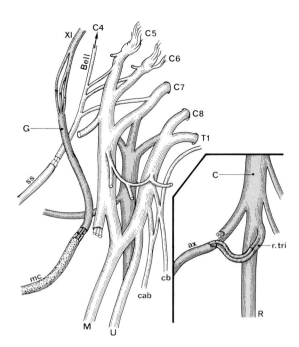

used it himself. Förster (1929), Steindler (1940), and the author transferred rami of the long thoracic (Bell's) nerve onto avulsed parts of the brachial plexus (Figs. 62–11, 62–12).

Plexoplexus neurotizations imply the connection of ruptured spinal nerves or even intact rami of the plexus with distal portions of nerve pathways whose origins have been destroyed or avulsed. Sacrifice of functional nerves in these cases has to be worth while. Lurje (1948) and the author (Narakas, 1977, 1982) have attempted this type of neurotization.

The use of some fascicles of the contralateral plexus has been discussed. The risk of jeopardizing function of the healthy side has limited such attempts. Only Gilbert has tried to connect rami to the pectoral muscles on the healthy side to a long graft, which was transferred in a two stage procedure to the musculocutaneous nerve on the affected side. The result in the unique case described by Gilbert at the time of this writing was not very convincing when seen in Uruguay by the author.

Numerous surgeons favor use of the intercostobrachial anastomoses and the upper intercostal nerves. Celli et al. (1978) have proposed neurotizations with the lower intercostal nerves, thus adding to the techniques proposed by Yeoman (1979), Seddon (1972),

Fantiš and Sezak (1967), Kotani et al. (1972), and Tsuyama (1972, 1980).

SURGICAL TECHNIQUES AND RESULTS

USE OF THE PHRENIC NERVE

In the Western world reports of this type of transfer, mentioned by Lurje (1948), have not been published and the author has never met a surgeon in the Occidental countries who had used it intentionally. According to information gathered when traveling in China in the autumn of 1982, a few Chinese surgeons have used this technique. The results were said to be good, and there were no marked complications following sacrifice of the phrenic nerve.

USE OF THE SPINAL ACCESSORY NERVE

The spinal accessory nerve has to be harvested distal to the sternocleidomastoid muscle in order to preserve innervation of the muscle. The terminal rami to the upper trapezius are generally used. They contain 800 to 1200 myelinated fibers, whereas the main trunk of the accessory nerve contains about 1700.

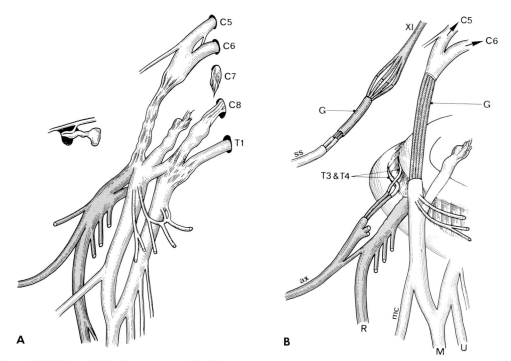

Figure 62–13. *A* and *B*, Attempt to avoid effects of mass reinnervation. This patient had rupture of the upper trunk C5-C6, avulsion of C7 and C8, and uncertainty with regard to the integrity of T1. In order to restore function of the shoulder independently from other functions of the limb, the entire upper trunk C5-C6 was connected with grafts (G) to the distal lateral cord to allow for flexion of the elbow, wrist, and perhaps fingers, while the accessory nerve (XI) was connected through an intermediate graft (G) to the suprascapular nerve (ss) and the intercostal nerves T3 and T4 were connected to the axillary nerve (ax). A result similar to that illustrated in Figure 62–8 was obtained but without the undesirable effect of mass reinnervation. The patient could abduct his arm without simultaneously flexing his elbow and wrist and vice versa. Additional abbreviations: see earlier drawings.

Kotani et al. (1972) tried to suture spinal accessory fibers directly to the musculocutaneous nerve. Allieu and his colleagues (1982) failed twice to do so; that is why they favor intermediate grafts in spinohumeral neurotizations. The author several times has sutured the spinal accessory nerve directly to the suprascapular nerve (Figs. 62–7, 62–8, 62–13).

According to Allieu et al. (1982) and Merle (1980), the best results with the use of the spinal accessory nerve are obtained when neurotizing the musculocutaneous nerve, because elbow flexion is an elementary movement depending on two antagonistic muscular groups, whereas shoulder motion is complex. Neurotization of any of the nerves to the shoulder girdle muscles with the accessory nerve has not been gratifying. The author has obtained on the average 30 degrees of true abduction of the humerus when neurotizing the suprascapular nerve. This angle combined with the tilting of the scapula out-ward gives about 45 to 50 degrees of abduction of the arm from the trunk. In successful cases about 40 degrees of external active rotation of the humerus can be obtained, starting from a position in which the limb, with the elbow flexed, is against the thorax.

Table 62–3 gives the results obtained by Allieu and other surgeons. They are equivalent to those obtained by Japanese surgeons. Although Millesi (1977) dislikes this type of neurotization, many European surgeons have obtained useful results with it.

The deficit caused by sacrifice of the spinal accessory nerve is minor. Only the upper trapezius is denervated and often incompletely. This denervation may even be useful, as we have seen previously.

USE OF THE DEEP CERVICAL PLEXUS

The transfer of the deep motor rami of the cervical plexus originating from C3 and C4 and innervating the muscles of the neck, as proposed by Tuttle (1913), reintroduced by Brunelli (1980), and used by Celli (1974, 1983) and the author, actually complements the use of the spinal accessory nerve. Careful dissection is necessary to find the muscular branches, and no results of this transfer have been published yet. So far, in my experience, they have been poor (Table 62–4). This transfer is justified only to reinnervate the long thoracic nerve when its cervical portion has been destroyed or when it cannot be repaired, as in avulsions of C5, C6, and C7 in order to restore some stability of the scapula that cannot be obtained by other means.

USE OF THE LONG THORACIC NERVE

The long thoracic (Bell's) nerve usually but not always originates from C4, from C5, C6, and C7, and rarely from C8. Therefore it cannot be considered as a source of axons in avulsions of the three upper roots or when all of them are avulsed.

Lurje (1948) used two terminal rami of this nerve to neurotize the suprascapular nerve in Erb-Duchenne palsy (Fig. 62–3) with partial success. Table 62–4 shows the results we obtained when using not more than two of its rami.

It seems logical to neurotize the branch to the long head of the triceps when trying to restore elbow extension; anterior projection of the shoulder, ensured by Bell's nerve, adds itself naturally to extension of the elbow in normal conditions.

The results obtained have been poor. Probably they could be better if more than two

rami would have been used, but the sacrifice of shoulder function would have been excessive. Even the use of two rami produces a partial scapula alata (Fig. 62–11).

Complete Bell's palsy represents a major handicap even when humeroscapular function is normal. There is no good palliative operation to retain the scapula against the thorax. Transfer of a functional teres major, detaching it from the humerus and inserting it on the fifth and sixth ribs, gives only equivocal results. In two patients operated upon in this way by the author, it was evident that the transfer contracted only partially when the arm was elevated and that it remained synchronous with adduction and internal rotation in the shoulder.

Scapulothoracic arthrodesis always implies the loss of about one third of the abduction available before operation; it is therefore justified only in exceptional cases.

USE OF THE INTERCOSTAL NERVES

This type of transfer, introduced by Yeoman and Seddon (1972) and used by Fantiš and Sezak (1967), has been widely used in brachial plexus surgery during the last 15 years.

Intercostal nerves contain 1200 to 1400 myelinated motor and sensory fibers. An intercostal nerve gives off about 35 per cent of its motor fibers along its course from the intervertebral foramen to the midaxillary line. There are, however, differences in this respect between the upper six and the lower six intercostal nerves.

The first intercostal nerve (as well as the

Table 62–4. NEUROTIZATION USING THE LONG THORACIC NERVE AND THE DEEP CERVICAL PLEXUS

	Number of Patients	Good	Fair	Poor or Nil
Thoracic nerve				
Narakas	7			
Onto C6	1	0	1	0
Onto the lateral part of lateral cord	2	1	0	1
Onto the suprascapular nerve	2	1	0	1
Onto the ramus for the triceps	1	0	1	0
Onto the motor nerve of a gracilis muscle transplanted into the arm to serve as an elbow extensor	1	0	1	0
Deep Cervical Plexus				
Morelli	12	0	0	12
Narakas	6	1	2	3

second, in postfixed plexuses) participates in the formation of the brachial plexus. The second intercostal nerve has only a few motor fibers and should not be used as a transfer because it innervates the skin of the axilla and the medial aspect of the arm. The third intercostal nerve gives off slightly anterior to the midaxillary line an important sensory branch, easily identified, which proceeds to the axillary skin, and a motor ramus, which is deep to the former. The latter can be identified and used as a single neurotizer, sparing the sensory ramus.

The fourth intercostal nerve below the axilla has a deep motor branch and two superficial sensory branches. The fifth and sixth intercostal nerves contain mostly motor fibers traveling anterior to the sternum. Because they innervate the mammary gland and the areolus, their sensory rami should be spared in women. The seventh and following intercostal nerves innervate, among other structures, some muscles of the abdomen. They should not be taken together in a row as neurotizers. Usually three to four intercostal nerves are harvested (Fig. 62–14) (in certain occasions five), starting from T3 down to T8, approaching them at the midaxillary line. Japanese surgeons expose them more anteriorly, almost at the level of the nipple, while

Celli et al. (1978) as well as Morelli (1983), in order to harvest a maximum of motor fibers, expose the intercostal nerves near their paravertebral origin and lengthen them with a graft that follows an extrapleural course to reach the plexus.

Celli et al. (1978) proposed the use of T8, T9, T10, and T11, lengthening them with a pedicled vascularized graft. In cases of C8-T1 avulsion he uses the ulnar nerve for this purpose, proceeding in two stages. First he transposes the ulnar nerve from the arm under the skin of the thorax, after transecting it at the elbow, and connects it to the donor intercostal nerves. When Tinel's sign has reached the axilla, in a second stage he severs the origin of the ulnar nerve at the plexus and transfers the distal end onto the nerve trunk he wants to reanimate.

In the same situation we use a similar technique, harvesting for the purpose the medial cutaneous nerve of the forearm. The terminal rami are cut at the level of the elbow and dissected upward to the axilla. Then the nerve with its terminal branches is transposed onto the lateral aspect of the thoracic wall. The terminal rami are connected by fascicular sutures to the fascicles of intercostal nerves T4 to T7 and sometimes to the motor ramus of T3. The proximal part of the medial cu-

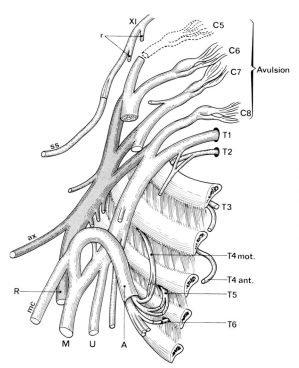

Figure 62–14. Selective motor neurotization of the lateral cord (A) with intercostal nerves T4 to T6. The motor rami are identified utilizing intraoperative stimulation. The sensory anterior rami are not used. T3 is not utilized, as its motor rami are very small whereas it gives off an important sensory ramus to the axilla. The suprascapular nerve (ss) is neurotized with the spinal accessory nerve (XI), and the two remaining rami (R) of the latter can be connected to fascicles of the axillary nerve (ax). Additional abbreviations: see earlier drawings.

taneous nerve of the forearm is identified at the plexus and endoneurolyzed cephalad to its origin within the medial cord to gain length; it is then cut. The distal stump is then swung toward the nerve to be neurotized. This technique allows maintenance of the vascularization of the medial cutaneous nerve of the forearm at the distal part of the plexus.

Approach to the Intercostal Nerves

The author exposes the intercostal nerves a few centimeters posterior to the midaxillary line. They are dissected 5 to 8 cm. anteriorly in order to be long enough to be connected directly to the nerve trunks to be neurotized. This is usually possible for the three to four upper intercostal nerves. The others are lengthened by intermediate grafts. Use of the medial cutaneous nerve of the forearm as an intermediate graft has been described. When several grafts have to be used, the quantity of connective tissue at the extremity of the grafts that will be connected to the receptor should be diminished. The musculocutaneous and axillary nerves at the level of the distal plexus when cut present an almost monofascicular aspect. The nerve tissue is tightly packed in several compartments with very thin connective tissue septa (internal epineurium). There is little sense in separating them into individual fascicles or fascicular groups. By contrast, individual grafts or terminal rami of a nerve such as the medial cutaneous nerve of the forearm, and even the main trunk of that nerve, are composed at least 50 to 60 per cent of connective tissue.

If several grafts are grouped together and put on the receptor nerve, an excessive amount of connective tissue will be apposed onto nerve tissue. Therefore epineurium is resected for 1 cm. at the end of the grafts to leave almost naked fascicles. These fascicles are then assembled with those of other grafts and glued together laterally with fibrin glue to form a cable. The cable will then be trimmed to present a clean-cut surface and is glued or sutured to the receptor nerve. Histological examination of slices taken from the cable has shown the presence of about 50 per cent connective tissue, whereas conventionally assembled grafts contain up to 80 per cent epineurium and adventitial non-nerve tissue.

This method cannot be applied as easily to the median, ulnar, and radial nerves at their origin at the plexus because most of the time they are multifascicular. Fascicles or fascicular groups have to be prepared to receive individually matching grafts or rami.

Results of Intercostohumeral Neurotization

In spite of the discrepancy between the few nerve fibers the intercostal nerves contain and the great number of fibers in the trunks to be colonized, effective results can be obtained with this type of nerve transfer, particularly when one seeks to restore elementary movements such as extension or flexion of the elbow and wrist and, to a lesser degree, of the fingers. Massive neurotization of the radial nerve implies some risk of failure: The radial nerve innervates antagonists of elbow flexion-extension. The triceps is an elbow extensor, while the brachioradialis and lateral third of the brachialis are elbow flexors. In cases of massive reinnervation, when the pathways of the regenerating fibers are mixed, a synkinesia will be created, limiting extension of the elbow (Fig. 62–15). The result is fair or good for extension of wrist and fingers.

Tsuyama and his coworkers, according to a report by Sugioka (1982, 1983), obtained useful results in about 70 per cent of the patients in whom an intercostohumeral nerve transfer was done. Our own good results were less numerous because of errors in our early cases, such as the use of T2, tight direct sutures not allowing ample movements of the limb and thorax, and coughing (Fig. 62–16, Table 62–5).

With regard to protective sensation, the results are impressive. Even light touch with cotton wool is perceived, but localization is poor. Tactile discrimination has been obtained only in children, but the static Weber test is over 3 cm. Nociceptive stimuli are usually referred first to the thorax and then with a delay of a second or so to the neurotized area (Fig. 62–16).

Various trunks can be neurotized. Only a few reports are available concerning neurotization of the median, ulnar, and radial nerves. Kotani et al. (1972), Millesi (1983), Morelli (1983), and the author (Narakas, 1982) have obtained a few positive results. Intercostal nerve transfer produces a movement that is a bit slow and lacks endurance, which seems paradoxical because this is the

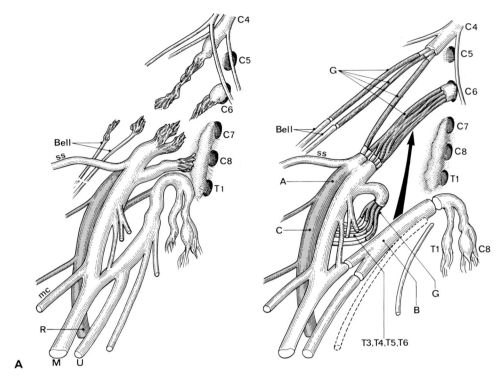

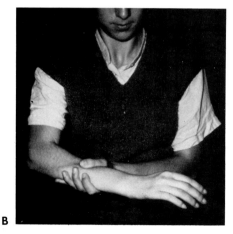

Figure 62–15. *A*, Utilizing autografts harvested from the antebrachial cutaneous nerve, C4 was grafted to the long thoracic nerve (of Bell) and some fascicles of the suprascapular nerve (ss). The medial cord (B) was stripped of its epineurium and utilized as an intermediate graft between C6 and the lateral cord (A), including one fascicle of the suprascapular nerve. Four intercostal nerves, T3, T4, T5, and T6, were transferred onto the distal stump of C7. *B*, Result 4 years after operation. Abduction in the shoulder occurs simultaneously with flexion of the elbow and extension of the wrist and fingers. The latter function is monitored by the intercostal nerve transfer. It is involuntary with deep breathing or coughing. In order to demonstrate that finger and wrist extension can be performed against gravity, the patient has to hold her forearm in pronation, as otherwise the biceps will supinate it. She has no valid pronators.

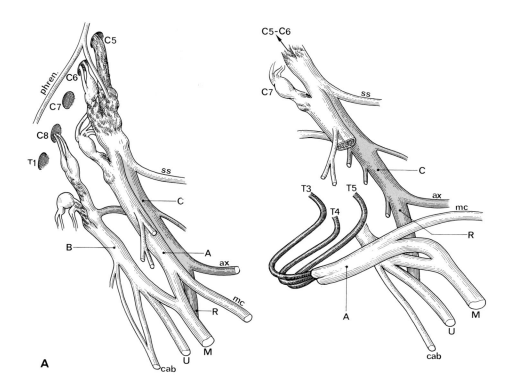

A

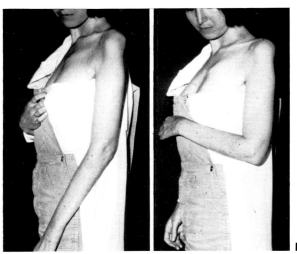

Figure 62–16. *A*, Avulsion of all roots of the brachial plexus. Neurotization of the lateral part of the lateral cord was performed with three intercostal nerves as an alternative to abandoning the extremity or amputating it in the upper humerus. *B*, The biceps and brachialis have recovered to M4. Protective sensibility is present on the lateral aspect of the forearm, thumb, index, and middle fingers. Slight touch with cotton wool is felt by the patient but the sensation is poorly localized. When asked, "which additional movement would you like to have if we could give you only one?" the patient answered, "adduction of the thumb."

B

Table 62–5. NEUROTIZATION WITH INTERCOSTAL NERVES

	Number of Cases	Good	Fair	Poor or Nil
A. Transfer onto the musculocutaneous or the lateral part of lateral cord				
Celli	About 20 cases		Success in about 50%	
Merle	A few cases		All failures	
Morelli	25	6	?	?
Tsuyama and Sugioka	64	43	8	13
Kotani	3	1	1	1
Millesi	7	4	0	3
Narakas	20	7	9	4
Sedel	10	5	3	2
B. Transfer onto the posterior cord, the axillary, suprascapular, and radial nerves				
Millesi	1	1	0	0
Morelli	1	1	0	0
Kotani	2	2	0	0
Narakas	11	0	7	4
Sedel	4	2	0	2
C. Transfer onto the medial cord, median and ulnar nerves				
Kotani	11	2	2	7
Millesi	?	1	?	?
Morelli	?	1	?	?
Narakas	12	0	4	8
Sedel	5	0	0	5
Tsuyama and Sugioka	?	1	?	?
D. Transfer onto C7 (post. or ant. division)				
Narakas	20	6	2	12

Note: H. Anderl (Innsbruck, Austria) has had several failures.

continuous function of the intercostal muscles. Finally it must be said that a complete flexion of the elbow, allowing the patient to reach his mouth with the hand, is exceptional in this type of nerve repair.

As with other types of nerve transfer, neurotization with intercostal nerves has to be localized; i.e., a maximal number of donor nerves must be concentrated on one receptor nerve. Usually about three years are required to evaluate the final result.

PLEXOPLEXUS NEUROTIZATIONS

When C5 is ruptured extraforaminally while C6 is avulsed from the spinal cord, and both upper spinal nerves C5 and C6 are ruptured at the interscalene level but C7 is avulsed, the nerve that has lost its connection with the spinal cord can be branched, after resection of the spinal ganglion, onto one of the proximal stumps. Because most plexus repairs are undertaken weeks or months after injury, the distal nerve trunks are partially atrophied. Therefore there is room enough on the proximal stumps to accept, in addition to the structures belonging normally to them, fascicles of an avulsed neighboring root. It is even possible to identify the motor rootlets

in the operative field and to neurotize them or follow the spinal nerve downward to its division into anterior and posterior portions (the latter goes to the posterior cord) and to undertake a selective neurotization favoring one or another function. Connections between the proximal and distal stumps are made either directly or by interposing grafts.

Whenever this type of nerve transfer is used, synkinesis will always be present. In about half the cases in which this technique has been used, a positive result has been obtained (Table 62–6).

In spite of synkinesis, this type of plexoplexus transfer yields results that seem qualitatively better and more natural than function obtained using extraplexus donors.

POSTOPERATIVE COURSE

When enough time has elapsed to allow the regenerating axons of the donor nerve to reach the muscles selected for reinnervation, a simple contraction (M1) is seen in the neurotized muscles or muscular groups when the patient tries to activate the ones belonging originally to the donor nerve. This means, for example, that in a case of transfer of intercostal nerves to the musculocutaneous

Table 62–6. PLEXOPLEXAL TRANSFERS

Narakas	Number of Cases	Good	Fair	Poor
C5 onto C5-C6	5	3	2	0
C5 onto C5-C6-C7	1	0	0	1
C6 onto C6-C7	9	4	2	3
C7 onto C5-C6	4	1	1	2
C6 onto the medial cord	3	1	1	1
Totals	22	9	6	7

The statistics of other authors are not available, but according to discussions favorable results were obtained in about half of the cases, while A. Gilbert has performed in obstetrical palsies more than 60 plexoplexal transfers obtaining convincing results in 65 per cent.

nerve, the biceps and later the brachialis will contract at the end of expiration. This happens at the earliest at the sixth postoperative month, usually at eight months. A few months later spontaneous activity of the biceps appears, synchronous with respiration. It persists for several months and represents an involuntary kind of physiotherapy. Voluntary contractions then appear and, if the case is a success, are reinforced gradually to reach M3 or M4. The function becomes independent of respiration and spontaneous activity disappears. Finally the patient can activate the neurotized muscles completely independently from the original function of the donor nerves. This usually requires about two years.

When the spinal accessory nerve has been transferred to the musculocutaneous nerve, the patient can eventually flex his elbow without elevating and pushing his shoulder backward. By contrast, if the suprascapular nerve was neurotized with the spinal accessory nerve, the synchronous shoulder movements persist. The original reflex arc is maintained, and the integration into the body image remains incomplete. The author has noted repeatedly that the function obtained by nerve transfer is not properly integrated into a sequence of muscular functions to create a gesture that would seem normal when the movement is ensured by intact or directly repaired nerves and one member of the chain depends on neurotization.

CONCLUSION

Neurotization is an adjunct in the treatment of traumatic brachial plexus lesions, particularly when radicular avulsions are present. It can restore a movement that cannot be obtained by other means. It can be useful in desperate cases when the alternatives are to fit the patient with a splint and give up treatment or to amputate the useless and paralyzed extremity, supplying a prosthesis, usually with a very disappointing result. It is well known that amputation has no effect on deafferentation pain.

In summary, the neuronerve transfer implies the following results: Synergism occurs in which the original movement linked with the donor nerve can be performed. The resulting movement often remains an isolated entity that is not properly, or not at all, integrated into the movement sequence. A synesthesia is established that modifies the body image. The sensation obtained is excellent in terms of protection, but tactile gnosis is poor. The original reflex arc is retained with inadequate retrieval in cases of nociception.

REFERENCES

Aguayo, A. J.: Neural graft and central nervous system regeneration. Communication, Scientific Meeting on Neuroplasticity and Repair in the Central Nervous System, OMS, Geneva, June 29, 1982.

Aitken, J. T.: Growth of nerve implants in voluntary muscle. J. Anat. (London), 84:38–49, 1950.

Allieu, Y., Privat, J. M., and Bonnel, F.: Les neurotisations par le nerf spinal. Neurochirurgie (Paris), 28:115–120, 1982.

Birch, R.: Review of types of lesions of the brachial plexus. Communication, Symposium sur les Lésions du Plexus Brachial, London, January 1983.

Bonnel, F., Allieu, Y., Sugata, Y., and Rabischong, P.: Bases anatomo-chirurgicales des neurotisations pour avulsions radiculaires du plexus brachial. Anat. Clin., 1:291–298, 1979.

Bonnel, F., and Rabischong, P.: Anatomie et systématisation du plexus brachial de l'adulte. Anat. Clin., 2:289–298, 1980.

Brunelli, G.: Neurotization of avulsed roots of the brachial plexus by means of anterior nerves of the cervical plexus (preliminary report). Int. J. Microsurg., 2:55–58, 1980.

Brunelli, G.: Les neurotisations directes. Communication, Hôpital Bichat, January 20–21, 1983.

Brunelli, G., Brunelli Monini, L., Antonucci, A., and Maraldi, N.: Neurotizzazione in zona aneurale di muscoli denervati (studio sperimentale). Policlin. Chir., 83:611–616, 1976.

Brunelli, G., and Fontana, G.: Risultati clinici e nuove esperienze sperimentali sulla neurotizzazione diretta. Communication, VIIe Congrès National de la Sté Italienne de Microchirurgie, Rome, November 19–20, 1982.

Celli, L.: Considérations sur les mécanismes avulsifs radiculaires. Communication, Symposium sur le Plexus Brachial, Lausanne, September 1978.

Celli, L.: Electromyographie per-opératoire des muscles cervicaux profonds dans l'évaluation des moignons proximaux du plexus. Third Symposium on Lesions of the Brachial Plexus. Internat. J. Microsurg., *1:*103–106, 1979 (abstract).

Celli, L., Balli, A., de Luise, G., and Rovesta, C.: La neurotizzazione degli ultimi nervi intercostali, mediante trapianto nervoso peduncolato, nelle avulsioni radicolari del plesso brachiale. Chir. Org. Movimento, *64:*461–464, 1978.

Celli, L., Mingione, A., and Landi, A.: Nuove acquisizioni di tecnica chirurgica nelle lesioni del plesso brachiale: indicazioni alla neurolisi, autoinesti et trapianti nervosi. LIX Congresso, Società Italiana di Ortopedia et Traumatologia, Cagliari, September 29-October 3, 1974.

Celli, L.: Personal communication, 1983.

Clark, J. M. P.: Reconstruction of biceps brachii by pectoral muscle transplantation. Br. J. Surg. *34:*180–181, 1946.

Clemente, C. D., and Windle, W. F.: Regeneration of severed nerve fibers in the spinal cord of the adult cat. J. Comp. Neurol., *101:*691–731, 1954.

Duval, P., and Guillain, G.: Pathogénie des accidents nerveux consécutifs aux luxations et traumatismes de l'épaule. Arch. Gen. Med., *8–10:*143–191, 1948.

Elsberg, C. A.: Experiments on motor nerve regeneration and the direct neurotisation of paralyzed muscles by their own and foreign nerves. Science, *45:*318–320, 1917.

Erlacher, P.: Ueber die motorischen Nervendigungen. Z. Orthop. Chir., *34:*561–585, 1914.

Fantiš, A., and Sezak, Z.: Kotazce chirurgické cécby poraneni brachialného plexu. Acta Chir. Orthop. Trauma, *34:*301–309, 1967.

Förster, O.: Die Therapie des Schussverletzungen der peripheren Nerven. *In* Lewandowsky (Editor): Handbuch der Neurologie. Berlin, Ergänzungsband, 1929, Ch. 3.

Fort, W. B.: An experimental study of the factors involved in the establishment of neuromuscular connections. Chicago, University of Chicago Libraries, 1940.

Fritsch, C.: Etude clinique des paralysies brachiales obstétricales. Thesis, Université de Lausanne, 1983.

Gersuny, A.: Eine Operation bei motorischen Lähmungen. Wien. Klin. Wochenschr., *10,* 1906.

Gilbert, A.: Personal communication.

Harris, R. I.: Treatment of irreparable nerve injuries. Can. Med. Assoc. J., *11:*833–836, 1921.

Harris, W., and Low, V. W.: On the importance of accurate muscular analysis in lesions of the brachial plexus and the treatment of Erb's palsy and infantile paralysis of the upper extremity by cross-union of nerve roots. Br. Med. J., *2:*1035–1038, 1903.

Heineke, H.: Die Direkte Einpflanzung des Nerven in den Muskel. Zbl. Chir. 1914, *41,* 465–467.

Jamieson, A. M., and Bonney, G.: Personal communication, 1983.

Jamieson, A. M., and Eames, R. A.: Reimplantation of avulsed brachial plexus roots: an experimental study in dogs. Int. J. Microsurg., *2:*75–80, 1980.

Jamieson, A. M., and Hughes, S.: The role of surgery in the management of closed injuries to the brachial plexus. Clin. Orthop., *147:*210–215, 1980.

Klumpke, A.: Contribution à l'étude des paralysies radiculaires du plexus brachial. Rev. Méd., *5:*591–790, 1885.

Kotani, P. T., Matsuda, H., and Suzuki, T.: Trial surgical procedures of nerve transfers to avulsion injuries of plexus brachialis. Excepta Med. (Int. 12th Congress Series 291), 348–350, 1972.

Landi, A.: The role of somatosensory-evoked potentials and nerve conduction studies in the management of brachial plexus injuries. J. Bone Joint Surg., *62B:*492–496, 1980.

Letievant, J. J. E.: Traité des Sections Nerveuses. Paris, Baillière, 1873.

Lurje, A.: Concerning surgical treatment of traumatic injury of the upper division of the brachial plexus (Erb's type) Ann. Surg., *127:*317–326, 1948.

Merle, M.: La chirurgie directe du plexus brachial traumatique. Rev. Réadapt. Fonct. Soc., *6:*42–52, 1980.

Merle d'Aubigné, R., and Deburge, A.: Traitement des paralysies du plexus brachial. Rev. Chir. Orthop. *53:*199–215, 1967.

Millesi, H.: Neurotisation lädierter Nerven unter Heranziehung gesunder Nervenstämme. *In* Nigst, D., et al. (Editors): Handchirurgie. Stuttgart, Georg Thieme Vorlag, 1983, Vol. 2, pp. 39.3–39.5.

Millesi, H.: Surgical management of brachial plexus injuries. J. Hand Surg., *2:*367–379, 1977.

Mira, J. C.: Dégénérescence et régénération des nerfs périphériques: observations ultrastructurales et électrophysiologiques, aspects quantitatifs et conséquences musculaires. *In* Aspects Biologiques de la Régénération du Nerf Périphérique. Paris, Volal, 1982, pp. 30–60.

Morelli, E.: Personal communication, 1983.

Narakas, A.: Paradoxes en chirurgie nerveuse périphérique au niveau du plexus brachial. Méd. Hyg., *35:*833–839, 1977.

Narakas, A.: The effects on pain of reconstructive neurosurgery in 160 patients with traction and/or crush injury to the brachial plexus. *In* Siegfried, J., and Zimmermann, M. (Editors): Phantom and Stump Pain. Berlin, Springer Verlag, 1981, pp. 126–147.

Narakas, A.: Les neurotisations ou transferts nerveux dans les lésions du plexus brachial. Ann. Chir. Main, *1:*101–118, 1982.

Nathaniel, E. J. H., and Nathaniel, D. R.: Regeneration of dorsal root fibers in the adult spinal cord. Exp. Neurol., *40:*333–350, 1973.

Peacock, E. E.: Restoration of sensation in hands with extensive median nerve defect. J. Bone Joint Surg., *54:*576, 1963.

Peterson, E. R., and Crain, S. M.: Regeneration and innervation in cultures of adult mammalian skeletal muscle, coupled with fetal rodent spinal cord. Exp. Neurol., *36:*136–159, 1972.

Privat, J. M., Malhe, D., Allieu, Y., and Bonnel, F.: Hémilaminectomie cervicale exploratrice et neurotisation précoce du plexus brachial. *In* Simon, L., and Allieu, Y. (Editors): Plexus Brachial et Médecine de Rééducation. Paris, Masson et Cie, 1982, pp. 66–73.

Sanjuanbenito, L., Esteban, A., and Gonzalez-Martinez, E.: Regeneration of the spinal ventral roots in cats. Acta Neurochir., *34:*203–214, 1976.

Seddon, H.: Surgical Disorders of the Peripheral Nerves. Edinburgh, Churchill Livingstone, 1972.

Sedel, L.: The results of surgical repair of brachial plexus injuries. J. Bone Joint Surg., *64B:*54–66, 1982.

Sjöstrand, J., Carlsson, C. A., and Thulin, C. A.: Regeneration of ventral roots in cats. Acta Anat., *74:*535–546, 1969.

Sorbie, C., and Porter, T. L.: Reinnervation of para-

lyzed muscles by direct motor nerve implantation. J. Bone Joint Surg., *51B*:156–164, 1969.

Steindler, A.: The method of direct neurotization of paralyzed muscles. Am. J. Orthop. Surg., *13*:33–45, 1915.

Steindler, A.: Direct neurotization of paralyzed muscles. Further studies of the question of direct nerve implantation. Am. J. Orthop. Surg., *14*:707–719, 1916.

Steindler, A.: Orthopedic Operations. Springfield, Illinois, Charles C Thomas, 1940, p. 129.

Steindler, A.: The Traumatic Deformities and Disabilities of the Upper Extremity. Springfield, Illinois, Charles C Thomas, 1946.

Sugioka, H.: Clinical study of brachial plexus traction lesions by intraoperative somatosensory evoked potentials and nerve action potential recording. J. Jpn. Orthop. Assoc., *57*:5–20, 1983.

Sugioka, H.: Rapport sur la neurotisation du musculo-cutané par les intercostaux (72 cas). Symposium on the Brachial Plexus, London, January 1983.

Sugioka, H., Tsuyama, N., Hara, T., Nagano, A., Tachibana, S., and Ochiai, N.: Investigation of brachial plexus injuries by intraoperative cortical somatosensory evoked potentials. Arch. Orthop. Traumat. Surg., *99*:143–151, 1982.

Sunderland, S.: Mechanisms of cervical root avulsion in injuries of the neck and shoulder. J. Neurosurg., *41*:705–714, 1974.

Sunderland, S.: Nerves and Nerve Injuries. Ed. 2. Edinburgh, Churchill Livingstone, 1978.

Thompson, N.: Investigation on autogenous skeletal muscle free grafts in the dog, with report on a suc-cessful free graft of skeletal muscle in man. Transplantation, *12*:353–356, 1971.

Tsuyama, N.: Further studies of nerve crossing in irreparably damaged peripheral nerve. Communication, Congrès de la Fédération Internationale des Sociétés de Chirurgie de la Main, Rotterdam, 1980.

Tsuyama, N., and Hara, T.: Intercostal nerve transfer in the treatment of brachial plexus injury of root avulsion type. Excepta Med. (Int. 12th Congress Series 291) 351–353, 1972.

Tuttle, H.: Exposure of the brachial plexus with nerve transplantation. J.A.M.A. *61*:15–17, 1913.

Umashev, G. S.: Conférence sur la Neurotisation dans les Lésions Médullaires, CHUV, Lausanne, March 1983.

Van Harreveld, A.: Re-innervation of denervated muscle fibers by adjacent functioning motor units. Am. J. Physiol., *144*:477–481, 1945.

Vulpius, O., and Stoffel, A.: Orthopädische Operationslehre. Ed. 2. Stuttgart, Enke, 1920.

Weiss, P.: Neue experimentelle Beweise für das Resonanzprinzip de Nerventätigkeit. Biol. Zbl., *50*:357–372, 1930.

Windle, W. F., and Chambers, W. W.: Regeneration in the spinal cord of the cat and dog. J. Comp. Neurol., *93*:241–257, 1950.

Wynn-Parry, C. B.: Pain in avulsion of the brachial plexus. Pain, *9*:41–53, 1980.

Yeoman, P.: Personal communication, 1979.

Zancolli, E., and Mitre, H.: Latissimus dorsi transfer to restore elbow flexion. J. Bone Joint Surg., *55A*:1265–1275, 1973.

Chapter 63

RESULTS OF MICROSURGICAL REPAIR OF BRACHIAL PLEXUS LESIONS

Laurent Sedel

This is a summary of our experience in 170 patients with brachial plexus palsy operated upon between 1972 and 1982 by the same surgeon. We shall concentrate our attention on the 63 cases that were followed for more than three years. In every case the decision to operate was made after a full clinical examination, electromyography, and cervical myelography. Surgical repair in all cases was attempted only if no sign of recovery was detectable at least two months after the injury.

We distinguish eight types of lesions. Each lesion was "labeled" only after surgical exploration. In our series sectioning of the clavicle was rarely necessary.

Type 1: All roots are avulsed from the cord.
Type 2: One or two roots are torn distally; the others are avulsed at the cord.
Type 3: Some roots are intact; others are avulsed from the cord.
Type 4: Some roots are intact; others are avulsed above the clavicle.
Type 5: Total rupture of the trunks or of their divisions.
Type 6: Complete rupture of the cords or of their main branches.
Type 7: Avulsion of the branches at their origin.
Type 8: The lesions are "in continuity."

The elements of surgical repair were as follows: When there was no loss of continuity, we carried out a neurolysis. Direct suturing usually proved impossible because of the loss of nerve tissue that usually accompanies avulsion injuries. Nerve grafts were often the only solution, using the sural nerve, which was sutured with 10/0 nylon under microscopic control. In a number of cases neurotizations (nerve transfers) were carried out using the intercostal nerves (as described by

Kotani et al.) or the lateral branch of the accessory nerve. Neurotization is indicated only in desperate cases when no other form of repair is possible.

In our original report of the results, we graded upper limb function as follows:

Grade I: Manual work can be performed with normal strength.
Grade II: The limb can perform everyday activities but lacks the power required for manual work.
Grade III: The limb can assist but not perform independently.
Grade IV: The limb is virtually useless although there is some movement of the elbow and the fingers; this is the esthetic animated arm.
Grade V: The limb is useless and inanimate.

In regard to returning to work, we differentiated four situations:

Grade I: Manual work is possible.
Grade II: The patient has resumed his normal occupation, which does not involve manual work.
Grade III: The patient has been forced to change his job.
Grade IV: The patient is unable to work.

The results in complete and partial palsies (at the time of surgery) are considered separately.

COMPLETE PALSY

Of the 32 patients, 27 were operated upon within one year after the injury and five between one and two years after the injury. Seven patients had type I lesions. In one exploration was carried out but no repair was attempted. The other six underwent neurotizations (nerve transfers)—from the intercostal nerves in three cases and from both

the intercostal and accessory nerves in the other three.

There was some improvement in all six cases, but in only four was there grade IV result, i.e., an esthetic animated arm with minimal mobility. Four patients recovered gross sensation as far down as the palm.

There were seven avulsions and one distal rupture (C5). These were treated by a nerve transfer from C5 in two cases and a combined transfer from C5 and intercostal nerves in six.

Three recovered usefulness of the limb to grade III and three to grade IV; two showed no improvement.

In seven cases there were two roots ruptured distally; the others avulsed from the cord. The usefulness of the limb was grade III in five patients and grade IV in one case; there was no recovery in one.

The remaining eight supraclavicular lesions were treated as follows: Three patients received a nerve graft (one or more) from C5, C6, or C7. Five were treated by neurolysis alone. Two neurolyses yielded good results, with a grade II recovery down to the hand in one case. Recovery in the remainder ranged between grades III and IV. There was no instance of failure in this group.

Finally, two patients with complete infraclavicular lesions were treated with long nerve transplants to make up for the long gaps. One patient recovered extension and flexion of the elbow and the other, extension only.

Thus, of the 32 patients with complete palsy, 26 were treated by nerve grafting, nerve transfer, or a combination of both. Eleven had a grade III recovery, 12 a grade IV recovery, and 3 a grade V recovery. Complete failure thus occurred in only three.

We also considered the surgical results in terms of the pain experienced by the patient, for this can be severe. Of the 21 patients who complained of pain preoperatively, only one was left with severe pain postoperatively. In most of the others, pain was relieved to some extent.

INCOMPLETE PALSY

The 31 patients with incomplete palsy initially had complete palsy but showed some degree of spontaneous recovery, especially in the hand. Ten of those were of the Erb type with involvement of C5 and C6. Two were treated with a nerve graft to the upper trunk, three with neurolysis of the upper trunk, and

one by direct suturing after excision of a schwannoma. Of these, three made a grade I recovery with good muscular function allowing return to manual work; three made a grade II recovery.

Nine patients had combined C5-C6-C7 palsy. All were treated with grafts from one or two roots. The result was good in eight cases, but three required further palliative surgery, such as arthrodesis of the shoulder or derotation of the humerus. Recovery was grade I in four cases, grade II in one, and grade III only in one.

Three patients presented slightly unusual supraclavicular lesions—either direct knife lesions to the roots or avulsion from the cord.

Finally, there were 13 infraclavicular lesions. Eight were complete and were treated by nerve grafting; five were partial and were treated by neurolysis only. Of these, six patients obtained a good or excellent result and one, a mediocre result. We recorded a grade I recovery in five patients and grade II recovery in three. Of the five patients with no break in continuity, all showed complete recovery, except one who is left with persistent weakness of the biceps.

CONCLUSIONS

Our results in 63 cases therefore provide answers to several important questions:

1. In none of the patients, and especially those with partial palsy, was there any worsening of the lesions.

2. Nerve grafts and nerve transfers, whenever possible, are always useful. The best results were obtained in partial palsies when grafting was limited to one root, one trunk, or one branch.

3. In complete palsy in which only one root can be treated by nerve transfer, the improvement is limited to flexion of the elbow, but muscle force is not always sufficient.

4. The effect on pain is often significant but unfortunately unpredictable.

Improvement in our techniques will, we hope, improve the quality of our results.

REFERENCES

Kotani, T., Matsuda, H., and Suzuki, T.: Trial surgical procedures of nerve transfer to avulsion injuries of plexus brachialis. Proc. 12th Congress of the International Society of Orthopaedic Surgery and Traumatology. Tel Aviv. Excerpta Medica, Amsterdam, 348, 1972.

Sedel, L.: The results of surgical repair of brachial plexus injuries. J. Bone Joint Surg., *64B*:1, 1982.

Chapter 64

SURGICAL INDICATIONS IN TRAUMATIC LESIONS OF THE BRACHIAL PLEXUS

Ezio Morelli
AND Pier Luigi Raimondi

With the experience of 318 traumatic lesions of the brachial plexus operated upon in our department between 1974 and 1981 (of which 142 were followed for two years or more), we feel able to define the indications for surgical treatment.

We divided our cases into four clinical groups—total paralysis, high plexus paralysis, low plexus paralysis, and lesions of the cords and distal branches of the plexus. In every case the clinical diagnosis was confirmed by electromyography and myelography.

The surgical repairs included neurolyses, direct suturing (when this proved possible), nerve grafts and neurotizations. In every patient a prolonged course of postoperative physiotherapy was prescribed.

Repeated reassessment of the results for two to five years after surgery helped us formulate a set of surgical indications. The difficulties in evaluating the function of individual muscles or muscle groups at different levels make it almost impossible to quantify the function of a limb in cases of complete brachial plexus palsy. Like Millesi, we find it more logical to evaluate a functional group. Thus we graded as "useful recovery" an M3 muscle contraction, i.e., contraction against gravity. We also interpreted Millesi's term "useful" as the recovery of minimal and not maximal function in a previously paralyzed limb. Thus, a supraspinatus muscle functioning at level M3 can raise the arm to 90 degrees and carry the hand to the mouth, but this remains inferior to full elevation of the limb, which also necessitates complete external rotation. The latter movement is possible only after full recovery of all the muscles supplied by the suprascapular nerve.

TOTAL PARALYSIS

Forty-eight patients were followed for three years or more. Useful functional recovery of the shoulder was obtained in 20 of the 48 cases, of the elbow in 25, of the wrist in 12, and of the hand in six.

Of the 48 cases, 41 involved preganglionic lesions of one or more roots, as follows: Four patients had one avulsed root, 12 had two, 11 had three, nine had four, and five had five avulsed roots.

Neurotization was carried out in 37 cases, as follows: neurotization from adjacent roots, 28 cases; neurotization from intercostal nerves, nine cases.

We were not always able to neurotize the whole plexus; hence, the discrepancy between the number of preganglionic lesions encountered (41) and the number of neurotizations carried out (37).

The "useful" results of our neurotizations were as follows: In operations using intact adjacent nerve roots, useful shoulder function resulted in one of 28 such patients and useful function of the elbow was restored in five of the 28. In two of the 28 patients useful wrist function was obtained. In the nine cases in which the intercostal nerves were used, shoulder function was restored in one patient and elbow function in two.

HIGH PLEXUS PARALYSIS

Fifty-one patients with high plexus paralysis were followed for two years or more. In 29 cases of paralysis of C5 and C6 useful functional results were obtained in the shoulder in 16 and in the elbow in 22.

Useful elbow flexion was achieved in two cases by neurotization—in one of three patients in whom intercostal nerves were used, and in the single patient in whom a spinal root was used.

Functional recovery in paralysis of C5, C6, and C7 (22 cases) was obtained in the shoulder in 12 cases, in the elbow in 16 cases (with triceps), and in the wrist and fingers in four cases (with, in addition, paralysis of the wrist and finger extensors).

In one of two cases useful abduction of the shoulder and elbow flexion were achieved by neurotization with intercostal nerves.

LOW PLEXUS PARALYSIS

The four patients with low plexus paralysis were followed for over three years. In two who underwent intercostal neurotizations there was no improvement, nor was there improvement in two who underwent repair using grafts from C8 and T1.

LESIONS OF THE TRUNKS AND CORDS OF THE PLEXUS

In this group, which included muscles involved in manual function, we were able to achieve M4 contraction in the following proportions of cases (follow-up over two years):

1. Posterior cord: six cases. In four there was a concomitant lesion of the musculocutaneous nerve. Useful results were obtained as follows: deltoid—six of six cases; triceps—four of six cases; carpal extensors—two of six cases; digital extensors—one of six cases; elbow flexion—four of four cases.

2. Circumflex and musculocutaneous nerves: 12 cases. Useful results were obtained as follows: deltoid—nine of 12 cases; biceps—11 of 12 cases.

3. Circumflex nerve alone: 12 cases. Eleven of 12 patients recovered useful deltoid function.

4. Trunk lesions in the axilla: nine cases. Individual nerves were involved as follows:

circumflex, seven cases; musculocutaneous, eight cases; radial, nine cases; median, nine cases; ulnar, seven cases. Useful results were obtained as follows: circumflex, five of seven cases; musculocutaneous, seven of eight cases; radial, four of nine cases; median, six of nine cases (two partial lesions); ulnar, two of seven cases (one partial lesion).

DISCUSSION

Taking into account the technical difficulties involved, the problems of age, the variable social background of the patients concerned, the possibility of long term reeducation, and the prosthetic alternatives available, we were able to draw the following conclusions from our results:

1. Patients sustaining traumatic lesions of the brachial plexus can benefit from surgical repair. Age and other factors affecting the life of the patient may constitute contraindications.

2. In total lesions of the brachial plexus with pre- and postganglionic rupture of the roots, the aim of surgery is to restore useful movement of the shoulder as well as some flexion-extension at the elbow. This is almost always possible by using the roots injured distal to the ganglion. If this is not feasible, neurotization from spinal or intercostal nerves often restores some mobility. In such cases manual function is seldom achieved: midforearm amputation and the fitting of a bioelectric prosthesis represent a somewhat desperate but potentially useful solution.

3. In lesions of the C5 and C6 roots, surgical repair should always be attempted.

4. Repair of C8 and T1 roots by grafts, or by neurotization in preganglionic lesions, has resulted in a high proportion of failures in our experience. Surgery can be justified, however, if protective sensation can be restored to the hand.

5. Our series indicates that an early repair has a much higher chance of success. After two months, improvement results only from spontaneous neurotizations, which are haphazard and insufficient. We believe that the longest delay compatible with a successful surgical repair is six to eight months.

Preliminary repair of only bone and vascular lesions must be avoided. In our experience this results in such distortion of the damaged nerve structures that secondary repair of the nerves is impossible. In more than one case we actually found additional iatrogenic lesions.

Age can constitute a relative contraindication: the older the patient, the lower the chances of recovery. However, we obtained a few surprising successes in patients over 45 years of age.

Pre- and postoperative re-education remains an essential part of the management of brachial plexus lesions. Improvement may occur only after several years of continuous and patient exercising. It is our impression that stimulation electrotherapy is an extremely useful adjunct.

Pain, which is always present after preganglionic lesions, can be relieved by neurotizations with the intercostal nerves even if function fails to improve. This is difficult to explain but is certainly worth mentioning.

Preganglionic avulsion of the whole plexus, especially in older patients, is a contraindication. However, partial recovery of some function has been achieved in such cases.

Chapter 65

MANAGEMENT OF BRACHIAL PLEXUS INJURIES

C. B. Wynn Parry

As more vehicles appear on the road, injuries to the brachial plexus are being seen with increasing frequency. During the years 1958–1974 we treated 164 patients with lesions of the brachial plexus, and 103 were followed from initial injury to final outcome (Wynn Parry, 1974). Of the 103 patients in the series, 80 had injuries caused by traffic accidents and 52 had been riding motorcycles when injured. The lesions were divided into two types: partial and complete. They can be further classified into those involving the upper trunk, those involving the lower trunk, and complete lesions of the entire plexus. With conservative treatment the prognosis for lesions of the upper trunk was good, some two-thirds of C5-C6 lesions recovering elbow flexion. The results of total lesions were poor, with only a few showing any functional recovery. The findings of Narakas (1977) that one-third of the patients he explored had ruptured nerve roots may account for the one-third of our C5-C6 lesions that did not recover, and his pioneer work in exploring the plexus revolutionized the management of plexus lesions.

From 1974 to 1983, 600 patients have been treated at The Brachial Plexus Service at the Royal National Orthopaedic Hospital at Stanmore. The severity of injuries has greatly increased as patients survive accidents owing to compulsory wearing of crash helmets and refinements of intensive care. The incidence of ruptures and avulsion lesions of the whole plexus are much higher.

One of the most devastating injuries that can affect a young person is complete avulsion of the brachial plexus from the cord, involving all spinal nerve roots from C5 to T1. The preganglionic nature of the lesion is confirmed by the normality of sensory action potentials in the presence of an anesthetic digit, a positive histamine test, and finally, by myelography. If the myelogram shows meningoceles for all roots, there is no chance for recovery. The presence of one or two meningoceles may not always mean avulsion of that root—myelography often overestimates the severity of the lesion. Horner's syndrome is not always a completely reliable indicator, for we have seen several cases in which a Horner's syndrome present at the earlier stages after the injury subsequently disappeared, and recovery occurred at a later date.

The histamine test is useful, although not entirely reliable, whereas sensory action potentials are extremely reliable and easy to determine. In this test, ring electrodes are placed over the little and index fingers and the digital nerve is stimulated; recordings are made over the nerves at the wrist. A normal sensory action potential in the presence of an anesthetic digit indicates that the posterior root ganglion is intact and that the lesion therefore must be preganglionic and the prognosis hopeless. Similarly, the radial nerve sensory action potential can be measured by stimulation over the superficial radial nerve in midforearm and recording over the first dorsal interosseous space with surface electrodes.

The radial nerve sensory action potential gives information concerning the C6 nerve root, the median nerve for C7, and the little finger for C8. Sensory evoked potentials have been used extensively in the past few years to provide a more accurate study of conduction in the brachial plexus. In this test the ulnar and median nerves are stimulated at the wrist with surface electrodes and recordings made with surface electrodes over the brachial plexus at the root of the neck, the spinous process of C2, and over the contralateral parietal cortex. The presence of a potential over the brachial plexus on stimulating the nerves at the wrist in the presence of total anesthesia of the hand must indicate a preganglionic lesion. Jones, Landi, and Wynn Parry (1981) found that the combination of sensory action potentials and sensory evoked potentials gave the most reliable results, but in the absence of complex equipment to measure sensory evoked potentials, the sensory action potentials give remarkably reliable and helpful information. At least two muscles supplied by each nerve root, C5-T1, should be sampled by electromyography in order to detect any surviving units, which of course will mean a lesion in continuity and therefore a much better prognosis. Table 65–1 shows the common clinical patterns of involvement in our series. It is distressing to note that total avulsion of all five roots is becoming almost the most frequent type of lesion. In the last 10 years the incidence of total lesions has exactly doubled in the patients referred to our service (Table 65–2). This represents the increasing number of motorcycles on the road with the increasing price of gasoline.

The great value of careful investigations such as electromyography and myelography means that as far as possible the lesion can be precisely determined and a prognosis offered. The most important feature is to decide those patients in which a ruptured nerve root may be present and which would be amenable to surgical grafting. Clearly the ideal treatment for all patients would be exploration of the plexus, for a definitive prognosis can be made with certainty and any ruptured nerves can be grafted. This is the ideal situation and whenever possible patients

Table 65–1. COMMON CLINICAL PATTERNS IN ORDER OF FREQUENCY OF PATIENTS WITH BRACHIAL PLEXUS LESIONS

C5, C6 lesions
Complete C5, C6, C7
Complete paralysis of the limb, with rupture of C5, C6, and C7, C8 and T1 being in continuity
Total paralysis of the arm with rupture of C5, C6, and avulsion of C7, C8, and T1
Avulsion of all five roots with a total and permanent flail arm

Table 65–2. INCREASING INCIDENCE OF TRACTION LESIONS OF THE BRACHIAL PLEXUS FROM 1977 TO 1981 AT THE ROYAL NATIONAL ORTHOPAEDIC HOSPITAL

	Number of New Patients	Total Lesions	
1977	58	14	24%
1978	73	17	23%
1979	102	32	31%
1980	117	48	40%
1981	110	54	49%

should be explored in the early stages. However, many patients suffer severe head injuries or chest injuries and are unfit for surgery. Moreover, there may not be ready access to a specialist unit. Consequently, a large number of patients are referred to the surgical team months or even years after the injury, and it is at this stage that careful investigations are valuable in trying to decide whether there is scope for surgery by grafting or whether the conservative approach should be adopted.

At one time it was the custom to amputate the arm and provide a prosthesis, having arthrodesed the shoulder. We have learned that few patients actually wear their artificial limbs, and that patients who have kept their flail arms prefer them to protheses—a stump attracts more attention on a beach or in a swimming pool than does a flail arm. Ransford and Hughes (1977) found that few patients used their artificial arms—and of course amputation never relieves pain, as some unfortunate patients have been led to believe.

We have also learned that amputation has often been done too early, for recovery can begin much later than realized, as long as two and one-half years after injury in a significant number of patients. It was initially believed that if one did not provide a limb within the first year, the patient would never become two-handed, but most people adapt to one-handedness in a few weeks. When a flail arm splint is provided, the argument is no longer valid, because the flail arm can be brought into patterns of movement. Amputation is indicated when the lost arm was completely dominant and the patient finds great difficulty in converting to nondominant arm use, and when the patient is very athletic and wants to continue participating in sports.

Because one cannot expect return of elbow flexion in less than one year (sometimes it takes 18 months whether treated surgically or not) and extension of the wrist and fingers cannot be expected for 18 months or possibly longer, the decision to undertake reconstructive surgery cannot be made until 18 months to two years have elapsed.

In patients with C5-C6 lesions only, i.e., who cannot abduct the arm or flex the elbow but have good wrist and finger extension, a simple elbow locking device is provided with a ratchet that allows fixation of the elbow in one of four positions. These modular splints are extremely light, worn under the clothing, unobtrusive, easy to clean, and cheap to provide. Being off the shelf they are readily available, and the patient only requires an hour or two to learn how to use them.

In patients who have lesions affecting C5, C6, and C7, the hand is nearly normal, in that the patient has good finger flexion and opposition of the thumb, with intrinsic activity but the patient cannot position the hand in the position of function; i.e., he cannot extend the wrist and fingers, and he cannot position the elbow in relation to the body for his work or hobbies.

A splint has been devised for these patients to allow them to position the arm and wrist for function. The splint consists of a shoulder piece with support on the opposite shoulder to prevent subluxation of the humerus, an elbow hinge joint with a ratchet device allowing the elbow to be maintained in one of five positions from extension to full flexion, and a cock-up piece attached to the distal end of the splint to put the wrist into dorsiflexion

and allow active flexion and extension of the digits (Fig. 65–1). There is also a facility for rotating the upper part of the splint so that the patient can effect internal or external rotation.

Recently we developed modular splints that can be fitted immediately, allowing patients to return to work quickly, for a custom built splint may take months to make. These splints are extremely valuable, for they allow a patient to position his elbow in more or less any position he wants, and allow him extension of the wrist so that he can use the hand fairly normally. We have had more than 50 patients with such splints, and all have found them invaluable.

The splints are, of course, only a temporary solution, for one hopes that the patient will regain sufficient active elbow flexion and extension of the wrist and fingers to dispense with the splint after 12 to 18 months. However, if recovery does not occur, the choice is between reconstructive surgery, or, if there are insufficient muscles for reconstruction to allow function, the splint may have to be worn permanently. We have a few patients who, indeed, are wearing this splint permanently, with a very good functional effect.

When the arm is totally flail, a splint is provided with the usual elbow lock but with a platform on the wrist to receive the standard artificial limb appliance. The patient operates these with the opposite shoulder. He is thus wearing an artificial arm over his flail arm. The arm is of some use, and movement patterns are preserved while recovery

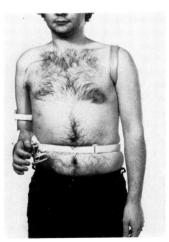 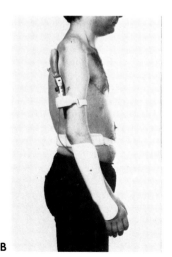 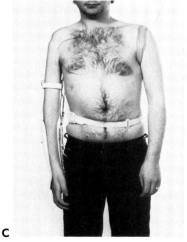

A   B   C

Figure 65–1. *A* to *C*, Flail arm splint with shoulder support, elbow locking device, and forearm piece for attachment of appliances.

is awaited. This is particularly important after surgical reconstruction, whether by use of grafts or neurotization. All the value of the surgery will be lost if the patient loses the image of his arm during the two years he is awaiting reinnervation and he will never make use of whatever muscle activity returns.

Over 200 patients have been provided with the complete flail arm splint for total paralysis. At a recent follow-up at two years after provision, 70 per cent were using the splint regularly either for work, for hobbies, or for recreation. It is important to ensure that the patient fully understands the use of the splints, and it is our practice to admit all our patients to our in-patient rehabilitation unit where the occupational therapist and the orthotist help the patient to learn to use the splint by training in the occupational therapy department in the workshops for 10 to 14 days. The patient cannot be expected to understand the splint or to use it if he is simply given it without training. Of supreme importance, as will be seen later, is the distraction from the severe pain that so many patients suffer from avulsion lesions of the plexus when they return to work, and in many of our patients the only way in which patients could be accepted for training or for full employment was by the demonstration that they had some function in their paralyzed arm by the use of a functional splint.

In our experience the most useful reconstructive procedure has been the Steindler operation for active elbow flexion. This requires good function in both the wrist flexors and the extensors, and after their origin has been transposed farther up the humerus, excellent powerful elbow flexion can be restored. When wrist extensors are not available, it may be better to do a Clarkes-Brooks transfer in which the pectoralis is inserted into the biceps. This is not as satisfactory a procedure as the Steindler operation, because there is inevitably some adduction of the arm across the chest wall, and in order to avoid this it may be necessary to perform an external rotation osteotomy of the humerus.

The standard procedures for permanent radial nerve paralysis are applicable for irrecoverable lesions of C7 when the C8 and T1 nerve roots are intact. Rarely one may see a patient in whom there has been a complete lesion of the brachial plexus, but the results of tests suggest that the majority of the lesion is postganglionic. Such a patient is described in the following case history.

ILLUSTRATIVE CASE

A Royal Air Force technician fell off his motorcycle and sustained a complete lesion of the right brachial plexus. Horner's syndrome was present from the start and persisted. It therefore looked as if the patient had sustained a total rupture of the plexus with preganglionic lesions of C5 to T1. However, the sensory action potentials were absent, and a myelogram showed a meningocele for T1 only. It was therefore decided to adopt a waiting policy, and the patient returned to work, using a special splint, which was, in effect, an artificial limb, over his paralyzed arm. This allowed him to position his elbow and to put the normal appliances for an artificial arm on the splints. He was able to return to his job as an armament fitter. Subsequently he gradually regained excellent elbow flexion, finger flexion, and sensation in the hand. He needed an external rotation osteotomy to prevent the elbow from flexing across the chest wall and an arthrodesis of the wrist to provide better stability of the wrist (Donal Brooks). Eventually, in order to provide some active abduction, he underwent a Zachary transfer, in which the latissimus dorsi was inserted into the infraspinatus. This allowed him 45 degrees of abduction. This patient, who is still serving in the Royal Air Force, has achieved the rank of sergeant and has passed at the top of his class in a demanding torpedo fitters' course.

Rehabilitation of patients who have brachial plexus paralyses, therefore, is concerned with the maintenance or restoration of the full passive range of the paralyzed joints, provision of dynamic or supportive splints to put the arm in the best position of function and allow spared muscles to work, and re-education of recovering function, or the function that results from reconstructive surgery when recovery clearly is not going to occur.

Certainly the most distressing feature of traction lesions of the brachial plexus is the appalling pain that so many patients with avulsion lesions suffer. In a series of 106 patients with known avulsion lesions studied in detail by our team, 90 per cent suffered severe pain at some stage of their illness. It is known experimentally that deafferentation of the spinal cord leads to spontaneous firing of the deafferented cells in laminas 1 and 5 (Loeser and Ward, 1967). It is postulated that this spontaneous firing is associated with pain. The more severe the degree of deafferentation, the more spontaneous firing is seen, and therefore, presumably more pain is felt.

It is certainly our experience that the severest pain is associated with avulsion of all five nerve roots, although we have seen very distressing pain in patients in whom only one nerve root has been avulsed. Classically these patients suffer two types of pain, one a continuous burning, crushing pain, usually felt in the paralyzed and insensitive hand, and the other severe paroxysms of shooting pain that may last only a few seconds but dart like lightning through the arm and can be devastating in their effect. Many patients shout out or grip their arm or turn away to the wall so painful are the paroxysms. The frequency of these paroxysms may vary from many times an hour to a few times a day. Their incidence is unpredictable and patients have no way of knowing when their next attack is going to come.

Paroxysmal pain is the most distressing for the patient and the most difficult to bring under control. The onset of this pain is usually immediate, but we have seen patients in which the pain has not developed for three months after the injury. The natural history of the pain is to subside within three years. Most patients find the pain tolerable within the first year. If the patient is still suffering significant pain at three years after injury, then he is likely to suffer the pain indefinitely. Moreover, in such patients the pain tends to get worse with time, particularly as they approach middle age, and it would seem that other nociceptive stimuli, such as pain from cervical spine arthritis, add to the already existing abnormal neuron pool in the spinal cord.

Analgesic drugs, including even the most powerful, and narcotics, are singularly unhelpful for this pain. There are only two ways in which this pain can be significantly controlled. The most important is by mental distraction. Here it would seem the patient is instinctively bringing his own inhibitory pain pathways into action. If he can return to an absorbing job or take up a meaningful hobby that occupies all his interest, then the pain may well be under control. That is why it is so important to help these young men to return to work as soon as possible or to retrain for a new job, and why the application of functional splinting may be so important.

The single most valuable modality is transcutaneous electrical nerve stimulation. In our service we insist on admission to our inpatient rehabilitation ward so that our skilled physiotherapists may try the stimulator in various different positions for many hours on end (Frampton, 1982). We try the stimulator for

at least two weeks before we abandon it as being unhelpful. Even if there is only a slight response, we persuade the patients to continue with the use of the stimulator throughout the day and sometimes throughout the night as well for a prolonged period, for at least a week, as the effect is known to be cumulative. Transcutaneous stimulation is an extremely valuable modality—it is unfortunately often abused, patients being given stimulators without proper instruction and told to use it for half an hour or an hour only at a time. This is wasteful and ineffective.

In patients with severe paroxysmal shooting pains it is always worth while trying the effect of anticonvulsant drugs, particularly carbamazepine or its analogues. Unfortunately, only 10 per cent of such patients in our series have responded significantly. In some patients the combination of aminotriptyline and perphenazine can be most helpful. This seems to be due to its central acting effect by potentiating the production of serotonin, stores of which are depleted in chronic pain. Dorsal column stimulation and thalamic stimulation appear to have no place in deafferentation pain. It is our practice to offer all patients with severe pain a prolonged trial of transcutaneous stimulation. If this is ineffective, then we will try Tegretol for the paroxysmal pain and Tryptofen for the chronic crushing pain. All patients will be helped to return to training or to work, through our resettlement and retraining service.

The vast majority of patients will learn to accept their pain and in many instances the pain will subside gradually over months or the first year or two. There remain a small but highly significant number of patients, perhaps 1 per cent of the total, who suffer severe continuous intractable pain that destroys their lives and that of their families. For them the dorsal root entry zone operation can be considered. Nashold et al. (1976) introduced this at Duke University and argued that by destroying that area where the spontaneous firing is taking place, pain should be relieved, the rationale being quite different from the normal destructive lesion in which tracts are cut or coagulated. This would be tackling the basic cause of the abnormal firing.

Nashold has reported 70 per cent success rate over a nine year period in patients with avulsion lesions of the brachial plexus, and similar findings have been reported by

Thomas and Jones (1984) from London, who have carried out such treatment of these lesions in a number of our patients. It has to be borne in mind that there are undoubtedly complications from this procedure. Some of our patients have had proprioceptive loss in the ipsilateral leg, many have unpleasant dysesthesia of the trunk, some have developed weakness of the ipsilateral leg, three have been rendered temporarily impotent and one permanently impotent, and in a few patients the pain is not affected at all.

It is therefore in only the psychologically most robust patient who is in a desperate state due to pain that this very serious operation should be considered. Certainly all other attempts to relieve the pain should have been tried over an extended period and it should have been explained in great detail to him and his relatives on several occasions what the implications may be. Having said this, we can report that a number of our patients have had their lives transformed by this procedure.

enable patients to make the most use of their weak or paralyzed arm. Unfortunately the employment situation in countries in which these lesions are common is poor, and it is becoming increasingly difficult to offer these patients a career. This inevitably means a high incidence of pain and a great deal of suffering.

Much can be done by careful diagnostic procedures, including myelography and electromyography, to establish which patients are going to benefit from surgery. Much can be done by intensive and skilled physiotherapy and occupational therapy to maintain good function and restore function to weak muscles and stiff joints. Much can also be done to help the pain, to improve function by splinting, by re-education, and by reconstructive surgery, but the most overriding problem is the prevention of such appalling injuries and the insistence that young men have proper training in managing these lethal motorcycles before they take to the road, and that they wear appropriate protective clothing.

SUMMARY

There has been a pronounced change in the pattern of involvement of brachial plexus lesions over the last 40 years. Forty years ago the most common lesion was a complete upper trunk lesion in which the prognosis for the return of elbow flexion was good. Now the most common lesion is a total avulsion of all roots of the brachial plexus. A significant proportion of patients have rupture of nerve roots, and these can be grafted surgically with the prospect of return of proximal function. The nature of the pain is now better understood, although unfortunately its incidence is much higher than heretofore.

There are ways of helping patients with such pain, and there is functional splinting to

REFERENCES

Fletcher, I.: *In* Wynn Parry, C. B. (Editor): Rehabilitation of the Hand. London, Butterworth & Co. (Publishers) Ltd., 1973.

Frampton, V.: Physiotherapy, *68*:77, 1982.

Jones, S., Wynn Parry, C. B., and Landi, A.: Injury, *12*:376, 1987.

Loeser, J. D., and Ward, A. A.: Arch. Neurol., *17*:629, 1967.

Narakas, A.: Rev. Chir. Orthop., *63*:44–54, 1977.

Nashold, B. S. Urban, B., and Zorab, D. S.: *In* Bonica, J. J., and Albe Fessard, D. (eds.): Advances in Pain Research and Therapy. Vol. 1. New York, Raven Press, 1976, p. 959.

Ramsford, A. O., and Hughes, S.: J. Bone Joint Surg., *59B*:417, 1977.

Thomas, D. G. T., and Jones, S. J.: Dorsal root entry zone lesions (Nashold's procedure) in brachial plexus avulsion. Neurosurgery, *15*:966, 1984.

Wynn Parry, C. B.: Proc. R. Soc. Med., *67*:488, 1974.

Part Three

SURGERY OF VESSELS

Chapter 66

INVESTIGATION OF THE CIRCULATION OF THE HAND

JEAN-PIERRE MELKI,
MARIE-CLAIRE RICHE,
C. FRANCHESCHI,
DANIEL REIZINE,
AND JEAN-JACQUES MERLAND

The circulation of the hand is investigated in a variety of conditions. Until recently arteriography was the most refined technique. More recent noninvasive methods, such as Doppler ultrasonography and capillaroscopy, now can aid in making a diagnosis, as in the so-called acrosyndromes.

It must be pointed out, however, that with the advent of less traumatizing puncturing devices and painless contrast media, arteriography itself has become a much less aggressive form of investigation. When used by an experienced operator, it has become simple and rapid and can be carried out without premedication on an outpatient basis. For these reasons arteriography remains highly popular not only as a diagnostic tool but to assist in determining the prognosis and to provide valuable preoperative information. It also is the only way of mapping out the detailed vascularization of the hand. Although arteriography may have lost some of its diagnostic value, it remains an essential adjunct in the endovascular treatment of some conditions such as angiodysplasias.

The recent introduction of digital angiography rendered arteriography even less aggressive through the reduced doses of contrast media and the use of still finer puncture needles. Its adaptation to the venous circulation could also help in studying the vascular anatomy of the hand.

RADIOANATOMICAL STUDY OF THE CIRCULATION OF THE HAND

THE ARTERIES OF THE HAND

The hand is supplied through two main arteries—the radial and the ulnar (Figs. 66–1, 66–2). Under normal circumstances these two vessels are responsible for virtually the entire arterial supply (Rouviere, 1962). Other important channels are the interosseous arteries (especially the anterior interosseous artery), which arise from the common interosseous branch of the ulnar artery. These vessels, which are relatively unimportant under normal circumstances, may assume a vital role if either of the main forearm arteries is injured. In 8 to 9 per cent of the cases the anterior interosseous artery gives off an artery that accompanies the median nerve; it is known as the median artery and usually anastomoses with the superficial palmar arch (Chermet, 1974). These arteries, through their anastomoses, form the arterial arches. The main ones are the superficial and deep palmar arches; the accessory ones are the dorsal and palmar carpal arches.

The Deep Palmar Arch

The deep palmar arch is formed by the terminal part of the radial artery and its

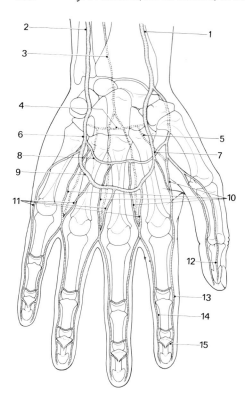

Figure 66–1. Diagram of the blood supply of the hand according to the classic description. 1 = radial artery, 2 = ulnar artery, 3 = anterior interosseous artery of the forearm, 4 = dorsal arcade of the carpus, 5 = dorsal metacarpal arteries, 6 = ulnar palmar artery, 7 = radial palmar artery, 8 = deep palmar arch, 9 = superficial palmar arch, 10 = palmar metacarpal artery, 11 = common palmar digital artery, 12 = radial collateral artery of the thumb, 13 = radial palmar collateral of the fingers, 14 = ulnar palmar collateral of the fingers, and 15 = subungual arch.

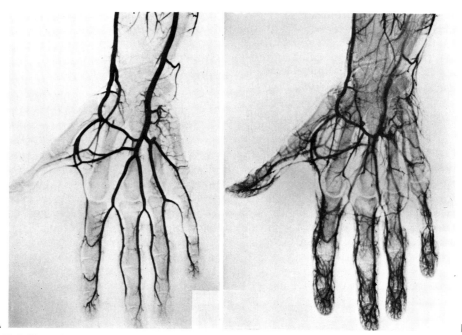

Figure 66–2. Normal computerized arteriogram of the hand. *A*, Early phase. *B*, Late phase. Anatomical variations: the palmar arches are present and small; a predominant ulnar artery supplying the last three fingers and the ulnar half of the index finger.

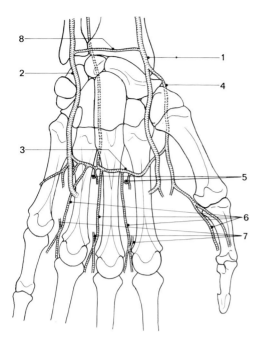

Figure 66–3. Deep palmar arch (Edwards-Chermet). 1 = radial artery, 2 = ulnar artery, 3 = deep palmar arch, 4 = radialis indicis, 5 = proximal perforating branch, 6 = palmar metacarpal artery, 7 = anastomosis between metacarpal and interosseous arteries, and 8 = palmar arch of the carpus.

anastomosis with the deep branch of the ulnar artery (Figs. 66–1, 66–3). It lies anterior to the upper extremity of the metacarpal shafts. It is seldom fully developed and the deep ulnar branch is often negligible. The dominance of the radial artery is readily demonstrable by the selective vascular compression test (Chermet, 1974).

The deep palmar arch gives rise to the interosseous (or metacarpal) arteries. These are, from lateral to medial, the interosseous artery of the first interspace (which ramifies into the ulnar palmar collateral and the radial palmar collateral, also known as the princeps pollicis, and the radial collateral artery of the index finger) and the interosseous arteries of the second, third, and fourth interspaces (Blonstein et al., 1977).

The Superficial Palmar Arch

The superficial palmar arch is formed from the anastomosis of the terminal branch of the ulnar artery with the superficial palmar branch of the radial artery (Fig. 66–4). On an arteriogram it is seen to lie under the deep

palmar arch and has a smaller caliber. It is fully developed in only 13 to 19 per cent of the cases. In 60 per cent of the cases it is formed from the ulnar artery alone and in 32 per cent from the superficial palmar branch of the radial artery. In 8 per cent of the cases it results from the anastomosis of the median with the ulnar artery (Chermet, 1974; Dijkstra, 1979; Dufour et al., 1981; Edwards, 1958, 1960). Often one arch and its branches are obviously dominant.

From its convex side the superficial palmar arch gives off four collaterals, known as the palmar digital arteries, which, from the ulnar to the radial side, are the first, second, third, and fourth digital arteries. There often is a fifth digital artery, which is of small caliber and anastomoses with the first palmar interosseous artery, itself a branch of the deep palmar arch.

The Carpal Arches

The dorsal carpal arch, when present, is formed by the union of homologous branches from the radial and ulnar arteries (Fig. 66–5). The interosseous dorsal arteries of the

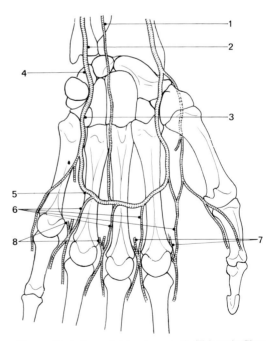

Figure 66–4. Superficial palmar arch (Edwards-Chermet). 1 = median artery, 2 = radial artery, 3 = radial palmar artery, 4 = ulnar artery, 5 = superficial palmar arch, 6 = palmar metacarpal artery, 7 = anastomosis between interosseous artery and digital artery, and 8 = distal perforating branches.

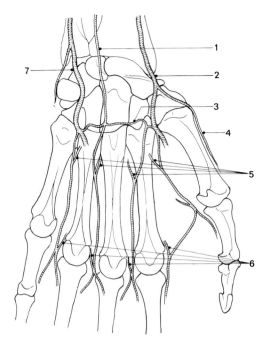

Figure 66–5. Dorsal arch of the carpus. 1 = dorsal interosseous artery (of the forearm), 2 = radial artery, 3 = dorsal arch of the carpus, 4 = radialis indicis, 5 = proximal perforating branches, 6 = distal perforating branches, and 7 = ulnar artery.

second, third, and fourth interspaces, as well as the medial collateral of the little finger, are formed from this arch. Each dorsal interosseous artery splits into two dorsal collateral branches that terminate on the lateral aspects of adjacent fingers. The dorsal carpal arch can function as a collateral channel between the radial artery and the deep palmar arch; it often receives a significant contribution from the radial artery.

Much less commonly found is a palmar carpal arch; it seldom forms a recognizable arcade and frequently consists of a loose collateral network known as the palmar carpal plexus. It usually connects the anterior interosseous artery with the radial and ulnar arteries.

Vascularization of the Fingers

The interosseous (or metacarpal) palmar and dorsal arteries anastomose with the palmar digital arteries and with one another through proximal and distal perforating channels to form the palmar collateral arteries of the fingers (Blonstein et al., 1977). Each finger has an ulnar and a radial collateral artery. Each pair is linked through transverse palmar anastomoses (digital arches) and ends up in the pulp and nail bed in terminal anastomoses (Fig. 66–6).

It should be noted that the palmar collateral arteries of the thumb and the radial collateral artery of the index finger usually come off the first interosseous branch of the deep palmar arch.

In addition to this major palmar network there is a dorsal supply arising from the dorsal carpal arch. The dorsal collateral vessels come off an inconstant dorsal arch that overlies the proximal phalanx of each finger (Chermet, 1974).

THE VEINS OF THE HAND

In both the hand and the fingers the superficial veins are well developed on the dorsal side while the palmar veins are limited to a network of small venules (Rouviere, 1962). The dorsal digital veins come off the subungual plexus, which in turn drains into the periungual vein. The latter in turn breaks into a dorsal plexus, which runs into a digital venous arch that overlies the proximal phalanx. The digital arches interconnect in the spaces between the metacarpal heads.

The metacarpal veins unite to form a dorsal

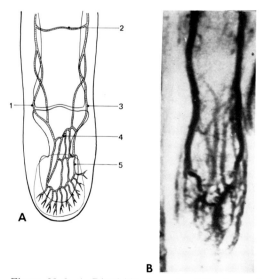

Figure 66–6. A, Distal blood supply of the finger. 1 = ulnar proper palmar digital artery, 2 = digital arch, 3 = radial proper palmar digital artery, 4 = subungual arch, 5 = arteries of the pulp. B, Normal arteriogram of a finger (enlargement).

venous arch into which drain the cephalic vein of the thumb and the vein of the little finger. The palmar veins likewise join the venous plexus of the fingers and the hand.

The venous plexuses of the hand give rise to three principal venous channels that drain into the forearm—the superficial radial or median vein, the superficial ulnar vein, and the accessory radial vein.

THE LYMPH VESSELS OF THE HAND

The lymph drainage of the hand is divided into a superficial and a deep system (Rouviere, 1962).

The Superficial Channels

The collecting vessels of the fingers run along the interdigital grooves toward the dorsum of the hand and forearm. The collecting channels of the palm travel on the anterior side of the forearm, where they are joined by the dorsal channels. Ultimately all the superficial lymphatics travel on the anterior aspect of the arm toward the axilla, where they drain into the central and axillary groups of lymph nodes.

The Deep Channels

The deep channels accompany the large blood vessels. In the hand they follow the palmar arches, and from there they run alongside the ulnar, radial, and interosseous vessels.

TECHNIQUES OF INVESTIGATION OF THE CIRCULATION OF THE HAND

The investigations requested and their order of selection depend on the primary clinical findings. Ultrasonography and capillaroscopy are so innocuous and yet so reliable that they are often the first choice. A logical sequence would start with noninvasive techniques (Doppler ultrasonography, capillaroscopy, isotope studies) before requesting the invasive ones (arteriography and phlebography). This order is by no means obligatory; when confronted with a congenital arteriovenous malformation or a severe hand injury, the surgeon is more likely to begin with an arteriogram whose arterial mapping he will use as a basis for his therapeutic strategy. As we shall see, the Doppler method can be a helpful diagnostic adjunct.

DOPPLER ULTRASONOGRAPHY AND ECHOTOMOGRAPHY

With Doppler ultrasonography it is possible to detect mobile structures and to measure their rate of movement. It is highly suitable, therefore, for blood flow measurements (Francheschi, 1979).

With a pulsed signal it is possible to measure the output (Levy et al., 1979; Martinaud et al., 1980). If a continuous signal is used, an echotomogram will give the section (S) of the vessel concerned, and the output is calculated as the product of $S \times V$ (where V is the flow rate). The echotomogram also can be used to study the vessel walls and vessel contents and can thus detect any lesion present (Francheschi, 1979).

The Doppler method can measure blood flow in different circumstances—at rest, during exertion, and in different positions and at different temperatures. Hence its relevance in functional studies of the circulation of the hand.

Arterial Studies

All the arteries of the upper limb can be studied by the Doppler method and echotomographic techniques, from the subclavian trunk down to the digital arteries.

Arteries in the Hand. Static studies are used to assess the patency of the radial and ulnar arteries, the palmar arches, and the digital collateral vessels. They also yield information regarding anatomical variations and blood flow through the pulp. Additional data can be obtained by capillaroscopy. The surgeon can thus be made aware of the eventual possibility of stenoses, arterial occlusions, and arteriovenous fistulas.

Dynamic studies make use of selective compression to evaluate the competence of the arterial arches and the capacity of the two main trunks to take over each other's territory in case of occlusion.

Thermal tests assess the capacity of the arterial network to adapt to temperature changes (vasodilation and vasoconstriction) and the resulting changes in arterial output.

Arteries Proximal to the Hand. If an associated lesion (multifocal vascular malformation) or a distant one (atheromatous plaque or other costoclavicular lesion) is present, this will be detected by the Doppler test.

STATIC TESTS. Static tests are used to detect changes in flow rate at a site of stenosis, occlusion, or an arteriovenous shunt. With the added help of echotomography, it is possible to measure the arterial output at rest and to determine the nature of a stenosis (e.g., an atheromatous plaque, a narrowing in the costoclavicular segment, or extrinsic compression). The Doppler test will also point out any abnormal arterial divisions and thus help in interpreting later angiograms.

DYNAMIC TESTS. Dynamic tests reveal alterations in blood flow in different positions of the limb, in selective compression, and in induced hyperemia, as well as the adaptability of the arterial network as a whole.

Venous Studies

Use of the Doppler method here permits recognition of the preferential channels of venous drainage and the detection of proximal lesions by means of static and dynamic testing. When used by an experienced operator, the Doppler and echotomogram can provide nearly as much anatomical information as an arteriogram, as well as evaluate the function of the afferent arteries.

CAPILLAROSCOPY

Capillaroscopy is a method of observing the microcirculation of the skin in vivo (Vayssairat and Housset, 1980). This original technique may be sufficient by itself or may prove a useful adjunct to the Doppler method.

The capillaroscope magnifies the cutaneous microcirculation 50 to 300 times. This microcirculation is made physiologically opaque by transillumination of the epithelium, which is almost transparent. The alignment of the capillary bed of the skin is mostly perpendicular to the epithelium, except in a few areas such as the nail bed where the capillaries can be examined as a horizontal network. Other areas where the capillaries can be readily visualized are the skin, the lips, and especially the ocular conjunctiva.

Normal Capillaroscopy (Color Plate V)

Static Study. In the nail bed the capillary appears as a continuous, smooth edged, orange-red, homogeneous filament (Fig. 66–7). Capillary loops vary in shape but most common is the hairpin configuration. There are an average of 10 parallel loops per millimeter, all evenly spaced. The pericapillary space is a uniform pink, the background color that indicates healthy tissue.

Dynamic Study. The capillary functions spasmodically: it fills and empties every 20 seconds. Venous compression improves visualization by causing slight dilation of the blood column. Arterial compression results in circulatory arrest, but the capillary remains wide open and clearly visible. Cold slows down the blood flow, but the loops remain visible and slightly dilated.

The Principal Capillaroscopic Anomalies

Quantitative Anomalies. Most forms of microangiopathy result in a reduction in the number of capillary loops; whole areas are bereft of capillaries, as in generalized scleroderma (Vayssairat and Housset, 1980).

Qualitative Anomalies. The megacapillary is a feature seen in dermatomyositis, scleroderma, and Sharp's syndrome. Capillary dystrophy (tortuous capillary with irregular walls and microaneurysms) suggests nonspecific microangiopathy. The regressive capillary is equally nonspecific.

Dynamic Anomalies. In sludging, the capillary loops are filled by a granular current, which indicates hyperviscosity of the blood.

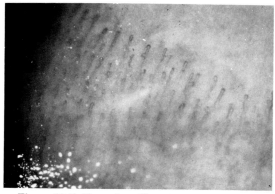

Figure 66–7. Normal capillaroscopy of the nail bed. (Kindly provided by Prof. Vaysserat.)

Closure on exposure to cold (the critical closing phenomenon) is seen in Raynaud's phenomenon.

Pericapillary Anomalies. Hemorrhage indicates a severe angiopathy. Edema is found in digital necrosis, but in the absence of trophic disorders it suggests scleroderma.

In summary, capillaroscopy is a simple technique permitting in vivo visualization of the microcirculation. It helps in the classification of the acrosyndromes and in the evaluation of any form of treatment.

ARTERIOGRAPHY

In this section we shall only consider arteriography as a diagnostic procedure. Selective arteriography and its therapeutic implications are dealt with in another chapter.

Equipment

The basic requirement is a standard room for vascular radiology with a fine focus radiogenic tube and facilities for immediate magnification. An arteriophlebograph capable of showing an arteriogram of the whole upper limb can prove extremely useful.

As a rule injections are delivered at a constant rate, and sequential films are taken to cover the arterial, capillary, and venous phases. Although arteriography is usually carried out in the circumstances just mentioned, on occasion it has to be done in much less favorable surroundings, i.e., in a routine radiology room, at the bedside or even in the operating room. Because only small amounts of contrast medium are required, manual injection is acceptable; only the timing of the vascular phases can be tricky.

Computerized angiography has now taken a large place in this type of exploration and allows the examiner to assess the dimensions of the part to be explored. Opacification in a flow state (2 to 4 cc. per sec.) is followed on the screen and covers all the vascular times until venous return.

Preparation of the Patient, Contrast Media, and Behavioral Changes

Arteriography of the hand in the past has rightly been regarded as a painful procedure. For this reason anesthesia was usually necessary. Since the introduction of low osmo-larity (600 mOsm.) 32 per cent hexaiodinated substances, anesthesia is seldom needed, except, of course, with children. The new contrast media are usually well tolerated by the patient and leave no traumatic memories, so that arteriography now can be performed on an outpatient basis.

When an anesthetic is deemed necessary, an axillary or supraclavicular (plexus) block is usually preferable to general anesthesia or even neuroleptanalgesia. (We shall come back to this choice in the context of therapeutic angiography.) It may be useful to alter the physical and chemical conditions during the examination.

The small amount of contrast medium used in computerized angiography reduces the risks, except in children in whom anesthesia is necessary; in the majority of adult cases no preparation is necessary.

Physical Conditions. The limb is frequently tested with heat and cold when investigating an acrosyndrome. Heat is of particular value, because there is a significant increase in arterial flow in the extremities at temperatures of 30 to 35° C. (Rosch et al., 1977).

Chemical Conditions. We are mostly interested here with the action of vasodilators. The arteries of the hand and their branches are particularly liable to spasm even after a single puncture. Indeed some operators advocate the systematic use of heparin, the appropriate dose being 60.5 mg. per kg. of body weight (Blonstein et al., 1977). We use one or two ampules of a vasodilator (Infenprodil) diluted, injected intra-arterially 2 to 5 min. before angiography.

The Puncture Site

If the mode of division of the brachial artery is not known, retrograde puncture of that vessel is preferred, for it is safer and gives consistently good results.

The humeral artery is punctured at the elbow crease with a catheter needle whose Teflon sheath is left in situ for the injection. Because the volumes involved are small (15 to 20 cc. at 3 to 5 ml. per sec.), a small bore atraumatic needle can be used. Arterial spasm can be reduced by keeping manipulation to a minimum. If subclavian angiography is indicated, a larger needle is preferred to accommodate the increased flow (15 to 20 ml. per sec.).

In the majority of cases the contrast medium is injected into the humeral artery at the elbow, with the arm extended and the hand in supination. In special circumstances (e.g., fixed flexion of the elbow, vein grafting, or humeral prosthesis), the injection is made more proximally, halfway up the arm or even at the axilla. Some physicians even prefer femoral catheterization using Seldinger's method; this may be the preferred technique if an arteriogram of the lower limb is required prior to a toe transfer, in which case the homolateral femoral artery is chosen (Blonstein et al., 1977).

The Arteriographic Study

An arteriogram may be required to illustrate the vascular tree of the hand alone or of the entire upper limb. In the latter case prior arteriophlebographic study is needed. This helps in timing the various phases of flow and can be used as a guide when programming the seriogram. In addition it can show an arterial spasm at the puncture site and thus help to explain a possible delay in distal flow. In computerized studies the progression of the flow of contrast material can be followed serially, and can be interrupted when the necessary information is obtained.

Whenever possible, magnified serial views of the hand are taken, and these can be repeated after radial or ulnar compression to test the efficacy of radioulnar anastomoses in the hand. Further information can be gleaned by carrying out the examination under Doppler control, especially when investigating arteriovenous malformations.

Incidents and Accidents

Accidents associated with puncture of the humeral artery are rare. Those associated with axillary puncture and femoral catheterization are well known. Their incidence is inversely proportional to the experience of the radiologist.

Arterial spasm is the most common incident and tends to occur in young patients after difficult or repeated punctures, emphasizing the importance of keeping the procedure as atraumatic as possible. Indeed arterial spasm can be so severe that blood flow is reduced to a trickle and the distal opacification is minimal, making it impossible to carry out a comprehensive study of the vascular lesions (Fig. 66–8). However, as a rule arteriography of the hand is a relatively simple investigation which needs little or no preparation and usually can be performed on outpatients.

DIGITAL SUBTRACTION ANGIOGRAPHY

Digital subtraction angiography is used to depict the arteries of the hand using either the venous or the arterial route. The images

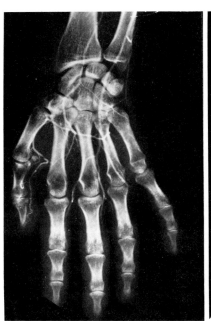 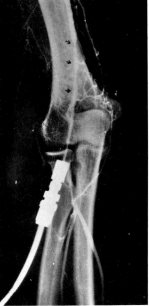

Figure 66–8. *A* and *B*, Spasm at humeral puncture site causing severe reduction of distal blood flow.

A   B

obtained are the result of a digital analysis of the variations in luminosity per unit of surface area; these are projected onto a screen, on which visualization by direct subtraction is possible.

Technique with Venipuncture

This technique consists of injecting 30 to 40 cc. (for an adult) of contrast medium into a peripheral vein (or into the vena cava) at a rapid rate (20 to 25 cc. per sec.) so that it reaches the left side of the heart and arteries in an adequate concentration.

Although this technique, which is not new, produces good visualization of the larger vessels (aorta, carotids, subclavians), it requires large amounts of contrast medium (80 cc. in an adult) and the results cannot compare in quality with the opacification obtained by direct intra-arterial injection. It is justified only in patients in whom arterial puncture is risky (polyarteritis, aortic disease).

Quantitative analysis of the images now allows amplification of the visual signal. The sensitivity of the technique has been further improved by direct subtraction, which can produce excellent visualization, especially of the larger vessels (aorta, carotid arteries, subclavian and iliac arteries). The results are less spectacular with the smaller arteries (arches of the hand, digital vessels). This method can provide useful information about the patency of the radial and ulnar arteries and the palmar arches, but cannot be relied upon to detect subtle lesions of the distal arteries.

The advantage of the technique lies in the fact that arterial puncture is avoided and that it can be carried out as an outpatient procedure. It has the additional advantage of providing information in cases in which the axillary artery cannot be utilized (e.g., traumatic lesions). It is unsuitable, however, in patients with an abnormal cardiac output, or if complete cooperation cannot be relied upon.

Technique with Arterial Puncture

The principles of quantitative analysis and direct subtraction are the same, but the volumes of contrast media injected are much smaller (3 to 4 cc. in all) than in conventional arteriography. This should encourage the use of even finer puncture needles and make arteriography possible as an outpatient procedure. The results are at least as good as in conventional arteriography, with the added advantage that one is able to transfer the results immediately onto the television screen.

OTHER TECHNIQUES

Other techniques can also provide useful information regarding the vascularization of the hand and can be considered as complementary to those already described.

Phlebography. Phlebography is more useful in study of the venous return in the arm and forearm than in the hand. By means of selective compression, more information can be gained, especially when investigating arteriovenous malformations. In addition, the late phases of an arteriogram can also help in studying the patterns of venous blood flow.

Lymphography. Lymphography is useful in the study of the lymphatic drainage of the upper limb but provides little information about the lymphatic network of the hand proper. The procedure can be difficult in the presence of lymphedema.

Phlebography and Lymphography Using Radioisotopes. These potentially useful techniques have the same drawbacks as their radiological equivalents, in that they have limited application in the study of the venous and lymphatic circulations of the hand. Their main advantage is that they are noninvasive, a major asset in the study of a lymphedematous limb (Gest, 1963; Hayt et al., 1977; Jacobson and Ostberg, 1973; Rees et al., 1980; Yun Ryo et al., 1977).

In practice, labeled colloids (usually with technetium) are injected subcutaneously for a lymphogram and intravenously for a phlebogram. The progress of the colloids is then followed using a gamma camera.

The Scanner. The scanner is particularly helpful in the study of angiodysplasias (Fig. 66–9). Indeed it may be useful in distinguishing between angiodysplasia and tissue hypertrophy, as well as in locating the exact site of the angiodysplasia (e.g., skin or muscle).

Thermography. Thermography is another complementary method of investigation that can be used in conjunction with the Doppler technique to follow the evolution of vascular lesions such as angiomas.

Plethysmography. Plethysmography remains useful in the study of acrosyndromes.

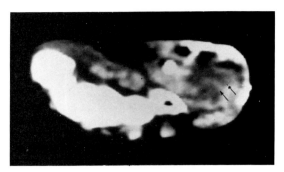

Figure 66–9. CT scan of pure venous angiodysplasia of the palm of the hand after sclerosis using Ethibloc plus Lipiodol. Ethibloc mixed with Lipiodol is visible especially at the surface (hyperdensity). Intramuscular venous lakes remain in the hypothenar eminence *(arrow)*.

TECHNIQUES OF SELECTIVE ANGIOGRAPHY AND THERAPEUTIC ANGIOGRAPHY

It is primarily in the context of therapeutic angiography that new techniques of selective angiography have developed. Here the operator must come very close to, or actually penetrate, the lesion. The main advantage of selective arteriography is its capacity to delineate a precise vascular territory, its arterial supply, and its venous channels.

The Arterial Route

Most endovascular therapeutic procedures, especially those dealing with emboli, are carried out via the arterial route. As a rule therapeutic arteriography is performed as a secondary procedure, after primary angiography and Doppler probing have established the distribution of the arterial tree and located the lesion.

Route of Access: Catheterization Equipment. The puncture site depends on the site of the lesion (Merland et al., 1979, 1980; Natali and Merland, 1976; Riche et al., 1981). The common approaches are downward puncture of the brachial proximal to its division, downward puncture of the radial or ulnar artery, puncture of a digital collateral, and direct puncture of a feeder artery in cases of arteriovenous angioma. The femoral approach is seldom used, being too far from the hand.

From these puncture sites a catheter can be introduced using Seldinger's method, or a fine catheter can be slipped in through the Teflon sheath of the needle and passed down to very small arteries. A variety of catheters can be used, including coaxial catheters, catheters with inflatable balloons to protect adjacent territories, and catheters with perforated balloons for embolization of less accessible vessels (Fig. 66–10).

Therapeutic Methods (Embolization). Whenever possible, we use nonabsorbable emboli, such as fragments of dura mater, Silastic spheres, or radiopaque microspheres. Polymerizing materials are more delicate to handle and require ample practice; they include the fast polymerizer Bucrylate, Silicone (which has no parietal adhesiveness), and the recently introduced Ethibloc.

If surgical excision is envisaged, we use fragments of Surgicel or autologous blood clots, provided the interval between embolization and surgery is 48 hours or less.

Substances injected intra-arterially for therapeutic purposes include vasoconstrictors and dilators, fibrinolytics and antimitotics. In the latter case a catheter can be left in situ for repeated or continuous perfusion.

Finally, we shall mention the technique of transluminal angioplasty, which may be useful in cases of stenosis of the radial or ulnar artery.

Preparation of the Patient. Anesthesia is more important here than in diagnostic

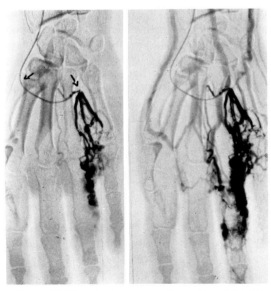

Figure 66–10. Arteriovenous malformation of the ring finger. Selective catheterization of the radial proper palmar digital artery at its origin. The catheter is inserted in the deep palmar arch *(arrow)*.

arteriography, because arterial spasm can jeopardize the treatment. We have a clear preference for brachial plexus block (supraclavicular or axillary), which produces excellent vasoplegia. General anesthesia in any case requires concomitant vasoplegia and is now seldom employed because the new hexaiodinated contrast media are so well tolerated. Vasodilators and anticoagulants are also frequently used preoperatively.

Equipment. It is possible to carry out the foregoing procedures in a room designed for routine vascular radiology, but we much prefer a room with the possibility of switching from the fluoroscope to the radiograph tube without continuously moving the patient. Also the direct magnification on the radioscopic screen improves the accuracy and safety of the catheterization.

The Direct Approach to Angiodysplasias

This procedure involves local puncture and no catheterization. It must be carried out, however, in the radiology department so that the architecture and connections of the malformation can be established before treatment begins. One must also ascertain that the tip of the catheter needle does not lie at the venous or efferent end of the malformation.

Sclerosing or fibrosing substances can be injected by this route in order to induce retraction of the malformation. Those most commonly used for this purpose are absolute alcohol and Ethibloc. The latter compound, owing to its viscosity, has the added advantage of progressively filling the malformation, which facilitates later surgical excision when this is indicated. Retraction occurs within two to three months, by which time the injected substance has been absorbed and replaced by fibrous tissue.

Lesions treatable by this method include the relatively localized, superficial capillarovenous malformations and cavernomas (which are usually accessible in surgery) as well as the deeper infiltrating lesions within muscular tissue.

RESULTS

PRIMARILY VASOMOTOR ARTERIOPATHIES

It is in this case that arteriography is increasingly less frequently employed, being replaced by the Doppler method and capillaroscopy as diagnostic tools. It can still be useful, however, to help in making a prognosis.

Raynaud's Disease

Raynaud's disease is primarily a functional (vasomotor) condition that in time can lead to organic lesions.

Capillaroscopy, performed at room temperature, is usually unremarkable, but when the hand is cooled, a critical closing phenomenon, with disappearance of the capillary loops, can be observed in 70 per cent of the cases. These features, which are typical of idiopathic Raynaud's disease, never develop into a collagen disease.

Doppler ultrasonography, carried out under dynamic conditions, shows the degree of arteriocapillary adaptation to temperature changes and can determine the stage of the disease.

The arteriographic changes also depend on the stage of the disease.

Early Stage. The slowing down of blood flow is constant and results from increased peripheral resistance. All the distal arteries go into spasm, and there is a tendency for the arteries of the hand and forearm to assume the same caliber, while the subclavian and axillary arteries remain unaffected.

At this stage the arteriogram can be of prognostic value, but the procedure must be carried out with and without vasodilators and at different temperatures (Rosch and Porter, 1977). The variations under the different conditions show the responses of the disease and help to determine the stage of the disease—purely functional, organicofunctional, or organic.

The Organic Stage. At this stage definite signs of distal arteritis are detectable in the digital arteries, the palmar arches, and even the distal ends of the radial or the cubital artery.

Other Conditions

Other conditions are also characterized by vasomotor disturbances (Raynaud's syndromes). Some authors believe that Raynaud's phenomenon has an organic cause, which can be detected by the relevant investigations. This is the case in neurovascular compression (cervical rib, costoclavicular and scalene syndromes) and in focal lesions of

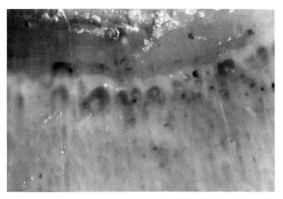

Figure 66–11. Capillaroscopy of the nail bed showing scleroderma and typical appearance of megacapillaries. (Kindly provided by Prof. Vayssairat.)

the subclavian artery (Huguet et al., 1980). The same applies to certain collagen diseases for which capillaroscopy represents an interesting diagnostic approach.

Thus, in systemic scleroderma cutaneous sclerosis is always preceded by a microangiopathy (Fig. 66–11). In 50 per cent of the cases capillaroscopy reveals the characteristic megacapillaries in the nail bed. These features are seen only in scleroderma, dermatomyositis, and Sharp's syndrome (Vayssairat and Housset, 1980; Vayssairat et al., 1981).

In other collagen diseases and in the inflammatory arteritides (lupus erythematosus, rheumatoid arthritis, Buerger's disease), capillaroscopy shows, in addition to a reduction in capillary loops, capillary dysmorphias as well as edema and microhemorrhages (Vayssairat and Housset, 1980).

Functional causes include neurological (poliomyelitis, syringomyelia), hormonal (hypothyroidism, Addison's disease), and cardiac disease (mitral disease, mitral stenosis, cardiac failure) and intoxications (ergot poisoning; Huguet et al., 1980).

Raynaud's phenomenon is also known to occur as a result of microtraumas, especially from vibrations, sustained at work. Thus, it is found in a high proportion of woodcutters who use electric saws, as well as in masons and tilers in whom the thenar eminence is subjected to repeated shocks (hammer syndrome). Patients in this group show the arteriographic, capillaroscopic, and Doppler changes characteristic of Raynaud's phenomenon in addition to signs of arterial dysplasia (aneurysms), which may be embolic in origin

and give rise to occlusion of the digital arteries.

Finally, industrial workers coming into contact with polyvinyl chloride are now known to show Raynaud-like changes, as well as finger clubbing, bone lysis of the distal phalanx, occlusion of the digital arteries, and hypervascularization of the metacarpophalangeal and interphalangeal joints.

ORGANIC ARTERIOPATHIES WITH INTERRUPTION OF ARTERIAL FLOW

The borderline between a vasomotor and an organic arteriopathy is often difficult to define, since, as we noted earlier, an initially vasomotor arteriopathy may in time become organic in type.

Arterial Emboli

Arterial emboli can be present in an acute or a chronic form.

Acute Form. The acute form occurs as acute ischemia in a patient with known mitral or aortic valve disease or one suffering from cardiopathy (endocarditis, left ventricular failure). The object of arteriography is to identify the site or sites of the emboli. These can lie at any level between the brachial and digital arteries and show up as "amputation" of an artery by a cup shaped embolus.

Chronic Form. Arterial occlusions can be more or less compensated for by a collateral circulation, and it may be difficult to differentiate between embolic and distal arteritis. In this group we find the causes proximal to the compression or obstruction—costoclavicular syndrome, cervical rib, and atheroma of the larger vessels with the attendant risk of embolization (Fig. 66–12). Thus, occlusion of a distal artery requires an investigation of the proximal larger vessels, and vice versa (Hayt et al., 1977). In every case the arteriogram and other tests must aim at identifying and locating all lesions while demonstrating the presence, if any, of collateral channels.

Distal Arteritis

Digital arteritis by definition affects the digital collateral vessels and takes the form of progressive thromboangiitis (Huguet et al., 1980). The arteries are narrowed and easily occluded. A collateral network of arterioles

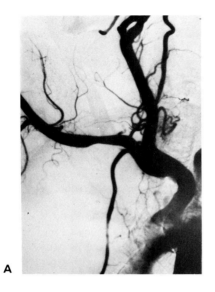
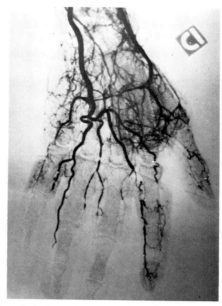

Figure 66–12. Costoclavicular stenosis. *A*, Stenosis of the subclavian artery appearing when the upper limb is in forced abduction. *B*, Distal arterial obstructions in the hand without apparent lesions of degenerative disease.

follows the course of the thrombosed artery, and microaneurysms may be present.

Buerger's arteritis is a recurrent, progressive, inflammatory thromboangiitis affecting mostly young males. There is associated phlebitis of the corresponding veins. The lesions are distal and readily diagnosed by angiography (Huguet et al., 1980).

Atheroma can affect all the arteries of the hand as well as the proximal trunks. It is usually recognizable angiographically by the irregular caliber of a vessel carrying one or more plaques (Fig. 66–13).

At first sight it may appear relatively easy to identify a pathological entity, but an angiographic diagnosis can be far from easy in intricate cases such as Raynaud's disease in a smoker with atheromatosis. In such cases it is important not to isolate the hand as a single pathological site, but to fully investigate the arterial tree of the whole upper limb.

VASCULAR MALFORMATIONS (ANGIODYSPLASIAS)

There are two main groups of vascular malformations—immature angiomas of the newborn, which tend to regress spontaneously, and mature angiomas of adults, which are "irreversible" (Enjolras et al., 1981).

Immature Angiomas; Hemangiomas

Immature angiomas are seen chiefly in the newborn or very young child; they appear within the first few weeks of life and go

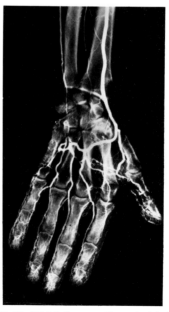

Figure 66–13. Distal degenerative arterial disease related to overload of the distal part of the ulnar artery, the deep palmar arch, and the proper palmar digital arteries. The axillosubclavian region is normal.

through a stage of rapid extension before slowly regressing over the next four or five years.

Several clinical forms are recognized. The "tuberose" angioma forms granular red plaques, which may be swollen. The "subcutaneous" angioma forms an elastic swelling covered by normal skin. The "mixed" angioma exhibits characteristics of the first two. Arteriography (which is seldom required to make a diagnosis) shows typical morphological and hemodynamic changes.

Most of these malformations are highly vascular and become opacified evenly, and they have a characteristic capillary pseudotumoral appearance (i.e., without early venous drainage). As a rule, no treatment is required, since the lesion disappears by the age of five, leaving virtually no trace. If, however, the angioma shows a tendency toward enlargement, ulceration, or hemorrhage, its evolution usually can be stopped by systemic or local steroid treatment. Embolization is not necessary.

Mature Angiomas

These lesions can be arteriovenous, capillarovenous, or purely venous.

Port Wine Stains. These appear clinically as geographic areas with various tints of red. They are present at birth and as a rule do not grow in size. They have little if any hemodynamic significance. There may be an underlying vascular malformation, or they may share the same metamere as a vascular malformation, one example of such being Cobb's syndrome, in which a port wine stain and a meningomedullary angioma may lie within the same metamere. If we exclude the port wine stain, there is a possible anatomical and hemodynamic classification that distinguishes the arterial and arteriovenous malformations from the purely venous malformations.

Arterial Malformations. Arterial malformations include arterial aneurysms, which are exceedingly rare in the hand except as a result of trauma, and pure arterial dysplasias, which show up upon arteriography as large tortuous arterial dilations. There is usually no arteriovenous shunt, but experience has taught us that they may eventually be converted into arteriovenous malformations.

Malformations with Arteriovenous Shunts. These are active vascular malformations.

ARTERIOVENOUS FISTULAS. Direct arteriovenous communications are usually trau-matic in origin. Clinically there is a detectable murmur and a thrill. Arteriography clearly demonstrates the fistula, as well as some degree of distal hypovascularization. Embolization, using a balloon or a coil, and surgery can both cure the condition, provided it is isolated.

ARTERIOVENOUS MALFORMATIONS. These are fed by several arterial pedicles and show an early venous return. Clinically the malformation appears as a warm swelling, which is pulsatile when superficial. There is also arterial hyperpulsatility and dilated veins.

Local complications are not uncommon; they include ulceration and hemorrhages due to trophic changes associated with diversion of flow and high venous pressure.

These malformations are rarely noticeable at birth, when they tend to be quiescent. Possible triggering factors in their progression include minor trauma, surgery for some other lesion, or hormonal changes (puberty, pregnancy, or delivery).

Arteriography demonstrates the malformation, its anatomy, and its feeding pedicles. Selective compression of the radial or ulnar artery clearly shows the arterial territories (Fig. 66–14), whereas compression slows the arterial flow. The latter maneuver makes possible progressive visualization of the ar-

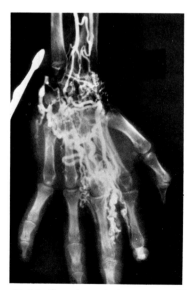

Figure 66–14. Complex arteriovenous malformation of the hand with involvement of the radial, ulnar, and interosseous arteries. The territory supplied by the interosseous arteries was investigated by compression of the radial and ulnar arteries under Doppler control. Associated venous compression results in progressive opacification of the malformation without superimposition of venous return.

terial and venous phases (without their being superimposed) and reduces the number of exposures required. A Doppler test at this stage not only helps to determine the degree of compression needed but provides information regarding the output of each pedicle and localizes the shunts.

The scanner, in conjunction with the Doppler and the arteriogram, should help in determining the relationship of the lesion to the adjacent tissues and its extent (i.e., whether it is localized to the hand or extends upward into the upper limb).

The behavior of these malformations is unpredictable. They may remain quiescent for years and yet go through phases of acute "activity." Apart from the accidental or surgical trauma mentioned earlier, other possible trigger factors are failed attempts at treatment and proximal arterial ligation; the latter not only are doomed to failure but even compromise later treatment. Surgery is often impossible and embolization is at best palliative. Even resorting to amputation has sometimes proved less radical than expected, for the malformation has been known to recur proximal to the level of amputation.

No definite program of treatment can therefore be advocated for these complex lesions. A quiescent malformation giving rise to no functional disturbance is probably best left alone and watched. Embolization followed by complete surgical excision can be attempted when possible—a rare occurrence in the hand. Palliative isolated embolization, under Doppler control, is worth considering in the event of hemorrhage or trophic changes or if there is evidence of extension of the lesion. Figure 66–15 sums up the possibilities of embolization for arteriovenous malformations in the hand.

Capillarovenous Malformations. The two main groups are capillary malformations and capillarovenous malformations.

CAPILLARY MALFORMATIONS. The telangiectasia of Rendu-Osler disease often occurs in the hand. It appears as multiple disseminated distal spots some 2 to 3 mm. across.

CAPILLAROVENOUS MALFORMATIONS. These are more voluminous lesions, which become turgescent when the limb is dependent (Fig. 66–16). The skin may look normal or show scattered bluish lesions. Palpable (radiopaque) phleboliths are common, as are other local changes such as bone or fatty tissue hypertrophy.

The Doppler method is of little assistance, but the scanner clearly shows the demarcation between the malformation and adjacent tissues. Only by hyperselective arteriography can one demonstrate the slow filling of the multiple and relatively stagnant loculi. The afferent arteries are not dilated.

Cavernomas or Phlebectasias. These appear as bluish, soft, pitting swellings, which increase in volume when the limb is dependent (Fig. 66–17). Venography shows either dilation of one venous trunk or of a stagnant saccular diverticulum. If they do not lie on an essential draining channel, they can be safely excised or embolized (Ethibloc).

Complex or Disseminated Malformations. It should always be remembered that some visible malformations may coexist with concealed ones, which may give rise to severe complications. Some patients of association are recognized, and we shall mention the most common.

SYSTEMIC AND REGIONAL ANGIOMATOSES. The Klippel-Trenaunay-Weber syndrome comprises a classic triad: cutaneous angioma, varicose dilation, and lengthening and hypertrophy of the limb concerned. Venography reveals the superficial venous trunks to be dilated while the deep ones appear abnormal. Proximal venous stenoses are sometimes seen. The visible venous dilations are the more obvious elements in a diffuse angiodysplasia. Arteriography may show areas of hypervascularization (microshunts). The true extent of the lesion can be measured only with the help of hyperselective arteriography.

The present tendency favors conservative therapy in the form of early elastic compression, which may or may not prevent lengthening of the limb. When the arteriovenous shunts predominate, the condition is labeled the Parkes-Weber syndrome or Klippel-Trenaunay-Weber syndrome.

Cobb's syndrome is an angiomatosis involving the various tissues of one metamere: skin, muscle, viscera, and the vertebromeningomedullary complex. Because the projection of a metamere can include an upper limb, angiomatosis of the hand of whatever type may be the only visible manifestation of Cobb's syndrome. In practice, any superficial angioma associated with cervical pain or a neurological syndrome should suggest this diagnosis.

SYSTEMIC DISSEMINATED ANGIOMATOSES. Rendu-Osler familial telangiectasia is a condition transmitted as an autosomal dom-

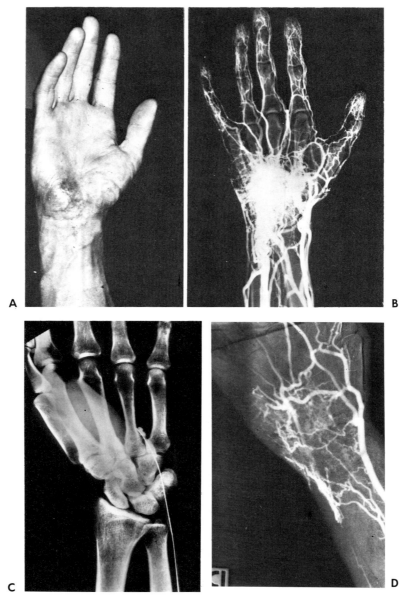

Figure 66–15. Arteriovenous malformation predominantly affecting the hypothenar eminence. *A*, Photograph of the hand before treatment. *B*, Arteriogram of the malformation showing massive opacification and numerous arteriovenous shunts. Early venous return coincides with the arterial phase. *C*, Protection of the ulnar artery and its territory using a balloon catheter before embolization. *D*, Result after embolization.

Figure 66–16. Capillarovenous malformation of the hand. *A*, Arterial phase: no abnormality. *B*, Late venous phase: multiple "grape seed" cavities filled with contrast medium.

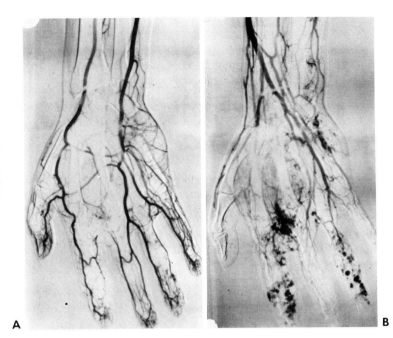

Figure 66–17. Pure venous angiodysplasia. *A*, Photograph of the hand showing both venous turgescence under the influence of gravity and blue subcutaneous zones. *B*, Phlebograph of the same extremity showing venous dilatation in the hand and forearm.

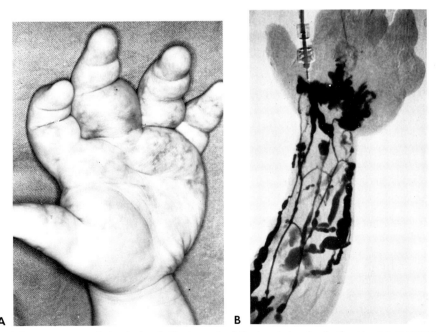

inant. It usually occurs at puberty with the onset of epistaxis, the source of which is the telangiectasia in the nasal fossas. The lesions can be found in any cutaneous area, including the hands and the face. Visceral involvement is not uncommon.

Bean's syndrome is characterized by the presence of disseminated cavernous, bluish skin angiomas, often associated with gastrointestinal angiomas.

Other syndromes include Maffucci's syndrome (angiomatosis with regional or disseminated chondromatosis) and Kaposi's sarcoma and related pseudosyndromes (angiokeratosis).

In a separate group, we include a number of ill defined malformations, encapsulated vascular swellings, lying halfway between benign tumors and dysplasias. Finally, there are the strange and rare lesions that appear as a diffuse vasodilation involving the whole limb. Unlike the case with the port wine stain, the skin is warm and pink. The arteriogram shows dilated veins and arteries, early venous return, and a rich intermediate plexus but no arteriovenous shunts. At present we know little of the natural course of these lesions.

INJURIES OF THE HAND

In cases of hand trauma, arteriography, whether carried out in an emergency or as a later investigation, remains an essential adjunct to surgical repair. Four main arteriographic pictures are recognized—interruption of flow, the "vascular desert," delayed flow, and arteriovenous shunts—or a combination of two or more.

1. Interruption of arterial flow indicates traumatic rupture of an important vessel. Arteriography can determine the type and level of the obstruction and helps in forecasting the potential for a collateral circulation.

2. The "vascular desert" is not uncommon. The vascular tree is still present, and yet a whole anatomical territory fails to opacify, indicating a drastic insufficiency in arterial flow. This picture is helpful, in that it guards against overambitious repairs and emphasizes the need for surgical improvement of the circulation.

3. Delayed flow is in itself a minor form of vascular lesion; it must be interpreted in comparative rather than absolute terms. It must be followed and recognized, for it is often caused by a subtle arterial lesion.

4. Arteriovenous shunts are suspected in cases showing early venous return in a given territory. They are usually found at the site of the injury. Arteriovenous shunts act as short circuits and result in distal hypovascularization.

Investigation of the circulation may be necessary in other circumstances, as in the presence of hemolymphangiomas, glomus tumors, bone tumors, and tumors of soft tissue. We cannot detail here the investigative routine, because this obviously varies with each type of lesion, but it is worth noting that hyperselective angiography is proving useful in an ever increasing variety of diseases.

CONCLUSION

Angiography remains an essential investigative technique in a high proportion of disorders of the hand. More recently developed techniques, such as the Doppler method and capillaroscopy, represent complementary rather than replacement investigations. In addition angiography has now taken on a therapeutic dimension; in its digital form its potential probably lies well beyond present expectations.

REFERENCES

Balas, P., Katsogiannis, A., Katsiotis, P., and Karaitanos, J.: Comparative study of evaluation of digital arterial circulation by Doppler ultrasonic tracing and hand arteriography. J. Cardiovasc. Surg., 21:455–462, 1980.

Blonstein, A., Doyon, D., and Harry, G.: L'artériographie de la main traumatique. Indications, méthode, résultats à propos de 150 observations. J. Radiol., 58:93–102, 1977.

Braun, J. B.: Les Artères de la Main. Thesis, University of Nancy, 1977.

Chermet, J.: Artériographie de la main. Encycl. Med. Chir. Paris Radiodiag., 3:12(32220 A-10), 1974.

Dijkstra, P. F.: The venous phase in hand angiography. Diag. Imag., 48:216–218, 1979.

Dufour, R., Merlen, J. F., Sarteel, A. M., and Vincent, G.: L'apport de la capillaroscopie dans l'étude des manifestations extra-articulaires de la polyarthrite rhumatoïde. J. Sci. Méd. Lille, T99:209–210, 1981.

Edwards, A. E.: Organization of the small arteries of the hand and digits. Am. J. Surg., 99:837, 1960.

Enjolras, O., Merland, J. J., Riche, M. C., and Melki, J. P.: Malformations vasculaires, angiomes, angiodysplasies cutanéo-muqueuses. Classification-explorations-indications thérapeutiques. Dermatol. Pratici., 10:13–41, 1981.

Franceschi, C.: L'investigation vasculaire par Ultrasonographie Doppler. In Collection de Médecine Ultra-sonore. Ed. 2. Paris, Masson et cie, 1979.

Gest, J.: La lymphographie isotopique. Bull. Acad. Suisse Sci. Med., *19:*97–113, 1963.

Hayt, D. B., Blatt, C. J., and Freeman, L. M.: Radionuclide venography: its place as a modality for the investigations of the thrombo-embolic phenomena. Semin. Nucl. Med., *VII:*3, July 1977.

Huguet, J. F., and Clerissi, J.: Artériographie du membre supérieur. Encycl. Méd. Chir. Paris Radiodiag., *3:*4(32215 A-10), 1980.

Huguet, J. F., Cecile, J. P., and Duquesnel, J.: L'artériographie du membre supérieur. Traité de Radiodiagnostic. Radiologie Cardio-vasculaire. Paris, Masson et cie, 1980, Vol. 30.

Jacobson, S., and Ostberg, G.: The axillary veins in postmastectomy edema of the arm. A gross and microscopical study. Vasa, 2, 1973.

Le Quentrec, P., Suterre, R., Coget, J. M., Sarteel, A. M., Franco, G., and Merlen, J. F.: Signal Doppler pulpaire. De son intérêt diagnostique. J. Mal. Vasc., *5:*285–287, 1980.

Levy, B. I., Valladares, W. R., Ghaem, A., and Martinaud, J. P.: Comparison of plethysmographic methods with pulsed Doppler blood flowmetry. Am. J. Physiol., *236:*899–903, 1979.

Martinaud, J. P., Valladares, W., Ghaem, A., and Levy, B.: Mesure du débit sanguin dans un segment de membre. Validation de la Vélocimétrie ultra-sonore Doppler à impulsion. Ann. Cardiol. Angeiol., *29:*117–123, 1980.

Merland, J. J., Natali, J., Riche, M. C., and Tricot, J. F.: L'embolisation artérielle au niveau des membres à propos de 49 cas. Act. Chir., *3:*96–100, 1979.

Merland, J. J., Riche, M. C., and Melki, J. P.: Selective arteriography and embolization in vascular malformations of the limbs. *In* Wilkins, R. A., and Viamonte, M. (Editors): Interventional Radiology. Oxford, Blackwell Scientific Publications Ltd., 1980, pp. 51–61.

Merlen, J. F., and Sarteel, A. M.: La capillaroscopie dans l'arthrite rhumatoïde. Phlébologie, *34:*165–169, 1981.

Mitz, V., Dardour, J. C., and Vilain, R.: Main et energie: l'Artériographie dans les traumatismes de la main, sa sémiologie, ses implications thérapeutiques. Ann. Chir., *28:*835–850, 1974.

Natali, J., and Merland, J. J.: Superselective arteriography and therapeutic embolization for vascular malformations. J. Cardiovasc. Surg., *17:*465–472, 1976.

Rees, W. V., Robinson, D. S., Holmes, E. C., and Morton D. L.: Altered lymphatic drainage following lymphadenectomy. Cancer, *45:*12–15, 1980.

Riche, M. C., Melki, J. P., and Merland, J. J.: l'Angiographie Thérapeutique. Paris, Editions Médicales Spécia, 1981.

Rosch, J., and Porter, J. M.: Hand angiography and Raynaud's syndrome. Fortschr. Rontgenstr., *127:*30–37, 1977.

Rosch, J., Antonovic, R., and Porter, J. M.: The importance of temperature in angiography of the hand. Radiology, *123:*323–326, 1977.

Rouviere, H.: Anatomie Humaine Descriptive et Topographique. (Revised by E. Cordier and A. Delmas.) Paris, Masson Editions, 1962, pp. 151–168.

Thulesius, O.: Exploration noninvasive et physiopathologie du phénomène de Raynaud. Rev. Prat., *31:*3981–3990, 1981.

Vayssairat, M., and Housset, E.: Place de la capillaroscopie dans les acrosyndromes. Rev. Prat., *30:*1923–1953, 1980.

Vayssairat, M., Fiessinger, J. N., Priollet, P., Goldberg, J., and Housset, E.: Intérêt de la capillaroscopie pour le diagnostic de la sclérodermie généralisée. Rev. Méd. Int., *2:*333–340, 1981.

Yun Ryo, V., Qazi, M., Srikantaswamy, S., and Pinsky, S.: Radionuclide venography: correlation with contrast venography. J. Nucl. Med., *18:*11–17, 1977.

Chapter 67

VASCULAR INJURIES IN THE UPPER EXTREMITY

JESSE B. JUPITER
AND HAROLD E. KLEINERT

Although more than 200 years have passed since Lambert (1762) reported the successful repair of a lacerated brachial artery, it is only in the past three decades that primary surgical repair of vascular injuries in the upper extremities has emerged as a routine procedure. Moreover, it was not until 1960, when Jacobson and Suarez demonstrated consistently patent anastomoses of vessels with diameters of 3 mm. or less, that the value of microvascular surgery was realized, with its resultant widespread application in surgery of the upper extremity. Vascular injuries must be considered significant if the involved extremity is deprived of blood supply sufficient to impair function and are of grave consequence if without vascular repair the viability of the extremity or part remains in jeopardy. With current refinements in vascular surgical principles and techniques, the hand surgeon should be equipped to deal with these problems just as he would other injured tissues in the upper extremity.

HISTORICAL ASPECTS

Although the control of hemorrhage following vascular injury has, by necessity, been a concern since the beginning of recorded history, it was Celsus who in 25 A.D. first described a limited use of the ligature (Harvey, 1929). Although this technique was soon expanded by Archigenes and later by Galen in the second century A.D. (Schwartz, 1958), its application was basically lost for the next 1200 years, being replaced by the brutal use of cautery. Paré is commonly credited with rediscovery of the ligature, although

Jerome of Brunswick preceded Paré in use of the ligature in 1497 (Schwartz, 1958).

The first recorded direct vascular repair, described by Lambert (1762), utilized a farrier stitch technique to close a brachial artery laceration. The laceration was transfixed by a pin placed through the arterial walls while a figure-of-eight suture woven around the pin approximated the lacerated edges. Another 124 year hiatus passed before a second instance of arterial repair by the lateral suturing of a human artery was reported by Postempski (1886). In 1897 Murphy reported the first successful end-to-end arterial anastomosis. The classic experimental studies of Carrel (1902) followed, and his triangulation method of direct arterial repair, careful intimal approximation, and the use of fine suture material remains fundamental to the tenets of vascular surgery. Goyanes in 1906 first reported the successful use of a vein graft to bridge an arterial defect following excision of a popliteal aneurysm. This event was followed one year later by Lexer's report (1907) of a saphenous vein interposition graft for the reconstruction of a post-traumatic axillary-brachial artery aneurysm.

In spite of the contributions of these early vascular surgeons, ligation remained the treatment of choice throughout both World Wars, associated with an amputation incidence of upward of 49 per cent in World War II (Debakey and Simeone, 1946). Improvements in anesthesia, antibiotics, blood replacement, and perhaps most importantly in the rapid evacuation of the injured patient made early vascular repair a reality during the Korean conflict (Hughes, 1949). It was further recognized that in addition to a marked decrease in limb loss, arterial repair enabled the injured limb to function in a more normal manner (Jahnke, 1958). The Vietnam conflict also stimulated considerable advances in the applications and techniques of primary vascular repair (Rich et al., 1970).

Although advances were made in revascularizing severely traumatized upper extremities (Kleinert and Kasdan, 1963), it remained for Malt (1964) to perform the first successful replantation of the completely severed upper arm of a 12 year old boy. None of the dreaded perioperative complications, so common in previous experimental replantations, ensued (Eiken et al., 1964; MacDonald et al., 1962; Mehl et al., 1964), and reports of successful extremity replantations soon followed from a number of centers, in particular, the Sixth People's Hospital in Shanghai (1967).

In the same era Kleinert and Kasden achieved the first clinically successful digital artery anastomosis in November 1962, joining the transected artery of an incompletely amputated thumb by use of a continuous suture of 8-0 Dacron. Buncke and Schulz (1965), using the rhesus monkey, reported successful digital replantation, demonstrating techniques applicable to the same clinical problem in man. The first successful microsurgical replantation of an amputated thumb occurred in the same year that Komatsu and Tamai (1968), using 8-0 microfilament nylon and 7-0 braided silk sutures, repaired two digital arteries and two dorsal veins. Numerous reports of successful digital replantations followed, along with the establishment of replantation centers, microsurgical research laboratories, and continued refinements in equipment, suture material, and techniques.

In light of the state of current knowledge and technical skills, we believe that restoration of vascular continuity in upper extremity arterial injuries, even in the face of inadequate collateral circulation, can and should be accomplished in most instances.

ANATOMY

Accurate knowledge of the relationships and pathways of the major arterial structures in the upper extremity, as well as their variational patterns, is of considerable relevance in the approach to and repair of vascular injuries.

Since Tiedman's treatise in 1831 on the variations of the arterial anatomy in the up-per extremities, a number of important studies have added to our understanding of normal and abnormal arterial configurations in the arm and hand.

The axillary artery demonstrates a fairly consistent anatomical pathway. It begins as the continuation of the subclavian artery at the lateral aspect of the first rib and ends as the brachial artery at the inferior border of the pectoralis major. The vessel anatomically may be divided into three parts by its relationship to the pectoralis minor muscle. The numerous branches of the axillary artery include the superior thoracic artery arising from the first segment, the thoracoacromial and lateral thoracic arteries from the middle section, and the subscapular and anterior and posterior circumflex humeral arteries, which anastomose freely with each other and provide an abundant collateral blood supply in the thoracic-scapular-humeral region. The close relationship with the brachial plexus and axillary vein contributes to the frequent association of nerve injuries in addition to occasional post-traumatic arteriovenous fistulas following axillary arterial trauma.

Beyond the lower border of the teres major, the brachial artery leaves the axilla medially and deep to the median nerve, coursing distally and laterally to terminate just beyond the antecubital fossa by dividing into the radial and ulnar arteries. The brachial artery has three major branches. The large profunda brachii passes downward between the medial and long heads of the triceps, branching to anastomose anteriorly with the radial recurrent artery and posteriorly with the posterior interosseous artery. A second branch, the superior ulnar collateral or inferior profunda artery, courses with the ulnar nerve, anastomosing distally with the posterior ulnar recurrent artery—all forming an extensive network of collateral vessels about the elbow (Fig. 67–1).

The brachial artery's anatomic variations of surgical significance involve the patterns of its termination (McCormack et. al., 1953; Strandness, 1969). The "superficial brachial artery" exists where the termination of the artery lies superficial to the median nerve and often serves as a "high origin" for either the radial or the ulnar artery (Keen, 1961). In fact, the high origin for the radial artery is perhaps the most common variation of the arterial anatomy of the upper extremity, involving approximately 77 per cent of all observed variations (McCormack et. al., 1953).

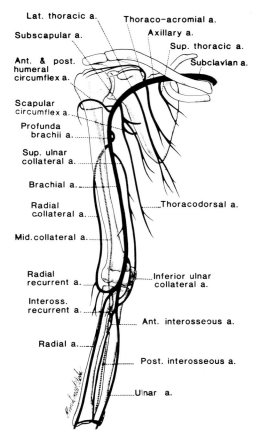

Figure 67–1. The arterial anatomy of the brachium and forearm. The collateral circulation passes longitudinally in the direction of the major vessels.

terior interosseous arteries. These, combined with the radial artery, establish an excellent collateral network in the forearm consisting of four parallel arterial pathways with numerous intercommunications.

The radial artery lies more superficial in the forearm, running just under the anterior aspect of the brachioradialis and across the supinator to enter the anterior and radial aspect of the forearm. At the proximal aspect of the wrist it generally is found between the flexor carpi radialis and the brachioradialis.

Although it is rare that both radial and ulnar arteries are absent in the forearm, when this situation does exist, the anterior interosseous artery frequently becomes the dominant vessel (Strandness, 1969). A persistent median artery, found in 10 per cent of limbs studied by Coleman and Anson (1961), contributes primarily to the superficial palmar arch, always passing deep to the transverse carpal ligament and often intimately associated with the median nerve (Edwards, 1960). Because a median artery normally may be found in the palmar arch of certain lower animals, the persistent median artery has been called an atavistic characteristic (Jaschtschinski, 1897). The possibility of a persistent median artery needs to be borne in mind in performing Allen's test to evaluate the patency of either the radial or the ulnar artery (Allen, 1929). Following exsanguination of the hand, 10 to 15 seconds are allowed to pass before releasing compression in order to rule out the presence of a functioning median artery.

A thorough understanding of the more conventional vascular patterns in the hand as well as the pertinent variations is a necessity in evaluating traumatic as well as chronic conditions affecting the hand (Fig. 67–2). At the level of the carpus lies an anterior and dorsal carpal rete formed from branches of the radial and ulnar arteries. The larger dorsal rete system also includes the terminations of the posterior branch of the anterior interosseous artery. Arising off this arch are the second, third, and fourth dorsal metacarpal arteries, which pass dorsally over their respective dorsal interosseous muscles and terminate by anastomosing with the digital arteries through the distal perforating arteries. The dorsal artery in the thumb-index interspace arises directly from the radial artery, while the fifth dorsal metacarpal artery is a direct branch of the ulnar artery.

The smaller anterior carpal rete is formed

Other less common anatomical observations include a superficial proximal origin for the ulnar artery and, even more unusual, an accessory brachial artery reflecting a proximal duplication of the brachial artery.

The collateral circulation about the elbow, and for that matter throughout the upper extremity, consists of vessels coursing relatively parallel to the path of the dominant vessel. This is in sharp contrast with the lower limb, in particular the knee where numerous collateral branches run in a virtually perpendicular plane to the popliteal artery. This anatomical feature is among the reasons for a much higher incidence of limb salvage with interruption of the brachial artery than with popliteal artery interruption.

In the forearm the ulnar artery ordinarily is the dominant artery. Proximally it gives rise to the large common interosseous artery, which bifurcates to either side of the interosseous membrane into the anterior and posterior

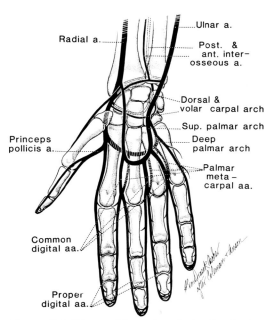

Figure 67–2. The arterial supply to the hand and wrist.

from branches of the radial, ulnar, and anterior interosseous arteries and recurrent branches from the deep palmar arch. This arch lies deep within the carpal tunnel and may be subject to increased pressures within the tunnel.

The superficial palmar arterial arch has been classically described as being formed by the termination of the ulnar artery distal to Guyon's canal, uniting with the superficial volar ramus of the radial artery. The arch lies just distal to the transverse carpal ligament at the level of the ulnar end of the proximal palmar crease. In the anatomical studies performed by Coleman and Anson (1961), 80 per cent of 650 specimens were found to have a complete arch while 20 per cent were incomplete. Each of these two groups was further subdivided, revealing that the classic pattern of the superficial palmar arch was present in only 34.5 per cent of the specimens with a complete arch. Thirty-seven per cent of the complete arches were derived entirely from the ulnar artery, while in 1 per cent of the cases, there was a three vessel arch, including the median in addition to both the ulnar and radial arteries.

Three common digital arteries, which supply adjacent sides of the four digits, arise from the superficial palmar arch and run distally to each web space. They lie superficial to the common digital nerves proximally but come to lie dorsal to the nerves more distally. At the level of the metacarpal heads, the common digital arteries anastomose with branches from the deep palmar arch. In some instances, where there is an absence of one or more common digital arteries, the vascular supply to the digital space may be maintained solely through the deep metacarpal arteries (Edwards, 1960).

The deep palmar arch, a continuation of the radial artery, is a more constant structure and is located more proximally in the hand. The arch lies on the proximal ends of the metacarpals and interosseous muscles. Proximally it sends branches to the anterior carpal rete, and distally three ulnar deep metacarpal arteries course from the arch, running on the interosseous muscles and anastomosing with the common digital arteries.

After passing through the anatomical snuffbox and between the two heads of the first dorsal interosseous muscle, the radial artery gives off the princeps pollicis artery. This is a relatively constant anatomical structure found in about 98 per cent of individuals. At the level of the metacarpophalangeal joint of the thumb, the artery usually terminates into the two palmar digital arteries of the thumb (Murakami et al., 1969; Parks et al., 1978). The radialis indicis artery, somewhat more variable, was found to arise from the princeps pollicis in approximately 50 per cent of dissections (Parks et al., 1978). When present, this artery supplies the radial side of the index finger, although it frequently also sends a branch to join the common digital artery to the index–long web space (Weathersby, 1955).

The digital arterial supply therefore is of triple origin, encompassing the common volar digital arteries from the superficial palmar arch, the deep volar metacarpal arteries arising from the deep palmar arch, and the dorsal metacarpal arteries coursing off the dorsal carpal rete. The large common digital arteries divide in the digital web spaces to form the proper digital arteries to the four fingers. The branches on the ulnar side of the index finger and the radial side of the little finger are usually larger than the opposite vessels (Edwards, 1960).

More distally on each digit the digital arteries themselves form dorsal and palmar retes with transverse digital branches found inherently related to the proximal joint capsule at the neck of the proximal and middle phalanges.

Table 67–1. RELATIVE INCIDENCES OF UPPER EXTREMITY VASCULAR INJURIES

Series	Year	Total Arteries	Axillary		Brachial		Forearm	
			No.	(%)	No.	(%)	No.	(%)
Military								
WW I: Makins	1919	1191	108	(9)	200	(16.8)	59	(4.9)
WW II: DeBakey and Simeone	1946	2471	74	(2.9)	601	(26.5)	168	(6.1)
Korean: Hughes	1958	304	20	(6.6)	89	(29.3)	—	—
Vietnam: Rich et al.	1971	1000	59	(5.9)	283	(28.3)	—	—
Civilian								
Kleinert and Kasdan	1963	79	3	(3.8)	14	(17)	62	(79)
Smith et al.	1963	61	3	(4.9)	13	(21.3)	7	(11.5)
Patman et al.	1964	271	24	(8.9)	46	(17.0)	51	(18.8)
Drapanas et al.	1970	226	12	(5.2)	39	(17.3)	46	(20.4)
Perry et al.	1971	508	38	(7.5)	78	(15.4)	97	(19.1)
Smith et al.	1974	285	10	(7.9)	28	(22)	26	(20)
Cheek et al.	1975	155	—	—	21	(13.5)	—	—
Kelley and Eiseman	1975	116	2	(1.7)	37	(31.9)	—	—
Hardy et al.	1975	360	23	(6.4)	75	(20.8)	—	—
Bole et al.	1976	126	2	(1.6)	14	(11.1)	9	(6.8)
Reynolds et al.	1979	191	14	(7)	40	(21)	—	—

INCIDENCE

Vascular injuries to the extremities have always been of great concern to military surgeons, and well documented accounts of relative incidences can be found in reports of both World Wars in addition to the Korean and Vietnam conflicts (Adar et al., 1980; DeBakey and Simeone, 1946; Hughes, 1954; Makins, 1919; Rich et al., 1970). Along with high speed motor vehicle accidents, increasing urban violence, major industrial accidents, and the increasing utilization of the upper extremity arterial system for diagnosis, monitoring, and access for drug abuse has come an ever increasing frequency of civilian cases of trauma to upper extremity macro- and small vessels.

The relative incidence of specific vascular injuries in previously reported series for a variety of reasons fails to reflect the true frequency of upper extremity vascular injuries. Anatomically, because the exact demarcation points between the axillary and brachial arteries may be difficult to determine, these vessels are listed together in some series. Isolated radial or ulnar artery lacerations repaired in forearms without vascular impairment are often not included, and the relative incidence of the large numbers of palmar or digital arterial repairs has never been accurately assessed.

In the accumulated series of peripheral vascular injuries, however, lesions of the brachial artery occur in 20 to 25 per cent of the patients who sustain major arterial trauma. These are associated with a variety of causes, including penetrating or blunt trauma, gunshot wounds, fractures and dislocations, arterial catheterization, and embolization (Table 67–1).

The number of complete upper extremity amputations that may be amenable to replantation has never accurately been determined. Experience in Vienna from 1974 through 1978 revealed that the incidence of replantation was one per 100,000 people per year (Berger et al., 1978). Despite numerous difficulties in obtaining true statistics, it may well be that the incidence lies between 1 and 10 per 100,000 people each year, the frequency of digital amputations being the highest (May and Gallico, 1980).

EVALUATION OF ARTERIAL INJURIES

Although vascular injuries associated with complete transection or limb severance may be quite apparent, contusion or vascular compression resulting from nonpenetrating trauma such as fractures or dislocations demands more astute observation and a search for the site of the injury. For example, by virtue of the close relationship between the axillary or brachial artery and the peripheral skeletal and nervous systems, the surgeon needs always to be wary of the potential for vascular injury in association with brachial plexus or skeletal injury. Similarly, when faced with apparent laceration of the ulnar nerve at the wrist, one must suspect injury to the ulnar artery, again by virtue of their close anatomical association.

The presence of pulsatile, bright red bleeding, even with a benign appearing wound, should arouse a high index of suspicion (Fig. 67–3). The mechanism of injury should be searched for, especially, for example, the type of missile or the nature of the crush. The duration of time from injury to presentation is especially important if the devascularized limb or severed part involves a considerable mass of skeletal muscle. The warm ischemic tolerance of skeletal muscle does not exceed four to six hours (Harman, 1948; Scully et al., 1961), although this has been significantly extended in digital amputations in which there is far less muscle mass.

Following a general physical examination to rule out associated injuries as well as skeletal or neural injury of the involved limb, a close evaluation of the wound under aseptic conditions is performed. The character of the bleeding, location of the injury, presence of a thrill or bruit, and nature of the surrounding hematoma may all provide additional evidence of an underlying significant vascular injury. In one large series of peripheral arterial injuries, only 13.5 per cent of 226 patients were actively bleeding at the time of admission to the hospital (Drapanas et al., 1970).

Upon examining the extremity distal to the injury, the five "P's" initially described by Griffiths (1948)—i.e., pulselessness, pallor, pain, paresthesia (or anesthesia), and paralysis—all reflect the lack of adequate distal arterial perfusion. A sixth "P," poikilothermia (coolness), should be added to this list. Vascular injuries in the upper extremity are often associated with injury to adjacent peripheral nerves, but deficits from nerve injury for the most part are segmental in nature, whereas the paresthesias associated with anoxia tend to be more diffuse; hence, the "stocking-glove" distribution.

The presence or absence of a peripheral pulse may have a variety of etiologies, which require precise evaluation. The loss of a pulse can be due to systemic hypotension, arterial injury, or peripheral vascular disease, but only rarely does it result from vascular spasm. In the absence of a normal arteriogram or surgical exploration, one cannot with confidence rely on the identification of vascular spasm as the cause of impaired distal perfusion. Even the presence of a palpable or audible distal pulsation does not rule out an associated vascular injury of significance, given the abundant collateral circulation of the upper extremity or the possibility of a tangential laceration of a major vessel.

The Allen test for patency of the ulnar and radial arteries at the wrist level should be an important part of the circulatory examination (Allen, 1929). The Allen test, modified somewhat from Allen's original description, in-

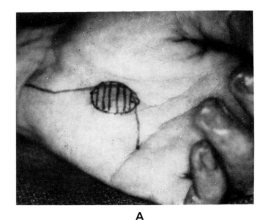

A

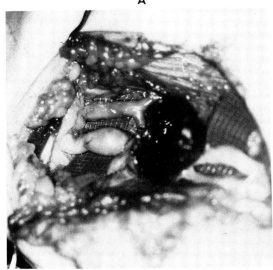

B

Figure 67–3. Following accidental laceration of his left palm on a piece of glass, this 28-year-old man noted pulsatile bleeding that was ultimately controlled and the wound closed in a local emergency room. He presented two months later with a painful mass in his palm (A), which at exploration proved to be an encapsulated hematoma in association with complete transection of the common digital artery and nerve to his fourth web space (B).

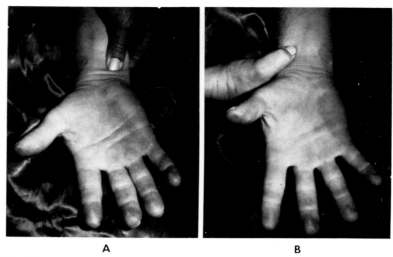

Figure 67–4. The Allen test can reveal occlusion of either the radial or the ulnar artery at the wrist. After exsanguination by repeatedly making a fist, with both arteries occluded, one artery at a time is released and the arterial inflow is observed *(A)*. A "positive" test occurs when no inflow is noted, as seen here with an ulnar artery thrombosis *(B)*.

volves compression of both the ulnar and radial arteries at the wrist while the patient makes a fist several times to exsanguinate the hand. Upon opening the hand and allowing a 15 second period to elapse in order to allow for the possibility of a patent median artery, one artery at a time is released and the rapidity of arterial inflow as well as the total area perfused is observed and carefully recorded. Perfusion usually is complete within 3 to 5 seconds; if no inflow is noted after a 10 to 15 second time period, this constitutes a "positive" test (Fig. 67–4). The digital Allen test may also be of use in more accurately assessing the integrity of the volar

digital arteries (Ashbell et al., 1967; Fig. 67–5).

A number of noninvasive methods have been developed to aid in the assessment of acute vascular injuries in the upper extremity. Battery operated and mobile, the Doppler flow directional probe provides a useful adjunct in the preoperative evaluation as well as in intraoperative and postoperative monitoring of the continuity of the arterial system. By evaluating the character of ultrasound waves reflected off moving blood cells, the direction and magnitude of flow can be estimated even into the digital arteries. The experienced listener can differentiate arterial

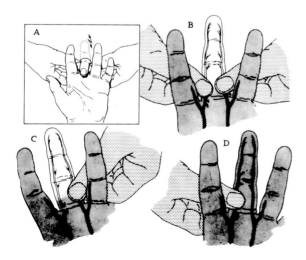

Figure 67–5. The digital Allen test is performed in a manner similar to that at the wrist level *(A and B)*. Release of one digital artery at a time may reveal a unilateral occlusion, demonstrated in this patient with a post-traumatic radial digital artery thrombosis *(C and D)*.

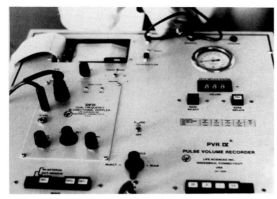

Figure 67–6. The impedance plethysmography or pulse volume recorder utilizes small digital pressure cuffs that can monitor arterial perfusion pressure on a continuous basis. The cuffs can be sterilized and used intraoperatively.

flow signals through patent as opposed to stenotic vessels and also can determine whether the arterial flow is secondary to collateral flow bypassing a proximal obstruction (Wilgis, 1980).

A second useful noninvasive technique for evaluating peripheral blood flow is the impedance plethysmography or pulse volume recorder (Raines et al., 1973). This system involves the use of one or two digital cuffs, one of which picks up the pressure changes while the other records the digital perfusion pressure. The cuffs can be sterilized and used intraoperatively to provide visible documentation of the adequacy of the circulation (Fig. 67–6).

ANGIOGRAPHY

Although in the majority of cases the nature of the wound or the physical findings distal to the injury are sufficient to ascertain the presence of a vascular injury, in some patients the signs of arterial injury are equivocal, the location of the wound is such that a major vascular structure could have sustained an injury, or the injury appears to be multileveled. This is especially the case in blunt trauma or in association with fractures or dislocations in which the presence of a fracture hematoma may raise concern about a vascular injury (Enge et al., 1975; McDonald et al., 1975; Wholey and Bocher, 1968).

Advances in angiographic techniques and equipment and experience in interpretation have made angiographic study an invaluable means for establishing the diagnosis of an arterial injury when the clinical diagnosis is not clearly defined. Even when there is an intact distal pulse and no surrounding hematoma, the angiogram may reveal injuries disrupting only the tunica intima and media (Gerlock et al., 1978; Fig. 67–7).

In most centers selective angiography of the involved extremity by way of the femoral artery (Seldinger's technique) has become the standard approach. Intraoperative studies, if necessary, may be conducted by direct puncture of the brachial artery proximal to the site of the suspected injury (Broudy et al., 1979). An 18 or 20 gauge arteriography needle is inserted into the artery and a three-way stop cock attached to plastic tubing is connected to the neeedle and to a 20 cc. syringe containing an appropriate contrast dye. As the last 5 cc. of dye is injected, radiographs are obtained. While awaiting development of the film, the tubing and needle are flushed with saline to prevent clotting and obstruction of the needle should further radiographs be required (Fig. 67–8).

The digital subtraction angiogram permits the arterial tree to be studied by a less invasive method of vascular imaging using venous injection of contrast material. Either a central venous catheter or even a short catheter in an antecubital vein provides a

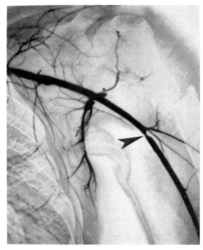

Figure 67–7. A 35-year-old man sustained a closed proximal humeral fracture and presented with a cool, although viable, hand. Distal pulsations were palpable but faint. A preoperative angiogram clearly demonstrated the focal zone of vascular injury (arrow), which proved, at surgery, to be an elevated intimal flap.

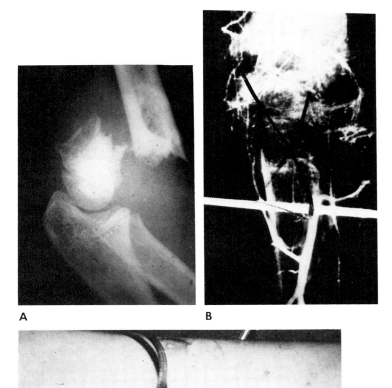

A

B

C

Figure 67–8. A brachial artery thrombosis in association with a closed supracondylar fracture in this five-year-old girl *(A)* was well demonstrated by means of an angiogram *(B)* performed through a direct arterial puncture of the artery proximal to the zone of trauma *(C)*. This avoided a more remote femoral arterial puncture and its attendant risks in a child. (Courtesy of Dr. J. W. May, Jr.)

satisfactory channel for the delivery of the contrast agent, thereby avoiding an arteriotomy. Temporal integration of several sequential video images provides a relatively accurate picture of the arterial anatomy, even to the level of the common digital arteries in the hand. By virtue of its low morbidity, this type of vascular study is also an excellent method of assessing patency following vascular repair (Fig. 67–9).

Although a valuable diagnostic tool, the arteriogram is an invasive study and fundamentally gives a static picture of the arterial anatomy, in contrast to the Doppler probe and impedance plethysmography, which provide a more dynamic picture of the circulation.

TYPES OF ARTERIAL INJURY

Laceration. A laceration may include anything from an isolated puncture wound of an artery to subtotal transection of a vessel wall. These injuries may be associated with the most extensive hemorrhage by virtue of the inability of the vessel ends to retract and thrombose.

Transection. While involving, by definition, the complete division of a vessel, a transection lesion can range from a sharp tidy wound to extensive vascular damage and loss of tissue substance, as in high velocity missile injuries.

Contusion. Injury to a vessel remaining in continuity may range from an adventitial he-

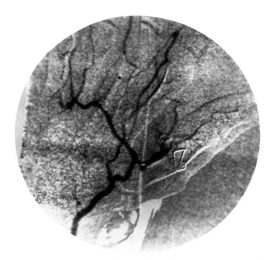

Figure 67–9. The digital subtraction angiogram utilizes a venous injection of contrast material that is enhanced by sequential video images to provide a relatively accurate picture of the arterial anatomy to the level of the mid-palm. In this case, an ulnar artery thrombosis is demonstrated.

matoma to a subintimal hemorrhage with a displaced intimal flap leading to stenosis or obstruction of the vascular lumen.

Spasm. Although truly an unusual occurrence, spasm may be a vascular myogenic response in the absence of true injury. As noted by Rich (1978), however, "the correct spelling for spasm is C-L-O-T."

Arteriovenous Fistula. Classically the arteriovenous fistula is the result of simultaneous injuries of an artery and an adjacent vein allowing blood to flow directly from the artery into the vein. Although most commonly the result of a penetrating injury, these lesions have been reported in association with closed fractures (Harris, 1963), human bites (Anthopoulos et al., 1965), and blunt trauma (Sako and Varco, 1970).

Aneurysm (False and True). A false aneurysm, commonly associated with a penetrating injury, involves a laceration or rupture of all three layers of the arterial wall that is sealed off by hematoma formation and eventually replaced by fibrous tissue and recanalized. True aneurysms involve injury to the elastic fibers of the tunica media and gradual saccular dilation of the vessel. These lesions may be idiopathic, traumatic, mycotic, or atherosclerotic.

Cavitational Effect. The impact of a missile in the surrounding soft tissues can lead to arterial spasm or even intimal disruption even though the missile does not actually touch the vessel wall (Amato et al., 1971). With high energy missiles, the expanding force from the associated shock wave is capable of completely disrupting the vessel.

THE MANAGEMENT OF VASCULAR INJURIES: GENERAL CONSIDERATIONS

Even though a cool, cyanotic, pulseless upper extremity or hand represents a serious emergency, specific efforts should always be taken preoperatively to determine the presence of associated injuries or intercurrent disease. This is especially the case in complete amputations in which instructions need be directed to the referring physician regarding the evaluation and stabilization of the patient prior to transportation to a replantation center. Major bleeding is best controlled by the use of direct pressure with a bulky dressing. Clamping of arterial bleeders is to be avoided because this will cause unnecessary vascular damage and may result in adjacent neural injury. Likewise, the use of a more proximal tourniquet, unless absolutely necessary, is best not done because it too can have a damaging local effect in addition to compromising any residual collateral circulation.

Completely severed parts should be placed in a dry polyethylene bag, which is then placed in regular ice for transport. The incompletely devascularized limb, however, may be rendered further ischemic by surface cooling; therefore sterile wound dressings and appropriate splintage are necessary prior to transport.

Tetanus prophylaxis as well as the parenteral administration of antibiotics should also be initiated at the primary care center, especially if the wound is contaminated or there is significant vascular insufficiency, such as with a completely amputated part.

We believe that arterial restoration should be attempted in all traumatic disruptions proximal to the wrist. There may well be no "safe" site for the ligation of a major vessel, because even if viability is preserved, the resulting arterial insufficiency may be disabling (Hughes, 1954; Jahnke, 1958). In addition to restoration of normal circulation to the peripheral tissues, arterial repair may avoid such late complications as a pulsating hematoma, false aneurysm, or arteriovenous fistula.

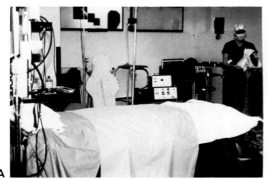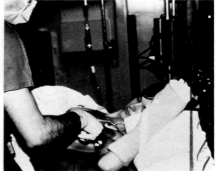

Figure 67–10. With the anticipation of a prolonged surgical procedure, the operating room should be fully prepared, including a water or foam mattress on the operating table, microscope and microvascular instruments, and a full complement of hand surgical equipment *(A)*. Axillary block anesthesia with a long-acting agent is preferred in the emergency patient (B).

The initial laboratory survey for all patients sustaining a major vascular injury or amputation should include a complete blood count, appropriate coagulation studies (such as prothrombin and partial thromboplastin times), a platelet count, and baseline renal function tests. A tube of blood should be obtained for typing and cross matching and in the case of a major arm replantation, fresh whole blood for transfusion is advantageous. Appropriate radiographs to assess skeletal integrity as well as the possibility of a foreign body are ordered in every instance of a vascular injury.

The use of an indwelling urinary catheter and central venous pressure catheter should be considered if a prolonged procedure or considerable blood loss is anticipated before the patient is prepared for surgery (Fig. 67–10).

Axillary block anesthesia using a long acting drug is preferred in the emergency patient because of its safety, efficiency in preventing muscle relaxation and analgesia extending into the postoperative period, and lastly its sympathetic blockade. In more proximal injuries general anesthesia may be required.

In injuries at or distal to the elbow, a pneumatic tourniquet permits preparation and exploration of the wound without excessive blood loss and permits the identification of small vessels with a minimum of tissue trauma. Although in the past concern was expressed over the possibility of thrombosis at anastomotic sites following reinflation of a tourniquet, we have not found this to be the case and, if necessary, do not hesitate to do this following completion of a vascular anastomosis.

In both civilian and military series, documented trauma to the radial and ulnar arteries has been frequently overlooked, no doubt in part because either the radial or the ulnar artery can be ligated in most circumstances without demonstrable immediate problems. Yet when both are involved, the magnitude of injury can threaten the viability of the hand (Gelberman et al., 1982). As a general principle, it is our opinion that repair of an injury to either artery should be undertaken to insure full distal circulation, if only for a brief period of time, in order to augment perfusion while a collateral circulation develops, prevent potential late complications, and maintain and improve proficiency in arterial repair.

With an associated nerve injury in the forearm, substantial evidence exists to show that concomitant unrepaired vascular injuries lead to poorer function and increased symptoms of cold intolerance (Bjorkesten, 1947; Seddon, 1972; Shumaker et al., 1953). In a more extensive injury the destruction of collateral channels similarly may lead to a poorer prognosis unless vascular repair is achieved (Kelley and Eiseman, 1976; Ortner et al., 1961). We also believe that both vessels should be repaired in the event that one later becomes thrombosed.

Extension of the existing wound and even additional incisions may be required in order to achieve adequate wound exposure and débridement. The proximal arterial inflow is usually not a problem following removal of the obstructing thrombus and resection of the damaged end to undamaged intima. In assessing the patency of the distal outflow tract, it is important to recognize that the incidence and extent of a distal thrombus may increase with the severity of the injury, the state of collateral flow, and the interval between injury and surgical repair. A distal thrombus usually can be removed by retrograde milking of the vessel or limb using an Esmarch bandage or, in the case of a very proximal lesion, a Fogarty ballooned vascular catheter. On occasion exposure of distal vessels and small arteriotomies may be required to remove small distal thrombi. Following thrombectomy, vessel closure can be achieved with 9-0 or 10-0 nylon sutures under appropriate magnification.

The state of distal perfusion and the duration of ischemic time influence the order of priority regarding vascular repair and skeletal stabilization. In injuries that have rendered skeletal muscle ischemic for periods beyond six hours, we advocate that revascularization precede the skeletal stabilization and consider external fixation advantageous. Some disagreement continues regarding internal versus external fixation in cases of extensive soft tissue injury (Connolly, 1970; Connolly

et al., 1969; Rich et al., 1971; Figs. 67–11, 67–12).

External fixation permits rapid rigid skeletal stabilization without additional soft tissue dissection and allows ready access in wound care. Its inherent disadvantages include pin tract infection and a higher incidence of nonunion than with rigid internal fixation.

Maintaining venous patency may be difficult in extensive injuries in which venorrhaphy has been performed. The low pressure venous system with its collapsible walls is susceptible to thrombosis. This can be offset to some degree by employing a long oblique anastomosis in the larger vein so that the sides of the circumferential suture line are not directly opposite each other.

One should never hesitate to perform a fasciotomy. Early fasciotomy enhances survival and is attended by minimal inherent complications. It is indicated in crushing injuries with extensive soft tissue trauma, in cases in which prolonged anoxia has occurred, and if significant swelling has occurred intraoperatively or is anticipated in the early postoperative period. In the crushed

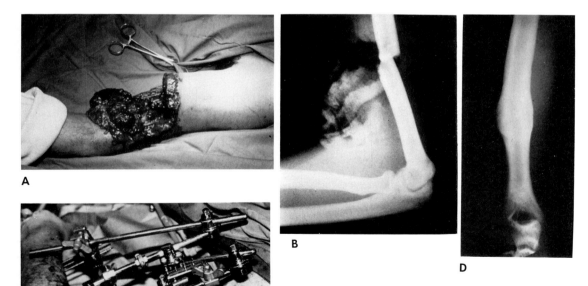

Figure 67–11. A 14-year-old boy sustained an incomplete amputation of his left arm through the mid-humerus in a motor cycle accident *(A).* The humerus fracture *(B)* was debrided, shortened, and stabilized with external fixation, after which the brachial artery and median and radial nerves were repaired *(C).* The humerus healed without difficulty *(D).*

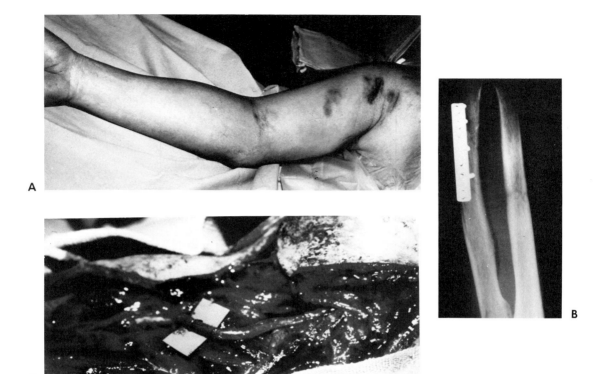

Figure 67–12. This 58-year-old fisherman had his right dominant arm caught in a winch and sustained closed fractures of his humerus, radius, and metacarpals, dislocation of his elbow, and disruption of his brachial artery *(A)*. The skeletal injuries were stabilized by internal fixation *(B)* following repair of his artery using an interposition reversed saphenous vein graft *(C)*.

hand, prophylactic release of the palmar fascia and canal of Guyon may enhance perfusion through the superficial palmar arch, and release of fascia over the distal interosseous muscles may prevent ischemic contractures. Loose or even delayed wound closure further accommodates swelling and diminishes the chance of venous obstruction. An open wound, in addition, enhances drainage and avoids potential compression (Fig. 67–13).

INSTRUMENTS

Specialized instruments are required for vascular surgery and even more so for microvascular surgery. The instrument ends must approximate accurately, be comfortably shaped to avoid intrinsic muscle fatigue, have a nonglare surface, and need to be kept separated from other instruments (Acland, 1977; Bright, 1979).

Vascular clamps should exert only gentle pressure and yet be capable of gripping the vessel securely. Double clamps with a sliding approximation adjustment are advantageous in the careful construction of a tidy anastomosis.

Hemostasis is mandatory for good microvascular work. The bipolar coagulator produces heat only in the small area between its jaws, with less chance of damage to the main vessel.

Magnification has greatly facilitated vascular repair in the upper extremity. The surgical telescope can be fitted to the surgeon. More complex surgery, especially with smaller vessels, requires use of the operating microscope. The requirements include a double head to permit the surgeon and assistant to view the same field, convenient focusing, and an easily controlled zoom lens.

Last, but of great significance, is the microvascular suture material. Axillary and brachial arteries may be repaired with 6-0 or 7-0 polyethylene sutures, ulnar and radial arteries with 8-0 or 9-0 monofilament nylon, and digital vessels with 9-0 or 10-0 monofilament nylon, depending upon the diameter of the vessel to be repaired.

VASCULAR REPAIR

THREE MILLIMETER DIAMETER OR GREATER

Attention to detail and careful preparation of the vessel ends are critical for successful vascular anastomoses. Débridement of damaged vessel ends until normal intima is revealed at both vessel ends is necessary to achieve a patent anastomosis. The adventitia need be resected only at the vessel end to eliminate the potential hazard of adventitia falling into the lumen to serve as a nidus for

platelet aggregation. With more proximal arterial injuries, the passage of a Fogarty catheter ensures that no distal thrombus will form. One must perform this maneuver with great care, in particular within the forearm in order to avoid arterial trauma.

Although an end-to-end suture line is the optimal repair, tension on the anastomotic line must be avoided and a reversed interposition autogenous vein graft (either saphenous or cephalic) should be employed. In most situations the use of adjacent venae comitantes is to be avoided, for these tend to be thin walled and may become aneurysmal under arterial pressure (Rich et al., 1970).

Prevention of narrowing at the suture line is important not only in the immediate res-

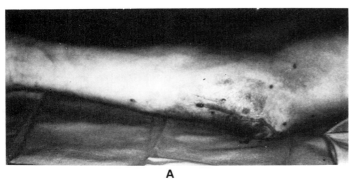

A

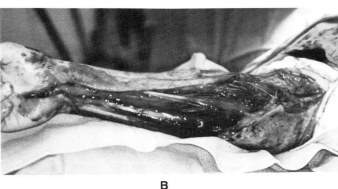

B

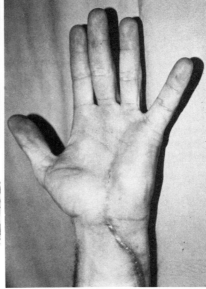

C

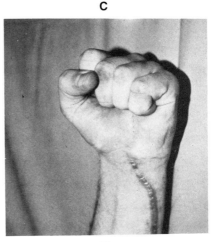

D

Figure 67–13. This 18-year-old male was shot at close range in his right dominant forearm and elbow with a shotgun. Arterial perfusion was only marginal and compartment pressures in his forearm measured 80 mm. Hg (A). Extensive fasciotomies of the forearm and palm, including release of Guyon's canal, dramatically improved the arterial circulation (B). Full hand function was restored (C and D).

toration of arterial flow but also to insure the long term patency of the reconstruction (Inahara, 1962). The modified end-to-end anastomosis, described by Linton (1973), lends itself to an intima-to-intima approximation with a running suture. A triangulation technique may also be effective, utilizing two stay sutures for control of the vessel ends. In small vessels these are placed one-third the circumference of the vessel apart and held with a delicate clamp to keep them taut without tearing. A running suture is continued between the two stay sutures for vessels larger than 3 mm. in diameter; interrupted sutures are used for smaller vessels and in pediatric patients. Prior to both initiation and completion of the anastomosis, the proximal and distal ends of the artery are irrigated with a heparinized solution (e.g., 10,000 units in 100 ml. of saline) to remove and prevent potential thrombus formation. Kinking or twisting of the anastomosis is avoided by meticulous pretesting and planning.

The low pressure distal clamp is removed prior to removing the proximal clamp, and gentle pressure is applied to the repair site until hemostasis is achieved. At times an additional suture may be required to secure adequate hemostasis. Segmental arteriospasm may occur; if it is not associated with localized vessel damage and thrombosis, treatment should consist of release of any mechanical pressure on the artery, 2 per cent Xylocaine irrigation, and the application of warm saline packs.

THREE MILLIMETER DIAMETER OR LESS

The operating microscope plays an integral role in the surgical repair of smaller vessels in the upper extremity, particularly those less than 1.5 mm. in diameter. The success of microvascular anastomoses is contingent upon the presence of undamaged vessel ends at the site of repair. The magnification afforded by the operating microscope permits careful inspection of the cut vessel ends for the characteristic signs of vascular damage both proximally and distally.

When assessing the proximal end, one should be aware that a pulsating vessel does not necessarily imply the absence of endothelial damage. After dissecting free an adequate length of vessel, dilating the lumen with a vessel dilator or microforceps, and bathing

the artery with 2 per cent Xylocaine, the vessel should be cut back until there is continuous spurting of arterial flow. On occasion a slight degree of distal traction on the cut end of the proximal artery will enhance good spurting (May and Gallico, 1980; Fig. 67–14).

In the evaluation of the distal vessel, local signs of vascular damage include telescoping or separation of the media from the adventitia, persistent white platelet aggregation consistent with endothelial damage, or areas of red cell extravasation through the adventitia (red streaking) indicative of distal vessel injury.

With the achievement of good arterial inflow from the proximal cut end in conjunction with an undamaged distal vessel, preparation can be made for either direct end-to-end primary anastomosis or the placement of an interposition vein graft. The surgeon must be able to perfectly visualize both vessel ends. Vessel mobilization is achieved by stripping the adventitia and its attached fat with a microforceps and microdissecting scissors. Additional mobility is gained by coagulating any restraining side branches with a bipolar microcoagulator.

Both vessel segments are carefully secured in an approximating clamp and irrigated with a warmed mixture of lactated Ringer's solution to which heparin (2000 units per 100 cc.) is added. It is critical for success that no undue tension be present at the anastomotic site (Fig. 67–15). Prior to constructing the anastomosis, the vessel ends are again gently dilated to one and one-half times their natural

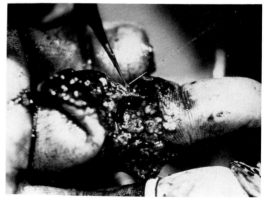

Figure 67–14. The surgeon must be assured of normal arterial inflow pressure prior to initiating the microvascular arterial anastomosis. On occasion, a slight degree of distal traction on the end of the proximal artery will enhance a good "spurt."

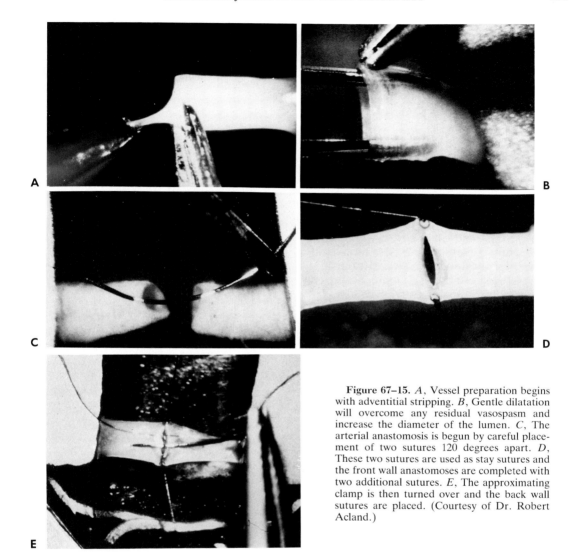

Figure 67–15. *A*, Vessel preparation begins with adventitial stripping. *B*, Gentle dilatation will overcome any residual vasospasm and increase the diameter of the lumen. *C*, The arterial anastomosis is begun by careful placement of two sutures 120 degrees apart. *D*, These two sutures are used as stay sutures and the front wall anastomoses are completed with two additional sutures. *E*, The approximating clamp is then turned over and the back wall sutures are placed. (Courtesy of Dr. Robert Acland.)

size to overcome any residual vasospasm, and proximal arterial inflow should again be demonstrated.

The arterial anastomosis is constructed, using 9-0, 10-0, or occasionally 11-0 nylon sutures, by placing two sutures 120 degrees apart, with one end of the suture from each knot left long to aid in control of the vessel. Special care is taken to carefully effect intima-to-intima suturing. Irrigation during knot tying should be done cautiously because it may force residual adventitia into the lumen. Two additional sutures are placed between the stay sutures, and the approximating clamp and vessel ends are turned over, exposing the back wall of each vessel end. A third triangulating suture is placed between

the original two sutures, and two additional knots are placed on either side of this, giving a total of at least nine sutures.

At this juncture the anastomosis should be bathed with 2 per cent Xylocaine and the approximating clamps released. Significant leaks can be overcome by placing an additional suture in the appropriate site. At times gentle massage of the vessel at the site of the clamp application may be required to overcome local spasm and initiate flow.

A patent anastomosis may be judged by the refill or patency test. Two microforceps are utilized, one to occlude the vessel just distal to the anastomosis and the second to milk the artery distally. The proximal microforceps is then released, and the quality of flow across the anastomosis is observed. One should avoid milking across the anastomosis.

There may be several explanations for inadequate flow across a constructed anastomosis. These include technical problems at the anastomosis such as a "through-stitch" that has caught the back wall of the vessel, poor arterial inflow, or physiological changes in the distal vascular bed, described by some as the no-reflow phenomenon (May et al., 1978). In this setting it has been suggested that prolonged ischemia produces endothelial cellular swelling and resultant obstruction of blood flow at the capillary level. The two major factors that appear to cause arterial spasm are cold and contact of the vessel with fresh blood (Acland, 1977). Because of the tendency for thrombosis to occur at the anastomosis, the anastomosis should be redone or an interposition vein graft placed.

When an excessive discrepancy exists between the sizes of the vessel ends, either an end-to-side anastomosis or an interposition vein graft is a consideration (Fig. 67–16). With the end-to-side anastomosis, success depends in part on making a tidy arteriotomy in the large vessel. The adventitia should be elevated at the proposed site with care to avoid cutting the vessel media. A pickup suture is then placed in the center of the arteriotomy site and tied, with one end left long. When placing this suture, care is taken to pass the needle into and out of the vessel wall. By pulling up on this suture, a cut is made in the vessel at a 60 degree angle with straight sharp pointed scissors. The depth of this cut is equal to half the diameter of the small vessel (Acland). A second cut is made at the same angle at a site opposite the first cut, creating a neat arteriotomy.

Construction of the anastomosis involves placing two stay sutures at opposite ends of the arteriotomy, followed by careful placement of individual sutures to complete each side of the anastomosis. The smaller vessel must be mobile enough to permit access for suturing the near and far walls (Fig. 67–17).

The end-to-side anastomosis is of special importance in injuries to the superficial palmar arch in which reconstruction may require anastomosis of the common digital arteries in an end-to-side manner to a long vein graft tied at the distal end and sutured end to end to the ulnar or radial artery more proximally (Fig. 67–18).

The indications for interposition vein grafts include gaps left after wide resection of dam-

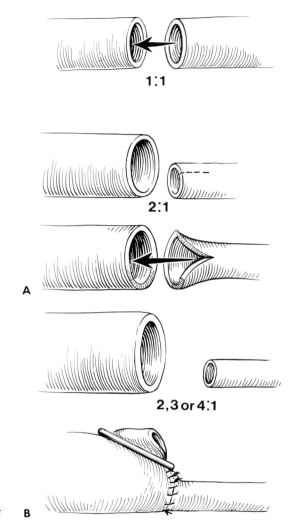

Figure 67–16. When faced with a size discrepancy between the ends of the vessels, one can enlarge the lumen of the smaller vessel by making a longitudinal cut, which increased the available lumen *(A)*. On occasion, one can also carefully narrow the end of the larger vessel with sutures or a small clip *(B)*.

aged vessels, inability to shorten the skeleton, as in cases when joint preservation is involved, and in cases in which access to the vessel may be difficult. The latter occasionally occurs in thumb replantations in which exposure of the digital arteries may be difficult. Vein grafts should be considered in preference to repeated anastomosing of damaged vessels, in particular in view of their well documented, excellent tendency to remain patent (Buchler et al., 1977). Conservatism should be the rule when the question arises whether to use an interpositional vein graft (Fig. 67–19).

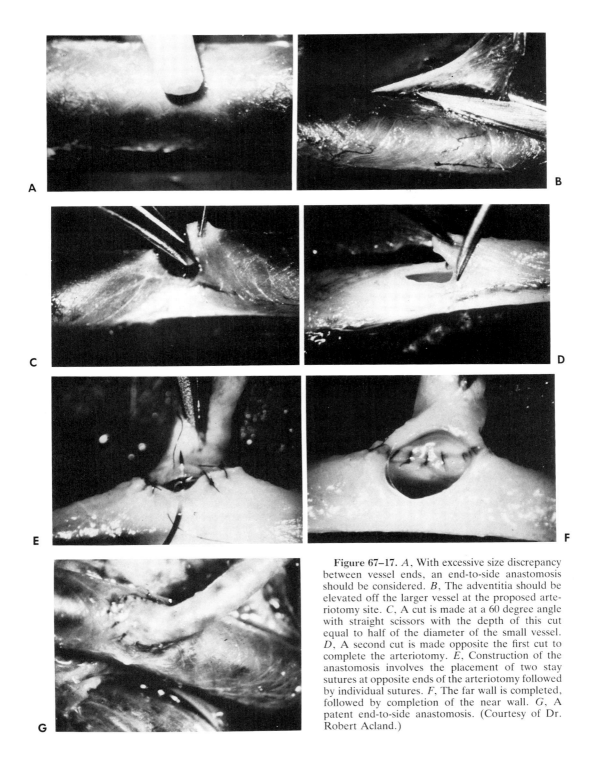

Figure 67–17. *A*, With excessive size discrepancy between vessel ends, an end-to-side anastomosis should be considered. *B*, The adventitia should be elevated off the larger vessel at the proposed arteriotomy site. *C*, A cut is made at a 60 degree angle with straight scissors with the depth of this cut equal to half of the diameter of the small vessel. *D*, A second cut is made opposite the first cut to complete the arteriotomy. *E*, Construction of the anastomosis involves the placement of two stay sutures at opposite ends of the arteriotomy followed by individual sutures. *F*, The far wall is completed, followed by completion of the near wall. *G*, A patent end-to-side anastomosis. (Courtesy of Dr. Robert Acland.)

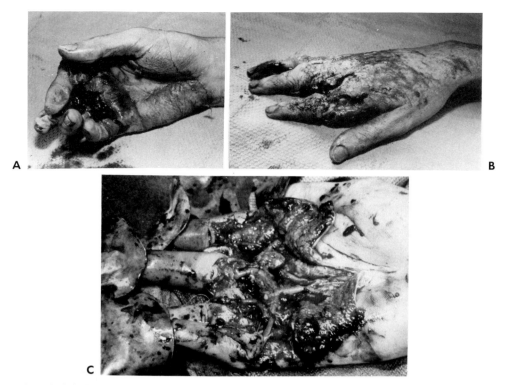

Figure 67–18. In injuries to the superficial palmar arch, vein grafts are frequently needed to reconstruct the vascular anatomy. As illustrated in this clinical case, several vein grafts were employed, utilizing both end-to-end and end-to-side anastomoses to revascularize four digits in this 18-year-old man who sustained a severe crushing injury to his right dominant hand *(A, B, and C)*.

For digital vessels, appropriate sized donor veins may be found in the distal forearm, foot, or the venae comitantes of the radial artery in the forearm (Tupper). The direction of the vein graft must be oriented for flow, i.e., reversed in arterial grafts and in its anatomical direction for venous grafting. The vein graft should be harvested under tourni-quet control with loupe magnification. Side branches are carefully ligated or coagulated with the bipolar microforceps coagulator. Marks are always placed to identify the prox-imal or outflow end. A vein graft when placed as an arterial graft may lengthen up to 10 per cent when distended under full blood pres-sure and may increase in diameter up to 50

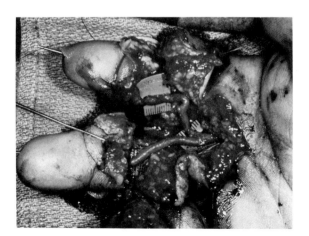

Figure 67–19. The forearm and the dorsum of the foot are excellent donor sites for size-matched vein graft. Y-shaped grafts can be obtained in instances in which two distal anastomoses are indicated, as seen in this case of a two-digit replantation.

per cent; thus careful planning is required to avoid ballooning or twisting (May and Gallico, 1980).

In most instances the distal anastomosis between the vein graft and the artery is performed first, care being taken to avoid excessive dilation of the vein lumen. Sutures are best placed from the vein into the artery to ensure proper placement of sutures in the artery. Care should be taken to suture the vein under some tension to avoid excessive dilation when the clamps are removed. Vein grafts placed between vein defects are not reversed and are generally easier to place because less dilation occurs as a result of the lower venous perfusion pressure (Fig. 67–20). When they are available, one can employ segments of artery for arterial grafts.

THROMBOSIS

Thrombosis as a result of trauma can occur at any level of the extremity. If not recognized early, symptoms of chronic ischemia, including paresthesias, coldness and cold intolerance, discoloration, blanching, and pain, may force the patient to seek surgical relief.

AXILLARY ARTERY

Thrombosis of the axillary artery may be found in association with a single trauma, such as a fracture or dislocation of the prox-

imal humerus, or repetitive insults, as when an axillary crutch is used (Brooks and Fowler, 1964; Calvet et al., 1942; Henson, 1956; Johnston and Lowry, 1962; Platt, 1930; Robb and Standeven, 1956; Stein et al., 1971; Theodorides and DeKeizer, 1976; Tse et al., 1980; Weile and Fjeldborg, 1971).

Although axillary artery thrombosis in the face of adequate collateral circulation may not place the upper extremity in immediate jeopardy, long term complications, including aneurysmal changes or distal thromboembolic events, are sufficient indications for surgical intervention. It is also important to recognize that shoulder girdle fractures or dislocations are common in the older population in whom the collateral circulation may be insufficient.

When axillary artery thrombosis is suspected, angiography should be undertaken in order to better establish the diagnosis as well as define the site and extent of injury.

Because the axillary artery is a vessel of substantial size and can be mobilized relatively easily, a high degree of success should be achieved with vascular reconstruction. Adequate exposure is important, especially in view of the close proximity of the brachial plexus. If added exposure is needed, the tendons of both pectoralis muscles can be divided. Routine use of a Fogarty balloon catheter both proximally and distally is helpful in eliminating thrombi, which may have migrated from the site of vascular injury. In many instances a direct end-to-end repair is

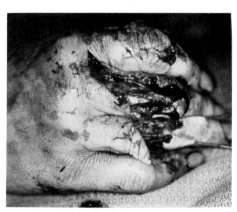 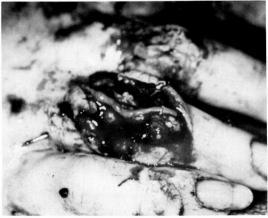

A B

Figure 67–20. Vein grafts are frequently needed in digital revascularizations for both arterial and venous reconstructions, as demonstrated in this case of a 23-year-old woman who had her long and ring fingers devascularized in a motor vehicle accident (A). Size-matched vein grafts from her foot were employed for both arterial and venous reconstructions (B). Satisfactory function resulted.

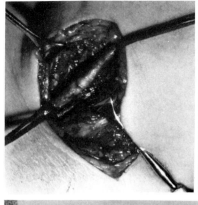

A

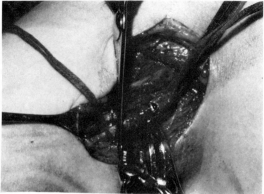

B

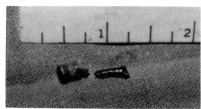

C

Figure 67–21. This patient developed arterial insufficiency after sustaining a gunshot injury to his thorax. The bullet migrated and lodged in the axillary artery *(A)*. The bullet and damaged arterial segment were excised and the artery was repaired primarily *(B and C)*.

possible following resection of the thrombotic segment.

Lastly, the surgeon must carefully assess the more distal muscle compartments. Depending upon the extent and duration of the ischemic period, compartment pressure monitoring may be beneficial in determining whether fasciotomy is required (Whitesides et al, 1975; Fig. 67–21).

BRACHIAL ARTERY

Laceration continues to be the most common form of injury to the brachial artery, but its close proximity to bone as well as overlying skin and subcutaneous tissue at the elbow places the artery at significant risk for thrombotic occlusions (Kerin, 1969; Lipscomb and Burleson, 1955; Louis et al., 1974; Myerding, 1936; Shaw, 1959). The increasing frequency of diagnostic procedures as well as inadvertent access to the arterial system through drug abuse has also accounted for an increasing incidence of brachial artery thrombosis (Barnes et al., 1974; Bolasny and Killen, 1971; Brener and Couch, 1973; Scott and Ochsner, 1948; Fig. 67–22).

The arterial tree at the elbow may also be subject to iatrogenic injury when an artery is mistaken for a vein (Gagnon, 1966; Hazlett, 1949). This has most frequently been de-

scribed following Pentothal injection into an ulnar artery located in a more superficial position than usual (Engler et al., 1964; Schanzer et al., 1979).

Arterial injury as a result of drug injections may vary from direct damage by the needle

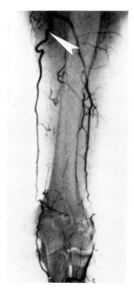

Figure 67–22. The use of the brachial artery for diagnostic procedures has led to an increasing incidence of brachial artery thrombosis. This patient had a left heart catheterization through her brachial artery with a resultant brachial artery thrombosis *(arrow)* requiring arterial reconstruction.

(ranging from production of an intimal flap to a through-and-through puncture with perivascular hematoma), a mechanical reaction from chemical endarteritis, or a blockade from precipitated crystals (Daniel, 1973).

The clinical presentation usually begins with intense burning discomfort extending from the point of injection to the finger tips ("hand trip") followed by blanching, severe pain, and later swelling and cyanosis. Some unfortunate patients may delay seeking medical attention until irreversible gangrenous changes have occurred (Engler et al., 1964; Hager and Wilson, 1967; Nathan, 1975; Petrie and Lamb, 1973).

Treatment of intra-arterial injection injuries is generally directed at maximizing tissue salvage. Perfusion is evaluated using a Doppler probe, plethysmography, and measurement of the digital temperature. Angiography is useful in excluding lesions that are amenable to operative intervention. These may include an intimal flap, a false aneurysm, or a mycotic aneurysm. Anticoagulation with heparin, the intra-arterial and systemic administration of vasodilators, stellate ganglion blockade, and thrombolysin have all been employed with varying degrees of success (Dellon et al., 1979; Fig. 67–23).

In a closed injury such as an elbow fracture or dislocation, the abundant collateral circulation in this region may minimize the symptoms and signs of not only acute but also late occlusions of the brachial artery. Noninvasive diagnostic procedures such as Doppler flow studies or impedance plethysmography may be of use in establishing the diagnosis in patients who have sustained blunt trauma (Broudy et al., 1979; Fig. 67–24).

In most cases fractures should be stabilized prior to arterial reconstruction. As with the axillary artery, resection of the involved segment and tension-free, direct repair by end-to-end approximation frequently may be accomplished by proximal and distal arterial mobilization (Tuzzeo et al., 1978; Wright et al., 1977). Consideration should always be given to shortening the skeleton at the fracture site to enhance the potential for a tension-free vascular repair. Ligation, even with an adequate collateral flow, cannot be recommended, with the possible exception of cases of multiple casualties or under adverse conditions. The "safety" of ligation is relative. Although the collateral circulation may offset acute ischemia and gangrene, the potential for later arterial insufficiency may prove most disabling.

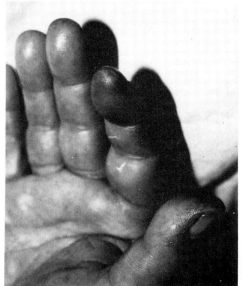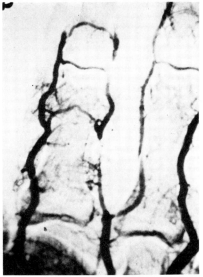

Figure 67–23. A 35-year-old drug addict inadvertently injected himself in his radial artery, resulting in thrombosis of the digital arteries at the level of the middle phalanx of his index finger *(A and B)*. The thrombotic segments were excised and interposition vein grafts were used to restore arterial flow.

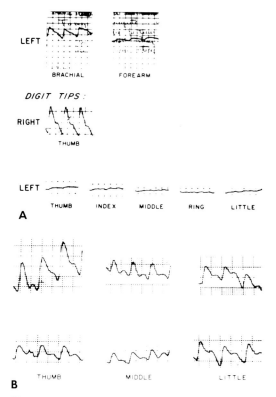

Figure 67–24. A five-year-old child presented with a closed supracondylar fracture of the humerus and no palpable distal pulsations. The cuff impedance plethysmograph demonstrated marginal arterial flow *(A)* and, at surgical exploration, a brachial artery thrombosis was noted. Following arterial reconstruction, the tracing demonstrated excellent blood flow *(B)*.

ULNAR ARTERY

Although thrombosis of the ulnar artery and its branches within the hand has been described by a number of authors under such labels as "hypothenar hammer syndrome," "post-traumatic digital ischemia," or "pneumatic tool disease" (Conn et al., 1970; Little and Ferguson, 1972), it was von Rosen (1934) who initially stressed the intimal injury differentiating this lesion from previously described ulnar artery aneurysms (Guattani, 1772; Maudaire, 1897; Middleton, 1933). A number of reports have followed, and the advent of microsurgical techniques now permits the resection and reconstruction of segments of thrombosed vessels (Given et al., 1978). Nevertheless the recognition and treatment of this disabling disorder remain ill defined and somewhat controversial.

More common in males, especially among manual workers, the presentation in ulnar artery thrombosis is often confused with that in a number of other disorders, including Raynaud's phenomenon, acrosclerosis, collagen vascular disorders, thoracic outlet compression, and ulnar nerve compression. A history of blunt trauma to the hypothenar eminence may be obtained in most instances, with repetitive trauma (such as employing the heel of the hand as a hammer) frequently found as the causative factor (Middleton, 1933). Occasionally a space occupying lesion, such as a ganglion extending into the confined space of Guyon's canal, may compress and eventually thrombose the artery.

The presenting signs of vascular involvement may include coolness or pallor of the ring and little fingers, evidence of distal trophic changes, and ulcerations. Cold intolerance in addition to pain or cramping is also prevalent with a clinical picture suggestive of Raynaud's phenomenon. The Allen test is positive in almost every instance, and commonly a palpable tender mass may be appreciated in the hypothenar region.

Symptoms may also include neurological complaints, such as aching or paraesthesias in the sensory distribution of the ulnar nerve to the little and ring fingers. In most instances intrinsic motor strength is intact (Zweig et al., 1969), and the results of objective testing, including electromyography, nerve conduction velocity, and two-point discrimination, are normal (Koman and Urbaniak, 1981).

The vulnerability of the ulnar artery to traumatic injury can be explained on an anatomical basis. At the wrist the artery passes lateral and slightly volar to the ulnar nerve and pisiform as it enters Guyon's canal (Guyon, 1861). In this location it lies anterior to the unyielding transverse carpal ligament and just beneath the volar carpal ligament. Just distal to this in the space of Guyon, the deep branches of the ulnar artery and nerve pass between the pisohamate and pisometacarpal ligaments while the superficial ulnar artery and nerve continue over the origin of the hypothenar musculature medial to the hamate hook covered only by the palmaris brevis, subcutaneous fat, and fascia and skin (Denman, 1978). By virtue of this anatomical arrangement, the artery, somewhat tethered in place, is subject to repeated trauma against the hook of the hamate.

The repetitive trauma leads to intimal damage with subsequent thrombosis and vascular occlusion. More extensive or prolonged trauma may also lead to subintimal hemorrhage, disruption of the internal elastic membrane, and ultimately dilation and aneurysmal changes (Green, 1973).

A number of diagnostic procedures, in addition to a confirmatory history and a positive Allen test result, can help in both confirming the diagnosis and defining the extent of the problem. These include digital impedance plethysmography, Doppler mapping, and angiography.

As a general rule, we believe, it is mandatory for the patient to discontinue usage of tobacco in any form. Following diagnosis we perform an angiogram in association with axillary block anesthesia, which not only defines the extent of the lesion but also provides a clearer picture of the extent of collateral circulation and distal "runoff." During the angiographic study, in addition, intra-arterial vasodilating drugs such as reserpine or tolazoline hydrochloride may be administered.

In patients who fail to respond to these measures and in whom threatened viability of one or more digits continues, operative intervention is indicated. Following identification and excision of the entire thrombosed segment—in particular, in the face of poor backflow from the distal vessels—a reversed interposition vein graft obtained from the forearm should be employed. The damaged vessel must be resected until normal intima, both proximally as well as distally, is visible under the microscope. The anastomoses are constructed with 9-0 nylon sutures in an interrupted fashion. We do not routinely use systemic heparinization postoperatively, but flush proximally and distally with heparinized irrigation prior to the anastomosis and often give a single parenteral bolus of 5000 units of heparin at the time of the anastomosis. Following completion of the anastomosis, the radial artery should be manually occluded for 10 to 15 minutes as arterial flow is re-established through the reconstituted ulnar artery. In a number of instances we have established permanent arterial patency as demonstrated by both the Allen test and follow-up angiography months and years after the repair (Fig. 67–25). When an extensive length of the artery is involved, the interposition vein graft can be brought through the carpal tunnel to avoid direct trauma.

Occasionally, in patients with extensive thrombosis extending into the digital vessels, symptoms of ischemia may persist despite resection of the thrombosed artery and adjuvant medical therapy. Additional relief of ischemic symptoms may be achieved by trans-axillary sympathectomy removing the lower third of the stellate ganglion and the thoracic ganglia of T2, T3, and T4 if prior stellate blocks provide some symptomatic, albeit temporary relief.

MEDIAN ARTERY

As noted, a persistent median artery may be present in 5 to 10 per cent of the population (Coleman and Anson, 1961; Pecket et al., 1973). Thrombosis of this vessel is rare and is nearly always related to a specific traumatic event. The clinical presentation reflects compression of the median nerve in the carpal canal; in fact, it is at the time of surgical decompression of the carpal tunnel that the thrombosed artery may be discovered (Burnham, 1963; DeAbrew and Godoy-moreira, 1958).

At the time of surgical decompression the thrombosed vessel should be ligated proximally and distally and resected because the median artery is rarely the primary supplier of the circulation to the palmar arch (Fig. 67–26). However, if one is unable to palpate a radial or ulnar pulse, the median artery should be reconstructed if it appears to be the major source of arterial supply. The transverse carpal ligament is incised in a zigzag manner, and the tips are sutured, which enlarges the tunnel as well as restores its roof.

RADIAL ARTERY

Just prior to entering the deep arch, the radial artery lies above the unyielding trapezium and is subject to thrombosis from repetitive trauma (Mays, 1970). In addition, its superficial location at the wrist makes the radial artery the most common site for arterial cannulation. The frequency of complications following cannulation may vary with the type of catheter used, the techniques of placement, and associated systemic complications. Thrombosis can occur either during cannulation or following removal of the catheter.

In a prospective study of 105 patients

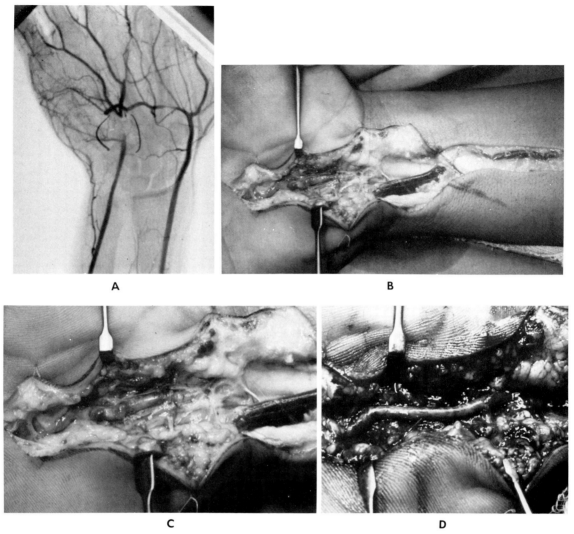

Figure 67–25. This 42-year-old mechanic presented with pain in the ulnar side of his hand. Physical examination revealed the little and ring fingers to be cooler than the other fingers, and an Allen test demonstrated no arterial perfusion through the ulnar artery. An ulnar artery thrombosis was confirmed on angiography *(A)*. At surgical exploration, an ulnar artery thrombosis was noted at the distal forearm, extending into Guyon's canal *(B and C)*. The thrombosis was resected and arterial restoration was achieved with an interposition vein graft *(D)*.

undergoing radial artery cannulation, Bedford and Wollman (1973) found evidence of arterial occlusion at the time of catheter removal in less than half the patients in whom thrombosis was eventually confirmed. Mandel and Dauchot (1977), using precatheter Doppler scanning and cannulations under aseptic conditions with 20 gauge needles, reported only two serious complications in a review of 1000 radial artery cannulations. In most series, however, prolonged cannulation, hypotensive episodes, and systemic diseases such as diabetes or vasculitis have been associated with a higher incidence of complications. Besides thrombosis, other complications of radial artery cannulation include hematoma, embolization of particulate matter, pseudoaneurysm or arteriovenous fistula formation, and the carpal tunnel syndrome (Downs et al., 1973; Mathieu et al., 1973; McLesky and Stehling, 1982; Saaman, 1971).

Prior to radial artery cannulation, the Allen test must be done to confirm the existence of a complete arterial arch system in the

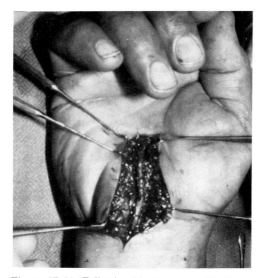

Figure 67–26. Following blunt trauma, this 31-year-old man presented with signs and symptoms consistent with compression of his median nerve in the carpal tunnel. At surgery, a large thrombosed median artery was discovered. Because a preoperative Allen test demonstrated intact blood flow to the radial and ulnar arteries, the thrombosed median artery was resected. The carpal ligament was incised in a zigzag manner and the tips were sutured to enlarge and yet restore the carpal tunnel roof.

hand. Doppler scanning may be useful in the unconscious patient. Although many thrombi recanalize and are of no clinical significance if there is an adequate collateral circulation, when the radial side of the hand is rendered ischemic, recanalization will likely be too late to prevent gangrenous changes (Falor et al., 1976; Fig. 67–27).

When faced with ischemic changes or impending gangrene, the hand surgeon should be prepared to explore the zone of arterial trauma, for the lesion, if well localized, is often amenable to surgical and vascular reconstruction—in most instances with an interposition vein graft (Katz et al., 1974).

DIGITAL ARTERY

Digital artery thrombosis often occurs in association with repetitive traumatic episodes, which may be occupational or recreational, for example, in sports such as baseball or handball (Lowrey et al., 1976; Teisinger, 1972; Telford et al., 1945).

The presenting symptoms for the most part are related to digital ischemia and include pain, paresthesias, coolness and cold intolerance, and not uncommonly swelling of the involved digit. Pain may be present in the absence of other signs of ischemia and most likely is related to stimulation of the periarterial sympathetic system by the distended thrombosed digital artery. In acute traumatic thrombosis a painful nodule may be palpated along the digital artery.

The diagnosis can be confirmed by a positive result in the digital Allen test as well as by noninvasive digital impedance phlethysmography. Angiography, in conjunction with stellate or brachial plexus block anesthesia, helps further in defining the anatomical lesion and the extent of the distal collateral circulation.

In the patient with a unilateral digital arterial thrombosis with adequate distal perfusion through the contralateral vessel, some recommend simply ligation and resection of the thrombosed segment. Our preference, however, is to consider interposition vein grafting if we can achieve both adequate arterial inflow and a suitable distal vessel (Fig. 67–28).

In bilateral digital arterial thromboses, more severe ischemic symptoms are often present, including fingertip ulceration. Conservative measures, including cessation of use of tobacco, avoidance of trauma or cold, and stellate ganglion blocks, may help to reduce the intensity of symptoms. In patients with

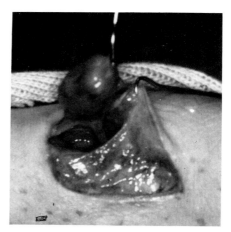

Figure 67–27. The radial artery is subject to thrombosis from repetitive trauma as well as from indwelling arterial cannulation. This patient presented with a pulsatile mass in the vicinity of the radial artery, which at surgical exploration proved to be a radial artery thrombosis. This was resected and an end-to-end repair of the radial artery was achieved.

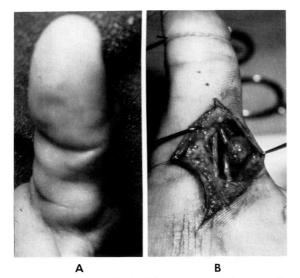

A   **B**

Figure 67–28. Following blunt trauma to the base of the thumb, this patient presented with a painful mass over the proximal phalanx *(A)*. The mass was pulsatile on examination and at surgery proved to be post-traumatic thrombosis of the digital artery to the thumb *(B)*.

thromboses of localized segments, resection and vein grafting have provided some measure of success. Consideration also should be given to digital arterial sympathectomy, as described by Flatt (1980). Under loop magnification or preferably with the operating microscope, the adventitia of the involved proper digital artery is circumferentially stripped for 3 to 4 mm. This should be done beyond the junction of the distal perforating artery with the common digital artery and should include the dorsal digital arterial branch arising off the digital artery proper.

ANEURYSMS

The surgical treatment of peripheral arterial aneurysms has paralleled the development of modern vascular surgery. Antyllus in the second century A.D. is reported to have treated small peripheral traumatic aneurysms by ligature proximally and distally and puncture of the center of the aneurysm (Schwartz, 1958). Guattani first described an aneurysm within the hand in 1772. In 1888 Matas published his method of endoaneurysmorrhaphy for the treatment of a brachial artery aneurysm. This approach, involving the opening of the aneurysm and closure of its communication into the arterial lumen, became the

standard for treatment during the succeeding 50 years. Resection of the traumatic aneurysm with arterial reconstruction by an interposition vein graft, initially described by Lexer in 1907, only began to come into popularity during the Korean conflict.

Acquired aneurysms in the upper extremity are for the most part traumatic and are considered as either false or true depending on the type and degree of the initial arterial injury (Kleinert et al., 1973; Spittel, 1958). False aneurysms are most commonly associated with penetrating wounds such as stab wounds and low velocity projectile injuries (Baird and Lajor, 1964; Cawley, 1947; Engleman et al., 1969; Louis and Simon, 1974; Milling and Kinmoth, 1977; Orhewere, 1966), but may also be secondary to closed skeletal fractures, diagnostic arterial puncture, and accidental arterial injury during surgery (Davis and Fell, 1951; Harris, 1963; Hentz et al., 1978; Hueston, 1973; Mathieu et al., 1973; Sterling and Haberman, 1975).

The arterial injury in a false aneurysm consists of a disruption of all three layers of the arterial wall. Arterial flow is usually maintained as the extravasated blood, contained by the surrounding soft tissues, organizes and seals the original point of injury. Eventually recanalization of the fibrosed hematoma results in an encapsulated false aneurysm whose lumen remains in continuity with that of the vessel. Histological examination reveals organized fibrous tissue without evidence of muscle or elastic fibers in the aneurysmal wall. Complications include false aneurysm and rarely consumption coagulopathy (May et al., 1982; Rhodes et al., 1973; Sachatello et al., 1974; Spittel, 1958).

The less frequent true aneurysm involves some part of all three layers of the arterial wall and is the result of nonpenetrating trauma, either a single event (Bradley, 1945; Fowler and Workman, 1964) or repetitive trauma such as that described by Middleton in 1933 as an "occupation aneurysm of the palmar arteries." More uncommonly true aneurysms have been reported to result from crutch compression of the axillary artery or traction (Abbott and Darling, 1973; Sharp and Hansel, 1967). As with traumatic thromboses, the most commonly involved areas in the hand are over bony prominences, such as the radial artery overlying the trapezium and the unprotected segment of the ulnar artery between the distal edge of the transverse carpal ligament and the medial edge of the palmar aponeurosis (Mays, 1970; Narsete, 1964). Involvement of the common or proper digital arteries has only infrequently been reported (Baruch, 1977; Hueston, 1973; Layman et al., 1982; Sanchez et al., 1982; Suzuki et al., 1980).

Within the dilated true aneurysm, in particular where the intima has also been damaged, laminated thrombi may develop that ultimately may occlude the vessel and serve as a nidus for more distal embolization (Green, 1973; May et al., 1982; Mays, 1970).

In most instances the diagnosis can be suspected on the basis of the physical examination, which must include palpation of all pulses and an Allen test. The angiogram provides a more definitive picture of the lesion as well as the adequacy of the distal circulation. Angiography should always be performed if surgical intervention is contemplated.

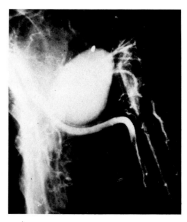

Figure 67–29. A 60-year-old woman presented with a nonunion of her left proximal humerus of one-year duration. A pulsatile mass was noted in the anterior aspect of the shoulder and the angiogram demonstrated a large false aneurysm of the axillary artery. The wall of the aneurysm was found to be compressing the nonunion site. The aneurysm was resected and reconstructed with an interposition saphenous vein graft.

TREATMENT

The treatment of axillary or brachial arterial aneurysms for the most part involves a limited arterial resection and reconstruction with an end-to-end anastomosis or vein graft. The surgical reconstruction should be performed soon after the diagnosis to avoid the potential complications of rupture, rapid expansion, and distal embolization (Fig. 67–29).

Within the hand and wrist, despite reports of success with resection and ligation of the involved artery (Carneiro, 1974), we believe that vascular reconstruction should be considered in most cases (Erskine, 1964; Kleinert et al., 1973). This is especially the case when the distal runoff or collateral circulation is marginal.

True aneurysms may be further subdivided, on the basis of etiology, into idiopathic, traumatic, atherosclerotic, and mycotic. Although reports exist of idiopathic aneurysms, such as that reported by Griffiths in 1897 involving the ulnar artery in a 23 year old female, there quite likely is a traumatic event associated with these. Whereas the traumatic aneurysm in the hand is virtually always located on the palmar side, the less common arteriosclerotic aneurysms tend to be located dorsally and occur in older patients (Malt, 1978; Thorrens et al., 1966). Recog-

nition of this form of aneurysm has important therapeutic implications because the collateral circulation in these circumstances may be insufficient to permit the use of excision and ligation alone as treatment. The even rarer mycotic aneurysm, almost always found in the smaller vessels in the hand, was more commonly seen prior to antibiotics and is associated with a more central focus of sepsis (Goadby et al., 1949; Poirier and Stansel, 1972; Weintraub and Abrams, 1968).

The most common clinical presentation of an aneurysm in the hand is as an enlarging, often painful mass. The mass may not be pulsatile, that characteristic being related to the amount of thrombus within the aneurysm. There may be evidence or a history of a penetrating wound. Although one should routinely auscultate for the presence of a systolic bruit that ceases with proximal obliteration of the parent vessel, this is not commonly present with aneurysms within the hand. That the aneurysm may be firm, warm, and tender to the touch can lead the unwary surgeon into incising it, thinking it to be an abscess (Hueston, 1973). Lastly, the initial presentation may consist solely of signs and symptoms of more distal digital ischemia related to intermittent distal embolization of thrombotic material (May et al., 1982; Sharp and Hansel, 1967).

ARTERIOVENOUS FISTULA

The acquired arteriovenous fistula, a direct communication between an artery and an adjacent vein, is for the most part the result of a penetrating injury to both vessels. In the upper extremity this may occur in association with an iatrogenic event such as a venipuncture or diagnostic studies performed in the antecubital fossa. Its recognition is fundamental because this form of vascular injury may not be associated with the more common signs of arterial injury (Beall et al., 1963; Freeman, 1946; Seeley et al., 1952). An acute arteriovenous fistula can be a subtle finding, for significant bleeding and hematoma formation may not occur. The persistence of a distal pulse and the absence of distal ischemia may also mask the presence of a more proximal arterial injury. On occasion the patient may be aware of a buzzing sound at the location of the fistula, and a murmur is always present, with the exception of low flow states. Branham's sign (slowing of the pulse) may be present with medium sized and larger arteriovenous fistulas.

As with other acute vascular injuries, immediate repair of acute arteriovenous fistulas is indicated. Early repair is technically far easier because permanent degenerative changes in the arterial wall will not have developed (Holman, 1965; Hughes and Jahnke, 1959; Lindenauer et al., 1969; Pate et al., 1965). Treatment consists of resection of the zone of arterial injury and either direct reanastomosis, if this can be accomplished without tension, or the use of an appropriate sized interposition vein graft. In most instances the involved vein can be ligated.

VENOUS INJURY

The importance of a patent venous system for the initial 24 to 72 hours following arterial repair, recognized in studies from the Korean and Vietnam Wars, has become a basic tenet of replantation and revascularization surgery (Chandler and Knapp, 1967; Gaspar and Treiman, 1960; Hughes, 1954; Rich et al., 1970). Hughes (1954) evaluated patients with concomitant arterial and venous injuries who had undergone arterial repair and venous ligation but ultimately required amputation despite the successful arterial repair. Patent arterial anastomoses were noted in the am-

putated specimens, but marked venous congestion was noted and judged to be secondary to venous thrombosis distal to the sites of ligation. This was confirmed by Barcia et al. (1972) in experimental studies in dogs.

One noteworthy isolated venous injury involves effort thrombosis of the axillary and subclavian vein, often called the Paget-Schroetter syndrome (Hughes, 1949). Most likely the result of a direct blow or prolonged exertional activity, it usually affects the dominant arm in young active males. The clinical presentation is a nonpitting edematous painful extremity in which the swelling may extend from the fingertips to the upper arm. Occasionally a palpable cord may be appreciated in the axillary vein. The differential diagnosis includes cellulitis and ascending lymphangitis, and venography is often necessary to establish the diagnosis.

The initial treatment consists of rest, elevation, and systemic anticoagulation therapy with the parenteral administration of heparin followed by the oral administration of Coumadin for eight to 10 weeks (Marks, 1956). Some have recommended venous thrombectomy during the acute phase, and this could be considered in patients in whom venography has demonstrated only a short segment of thrombosed vein (Drapanas and Curran, 1966).

In most cases, following the initiation of treatment, the symptoms abate over a short period of time; however, 70 per cent of the patients left untreated have chronic symptoms of venous insufficiency, including swelling and exertional pain (Tilney et al., 1970). The treatment of chronic symptoms includes elevation, diuretics, and compression with elastic wraps (Fig. 67–30).

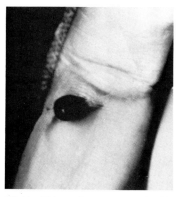

Figure 67–30. This patient presented with a painful mass in her digit. Surgical exploration revealed a thrombosed digital vein that was resected successfully.

ELECTRICAL INJURY

Since electrical injury frequently results from grasping an electrically charged object, the hand is more commonly involved than any other part of the body (Sullivan et al., 1981). Vascular damage often proves to be the most serious aspect of the electrical injury because the blood in the vascular tree offers minimal resistance to the electrical charge, thereby providing an accessible pathway for the current. As a result of the extreme temperature of the high voltage, the vessels themselves may be damaged with progressive intimal and media necrosis and resultant thrombosis (Hunt et al., 1974). As the vessel wall damage progresses, one frequently sees progression of thrombosis extending into the smaller vessels. If both veins and arteries are damaged, potential irreversible gangrene becomes a reality. The continuing vascular thrombosis and resultant ischemia lead to soft tissue loss, which in the hand and forearm creates a severe problem with the exposure of vital neurovascular and tendinous structures.

In addition to the overall emergency care to prevent the potential systemic complications of myoglobinuria and acidosis, emergency forearm and hand fasciotomy may be critical in reducing the ischemia in the extremity (Butler and Gant, 1977). Early fasciotomy not only enhances distal perfusion but also permits a closer inspection of the muscle compartments of the forearm and hand. Aggressive débridement of devitalized tissue may help to offset resultant scar formation, contracture, or stiffness. This is particularly a problem in electrical injuries in which ischemia resulting from progressive small vessel thrombosis leads to poor nutrition of the soft tissues, tendons, and muscles in the upper extremity.

As a result of advances in microvascular surgery and free tissue transfer, some electrical injuries in the hand and upper extremity are amenable to free flap reconstruction to provide wound coverage and to enhance vascularity and at times to restore sensibility (May et al., 1977; Morrison et al., 1978; Ohmori and Hari, 1976). Because of the pathophysiological effects of the electrical current on the vascular system, it is crucial that the surgeon construct anastomoses in uninjured vessels, for unrecognized vascular damage may lead to thrombosis at the anastomotic site. Angiography should be performed to better delineate the zone of vascular trauma and accessible uninjured recipient vessels. In electrical injuries with marginal viability, early revascularization using free flap transfers enhances limb or digit salvage (Fig. 67–31).

THORACIC OUTLET SYNDROME

The term thoracic outlet syndrome describes a disease complex characterized by compression of the neurovascular structures between the intervertebral foramina and the axilla. The clinical presentation may vary depending upon the degree of compression of the axillary contents, but the vascular complications, although infrequent, may be severe.

The vascular presentations in the thoracic outlet syndrome have attracted the interest of surgeons for some time (Coote, 1861; Poland, 1869). Halstead (1909) described a patient who had developed an aneurysm suddenly after resection of a cervical rib. Symonds (1927) clarified the thromboembolic origin of a number of the peripheral vascular symptomatology and this was further described by Lewis and Pickering (1934).

The fundamental arterial lesion involves compression of the second portion of the subclavian artery with resultant poststenotic dilation and associated turbulence with mural thrombus formation and degeneration (Judy and Heymann, 1972; Schein et al., 1956).

With this sort of vascular lesion, distal embolization of an incomplete thrombus is always a threat. The patient may present with signs and symptoms consistent with a unilateral Raynaud's phenomenon, including pain and coolness of the digits, fingertip ulceration, or subungual hemorrhages. There may be a history of recent exercise claudication. On occasion the patient may present with severe distal ischemia secondary to acute occlusion of the brachial artery (Baird and Lajor, 1964).

In the physical examination careful attention must be paid to the arterial pulses and blood pressures, in particular with the shoulder hyperabducted and externally rotated. Auscultation in the supraclavicular fossa may reveal an arterial bruit. Ipsilateral muscle atrophy or coolness to touch may also be found in association with a vascular lesion.

Routine radiographs of the cervical spine and upper chest may reveal a cervical rib, a

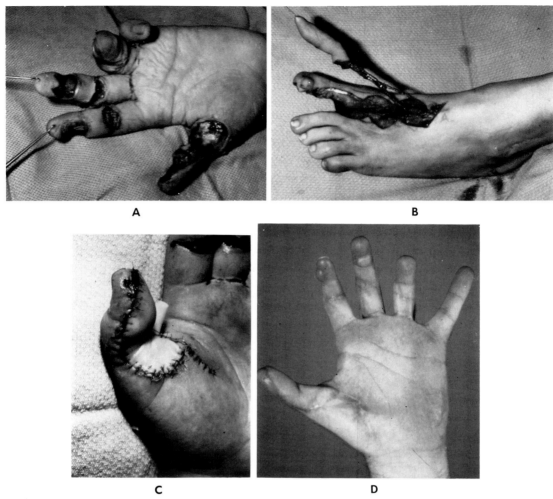

Figure 67–31. An electrical contact burn left this patient's thumb partially degloved and without sensibility on the contact surface *(A)*. Following debridement, a free innervated first web transfer from the foot was utilized to provide durable and sensate skin. The vascular transfer also enhanced the local vascularity, which is crucial in the reconstruction of electrical injuries *(B, C, and D)*.

clavicular exostosis or deformity, or anomalous thoracic ribs. When concern exists regarding a possible vascular lesion, consideration must be given to selective angiography including not only the subclavian and axillary vessels but also the entire arterial system of the arm and hand.

Although the transaxillary route for the surgical approach to thoracic outlet compression, as advocated by Roos (1966), has gained widespread popularity, if a vascular lesion is suspected, we prefer the supraclavicular approach with clavicular osteotomy or resection if additional exposure is required. In addition

to resecting any offending structure, such as a cervical rib or clavicular exostosis, the first rib and anterior scalene muscles are resected or released. The subclavian artery should be inspected, and if thrombosis is present, either an arteriotomy and arterioplasty or resection and reconstruction are warranted. Careful attention must be paid to identifying and preserving collateral vessels, especially if the vascular lesion is not amenable to surgical reconstruction. In addition, cervicodorsal sympathectomy has been recommended to help augment distal flow (Judy and Heymann, 1972).

REPLANTATION

The term replantation must be reserved to describe the restoration of limbs or parts that have been completely severed without any residual attachment, whereas revascularization is more appropriate in describing incompletely amputated parts whose circulation has been so disrupted that immediate vascular repair is necessary for survival of the part.

Because of continued improvements in technique and incidence of survival, success must be measured in terms of the ultimate function of the replanted part. Proper selection of the patient therefore is fundamental. The patient's age, occupation, and hand dominance, the level of the amputation, the condition of the amputated part, and associated injuries are determining factors in the decision to attempt replantation. Extensive degloving, crush, or multiple level injuries of the amputated part are contraindications to replantation. Although the operation is technically more difficult in pediatric patients, the inherent suppleness of their joints and unique regenerative capacity, especially with neural repair, favor greater functional success.

The levels of amputation in the hand may be divided for simplicity into three zones. In zone 1, extending distally beyond the sublimis insertion, replantations in clean guillotine amputations have proved functionally rewarding with little morbidity and good overall reinnervation. Zone 2 injuries, extending from the level of the metacarpophalangeal joint distally to the insertion of the sublimis tendon, are true digital amputations, and consideration of replantation must include the type of injury and the number and location of the digits. In amputations of the thumb, multiple digits, and single digits in children, replantation should be performed, although selectivity may be required with multiple digital amputations. A single digital replantation in an adult, especially of the index or little finger, may prove functionally unrewarding, yet in individuals whose motivation may be esthetic or psychological rather than economic, a single digit replantation may be well accepted.

In zone 3 and more proximal amputations, the indications for replantation widen. In most cases transmetacarpal, transcarpal, and distal forearm replantations should be attempted, whereas increased selectivity is necessary in upper arm and lower limb replantation because these hold a greater potential for more profound complications.

The mechanism of injury and the integrity of the severed part are of fundamental importance to both the technical feasibility of a successful replantation and functional success. A clean-cut amputation has afforded the best prognosis in all series, extending to a 94 per cent survival incidence in the Sixth People's Hospital series. A crush amputation, often the result of blunt trauma, requires more extensive débridement and carries a somewhat less favorable prognosis—87 per cent survival in the same Chinese series. Avulsion injuries have even a more unfavorable outcome because they frequently involve extensive damage to the neurovascular structures along with avulsion of the flexor tendons at their musculotendinous junctions.*

---

*For details on technique of replantation, see Chapters 85 to 89.

REFERENCES

Abbott, W. M., and Darling, R. C.: Axillary artery aneurysms secondary to crutch trauma. Am. J. Surg., 125:515–520, 1973.

Acland, R.: Instrumentation for microsurgery. Orthop. Clin. N. Am., 8:281–294, 1977.

Acland, R.: Personal communication.

Adams, J. T., DeWeese, J. A., Mahoney, E. B., and Rob, C. G.: Intermittent subclavian vein obstruction without thrombosis. Surgery, 63:147–163, 1968.

Adar, R., et al.: Arterial combat injuries of the upper extremity. J. Trauma, 20:297–302, 1980.

Allen, E. V.: Thromboangiitis obliterans: methods of diagnosis of chronic occlusive arterial lesions distal to the wrist with illustrative cases. Am. J. Med. Sci., 178:237–244, 1929.

Amato, J. J., et al.: High velocity arterial injury: a study of the mechanism of injury. J. Trauma, 11:412–416, 1971.

Antal, C. S., Conforty, B., Engleberg, M., and Reiss, R.: Injuries to the axillary artery due to anterior dislocation of the shoulder. J. Trauma, 13:564–566, 1973.

Anthopoulous, L. P., Johnson, J. B., and Spellman, M.: Arteriovenous fistula in multiple saccular arterial aneurysms of a finger following childhood human bite. Angiology, 16:89–92, 1965.

Ashbell, T. S., Kutz, J. E., and Kleinert, H. E.: The digital Allen test. Plast. Reconstr. Surg., 39:311–312, 1967.

Baker, N. W., and Hines, E. A., Jr.: Arterial occlusions in the hands and fingers associated with repeated occupational trauma. Proc. Mayo Clin., 19:345–349, 1944.

Baird, R. J., and Doran, M. L.: The false aneurysm. Can. Med. Assoc. J., 91:281–284, 1964.

Baird, R. J., and Lajor, T. Z.: Emboli to the arm. Ann. Surg., 160:905–909, 1964.

Barcia, P. J., Nelson, T. G., and Whelan, T. J., Jr.: Importance of venous occlusion in arterial repair failure: an experimental study. Ann. Surg., 175:223–227, 1972.

Barnes, R. W., Petersen, J. L., Krugmirer, R. B., and Strandness, D. E.: Complication of brachial artery catheterization. Chest, 66:363–367, 1974.

Baruch, A.: False aneurysm of the digital artery. Hand, 9:195–197, 1977.

Beall, A. C., Jr., Harrington, O. B., Crawford, E. S., and DeBakey, M. E.: Surgical management of traumatic arteriovenous aneurysms. Am. J. Surg., 106:610–618, 1963.

Bedford, R. F., and Wollman, H.: Complications of percutaneous radial artery cannulation. Anesthesiology, 38:228–236, 1973.

Berger, A., et al.: Replantation and revascularization of amputated parts of extremities: a three year report from the Viennese replantation team. Clin. Orthop., 133:212–214, 1978.

Bertelsen, S., Mathiesen, F. R., and Ohlenschlager, H. H.: Vascular complications of cervical rib. Scand. J. Thorac. Cardiovasc. Surg., 2:133–139, 1968.

Bjorkesten, G.: Suture of war injuries to peripheral nerves. Clinical studies of results. Acta Chir. Scand., 95:(Suppl. 119):1, 1947.

Bolasney, B. L., and Killen, D. A.: Surgical management of arterial injury secondary to angiography. Ann. Surg., 174:962–964, 1971.

Bole, P. V., et al.: Civilian arterial injuries. Ann. Surg., 183:13–23, 1976.

Bradley, R. M.: Aneurysms of the palmar arteries. Milit. Surg., 97:486–489, 1945.

Branham, H. D.: Aneurysmal varix of the femoral artery and vein following a gunshot wound. Int. J. Surg., 3:250, 1890.

Brener, B. J., and Couch, N. P.: Peripheral arterial complications of left heart catheterizations and their management. Am. J. Surg., 125:521–526, 1973.

Bright, D. S.: Techniques of microsurgery. A.A.O.S. Symposium on Microsurgery. St. Louis, The C. V. Mosby Company, 1979, ch. 4.

Brooks, A. L., and Fowler, J. B.: Axillary artery thrombosis after prolonged use of crutches. J. Bone Joint Surg., 46A:863–864, 1964.

Broudy, A., Jupiter, J., and May, J. W., Jr.: Management of supracondylar fracture with brachial artery thrombosis in a child. Case report and literature review. J. Trauma, 19:540–543, 1979.

Buchler, U., Phelps, D. B., and Boswick, J.: The influence of experimentally induced anemia on the patency of microvascular anastomoses. J. Hand Surg., 2:29–30, 1977.

Buncke, H. J., Jr., and Schulz, W. P.: Experimental digital amputation and replantation. Plast. Reconstr. Surg., 36:62–70, 1965.

Burnham, P. J.: Acute carpal tunnel syndrome. Arch. Surg., 87:645–646, 1963.

Butler, E. D., and Gant, T. D.: Electrical injuries with special reference to the upper extremities. Am. J. Surg., 134:95–102, 1977.

Butsch, J. L., and James, J. M.: Injuries of the superficial palmar arch. J. Trauma, 3:505–516, 1963.

Calvet, J., Leroy, M., and Lacroix, L.: Luxations de l'épaule et lésions vasculaires. J. Chir., 58:337–348, 1941–1942.

Carneiro, R. O. S.: Aneurysm of the wrist. Plast. Reconstr. Surg., 54:483–489, 1974.

Carrel, A.: Suture of blood vessels and transplantation of organs. Nobel Lecture, 1912. In Nobel Lectures in Physiology-Medicine. New York, American Elsevier Publishers, Inc., 1967, p. 442, Vol. 1.

Cawley, J. J.: Acute traumatic aneurysm of the palm. Am. J. Surg., 74:98–99, 1947.

Chandler, J. G., and Knapp, R. W.: Early definitive treatment of vascular injuries in the Vietnam conflict. J.A.M.A., 202:960–966, 1967.

Cheek, R. C., et al.: Diagnosis and management of major vascular injuries. A review of 200 operative cases. Am. Surg., 41:755–760, 1975.

Ch'en, C. W.: Personal communication.

Coleman, S. S., and Anson, B. J.: Arterial patterns in the hand based upon a study of 650 specimens. Surg. Gynecol. Obstet., 113:409–424, 1961.

Conn, J., Jr., Berigan, J. J., and Bell, L.: Hypothenar hammer syndrome. Surgery, 68:1122–1127, 1970.

Connolly, J.: Management of fractures associated with arterial injuries. Am. J. Surg., 120:331, 1970.

Connolly, J., Williams, E., and Whittaker, D.: The influence of fracture stabilization on the outcome of arterial repair in combined fracture-arterial injuries. Surg. Forum, 20:450–452, 1969.

Coote, H.: Pressure on the axillary vessels and nerve by an exostosis from a cervical rib. Interference with the circulation of the arm. Removal of the rib. Recovery. Med. Times Gaz., 2:108, 1861.

Costigan, D. G., Riley, J. M., Jr., and Coy, F. E., Jr.: Thrombofibrosis of the ulnar artery in the palm. J. Bone Joint Surg., 41A:702–704, 1959.

Daniel, D. D.: The acutely swollen hand in the drug user. Arch. Surg., 107:548–551, 1973.

Davis, C. B., and Fell, E. H.: Traumatic aneurysm as a complication of supracondylar fracture of the humerus. Arch. Surg., 62:358–364, 1951.

DeAbrew, L. B., and Godoymoreira, R.: Thrombosis of median artery. J. Bone Joint Surg., 40A:1426–1427, 1958.

DeBakey, M. E., and Simeone, F. A.: Battle injuries of the arteries in WW II.: an analysis of 2471 cases. Ann. Surg., 123:534–539, 1946.

Dellon, A. L., Curtis, R. M., and Chen, C.: Prevention of femoral vein occlusion by local injection of Thrombolysin in the rat. J. Hand Surg., 4:121–128, 1979.

Denman, E. E.: The anatomy of the space of Guyon. Hand, 10:69–76, 1978.

Downs, J. B., et al.: Hazards of radial artery catheterization. Anesthesiology, 38:283–286, 1973.

Drapanas, T., and Curran, W. L.: Thrombectomy in the treatment of "effort" thrombosis of the axillary and subclavian veins. J. Trauma, 6:107–119, 1966.

Drapanas, T., Hewitt, R. L., Weickert, R. F., and Smith, A.: Civilian vascular injuries. Ann Surg., 172:351, 1970.

Edwards, E. A.: Organization of the small arteries of the hand and digits. Am. J. Surg., 99:837–846, 1960.

Eiken, O., Nabseth, D. C., Mayer, R. F., and Deterling, R. A.: Limb replantation. I. The technique and immediate results. II. The pathophysiological effects. III. Longterm evaluation. Arch. Surg., 88:48, 54, 66, 1964.

Enge, I., Aakhus, T., and Evensen, A.: Angiography in vascular injuries of the extremities. Acta Radiol. (Diagn.), 16:193–199, 1975.

Englemen, R. M., Clements, J. M., and Herrman, J. B.: Stab wounds and traumatic false aneurysms in the extremities. J. Trauma, 9:77–87, 1969.

Engler, H. S., Freeman, R. A., Kanavage, C. B., et al.: Production of gangrenous extremities by intra-arterial injection. Am. Surg., *30*:602–607, 1964.

Equoro, H., and Goldner, J. C.: Bilateral thrombosis of the ulnar arteries in the hands. Case report. Plast. Reconstr. Surg., *52*:573–578, 1973.

Erskine, J. M.: Case report: a true traumatic aneurysm of the radial artery at the wrist treated by resection and arterial repair. J. Trauma, *4*:530–534, 1964.

Falor, W. H., Hansel, J. R., and Williams, G. B.: Gangrene of the hand: a complication of radial artery cannulation. J. Trauma, *16*:713–716, 1976.

Field, J. R., and McBurney, R. F.: Complications of 1000 brachial arteriograms. J. Neurosurg., *36*:374–379, 1972.

Flatt, A. E.: Digital artery sympathectomy. J. Hand Surg., *5*:550–556, 1980.

Fowler, I. C., and Workman, C. E.: Aneurysms of the ulnar artery due to blunt trauma of the hand. Mo. Med., *61*:927–929, 1964.

Freeman, N. E.: Arterial repair in the treatment of aneurysms and arteriovenous fistulae. A report of eighteen successful restorations. Ann. Surg., *124*:888–919, 1946.

Gagnon, R.: Superficial arteries of the cubital fossa with reference to accidental intra-arterial injections. Can. J. Surg., *9*:57–65, 1966.

Gaspar, M. R., and Hare, R. R.: Gangrene due to intra-arterial injections of drugs by drug addicts. Surgery, *72*:573–577, 1972.

Gaspar, M. R., and Treiman, R. L.: The management of injuries of major veins. Am. J. Surg., *100*:171–175, 1960.

Gelberman, R., Blasingame, J. P., Fronek, A. and Dimick, M.: Forearm arterial injuries. J. Hand Surg., *4*:401–408, 1979.

Gelberman, R. H., et al.: The results of radial and ulnar arterial repair in the forearm. J. Bone Joint Surg., *64A*:383–387, 1982.

Gerlock, A. J., Mathis, J., Goncharenko, V., and Maravilla, A.: Angiography of intimal and intramural arterial injuries. Radiology, *129*:357–361, 1978.

Given, K. G., Puckett, C. L., and Kleinert, H. E.: Ulnar artery thrombosis. Plast. Reconstr. Surg., *61*:405–411, 1978.

Goadby, H. K., McSwiney, R. R., and Rob, C. G.: Mycotic aneurysm. St. Thomas Hosp. Rep., *5*:44–52, 1949.

Goren, M. L.: Palmar intramural thrombosis in the ulnar artery. Calif. Med., *89*:424–427, 1958.

Goyanes, D. J.: Substitution plastica de las arterias por las venas, o arterioplastia venosa, aplicada, como nuevo metodo, al tratamiento de los aneurisimas. El Siglo Medico, 345, 561, 1906.

Green, D. P.: True and false aneurysms in the hand. J. Bone Joint Surg., *55A*:120–128, 1973.

Griffiths, D. L.: The management of acute circulatory failure in an injured limb. J. Bone Joint Surg., *30B*:280–289, 1948.

Griffiths, J. A.: A case of spontaneous aneurysm of the ulnar artery in the palm. Excision of the artery. Recovery Br. Med. J., *2*:646–647, 1897.

Guattani, C.: De externis aneurysmatibus manu chirurgica methodice pertractandis. Rome, 1772. (Translated by J. E. Erichsen. London, Sydenham Society, 1844, p. 268.)

Gunning, A., Pickering, G., Robb-Smith, A., and Rus-

sell, R.: Mural thrombosis associated with cervical ribs and surgical consideration. Surgery, *40*:428–443, 1956.

Guyon, F.: Note sur le disposition anatomique propre à la face antérieure de la région du poignet et non encore d'ecovte. Bull. Soc. Anat. Paris, *6*:184–186, 1861.

Hardy, J. D., Raju, S., Neeley, W. A., and Berry, D. W.: Aortic and other arterial injuries. Ann. Surg., *181*:640–651, 1975.

Harmon, J. W.: A histological study of skeletal muscle in acute ischemia. Am. J. Pathol., *23*:551–565, 1948.

Harris, J. D.: A case of arteriovenous fistula following closed fracture of tibia and fibula. Br. J. Surg., *50*:774–776, 1963.

Harvey, S. C.: The History of Hemostasis. New York, Paul B. Hoeber, 1929.

Henson, G. F.: Vascular complications of shoulder injuries. J. Bone Joint Surg., *38B*:528–531, 1956.

Hentz, V., Jackson, I., and Fogarty, D.: Case report: false aneurysm of the hand secondary to digital amputation. J. Hand Surg., *3*:199–200, 1978.

Holman, E.: Abnormal arteriovenous communications. Great variability of effects with particular reference to delayed development of cardiac failure. Circulation, *32*:1001–1009, 1965.

Hueston, J. T.: Traumatic aneurysm of the digital artery. A complication of fasciectomy. Hand, *5*:332–334, 1973.

Hughes, C. W.: Acute vascular trauma in Korean War casualties: an analysis of 180 cases. Surg. Gynecol. Obstet., *99*:91–100, 1954.

Hughes, C. W.: Arterial repair during Korean War. Ann. Surg., *147*:555–561, 1958.

Hughes, C. W., and Jahnke, E. J., Jr.: The surgery of traumatic arteriovenous fistulas and aneurysms. A five year follow-up of 215 lesions. Ann. Surg., *148*:790–797, 1959.

Hughes, E. S. F.: Venous obstruction in the upper extremity (Paget-Schroetter syndrome); a review of 320 cases. Surg. Gynecol. Obstet. Int. Abst. Surg., *88*:89, 1949.

Hunt, J. L., et al.: Vascular lesions in acute electrical injuries. J. Trauma, *14*:461–473, 1974.

Hunter, D., McLaughlin, A., and Petty, K. M. A.: Clinical effects of the use of pneumatic tools. Br. J. Industr. Med., *2*:10–16, 1945.

Inahara, T.: Arterial injuries of the upper extremity. Surgery, *51*:605–610, 1962.

Jackson, J. P.: Posttraumatic thrombosis of the ulnar artery in the palm. J. Bone Joint Surg., *36B*:438–439, 1954.

Jacobsen, J. H., II, and Suarez, E. L.: Microsurgery in anastomosis of small vessels. Surg. Forum, *11*:243–245, 1960.

Jahnke, E. L., Jr.: Late structural and functional results of arterial injuries primarily repaired. Surgery, *43*:175–183, 1958.

Jaschtschinski, S. N.: Morphologie und topographie des arcus volaris sublimis und profundus. Anat. Hefte, *7*:163–188, 1897.

Johnston, G. W., and Lowry, J. H.: Rupture of the axillary artery complicating anterior dislocation of the shoulder. J. Bone Joint Surg., *44B*:116–118, 1962.

Judy, K. L., and Heymann, R. L.: Vascular complications of thoracic outlet syndrome. Am. J. Surg., *123*:521–531, 1972.

Katz, A. M., Birnbaum, M., and Maylass, J.: Gangrene

of the hand and forearm: a complication of radial artery cannulation. Crit. Care Med., 2:370–372, 1974.

Kaufer, H., Spengler, D. M., Noyes, F. R., and Louis, D. S.: Orthopedic implications of the drug subculture. J. Trauma, 14:855–867, 1974.

Keen, J. A.: A study of the arterial variations in the limbs with special reference to symmetry of vascular patterns. Am. J. Anat., 108:245–261, 1961.

Kelley, G., and Eiseman, B.: Civilian vascular injuries. J. Trauma, 15:507–514, 1975.

Kelley, G. L., and Eiseman, B.: Management of small arterial injuries: clinical and experimental studies. J. Trauma, 16:681–685, 1976.

Kerin, R.: Elbow dislocation and its association with vascular disruption. J. Bone Joint Surg., 51A:756–758, 1969.

Kleinert, H. E., et al.: Aneurysms of the hand. Arch. Surg., 106:554–557, 1973.

Kleinert, H. E., and Kasdan, M. L.: Restoration of blood flow in upper extremity injuries. J. Trauma, 3:461–474, 1963.

Kleinert, H. E., and Kasdan, M. L.: Salvage of devascularized upper extremities including studies on small vessel anastomosis. Clin. Orthop., 29:29–38, 1963.

Kleinert, H. E., Kasdan, M. L., and Romero, J. L.: Small blood vessel anastomosis for salvage of severely injured upper extremity. J. Bone Joint Surg., 45A:788–796, 1963.

Kleinert, H. E., Kutz, J. E., and Cohen, M. J.: Primary repair of zone 2 flexor tendon lacerations. A.A.O. Symposium on Tendon Surgery in the Hand. St. Louis, The C. V. Mosby Company, 1975, pp. 91–103.

Kleinert, H. E., and Volianitis, G. J.: Thrombosis of palmar arterial arch and its tributaries, etiologies, and newer concepts in treatment. J. Trauma, 5:446–457, 1965.

Koman, L. A., and Urbaniak, J. R.: Ulnar artery insufficiency: a guide to treatment. J. Hand Surg., 6:16–24, 1981.

Komatsu, S., and Tamai, S.: Successful replantation of a completely cut off thumb. Plast. Reconstr. Surg., 42:1374–1377, 1968.

Lambert, J.: Extract of a letter from Mr. Lambert, surgeon at New Castle-Upon-Tyne to Dr. Hinger: giving an account of new method of treating an aneurysm. Med. Observ. Ing. (Lond.), 30:360, 1762.

Laurence, R. R., and Wilson, J. N.: Ulnar artery thrombosis in the palm. Case reports. Plast. Reconstr. Surg., 36:604–608, 1965.

Layman, C. D., Ogden, L. L., and Lister, G. D., True aneurysm of digital artery. J. Hand Surg., 7:617–618, 1982.

Leriche, R., Fontaine, R., and Dupertin, S. M.: Arterectomy with follow-up studies on 78 operations. Surg. Gynecol. Obstet., 64:149–155, 1937.

Levy, M., and Parker, M.: Carpal tunnel syndrome due to thrombosed persisting median artery. A case report. Hand. 10:65–68, 1978.

Lewis, T., and Pickering, G. W.: Observations upon maladies in which the blood supply to the digits ceases intermittently or permanently and upon bilateral gangrene of the digits: observations relevant to so-called Raynaud's disease. Clin. Sci., 1:327, 1934.

Lexer, E.: Die ideale operation des arteriellen und des arterielluenosen aneurysma. Arch. Klin. Chir., 83:459, 1907.

Lindenauer, S. M., Thompson, N. W., Kraft, R. O., and Fry, W. J.: Late complications of traumatic arteriovenous fistulas. Surg. Gynecol. Obstet., 129:525–532, 1969.

Linton, R.: Atlas of Vascular Surgery. Philadelphia, W. B. Saunders Company, 1973, p. 433.

Lipscomb, P. R., and Burleson, R. J.: Vascular and neural complications in the supracondylar fractures of the humerus in children. J. Bone Joint Surg., 37A:487, 1955.

Little, D. M., and Ferguson, D. A.: The incidence of hypothenar hammer syndrome. Arch. Surg., 105:684–685, 1972.

Louis, D., Ricciardi, J. E., and Spengler, D. M.: Arterial injury: a complication of posterior elbow dislocations. A clinical and anatomical study. J. Bone Joint Surg., 56A:1631–1636, 1974.

Louis, O., and Simon, M. A.: Traumatic false aneurysms of the upper extremity. J. Bone Joint Surg., 56A:176–179, 1974.

Lowrey, C. W., Chadwick, R. O., and Waltman, E. N.: Digital vessel trauma from repetitive impact in baseball catchers. J. Hand Surg., 1:236–238, 1976.

MacDonald, G. L., Jr., Tose, L., and Deterling, R. H., Jr.: A technique for reimplantation of the dog limb involving the use of a mechanical stapling device and a rapid polymerizing adhesive. Surg. Forum, 13:88, 1962.

Makins, G. W.: Gunshot Injuries to the Blood Vessels. Bristol, John Wright and Sons, Ltd., 1919.

Malloch, J. D.: Palmar-arch thrombosis. Br. Med. J., 2:28, 1962.

Malt, R. A., and McKhann, C. F.: Replantation of severed arms. J.A.M.A., 189:716–722, 1964.

Malt, S.: An arteriosclerotic aneurysm of the hand. Arch. Surg., 113:762–763, 1978.

Mandel, M., and Dauchot, P. J.: Radial artery cannulation in 1000 patients: Precautions and complications. J. Hand Surg., 2:482–485, 1977.

Marks, J.: Anticoagulation therapy in idiopathic occlusion of the axillary vein. Br. Med. J., 1:11–13, 1956.

Martin, A. F.: Ulnar artery thrombosis in the palm. Clin. Orthop., 17:373–376, 1960.

Matas, R.: Traumatic aneurysm of the left brachial artery. Incision and partial excision of sac; recovery. Phila. Med. News, 53:462, 1888.

Mathieu, A., et al.: Expanding aneurysm of the radial artery after frequent puncture. Anesthesiology, 38:401–403, 1973.

May, J. W., Jr., et al.: Free neurovascular flap from the 1st web of foot in hand reconstruction. J. Hand Surg., 2:387–1977.

Maudaire: Anéurisme de l'artere cubitale dans sa portion carpometacarpienne. Bull. Soc. Anat. Paris, 72:208–209, 1897.

Maxwell, T. M., Olcott, C., and Blaisdell, F. W.: Vascular complications of drug abuse. Arch. Surg., 105:875–882, 1972.

May, J. W., Jr., et al.: The no-reflow phenomenon in experimental free flaps. Plast. Reconstr. Surg., 61:256, 1978.

May, J. W., Jr., and Gallico, G. G.: Upper extremity replantation. In Current Problems in Surgery. Chicago, Year Book Medical Publishers, 1980.

May, J. W., Jr., Grossman, J. A., and Costas, B.: Cyanotic painful index and long fingers associated with an asymptomatic ulnar artery aneurysm. Case report. J. Hand Surg., 7:622–625, 1982.

Mays, T. C.: Traumatic aneurysm of the hand. Am. Surg., 36:552–557, 1970.

McCormack, L. J., Cauldwell, E. W., and Anson, B. J.: Brachial and antebrachial arterial patterns. Surg. Gynecol. Obstet., 96:43–54, 1953.

McDonald, E. J., Goodman, P. C., and Winestock, D. P.: Clinical indications for arteriography in trauma to the extremity. Radiology, 166:45–47, 1975.

McLesky, C. H., and Stehling, L.: Complications of radial artery cannulation. Orthop. Rev., 11:105–107, 1982.

McNamara, J. J., et al.: Management of fractures with associated arterial injury in combat casualties. J. Trauma, 13:17–19, 1973.

Mehl, R. L., Paul, H. A., Scheewind, J., and Beattie, E. J.: Treatment of "toxemia" after extremity replantations. Arch. Surg., 89:871–879, 1964.

Middleton, D. S.: Occupational aneurysm of the palmar arteries. Br. J. Surg., 21:215–218, 1933.

Mignard, J. P., et al.: Emergency treatment of traumatic lesions of the digital arteries of the limbs. Ann. Chir. Thorac. Cardiovasc., 30:245–248, 1976.

Millender, L., Nalebuff, E., and Kasden, E.: Aneurysms and thrombosis of ulnar artery in the hand. Arch. Surg., 105:686–690, 1972.

Milling, M. A. P., and Kinmoth, M. H.: False aneurysm of the ulnar artery. Hand, 9:57–59, 1977.

Morrison, W. A., O'Brien, B., and Hamilton, R. B.: Neurovascular free foot flaps in reconstruction of the mutilated hand. Clin. Plast. Surg., 5:265–272, 1978.

Muramaki, T., Takaya, K., and Outi, H.: The origin, course and distribution of the arteries to the thumb, with special reference to the so-called princeps pollicis. Okajimas Folia Anat. Jap. 46:123–127, 1969.

Murphy, J. B.: Resection of arteries and veins injured in continuity, end-to-end suture. (Exp. Clin. Res.) Med. Res., 51:73, 1897.

Myerding, H. W.: Volkmann's ischemic contracture associated with supracondylar fracture of the humerus. J.A.M.A., 106:1139–1144, 1936.

Narsete, E. G. Traumatic aneurysm of the radial artery. Am. J. Surg., 108:424–427, 1964.

Ohmori, K., and Hari, K.: Free dorsalis pedis sensory flap to the hand with microvascular anastomosis. Plast. Reconstr. Surg., 58:546–554, 1976.

Orhewere, F. A.: Post-traumatic aneurysm of the radial artery at the wrist. Br. Med. J., 2:1501–1502, 1966.

Ortner, A. B., Berg, H. F., and Lebendigen, A.: Limb salvage through small vessel surgery. Arch. Surg., 83:414–419, 1961.

Paaby, H., and Stadil, F.: Thrombosis of the ulnar artery. Acta Orthop. Scand., 39:336–345, 1968.

Parks, B. J., Arbelaez, J., and Horner, R. L.: Medical and surgical importance of the arterial blood supply of the thumb. J. Hand Surg., 3:383–385, 1978.

Pate, J. W., et al.: Cardiac failure following traumatic arteriovenous fistula: a report of 14 cases. J. Trauma, 5:398–403, 1965.

Patman, O. R., Poulos, E., and Shires, G. T.: The management of civilian arterial injuries. Surg. Gynecol. Obstet., 118:725–738, 1964.

Pecket, P., Gloobe, H., and Nathan, H.: Variations in the arteries of the median nerve with special considerations on the ischemic factor in the carpal tunnel syndrome. Clin. Orthop., 97:144–147, 1973.

Perry, M. O., Thal, E. R., and Shires, G. T.: Management of arterial injuries. Ann. Surg., 173:403–408, 1971.

Peters, F. M.: A disease resulting from the use of pneumatic tools. Occup. Med., 2:55–66, 1946.

Petrie, P. W. R., and Lamb, D. W.: Severe hand problems in drug addicts following self-administered injections. Hand, 5:130–134, 1973.

Platt, H.: Occlusion of the axillary artery due to pressure by a crutch. Report of 2 cases. Arch Surg., 20:314–316, 1930.

Poirier, R. A., and Stansel, H. C., Jr.: Arterial aneurysms of the hand. Am. J. Surg., 124:72–74, 1972.

Poland, A.: On a case of fusiform and tubular aneurysm of the subclavian artery and its successful treatment by indirect digital compression. Medico-Chi-Trans., 52:288, 1869.

Postempski, P.: La sutura dei vasi sanguigni. Arch. Soc. Ital. Chir. Roma, 3:391, 1886.

Raines, J. K., Jeffrin, M. Y., and Rao, S.: A noninvasive pressure pulse recorder development and rationale. Med. Instrum., 7:245, 1973.

Reynolds, R. R., McDowell, H. A., and Diethelm, A. G.: The surgical treatment of arterial injuries in the civilian population. Ann. Surg., 189:700–708, 1979.

Rhodes, G. R., Cox, C. B., and Silver, D.: Arteriovenous fistula and false aneurysm as the cause of consumption coagulopathy. Surgery, 73:535–540, 1973.

Rich, N. M., Baugh, J. H., and Hughes, C. W.: Acute arterial injuries in Vietnam: 1,000 cases. J. Trauma, 10:359–369, 1970.

Rich, N. M., Hughes, C. W., and Baugh, J. H.: Management of venous injuries. Ann. Surg., 171:724–730, 1970.

Rich, N. M., et al.: Internal vs. external fixation of fractures with concomitant vascular injuries in Vietnam. J. Trauma, 11:463–473, 1971.

Rich, N. M., and Spencer, F. C. (Editors): Vascular Trauma. Philadelphia, W. B. Saunders Company, 1978, p. 372.

Robb, C. G., and Standeven, A.: Closed traumatic lesions of the axillary and brachial arteries. Lancet, 1:597–599, 1956.

Robb, C. G., and Standeven, A.: Arterial occlusion complicating thoracic outlet compression syndrome. Br. Med. J., 2:709–712, 1958.

Robb, D., McKechnie, W. R., and Guthrie, D. W.: Peripheral aneurysms of traumatic origin. Cases occurring in brachial, radial, and ulnar arteries. Aust. N.Z. J. Surg., 12:147–148, 1942.

Roos, D. B.: Transaxillary approach for first rib resection to relieve thoracic outlet syndrome. Ann. Surg., 163:354–358, 1966.

Saaman, H. A.: The hazards of radial artery pressure monitoring. J. Cardiovasc. Surg., 12:342–347, 1971.

Sachatello, C. R., Ernst, C. B., and Griffen, W. O., Jr.: The acute ischemic upper extremity. Selected management. Surgery, 76:1002–1009, 1974.

Sako, Y., and Varco, R. L.: Arteriovenous fistula: results of management of congenital and acquired forms, blood flow measurements and observations on proximal arterial degeneration. Surgery, 67:40–61, 1970.

Sanchez, A., Archer, S., Levine, N. S., and Buchanan, R. T.: Traumatic aneurysm of a common digital artery—a case report. J. Hand Surg., 7:619–621, 1982.

Schanzer, H., Gribetz, I., and Jacobsen, J. H., II: Accidental intra-arterial injection of penicillin G. J.A.M.A., 242:1289–1290, 1979.

Schein, C. J., Haimovici, H., and Young, H.: Arterial thrombosis associated with cervical ribs and surgical considerations. Surgery, 40:428–443, 1956.

Schwartz, A. M.: The historical developments of methods of hemostasis. Surgery, 44:604–610, 1958.

Scott, M. L., and Ochsner, J. L.: Thrombosis of the

brachial artery following cardiac catheterization. Etiology and treatment. South. Med. J., *65:*1095–1948.

Scully, R. E., Shannon, J. M., and Dickerson, G. R.: Factors involved in recovery from experimental skeletal muscle ischemia produced in dogs. Am. J. Pathol., *39:*721–737, 1961.

Seddon, H. J.: Surgical Disorders of the Peripheral Nerves. Edinburgh, Churchill-Livingstone, 1972.

Seeley, S. F., Hughes, C. W., Cook, F. N., and Elkin, D. C.: Traumatic arteriovenous fistulas and aneurysms in war wounded. Am. J. Surg., *83:*471–479, 1952.

Sharp, W. V., and Hansel, J. R.: Aneurysm of the brachial artery: case report of an unusual pathogenesis. Ohio State Med. J., *63:*1177–1178, 1967.

Shaw, R. S.: Reconstructive arterial surgery in upper extremity injuries. J. Bone Joint Surg., *41A:*665–673, 1959.

Shumaker, H. B., Jr., and Carter, K. L.: Arteriovenous fistulas and false aneurysm in military personnel. Surgery, *20:*9, 1946.

Shumaker, H. G., Boone, R., and Kunbler, A.: Studies of combined vascular and neurological injuries. Arch. Surg., *67:*755, 1953.

Sixth People's Hospital, Shanghai: Reattachment of traumatic amputations: a summing up of experience. Chin. Med. J., *1:*392–401, 1967.

Smith, F., et al.: Acute penetrating arterial injuries of the neck and limbs. Arch. Surg., *109:*198–205, 1974.

Smith, L. L., Foran, R., and Gaspar, M. R.: Acute arterial injuries of the upper extremity. Am. J. Surg., *106:*144–151, 1963.

Smith, J. W.: True aneurysm of traumatic origin in the palm. Am. J. Surg., *104:*7–13, 1962.

Spittel, J. A., Jr.: Aneurysms of the hand and wrist. Med. Clin. N. Am., *42:*1007–1010, 1958.

Stein, R. E., Bono, J., Korn, J., and Wolff, W. I.: Axillary artery injury in a closed fracture of the neck of the scapula. A case report. J. Trauma, *11:*528–531, 1971.

Sterling, A. P., and Haberman, E. T.: Traumatic aneurysms of the radial artery. Hand, *7:*294–296, 1975.

Strandness, D. E., Jr. (Editor): Collateral Circulation in Clinical Surgery. Philadelphia, W. B. Saunders Company, 1969.

Suzuki, K., Takahashi, S., and Nakagawa, T.: False aneurysm in a digital artery. J. Hand Surg., *5:*402–403, 1980.

Symonds, C. P.: Two cases of thrombosis of subclavian artery with chondrolateral hemiplegia of sudden onset, probably embolic. Brain, *50:*259, 1927.

Teisinger, J.: Vascular disease disorders resulting from vibratory tools. J. Occup. Med., *14:*129–133, 1972.

Telford, E. D., McCann, M. B., and MacCorma, D. H.: "Dead hand" in users of vibrating tools. Lancet, *2:*359–360, 1945.

Theodorides, T., and DeKeizer, G.: Injuries of the axillary artery caused by fractures of the neck of the humerus. Injury, *8:*120–123, 1976.

Thorrens, S., Trippel, D. H., and Bergan, J. J.: Arteriosclerotic aneurysms of the hand. Arch. Surg., *92:*937–939, 1966.

Tiedman, F.: Manual of Angiology. (Translated by Robert Knox.) Edinburgh, Maclachlan and Stewart, 1831.

Tilney, N. L., Griffiths, H. J., and Edwards, E. A.: Natural history of major venous thrombosis of the upper extremity. Arch. Surg., *101:*792–796, 1970.

Tse, D. H., Slabaugh, P. B., and Carlson, P. A.: Injury to the axillary artery by a closed fracture of the clavicle. J. Bone Joint Surg., *62A:*1372–1373, 1980.

Tupper, J.: Personal communication.

Tuzzeo, S., Saad, S. A., Hastings, D. M., and Swan, K. G.: Management of brachial artery injuries. Surg. Gynecol. Obstet., *146:*21–24, 1978.

Volkmann, J.: Über traumatische arterielle aneurysme der hohl Handbogen. Dtsch. Z. Chir., *227:*151, 1930.

Von Rosen, S.: Ein fall von thrombose in der arteria ulnaris nach ein wirkung von stumpfer gewalt. Acta Chir. Scand., *73:*500–506, 1934.

Weathersby, H. T.: The artery of the index finger. Anat. Rec., *122:*57, 1955.

Weile, F., and Fjeldborg, O.: Lesions of the axillary artery associated with dislocation of the shoulder. Acta. Chir. Scand., *137:*279–281, 1971.

Weintraub, R. A., and Abrams, H. L.: Mycotic aneurysms. Am. J. Roentgenol. *102:*354–362, 1968.

Whitesides, T. E., Haney, T. C., Morimoto, K., and Harada, H.: Tissue pressure measurements as a determinant for the need of fasciotomy. Clin. Orthop., *113:*43–51, 1975.

Wholey, M. H., and Bocher, J.: Angiographic features of aortic and peripheral arterial trauma. Arch. Surg., *97:*68–74, 1968.

Wilgis, E. F. S. Special diagnostic studies. *In* Omer, G., and Spinner, M. (Editors): Management of Peripheral Nerve Problems, Philadelphia, W. B. Saunders Company, 1980, Ch. 5.

Wright, C. B., Geelhoed, G. W., and Hobson, R. E.: Acute vascular insufficiency due to drugs of abuse. *In* Rutherford, R. B. (Editor): Vascular Surgery. Philadelphia, W. B. Saunders Company, 1977.

Zweig, J., Lie, K. K., Posch, J. L., and Larsen, R. D.: Thrombosis of the ulnar artery following blunt trauma to the hand. J. Bone Joint Surg., *51A:*1191–1198, 1969.

Part Four

SPECIAL INJURIES

Section 1

BURNS

INTRODUCTION

Raoul Tubiana

Burns of the hand are a special entity because of their multiple clinical aspects and their gravity from an esthetic and functional standpoint. The vital prognosis is in question when burns affect more than 20 per cent of the body surface area. Although there has been great progress in general treatment, for patients with 70 to 80 per cent of their surface area burned may now be saved, local treatment has not advanced in the same way. During my career I have seen suggested, then rejected, then rediscovered a whole range of local treatment techniques: baths, exposure to air, antiseptic dressings, surgical or chemical débridement, sealed plastic bags allowing movement such as the "Banyan bags" used in the British army during the Second World War, etc. The controversy between early excision grafting and late grafting still continues.

In my opinion, the only real progress in local treatment of burns of the hand since the last world war involves the following:

1. Protective positioning of the joints of the hand, applied very early to burnt hands, the wrist in extension, the metacarpophalangeal joint flexed and the interphalangeal joints in extension.

2. The need to cover unhealed burnt areas by skin grafts before the twenty-first day.

3. Rehabilitation together with the wearing of compressive splints to avoid abnormal positions and retraction. Such physical therapy must be started early and continued long after healing.

4. Finally, the early use of skin flaps with good blood supply to protect threatened joints as well as neurovascular bundles. Such flaps may sometimes be taken in the region, particularly the new generation of forearm flaps: the radial artery flap, the ulnar artery flap, the posterior interosseous artery flap, the dorsoulnar artery flap, etc. Free skin flaps may also be used early, e.g., after an electrical burn of the wrist.

In this section, an international group of surgeons, each with extensive experience, will describe the different aspects of these burns. My thanks are due to Dr. J. Grossman for his help in bringing these contributions together.

Chapter 68

THERMAL AND CHEMICAL BURNS

SERGE BAUX

Hand burns can be the result of thermal, electrical, chemical, or radiation injury.

THERMAL BURNS

Thermal burns are by far the commonest and account for 89 per cent of all burn injuries, according to Kenesi (1965). They occur in a number of ways:

1. Contact with a heated body, resulting in deep but localized lesions. Included in this group are lesions caused by hot presses in which thermal and crush injuries are combined with disastrous effects.

2. Contact with a liquid (e.g., water, milk), when the severity of the lesions is proportional to the temperature of the liquid and its viscosity.

3. Explosions that result in injuries to the dorsum of the hands and often the face.

4. More frequently still, the direct effect of flames from burning solids or liquids (usually gasoline).

The circumstances of the injury vary, burns at work and in the house occurring in about equal numbers. The majority of the former affect men and the majority of the latter, women. A small percentage are due to traffic accidents in which a vehicle catches fire.

The countless varieties of hand burns differ in terms of three factors—the depth of the burn, its location, and the presence of burns elsewhere on the body.

DEPTH OF THE BURN

Defining the depth of a burn implies making a pathological diagnosis, prejudging the clinical course, and deciding about the treatment. Such a definition is therefore an essential step. To avoid confusion, let us review some basic concepts (Fig. 68–1):

1. A first degree (superficial) burn involves only the horny layer of the skin; it heals with only slight desquamation.

2. In a second degree (dermal) burn the basal layer is spared. Since the main function of this layer is to form the epidermis, one can expect these lesions, if superficial, to heal rapidly by epidermalization in situ whatever the treatment and often in spite of it. Deep dermal burns have consequences similar to those of full thickness injuries.

3. A third degree burn destroys both epidermis and dermis. Spontaneous healing can occur, therefore, only from the edges, i.e., by epithelialization and contraction. This process is obviously unacceptable in the hand (unless the affected area is minute) because of the inevitable functional sequelae.

There remain the more extreme burns defined by Dupuytren as fourth degree (subcutaneous), fifth degree (aponeurotic), and sixth degree (osseous burn); these are now usually collectively referred to as carbonization.

One must distinguish between burns that only expose the tendons and those that result in their partial or total destruction. An accurate diagnosis is important, since early grafting will save the tendons in the first case while they are doomed in the second. The distinction must be made early because prolonged exposure leads to necrosis of the tendons regardless of whether they have been damaged by the burn.

In clinical practice the temptation is to evaluate the anatomical lesion on the basis of the appearance alone; i.e., erythema means first degree, blisters second degree,

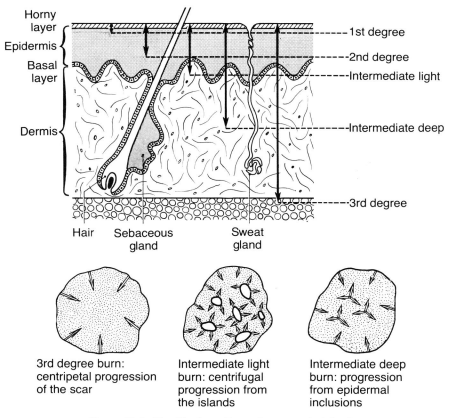

Figure 68–1. Classification of burns by anatomical depth.

and eschar third degree. This approximation may be convenient but is unsatisfactory in practice. Paradoxically the more burns one sees, the less one is prepared to judge from a first visual impression.

Admittedly some lesions are easier to evaluate on the basis of their etiology and appearance, but in many others an early error of diagnosis is possible, which may have repercussions on the whole clinical course and treatment of the burn.

There is also the problem of damage "beyond the skin" that is not necessarily visible and can progress. This damage includes edema, contraction, and connective tissue fibrosis. Their presence invariably influences the functional future of the hand, especially if secondary infection sets in.

Skin thickness varies in different parts of the hand. In this respect there are three distinct zones or regions (Fig. 68–2):

In the palmar region the skin is thick and heavily keratinized, especially in manual workers. There is an abundance of sebaceous glands, which form well protected recesses

that can be the starting points for epithelialization in intermediate burns. There is in addition a thick lining of dense fatty tissue. The tendons and neurovascular bundles are protected by their depth in the palm and to a lesser extent in the fingers.

In the dorsal metacarpal region the skin is thin but hairy and therefore has a regenerating potential. The dorsal aponeurosis and subcutaneous cellular layer, though slender, exist as definite entities.

The extensor tendons possess a wide paratendon, but the neurovascular elements are slender. The tendons are at risk but not unprotected, and total destruction is rare.

The dorsal digital region incurs the greatest risks. The skin is extremely thin, the subcutaneous tissue is virtually nonexistent, the extensor tendon apparatus is flattened, and at the joints the capsule is dangerously superficial.

For a given degree of burn, therefore, the risks are quite different in different regions of the hand.

Total burns of the palm are rare, while on

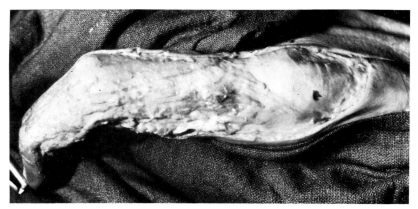

Figure 68–2. Anatomical preparation showing the different skin thickness of the palm and dorsum of the hand.

the dorsum, the tendons are readily exposed. Beyond the metacarpal zone, a protective layer of skin or paratendinous tissue usually persists and forms a useful graft bed. In the fingers, by contrast, the tendons are frequently involved and the capsule is definitely at risk. At the interphalangeal joints, flexion interferes with the blood supply: this is demonstrated by the obvious blanching that occurs when the fist is closed. The risk of tendon or capsular destruction is therefore very real, and the deep tissues at that level form an inhospitable graft bed.

The concept of danger zones is a useful one, and the greatest risks lie at the proximal interphalangeal joint level as well as at the interdigital clefts where retraction and coalescence are possible dangers.

Finally, there is carbonization of the extremities, which can be regarded as thermal amputations, and deep dorsal burns of the distal interphalangeal joints, which can expose the joints and lead to amputation by osteoarthritis.

THE SITE OF THE BURN

Other parts of the body can be involved in the burn injury. We can, for simplicity, consider three main groups:

Burns Involving Only the Hands. These burns carry the most favorable prognosis because from the start there are no therapeutic restrictions. The patient's general condition may not be affected, but manual function is very much at risk. Burns by direct contact are the commonest and, when caused by a hot press, are complicated by crush injury.

The Face-Hands Syndrome. The face-hands syndrome, common in explosion injuries, combines burns of the face and neck with burns of the dorsum of the hands, which are reflexly brought up in a vain attempt to protect the face. The lesions are seldom very deep, usually second degree or intermediate. Associated burns of the neck and upper limbs may require immediate intravenous rehydration. Facial burns also carry the risk of early or delayed (sixth to tenth day) hypoxia, involvement of the upper respiratory tract, while also limiting the possibilities for anesthesia. All these factors therefore plead in favor of conservative or expectant treatment.

Severe Multiple Burns. As soon as the burn covers more than 20 per cent of the body surface in the adult (and 10 per cent in the child), the problem becomes quite a different one. Treatment must be timed and chosen in the context of the patient's overall condition. Although the hand retains priority from a functional standpoint, it should be remembered that plastic repairs require prolonged operating sessions and are very demanding. Excision and grafting can be undertaken only with consideration for the more vital requirements. It is in such cases of multiple burns that treatment is most restricted and sequelae are often the most severe.

INITIAL TREATMENT

The initial treatment includes all forms of treatment undertaken between the moment of the burn and the application of a skin cover. There is still some disagreement about the methods of choice. We shall consider first the types of treatment available and their precise applications.

Escharotomy Incisions

Escharotomy incisions (Fig. 68–3) usually constitute the first therapeutic maneuver. They can be made soon after the patient's arrival to relieve the strangling effect of the burnt tissues that restricts expansion of the edema. The incisions are made on the laterodorsal aspects of the hands and can be lengthened as required into the fingers and toward the forearm (Fig. 68–3). It is often useful to make another incision on the palmar side that crosses the crease of the wrist.

The incisions are made with a knife as delicately as possible without anesthesia; they should not be so deep as to induce pain or bleeding. In theory they are indicated in deep circular burns of the forearms and hand. In practice they are also necessary in dorsal hand burns because the dorsal side is the only area into which edematous fluid can escape. It is not essential first to make an accurate diagnosis of the degree of the burn because the presence or absence of pain can serve as a guide to the depth and extent of the incision.

Some surgeons condemn the use of escharotomies because of the risk of infection. We believe that this risk is minor and is far outweighed by the benefits of the incision, which not only assists the distal circulation but probably also improves the circulation of the burned area.

Débridement

The two methods available are surgical and mechanical débridement.

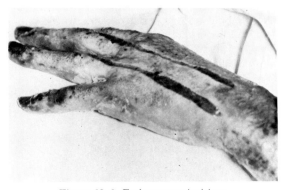

Figure 68–3. Escharotomy incisions.

Surgical Débridement. Surgical débridement consists of the removal of all damaged nonviable tissue. Its aim is to obtain a healthy surface that can be grafted over at once or after a few days. For this reason débridement should be carried out as soon as possible, usually within days after the actual injury. If performed within 48 hours, the right plane of cleavage is found more readily while the edema is still present.

As a rule, the shorter the healing time, the less the risks of infection, sclerosis, and stiffness and the fewer the complications. In practice, however, surgical débridement is not as simple as it might seem. It should be preceded by accurate mapping of the depths of the burned areas. Although its benefits are undisputable in third degree burns, it is obviously unnecessary in superficial lesions. The problem arises in intermediate burns. Some authors, such as Millesi (1974), have suggested injecting a dye to assess with precision the depth and extent of the lesions. The most difficult area is the dorsum of the fingers, especially the part overlying the interphalangeal joints: excessive débridement is unnecessarily mutilating and insufficient cleansing dooms the treatment to failure. It goes without saying that surgical débridement must be followed by skin grafting immediately or within a few days.

TECHNIQUE OF SURGICAL DÉBRIDEMENT. Early excision grafting consists of the removal of nonviable tissue and immediate covering. The first phase thus involves complete removal of burnt tissue to reach healthy tissue, which is possible by the following methods:

1. Either by single-layer excision using an ordinary scalpel or in the opinion of some by coagulation diathermy. This may be carried out using a tourniquet to limit bleeding. This method is obviously used in cases of true third degree burns.

2. By tangential excision (method of Janzekovic, 1970) using a hand dermatome to remove successive layers of burnt tissue until bleeding, viable tissue is reached, free of venous thromboses and with a typical appearance of spotted dermal hemorrhage. This is the method of choice for intermediate burns. Many authors suggest that this should be carried out using a tourniquet. I prefer to work with a tourniquet, thereby ensuring better stepwise hemostasis and also a better visual impression of the quality of the tissue exposed.

Laser excision has the theoretical advantage of being less hemorrhagic but the disadvantage of potentially interfering with the success of subsequent grafting (Fidler, 1974). As previously stated, surgical débridement must be followed by skin grafting immediately or within a few days if all the advantages gained are not to be lost. Difficulties result from bleeding, which cannot be permitted under a graft. After single-layer excision, hemostasis must be done carefully. It is lengthy and difficult, but possible. After tangential excision some oozing persists which cannot be coagulated because of its multiple sources. Application of a compressive dressing with thrombase for 10 to 15 min. is often successful. Two or three successive compressions may be necessary before application of the graft. A nonexpanded mesh graft may be very useful, because it allows for drainage of any possible oozing of blood. Rarely, and in case of difficulty, a biological dressing may be used (homograft, pig skin, synthetic skin substitution) to delay to autograft by 24 or 48 hours.

The attractive nature of early excision grafting should not be allowed to hide its difficulties. It requires accurate evaluation of the thickness of the burn, and above all, the precision of the excision is of primary importance. Any excess is unnecessarily mutilating, even if it is sometimes useful to sacrifice healthy skin to comply with the borders of functional skin units. Any insufficiency in excision will result in failure of the graft, thereby eliminating all the advantages of the method. It must be stressed that early excision grafting of one hand, and even more of both, is not a benign procedure. The operation is lengthy, bleeding for excision and the taking of grafts is heavy, and in those patients in a precarious hemodynamic state, it requires skilled and appropriate postoperative management. Technical difficulties require a trained team, and when both hands are affected, we prefer to operate as two teams. In view of the potential shock resulting from the operation, it is obvious that its use is restricted by age, general condition, and the extent of the burns involved. When excision exposes major structures such as tendons or joints incapable of accepting a graft, the question arises of skin flaps with their own blood supply.

Mechanical Débridement. Mechanical débridement consists of cleansing the burns without having recourse to surgical means. The first maneuver is to clean with water and acid soap and to remove scabs. This is done while the patient is in bed without anesthetic; pain and bleeding indicate the limits of the débridement.

Next comes the dressing, which is adapted to the stage of the burn. A petrolatum dressing is used to detach the scabs and induce granulation. Atonic surfaces are treated with normotonic or hypertonic saline baths with or without enzyme sprays.

The main criticism leveled at mechanical débridement is that it is slow and increases the risks of infection and fibrosis. There is no doubt that permanent necrosis favors bacterial growth, but we believe that if the treatment is properly applied, the burns can be treated as open wounds (bacteriocycle of Vilain, 1971) and infections by virulent strains can be avoided.

Fibrosis represents a very real danger to which other factors contribute, such as the initial "lesions beyond the skin" mentioned earlier. This can be minimized, however, if strict time limits are observed. Thus dressings should not be continued indefinitely; the twenty-first day is the limit, by which time there should be a healthy covering layer, which may be obtained spontaneously by grafting. It is to hasten the process that the therapeutic adjuncts mentioned earlier are suggested. On the whole the conservative nature of the treatment makes up for its slowness while reducing the likelihood of excessive and pointless loss of tissue.

DRESSINGS

We have already mentioned the various types of dressings that are an essential part of mechanical débridement. In addition to the medication, chosen according to the clinical condition of the burn, the dressings consist of a layer of moist gauze held in place by a bandage or elastic netting. It is important that the fingers be kept apart. Being semirigid, the dressings provide relative immobilization (Fig. 68–4).

A rival school of thought advocates exposure of the burn to air, the two main advantages being easier mobilization and absence of maceration. As a rule a crusty coagulum tends to form on the surface, which must be removed later. However, these advantages

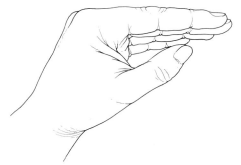

Figure 68–4. Position of immobilization for the burned hand.

are more theoretical than real: The crusts can hinder active mobility and make movements painful with the result that the hand and fingers are effectively immobilized, sometimes in a faulty position. It is not uncommon for pus to form under the crust. Finally, the patient may become psychologically disturbed by the sight of the lesions.

Some authors, such as Michon, have suggested exposing the burn to oxygen-rich air or to pure oxygen, which would provide better control of infection. However, the equipment must be carefully set up to avoid the risk of explosion. This method does not seem to have gained favor.

Alternatives to dressings and exposure consist of the application of various antiseptic products. Silver nitrate after a brief vogue fell into relative disuse for two reasons—soiling and toxicity.

Sulfamylon has been blamed for inducing metabolic acidosis, at least in cases of extensive burns with pulmonary complications. It also is uncomfortable to the patient.

Silver sulfadiazine is the most popular drug at the present time.

In fact, all these methods provide excellent protection against infection but have no curative action on scabs and deep burns. They have no logical place, therefore, except for the treatment of superficial burns, which can be expected to heal spontaneously. Alternately they can be used as a temporizing measure prior to surgical excision or skin grafting.

SKIN COVERING

If we exclude cases in which regeneration occurs spontaneously or after assisted débridement and dressings, fresh skin must be provided by grafts or flaps. This can be performed early after surgical débridement.

Skin Grafts

As a rule, only full or partial thickness autografts are utilized.

Heterografts (pigskin) and homografts (cadaver skin) have a place in the treatment of hand burns. They are biological dressings used to cover large surface areas. Their application to the hand is only accessory. It is possible to use pigskin or homograft as a test of the graft bed and of its capacity to accept an autograft. Thus, when there is some doubt concerning the completeness of the excision, a heterograft can be justified on a short term basis.

As for pinch grafts, they can be considered, but hand burns are not the best indication since the small area to be covered offers little scope for their expansion potential. Besides, the quality and cosmetic appearance of the cover obtained are less satisfactory than with full grafts. Their main advantage, therefore, remains their capacity to take in poor quality graft beds.

Full thickness grafts, the classic treatment of palmar burns, are only indicated initially in the rare cases of superficial burns with a perfect graft bed. On the whole, they should be used as secondary treatment because the almost perfect conditions required for their successful use are seldom encountered in practice.

The therapeutic mainstay, therefore, remains the split thickness or Tiersch graft (Fig. 68–5). We like to use this graft with a plastic lining, especially for the dorsum of the hand; its rigidity makes it less adaptable to digital surfaces, especially for less experienced surgeons.

The graft, 0.3 to 0.4 mm. thick, is applied and fixed to the edges of the defect by a few stitches. It is always preferable to respect functional units by avoiding longitudinal sutures and using Z incisions, as with all grafts in the hand and fingers. These principles, however, may have to be bypassed in patients with multiple burns in whom economy of tissue becomes a priority.

If some surgeons still prefer to rely on exposure to air, the majority prefer treatment by dressings and immobilization for four to eight days.

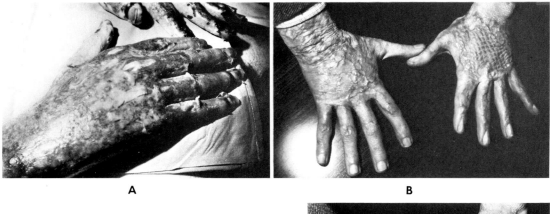

A

B

Figure 68–5. Example of débridement and grafting. *A*, At two weeks. *B* and *C*, Functional result.

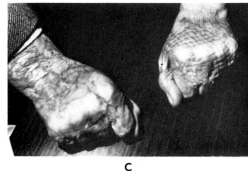

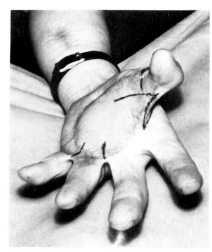

C

The main advantage of the partial thickness graft is the readiness with which it takes; the disadvantages are future fragility and the possibility of contraction. Its reinnervation potential is still under study.

Skin Flaps

Flaps can be used in the first instance to protect structures such as tendons and joints that will not tolerate a graft (Fig. 68–6). In theory they must carry their own blood supply via the pedicle. Their revascularization will come from the skin edges of the defect and not from the substratum. For this reason one has recourse to thick flaps rather than to Colson's flap grafts,* which are more useful in secondary treatment.

The flaps are mostly abdominal in origin, preferably centered on the circumflex iliac or subcutaneous vessels—flat flaps with an inferior pedicle. They adapt better to the dorsal aspects of the hand and fingers. They are harder to design for the palm where the results are usually mediocre anyway. A viable alternative is Negri's pocket flap.

The pedicle is divided as a rule at 21 days.

The disadvantages of flaps are multiple. The cosmetic appearance is unsatisfactory, and the thick flap can be cumbersome and may require thinning later. Pluridigital burns using the same flap are temporarily syndactylized; separation and commissural reconstruction necessitate further surgery later. Prolonged immobilization is necessary and may lead to stiffness.

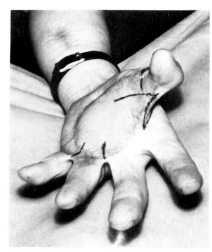

Figure 68–6. Abdominal flap for a palmar burn. Its thickness necessitates later defatting.

---

*See the chapter on flap grafts in Volume II.

Flaps must be regarded, therefore, more as a necessity than as a solution of choice.

MOBILIZATION AND IMMOBILIZATION

The risk of joint stiffness should be kept in mind throughout the initial treatment. It inevitably influences the choice of débridement and skin covering method. Preference is usually given to the method that will allow early physiotherapy, since re-education remains difficult as long as cicatrization is incomplete. However, most authors advocate early mobilization of the hand, whether exposed or under dressings, within the limits of possibility and by taking advantage of the sessions of mechanical débridement, especially if this is conducted under immersion. This attitude can be criticized to the extent

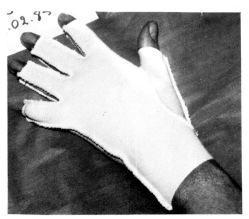

Figure 68–8. Compressive gloves.

that, at some stage, complete immobilization is preferable. It is generally agreed that immobilization is indicated during the days that follow grafting, but few would advocate it during the period of débridement. It is conceivable that mobilization might favor inflammation and thus promote the spread of infection, both of which can induce cicatricial sclerosis. Besides, pain may be indicative of sympathetic dystrophy. For these reasons we believe that early re-education should be undertaken only with the greatest prudence. During this period, therefore, we prefer immobilization of the hand in a correct position. Active mobilization is allowed only if it is painless and only under immersion between dressings.

The hand is immobilized with the metacarpophalangeal joints in 60 to 90 degrees of flexion with the interphalangeal joints extended or very slightly flexed. When the lesions are so deep that the joints are bared or at risk of exposure, we prefer to immobilize them by means of Kirschner wires. Physiotherapy is resumed fully as soon as healing is complete.

Hypertrophic scarring is common and often can be prevented by the early use of compressive gloves (Figs. 68–7, 68–8). Later reconstruction in cases of severe hypertrophic scarring and contractures is discussed elsewhere (see Chapters 73 and 74).

SUMMARY AND CONCLUSION

It is difficult to outline a standard approach to treatment because of the multiplicity of the parameters involved. However, a number of broad pictures may be used as a guide.

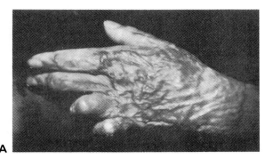

A

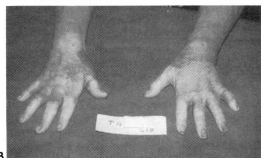

B

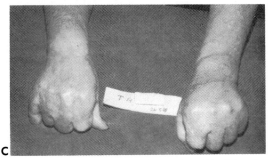

C

Figure 68–7. A, Hypertrophic scarring of both hands. B, Bilateral Colson's flap grafts done in one stage. C, Complete flexion of the fingers.

When initial clinical evaluation of the lesions indicates the slightest doubt of deep burns of the dorsum of the hand then releasing incisions are necessary. Apart from their therapeutic action they are the best method for testing the depth of the lesion.

In *isolated hand burns*, the depth and site of the lesion are the principal guides in management.

Palmar burns are most often treated by mechanical débridement. Dorsal burns are treated by tangential excision for intermediate burns and by single-layer excision for third degree burns. Covering usually involves split thickness graft. In rare cases, skin flap may be needed for a burn extending beyond the skin. When there is carbonization of the extremities, amputation should be delayed until the precise limits of the lesions become evident.

In the major burns patient the indication for early excision grafting of the hand must be viewed with great caution.

CHEMICAL BURNS

Chemical burns are skin lesions resulting from the caustic action of an acid or a strong base. Chronic irritation due to repeated chemical contacts will not be discussed here.

ETIOLOGY

Causative agents include strong acids (such as hydrochloric, sulfuric, nitric, and hydrofluoric acid) and strong bases (such as sodium and potassium salts). Most accidents occur at work. The chemical agent may be hot, in which case the result is a mixed chemical and thermal lesion. This is also true of burns caused by phosphorus, which ignites by simple contact with air.

PATHOPHYSIOLOGY

A "chemical burn" is the result of a simple chemical reaction between the causal agent and the tissues. The immediate reaction, whether the agent is an acid or a base, is that of combining with tissue water and the resultant liberation of heat. Acids react with alkaline salts and coagulate albumin; bases coagulate proteins.

A very important aspect is the depth of penetration of the chemical, which produces lesions that progress with time. Thus, the fluorine ion of hydrofluoric acid shows a great affinity for the Ca^+ ion. It penetrates into the tissues and induces more deep necrosis than is apparent on the surface. Progression can continue for up to one week.

However, even if the pathophysiological changes are different, the ultimate result is a loss of skin and soft tissue (as with heat burns), and the treatment is similar except for differences in the immediate post-traumatic period.

TREATMENT

As the chemical agent penetrates, it becomes progressively less accessible and more difficult to remove. Therefore, first aid measures must be applied rapidly.

The first step is to wash the burn at once, and for a long time, in water. This may influence the course of the injury. The importance of this emergency measure is stressed by all authors who suggest that it be widely taught and that all facilities and equipment be readily available on the spot wherever such accidents are likely to happen. The need for abundant washing is obvious, as the aim is to dilute the chemical. The lesions and surrounding areas should be liberally flooded by a water shower or water jet, especially in the creases and interdigital clefts, for at least 30 minutes (some authors even suggest 24 hours).

Water baths have replaced "neutralization," which is usually time-consuming and can be attempted later (if possible after measuring the pH). Acid burns are usually sprayed with 5 per cent or 10 per cent sodium bicarbonate and alkaline burns with 5 per cent boric acid.

For acid burns, 5 per cent to 10 per cent triethanolamine has been suggested. This agent is said to have better penetration, and administration can be continued for 48 hours by the application of triethanolamine stearate ointment. Some authors believe that triethanolamine also has a beneficial effect in alkaline burns. The mechanism then would not be one of neutralization but of reduction of cellular acidosis in the burned tissues.

A few special cases require additional discussion. In cases of burns by hydrofluoric acid, the following procedure is recommended: Wash the area with water, bathe it in an ice-cold solution of 3 per cent magnesium sulfate, and use a dermo-jet infiltration with 10 per cent calcium gluconate. This treatment has been shown to reduce the severity of the burn, which in the pulp produces a purulent blister overlying necrosis of the dermis. For phosphorus burns, the treatment recommended is alternating baths in alkaline bicarbonate solution with exposure to air until phosphorescence has disappeared.

Apart from these emergency measures, which are of vital importance, the long-term treatment is the same as with other types of burns, except that grafting is notoriously difficult in chemical burns.

REFERENCES

Baux, S., and Colson, P.: Brûlures de la main. 10e Congrés de la SICOT Bruxelles, Imprimerie des Sciences, Vol. 2, 1972, pp. 106–114.

Colson, P., Houot, R., Gandolphe, M., de Mourgues A., Laurent, J., Biron, G., and Janvier, M.: Utilisation des lambeaux dégraissés (lambeaux-greffes) en chirurgie réparatrice de la main. Ann. Chir. Plast., 12:298–310, 1967.

Colson, P., Janvier, H., and Gangolphe, M.: Un procédé de Sterling Bunnel pour réfection des commissures digitales par rotation de lambeaux. Ann. Chir. Plast., 5:205–211, 1960.

Davies, J. W. L.: Prompt cooling of burned areas: a review of benefits and the effector mechanisms. Burns, 91–6, 1982.

Edstrom, L. E., Robson, M. C., Macchiaverna, J. R., and Scala, A. D.: Prospective randomized treatment for burned hands, nonoperative vs. operative. Scand. J. Plast. Reconstruct. Surg., 13:131–135, 1979.

Fidler, J. P., Rockwell, R. J., Siler, V. E., MacMitten, B. G., and Altemeier, W. A.: Early laser excision of thermal burns in the white rat and miniature pig. Burns, 1:5–12, 1974.

Frist, W., Ackroyd, F., Burke, J., and Bondoc, C.: Long term functional results of selective treatment of hand burns. Am. J. Surg., 149:516–521, 1985.

Gate, A., and Deleuze, R.: Traitement desbrûlures profondes du dos de la main. Ann. Chir. Plast., 6:211–222, 1961.

Goodwin, C. N., Maguirre, M. S., MacManus, W. F., and Pruitt, B. A.: Prospective study of burn wound excision of the hands. J. Trauma, 23:510–517, 1983.

Jansekovic, Z.: A new concept in the early excision and immediate grafting of burns. J. Trauma, 10:1103–1108, 1970.

Kenesi, C.: Brûlures récentes de la Main. Thesis, Paris, 1965.

Leung, P. L., and Chow, Y. Y. N.: Treatment of burned hands. Burns, 8:338–344, 1982.

Lowbury, E. J. L.: Fact or fashion? The rationale of exposure method vaccination and other anti-infectious measures. Burns, 5:149–159, 1978.

Michon, J., and Masse, P.: L'exposition des mains brulées som cloche à oxygène. Ann. Chir. Plast., 6:269–285, 1961.

Millesi, H., Berger, A., and Meissl, G.: Estimation of burned depth for primary excision by enzymatic method. 4th Congress I.S.B.I., Buenos Aires, 1976.

Muhlbauer, W., Herndl, E., Stock, W., and Song, R.: Plast. Reconstr. Surg., 70:336–344, 1982.

Razemon, J. P.: Séquelles de brûlures traitées par lambeau-greffe de Colson. Ann. Chir., 22:682, 1968.

Tubiana, R., Baux, S., and Kenesi, C.: A propos de 300 brulures récéntes des mains. Ann. Chir., 23–24:1387–1395, 1967.

Vilain, R.: Le bacteriocycle infectieux de la brulure: infection et surinfection. Therapie, 26(2):339–344, 1971.

Vilain, R., and Perdu, J. C.: Etude critique du pansement-greffe à l'hydrocortisone sur le bourgeon charnu. Ann. Chir. Plast., 4:197–215, 1959.

Chapter 69

MANAGEMENT OF ACUTE THERMAL HAND INJURIES

Conrado C. Bondoc,
William C. Quinby, Jr.,
John Siebert,
John A. I. Grossman
and John F. Burke

The management of thermal hand injuries continues to be a difficult and complicated problem. Such injuries often result in a distressingly high morbidity. Although the skin surface of the hand constitutes less than 5 per cent of the body surface area, deep cutaneous burns of the dorsum of the hand, if not managed accurately and promptly beginning in the immediate postburn period, can result in severe crippling deformity and permanent physical disability.

INITIAL EVALUATION OF HAND INJURY

Initially the extent and depth of burns, as well as the circulatory status of the hand and fingers, must be determined by examination.

The depth of skin involvement may vary from second degree burns to deep burns involving the whole thickness of the skin. Second degree burns may be superficial second degree, or they may be deep second degree mixed with areas of full thickness loss or uniformly involve the whole thickness of the skin.

The term third degree burn implies that the whole thickness of the skin is involved down to the level of the fascia, even including the deep veins or the tendons of the dorsum of the hand.

The foregoing classification is of great significance in choosing the appropriate therapeutic approach, as will be discussed.

EXTENT OF THERMAL INJURY

The extent of the burn is an important consideration in the clinical approach to the therapy of the burn patient. For severe and extensive thermal burns of the body, the rational approach is quite different from that for burns involving or limited to the hand alone. In such instances the primary objective is to encourage the wound to heal as early and as quickly as possible in order to save the patient's life; care of the hand receives secondary consideration. When the extent of burn injury is not life threatening, however, hand burns assume early priority for operative treatment.

COMPLICATIONS AND ASSOCIATED INJURIES

It must be emphasized that initially close attention must be directed to the circulatory status of the hand and fingers. Deep circumferential burns involving the hand, as well as those proximally in the forearm or at the wrist, can lead to serious ischemic complications involving the hand and fingers. Accumulation of edema fluid in the early postburn period, under the unyielding circumferential eschar, may lead to vascular compromise. If there is evidence of ischemia of the hand or fingers by physical examination or by Doppler ultrasound testing, decompression of the hand and fingers must be carried out imme-

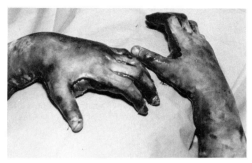

Figure 69–1. Deep circumferential burns of the forearms and hands with absent pulses. Escharotomies were performed to re-establish circulation.

diately by performing adequate escharotomies until the circulation has been re-established (Fig. 69–1).

HAND DEFORMITY SOON AFTER BURN INJURY

Acute deformities of the hand occurring soon after burn injury involve the skin, fascia, ligaments, tendons, muscles, and joints. As with any soft tissue injury, particularly of the hand, the degree of functional recovery and the cosmetic result depend to a large extent on the anatomical extent of the injury and the results of scar formation during the healing process. Fibrosis and hypertrophic scarring cause deformity by contracture, and additionally improper immobilization, edema, and disuse can give rise to joint stiffness, muscle wasting, and deformity. The ensuing deformities include hyperextension at the metacarpophalangeal joints, flexion at the proximal and distal interphalangeal joints, adduction of the thumb, and volar flexion of the wrist, finally resulting in the so-called "claw hand deformity." The most common deformities encountered are web space and thumb contractures, proximal and distal joint contractures, hypertrophic scars and extension contractures, and the boutonnière deformity.

These anatomical and functional impairments in deep thermal hand injuries may be avoided and do not result in permanent fixed deformities if managed properly and promptly. Over the years our clinical experience in treating over 900 patients with hand injuries has shown that serious anatomical

and functional impairment occurring after deep burn injury can best be avoided by early and accurate excision of the burn eschar, immediate wound closure, and adherence to certain therapeutic principles:

1. Immobilization of the hand and fingers in a functional position
2. Control of edema by elevation
3. Prevention of infection by use of antibacterial drugs and biological dressings
4. Early excision of burn eschar with immediate wound closure by grafting
5. Early restoration of motion

IMMOBILIZATION IN POSITION OF FUNCTION

To prevent the development of deformities, it is important to immobilize the hand and fingers in a position of function beginning in the immediate postburn period. This includes positioning the wrist in 45 degrees of dorsiflexion, the metacarpophalangeal joint in 70 degrees of flexion, the proximal and distal interphalangeal joints in slight flexion, and finally the thumb in radiopalmar abduction (Fig. 69–2). The splinted hand must be kept constantly elevated to control edema and minimize swelling. These steps must be carried out during the immediate postburn period as well as during the postoperative period until the wound has healed completely.

MANAGEMENT OF THE BURNED HAND

A number of methods have been advocated for the care of the burned hand, including the topical application of antibacterial drugs alone to facilitate spontaneous healing, late skin autografting after eschar separation, primary excision and grafting only for full thickness burns, primary fascial excision for deep second degree as well as third degree burns, and tangential excision with skin grafting of the hand for full thickness injury (Boswick, 1974; Brown, 1967; Earle and Fratianne, 1979; Huang et al., 1975; Krizek et al., 1973; Mahler and Hirschowitz, 1976; Moncrief et al., 1966; Peacock et al., 1970; Wexler et al., 1974; Whitson et al., 1971).

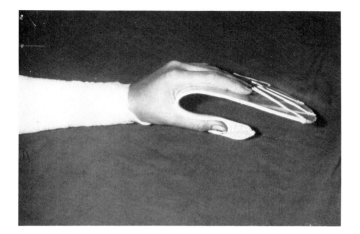

Figure 69–2. Hand immobilized in a functional position with thermoplastic splints.

TOPICAL APPLICATION OF ANTIBACTERIAL DRUGS

Several topically applied antibacterial drugs such as 0.5 per cent silver nitrate, Silvadene, and Sulfamylon have been effective in controlling bacterial proliferation in burn wounds (Fox, 1969; Moncrief et al., 1966; Moyer et al., 1965). This treatment has resulted in a significant decrease in the conversion of superficial burns to deeper injuries by sepsis, and thus promotes spontaneous healing of burn wounds. Clinical studies have also shown that biological materials, such as viable cadaver allografts, heterografts, and amniotic membranes, have been most effective as temporary wound covers and have prevented bacterial colonization of wounds (Shuck et al., 1969). The topical use of antibacterial drugs and biological dressings, especially viable allografts, has been most effective in accelerating the healing of superficial second degree burns. Clinical studies have demonstrated that allografts, when applied over superficial second degree burns, stimulate and promote the rapid growth of epithelial elements under the allografts, leading to spontaneous healing of the wound (Zaroff et al., 1966). It is clear, therefore, that in the treatment of superficial second degree burns, the topical application of antibacterial drugs and the use of biological dressings like allografts are the most effective methods of treatment and result in excellent healing without hypertrophic scarring or contracture (Burke and Bondoc, 1968). For deeper burn injuries (deep second degree and full thickness skin loss), however, this approach has not been effective because the use of antibacterial drugs and biological materials does not deal with the basic problems of deep burns, i.e., the presence of necrotic burn tissue and the open wound.

PRIMARY EXCISION AND IMMEDIATE GRAFTING

At the Massachusetts General Hospital and Shriners Burns Institute in Boston, operative excision has been used as routine therapy for deep thermal burns based on the surgical principle of early eschar excision and immediate wound closure (Burke et al., 1974, 1976; Cope et al., 1947). Since the anatomy of the dorsum of the hand is not unlike that of other parts of the body, the same approach of routine surgical excision and immediate wound closure is utilized for the expeditious care of deep thermal hand injuries.

The importance of early eschar excision and prompt wound closure in deep thermal injuries should not be overlooked simply because the topical use of antimicrobial drugs can effectively reduce the incidence of superficial infection. Although these drugs have been shown to reduce substantially the incidence of conversion of superficial second degree burns to full thickness injury by bacterial invasion, the advantages of achieving early wound healing by excision in deep burns are so great that patients should not be denied the definitive therapy designed to attain this objective.

Primary excision and immediate grafting therefore are employed as routine therapy only for deep thermal hand injuries (Bondoc et al., 1976, 1977; Burke et al., 1976). These steps are carried out after immediate physiological needs have been met and the patient's condition is stable. The earlier the excision is performed, the easier the excision is, and tissue planes are easier to identify. Additionally, the burn wound is relatively sterile and significant bacterial colonization of the wound has not set in. In the operative management of the burned hand, primary excision of all necrotic burned tissue is carried out using one of two surgical techniques (Bondoc et al., 1976, 1977; Burke et al., 1976).

Sequential Excision

The first technique makes use of sequential eschar excision (Jackson and Stone, 1972; Janzekovic, 1970). A free-hand guarded knife (Watson-Edwards or Goulian knife) is used when burns of the hand consist of irregular areas of deep dermal and full thickness injury, as well as when a definite clinical decision concerning the presence or extent of third degree burns cannot be made in the early postburn period (Fig. 69–3B). In carrying out this excision, the knife guard is set at 0.006 to 0.008 inch. The exact depth of the burn can be established by observing the area excised after each débriding slice. The burn eschar is removed by successive débriding slices until viable dermis with a uniform bleeding base is encountered. Thrombosed subdermal veins as well as dead fat must be excised sharply.

After all devitalized tissue has been sharply excised, complete hemostasis must be accomplished by pressure dressings and electrocoagulation of bleeding points. It is extremely important to achieve complete hemostasis before grafting to ensure a 100 per cent graft take. Sheets of previously harvested autograft skin of appropriate thickness should be fitted carefully over the excised wound and sutured

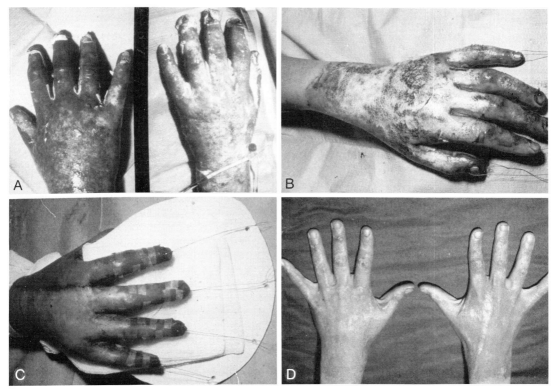

Figure 69–3. A four-year-old boy sustained mixed deep second and third degree burns over the dorsum of both hands. *B*, Left hand after sequential excision of the dorsum of the hand, with areas of deep second degree burns and a few areas of third degree burns. *C*, Hand immobilized in a position of function with a thermoplastic splint after sequential excision and grafting. *D*, Both hands one year after excision and grafting. Excellent function and cosmetic appearance resulted.

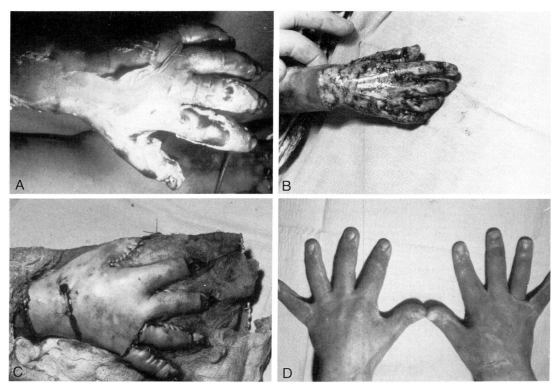

Figure 69-4. A two-year-old boy sustained deep burns of both hands. *A*, Left hand, showing full thickness or persistent waxy white eschar over dorsum of hand. *B*, Whole thickness of burned skin excised down to the level of the deep fascia and over the tendons of the right hand. *C*, Right hand grafted with thick split thickness graft and immobilized in a volar splint. *D*, Both hands two years after excision and grafting, showing excellent function.

in place with interrupted 5-0 chromic catgut sutures and Steri-strips (Fig. 69-3*C*). Grafting of the excised wound is carried out during the same operative procedure as excision to achieve immediate wound closure.

Excision of Full Thickness Burns

The second operative technique utilizes direct excision of the entire thickness of the burned skin down to the areolar layer surrounding the deep veins lying on the deep fascia. This technique is used for burns of the hand that are unquestionably and uniformly full thickness (Fig. 69-4*B*). In carrying out this excision, it is important to preserve the dorsal venous network, if this is not thrombosed, to provide adequate venous drainage during the immediate postburn period (Fig. 69-5*B*). In patients whose injuries extend down to the deep fascia, débridement must include all devitalized tissues, including muscle if indicated, before grafting can be done.

Excision down to fascia is carried out using a sharp scalpel or an electrocautery knife. During the excisional procedure, care is taken to remove all burned tissues in and around the thenar and hypothenar areas, as well as the lateral aspects of the involved fingers to prevent areas of slow secondary healing and subsequent scar formation.

A pneumatic tourniquet may be used at times to minimize blood loss. Again complete hemostasis must be accomplished before the wound is grafted in order to achieve the complete take. Autografts used to cover the excised wound over the dorsum of the hand and fingers are harvested using the Padgett air-driven dermatome from available donor areas, preferably the back or buttocks; the thickness of the grafts harvested may vary according to the depth of the excised wound. Skin autografts in sheets are fitted over the dorsum of the hand and fingers and sutured in place using interrupted 5-0 chromic catgut sutures and Steri-strips. The grafted hand is immobilized and treated in an open fashion (no dressings over the grafted areas) in order to be able to observe the grafted hand (Fig. 69–4C). In certain instances careful rolling of grafts with cotton swabs in the immediate postoperative period may be necessary to effectively remove collections of serum or blood under the grafts.

MANAGEMENT OF THERMAL INJURIES OF THE PALM

The palmar area of the hand is the triangular space bounded by the lateral border of the hypothenar eminence, the opposition crease of the thumb, and the transverse palmar crease.

Unlike the skin covering the dorsum of the hand, the palmar skin is anchored to the underlying deep fascial plane by numerous perpendicular fibrous tracts. These fibrous septa transverse the underlying deep fat pads, separating them into bundles. The result is the absence of a distinct subcutaneous tissue plane, and the most distinct characteristic feature of the palmar skin is its tethering to the deep fascial plane.

Because of this special characteristic anatomical feature, the management of deep

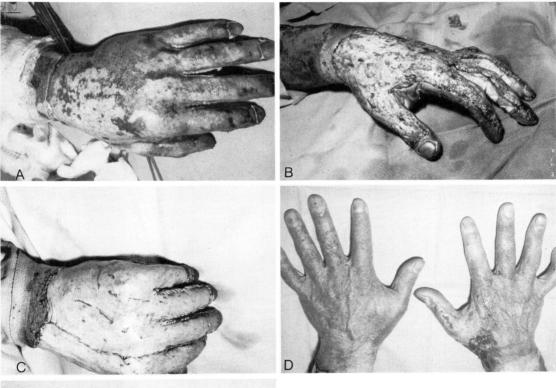

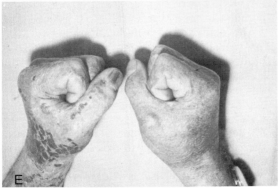

Figure 69–5. A 46-year-old male sustained third degree burns of the dorsum of both hands. A, Left hand with persistent waxy white eschar. B, The whole thickness of burned eschar was excised down to the fascia over the dorsal veins of the hand. C, Left hand grafted with thick autografts and hand immobilized in position of function using Kirschner wire. D, Both hands two years after excision and grafting, showing excellent results. E, Both hands with full range of motion and good grasp.

burns of the palm become complicated and difficult. Since there is no distinct fascial plane, the surgical technique employed is sequential excision. A free-hand guarded knife set at 0.006 to 0.008 inch is used to excise the burned eschar. The burn eschar is excised in sequential fashion, observing after each débriding slice until viable dermis and uniform bleeding are encountered over the underlying tissues. After all nonviable tissues have been sharply excised, complete and thorough hemostasis must be accomplished. Previously harvested thick (0.018 to 0.020 inch) split thickness skin is fitted over the excised area and sutured in place with interrupted 4-0 chromic catgut sutures. In addition, it is important to anchor the skin along the different palmar creases by applying several interrupted sutures to stabilize the skin in place and maintain the normal palmar creases (Fig. 69–6). Palmar pressure dressings are applied. The hand is immobilized by splinting in 45 degrees of dorsiflexion.

SPLINTING AND INTERNAL FIXATION

In the immediate postoperative period the hand is immobilized in a functional position using thermoplastic volar splints (Fig. 69–3C) or by internal fixation with Kirschner wires (Fig. 69–5C).

In general, internal Kirschner wire fixation is used when the burn is deep and involves the tendons and joints. However, regardless of the type of immobilization employed, it is necessary that the hand is kept in slight dorsiflexion with the metacarpophalangeal

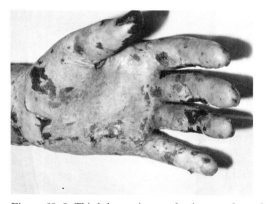

Figure 69–6. Third degree burns of palmar surface of the left hand were repaired by sequential excision and grafting using thick grafts (0.02 inch).

joints in 70 degrees of flexion and the proximal interphalangeal and distal interphalangeal joints in slight flexion. When the patient's hand is maintained in a functional position with thermoplastic dynamic volar splints during the immediate postoperative period, it is necessary to keep the splinted hand elevated to prevent the development of dependent edema. After the sixth postoperative day, the patient in a dynamic splint is encouraged to gradually increase motion over the joints, and in about 12 to 14 days a progressively vigorous program of active and passive exercises of the hand and fingers is initiated.

Again it must be emphasized that the operative procedure is usually carried out as soon after the injury as possible. However, there are instances when excision of the hand must be delayed, and this is the case in patients with extensive burns. In such instances the primary objective is the patient's survival, and thus donor skin is used to include as wide an area of wound coverage as possible. Excision and grafting of the hand therefore must receive secondary priority.

Clinical experience accumulated through the years in the management of 959 patients (adults and children) has clearly demonstrated that early excision and immediate autografting have resulted in results far superior to those in patients treated with topically applied antibacterial drugs, spontaneous separation of eschar, and late grafting of a granulating base. Far fewer anatomical hand deformities were encountered in the patients who underwent excision, as shown by the number of patients who required secondary reconstructive procedures to correct hand deformities (Bondoc and Burke, 1982; Frist et al., 1985). Hypertrophic scarring and flexion contractures at the interphalangeal joints, the classic "clawing," and the boutonnière deformity have been seen less frequently. The patients treated with early excision have had a low incidence of complications.

Evaluation of the long term status of patients with deep thermal hand injuries has shown that early direct surgical excision and immediate grafting have produced superior and impressive functional as well as cosmetic results (Table 69–1). Even in patients who needed secondary reconstructive procedures, the results were good to excellent except for a few in whom the outcome was poor. These were patients whose injuries were massive,

Table 69–1. LONG TERM STATUS OF HANDS IN PATIENTS EXCISED AND GRAFTED*

	Results	Functional NO. PATIENTS	%	Cosmetic NO. PATIENTS	%
No reconstructive procedure done	Excellent	224	63	178	50
After reconstruction	Very good	78	22	89	25
	Good	27	7	35	9
	Fair	17	5	38	11
	Poor	11	3	17	5

*Excisions in 357 patients, July 1974 to December 1980.

and the hand injuries were treated later in the course of their illness because of the extent of the injury.

The concept of direct excision of burned tissue and immediate wound closure is based on sound biological and surgical principles, particularly when applied to uniform full thickness injuries. Excision of burns of the hand should be carried out as soon after injury as possible and the wound should be closed immediately after excision. If the burn eschar is excised early and the wound closed immediately, one can achieve primary healing and avoid inflammatory reaction and the production of granulations leading to the development of hypertrophic scars. The reduction in time between the injury and excision and wound closure has a marked effect on the quality of the repair and the functional as well as cosmetic results. It must be emphasized that the wound must be closed completely with sheet grafts (not meshed grafts), avoiding gaps between grafts where secondary healing and scars eventually develop.

There has been a great reluctance to excise burns of the hands if the burn is only a deep second degree injury mixed with small areas of third degree burns, i.e., if the injury does not involve the whole thickness of the skin uniformly. Clinical experience has repeatedly shown that many hypertrophic scars over the dorsum of the hand and joint capsules are related to deep dermal burns that were allowed to heal spontaneously over a period of many weeks. The prolonged immobilization and absence of motion in the joints during the many weeks of slow healing in those hands that were not grafted early can result in joint stiffness, marked deformity, and significant impairment of function. When deep dermal burns with areas of third degree burn were excised early and the wound grafted immediately, healing occurred without the development of abnormal hypertrophic scars and with excellent functional and cosmetic results.

The development of methods of burn excision, both primary fascial and sequential eschar excision, has brought about significant improvement in the final outcome in the care of the burned hand. The introduction of sequential eschar excision in the management of deep dermal burns has introduced a new dimension in the primary care of deep dermal burns of the hands. This approach makes it possible to deal with thermally injured tissue by direct excision of all necrotic burn eschar without sacrificing normal viable tissue.

REFERENCES

Bondoc, C. C., and Burke, J. F.: Early excision of the burned hand. Follow-up evaluation. Presented at Symposium on Burned Hand, American Society for Surgery of the Hand, Boston, September 1982.

Bondoc, C. C., Quinby, W. C., Jr., and Burke, J. F.: Primary surgical management of the deeply burned hand in children. J. Pediatr. Surg., 11:355–362, 1976.

Bondoc, C. C., Quinby, W. C., Jr., Schefflan, M., and Burke, J. F.: Expeditious primary excision and grafting of the deeply burned hand. Orthop. Rev., 6:99–102, 1977.

Boswick, J. A., Jr.: The management of fresh burns of the hand and deformities resulting from burn injuries. Clin. Plast. Surg., 1:621–631, 1974.

Brown, R. F.: Care of the burnt hand. Proc. R. Soc. Med., 69:862, 1967.

Burke, J. F., and Bondoc, C. C.: Combined burn therapy utilizing immediate skin allografts and 0.5 per cent AgNO₃. Arch. Surg., 97:716–721, 1968.

Burke, J. F., Bondoc, C. C., and Quinby, W. C., Jr.: Primary burn excision and immediate grafting. A method of shortening illness. J. Trauma, 14:389, 1974.

Burke, J. F., Bondoc, C. C., Quinby, W. C., Jr., and Remensnyder, J. P.: Primary surgical management of the deeply burned hand. J. Trauma, 16:593–598, 1976.

Burke, J. F., Quinby, W. C., Jr., and Bondoc, C. C.: Primary excision and prompt grafting as a routine therapy for the treatment of thermal burns in children. Surg. Clin. N. Am., 56:477–494, 1976.

Cope, O., Langhor, J. L., and Moore, F. D.: Expeditious care of full thickness burn wounds by surgical excision and grafting. Ann. Surg., 125:1, 1947.

Earle, A. S., and Fratianne, R. B.: Delayed definitive reconstruction of the burned hand: evolution of a program of care. J. Trauma, 19:149–152, 1979.

Fox, C. C.: Clinical experience with silver sulfadiazine.

A new topical agent for control of Pseudomonas in burns. J. Trauma, 9:377, 1969.

Frist, W., Ackroyd, F., Burke, J., and Bondoc, C.: Long term functional results of selective treatment of hand burns. Am. J. Surg., 149:516–521, April 1985.

Huang, T. T., Larson, D., and Lewis, S.: Burned hands. Plast. Reconstr. Surg., 56:21, 1975.

Jackson, D. W., and Stone, P. A.: Tangenital excision and grafting of·burns: the method and report of 50 cases. Br. J. Plast. Surg., 4:416, 1972.

Janzekovic, Z.: A new concept in the early excision and immediate grafting of burns. J. Trauma, 10:1103, 1970.

Krizek, T. J., et al.: Delayed primary excision and immediate grafting of the burned hand. Plast. Reconstr. Surg., 51:524–529, 1973.

Mahler, D., and Hirschowitz, S.: Tangential excision and grafting for burns of the hand. Br. J. Plast. Surg., 29:78–81, 1976.

Moncrief, J., Lindberg, R., Switzer, W., and Pruitt, B.: Use of topical sulfonomide in burn wound sepsis. J. Trauma, 6:407–419, 1966.

Moncrief, J., Switzer, W., and Rose, L.: Primary exci-

sion and grafting treatment of third degree burns of the dorsum of the hand. Plast. Reconstr. Surg., 33:305, 1964.

Moyer, C. A., Brentano, L., Gravens, D. L., Margraf, H., and Monafo, W.: Treatment of large human burns with 0.5 per cent silver nitrate solution. Arch. Surg., 90:812, 1965.

Peacock, E. E., Madden, J. W., and Tier, W. C.: Some studies on the treatment of burned hands. Ann. Surg., 171:903, 1970.

Shuck, J. M., Pruitt, B., and Moncrief, J.: Homograft skin for wound coverage. Arch. Surg., 98, 1969.

Wexler, M. R., Yoschua, Z., and Newman, Z.: Early treatment of burns of the dorsum of the hand by tangential excision and skin grafting. Plast. Reconstr. Surg., 54:268–274, 1974.

Whitson, T. C., Major, M. C., and Allen, B.: Management of the burned hand. J. Trauma, 11:606–614, 1971.

Zaroff, L., Mills, W., Duckett, J., Jr., Switzer, W., and Moncrief, J.: Multiple uses of viable cutaneous homografts in burned patients. Surgery, 59:368–372, 1966.

COLOR PLATES

PLATE I

Blood Supply of the Extensor Apparatus of the Fingers (Microangiographic Study by Maeda and Matsui).

The vascularization of the extensors differs from that of the flexors. The vessels arise from dorsal branches of the proper digital arteries. Their branches anastomose to form a terminal network on the superficial and deep surfaces of the aponeurosis. The superficial network is clearly more abundant than the deep network, which corresponds to the gliding surface. The zones of contact with the interphalangeal articulations are virtually avascular. The vascular supply, both to extensors and flexors, diminishes with age, and the reduction becomes marked by the beginning of the sixth decade.

Figure 1. The blood supply of the extensor apparatus is provided by dorsal branches of the proper digital arteries.

Figure 2. Dorsal view of the extensor apparatus, showing the longitudinal vessels on each side of the extensor digitorum communis and the terminal anastomotic plexus.

Figure 3. Palmar view of the extensor apparatus. The vessels are visible at the level of the metacarpal and proximal phalanges, but they are markedly reduced distally.

Figure 4. Terminal vessels not detectable by microangiography may be seen on this print.

Figure 5. The terminal vessels cross the central slip of the common extensor and lateral bands. Others anastomose with the vessels of the interosseous and lumbrical muscles.

Figure 6. The extensor apparatus of the thumb. Although the anatomical structure of the thumb differs from that of the fingers, the blood supply is similar.

Figure 7. The vascular network extends throughout the length of the extensor apparatus in the thumb.

Figure 8. Diminished vascular supply to the extensor apparatus in the left index finger of a 52-year-old man.

Figure 9. Same as the preceding illustration following clarification.

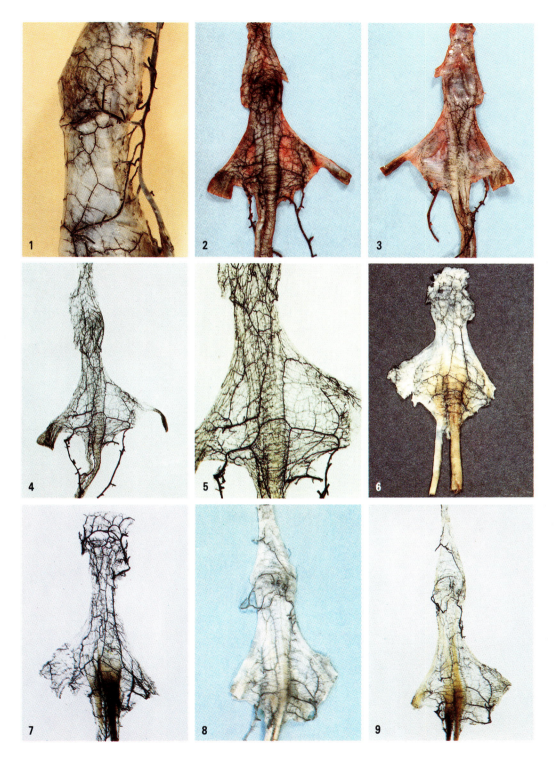

PLATE I

PLATE II

Blood Supply of the Flexor Tendons. Influence of Age and Variations of the Vincula (Matsui and Hunter).

Two vascular systems are evident at the level of the deep flexor tendon. The proximal system, as far as the base of the proximal phalanx, is made up of longitudinal vessels originating in the palm that are joined by vessels supplying the synovial membrane. This system supplies the anterior and central portions of the tendon. The distal system supplies the vincula of the dorsal portion of the tendon.

The blood vessels change orientation at the boundary between the proximal and distal systems, which is located at the base of the proximal phalanx. There is an avascular zone in the distal anterior part of the deep tendon. Although the short vincula have a consistent morphology, the same is not true of the long vincula. In most cases the long vinculum of the deep flexor tendon is supplied by vessels from the short vinculum of the superficial flexor tendon at the level of Camper's chiasm. In some instances, however, the long vinculum of the deep flexor is fed directly from the long vinculum of the superficial flexor. In other instances the long vinculum of the deep flexor is supplied by vessels from the synovial membrane between the two slips of the superficial flexor tendon proximal to the chiasm. Rarely, the long vinculum is absent. Progressive diminution of the blood supply with age is clearly visible in the specimens shown here.

Figure 1. Blood supply of the flexor tendons in a newborn, 10 hours old.

Figure 2. Good blood supply to the flexor tendons of the middle finger in a 26-year-old woman.

Figure 3. Diminished blood supply to the flexor tendons of the index finger in a 52-year-old man.

Figure 4. Variations in the long vinculum of the deep flexor tendon of the little finger in a 52-year-old subject.

Figure 5. The index finger of a 52-year-old subject.

Figure 6. The ring finger of a 40-year-old subject.

Figure 7. Absence of a deep flexor tendon vinculum in the right finger of a 26-year-old subject.

Figure 8. A large vinculum, resembling a mesotendon, in the fifth finger of an 8-year-old child.

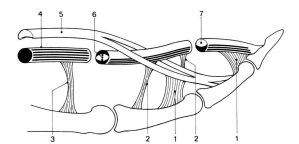

Diagram of the blood supply of the flexor tendons. *1,* Short vinculum; *2,* long vinculum; *3,* synovial membrane; *4,* deep flexor tendon; *5,* superficial flexor tendon; *6,* crossover zone; *7,* avascular zone.

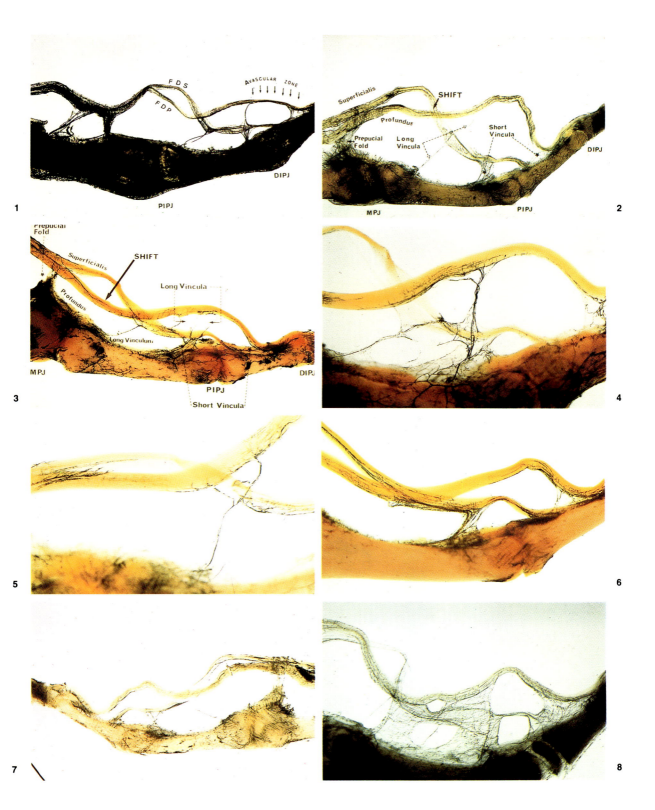

PLATE II

Top: Radial nerve. *1*, Anterior sensory branch; *2*, branch of extensor carpi radialis brevis; *3*, extensor carpi radialis longus; *4*, brachioradialis; *5*, posterior interosseous nerve; *6*, posterior sensory branches; *A*, intraneural fasciculation of the superficial (sensory) radial nerve. *B*, intraneural fasciculation of the posterior interosseous nerve.

Middle: Median nerve. *1*, Pronator teres; *2*, anterior interosseous nerve (pronator quadratus); *3*, palmar cutaneous branch; *4*, flexor digitorum superficialis; *5*, thenar muscular branch; *6*, common palmar digital nerves; *A*, intraneural fasciculation of the pronator teres; *B*, intraneural fasciculation of the flexor digitorum superficialis; *C*, intraneural fasciculation of the pronator quadratus; *D*, intraneural fasciculation of the thenar muscular branch; *E*, intraneural fasciculation of the palmar cutaneous branch.

Bottom: Ulnar nerve. *1*, Flexor carpi ulnaris; *2*, flexor digitorum profundus; *3*, dorsal cutaneous branch; *4*, deep terminal motor branch; *5*, palmar sensory branches; *A*, intraneural fasciculation of the deep terminal motor branch; *B*, intraneural fasciculation of the flexor digitorum profundus; *C*, intraneural fasciculation of the flexor carpi ulnaris; *D*, intraneural fasciculation of the dorsal cutaneous branch.

PLATE III

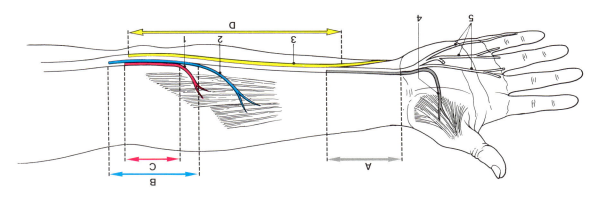

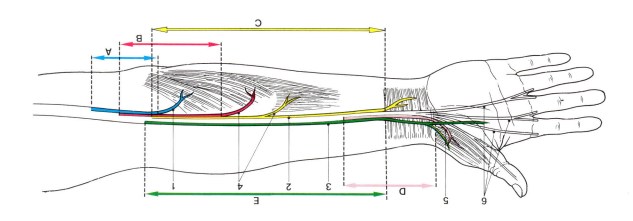

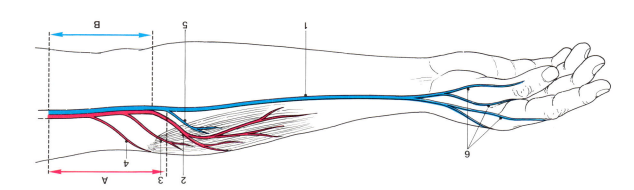

PLATE IV

The Brachial Plexus

1. C4
2. C5
3. C6
4. To phrenic nerve
5. C7
6. Phrenic nerve
7. C8
8. T1
9. Subclavian artery
10. Subclavian vein
11. Subclavius muscle
12. Long thoracic nerve
13. Second rib
14. Superior subscapular nerve
15. Second intercostal nerve
16. Subscapular artery
17. Thoracodorsal nerve
18. Inferior subscapular nerve
19. Pectoralis minor
20. Pectoralis major
21. Serratus anterior
22. Subclavius nerve
23. Suprascapular nerve
24. Subscapular artery
25. Trapezius
26. Acromiothoracic artery
27. Pectoralis minor

28. Upper subscapular nerve
29. Cephalic vein
30. Musculocutaneous nerve
31. Pectoralis major
32. Deltoid
33. Coracobrachialis nerve (branch of musculocutaneous)
34. Median nerve
35. Coracobrachialis
36. Biceps brachii
37. Axillary nerve
38. Radial nerve
39. Deep brachial artery
40. Axillary artery
41. Branch of musculocutaneous nerve to long head of biceps
42. Ulnar nerve
43. Axillary vein
44. Medial cutaneous nerve of forearm (medial antebrachial cutaneous nerve)
45. Medial cutaneous nerve of arm (medial brachial cutaneous nerve)
46. Latissimus dorsi
47. Accessory nerve
48. Branch to rhomboideus from dorsal scapular nerve
49. Scalenus anterior

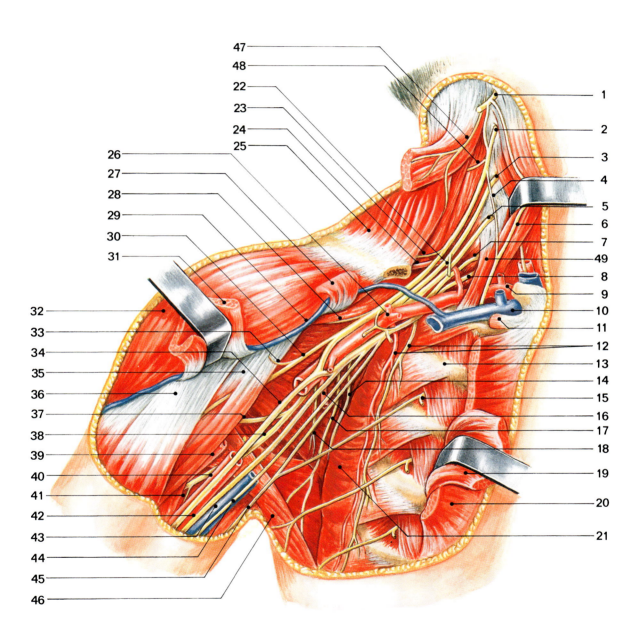

PLATE IV

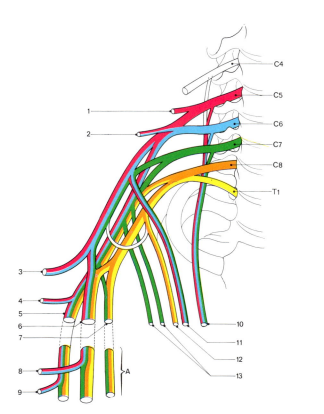
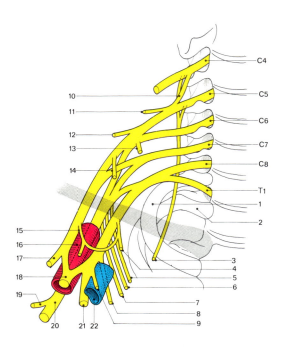

Upper left: Diagram of the brachial plexus. *1*, Dorsoscapular nerve; *2*, suprascapular nerve; *3*, musculocutaneous nerve; *4*, axillary nerve; *5*, radial nerve; *6*, median nerve; *7*, ulnar nerve; *8*, pronator teres and flexor carpi radialis nerve; *9*, brachioradialis and extensor carpi radialis nerve; *10*, serratus anterior nerve; *11*, lateral pectoral nerve; *12*, medial pectoral nerve; *13*, latissimus dorsi and teres major nerves; *A*, distal to elbow.

Upper right: Distribution of the brachial plexus. *1*, First rib; *2*, second rib; *3*, long thoracic nerve; *4*, medial pectoral nerve; *5*, superior subscapular nerve; *6*, thoracodorsal nerve; *7*, inferior subscapular nerve; *8*, medial cutaneous nerve of arm; *9*, medial cutaneous nerve of forearm; *10*, to C5; *11*, branch to rhomboideus from dorsal nerve; *12*, suprascapular nerve; *13*, subclavian nerve; *14*, lateral pectoral nerve; *15*, to pectoralis major; *16*, axillary artery; *17*, musculocutaneous nerve; *18*, median nerve; *19*, axillary nerve; *20*, radial nerve; *21*, ulnar nerve; *22*, axillary vein.

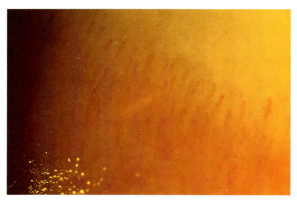
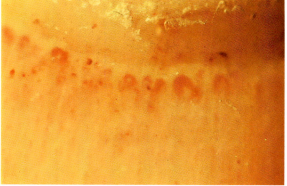

Bottom: Capillaroscopy of the nailbed. *Left*, Normal. *Right*, Scleroderma. (Courtesy of Prof. M. Vayssairat.)

PLATE V

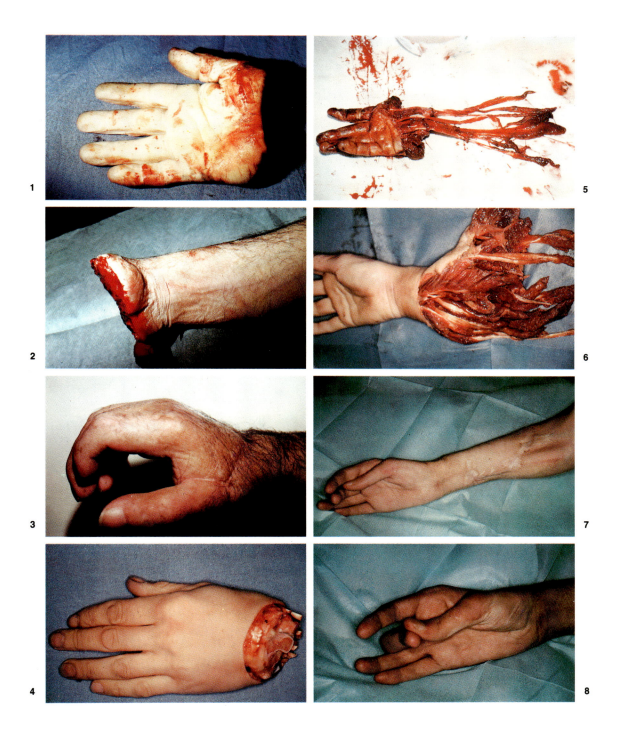

PLATE VI

Replantation

Figures 1 and 2. Cut section of the hand at the proximal part of the palm.

Figure 3. Result after 2 years.

Figure 4. Hand amputation by a saber.

Figure 5. Avulsion of four fingers with stripping of tendons.

Figure 6. Avulsion of the muscles of the forearm.

Figures 7 and 8. Results in the patient shown in Figure 6. Extension of the fingers and restoration of a thumb-to-third finger pinch by opposition plasty of the thumb.

PLATE VII

Toe Transfer for Traumatic Amputation of the Left Thumb with Preservation of the Base of the First Phalanx in a 21-Year-Old Man.

Figure 1. Appearance just before toe transfer.

Figure 2. Radiographic appearance.

Figure 3. The hand is prepared and the structures identified.

Figure 4. The donor toe. The profundus tendon has been retained in order to allow its anastomosis at the wrist.

Figure 5. The area of skin loss is covered by a rotation flap.

Figure 6. Six months after operation: the foot.

Figure 7. The thumb.

Figure 8. Opposition of the thumb.

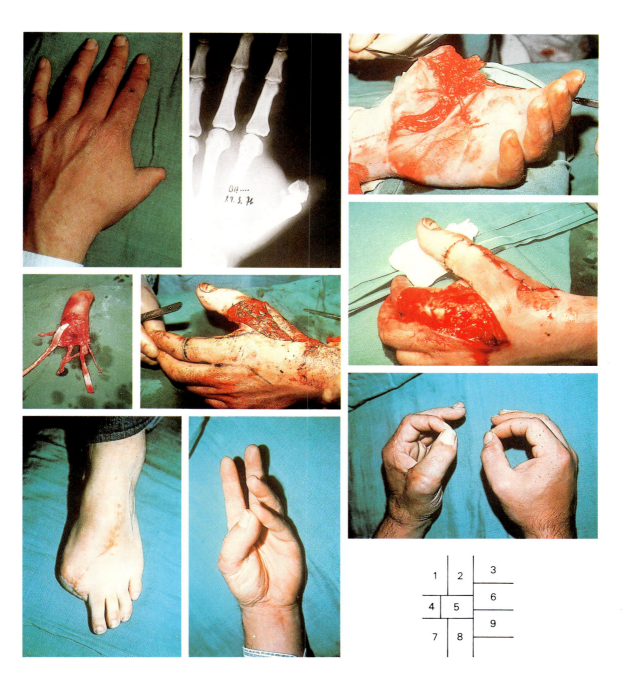

PLATE VII

PLATE VIII

Partial Toe Transfers.

Figures 1 to 4. Large soft tissue loss from the distal phalanx of the index finger of the dominant hand in a 9-year-old child following a lawn mower accident. *Figure 1.* Free flap of pulp from the second toe to cover the defect. *Figure 2.* The common digital artery was chosen to supply the transplanted tissue, and the collateral digital nerve was sutured as far distally as possible. *Figure 3.* Minimal sequelae in the toe. *Figure 4.* Good esthetic and functional result; two-point discrimination was 8 mm.

Figures 5 to 7. Distal amputation of the thumb of the dominant hand in a young woman. *Figure 5.* Two painful distal neuromas hinder use of the hand. *Figure 6.* Composite transfer of one piece of pulp, a fragment of vascularized bone taken longitudinally from the phalanx of the great toe, and the ungual complex. *Figure 7.* Good esthetic and functional result provided by reconstruction symmetrical to the normal hand.

Figures 8 to 11. Proximal amputation of the thumb in a child. *Figures 8 and 9.* The vascularized skeleton and the flexor and extensor tendons of the second toe were transferred with the skin and nail of the first toe. *Figure 10.* The foot was reconstructed by covering the skeleton of the first toe with the skin of the second. *Figure 11.* The advantage of this composite transfer is that it supplied vascularized bone (avoiding resorption), tendons, a joint (with interphalangeal mobility limited to 20 degrees in this case), and epiphyseal cartilage.

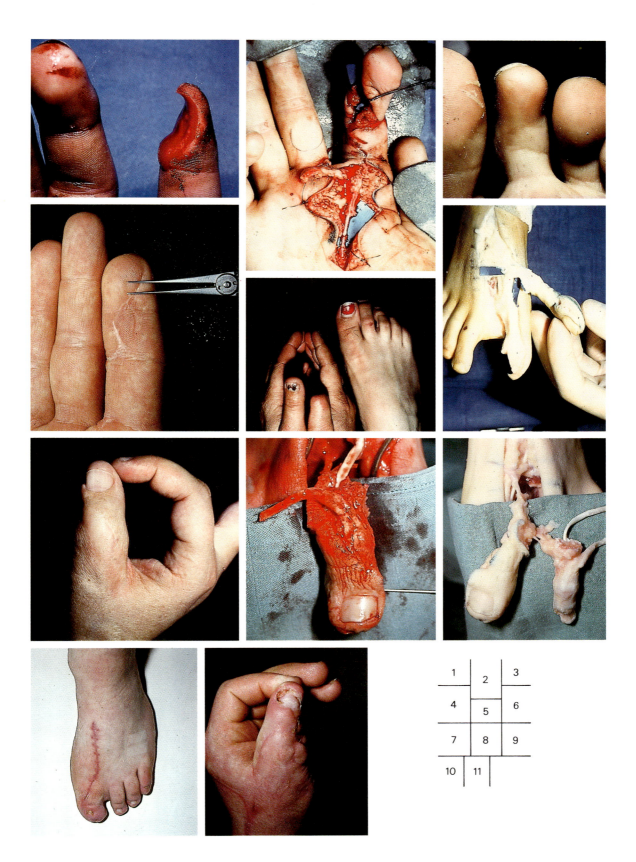

PLATE VIII

THE MANAGEMENT OF HAND BURNS: A CONSERVATIVE APPROACH WITH PRESERVATION OF MAXIMAL FUNCTION

GUY TRENGOVE-JONES

Conservative treatment distinguishes management from active early surgical intervention, but does not imply inactivity. It embraces the concept that the immobilization of a hand after injury can have permanent consequences in terms of limitation of movement. Therefore, an approach to hand burns in which function is maintained throughout permits a better end result. However, this does not preclude surgical intervention, but permits healing to continue in the more equivocal cases in some instances and therefore obviates surgery without losing function. When surgery is indicated, nothing is lost, because a full range of motion is maintained throughout. In essence, conservative management is synonymous with preservation of function and depends entirely on dressing technique. The ideal method in our experience is the use of a plastic bag or glove and the topical application of an antimicrobial drug.

BACKGROUND

The concept of two to three weeks of splintage for burned hands was proposed by Robertson in 1958. This concept has now been seriously questioned (Boswick, 1974; Labanter et al., 1966). Indeed there is good evidence that the optimal functional result for a given burned hand is dependent on the preservation and maintenance of motion.

This is not to say that tangential excision and grafting or formal excision and grafting that are appropriate to the depth and area of the burn are not performed as indicated (Boswick, 1970; Scovich, 1917), but continual physical therapy is the key in the cooperative patient (in contradistinction to the unconscious and the young patient). Principal difficulties in maintaining motion are pain, swelling, restrictive dressings, and hard eschar or coagulum.

A number of mobilization regimes have been proposed, all requiring major active patient cooperation and a great deal of help from the physical therapy and nursing staff (Boswick, 1974; Labanter et al., 1966). We have found that the technique to be detailed, by reducing all these factors, has helped dramatically in the mobilization of patients with burned hands. We have also found it of particular help in the overall management of bilateral hand burns, because the hands can be practically functional in terms of feeding and other daily activities. We use the technique in association with elevation, splintage, positioning, active and passive range of motion exercises, and surgery, when indicated.

TECHNIQUE

1. All burns in conscious adults are dressed by this method.
2. Depending on the total area and depth

of burn and the patient's general condition, the burn is treated on an inpatient or outpatient basis.

3. Standard, suitably sized sterile surgical gloves or plastic bags are used. The starch powder should be washed out from the gloves with the sterile saline.

4. Silver sulfadiazine is usually used topically as an antibiotic and lubricant inside the glove.

5. The nonpermeable covering is applied as soon after the burn as possible, usually within 24 hours.

The initial patient and attendant apprehension is overcome by the use of analgesics and by the obvious rapid gain in comfort when the patient is safely within this plastic microcosm. The frequency of glove change is dictated by the nature of the burn. This usually means that the glove is changed every four to six hours. The patient's hand is cleaned completely by irrigation and débrided when necessary between glove changes. Scrupulous observation of the cleansing irrigation is necessary, for if the surface is not fully clean, superinfection and conversion in terms of depth can result. Fresh silver sulfadiazine is then applied and the hand is replaced within the hand bag. The early regimen of absolute elevation is observed for 24 to 48 hours, or longer if required. The patient is encouraged to feed himself and perform his own toilet needs; this is particularly valuable in bilateral burns. The patient is also encouraged to undertake his own hourly active physical therapy (for an inpatient attended by a physical therapist, two to three times a day). Both active and passive range of motion exercises are performed within the gloves. Outpatients are given a regimen by the physical therapist to follow at home. Night splintage is, in fact, facilitated because the hand can more easily conform to molded plastic splints, maintaining an "Edinburgh position" (Boswick, 1970). Thus, accurate splintage is facilitated.

Surgery, if indicated, is performed at the earliest possible moment, but postoperative splintage is limited to 72 to 96 hours. The patient's hands can then be placed back into the gloves. The indication for this conservative approach is first degree hand burns, which invariably infect the dorsum only and are eminently suitable for this method of treatment; the blistering and rupturing are well facilitated by a loose plastic dressing.

Second degree burns have to be assessed on their own merits. The initial assessment is the most accurate. The general condition of the patient, the patient's age, and the overall extent of the burn play a large part in the decision making process. All second degree superficial and intermediate burns must be kept sterile and are fully functional in this type of dressing. The risks of conversion are probably less. If the wound does appear to be slow to heal and function has not been lost, in our experience the excision and skin grafting procedure can be delayed beyond the first week without compromising the long term result. Thus, it is in this group that unnecessary surgery can be avoided, without loss of function.

In the deep second degree burn or deep dermal burn, in which the chances of primary healing are greatly reduced, early tangential excision or total excision and grafting constitute the treatment of choice. However, while awaiting surgery a light mobile dressing not only maintains the correct environment but while providing early motion facilitates subsidence of the edema. This not only improves the ultimate take of the skin graft but by improving circulation perhaps will serve to reduce the risk of infection.

The clinical indicators of burn depth are capillary refill, sensation, and skin turgor. The latter is most helpful when one is trying to decide whether to do an escharotomy. In the full thickness burn, with or without escharotomies, motion can be maintained, edema reduced, and the burns kept sterile in this type of occlusive dressing. Here early surgery is without doubt the treatment of choice, followed by early mobilization. Figures 70–1 and 70–2 demonstrate how a plastic bag dressing is used. The range of motion within the range of motion is also demonstrated.

DISCUSSION

There have been previous descriptions of the use of plastic bags and silicone bags containing silcone gel as dressings for burned hands (James, 1970). The latter have the disadvantage of bulk and possible dependency. The rubber glove, which can be applied if there is minimal edema, gives the patient the most dexterity. It is important to stress, however, that the humidity within the bag, while making the normal skin and eschar

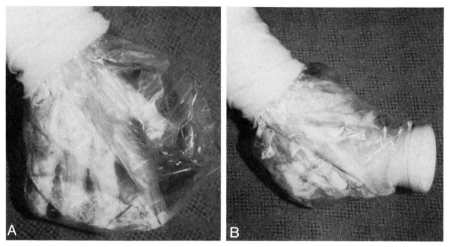

Figure 70–1. *A* and *B,* The burned hand in extension and functionally active in a plastic bag.

supple, does produce considerable "wrinkling" and a somewhat unhealthy appearance. I do not believe that anything is lost by this phenomenon. It is essential to maintain initial adequate levels of analgesia so that the patient can go through the range of motion exercises without unreasonable pain. With encouragement, the pattern will be self-propagated. We have used this approach for all burns, with the exception of deep second and third degree burns during the immediate postgraft period, to objectively assess and compare the treatment of hand burns with the many variables of age, constitution, depth of burn, and overall patient condition. The intangibles of patient cooperation and pain tolerance are extremely difficult to judge. It

is my opinion that patients managed by this form of nonrestrictive dressing have maintained an excellent if not better range of motion than they would have with more conventional dressings. It is also possible to visualize the wound through a transparent covering. The physical therapy is essential and facilitative, and the patient has a greater appreciation of his progress.

After skin grafting, the shearing forces so damaging to the take of a skin graft are minimized. In full thickness burns, the sloughing skin softens and separates quickly. In mixed partial full thickness burns, granulation tissue flourishes and marginal epithelialization proceeds.

It must be stated that the appearance of

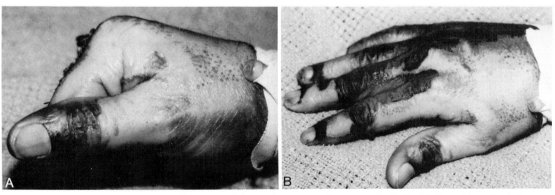

Figure 70–2. *A* and *B,* An intermediate second degree burn treated conservatively for 10 days. Note the full range of movement.

rapid healing of the mixed partial full thickness burn can mislead one into continuing conservative management in patients who will ultimately need grafting. However, I think that the absolute necessity for surgical intervention is less. The possible increased chance of hypertrophic scarring can now be judged by the widespread usage of pressure therapy. Possibly time out of work could be extended from seven to 10 days if skin grafting is needed ultimately. This must be balanced against the cases in which surgery is implemented in burns that could possibly have healed spontaneously. It is possible that the overall cosmetic effect may be less optimal than with excision and grafting of the entire cosmetic unit of the dorsum of the hand. However, the perimeter scarring and possible "overgrafting" effects can be fairly prevalent with this more radical surgical approach. I do not think, therefore, that cosmesis should enter into the decision. Function is the most important determinant.

REFERENCES

Boswick, J. A.: 1970. Management of the burned hand. Orthop. Clin. N. Am., *1:*311, 1970.

Boswick, J. A.: Rehabilitation of the burned hand. Clin. Orthop., *104:*162–174, 1974.

James, J. I. P.: Common problems in the management of injuries. Proc. R. Soc. Med., *63:*69, 1970.

Labanter, H., Kaplan, I., and Sharitt, C.: Burns of the dorsum of the hand. Conservative treatment with intensive physical therapy versus tangential excision and grafting. Br. J. Plast. Surg., *29:*352–354, 1966.

Robertson, D. C.: The management of the burned hand. J. Bone Joint Surg., *40A:*625, 1958.

Scovich, I.: New concepts in the early excision and immediate grafting of burns. J. Trauma, *10:*1103, 1917.

Chapter 71

ELECTRICAL INJURIES OF THE UPPER LIMB

John A. E. Hobby

and James Ellsworth Laing

Electrical burns account for about 3 per cent of the admissions to major burns units (DiVincenti et al., 1969). In our unit 169 electrical burns in a total of 3357 admissions were treated between 1960 and 1979. Seventy per cent of these burns involved the upper limb. This clinical problem is uncommon, but the local and distant effects of electrical injury make this a difficult area for treatment.

Electrical injury to the upper limb is of two main types—low tension injuries (less than 400 volts) resulting from accidents in the home with domestic appliances and industrial high tension injuries (more than 400 volts).

The wounds resulting from electrical injury are extremely variable, but are of four main types:

1. A true electrical injury is caused by the passage of an electric current through the skin to the tissue from the conductor.

2. "Arc" burns are produced by current passing external to the body from the contact point to the ground. These burns are associated with high tension injuries and may be severe and deep because the arc temperature can be as high as 11,000° C. at its center. The existence of the current arc means that the patient does not have to be in direct contact with the conductor to suffer injury, because the current can arc in ordinary atmospheric conditions up to 1 inch (2.5 cm.) for every 20,000 volts. Once in contact, the patient can draw the arc away from the conductor for up to 10 feet (3 m.) from the highest live voltages.

3. Flame burns may result from ignition of clothing in high tension injuries associated with arcing. These burns may be more serious than the original electric burn, and they are often full thickness burns owing to the prolonged exposure time.

4. Direct contact with the bars of electrical heating appliances, particularly in children, may result in burns. The effects of electrical current in these burns is negligible, but the temperatures of the red hot elements may be as high as 600 to 800° C. and result in deep full thickness burns.

THE EFFECTS OF ELECTRICAL CURRENT

The effects of electrical current have been elucidated by Kouwenhoven (1949) and Hodgkin (1974). Electrical energy generates a potential difference or voltage (V) between two points, which results in a flow of current (I) between them, measured in amperes. It is the flow of current that damages tissues, and the intensity of the current may be life threatening. As current flows through tissues, electrical energy is converted to heat (the Joule effect). The strength of a current passing through the tissues depends on the voltage applied and the resistance of the tissues (R): $I = V/R$. Insulating materials have a high resistance, which reduces current and therefore provides protection from electrical shock. Current flow may be unidirectional or direct or alternating.

Alternating current causes tetanic muscular contraction, which, if the flexor muscles of the upper limb are involved, may "lock" the victim's hand to the electrical conductor, allowing prolonged contact and therefore more severe damage. Conversely, on the dorsum of the hand or forearm, extensor muscle contraction tends to throw the limb away from the conductor, thereby minimizing injury.

Direct current does not produce the same contraction of muscles. Low tension direct current is not so dangerous as the same voltage of alternating current. However, contact with high voltage direct current is more likely to prove fatal than contact with alternating current of an equivalent voltage.

In many accidents only the voltage may be known. It is impossible to calculate the current, because the resistance at the time is unknown and may vary. That current intensity is important is shown by the Joule effect; the heat generated (calories, Q) is proportional to the current squared, multiplied by the tissue resistance ($Q \propto I^2 \times R$).

The resistance of various body tissues traversed by electrical current influences the amount of injury. Body resistance has two main components—high resistance of skin and internal resistance, which because of the body's salinity tends to be low except for bone and tendon, which have a relatively high resistance.

Dry epidermis has a high resistance, which varies depending on skin thickness and vascularity, but on average is about 40,000 ohms per square centimeter; callouses on the palms in manual workers may have a resistance value of 1,000,000 ohms per square centimeter. The dorsum of the hand offers less resistance to the passage of electrical current because the skin is thinner. Moisture, however, can have a profound effect on skin resistance, reducing it to only 300 ohms per square centimeter. The resistance of the skin may vary, depending upon the applied voltage and temperature, as well as moisture. High tension injuries tend to char and coagulate the skin, leading to increased resistance, whereas low tension injuries if prolonged may result in blister formation with a resulting fall in resistance. At 50 volts blister formation occurs in six to seven seconds and, because I = V/R, there is a resultant increase in current strength, which may have catastrophic cardiac or respiratory effects.

In the upper limb, bone also has a high resistance, whereas nerve tissue, blood vessels, and tissue fluid are good conductors because of their salinity. The internal resistance, except for bone, is therefore small. The greater the resistance of tissue, the greater the heat produced when current flows

and the greater the local tissue damage. In high tension injuries heat is the principal mediator of tissue damage and is inversely proportional to the unit cross sectional area of the tissue involved. This accounts for the frequency of severe injuries to the upper limb and the rarity of severe injuries to the main body trunk.

Resistance to current in the upper limb is a characteristic of the skin and internally of bone. In high tension injuries, severe tissue damage occurs in association with these two structures, resulting in charring of the skin and periosseous tissue damage. Cooling then follows, heat loss being greater in the superficial tissues. In the deep tissues around bone, heat loss is delayed, and because tissue damage depends not only on absolute temperature but also on the length of contact with the heat source, severe injuries may occur around bone despite apparently normal superficial muscle.

This fact must be kept in mind in performing escharotomy, fasciotomy, and débridement (to be discussed). As already mentioned, the power of alternating current that flows through the body is extremely important, as is the direction of the flow. Hodgkin (1974) has demonstrated that 60 hertz (cycles per second) shocks one second or more in duration from limb to limb have the following effects: perception at 1 milliampere, a sensation of pain at 5 milliamperes, and tetanic muscle contraction at 15 milliamperes, which, if it affects the flexor muscles, results in the "no let go" phenomenon already described. At twice this current (30 milliamperes) the respiratory muscles tetanically contract, resulting in respiratory failure. Similarly, at twice this current (60 milliamperes), current density in the heart is enough to cause ventricular fibrillation. Currents between 60 and 5000 milliamperes likewise cause cardiac fibrillation. Above this level, current causes respiratory failure, convulsions, and burns.

The area and site of contact affect the outcome of electrical shock. Large areas of contact result in low contact resistance and consequently large current levels. If contacts are on the same limb, current flows only through that limb and vital centers, such as the heart, brain, and lungs, are unaffected. If contacts are from limb to limb, the limbs provide resistance to flow, but the current is distributed throughout the volume between the contact points. The most dangerous areas of contact are obviously from upper limb to upper limb, circuiting straight across the chest. Electrical contact over a small area increases the contact resistance, resulting in greater local tissue destruction.

THE APPEARANCE OF ELECTRICAL WOUNDS

Burn wounds occur at the entrance and exit sites of electrical current. The hands are a common entrance site because of the nature of electrical work, and the soles of the feet often transmit current to the ground. When the entrance and exit wounds both occur on the same upper limb, severe internal destruction in the limb is likely (Fig. 71–1). In general, greater damage occurs at the entrance site.

The burns vary from small circular spots a few millimeters across to areas many centimeters wide. They tend to have raised, well defined edges and irregular excavated centers. As already emphasized, they are not a good guide to the deep damage that may have occurred. The initial examination may reveal very little, but after a few days, areas of necrosis become obvious (Fig. 71–2). The usual entrance site appears as an ischemic, dry, white or yellow coagulated area, slightly depressed and painless; some charring may be present (Fig. 71–3). Fragments of metal wire or the imprint of a metal wire may be present in the wound.

Exit lesions, in contrast, tend to be of the "blowout" or "gunshot" type; the skin is often scorched and marked by radiating tears (Fig. 71–4). Blister formation at entrance and exit wounds is rare because heat coagulation prevents any inflammatory reaction in the tissues, although after 24 to 48 hours, an area of erythema and edema appears around and deep to the burn.

The burns are deep and extend into the subcutaneous tissues where tendons, muscles, nerves, cartilage, and bone may be destroyed. Coagulation necrosis from heat results in the initial damage to skin and deep structures, but this may subsequently spread as a result of arterial lesions. The internal destruction may be extensive and progressive.

Tissues are destroyed not only deep to the entrance wound but along the path of the current, particularly in the "resistance" tissues, such as bone and tendon. Muscles may be paralyzed as a result of nerve lesions. Blood vessels are good conductors of electrical current, and as a result vascular and other damage may occur at a distance from the original injury. Marked arterial spasm and vessel wall necrosis may extend the area of necrosis, producing uneven ischemic necrosis of muscles. Sometimes palpable pulses are present in the main arteries of the upper limb, although nutrient vessels to the muscles are occluded. Uneveness of muscle injury is characteristic of electrical injury. Gangrene of part or all of the upper limb may be related to the entrance or exit sites if they both occur on the same limb, as stated previously (Fig. 71–1). A further hazard of medial necrosis of the vessel wall, if not followed by thrombosis, may be delayed hemorrhage.

Flame burns resulting from the ignition of

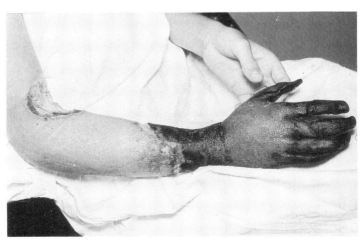

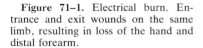

Figure 71–1. Electrical burn. Entrance and exit wounds on the same limb, resulting in loss of the hand and distal forearm.

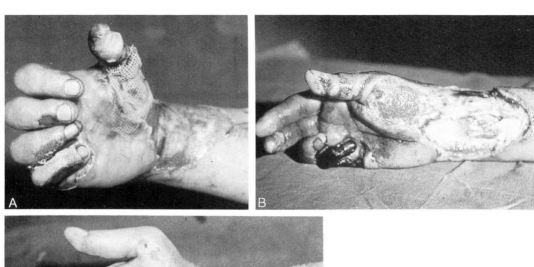

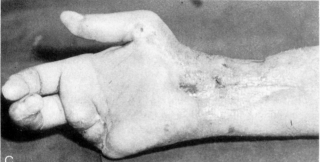

Figure 71–2. *A*, Initial burn injury. *B*, Necrosis obvious at 14 days. *C*, Resultant amputation of the fourth and fifth digits of the hand.

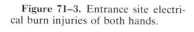

Figure 71–3. Entrance site electrical burn injuries of both hands.

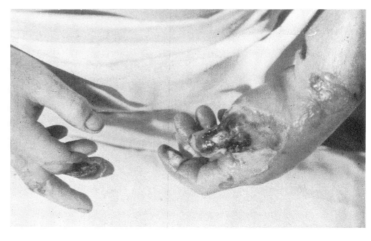

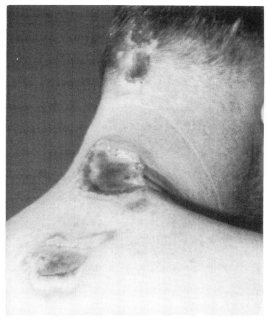

Figure 71–4. Exit site lesions of patient shown in Figure 71–3.

clothing or from current arcing may be associated with electrical burns, particularly of the high tension type. These burns are often more extensive than the true electrical injuries and are similar to normal thermal burns. However, they do tend to be deep burns because of the prolonged burning time, especially if any cerebral confusion follows the electrical injury.

Thermoelectrical contact burns are not true electrical injuries. They occur mainly in young children and are described, together with their treatment, in other chapters in this section.

TREATMENT PLAN

Those first on the scene must ensure that the patient is disconnected from the electrical supply, either by switching off the current or by cutting the supply cable using insulated pliers or a wooden handled axe.

The electrical phenomena associated with cardiac fibrillation and respiratory arrest have already been described. They deserve emphasis, because mouth to mouth resuscitation and external cardiac massage may be life saving in these cases, prior to the patient's transfer to a hospital where facilities for cardiac defibrillation and endotracheal intubation are available. Respiratory arrest may necessitate endotracheal intubation, oxygen administration, and mechanical ventilation. Cardiac fibrillation requires cardiac defibrillation, although minor cardiac arrhythmias, which are not uncommon, last for 48 to 72 hours and invariably resolve spontaneously.

Patients subject to electrocution may lose consciousness or fall, sustaining associated fractures, dislocations, or head injuries. These must be looked for and appropriate treatment instituted.

FLUID RESUSCITATION

During the past 20 years, 3357 burn patients, including those with electrical burns, were treated in our unit. It is our practice to institute intravenous infusions in adult patients with burns involving more than 15 per cent of the body surface and in children in whom the burns involve more than 10 per cent of body surface area. Intravenous infusion has been necessary in 780 patients, i.e., 23.2 per cent of the total. We use colloid, not crystalloid, solutions. In the first 15 years of this period, plasma was used, and during the last five years plasma protein fraction has been used. During this period no patients have received a volume of fluid greater than their own blood volume (which can easily be calculated by multiplying the body weight in kilograms by 75) during the first 36 hours following the burn injury. To this must be added the insensible loss and loss from vomiting should fluids not be tolerated by mouth. No central venous pressure lines or urinary catheters are used, although 24 hour urine specimens are collected for analysis. We regard the urine concentrating power as particularly important. This regimen has the great value of simplicity. Throughout this period there have been four deaths associated with renal failure, although no deaths due to this cause have occurred in our electrical burn patients.

This philosophy is at variance with that described in the American literature. Hunt and Sato (1980) and Baxter et al. (1967) believe that the minimal fluid requirement for a patient with a high tension electrical burn is 4 ml. of Ringer's lactate per kilogram per percentage of body surface area burned. When there is underlying muscle damage, they increase the volume of intravenous fluids in order to maintain a urine output of 100 ml. per hour until hemoglobin and hemochromogens disappear from the urine. They also recommend that 44.5 mEq. of sodium bicarbonate be added to each liter of fluid until an alkaline urine pH is established. Mannitol (12.5 gm.) as a bolus or continuous infusion is recommended at the start of resusitation. They recommend this regimen in order to prevent the development of acute tubular necrosis and renal failure.

Acute tubular necrosis in these circumstances is probably due to a combination of factors, among which are hypotension, dehydration, thermal damage, hypokalemia, rhabdomyolysis, myoglobinuria, and hemoglobinuria (Editorial, 1978). However, the use of this regimen is not universally successful, Hunt (1976) reported 84 patients with electrical injuries of the upper limb, of whom four developed acute tubular necrosis and renal failure; there was a fatal outcome in three. Similar cases have been reported by Baxter et al. (1967) and Butler and Gant (1977). Refractory oliguria in some of these patients has been corrected by removal of large amounts of necrotic tissue or limb amputation.

We have presented the two philosophies but recommend the former "simple" approach. As already described, the development of acute tubular necrosis is multifactorial, one of the major causes being oligemia, which in our series has been rare. This may be because we operate within a small geographical area and intravenous plasma infusions are instituted prior to the admission of patients being sent us.

Patients normally arrive at our hospital within three hours after the electrical burn injury. When there is massive muscle necrosis, we perform an early excision of necrotic muscle and other dead tissue, because we believe that the presence of dead muscle is a significant cause of subsequent renal problems.

WOUND MANAGEMENT

Low tension electrical entrance and exit wounds should be kept clean and dry. We routinely use the exposure method of treatment. Hand burns are treated in plastic bag occlusive dressings. Active hand exercises in elevation are encouraged, because we believe this to be of greater value than static splinting in a functional position. However, if splinting and dressings are necessary, particularly in the unconscious patient, correct hand positioning can be achieved by placing the wrist in 30 degrees of extension. This automatically flexes the metacarpophalangeal joints to a right angle, the proximal interphalangeal joints to 30 degrees, and distal interphalangeal joints to 15 degrees of flexion. If full thickness burns occur over the flexor or extensor tendons, particularly over the metacarpophalangeal joints, we splint the hands straight. We believe that some shortening in the metacarpophalangeal joint collaterals is preferable to a contracted flexor tendon or a ruptured extensor tendon with exposure of the dorsal metacarpophalangeal joints. The majority of postburn contractures in the fingers tend to follow ischemia and shortening in the intrinsic muscles. Reversal of ischemia in the intrinsic muscles is aided by the early resolution of edema by exercises in elevation and intermittent positive pressure compression therapy combined with escharotomy over the intermetacarpal spaces. The nonburned areas are cleaned with normal saline, and any adjacent blisters associated with deep dermal burns are deroofed and treated by the exposure method. If for any reason dressings need to be applied to the burned areas, we use nitrofurazone impregnated gauze dressings.

Edema of the upper limb may be marked in burns of the upper limb, this is a physiological response to injury.* Elevation and exercises are essential to reduce this edema. Salisbury (1973) has shown that intermittent positive pressure compression can reduce edema in the burned upper limb more quickly than elevation alone. Postoperative edema of the hand can also be reduced by using this method (Hobby, 1978).

The timing of surgery in these cases is as follows:

1. If small discrete full thickness burns are present, provided they do not overlie digital nerves or vessels, or the dorsal aspects of the metacarpophalangeal or interphalangeal joints, early excision and grafting are performed between the third and fifth days after the burn.

2. For larger burns we prefer to delay

---

*See Chapter 12 in Volume II on edema by Hobby.

surgery, particularly in children, until the tenth to fourteenth day in order to allow full thickness skin loss to declare itself.

High tension electrical injuries must be treated differently, because one's appraisal of tissue damage at the site of electrical contact often underestimates deep tissue damage. Immediate decompression by escharotomy and fasciotomy must be followed by full débridement. Escharotomy is often necessary to decompress circumferential burns in the upper limb. Venous compression appears to be the main factor in the development of edema and circulatory insufficiency.

The indications for escharotomy follow:

1. Cyanosis of distal unburned skin.

2. Impaired capillary filling, which is best judged by compression of the fingernails.

3. Progressive hypoesthesia, anesthesia, or paralysis of the distal upper limb.

4. As a clinical aid, the Doppler flow meter may be employed. Moylan et al. (1971) noted the return of palmar arch arterial flow immediately following escharotomy in the upper limb in 18 cases. They also treated 25 patients with the clinical indications for escharotomy who had an intact distal flow as determined by Doppler studies. These patients were treated only by elevation and exercises with good results. The need for escharotomy occurs within the first 72 hours, after which the edema tends to subside.

In the upper limb and fingers we prefer to make our escharotomy incisions along the medial or lateral midaxial lines, including the wrist and elbow joints when indicated. Care should be taken to make the medial escharotomy incision anterior to the medial condyle at the elbow, in order to avoid damaging the ulnar nerve.

This procedure is necessary only in full thickness or deep thermal burns, rendering anesthesia unnecessary. Some blood loss invariably occurs following this procedure, and we dress the limbs in nitrofurazone tulle gauze dressings and bandages and place the limb in elevation. The procedure may be performed as an emergency in the patient's bed. In extensive burns it may be combined with escharotomies of the chest or abdomen to relieve respiratory embarrassment. In high tension injuries when deep muscle damage is suspected, fasciotomy and débridement must be performed early in order to decrease the amount of muscle necrosis and to decrease damage to vital tendons and nerves.

Progressive muscle necrosis is not due to the high tension injury itself but to hypoxia and infection, particularly around bones, as previously described. Both these complications can be prevented by thorough débridement of all dead muscle and decompression of deep muscle compartments by fasciotomy. These procedures require general anesthesia and blood replacement. In performing débridement one should be aggressive as far as muscle is concerned but conservative where tendon and nerve tissue are concerned. Although they may seem in jeopardy, provided a biological cover is provided, remarkable recovery is sometimes possible, particularly in children. A biological cover can be provided by autoskin grafts, homografts, or flap cover (Fig. 71–5). We prefer to use the flap cover as a delayed procedure and use split skin grafts until we are sure that all nonviable muscle has been excised. This sometimes requires more than one procedure.

The extent of surgical débridement depends upon clinical judgment. The assessment of the extent of muscle damage can be aided, when facilities are available for scanning, by the use of technetium ^{99m}Tc pyrophosphate (Hunt and Sato, 1980), or enzyme studies can be performed (Coombes et al., 1978).

As with any crush or compression injury in which ischemic necrotic tissue results, there is the ever present danger of anaerobic wound infection. Tetanus immunization is essential in electrical injuries. Patients who have already been immunized require 0.5 ml. of tetanus toxoid. Patients who have not had prior immunization require 250 units of hyperimmune globulin and 0.5 ml. of tetanus toxoid, followed by 0.5 ml. of toxoid at two six-week intervals. In any suspected case of anaerobic wound infection the patient is treated with large doses of crystalline penicillin and metronidazole.

It is not our practice to give prophylactic antibiotics routinely to any burn patient. We prefer to await bacteriological and sensitivity tests, so that the appropriate antibiotics can be administered.

COMPLICATIONS

Apart from the points already mentioned, the following are of importance:

Sepsis. Local sepsis in the upper limb burn

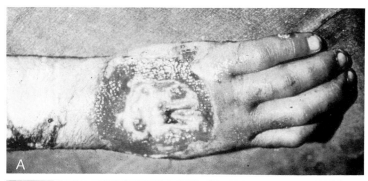

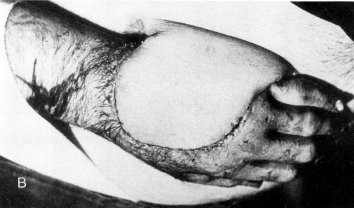

Figure 71–5. *A*, Full-thickness burn on dorsum of hand. *B*, Full-thickness skin cover obtained using a pedicled groin flap.

and systemic sepsis constitute the major cause of late morbidity and mortality in the burn patient. Aseptic technique, meticulous surgery, and the judicious use of antibiotics lessen the frequency of this complication.

Peripheral Nerve Injuries. Peripheral nerve injuries occur in about 10 per cent of the cases of high tension electrical injuries of the upper limb. Most often the median nerve in the forearm or wrist is affected, and occasionally this nerve is damaged in the palm. The ulnar nerve is next commonly affected and the radial nerve rarely so. Provided the nerves are not further damaged during surgical procedures, most patients with peripheral nerve lesions recover useful function.

Amputations. Part of a digit or single or multiple digits may be lost, or even whole limbs, depending on the severity of injury. Hunt (1976) reported an amputation rate of 43 per cent in high tension injuries, and Luce et al. (1978) reported the loss of 11 upper limbs in 18 young male patients.

Fractures. Fractures that occur in association with electrical injuries should be secured by external fixation only. Internal fixation carries a high risk of local sepsis.

Contractures. Contractures occur in skin, ligaments, tendons, and joints. They and their treatment are comprehensively dealt with in other chapters in this volume. With regard to skin contractures, however, we would like to emphasize the gratifying results obtainable with the use of pressure dressings, which are applied when primary healing has taken place. The garments are worn for a minimum of 12 months.

SUMMARY

Electrical burns of the upper limb occur infrequently but may have a devastating effect on hand and upper limb function.

The effects of electrical current on tissues and vital organs are reviewed. The beneficial effects of early resolution of edema and relief of tension in muscle compartments are outlined.

The importance of radical débridement in

high tension injuries and minimal interference in dealing with nerves and tendons is stressed. Provided all devitalized muscle is removed, one may then adopt an expectant approach. Surviving muscle may function satisfactorily with the aid of synergistic muscle groups. Bone usually recovers satisfactorily provided a local soft tissue cover can be found or distant flap tissue introduced.

The late sequelae of burns of the upper limb are enumerated. All these factors are important in the total rehabilitation of the patient and his hand function.

REFERENCES

Baxter, H., Drummond, J. A., and Dossetor, J. B.: Transactions of the Fourth International Congress. Plast. Reconstr. Surg., 196–202, 1967.

Butler, E. D., and Gant, T. D.: Injuries with special reference to the upper extremities. Am. J. Surg. 134:95–101, 1977.

Coombes, E. J., Batstone, G. F., Levick, P. L., and Shakespeare, P. G.: Serum enzymes: a guide to the aetiology of burn injury. Burns, 6:42–44, 1979.

DiVincenti, F. C., Moncrief, J. A., and Pruitt, B. A., Jr.: Electrical injuries: a review of 65 cases. J. Trauma, 9:497–507, 1969.

Editorial: Acute renal failure, hyperuricaemia, and myoglobinuria. Br. Med. J., 1233–1234, 1979.

Grossman, R. A., Hamilton, R. W., Morse, B. M., Penn, A. S., and Goldberg, M.: Nontraumatic rhabdomyolysis and acute renal failure. N. Engl. J. Med., 291:807–811, 1974.

Hobby, J. A. E.: Diminution de l'oédeme post opératoire de la main par utilisation de massages intermittents en pression positive. Groupe d'Etude de la Main. Paris, 1978.

Hodgkin, B. C.: Some consequences of electrical shock. J. Maine Med. Assoc. 65:1–3, 1974.

Hunt, J. L. In Salisbury, R. E., and Pruitt, B. A. (Editors): Burns of the Upper Extremity. Philadelphia, W. B. Saunders Company, 1976, pp. 72–83.

Hunt, J. L., and Sato, R. M.: Acute electric burns. Arch. Surg., 115:434–438, 1980.

Kouwenhoven, W. B.: Effects of electricity on the human body. Electr. Eng. 68:199–203, 1949.

Editorial: High tension electrical injury. Lancet, 2:978, 1978.

Luce, E. A., Dowden, W. L., and Hoopes, J. E.: High tension electrical injury of the upper extremity. Surg. Gynec. Obstet., 147:38, 1978.

Moylan, J. A., Inge, W. W., and Pruitt, B. A.: Circulatory changes following circumferential burns evaluated by the ultrasonic flowmeter. J. Trauma, 11:763–770, 1971.

Platts, M. M., and Rozner, L.: Survival after high tension electrical burns complicated by acute tubular necrosis. Br. Med. J. 1:781–782, 1966.

Pruitt, B. A., Dowling, J. A., and Moncrief, J. A.: Escharotomy in early burn care. Arch. Surg., 96:502–507, 1968.

Salisbury, R. E.: Post burn oedema of the upper extremity: evaluation of present treatment. J. Trauma, 13:857–862, 1973.

Sevitt, S.: Burns: Pathology and Therapeutic Applications. Louder, Butterworth & Co. (Publishers) Ltd., 1957, pp. 321–330.

Week, R. S.: The crush syndrome. Surg. Gynec. Obstet., 127:369–375, 1968.

Wilkinson, C., and Wood, M.: High voltage electric injury. Am. J. Surg., 136:693–696, 1978.

Chapter 72

ACUTE HAND BURNS IN CHILDREN—SPECIAL CONSIDERATIONS

John A. I. Grossman
and P. Esteve

As many as 30 per cent of the total number of burn victims in the United States each year are estimated to be children. Burns of the hand are often seen in combination with extensive flame or scald injuries, but can also occur in isolation. Contact and scald burns of the hands of toddlers are not uncommon (Fig. 72–1).

First-degree and superficial second-degree burns can be managed with any number of techniques, as outlined in earlier chapters. Initial assessment of the depth of injury can be particularly difficult in children. Clinical judgment remains the best guide. With deep dermal and full thickness burns, appropriate escharotomy incisions should be undertaken at the earliest signs of circulatory compromise (Fig. 72–2).

Dressings, splinting, and physical therapy are consistently more difficult with children. If incision and grafting are used, great care must be taken to obtain absolute immobilization of the hand postoperatively, as no cooperation can be expected from the patient. In general, we have found that a dressing that completely wraps the hand in multiple layers of Dacron wool works well. Although some surgeons advocate the use of Kirschner wire fixation of the metacarpophalangeal joints, this is usually not necessary, is difficult, and can lead to complications. Likewise, dressing changes can be difficult and often require heavy sedation. Thus, if one is to obtain good graft take and limit areas of secondary healing, great attention must be given to dressing changes.

Generally, we advocate early excision and unmeshed split thickness skin grafting of deep dermal and full thickness burns of the hand in children (Fig. 72–3). For excision of these

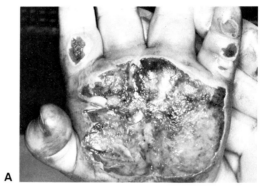

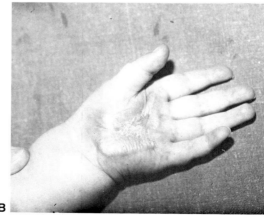

Figure 72–1. *A*, Palmar burn from touching an oven door. *B*, Scarring at one month.

788

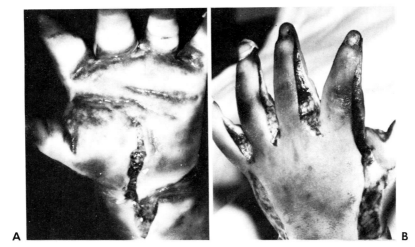

Figure 72–2. Third-degree flame burn. *A*, Palmar view, escharotomy incisions. *B*, Closed view.

burns within the first two to three days following injury, intravenous fluorescein dye has proved useful in certain patients, particularly in the age group in whom there is a large amount of subcutaneous fat (Figs. 72–4 to 72–7).

As with all hand and face burns, there is a limited application for meshed skin grafts, and graft application to the digits and hands must conform if possible to both functional and esthetic units. Failure to adhere to these basic reconstructive principles leads to unsat-

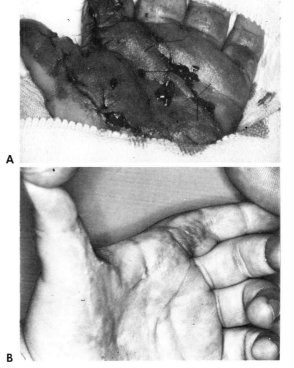

Figure 72–3. *A*, Early excision and grafting for a deep palmar burn. *B*, Result at nine months.

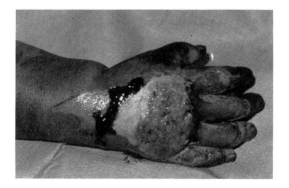

Figure 72–4. Full thickness scald burn of the dorsum of the hand and digits in a young child.

Figure 72–5. Tangential excision using intravenous fluorescein as a guide three days after the burn. Note that the dye is visible even without an ultraviolet light.

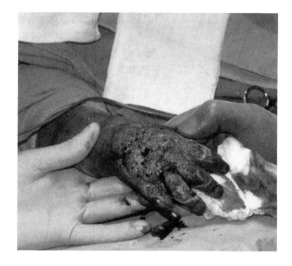

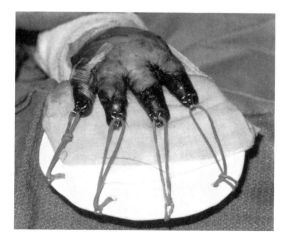

Figure 72–6. Split thickness skin grafting. We immobilize the hand using curtain hooks glued to the finger nails. This allows open treatment of the graft and improved graft take.

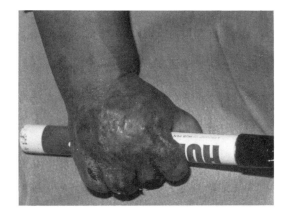

Figure 72–7. Result at two months after burn.

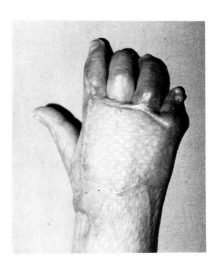

Figure 72–8. With excision and grafting one must avoid dorsal meshed grafts that do not follow functional units.

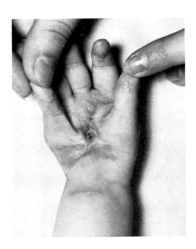

Figure 72–9. Palmar scar contracture between the thenar and the hypothenar eminences.

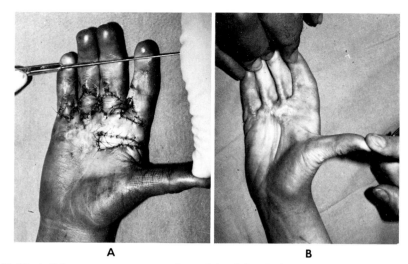

Figure 72–10. *A*, Palmar contracture at one base of the digits. *B*, Correction using full thickness grafts.

isfactory results requiring secondary revision (Fig. 72–8).

The burn specialist will often be asked to treat children with an eight to ten day old hand burn that was washed, dressed, and thought not to be "too deep" by a less experienced physician. He is then faced with a child with a stiff, edematous hand covered by thick, often infected eschar. In these cases we prefer prompt excision, homografting, and subsequent skin grafting. Prompt excision allows avoidance of progressive infection and abscess formation accompanied by deep soft tissue destruction. It also allows an opportunity to put the hands through a range of motion under anesthesia. The hands can be manipulated with homografts for an additional five to seven days without worrying about graft loss. Definitive skin grafting is then done on a healthy recipient bed.

The postoperative management of the burned hand in the child requires the understanding that one is dealing with a growing extremity. Attention must be given not only to long-term physiotherapy with frequent fittings of new pressure garments but also to the need for prompt intervention by the surgeon to release scars and contractures that inhibit normal development (Figs. 72–9 to 72–11). As Colson has pointed out, this can result from both dorsal and palmar contractures, is rapid in onset, and requires prompt relief.

The secondary reconstruction of these contractures can be difficult. The choice of skin grafts, Z-plasty, or local flaps depends in large part on a careful analysis of the quality and quantity of adjacent tissues and the size and location of the defect. Although the Z-plasty or local flap can be useful for releasing contractures of the dorsal or web spaces, palmar contractures generally do better with a skin graft or occasionally a heterodigital flap. The secondary reconstructive procedures are discussed elsewhere in this text.

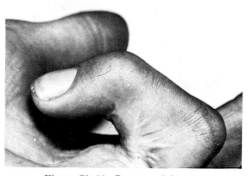

Figure 72–11. Contracted finger.

REFERENCES

Chait, L. A.: The treatment of contact burns of the palm in children. S. Afr. Med. J., *49*:1839–1842, 1975.

Colson, P.: Les brûlures de la face palmaire chez l'adolescent. *in* Tubiana, R. (Ed.): Traité de Chirurgie de la Main. Paris, Masson, 1986, pp. 683–691.

Corlett, R. J.: The treatment of deep burns of the hand. Aust. N.Z. J. Surg., *49*:567–572, 1979.

Davies, D. M., and Yiacoumettis, A. M.: A method of grafting hand burns following early excision. Br. J. Surg., 65:539–542, 1978.

Edstrom, L. E., Robson, M. C., Macchiaverna, J. R., and Scala, A. D.: Prospective randomized treatments for burned hands: Nonoperative vs. operative. Preliminary report. Scand. J. Plast. Reconstr. Surg., 13:131–135, 1979.

Gant, T. D.: The early enzymatic debridement and grafting of deep dermal burns to the hand. Plast. Reconstr. Surg., 66:185–190, 1980.

Hunt, J. L., and Sato, R. M.: Early excision of full-thickness hand and digit burns: Factors affecting morbidity. J. Trauma, 22:414–419, 1982.

Hunt, J. L., Sato, R. M., and Baxter, C. R.: Early tangential excision and immediate mesh autografting of deep dermal hand burns. Ann. Surg., 189:147–151, 1979.

Krizek, T. J., Flagg, S. V., Wolfort, F. G., and Jabaley, M. E.: Delayed primary excision and skin grafting of the burned hand. Plast. Reconstr. Surg., 51:524–529, 1973.

Labandter, H., Kaplan, I., and Shavitt, C.: Burns of the dorsum of the hand: Conservative treatment with intensive physiotherapy versus tangential excision and grafting. Br. J. Plast. Surg., 29:352–354, 1976.

Magliacani, G., Bormioli, M., and Cerutti, V.: Late results following treatment of deep burns of the hands. Scand. J. Plast. Reconstr. Surg., 13:137–139, 1979.

Mahler, D., and Hirshowitz, B.: Tangential excision and grafting for burns of the hand. Br. J. Plast. Surg., 28:189–192, 1975.

Malfeyt, G. A.: Burns of the dorsum of the hand treated by tangential excision. Br. J. Plast. Surg., 29:78–81, 1976.

Miller, S. H.: Burns of the upper extremity and hand. In Serafin, D., and Georgiade, N. (eds.): Pediatric Plastic Surgery. St. Louis, The C. V. Mosby Company, 1984.

Nielsen, A. B., and Sommer, J.: Surgical treatment of the deeply burned hand. Burns Incl. Therm. Inj., 9:214–217, 1983.

Salisbury, R. E., and Pruitt, B. A. (eds.): Burns of the Upper Extremity. Philadelphia, W. B. Saunders Company, 1976.

Salisbury, R. E., and Wright, P.: Evaluation of early excision of dorsal burns of the hand. Plast. Reconstr. Surg., 69:670–675, 1982.

Wexler, M. R., Yeschua, R., and Neuman, Z.: Early treatment of burns of the dorsum of the hand by tangential excision and skin grafting. Plast. Reconstr. Surg., 54:268–273, 1974.

Chapter 73

BURNS OF THE UPPER LIMB: MEDICAL AND SURGICAL TREATMENT

MAURICE ROUSSO
AND MENACHEM RON WEXLER

The untreated or incompletely treated burn of the upper limb often results in deformity and dysfunction. Presented here is an alternative approach to the classic methods for the prevention and correction of such deformities. This approach is a complementary and often radical departure in both classification and method that has been systematically and successfully used by the authors since 1971.

The concepts on which this approach is based are the division of the limb into anatomofunctional topographical units specifically for burns, the identification in the majority of cases of specific patterns of deformity related to each unit, and the knowledge that deformity and dysfunction are not always inevitable but rather complications resulting from incorrect treatment. These new departures in medical and surgical methods of treatment for the prevention or correction of these complications lead to a more desirable cosmetic and functional result.

ANATOMOFUNCTIONAL TOPOGRAPHICAL UNITS OF THE UPPER LIMB

In dealing with burns of the upper limb we look at the limb in a different way from that of accepted anatomy. We visualize the soft tissues–skin and subcutaneous–of the limb as in several circumscribed areas or units, dorsal and ventral, each one with a transverse or longitudinal diameter, which is the "geometrical lieu" of a specific movement. The center of each movement is also the center of a given anatomofunctional topographical unit. That is, the limb can be divided into transverse and longitudinal anatomofunctional topographical units, the emphasis here being on the direction of their movement (Fig. 73–1).

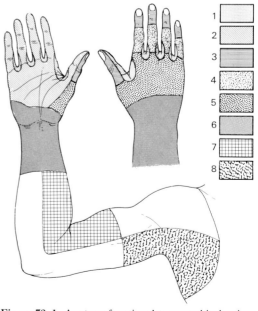

Figure 73–1. Anatomofunctional topographical units.

794

Transverse Anatomofunctional Topographical Units

Transverse anatomofunctional topographical units are always both volar and dorsal in their distribution. The skin and subcutaneous tissue of the interdigital web spaces—concave and transversely situated dorsally and ventrally in the same unit between two adjacent metacarpophalangeal joints—form the transverse metacarpophalangeal arch, which is concave towards the anterior side of the palm. Normal soft tissues, as a result of their elasticity, permit digital abduction and thumb anteposition and opposition; they also intervene in the sagittal movements of the first phalanx of the fingers. All these movements are transversely related to the longitudinal axis of the hand.

Longitudinal Anatomofunctional Topographical Units

Longitudinal anatomofunctional topographical units are either volar or dorsal in their distribution. During flexion-extension of the distal interphalangeal, interphalangeal, metacarpophalangeal, wrist, and elbow joints, the volar and dorsal skin moves longitudinally in a reciprocal way; i.e., when the skin is stretched on the volar side of a joint during flexion or extension, it is always relaxed on the dorsal aspect of the same joint, and vice versa. The same happens at the inner and external sides of the axilla during aduction-abduction movements of the arm. Another characteristic of these units, which is of special significance in understanding the dynamics of deformity, is that some units have a tendency to concavity, and others to convexity, during flexion-extension.

The periungual area is a special part of the dorsal distal interphalangeal unit. This is so because the treatment of burns, considered in the light of pathogenic factors, requires that (for longitudinal anatomofunctional topographical units) the limb be divided into anatomical areas that have joints at their centers, joints that are responsible for flexion-extension.

The transverse anatomofunctional topographical units compose the areas of soft tissues (web space) between adjacent metacarpophalangeal joints, which are the center of lateral movements of the respective digits.

PATTERNS OF DEFORMITY

Thermal injury generally involves only part of the thickness of the skin, except of course in severe burns. However, the primary inflammatory response is global, involving in different degrees adjacent tissues at the surface and at the deeper levels.

The severity and duration of this response differ for each patient, but the clinical expression is predictable, depending on the severity of the thermal injury, its topography related to the anatomofunctional topographical units involved, and the treatment performed.

A general feature of all burns, regardless of site, is that the center of the burned area is more damaged than its periphery, therefore sustaining more severe scarring and dysfunction. It is also important to note that a given anatomofunctional topographical unit can be burned partially or several units can be affected together.

Local Pathogenic Factors

At any given locale we can distinguish seven distinct yet interacting dynamic pathogenic factors (some single, others grouped) that can lead to deformity and dysfunction following burns: edema, pain and acute dystrophy, infection,[*] stiffness, joint deformity, skin contractures, and hypertrophic scars, the latter four being associated with fibrosis. Edema and pain with acute dystrophy are part of the immediate inflammatory response in all burns. In minor burns, in which they constitute the only response, no specialized treatment is required. The remaining factors are a consequence of more serious burns, after variable periods of delay, and if left untreated most probably will become permanent.

The Special Role of Fibrosis

Fibrosis is an important element in all lesions that tend to result in permanent disability. Left to itself, edema fluid organizes into fibrous tissue, which is also the common denominator in stiffness, contracture, and hypertrophy.

---

[*]Infection of course plays a role but is not dealt with here.

PREDOMINANT FACTORS

Over the course of time, one or more of these responses may become predominant as well as chronic. When this happens, the response or responses (e.g., chronic edema, dystrophy, and pain) become diseases in their own right with the need for their own particular treatment.

THE SITE OF THE LESION

Some sites lend themselves to the development of permanent scarring and deformity. These are the sites of movement—i.e., the joints, their surrounding tissues, and the interdigital web spaces. In these places maximal skin contractures and hypertrophic scars occur, especially if the anatomofunctional topographical unit involved is situated at a concave site.

The lines of contracture are generally parallel to the direction of the original movement and so impose limitation on that movement. This directional pull exacerbates hypertrophy of the scar. Therefore maximal contracture occurs at the site of maximal movement (Fig. 73–1). Contractures of the web spaces are transverse, are more frequently dorsal, and interfere with digital abduction, especially at the first web level where they also limit anteposition and opposition.

Longitudinal contractures of the dorsal skin of the metacarpophalangeal joints hyperextend them, leading also to clawing of the involved digit. If the dorsal aspect of metacarpophalangeal joints is involved, the transverse arch of the hyperextended metacarpophalangeal joints reverses to become a dorsal concavity; the thumb is kept in permanent adduction-retroposition. Grasping is therefore impossible (Fig. 73–2).

At dorsal proximal interphalangeal joint level, untreated burns often result in permanent and progressive tendon and joint damage, with volar drop of the midphalanx, boutonnière deformity, or ankylosis, even though the original injury did not penetrate beneath the skin.

Sometimes the opposite deformity occurs, and a dorsal hypertrophic scar of the skin and extensor tendon hyperextends the proximal interphalangeal joint area. Only deep burns at the volar aspect of the digit or palm produce permanent contractures at these

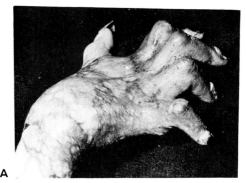

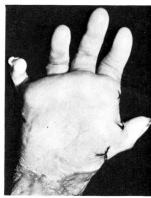

Figure 73–2. *A* and *B*, Dorsal and palmar views. The metacarpophalangeal joints are hyperextended and the transverse metacarpophalangeal arch is reversed following an incorrectly treated burn of the dorsum of the hand.

sites. When there are such contractures, they are longitudinal in their direction and hence limit extension of the digit or the palm. When two or more digits are involved, there is an associated volar interdigital web contracture with the digitopalmar scar.

Even the most longstanding joint deformities (at all sites, except the dorsal proximal interphalangeal joint) have proved surprisingly reversible after medical or surgical treatment. Because they are actually due to skin contracture alone, the joint retains latent function throughout.

Deep burns of the dorsal distal interphalangeal joint area frequently produce hyperextension associated with periungual distortion, and sometimes with a boutonnière deformity. By contrast, weakness of the terminal extensor tendon causes the distal interphalangeal joint to drop and a mallet finger results. The mallet finger deformity in turn predisposes to hyperextension of the proximal interphalangeal joint and an even more disabling swan-neck deformity. Contractures at any other site have a tendency to be longitudinal.

Worthy of emphasis with respect to the frequency of burns, importance of function, and a special tendency to develop contractures, are the dorsum of the proximal interphalangeal joints, metacarpophalangeal areas with web spaces, the anterolateral side of the elbow, and the anterior and posterior sides of the axilla (Fig. 73–1). Concave areas tend to be protected at the moment of injury by flexion, leaving the central area of skin intact, even in severe burns, a fact utilized in the surgical treatment to be described (Rousso, 1975a, b).

In contrast, burns over flat areas, distant from joints, have less tendency to produce contractures, hypertrophy, and deformity.

We are now in a position to define the limits of the longitudinal anatomofunctional topographical units. Their proximal and distal limits are at the transverse neutral line midway between two adjacent joints situated along the same longitudinal axis, their lateral limits are situated at the lateral longitudinal neutral lines of every segment of the upper limb, and their respective centers are at the anterior or posterior joint projections.

PREVENTION OF COMPLICATIONS

Prevention of complications is often possible and much easier to effect than correction of established sequelae. In the majority of cases correct medical treatment can avoid the necessity for painful, difficult, prolonged, multistaged secondary surgical treatment. Definitive injury often results from incorrect treatment.

What constitutes incorrect treatment of burns of the upper limb?

NONINTERVENTION

Spontaneous healing (i.e., nonintervention) leads to different degrees of deformity and dysfunction even in partial thickness skin burns of the hand. Therefore there is no such thing as a "wait and see" attitude. Some procedure is always necessary, commencing as already stated with medical procedures, which are generally quite simple.

FAULTY TIMING

Knowledge of the dynamic pathogenic factors helps in guiding the treatment program. Because we know that edema and pain with acute dystrophy are early manifestations and stiffness, joint deformity, and contractures and scarring are late manifestations, we plan an immediate as well as a long term strategy to ensure control of the healing process. Gaining control is of paramount importance in burns of the upper limb (and especially of the hand) because of the complex and delicate system of biological and biomechanical forces constantly interacting there, forces that are apt to produce undesirable effects.

Prevention of one dysfunction may produce another complication. For example, active movements combat edema, disuse atrophy, and stiffness, but may exacerbate pain. Rest decreases pain, contractures, and hypertrophic scars but increases stiffness. The earlier and more comprehensive the program of treatment, the shorter the morbidity, the smaller the permanent disability, and the better the long-term result.

When burns are extensive and involve several anatomofunctional topographical units, simultaneous treatment to avoid potential complications of all the units is not always possible. For example, the functions of two anatomofunctional topographical units can be antagonistic because they are situated at opposite sides of the same joint. It has already been stressed that incorrect treatment of some of the units will lead to more marked disability than that of others. Therefore, the treatment of the more important units takes priority so that they will receive the major portion of treatment time, and the anatomofunctional topographical unit side at lesser risk is treated second.

MISTAKE IN CHOICE OF TREATMENT

A mistake in treatment may involve either timing or an actual procedure. Most frequent is the overtreatment of simple although often extensive superficial burns in which the surgeon overuses topical drugs and prescribes too many changings of dressings, instead of finding the best way to clean the wound as quickly as possible, avoiding potential infection, and providing splints to protect and guide epithelial regrowth during healing and to maintain the joints in a desired position during rest periods and between exercises in order to prevent joint imbalance. He must also apply uniform soft compression to the injured area to avoid edema and pain (Larson et al., 1971, 1974; Rousso and Wexler, 1978, 1980).

Less frequently the mistake in treatment occurs in the contrary situation—failure to recognize the need for early amputation of an irreparably damaged digit and selecting instead long continued conservative treatment that interferes with function. Some cases are borderline, e.g., deep second degree burns of the dorsum of the hand and digits. We elect earlier and more aggressive treatment, but of course each case must be treated individually.

Sometimes the major difficulty in incorrect treatment is that procedures are undertaken and strategies planned that require an abundance of medical and occupational services, which may not exist in a small hospital. Thus judgment must be exercised whether to continue to treat the patient or, after rendering first aid and resuscitation, to send him on to a larger specialized burn center. This is especially true when surgical treatment is indicated. In the case that requires purely medical treatment, one of the advantages of our method is that it can be carried out by a minimal staff. Another factor that can determine the outcome of treatment is the patient's motivation. The social worker and psychiatrist on the team are in the best position to make this judgment.

MEDICAL AND SURGICAL METHODS OF TREATMENT

We do not describe here accepted methods of treatment, which we continue to use in part, but will describe other methods that in our experience in recent years have led to a different evolution and prognosis for burns of the upper limb. Treatment is divided into primary and secondary stages according to the time that has elapsed after the burn,* the presence of epithelial healing, and the presence of complications associated with fibrosis.

---

*The time lapse is subject to the variations imposed by such factors as age, disease, the patient's occupation, and partial treatment.

TREATMENT IN THE PRIMARY STAGE

In the primary stage one object of treatment is to achieve complete epithelial healing by the immediate and early persistent use of medical treatment and such surgical procedures as may be indicated. By the same means one prevents complications associated with fibrosis and deformity. We believe that when primary treatment meets these two goals, secondary stage treatment will not be necessary. This applies to the majority of burns in civilian life.

Immediate Medical Treatment

Initial Sterile Dressing. This initial basic and essential step applies in all cases, with the exception of extremely severe burns complicated by distal ischemia. Given stable general conditions, evaluation and preliminary mapping of the burned areas are done to determine the surface area and depth of tissue involved. If the burned hand is seen during the first hour, pain is not yet severe, and analgesia and sedation are not necessary. Because the burn is contaminated on the surface but not yet infected, the aim of the initial dressing is to clean the burned area as early and as effectively as possible, avoiding unnecessary trauma (mechanical as well as chemical).

In the usual burn case this conservative treatment—i.e., dressings and simple but individualized splinting—will be the only treatment needed. In extensive deep second degree burns of the dorsum of the hand, we plan the early surgical treatment for the first week, as we do for deeper burns.

After preparation of a sterile table, with the required materials already prepared, we proceed with gentle but thorough cleansing of the burn and its surrounding area under tap water. Repeated water and soap washings and rinsings are carried out with gloved hands to avoid trauma and pain. We strip off only the epidermis that is lacerated and heavily contaminated. No antiseptic solutions are used at any time during this stage of treatment. Sterile longitudinal pieces of polyurethane foam enveloped with hydrophilic gauze are placed between the digits as well as one layer of a conventional ointment gauze that has already been prepared.

Next we dress both the volar and dorsal sides of the hand and other burned areas with

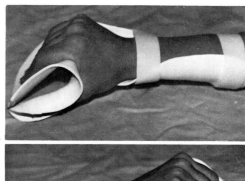

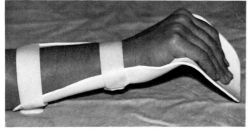

Figure 73–3. *A* and *B*, Michigan splint position. The 90 degree flexed volar splint keeps the metacarpophalangeal joints at approximately 70 degrees of flexion.

one layer of ointment gauze, cotton, and foam, working from distal to proximal. We carefully mold the web spaces, and then the hand is gently compressed against a volar splint. The dressing is completed by application of a sterile elastic bandage, so that mild compression is uniformly transmitted to the soft tissues through the polyurethane foam.

Positioning. A plaster of Paris splint is placed on the volar aspect of hand and wrist in the functional position appropriate to the anatomofunctional topographical unit that is burned. In the primary or secondary treatment of the burned upper limb, as a rule positioning must be maintained in the position opposite that of the expected deformity.

In burns of the dorsum of the hand (the most frequent of all burns) the Michigan splint position achieves the most effective results (Fig. 73–3). The wrist is kept in 20 degrees of dorsiextension, the metacarpophalangeal joints of the fingers in 70 degrees of flexion, the interphalangeal joints in almost complete extension, and the thumb in abduction-anteposition (Feller, 1964; Koepke, 1967; Koepke et al., 1963; Koepke and Feller, 1967). That is, the hand is kept in a moderate intrinsic plus position to avoid clawing of the fingers due to edema of the dorsum of the hand and progressive weakness of the dorsal proximal interphalangeal joint structures.

If the predominant injury is volar (palmar, digital, digitopalmar, or interdigital), a supportive volar splint is used to position the metacarpophalangeal and finger joints in almost complete extension during most of the immediate and early treatment period. This applies to both second and deep second degree burns.

In second degree burns of both the dorsum and the volar aspect of the hand and fingers, treatment of the dorsum has priority in positioning and early surgical treatment (deep second degree burns). In small children, positioning and immobilization are difficult, and we prefer a boxing glove type of dressing, using the same technique and in the position already mentioned (Fig. 73–4). A light clean cheap splint can be prepared in advance by molding four to six layers of plaster of Paris and painting the splint with plastic glue. In the case of mass casualties, it is essential to be prepared with a stack of this or another kind of ready-to-use splint in a position of function for dorsal burns, preferably in three different sizes.

Immobilization. Good results have been obtained by different methods. Elevation and joint rest in a mild compressive splint dressing give the same result during the first days as elevation with active physiotherapy, and are better tolerated. Passive stretching of the burned tissues and surrounding area of inflammatory response should be avoided at this stage, because this causes pain, additional trauma, scarring, and stiffness. Iso-

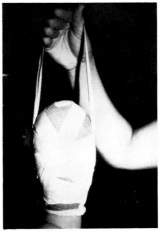

Figure 73–4. "Boxing glove" compression splint dressing for children. The inner dressing is the same as for adults; the splinting is by polyurethane foam alone.

metric active exercises are encouraged inside the dressing as early as possible. Usually the initial sterile dressing should remain undisturbed for 10 days, by which time sufficient epithelialization has occurred in the majority of cases (superficial second degree burns).

Early Medical Treatment

We use three types of early medical treatment, not including cases in which deep second degree burns of the dorsum of the hand are predominant.

Open Treatment. On removal of the dressing after 10 days, the major part of the burn area has healed satisfactorily and only small islands of deep second degree burn remain. More vigorous active exercises of the fingers and wrist, or any other burn area, can begin. No conventional dressings are used, but soap and water baths are continued with appropriate ointments, and a polyurethane soft splint-dressing is applied during the night and as much as possible during the waking hours.

Closed Treatment: The Second Dressing. If on removal of the initial dressing it is found that a considerable amount of deep second degree burned tissue has not yet epithelialized (as seen by the strong adherence of the petroleum gauze to the healing area), a second dressing is applied without any cleansing or stripping of any tissues. Instead of forcefully removing the last adhering layer of dressing, we let it remain in situ, thus avoiding trauma to the new epithelium. Close attention is paid to sterility, positioning, compression, and immobilization. This is maintained for another 10 days, and isometric active exercises are continued throughout. Unless there has been an error of judgment about the depth of the burns, at the end of this period, all the area will have healed. The deepest layer of ointment gauze can be removed easily and without trauma, and open treatment can follow.

If the patient comes to our attention after an initial treatment in which cleansing was not sufficiently thorough, but still within the first week after the burn, a thorough cleaning is performed—but most likely under regional or general analgesia-anesthesia because of pain, some edema, infection, and malposition. The aim is to establish the correct path of the healing process. In these cases the frequency of dressing change varies depending on the severity of the local infection. Repeated wet dressings are used in the most severe cases. Antibiotic therapy is added that is appropriate for the micro-organism culture. The limb is maintained elevated and at rest.

Semiopen Treatment. A removable splint-dressing can be used that permits movement of the different segments of the fingers and that simultaneously supports the functional position of the hand and wrist. This is useful when moderate deep second degree burns are present on the dorsum of the hand. It permits easy removal of the splint for bathing, occupational therapy, and dressing changes (Fig. 73–5).

Deep second degree burns of the volar aspect of the hand are maintained in extension in a supportive splint during most part of the primary treatment, but assisted exercises are performed twice a day in flexion to avoid joint stiffness.

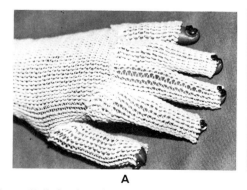
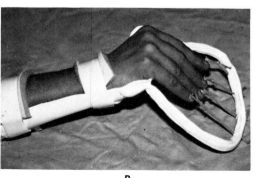

A	**B**

Figure 73–5. Semi-open treatment. *A,* Each segment has its individual dressing. Hooks are strongly glued to the fingernails. *B,* Banjo thermoplastic splint is an alternative possibility.

Polyurethane Foam Soft Splint-Dressing System

Interdigital Web Level. For burns in this area, we devised a special sagittal splint-dressing to be applied during and after early open and semiopen medical treatment, as well as during and after early or secondary surgical treatment using grafts or flaps (Rousso and Wexler, 1978, 1980). An essential innovation in our method is the use of sagittal polyurethane foam strips, varying in size and width according to the anatomofunctional topographical units involved, that firmly mold the concavity of the web spaces and the anterior and posterior metacarpal areas. As they are stretched along the sagittal plane, the strips of polyurethane foam are anchored to a polyurethane foam–Velcro wrist strap. Depending on the stage of healing, conventional medicated gauze dressings may or may not be used. The sequence therefore is: skin or dressings, wrist strap, and sagittal foam strips. If epithelial healing is complete, the foam is placed directly on the skin, which has been treated topically with an antibiotic-hydrocortisone ointment (Fig. 73–6A, B). If several webs are involved, the following variant is of a simple design and very useful (Fig. 73–6C, D).

First Web Level. An important goal of the sagittal soft splint-dressing is to make possible abduction-antepositioning of the thumb by use of a wider and thicker strip of polyurethane and by attaching the sagittal strip to the wrist strap at the desired angle. Because the volar aspect of the fingers is free, this method for sagittal splinting of the web spaces does not interfere with grasping and other delicate tactile or prehensile functions of the thumb and fingers. Therefore, the patient can return earlier to his occupation.

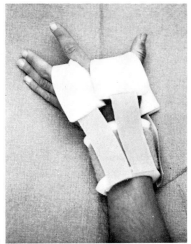

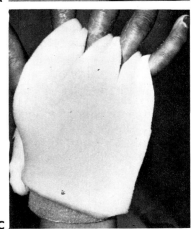

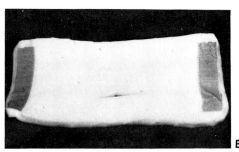

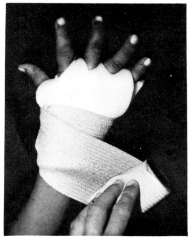

Figure 73–6. *A,* Sagittal polyurethane foam soft splint dressing for webs. *B,* Splint is improvised. *C* and *D,* "Golf glove" foam splint dressing when several webs are involved. This is also very useful in children.

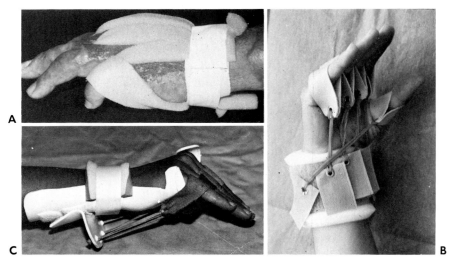

Figure 73–7. *A* and *B*, Elastic flexion of the metacarpophalangeal joints by polyurethane foam or elastic bands. *C*, Thermoplastic splint with higher volar profile (fixed or detachable) improves flexor metacarpophalangeal movement. Splinting can be combined with sagittal soft web splinting.

During the early stages of the treatment the foam must always be sterile. When new skin is well established, medicated ointment is applied to this skin, and unsterilized but clean polyurethane foam strips are positioned and anchored to the wrist strap as before.

Flexion of the Metacarpophalangeal Joints. When assisted flexion of the metacarpophalangeal joints is indicated, a soft loop (preferably of polyurethane foam) is wound around the first phalanx of the corresponding finger and attached volarward to the wrist directly or with a rubber band. This flexes the metacarpophalangeal joints, avoiding imbalance or contracture in hyperextension and clawing of the finger (Fig. 73–7).

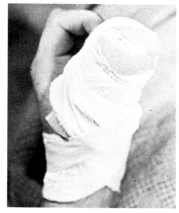

Figure 73–8. "Sandwich" dressing.

Dorsal Distal Interphalangeal–Periungual Anatomofunctional Topographical Unit. After reconstruction of this area the splint-dressing makes a "sandwich" of the finger section with its dressing between two transverse layers of polyurethane foam (Fig. 73–8).

Circular Areas. A circular soft splint-dressing can also be applied with great advantage on any other area where a circular bandage is possible. After burns of the external side of the first ray (from wrist to thumb), a splint-dressing around both anatomofunctional topographical units prevents the development of hypertrophic scars and progressive radial deviation, without limiting grasp. One can use a specially designed foam splint or more simply a figure of eight foam bandage (Fig. 73–9). Joint deviation can be prevented by positioning the cross part of the figure of eight over or opposite the burned area. A soft splint-dressing can be used with any type of supportive or elastic splint (Figs. 73–7C, 73–10).

At the interphalangeal joints, wrist, elbow, or axillary level during early or secondary medical treatment or after surgery (grafts or flaps), the simplest and ideal dressing is, in our opinion, a circular bandage of polyurethane foam, which gently compresses the area. Also, because it permits relative movement of the involved joint instead of prolonged extension-immobilization, there is no interference with function, making possible

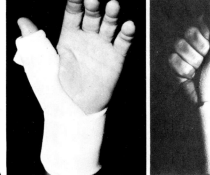
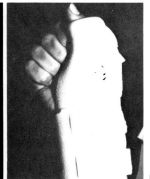

Figure 73–9. *A* and *B*, Circular foam splint dressing.

prolonged periods of use (even more than one year if indicated). It also has the advantage of insuring automatic continuous massage of the healing tissues (Figs. 73–30*E*, 73–31*E*).

The soft splint-dressing is used continuously throughout the primary treatment period. During this time the central part of the foam strips push firmly in a sagittal or transverse direction perpendicular to each predicted line of scar, thus preventing contracture. After this period the splint-dressing is used during the night and as much as possible during the day until completion of the remodeling of fibroplastic collagen tissue and until all signs of hypertrophy disappear.

Protection against the sun and corticoid ointment must also be provided until the end of the secondary period and stabilization of the healing process, which often takes one year or more.

Occupational Therapy

The following exercises are especially useful in assisting or resisting sagittal or lateral movements of metacarpophalangeal and proximal interphalangeal joints and in massaging the web spaces (Fig. 73–11).

Special Methods of Treatment

Pain. Sometimes pain is the predominant symptom, often associated with sympathetic dystrophy. The site of the pain can be the burn area or the donor site of a split thickness skin graft. The application of modulated transcutaneous electrical nerve stimulation provides analgesia, relieves muscular spasm, and improves the cooperation of the patient during active or passive exercises.

Pneumatic Intermittent Compression for Edema. Pneumatic compression is needed only if there was no early treatment with the polyurethane foam splint-dressing system to control and prevent the formation of chronic edema or hypertrophic scars. If the burn patient is seen late with chronic edema of the dorsum of the hand, hyperextension of the metacarpophalangeal joints, and variable degrees of hypertrophy, active and passive physiotherapy and occupational therapy will be painful and prolonged. This situation can be improved, and may even be reversed, if

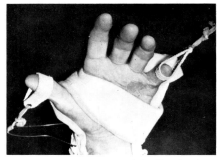
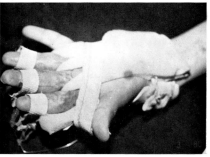

Figure 73–10. *A* and *B*, Circular foam dressing combined with elastic splint.

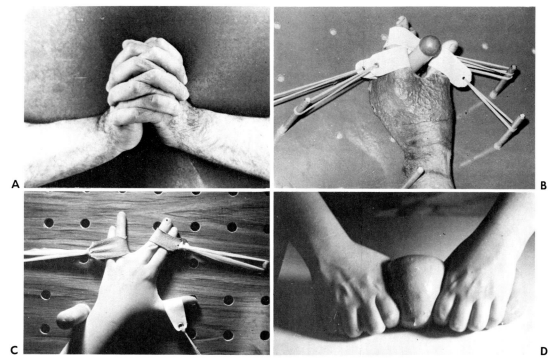

Figure 73–11. *A*, Exercises to massage the webs and to move the metacarpophalangeal joints (after Weinberg). *B* and *C*, With the hand centered around the "broom handle," the fingers are anchored by rubber bands to a pegboard to assist or resist finger joint movement. *D*, Exercises using dough for webs, digitopalmar region, and wrist (after Ben Porath, O.T.).

the following round-the-clock program is instituted:

During the hours when the occupational therapist is available, the soft splint-dressing is used to encourage healing of the interdigital web spaces and the flexion of the metacarpophalangeal joints. Other related procedures are also carried out.

During all the other hours, automatic intermittent (two to five minutes) gentle compression (20 to 90 mm. Hg) of the limb takes place inside a sleeve connected to an alternating pneumatic pump (Fig. 73–12). The treatment reduces edema and hypertrophic scars and decreases pain. It also improves the circulation of the limb, acting directly to prevent venous stasis and probably also on arteriocapillary components.

Automatic Exercises. Because of its analgesic effect, the treatment we have described permits the placement (within the sleeve) of a small air filled bag in the palm of the hand that is also connected to the pump. This bag inflates and opens the metacarpophalangeal joints and abducts the thumb in anteposition

during the alternative phase when the sleeve is decompressed.

If the patient is seen during the secondary stage and already has severe stiffness and deformity of the wrist and metacarpophalangeal and proximal interphalangeal joints, a special pneumatic exerciser can be used to progressively decrease stiffness of wrist and

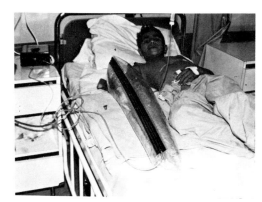

Figure 73–12. Pneumatic intermittent compression of upper limb.

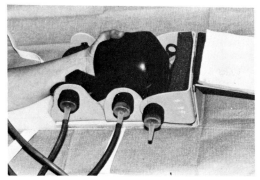

Figure 73–13. Pneumatic exerciser for finger and wrist joints.

adduction contracture of the thumb and to improve movement of the joints (Fig. 73–13). Since this machine does not affect pain, modulated analgesia is required prior to and simultaneously with the use of the pneumatic exerciser.

Surgical Treatment in the Primary Stage

Special attention is given here to deep second degree burns of the dorsum of the hand and digits. Usually they are interspersed with small islands of third degree burns.

The Classic Approach. Repeated wet or ointment dressings permit spontaneous healing of the more superficially burned areas by islands of epithelium growing up from the deep dermis. There will remain patches of eschar at the third degree sites, which are removed with continued application of the dressings or surgical excision. In either case the result is granulation tissue, which must be covered by split thickness skin grafts.

The disadvantages of the classic approach are that the procedure is drawn out, taking at least three to six weeks. An enormous amount of staff time is involved—several surgical stages, anesthesia, dressings—and suffering is imposed on the patient because of anesthesia risk, fasting, and pain. Uncertainty about the readiness of the granulation tissue (the recipient bed) means that different patches of skin grafts will have different ages, and therefore physiotherapy and occupational therapy will be delayed, incurring the risk of local infection, pain during exercise, malpositioning, stiffness, or atrophy. Moreover, spontaneous healing of deep second degree burns leads to skin contracture and

hypertrophy. All these prolong treatment time and often yield results that are disappointing both aesthetically and functionally.

Early Tangential Excision and Immediate Skin Grafting. The cornerstone of this more aggressive surgical treatment is the technique of Jancekovic (1970), who coined this descriptive title for her innovative technique for the treatment of deep second degree burns.

There have been other contributions that recognized the importance of early excision and prompt cover with skin grafts. Peacock et al. (1970) stressed the importance of early excision. Grafting with split thickness skin before edema fluid is fixed in the connective tissue halts the inflammatory process and prevents fibrosis. The resultant skin regains its elasticity in a shorter period of time, thus avoiding joint stiffness and deformity. Derganc and Zdravic (1963) emphasized the role of the dermis in the prevention of hypertrophic scar formation during the healing of burns. Jackson (1969) stressed the importance of using large sheets of skin without leaving exposed dermis, which could necrose instead of heal.

TECHNIQUE. Two to five days after the burn, with adequate anesthesia (without regional ischemia but with a tourniquet in place), the eschar is shaved tangentially layer by layer with a Humby type of hand dermatome until punctiform bleeding appears in remaining healthy dermis (Fig. 73–14). This is followed by immediate application of a split thickness skin graft with the hand already in a functional position. Many burns include patches of deep second and third degree burns, and this method preserves and utilizes viable tissue. If it is necessary to delay the autograft because the area is not yet ready on account of excessive depth, a wet saline dressing is maintained for 48 hours more, followed by a new tangential excision, after which the autograft may be performed. The skin-grafted hand is dressed, positioned, elevated, and treated as already described in the section on primary medical treatment. (Temporary coverage with lyophilized xenografts has not proved to be of any immediate or long term advantage in our extensive series of patients.)

Special Situations. Arthrodesis of proximal interphalangeal joints that have been irreparably damaged by deep burns of the dorsum can be performed at the same time as the skin grafting, or during the secondary

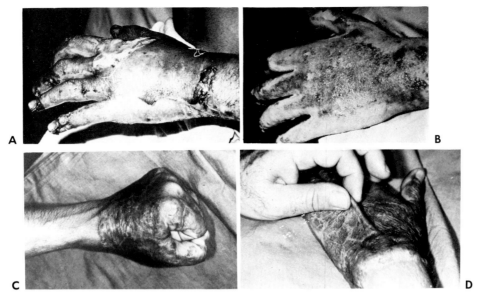

Figure 73–14. *A,* Deep second degree burns of dorsum of hand. *B,* Following tangential excision. *C* and *D,* End result after skin graft.

surgical treatment. Koepke (1970) recommended Kirschner wire immobilization during the primary treatment. We recommend the dorsal approach, wedge excision, and longitudinal Kirschner wire fixation as the simplest solution with almost no risk of infection during the primary treatment (Rousso and Wexler, 1978, 1980; Fig. 73–15). If temporary Kirschner wire fixation of joints is indicated, infection of the joint can be prevented by placing a single Kirschner wire transarticularly between both phalanges. Sometimes the proximal interphalangeal joint is so greatly flexed that the metacarpophalangeal joint can be positioned only after arthrodesis of the proximal interphalangeal joint (Figs. 73–16, 73–19*F*).

It is important to cover exposed tendons immediately with temporary skin grafts to enhance their survival. Although skin flaps are the accepted permanent cover, in our experience exposed dorsal extrinsic tendons are seldom irreversibly damaged, and cross flaps are infrequently needed.

On the dorsum of the metacarpophalangeal and metacarpal area we have obtained satisfactory functional results by applying thick split thickness skin grafts directly over the extrinsic extensor tendons, after early deep excision of the eschar (Figs. 73–2*A*, 73–16*A*, 73–19). If one of the digits is severely damaged and will interfere permanently with grasping (e.g., irreversible damage of the extensor tendons and metacarpophalangeal

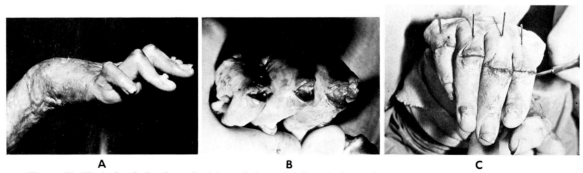

Figure 73–15. Arthrodesis of proximal interphalangeal joint. *A,* Severe irreversible flexion deformity. *B,* Dorsal wedge excision. *C,* Longitudinal single Kirschner wire fixation of arthrodesis.

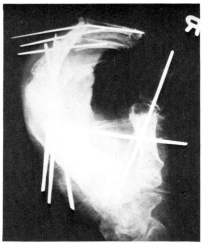

Figure 73–16. Pre-articular temporary metacarpophalangeal fixation. X-ray showing the arthrodesis of the proximal interphalangeal joints and fixation of the metacarpophalangeal joints performed at the same time.

and proximal interphalangeal joints of the little finger), we proceed to fillet it after a short delay and use its remaining dorsal or volar flap of viable skin as a filling for open areas at the volar or dorsal metacarpal level. This skin flap usually has all its sensation, assuring quick and complete rehabilitation of the hand (Fig. 73–17). We have found this approach especially useful (as compared to more conservative methods) in deep electrical burns of the metacarpophalangeal joints and volar or dorsal metacarpal areas. The filleting is carried out by the end of the first week, for by that time all the areas of necrosis are clearly defined.

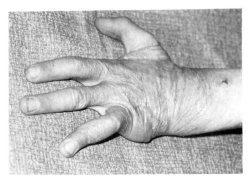

Figure 73–17. Filleted fifth finger to fill a large defect of the dorsum at metacarpals 3, 4, and 5. As delayed primary treatment, this method is especially indicated after deep electrical burns of the metacarpophalangeal and metacarpal region, volar and/or dorsal.

TREATMENT IN THE SECONDARY STAGE

The major goal in the secondary stage is the surgical treatment of permanent complications, i.e., reconstruction after the occurrence of joint deformity and stiffness, skin contractures, and hypertrophic scars. In contrast to what is done during the early stages of treatment, secondary stage surgical treatment is seldom performed on both hands at the same time, because the patient would be completely incapacitated. Therefore we program the secondary reconstruction to alternate sites of surgery so that one of the hands is always free of dressings.

The strategy in secondary surgical treatment is that at any given transverse level of the anatomofunctional topographical units involved we try to perform all the corrections together. This enables all the steps of occupational therapy to be carried out synergistically, e.g., active and passive exercises and splinting.

In our opinion the sequence and priority of surgical repair of severe contractures during this secondary stage treatment should be as follows:

1. Repair of metacarpophalangeal joint hyperextension.

2. At the same stage, repair of the adduction-retroposition of the thumb.

3. Repair of digitopalmar contractures.

4. Repair of longitudinal axillary, elbow, or wrist contractures (in that order).

5. Reconstruction of transverse dorsal interdigital contractures.

We seldom excise scar tissue, preferring its release by incision, repositioning of structures, and immediate skin resurfacing. We avoid as much as possible the utilization of skin grafts, which interfere with early mobilization and have a strong and prolonged tendency to contract and hypertrophy.

If the contracture is very tight, we use triangular split thickness skin grafts at the extremities of the line of reconstruction. The more linear and prominent the contractures, the easier the geometrical and surgical solution, in one or two stages, by the use of combinations of Y-V and Z-plasties (Fig. 73–18) (Rousso, 1975a,b; Rousso and Wexler, 1978, 1980). If a second revision becomes necessary at a given anatomofunctional topographical unit, we try to wait at least five to six months to enable remodeling of the healing collagen tissue to take place. The latter

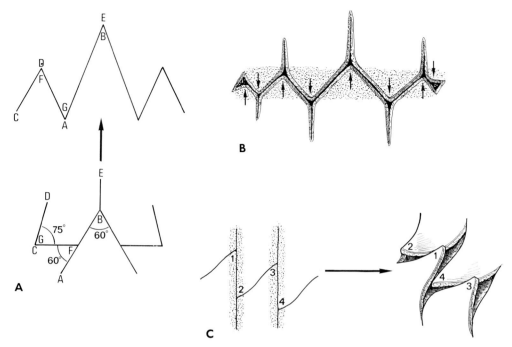

Figure 73–18. Redistribution of scarred and healthy tissue by different Y-V and Z-plasty combinations. *A,* Five-flap technique, in which a central Y-V plasty separates two opposed Z-plasties. *B,* Multiple Y-V plasty, used in the primary repair or as revision of previous five-flap procedure. *C,* Z-plasty combination to overcome the problem of two parallel lines of contracture; scar is elongated by a common limb Z-plasty.

process is greatly enhanced and guided by the uniform compression provided by the polyurethane soft splint-dressing, as well as by the redistribution of scars and healthy tissues by means of our five-flap technique and their possible revision by five Y-V plasty, methods that will be presented in detail (Rousso and Wexler, 1980). Any surgical step (grafts or flaps) is preceded and followed by appropriate soft splinting.

Dorsal Contractures of the Hand

Extensive Contractures of the Dorsum of the Metacarpophalangeal and Metacarpal Areas. Such contractures are best treated, in our opinion, by a comprehensive program that corrects, in a single stage, hyperextension of metacarpophalangeal joints 1, 2, 3, 4, and 5 and adduction-retroposition contracture of the thumb and the first web. Release of these contractures restores the normal anterior concavity of the transverse arch of the metacarpophalangeal joints.

This program is accomplished by the following:

1. A dorsal transverse incision is made across metacarpals 2 to 5, proximal to the metacarpophalangeal joints, to the volar sides of metacarpals 2 and 5 (Fig. 73–19).

2. At the volar and dorsal metacarpal level of the thumb, a racquet incision (with two handles) is made in the sagittal direction, and the thumb is transposed anteriorly in abduction.

3. The strong flexion of metacarpophalangeal joints 2 to 5 is maintained for three weeks by the prearticular insertion of single longitudinal Kirschner wires.

4. The reconstruction of the first web is accomplished by interlacing two metacarpal skin flaps—one dorsal and one volar.

5. Thick split thickness skin grafts are placed on the resulting extensive raw areas, even over denuded tendons. The skin is anchored by small pieces of Steri-strips instead of stitches to expedite the procedure.

Dorsal Contractures of the Proximal Interphalangeal Joints. Contractures in flexion with permanent damage to the skin, extensor apparatus, and joint cartilage have already been discussed. If contracture of the skin and extensor apparatus limits flexion of the proximal interphalangeal joint, producing hyperextension and a swan-neck deformity, we do the following:

1. Skin release by a transverse dorsal approach.

2. Distal extensor dissociation (Fig. 73–20). The central slip of the extrinsic extensor tendon is separated from the lateral bands, and the proximal interphalangeal joint is flexed. If the central slip is shortened, a controlled release is effected by multiple transverse incomplete incisions.

3. Thick split thickness skin grafts to cover the raw area, even over denuded tendon.

4. After the graft takes, soft splinting in flexion is instituted for several months whenever the hand is not in use—a position that must be strictly maintained, since this contracture deformity has a strong tendency to recur.

Dorsal Contractures of the Distal Interphalangeal Joint and Periungual Region. Three deformities are associated with this area—periungual distortion, hyperextension of the distal interphalangeal joint (frequently associated with a boutonnière deformity), and mallet finger (the opposite situation) due to weakness of the burned terminal extensor tendon.

The technique for correction of periungual distortion improves the trophicity of the nail (Figs. 73–21, 73–22). Care must be taken not to undermine too far or to crush the delicate periungual flaps.

A hyperextension deformity of the distal interphalangeal joints is due to skin and tendon contracture and is frequently associated with periungual distortion. Both deformities can be treated at the same time, in the following sequence:

1. Design and delicate elevation of two periungual flaps.

2. Dissection and controlled release of the terminal extensor tendon by multiple transverse incomplete incisions until free flexion of the distal interphalangeal joint is achieved.

3. Closure of the periungual area by rotation, followed by a thick split thickness skin graft placed directly on the raw area and exposed tendons.

If a mallet finger deformity is interfering with hand function, application of the terminal extensor tendon corrects the problem.

Dorsal Interdigital Web Contractures. Such contractures are the most frequent permanent deformity following burns of the upper limb.

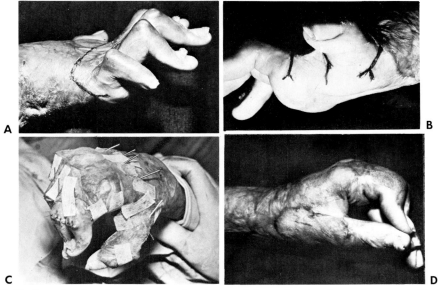

Figure 73–19. Extensive dorsal contractures of metacarpophalangeal and metacarpal areas. *A*, Typical bilateral established deformity following deep burns. Transverse incision for release of hyperextended metacarpals 2 to 5. *B*, Racquet incision to permit thumb to return to normal position. *C*, Pre-articular temporary Kirschner wire fixation and skin grafting after metacarpophalangeal joint flexion. Arthrodesis of the proximal interphalangeal joints by dorsal wedge excision may be a necessary prerequisite to permit strong metacarpophalangeal flexion. *D*, Bilateral long-term result.

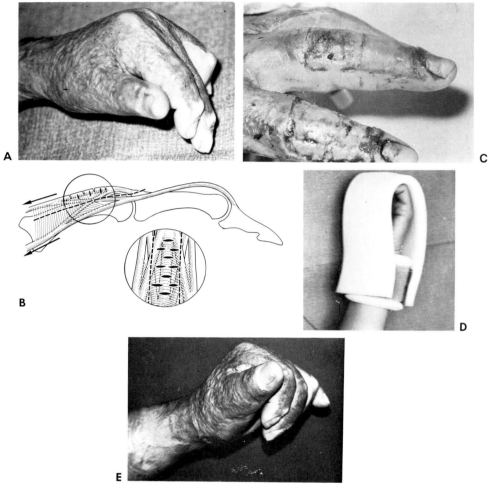

Figure 73–20. Dorsal contracture in extension of proximal interphalangeal joint. *A,* Patient is attempting to make a fist. Fingers 2 and 3 are in strong extension because of skin scar. Sometimes, as in this case, there is also contracture of the central slip, i.e., "distal extrinsic extensor plus," leading to a swan neck deformity. *B,* Diagram of controlled release of contracted central slip by multiple incomplete transverse incisions. *C,* Skin grafts over raw areas, carried out with the proximal interphalangeal joint in flexion. *D,* Polyurethane soft splint dressing to flex the proximal interphalangeal joint gently but firmly. *E,* End result, one year later. Fingers 2 and 3 are now flexible.

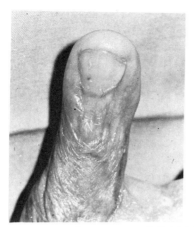

Figure 73–21. Dorsal contracture of distal interphalangeal and periungual region.

We devised the five flap technique (and its variations) as the best method of repair for this deformity in its several degrees of severity (Rousso, 1975a,b; Rousso and Wexler, 1978, 1980; Fig. 73–18). This geometrical method influences the biology of the scar formation. Change is imposed on the direction of the collagen fibers, and healthy flaps are interposed within the scarred area, which in turn halts the tendency to hypertrophy. The scar flattens progressively, and there is blending between it and the healthy skin flaps (Fig. 73–23). One gains the impression that there is growth in all five skin flaps, scarred as well as healthy, probably as a result of the recovery of elasticity of the scarred tissue. Gentle compression by a polyurethane soft splint-dressing helps to shape this process.

If the contracture is severe and involves several webs, repair of alternative sites (e.g., webs 1 and 3 followed by webs 2 and 4 at a different time) avoids cyanosis and edema of the central digits, which will probably occur if all webs are reconstructed together. The five Y-V plasty carried out six months after the first repair greatly improves the result in severe contractures in both sagittal and transverse directions (Fig. 73–24).

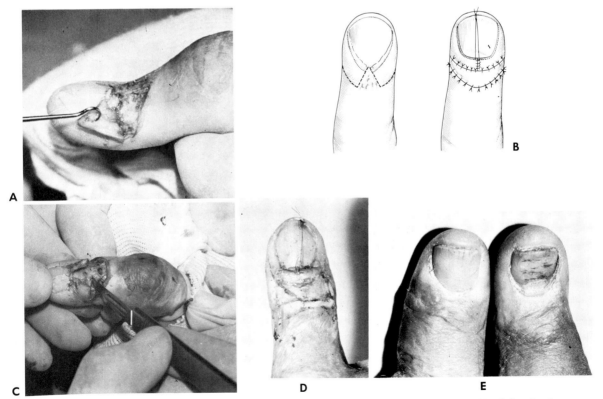

Figure 73–22. *A,* Typical mallet fingers 3 and 4 after deep burn of dorsum. *B,* Diagram of mallet deformity due to weakness of the terminal extensor tendon, overstretching, and tendinous callus formation. *C,* Dissection of terminal extensor with its tendinous callus. *D,* Plication of tendon restores normal position of the interphalangeal joints. *E,* End result.

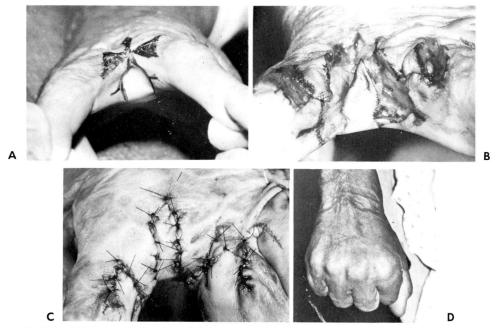

Figure 73–23. *A*, Typical transverse interdigital web contracture associated with contracture of all AFT units to elbow level. *B*, Modified five-flap procedure (see also Fig. 73–18*B*). *C*, Closure of the repair after redistribution. Three healthy volar flaps interdigitate with two dorsal cicatricial flaps. Undermining is necessary only at the sides of the Z-plasties for transposition. *D*, Hypertrophy diminishes after surgery, assisted by sagittal soft splint dressing.

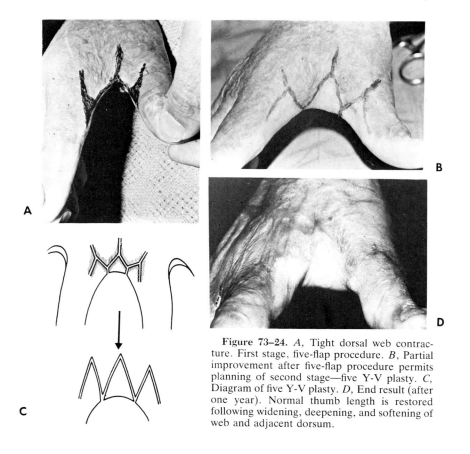

Figure 73–24. *A*, Tight dorsal web contracture. First stage, five-flap procedure. *B*, Partial improvement after five-flap procedure permits planning of second stage—five Y-V plasty. *C*, Diagram of five Y-V plasty. *D*, End result (after one year). Normal thumb length is restored following widening, deepening, and softening of web and adjacent dorsum.

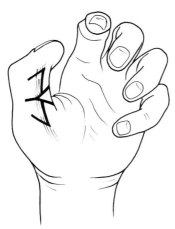

Figure 73–25. Diagram of a digitopalmar skin contracture and its correction by the five-flap technique. Distal Z-plasty reconstructs the pulp.

Volar Contractures of the Hand— Digitopalmar, Interdigital, and Volar Mutilation

The general pattern of volar contractures is longitudinal, palmar, or digital. The treatment in the typical case is shown in Figures 73–25 and 73–26. If despite persistent splinting the volar digitopalmar contracture has a "malignant" tendency to recur, we find it best to resort to a shortening-arthrodesis of the proximal interphalangeal joint, excising the distal half of the proximal phalanx.

Injury that involves adjacent fingers and the palm will also include a transverse volar interdigital web scar (Fig. 73–27). Various five flap combinations have been devised to solve the problem of the restoration of the triple dihedral shape of the normal volar interdigital webs in one single operation.

The most severe volar injuries take the clinical form described as "volar mutilation

of the hand by fire" (Rousso and Wexler, 1980). In this situation there are two solutions possible, depending on the severity of contracture:

1. For the most severe cases in which there is shortening of the digital neurovascular bundles, we release and reposition structures as much as this shortening permits. The pneumatic tourniquet is released, and maximal extension of the proximal interphalangeal joint is regulated according to the vascular supply to the finger tip. Skin grafting is carried out with maximal extension of the digit, but the hand is positioned in semiflexion inside a mild compression dressing.

2. The digitopalmar and interdigital five flap combination can be used with the addition of triangular skin grafts at the extremities of the five flaps. In severe interdigital web cicatricial syndactylies, double anterior and posterior proximally based flaps in addition to skin grafts of raw areas are useful in restoring depth to the web and length to the fingers (Fig. 73–28).

All these programs can be carried out in one or more stages, in which case reconstruction is best carried out from proximal to distal, in the same transverse line of the anatomofunctional topographical units, line after line. This permits the most efficacious use of occupational therapy.

Hypothenar Graft. We have found that, if available, the skin of the hypothenar area provides the best means for resurfacing raw areas on the volar aspect of the hand.

Burns of the Wrist, Elbow, and Axilla

Extensive or circumferential contractures can be repaired by transverse division of scars and repositioning of structures, followed by

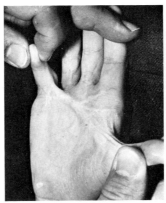
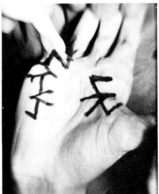

Figure 73–26. *A,* Severe digitopalmar contracture after electrical burn. *B,* Five-flap combination for fifth digitopalmar ray and five-flap plasty for repair of first web.

A

B

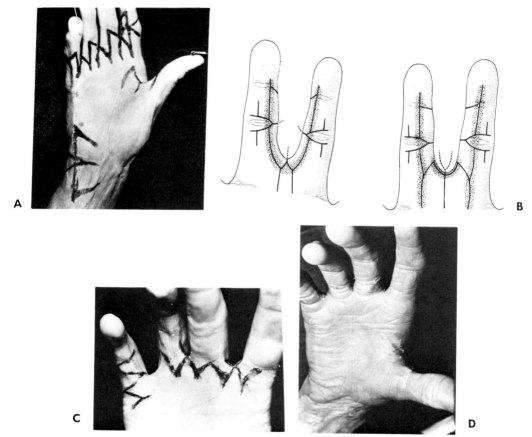

Figure 73–27. *A*, Typical extensive digitopalmar and volar interdigital skin contracture. The normal square of the palm is distorted and lengthened into a rectangle. Surgery is actually performed in two stages, taking alternate webs. *B*, Five-flap combinations recommended for different types of digitopalmar plus volar interdigital skin contractures. *C*, Second stage in surgical revision after six months of soft splint dressing of webs. *D*, End result. Note square palm restoration (by deepening of webs) and quality of skin improvement, as well as normal triple dihedral shape of volar interdigital webs.

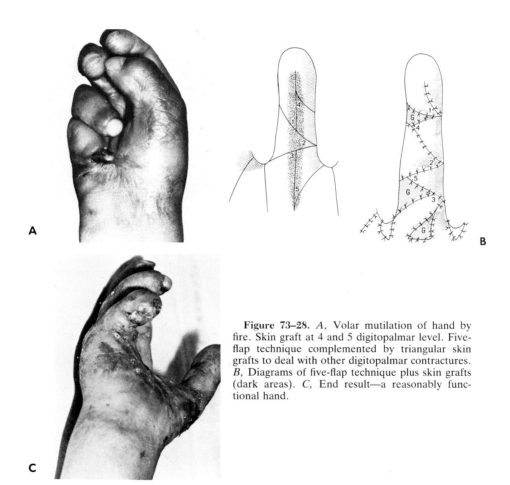

Figure 73–28. *A*, Volar mutilation of hand by fire. Skin graft at 4 and 5 digitopalmar level. Five-flap technique complemented by triangular skin grafts to deal with other digitopalmar contractures. *B*, Diagrams of five-flap technique plus skin grafts (dark areas). *C*, End result—a reasonably functional hand.

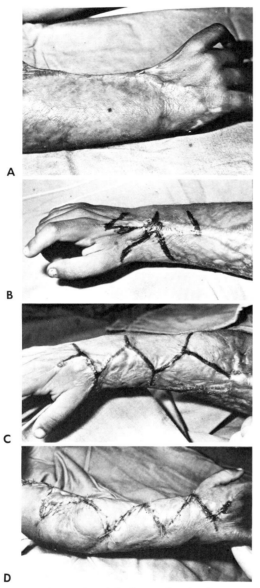

Figure 73–29. *A* and *B*, Severe dorsal wrist contracture necessitating transverse release plus skin grafting. There is a persistent tendency to recurrence.

the use of skin grafts or even better by different combinations of Y-V and Z-plasties in one or more steps (Figs. 73–29 to 73–31).

REGIONAL ANESTHESIA

In secondary reconstruction of the upper limb, regional anesthesia is recommended. This is especially important when several stages of surgery are necessary (Rousso,

1978; Rousso et al., 1981; Vatashsky, 1980). Intravenous regional anesthesia effected with Marcaine and a double tourniquet at arm or forearm level has been especially useful in repeated secondary treatment of burns of the upper limb, up to and including the elbow.

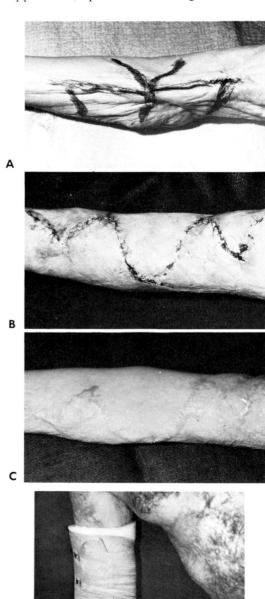

Figure 73–30. *A,* Typical anterolateral contracture of elbow. *B* and *C,* Five-flap technique demonstrates progressive improvement of hypertrophy and collagen remodeling. No scar excision was done. *D,* Circular soft splint dressing.

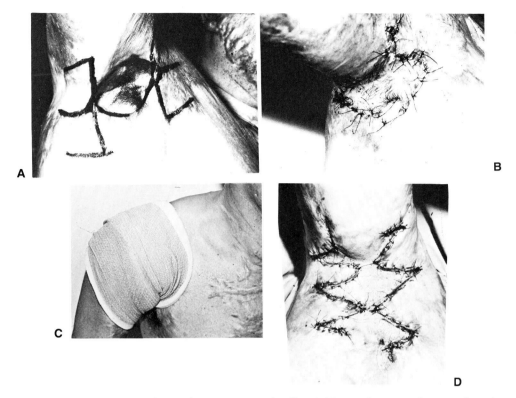

Figure 73–31. Severe anterior and posterior contracture of axilla. *A,* The total program is mapped out but only the central portion is carried out as a first stage (double opposed Y-V plasty). *B,* End of first stage—a pocket of healthy central skin is revealed. *C,* After several months of circular soft splint dressing, hypertrophy lessens. *D,* At the second procedure, the technique of double opposed five-flaps is possible.

ACKNOWLEDGMENTS

We thank Mrs. Rivka Ben Porath, Occupational Therapist, for her assistance in the preparation of the material on splinting and Dr. Miriam Gavarin for correction of the English manuscript.

REFERENCES

Derganc, M., and Zdravic, P.: Advantages of early and active treatment of the deep dermal burn. *In* Transactions of the Third International Congress of Plastic Surgery, 1963. Amsterdam, Excerpta Medica Foundation, 1964, pp. 142–145.

Feller, I.: Differential diagnosis of depth of burn. Univ. Michigan Med. Center J., *30:*297–300, 1964.

Jackson, D. M.: Second thoughts on the burn wound. J. Trauma, *9:*839–862, 1969.

Jancekovic, Z.: A new concept in the early excision and immediate grafting of burns. J. Trauma, *10:*1103–1108, 1970.

Koepke, G. H.: Treatment of burned patients by physical means. J. Trauma, *7:*120–122, 1967.

Koepke, G. H., and Feller, I.: Physical measures for the prevention and treatment of deformities following burns. J.A.M.A., *199:*791–793, 1967.

Koepke, G. H.: The role of physical medicine in the treatment of burns. Surg. Clin. N. Am., *50:*1385–1399, 1970.

Koepke, G. H., Feallock, B., and Feller, I.: Splinting the severely burned hand. Am. J. Occup. Ther., *17:*147–150, 1963.

Larson, D. L.: The Prevention and Correction of Burn Scar Contracture and Hypertrophy. Galveston, Shriners Burns Institute, University of Texas Medical Branch, 1973.

Larson, D. L., Abston, S., Evans, E. B., Dobrkovsky, M., and Linares, H. A.: Technique for decreasing scar formation and contractures in the burned patient. J. Trauma, *11:*807–823, 1971.

Larson, D. L., Abston, S., Willis, B., Linares, G., Dobrkovsky, M., Evans, E. B., and Lewis, S. R.: Contracture and scar formation in the burn patient. Clin. Plast. Surg. *1:*653–666, 1974.

Larson, D. L., Baur, P., Linares, H. A., Willis, B., Abston, S., and Lewis, S. R.: Mechanisms of hypertrophic scar and contracture formation in burns. Burns, *1:*119–127, 1973.

Peacock, H. A., Madden, J. W., and Trier, W. C.: Some studies on the treatment of burned hand. Ann. Surg., *171:*903–914, 1970.

Rousso, M.: Brûlures dorsales graves de la main. Reconstruction de la commissure. Technique à cinq lambeaux. I. La premiere commissure. Ann. Chir., *29:*475–479, 1975a.

Rousso, M.: Brûlures dorsales graves de la main. II. Reconstruction des commissures 2-3 et 4. Modification à la technique à cinq lambeaux. Ann. Chir., 29:1014–1015, 1975b.

Rousso, M., and Wexler, M. R.: Secondary reconstruction of the burned hand. Prog. Surg. 16:182–206, 1978.

Rousso, M., Wexler, M. R., Weinberg, H., and Magora, F.: Regional anesthesia for hand surgery. Prog. Surg. 16:44–52, 1978.

Rousso, M., and Wexler, M. R.: Management of the burned hand. In Goldwyn, R. M. (Editor): Long-Term Results in Plastic and Reconstructive Surgery. Boston, Little, Brown and Company, 1980, Vol. 2, pp. 892–907.

Rousso, M., et al.: Low IV regional analgesia with bupivacaine for hand surgery. Br. J. Anaesth., 1981.

Vatashsky, E., Aronson, H. B., Wexler, M. R., and Rousso, M.: Anesthesia in a hand surgery unit. J. Hand Surg. 5:495–497, 1980.

Wexler, M. R., Yeschua, R., and Neuman, Z.: Early treatment of burns of the dorsum of the hand by tangential excision and skin grafting. Plast. Reconstr. Surg., 54:268, 1974.

Wexler, M. R., and Neuman, Z.: The immediate management of the burns of the dorsal hand surface (emphasis on early tangential excision). In Converse, J. M. (Editor): Reconstructive Plastic Surgery. Philadelphia, W. B. Saunders Company, 1977, p. 338.

Wexler, M. R., and Rousso, M.: The immediate treatment of the burned hand. Prog. Surg., 16:165–179, 1978.

Chapter 74

THE FOREARM FLAP IN RECONSTRUCTION OF BURNS OF THE HAND

Ti-Sheng Chang

Since the introduction of the forearm flap by Chinese military surgeons Yang Guo-Fan, Chan Bao-qui, and Gao Yu-zhi in Shengyang Military Hospital in March 1979, this flap has become widely used in repairing soft tissue defects or in organ reconstruction in plastic and reconstructive surgery, maxillofacial surgery, urology, and otorhinolaryngology, including one-stage reconstruction of the penis, one-stage reconstruction of the hypopharynx after its excision, and one-stage reconstruction after combined cranio-maxillofacial resection in cancer patients.

One special feature is the use of the forearm flap for skin coverage in soft tissue defects of the hand after acute complicated injuries or in reconstruction of postburn hand deformities with exposed deep structures, including tendons, vessels, nerves, and joints.

In the Plastic and Reconstructive Department of the Ninth People's Hospital of Shanghai Second Medical College in China, during a period of six years experience accumulated in the surgical practice of use of the forearm flap in hand reconstruction. A procedure evolving from use of a free forearm flap by microsurgical technique to a reversed forearm flap and forearm fascial flap (which are conventional plastic surgical techniques) was developed with good postoperative results.

ANATOMY

Injection studies on 70 adult cadaver forearms revealed:

1. The forearm skin is nourished by radial and ulnar cutaneous branches. Abundant anastomoses exist between these branches subcutaneously in such a way that the dermal and hypodermal vascular networks can be clearly delineated by injection in either the radial artery or the ulnar artery (Fig. 74–1). This means that either artery can be used as a forearm flap arterial pedicle; however, the radial artery, being more superficially located, is the ideal donor artery.

2. The radial artery, measuring 215.3 ± 2.7 mm. in average length, can be grossly divided into two portions (Fig. 74–2). The upper portion, 111.7 ± 3.4 mm. in average length, is covered by the brachioradialis muscle, and lower portion, 101.4 ± 2.8 mm. in average length, is exposed in the sulcus formed by the tendons of brachioradialis and flexor carpi radialis. Its caliber averages 2.7 ± 0.5 mm. in the upper part, 2.3 ± 0.1 mm. in mid-portion, and 2.4 ± 0.1 mm. in the lower part. Two arterial branches can be recognized, the anterior radial recurrent artery and the superficial palmar artery. Occasionally an interrosseous artery can be found in the upper extremity in 6.6 per cent of cases. G. Foucher, in reviewing composite forearm flaps, described two constant fine arterial branches emerging from the distal radial artery, one is destined to the tendinous portions of the brachioradialis and flexor carpi radialis and the other runs directly to the radial styloid process.

3. The cutaneous branches of the radial artery, numbering four to eight in its lower exposed portion, have calibers ranging from 0.2 to 0.4 mm., whereas the cutaneous branches of this artery, numbering 0 to 10 in its covered upper portion, have calibers ranging from 0.3 to 0.4 mm.

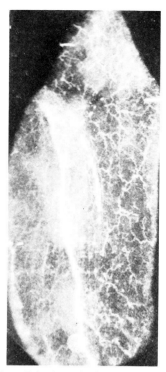

Figure 74–1. Injection of a forearm flap utilizing the complete ulnar and radial arteries. Injection of contrast medium in the radial artery clearly delineates the dermal and hypodermal vascular networks including the ulnar artery. (Courtesy of Yang Gaofan.)

4. The cutaneous branches of the ulnar artery arise from both sides of the artery in its two lower thirds. The radial side branches, numbering four to eight, are anastomosed with the cutaneous branches of the radial artery, and the cubital side cutaneous branches, numbering two to six, are destined to vascularize the dorsal forearm skin.

5. Venous return of the forearm skin flap. Two satellite veins to the radial artery, with many communications between them and an average caliber of 1.3 ± 0.1 mm., can be used for anastomosis. The cephalic vein originates from the radial side of the dorsum of the hand and ends at the basilic vein in 68.18 ± 8.22 per cent of cases and at the brachiocephalic vein in 18.18 ± 8.22 per cent. Its caliber averages in 2.8 ± 0.2 mm.

6. Nerve of the forearm flap. To have a sensory flap, the lateral cutaneous nerve, a continuation of the musculocutaneous nerve, can be used. The superficial branch of the radial nerve must be preserved intact in order to prevent a neuroma and the problem of a residual anesthetic area on the hand.

SURGICAL TECHNIQUE

FLAP DESIGN

1. The Allen test and Doppler determination of the radial and ulnar arteries are indispensable to assure the patency of these vessels.

2. The courses of the radial artery and the cephalic vein are traced dermographically.

3. The edge of the forearm flap must be 0.5 to 1.0 cm. beyond that of the recipient area.

4. The maximum area (35 × 15 cm.) of the flap can theoretically involve the whole forearm and the skin of the inferior third of the arm. In practice, the basilic vein and its skin covering must remain intact for easy venous return of the hand.

5. To have a sensory flap the lateral cutaneous nerve can be included in the flap.

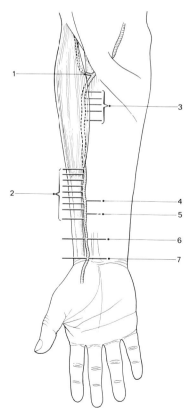

Figure 74–2. Schematic representation of cutaneous branches of the radial artery. 1 = Anterior recurrent radial artery, 2 = cutaneous branch of superficial radial artery, 3 = cutaneous branch of deep radial artery, 4 = dorsal branch to the wrist, 5 = palmar branch to the wrist, 6 = branch to the scaphoid, and 7 = distal radial artery.

6. The tendon of the brachioradialis or palmaris longus and a segment of bone from the radial styloid can be excised en bloc to make a composite flap.

Raiging the Free Forearm Flap

1. Using an Esmarch tourniquet without exsanguination, the skin incision is deepened down to the subcutaneous fascia.

2. The flap is developed by sharp dissection between the superficial and deep layers of the fascia to meet the flexor carpi radialis tendon medially and the brachioradialis tendon laterally. The paratenon should remain intact for easy "take" of the free skin graft put upon them and for prevention of tendon adhesions. The dissection is delicate in that the fine cutaneous branches derived from the radial artery should be protected from injury.

3. The distal radial artery, cephalic vein, and radial satellite veins are divided and ligated. The superficial branch of the radial nerve beneath the dorsal aspect of the cephalic vein should be preserved.

4. The flap is elevated disto-proximally at the deep aspect of the radial artery, and its muscular branches are cut and coagulated. The distal flap is thus developed and the proximal radial artery and its venae comitantes remain attached.

5. The tourniquet is released and meticulous hemostasis is maintained. The flap pedicle remains intact until the recipient vessels have been prepared for anastomosis, the ischemic time of the flap thus being reduced to a minimum.

6. The radial artery defect is reconstructed by an interposing vein graft, and a partial thickness skin graft is used to cover the forearm skin defect.

FOREARM FLAP

One-stage reconstruction is a new trend in surgical repair of acute complicated hand injuries or in postburn hand deformities, especially those associated with plastic repair of important deep structures such as tendons, nerves, bones, and joints in which a well-vascularized, high-quality skin flap is absolutely necessary for a useful hand both esthetically and functionally.

The forearm skin flap is the flap of first choice in hand reconstructive surgery, as it is a good color match and has a long vascular pedicle, large vascular caliber, large skin flap area, and thin subcutaneous tissue. Since April 1979 (a few months after Yang's first introduction of the flap) in a period of less than five months, 37 forearm flaps were successfully transplanted for hand reconstruction in our clinic with very good esthetic and functional results. It goes without saying that the flap is taken from the opposite forearm to repair the contralateral mutilated hand.

Case Reports

Case No. 1. A 37-year-old man was admitted on July 25, 1979 for treatment of a dorsal scar contracture of both hands resulting from a severe burn one year ago. Examination revealed hypertrophic scar formation over the dorsal surface of the right hand with little disturbance of its function. On the right side, deep-seated scar tissue with underlying adhesions of the digital extensors caused a moderate degree of claw-hand deformity (Fig. 74–3A). A split thickness skin graft was sufficient to correct the left hand deformity, whereas a free forearm flap was necessary to reconstruct the right claw-hand deformity.

After thorough excision of scar tissue and reduction of the hyperextended metacarpophalangeal joints, a 10 × 15 cm. left forearm flap was used to cover the skin defect by microsurgical technique, the donor site being skin grafted. Both forearm flap and skin graft survived without delay (Fig. 74–3B).

Follow-up study two years after the operation showed good quality of the transplanted forearm flap (Fig. 74–3C). The functional recovery was good except for a mild degree of radial deviation of the metacarpophalangeal thumb joint (Fig. 74–3D).

Case No. 2. A 20-year-old woman was admitted on January 16, 1980 for treatment of a hyperextension deformity and limited movement of the right wrist due to postburn adhesions of the digital extensor tendons. On examination, the wrist was fixed in 120 degrees of dorsiflexion and 30 degrees of ulnar deviation. The extensors were fixed and digital flexion limited (Fig. 74–4A). Next, 6 × 12 cm. scar tissue was excised, followed by tenolysis of the scarred extensors. A 6.5 × 19 cm. skin defect was created and covered by a opposite side free forearm flap. Excellent postoperative functional result was obtained (Fig. 74–4B, C, D).

REVERSED DISTAL ISLAND FOREARM FLAP

The good quality of the forearm flap in hand reconstructive surgery has made its use

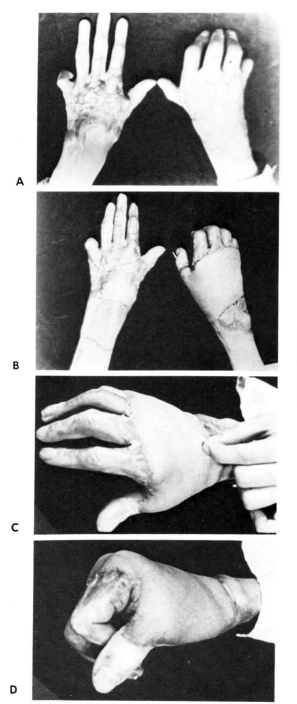

Figure 74–3. Case No. 1. *A*, Postburn dorsal scar contracture of both hands. *B*, Both the free forearm flap on the right hand and the skin graft on the left forearm survived without complications. *C*, The forearm flap is soft and pliable. *D*, The postoperative functional result was good. There was a mild degree of radial deviation of the metacarpophalangeal joint of the thumb.

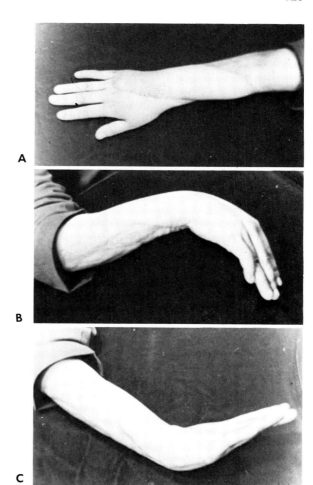

Figure 74–4. Case No. 2. *A*, Postburn hyperextension deformity of the right wrist, which was fixed in 120 degrees dorsiextension and 30 degrees ulnar deviation. *B* and *C*, Excellent postoperative results.

popular in our clinic. The technique is complicated by microsurgical rebranching of donor vessels to the recipient vessels and the need to sacrifice the contralateral forearm skin and its radial artery. To simplify the technique we had the idea of changing the free forearm flap to a pedicle one. The distal radial artery, which has a rather high retrograde blood flow, is quite sufficient to nourish the distal island flap. The problem that remains unsolved is the venous return of the flap. To test the feasibility of the technique, a forearm flap pedicled on the distal radial artery with its venae comitantes remaining intact was tried, the distal island flap being elevated and twisted 180 degrees (Fig. 74–5). No problem with circulation of the island flap was encountered during a 2-hour period of observation, and the flap was accordingly used to cover the skin defect of the hand. The flap survived and the postoperative course was uneventful. Since our first such

procedure (accomplished in September 1980) to September 1984, more than 80 procedures in our clinic and another total of 161 procedures (reported by many authors at the Conference of Hand Surgery held at Anhui, China in October, 1984) were done without one failure. The technique is therefore feasible and safe.

ANATOMICAL BASIS OF THE DISTAL ISLAND FOREARM FLAP

The flap based on the distal segment of the radial artery, after its division, receives a retrograde blood flow from the ulnar artery by way of the superficial and deep palmar arterial arches. The venous return is completed through venae comitantes of the radial artery for the small area island flap; for the large flap, the cephalic vein should be included inside to ensure adequate venous

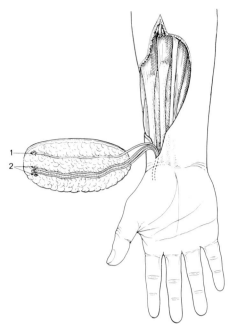

Figure 74–5. The reversed forearm flap. The venous return is via the venae comitantes. In the case of a problem with venous return, the cephalic vein can be used to anastomose the recipient veins. 1 = cephalic vein and 2 = venae comitantes of radial artery.

drainage. There are valves in the venae comitantes of the radial artery that receive valveless tributaries. As the valveless tributaries communicate closely with each other, the blood flow in the veins of the reversed flap could return in a retrograde zigzag fashion without difficulty (Fig. 74–6).

With regard to the venous blood return of this flap, some surgeons questioned the possible presence of the venous valves that might interfere with the venous return. However, in our clinical cases, we have not observed any flaps complicated by venous return.

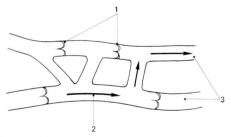

Figure 74–6. Retrograde venous return in zigzag fashion in two venae comitantes of the radial artery. 1 = valves in venae comitantes, 2 = venous return is assured by use of zigzag, and 3 = venae comitantes of radial artery.

Moreover, in October 1983, the Department of Anatomy of the First Military Medical School of the Chinese Army reported their research work on cadavers. They found a total of 241 valves in 66 radial veins of the forearm. The average number of valves was 3.7. In the distal part of the forearm, 24 of these 66 veins had no valve at all. In the other 42 veins, there was only one valve present on average, some of which showed hypoplasia. Moreover, there were many tiny communicating branches in between the radial artery and the venae comitantes. Therefore, during the dissection of this flap, if we can carefully preserve the vascular bundle as a whole, there will be no problem concerning venous return postoperatively. However, if the flap is larger than 10 × 12 cm., it is better to simultaneously preserve both the cephalic veins and venae comitantes of the radial artery in order to prevent any disturbance of venous return.

Timmons used experimental injection of 1 per cent lidocaine into the tissues around venous valves that had become incompetent, immediately allowing reverse flow to occur, to indicate that local anesthesia following surgical elevation of a flap is responsible for immediate retrograde venous flow in reversed forearm flaps.

SURGICAL TECHNIQUE

The courses of the radial artery and cephalic vein are drawn demographically. The cephalic vein is clearly visible with the arm in the dependent position, and the superficial skin projection of the radial artery can be marked by tracing a line passing through the point of tendon insertion of the biceps brachii superiorly and the palpable pulse of the radial artery at the wrist.

The reversed pedicle forearm flap technique is simple and easy, in that microsurgical rebranching of the vascular pedicle is omitted. A preoperative Allen test in emergency cases and arteriography in selected cases are desirable. The largest of our island flaps was 15 × 9 cm.; theoretically, the flap can be further enlarged. In the latter case, the proximal cephalic vein must be kept within the flap and anastomosed to the recipient vein in order to encourage venous return.

The dissection begins by approaching the radial artery on both the superior and inferior borders of the flap. The proximal radial artery is ligated and severed, and the proximal cephalic vein is dissected for a length of 2 to 3 cm. beyond its margin for anastomosis to the recipient vein if necessary. The musculocutaneous nerve remains untouched.

The flap is developed by dissection between the superficial and deep layers of the forearm fascia, centered on the radial artery as an axis. Care should be taken in dissecting the radial pedicle near the radial pulse gutter, where the venae comitantes should be protected from injury.

The island flap pedicled on the wrist can be mobilized to cover the skin defect of the hand.

The dissection can proceed further by crossing the radial pedicle under the abductor longus, extensor brevis, and extensor longus tendons of the thumb to reach the first metacarpal space. In such cases, the length of the pedicle is greatly increased, and the flap can be used to cover any skin defect of the hand, including the thumb and long fingers.

Reinnervation of the flap by anastomosing the lateral cutaneous nerve to the collateral nerve of the recipient site was tried, but the long-term results are not yet available. Furthermore, forearm island composite flaps and osteocutaneous flaps were used to reconstruct the missing thumb in four cases, as reported by G. Foucher.

Case Reports

Case No. 3. A 25-year-old man was hospitalized on June 25, 1980 for correction of traumatic narrowing of the first web space of the right hand. Two years earlier, an injury resulted in partial loss of the adductor pollicis and interosseous muscles of the right hand; the thumb opposition was lost and the index finger was radially deviated (Fig. 74–7A). The reconstruction consisted of thorough excision of scar tissue over the first web space followed by web contracture release (Fig. 74–7B). A 16 × 5 cm. distal forearm flap with a 3-cm. radial vascular pedicle was elevated. The skin bridge interposed between the forearm and web space wounds was cut to make them into one incision. The vascular pedicle was carefully dissected and mobilized (Fig. 74–7C) and then turned 180 degrees to cover the web space skin defect (Fig. 74–7D). The reversal forearm flap survived completely without any problems of venous return. The postoperative opposition between the thumb and index finger recovered quite well (Fig. 74–7E).

Case No. 4. A 36-year-old woman had a gas burn over the palm of her right hand eight months earlier, resulting in a flexion contracture of the thumb against the palm and severe contracture of the little finger (Fig. 74–8A). The operation (done on September 25, 1981) consisted of release of the thumb from the palm by scar excision, leaving a skin defect over 75 per cent of the palmar surface (Fig. 74–8B). A 7.5 × 13.5 cm. reversed forearm flap with 2-cm. long radial vascular pedicle was developed (Fig. 74–8C). The flap was then turned in a reverse direction to cover the skin defect over the palm (Fig. 74–8D). The donor site was skin grafted. Good functional recovery of the reconstructed hand was obtained.

REVERSED FOREARM FASCIAL FLAP

A skin flap is always necessary to cover soft tissue defects of the hand, especially those with exposure of deep structures. The forearm island flap is ideal for this purpose, but a free skin graft on the donor forearm causes an unacceptable cosmetic defect for the patient. Our goal therefore was to have an acceptable donor site scar and to simplify the technique. Based on our experience in using the temporal fascia to cover deep structures of the hand in surgical treatment of claw-hand deformities, a synthetic skin flap (distal island forearm fascial flap with a skin graft placed on top of it) was developed by one of my senior staff. The technique was used to cover the exposed deep structures of the hand 18 times in 17 postburn cases, with satisfactory results both esthetically and functionally during the 4 to 16 months of follow-up.

SURGICAL TECHNIQUE

A preoperative Allen test and Doppler flowmetry to determine the patency of the radial artery as an axis of the flap are indispensable. With the radial artery marked out as an axis, the fascial flap is shaped on the forearm, conforming to the size and shape of the skin defect of the hand.

As soon as the recipient site dissection in the hand is ready, an S-shaped skin incision is made on the ventral forearm skin along the radial artery, and two skin flaps are developed and retracted laterally. The fascia is exposed, and the radial artery, accom-

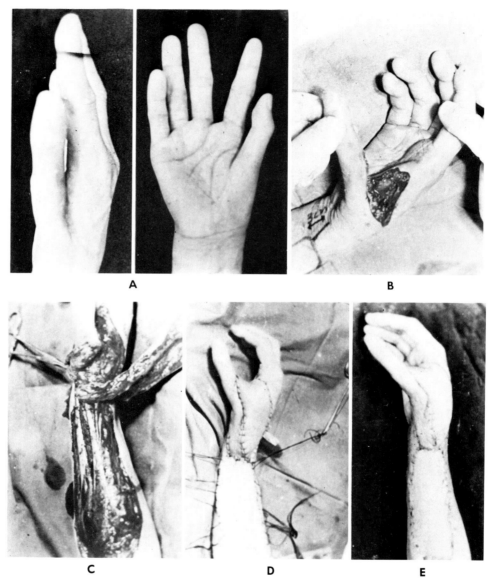

Figure 74–7. Case No. 3. *A*, Traumatic narrowing of the first web space with loss of opponent function between the thumb and index finger. *B*, Skin defect after web contracture release. *C*, Elevation of distal forearm flap. *D*, Web skin defect is covered by reversed forearm flap and the donor skin is grafted. *E*, Opponent function recovered quite well.

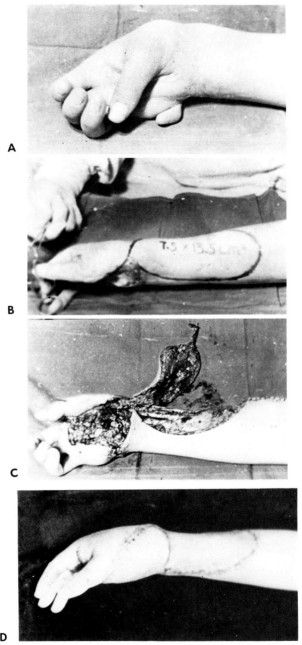

Figure 74–8. Case No. 4. *A*, Flexion contracture of the thumb against the palm and severe distortion of the little finger. *B*, Release of the thumb from the palm, leaving a palmar skin defect. *C*, A 7.5 × 13.5 cm. reversal forearm flap was developed. *D*, The distal forearm flap was mobilized to cover the palmar skin defect. Good functional recovery of the reconstructed hand was obtained.

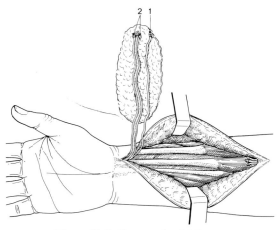

Figure 74–9. Forearm fascial flap.

panied by its venae comitantes, is dissected out proximally and distally to the flap. Having ligated and cut the proximal radial artery, an incision is made at the periphery of the desired fascial flap, and the flap is developed in a retrograde fashion by dissection at a plane just superficial to the perimysium, with the distal radial artery and its venae comitantes intact as a pedicle (Fig. 74–9).

The island fascial flap is either transferred through a subcutaneous tunnel or just turned over distally to cover the exposed tendons and metacarpophalangeal joints of the hand. Its margin is sutured to the edge and the entire raw surface of the hand, and the fascial flap is resurfaced with a split thickness skin graft, which is secured by a tie-over dressing.

The donor site on the forearm is approximated. If there is extensive scar formation on the donor forearm, the scar can first be excised to an extent that conforms to the size of the required fascial flap. Then the fascial flap is raised, as mentioned earlier. The donor site is covered with a skin graft.

Case Reports

Case No. 5. A 22-year-old woman suffered from severe burns over both hands (Fig. 74–10A). It

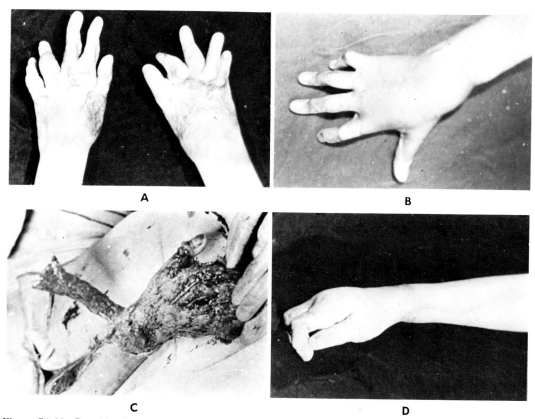

Figure 74–10. Case No. 5. *A*, Postburn hand deformities. *B*, A 5.5 × 15 cm. reversal forearm fascial flap was raised. *C*, Good esthetic and functional results after operation. *D*, The S-shaped linear incision scar on the forearm is esthetically acceptable.

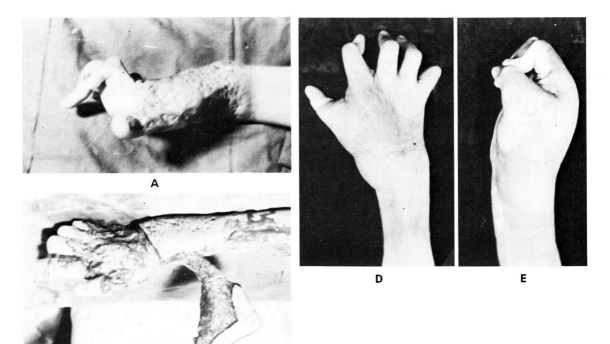

A

B

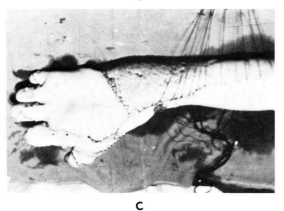

C

D

E

Figure 74–11. Case No. 6. *A*, Postburn right claw-hand deformity. *B*, A 5 × 8 cm. reversal forearm island fascial flap, together with a flap attached to its distal end, was raised. *C*, The skin portion of the flap was used to cover the thumb and the first web space defects, while the fascial flap covered the exposed extensor tendons and metacarpophalangeal joints of the index and long fingers. *D*, The entire raw surface was covered with a split thickness skin graft. *E*, One year after the operation, a good functional result was obtained.

was decided that the right hand would receive a flap repair, whereas the left hand would receive only a free skin graft. The operation was undertaken in May 8, 1982, under cervical epidural block anesthesia. Following excision of the scar tissue over the dorsum of the right hand, the metacarpophalangeal joints of index and middle fingers were reduced, after lengthening of the extensor tendons, resection of the collateral ligaments, and release of adhesions in the joint cavities. However, the metacarpophalangeal joints of thumb, ring, and little fingers were reduced by manipulation only. The proximal interphalangeal joint of the index finger was fused.

Through an S-shaped incision over the forearm, the fascial flap was raised based on the distal radial artery with its venae comitantes and on the cephalic vein. The flap measured 5.5 × 15 cm. It was turned over at 180 degrees to cover the exposed tendons and metacarpophalangeal joints of the index and middle fingers (Fig. 74–10*B*).

The entire raw surface on the dorsum of the hand and the wrist was covered with a medium split thickness skin graft of 15 × 15 cm. The forearm donor wound was closed directly. The postoperative course was uneventful and stitches were removed on the tenth postoperative day. The skin graft took completely and the donor site healed primarily. Follow-up study 16 months later showed satisfactory results (Fig. 74–10*C*). The S-shaped incision linear scar over the forearm is acceptable (Fig. 74–10*D*).

Case No. 6. A 29-year-old woman presented with a right postburn claw-hand deformity and an extensive scar on the forearm (Fig. 74–11*A*). The operation was done in May 13, 1983, under brachial plexus block anesthesia. Excision of the scar on the hand and correction of the metacarpophalangeal joints were performed, but this led to exposure of the extensor tendons and joint cavity in the radial three fingers. The scar in the forearm was also excised, leaving the underlying intact fascia. A reversed island fascial flap measuring 5 × 8 cm. was raised and transferred, together with a small two wing–shaped skin flap attached to its distal end; both were based on the radial artery and its venae comitantes (Fig. 74–11*B*). The skin portion of the flap was used to cover the thumb and the first web space, while the fascial flap covered the exposed extensor tendons and metacarpophalangeal joints of the index and middle fingers (Fig. 74–11*C*). The entire raw surface extending from the back of the hand to the donor site of the forearm was resurfaced with a split thickness skin graft 250 cm. in size (Fig. 74–11*D*). A light pressure dressing was applied to secure the graft. The sutures were removed on the tenth postoperative day and the skin graft took completely. Follow-up study one year late showed good functional restoration of the hand (Fig. 74–11*E*).

CONCLUSION

The one-stage operation is a modern trend in surgical treatment of postburn claw-hand deformity or complicated acute hand injuries. It can be carried out either by a free forearm flap transfer or by the use of a reversed forearm pedicle flap and reversed forearm fascial pedicle flap with excellent results.

Microsurgery is a modern progression in the field of plastic and reconstructive surgery; however, microsurgery should not replace all forms of traditional plastic surgery. The practice of these two reversed forearm tissue pedicled flaps is an example of the relationship between microsurgical and traditional plastic surgery techniques.

COLD INJURIES

Chapter 75

COLD INJURIES IN THE ADULT PATIENT

JOHN A. BOSWICK, JR.

It is a common misconception that cold injuries are unusual except in times of war or under unusual circumstances. Those who have worked in institutions where large numbers of patients with cold injuries are treated are aware that cold weather alone is not the cause of most cold injuries. The personal and social factors in the epidemiology of cold injuries are extremely important.

MECHANISM AND CAUSES OF COLD INJURY

The primary factors that contribute to a cold injury are a low temperature and adequate exposure time. A cold injury will not occur unless an individual is exposed to a sufficiently low temperature for an adequate period. In addition to temperature and duration of exposure other factors contribute to the development of a cold injury. As would be expected, some factors are more important than others. One of the most significant is wind velocity, which is so important that the term "wind chill factor" has been coined to describe the combination of its effect with that of temperature. Since many, if not most, cold injuries occur when the wind velocity is an important consideration, the time–wind chill factor is much more significant than the time and temperature.

Another major contributor to the development of cold injury is humidity, or wetness. Increased humidity in the environment or locally on a part of the body aggravates a cold injury. The significance of wetness in contributing to a cold injury is most evident in patients who develop cold injuries through openings in gloves or boots. A small amount of moisture may enter a glove or a boot without the wearer's noticing it until hours later, when the glove or boot is removed and the injury is obvious. In some cases significant cold injury has occurred in an extremity covered by a glove or boot with a break in it, while in the opposite extremity, on which the glove or boot was intact, there was no demonstrable injury.

The cold injury that occurs when living tissue is in contact with a cold object (especially metal) is more severe than that which occurs when the tissue is merely exposed to a cold environment. When the skin is in contact with a cold object, there is a more rapid transfer of heat than occurs when it is surrounded by cold air. This is often noticeable in cases in which the patients became unconscious or comatose and sustained cold injuries. An exposed hand or foot is often in contact with a park bench, railroad track, steering wheel, or other cold object. The most significant area of injury is invariably the part in contact with the cold object, compared with the adjacent tissue. The contribution of direct contact with a cold object to a cold injury is most significant when humidity is also a factor. This is seen when a cold object contributes to a cold injury through a wet glove.

A cold injury can be most dramatic when there is lack of even minimal protection. Conversely stated, a minimal amount of protection may prevent a cold injury. The protection or lack of protection as it applies to a cold injury is also related to the factors of duration of exposure, temperature, and wind velocity.

Minimal protection is so important in preventing cold injury that it deserves special emphasis. We have had patients suffering from cold exposure of both hands in whom one was protected by a thin glove. The protected hand would have sustained a slight or undetectable cold injury, and the unprotected hand would have a cold injury necessitating amputation of several centimeters of tissue. The amount of clothing needed to protect against a cold injury is unknown, but obviously is related to ambient temperature, duration of exposure, wind velocity, humidity, and whether the part is in contact with a cold object.

Several other factors questionably contribute to the mechanism or significance of a cold injury. Elderly patients are thought to sustain more severe cold injuries than younger patients exposed to the same conditions. This is difficult to evaluate because the elderly are more likely to have preexisting vascular disease that would complicate a cold injury. Younger patients are more likely to be alert and to be able to move out of the cold and to detect cold or wet clothing. In addition to preexisting disease that may complicate a cold injury, elderly patients are more likely to have associated conditions that would prevent them from getting out of the cold. We have seen this in the arthritic patients and in patients with central nervous system disorders.

Another possible or questionable factor that may contribute to the significance of a cold injury is circulatory impairment or decreased vascularity of an extremity. Patients who have arterial or venous disease of the lower extremities appear to have more significant reactions to a cold injury than do those with normal circulatory systems. This is observed frequently enough to give a strong clinical impression that it is correct. However, it must be remembered that the natural progression of most circulatory disorders results in tissue loss without an added cold injury.

Military studies of the incidences of cold injuries suggest that racial and geographic backgrounds may be contributing factors.

Compared with burns and other types of trauma, the incidence of cold injuries to the hands is extremely low. Although thousands of patients with burn injuries of the hand are seen annually, only a few hundred patients with cold injuries are seen. In treating patients with cold injuries of the hands, it is important to keep in mind the difference between the incidences of cold injuries and the opposite thermal injury—burns of the hand. It is often said that cold injuries are similar to burns, and this might suggest that the treatments are similar. In many ways the treatments differ considerably. An accepted technique for treating full thickness burns of the hand is early excision and grafting. Minimal debridement with late amputation is a more accepted policy in treating cold injuries.

Three factors need to be considered in treating patients with cold injuries of the hand, especially before instituting local care: the general or systemic condition of the patient, including his general response to cold and the effects of lowered temperature on other areas of the body; the condition of the tissue when the patient is first seen; and the amount of tissue injured.

MANAGEMENT OF THE SYSTEMIC RESPONSE TO COLD

Patients who have cold injuries of the hands have variable systemic responses and therefore need individualized management. There is only a slight systemic response when only the hands are involved, especially if the injury is of short duration and superficial in depth. A review of our experience in treating more than 400 patients who had sustained cold injuries of both hands showed that more than 250 had involvement of one or both lower extremities, and 22 had cold injuries extensive enough to necessitate bilateral below the knee or more proximal amputation. As the extent and depth of a cold injury increase, the significance of the systemic response usually increases. This includes generalized hypothermia, hypovolemia, acidosis, and hypoxemia. Alcoholic withdrawal symptoms and malnutrition are common complications in patients who have cold injuries. Treatment must be directed toward the total patient and not just the injured tissue.

Generalized hypothermia rarely occurs in a patient who has a cold injury involving only the hands. However, extensive cold injuries of the hands commonly occur in patients with generalized hypothermia. It is generally agreed that rapid rewarming is the method of choice for treating a localized cold injury. However, there is some question as to the most effective method of rewarming a patient with generalized hypothermia. The most accepted technique today in severe hypothermia is rapidly rewarming the blood with an external heating device and a pump.

Following an extensive hot thermal injury (a burn), hypovolemia may be a significant complication. In cold injuries hypovolemia frequently occurs, but it is rarely significant. Extensive tissue damage and fluid loss are unusual in cold injuries when compared with burns. When there is a cold injury involving several extremities with the tissue cold or frozen, the hematocrit level may reach 60 per cent or higher. Most patients under these circumstances have had prolonged exposures, and dehydration as well as fluid loss may play a role in the development of hypovolemia. The relatively moderate hypovolemia that occurs with a cold injury presents no problem in management. Administration of a balanced electrolyte solution in amounts twice the daily fluid requirements usually correct the situation in 24 to 48 hours.

In patients with cold injuries of the hands, if the tissue is cold or frozen, some acidosis is usually present. The extent of the acidosis depends upon the extent and depth of the injury and what has occurred from the time of injury to the time the patient is seen. When only the hands are involved, arterial blood pH levels may be as low as 7.24; with a more extensive injury an arterial blood pH of 7.16 has been recorded.

Patients who have sustained cold injuries of the hands and in whom the tissue is cold or frozen at the time of admission are likely to have decreased arterial blood oxygen tensions. The duration of exposure and level of metabolism usually correlate with the arterial blood Po_2. The administration of oxygen by nasal catheter or by mask usually restores the arterial blood Po_2 to normal in eight to 12 hours.

A significant problem in the management of patients with cold injuries is the treatment of alcoholic withdrawal symptoms. In most series high percentages (50 to 85 per cent) of patients with cold injuries sustained the injuries while under the influence (chronic or acute) of alcohol. Early treatment is recommended when the history or findings suggest that this might be an actual or potential problem. A part of the treatment is the use of sedatives (barbiturates, promazine, chlordiazepoxide) and the antitremor drugs (diphenylhydantoin and magnesium sulfate), along with appropriate nutritional and vitamin replacement.

Patients who sustain cold injuries are often suffering from malnutrition. As soon as practical after injury, an adequate dietary intake should be provided along with appropriate vitamin replacement. Although this may be very important, the early systemic management of a patient with a cold injury should not detract from the local care of cold injured tissue. Patients with cold injuries may have tissue that is frozen, cold, blistered, cyanotic, and occasionally gangrenous.

THE CARE OF COLD INJURED TISSUE

The condition of the tissue at the time the patient is seen at the facility where definite care can be rendered is the most significant factor influencing local care. The most serious condition in a cold injury is frozen tissue. Less than 1 per cent of all patients sustaining cold injuries reach the hospital with tissue that is frozen. Some patients who sustain cold injuries severe enough to result in the tissue's becoming frozen are also hypothermic: i.e., core temperature will be below 32° C. (89° F.). (The complete treatment of generalized hypothermia is beyond the scope of this chapter.)

The care of frozen tissue requires concurrent systemic therapy, since the management of frozen tissue is rapid rewarming, a process that can compound the problem of acidosis. A most effective method of treating frozen tissue in a patient who does not have generalized hypothermia is total body rewarming. After obtaining a specimen of arterial blood for P_{O_2}, P_{CO_2}, and pH determinations, an infusion of lactated Ringer's solution with appropriate amounts of sodium bicarbonate (100 mEq./liter of fluids) should be started. The patient should be placed in a tub or body whirlpool with the water at 38° C. (100° F.). The temperature of the water may be slowly raised to 40° C. (105° F.). It usually takes 15 to 20 minutes for the skin temperature to reach a normal level. If the skin temperature has not reached normal after 25 to 30 minutes, further rewarming should be done cautiously. Systemic changes may occur rapidly after this time. Following rewarming, the management of the injured tissue should proceed according to its condition.

The early management of a patient with cold injury who reaches the hospital with cold tissue is the same as that of a patient with frozen tissue. The time needed for rewarming is usually not as long as with frozen tissue. Since cold tissue does not lower the temperature of the water as rapidly as does frozen tissue, it is not necessary to increase the temperature of the water. Blistering occasionally occurs after cold or frozen tissue is rewarmed.

It is not unusual for patients who have cold injuries to have tissue that is cyanotic or blistered when they are admitted to the hospital. The immediate or early care of blistered tissue and that of cyanotic tissue are basically the same. Frequent washings are indicated to keep the tissue clean. Active motion should be started as early as possible, with appropriate positioning and splinting during periods of rest. Washing and cleansing of the injured tissue can be accomplished in many ways, depending upon the patient's general condition, other injuries, and his ability to cooperate. Patients are encouraged to wash and actively move their hands frequently. The amount of motion in the metacarpophalangeal and interphalangeal joints in a patient who has sustained a cold injury is considerably less than that in the joints of an uninjured hand. Having the patient sit in a body whirlpool and wash his hands at face or shoulder level is an effective means of accomplishing cleansing and active motion. This provides the patient the opportunity of seeing the hands move and, it is hoped, increase in range of motion each day. As motion in-

creases, the patient is usually motivated to increase the time spent moving the hand.

The same program can be accomplished by use of a wash basin when a whirlpool is not available. Caution must be exercised in allowing the feet to be dependent if they are also involved with a cold injury.

It is important that the program of frequent washing and active motion be continued until there is optimal healing of partial thickness wounds and demarcation of the full thickness areas. This phase of care often extends for 12 to 15 weeks. The amount of full thickness injury is usually overestimated, and the partial thickness areas show progressive healing for several weeks. Within a few days after injury most of the care can be rendered on an outpatient basis when only the hands are involved.

The management of blebs and blisters presents a problem in the treatment of cold injured tissue. Blisters may have developed at the time of hospitalization, or they may develop after the rewarming of cold or frozen tissue. In either situation the care is the same. Blebs or blisters are left intact unless they interfere with hand function and appear taut, and it is believed that the pressure will produce further injury to the underlying tissue, or the blister fluid appears purulent and could result in local or systemic infection.

The prevention of functional loss and the development of anatomical deformities is a significant problem from the time a cold injury is sustained until wound closure is accomplished by spontaneous healing, skin grafting, or amputation.

A well-organized program of active motion, positioning, and splinting can minimize these problems. The advantages and technique of active motion have been described. Equally important is correct positioning of the hands. The wrist should be maintained in an extended position both at rest and while moving. When the wrist is extended, the metacarpophalangeal joints tend to flex owing to the effects of gravity and the pull of the intrinsic muscles. When the metacarpophalangeal joints are flexed, the proximal interphalangeal joints are more supple and are less likely to develop a flexion deformity, since the pull of the flexor tendons is not so great as when the metacarpophalangeal joints are extended. If the wrist is allowed to assume a flexed position, which is usually a position of rest or comfort, the metacarpo-

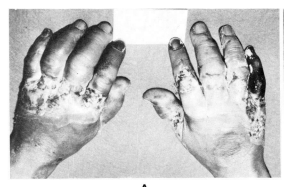
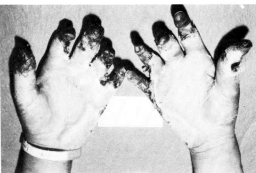

A

B

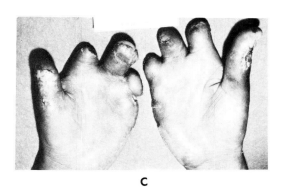

C

Figure 75–1. *A*, Ten days after injury there is healing of the superficial partial-thickness wounds and obvious gangrene of the right little finger. *B*, Twenty-five days after injury there is demarcation between the viable and nonviable tissue with an area of granulation suggesting that there has been optimal healing of the partial-thickness wounds. *C*, Seventy days after injury the amputation stumps are well healed; however, the tissue is still firm and tender.

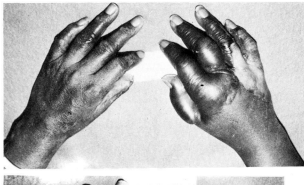

A

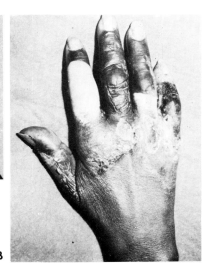

B

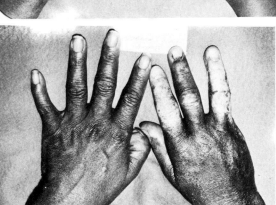

C

Figure 75–2. *A*, Twenty-four hours after injury, with blisters intact on the thumb and the index and long finger. The blisters on the ring and little finger were traumatically ruptured and the loose tissue removed. *B*, Twenty-one days after injury the partial-thickness wounds are healing and the full-thickness areas on the little finger show gangrenous changes. *C*, Fifty-six days after injury the gangrenous tissue has been amputated and the partial-thickness areas have re-epithelialized. Depigmentation is still present in the area of the injury.

phalangeal joints will tend to assume an extended or hyperextended position with a compensatory flexion deformity of the interphalangeal joints. A wrist extension splint is commonly employed to prevent wrist flexion. When a splint is used for this purpose, it should be worn at night during periods of rest but it should not be worn at times that would interfere with actively moving the hand. In some patients the use of a wrist extension splint will not prevent the development of metacarpophalangeal, interphalangeal, and thumb adduction deformities. If these deformities develop when a wrist extension splint is worn, the splint should be extended in a manner such that the metacarpophalangeal joints can be pulled into flexion, the interphalangeal joints pushed into extension, and the thumb pulled or pushed into abduction.

Although it is important to institute measures that maintain function and prevent the development of deformities in the hand with a cold injury, it is also important to properly treat the tissue that has sustained the cold injury. During all phases of care it is important to handle the injured tissue gently. This can be accomplished by frequent washings, gentle motion, and minimal tissue manipulation. The injured extremity should be elevated as much as possible and the loose crusts or dead tissue removed every two to three days. This is best accomplished after the hands have been washed and while the tissue is moist and easily separated. With tissue forceps and scissors the loose tissue is trimmed to the point of firm attachment. This allows the new epithelium to regenerate more rapidly in areas where the wounds are of partial thickness. The full thickness wound will tend to contract or shrink. Between areas of partial and full thickness injuries, areas of granulation tissue usually develop. When this occurs, amputation distal to the level of the granulation is indicated (Fig. 75–1).

When blisters are present early after a thermal injury, they are left intact unless there is an indication for their removal. Figure 75–2 illustrates the case of a patient who had blisters on admission following a cold injury.

SUMMARY

Patients who sustain cold injuries of the hands may need only minimal care if the injuries are limited and the systemic responses are not too significant. When such an injury is extensive and the systemic response is significant, patient care may be complex. When a cold injury involves more than one extremity and the systemic response is significant, both local and systemic care will be necessary.

Preservation of tissue and function of the involved parts is an important goal of treatment. Important guidelines of care are minimal daily debridement and late amputation.

REFERENCES

Blair, J. R.: Follow-up on cold injury cases from the Korean War. In Ferrer, I. M. (Ed.): Fourth Conference on Cold Injury. New York, Josiah Macy, Jr., Foundation, 1955.

Golding, M. R., DeJong, P., Hennigar, G. R., Sawyer, P. N., and Wesolowski, S. A.: Protection from early and late sequelae of frostbite by regional sympathectomy: mechanism of "cold sensitivity" following frostbite surgery. Surgery, 53:303, 1963.

Golding, M. R., Mendoze, M. F., Hennigar, G. R., Fries, C. C. and Wesolowski, S. A.: On settling the controversy on the benefit of sympathectomy for frostbite. Surgery, 56:221, 1964.

Hermann, G., Schechter, D. C., Owens, J. C., and Starzl, T. E.: The problem of frostbite in civilian medical practice. Surg. Clin. N. Am. 43:519, 1963.

Knize, D. M., Weatherley-White, R. C., and Paton, B. C.: Use of antisludging agents in experimental cold injuries. Surg. Gynecol. Obstet., 129:1019, 1969.

Knize, D. M., Weatherley-White, R. C., Paton, B. C., and Owens, J.C.: Prognostic factors in the management of frostbite. J. Trauma, 9:749, 1969.

Meryman, H. T.: Tissue freezing and local cold injury. Physiol. Rev., 37:233, 1957.

Chapter 76

COLD INJURIES IN CHILDREN

Robert W. Harris

The effects of cold on most tissues are the same in the child as in the adult. An exception occurs at the skeletal level, where the effects of cold injury differ greatly between the growing and the adult hand. Although in children's fingers frostbite may produce the same acromutilation and late osteoporotic changes as seen in adults, the principal injury in childhood occurs at the digital growth areas, which are situated in the juxta-articular position. The structures involved include the bony and cartilaginous epiphyses, the articular cartilages, and the metaphyses (Fig. 76–1).

CLINICAL ENTITY

Although it is clear that cold injury as an etiological factor produces a distinct clinical entity in childhood, the incidence of cold induced digital epiphyseal necrosis is unknown, and the frequency of this condition in frostbite cases has not been established. Because of the six to eight month interval between exposure and the onset of changes in the finger, the cause and effect relationship is seldom determined, and very few cases have been documented in the literature. Lohr (1930) recorded one of the earliest descriptions of this lesion, based on findings in three cases. Bennett and Blount (1935), Thelander (1950), Dreyfuss and Glimcher (1955), and Florkiewicz and Kozlowski (1962) each reported single cases; Bigelow and Ritchie (1963) documented 13 cases.

These young patients are usually between four and nine years of age. Incidences in boys and girls appear to be equal. The patients have complaints of dull, aching finger joint pain and a slight decrease in cold tolerance. They are brought for examination because of the angulatory deformities of some digits

noticed by the parents. Clinically the pain is in the finger joints, particularly the distal interphalangeal joint, and it is worse when the barometer is falling. The index, ring, and little fingers are most often involved. The middle finger is less frequently involved because of its more protected position, and the thumb, because of its strong circulation, virtually never.

The early clinical findings are of terminal phalanx deviation laterally or medially and volar angulation (Fig. 76–2). The hands are weak and finger dexterity is poor. Later examination reveals that growth is retarded. The involved fingers are shorter and also stubbier than normal (Fig. 76–3). Evolution of the condition is slow, with occasional flare-ups of pain severe enough to necessitate oral administration of an analgesic and voluntary diminution of manual activity. Eventually the pain resembles that of osteoarthritis. There are no neurological symptoms or signs. There is limited usefulness of the hands, and these patients have restricted digital skill capacity because of reduction of joint amplitude and loss of stability (Fig. 76–4).

RADIOLOGICAL APPEARANCE

The radiological image is typical, and has been well described by Caffey (1967), Werzl et al. (1967), Lindholm et al. (1968), and Selke (1969). It includes an accentuation of the trabecular pattern and slight generalized bone atrophy, especially at the extremities of the fingers. The most marked lesions are at the distal interphalangeal joint level, where the bony epiphyses of the distal phalanges may be partially or completely absent. A tiny fragment of this secondary ossification center may remain. The head of the middle phalanx appears widened and flattened and may show

837

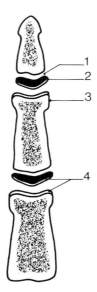

Figure 76–1. Diagrammatic representation of the phalangeal components of the finger in childhood. 1 = physis (cartilaginous epiphysis, epiphyseal plate), 2 = epiphysis (bony epiphysis, secondary ossification center), 3 = phalangeal head (middle phalanx), and 4 = articular cartilage.

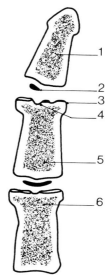

Figure 76–3. Diagram of the various changes resulting from cold injury to the growth elements of the digital phalanges. Greater cartilaginous and bony destruction is sustained distally than proximally. 1 = deviation of distal phalanx, 2 = necrosis of bony epiphysis, 3 = erosion of articular cartilage, 4 = erosion of subcartilaginous bone, 5 = shortening of phalanges, and 6 = widening of metaphysis.

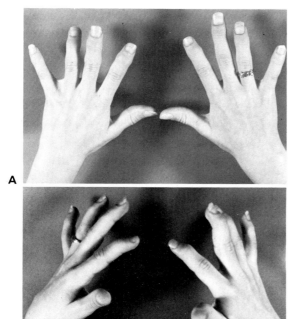

Figure 76–2. *A*, Cold-induced digital epiphyseal necrosis in an 8-year-old girl who had sustained the injury a year and a half previously. Lateral deviations of the index fingers at the distal interphalangeal joints are evident. Shortening and juxta-articular widening are particularly evident in the left middle finger. *B*, In the lateral view the mallet finger deformity is clearly visible. This is due to loss of length of the bony components, particularly at the level of the distal phalanx base and at the middle phalanx head. The swan-neck deformity is not, however, due to intrinsic muscle contracture.

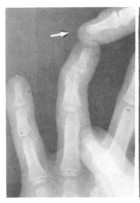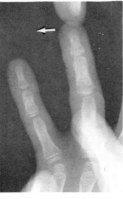

Figure 76–4. Stress radiographs demonstrating the lack of collateral support as the capsular structures become relatively too long secondary to destruction within the joint.

punched-out irregularities or even complete destruction (Fig. 76–5). A similar image is seen at involved proximal interphalangeal joints, but the changes are less severe. Lesions at this level never develop without distal interphalangeal joint involvement. The basal epiphysis of the middle phalanx may be smaller than normal, but the metaphysis is wider. There may be irregularities in the proximal phalanx head, indicating bone necrosis deep to the articular cartilage.

Later radiographs demonstrate the varus or valgus deviation and volar angulation seen clinically (Fig. 76–6A, B). These may be

associated with premature fusion of a part of the epiphyseal line. The interphalangeal joint spaces, particularly the distal space, are often narrowed, and the margins of bone are flared. A compensatory hyperextension deformity develops at the proximal interphalangeal joint level (Fig. 76–6C).

PATHOGENESIS

The results of laboratory investigations in these patients are virtually useless. Cold agglutinins, cryoglobulins, and cryofibrinogens have not been demonstrated. Werzl et al. (1967) found that the sedimentation rate was normal and the rheumatoid factor reaction negative. Arteriographs do not show any pre-existing abnormality, although Bigelow and Richie (1963) found tortuosity of the terminal digital arteries in some cases.

The present consensus in that there is a dual effect of prolonged exposure to severe cold in childhood. The first is a direct lethal effect on the chondrocytes of the cartilaginous epiphysis and those of the articular cartilage. The evidence for this is in the loss of staining properties of the chondrocytic nuclei, darkening, shriveling, and finally absorption of the cartilage. Added to this is the delayed secondary effect of ischemia, which produces death of osteocytes and bone necrosis of the epiphyses per se. Kulka (1964) demonstrated that in cold injury to the ex-

Figure 76–5. *A*, Radiographic appearance of joints two years after sustaining cold injury. The bony epiphyses of the distal phalanges are almost completely destroyed. Bony irregularities of the juxta-articular components reflect the ischemic necrotic process. New bone is formed in an irregular manner. *B*, Destruction of the cartilaginous elements, including the epiphyseal cartilage (physis), and erosion of the juxta-articular bone are evident at the distal interphalangeal joint level in this radiograph. The head of the middle phalanx appears widened and flattened.

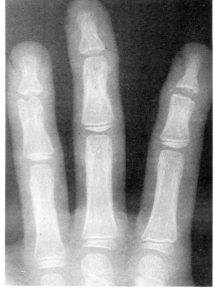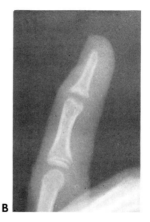

A   B

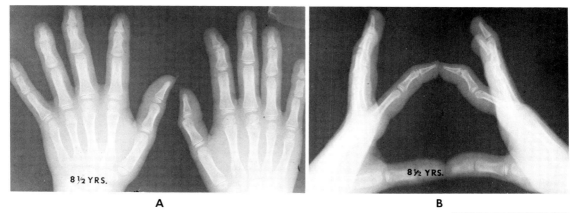

A   B

Figure 76–6. *A*, Lateral deviation of the distal phalanges is especially evident in the
radiograph taken one and a half years after a cold exposure incident. The angulation is
due to uneven growth secondary to partial destruction of the cartilaginous epiphysis.
Radial deviation results from destruction of the radial part of the physis. Growth
continues in the ulnar portion. *B*, Radiograph showing volar angulation. The mechanism
is similar to that seen in the mallet finger deformity. There is relative lengthening of the
extensor tendon, whereas the profundus flexor is able to accommodate and even aggravate
the deformity. In these cases, loss of bony length contributes to the relative elongation
of the extensor tendon. The dorsal extensor mechanism moves proximally as a compensatory action, and a hyperextension deformity appears at the proximal interphalangeal
joint level. *C*, The primary distal interphalangeal and secondary proximal interphalangeal
deformities can be clearly seen. The middle phalanx is the intercalated segment.

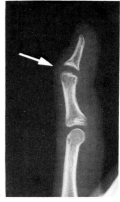

C

tremities the microcirculation fails rapidly,
capillary venular blood flow stops, and
thrombi form and produce osteocytic necrosis, especially in areas that do not have an
extraosseous circulation. Interference with
the epiphysis by direct chondrocytic death
alters both appositional and interstitial
growth patterns and produces the angulatory
and increased bone width deformities evident
clinically and radiologically. If all the cartilaginous epiphysis dies, there will be premature fusion of the primary and secondary
epiphyses, with resulting shortening of the
phalanx and total digit. If only part of the
epiphyseal cartilage is destroyed, there will
be a progressive angulation toward this side
of the phalanx as growth continues on the
other side. Loss of the bony epiphysis on one
side of the distal interphalangeal joint and of
the subchondral (articular) bone on the corresponding phalangeal head causes an overall
juxta-articular shortening. Incomplete extension of the distal phalanx results from the
relatively lengthened extensor tendon, and
the flexion deformity so created is further

aggravated by the strong pull of the flexor
profundus tendon. Extension effort is transferred to the middle phalanx, where a hyperextension deformity may develop (Fig. 76–
6C).

DIFFERENTIAL DIAGNOSIS

Most dysplasias and dystrophies of bone
involve most of the skeleton, or at least most
of the tubular bones and not just the extremities. Therefore, such conditions—described
by Aegerter and Kirkpatrick (1968) as multiple epiphyseal dysplasia, physiological sclerosis of the epiphyseal ossification centers,
and dietary deficiency diseases affecting the
epiphyses—may be easily ruled out. Among
the dystrophies that may resemble cold induced digital epiphyseal necrosis one must
consider osteochondrosis, Kirner's deformity, Thiemann's disease, and irradiation induced epiphyseal necrosis (Fig. 76–7).
Osteochondrosis or osteochondritis is a
form of avascular necrosis, and the process

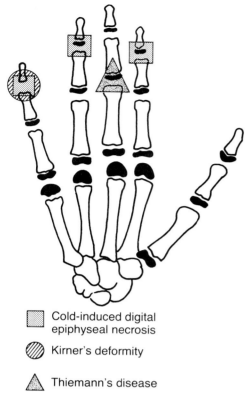

■ Cold-induced digital epiphyseal necrosis

◐ Kirner's deformity

▲ Thiemann's disease

Figure 76–7. Diagrammatic representation of the sites of predilection in three finger joint lesions. Kirner's deformity always involves the distal interphalangeal joint of the little finger. Thiemann's disease most often attacks the proximal interphalangeal joints and, in particular, that of the middle finger. Cold-induced digital epiphyseal necrosis involves particularly the distal interphalangeal joints of the index, ring, and little fingers.

in the digital phalangeal epiphyses, according to Staples (1943), is similar to that seen in other body sites such as the femoral head in Legg-Perthes disease. The cause is a decreased blood supply secondary to either trauma with sustained vessel spasm or even interruption, vascular disease, or thrombosis. The distribution of the lesions seems to depend on some special vulnerability of the vasculature or on an increased tissue demand, which is unsatisfied at a particular moment. Most such cases occur in late childhood. This condition must be differentiated from cold induced digital epiphyseal necrosis on the grounds that the cartilaginous epiphysis is not involved, and hence growth as such is not disturbed.

Kirner's deformity was first described in 1927. Kaufmann and Taillard (1961) considered it to be the result of nontraumatic epi-

physeal cartilage necrosis (epiphysiolysis). It affects girls twice as often as boys. The onset is after eight years of age as a rule, and Blank and Girdany (1965) found that the involvement is usually bilateral. There is a slowly progressive deformity of the little fingers with volar and radialward angulation of the distal phalanges. The distal interphalangeal joints appear clubbed and there is diminished amplitude of movement. Radiologically a broadened distal phalanx bony epiphysis is seen that does not fuse with the primary ossification center. The diaphyseal cortex is thin on the radial and volar aspects. This condition is thought to be due to an inherited defect.

Thiemann's disease was thought by Greenfield (1969) to be simply the digital form of epiphyseal avascular necrosis, but careful appraisal indicates that there is probably a dual lesion, viz., a primary lethal epiphyseal plate effect and a secondary vascular impoverishment of the bony epiphysis and other bony elements of the joint. Shaw (1964) considered that it also may be an inherited disease, because a familial tendency exists. Clinical signs include slight finger joint swelling and mild pain beginning in late childhood (12 to 13 years of age). The condition is usually bilateral and most frequently involves the middle fingers. The most common sites are proximal interphalangeal joints of the middle fingers. Therefore, a pattern exists that is just the opposite of that seen in cold induced digital epiphyseal necrosis. Growth is retarded and the affected digits are shortened and widened. Joint function is maintained and angulation is uncommon. The radiographical image indicates a deformity at the site of the epiphyseal cartilage. Thiemann himself (1909) found that instead of having the usual form, the epiphysis is meniscus shaped (thin centrally and thicker at the edges).

Finally, irradiation injury of the hands produces an appearance almost identical to that seen in cold induced necrosis. There should be little difficulty in establishing the relationship between the onset of the phalangeal lesions and the exposure to radiation. This entity was well described by Rubin and Casarett (1968).

TREATMENT

In the early stages of cold induced digital epiphyseal necrosis, the oral administration of mild analgesics and the use of night splints to passively correct the angulatory deformities may be needed. Dynamic daytime splints are poorly tolerated by children as a rule. There is a place for corrective exercises, however, for these help avoid excessive stresses on the involved joints by reinforcing weak muscle groups.

Surgery may be necessary to correct marked deviations. Epiphysiodesis of the functioning portion of the epiphysis before growth is complete will prevent further angulation. This procedure should be delayed as long as possible to allow maximal growth. Later management should include surgery to correct volar angulation and valgus and varus deviations. For the purpose of follow-up it is important to record the degree of arthritis in the involved joints and the amount of painless passive and active movement. Extensor tenorrhaphy may be needed to overcome mallet finger deformities of the distal phalanges. Sectioning of the median band of the extensor apparatus at the base of the middle phalanx should at least partially correct the dropped tip and hyperextension at the proximal interphalangeal joint level. Palmar proximal interphalangeal joint capsulorrhaphy may also be indicated. Angulatory deviations must be corrected either by wedge osteotomy or by arthrodesis, depending on the state of the joints and the juxta-articular structures. Severely damaged joints and arthritic joints are best dealt with by fusion in the best possible position for the particular digit.

REFERENCES

Aagerter, E., and Kirkpatrick, J. A., Jr.: Orthopedic Diseases. Philadelphia, W. B. Saunders Company, 1968.

Bennett, R. B., and Blount, W. P.: Destruction of Epiphyses by freezing. J.A.M.A., *105:*661, 1935.

Bigelow, D. R., and Ritchie, G. W.: The effects of frostbite in childhood. J. Bone Joint Surg., *45B:*122, 1963.

Blank, E., and Girdany, B. R.: Symmetric bowing of the terminal phalanges of the fifth fingers in a family (Kirner's deformity). Am. J. Roentgenol., *93:*367, 1965.

Caffey, J.: Pediatric X-ray Diagnosis. Chicago, Year Book Medical Publishers, Inc., 1967.

Dreyfuss, J. R., and Glimcher, M. J.: Epiphyseal injury following frostbite. N. Engl. J. Med., *253:*1065, 1955.

Florkiewicz, L., and Kozlowski, K.: Symmetric epiphyseal destruction by frostbite. Arch. Dis. Child., *37:*51, 1962.

Greenfield, G. B.: Radiology of Bone Diseases. Philadelphia, J. B. Lippincott Company, 1969.

Kaufmann, J. H., and Taillard, W. F.: Bilateral incurving of the terminal phalanges of the fifth fingers. An isolated lesion of the epiphyseal plate. Am. J. Roentgenol., *86:*490, 1961.

Kulka, J. P.: Experimental injuries produced by prolonged exposure to cold air. *In* Procedures of the Symposium on Arctic Medicine and Biology. New York, Corlies, Macy & Company Inc., 1964, Vol. IV.

Lindholm, A., Nilsson, O., and Svartholm, F.: Epiphyseal destruction following frostbite. Acta Chir. Scand., *134:*37, 1968.

Lohr, W.: Die Verschiedenheit der Auswirkung Gleichartigenbekannter Schoden. Zentralbl. Chir., *57:*898, 1930.

Rubin, P., and Casarett, G. W.: Clinical Radiation Pathology. Philadelphia, W. B. Saunders Company, 1968.

Selke, A. C., Jr.: Destruction of phalangeal epiphyses by frostbite. Radiology, *93:*859, 1969.

Shaw, E. W.: Avascular necrosis of the phalanges of the hands (Thiemann's disease). J.A.M.A., *156:*711, 1964.

Staples, O. S.: Osteochondritis of the epiphyses of the terminal phalanges of the fingers. J. Bone Joint Surg., *25:*917, 1943.

Thelander, H. E.: Epiphyseal destruction by frostbite. J. Pediatr., *36:*105, 1950.

Thiemann, H.: Juvenile Epiphysenstorungen. Fortsch. Gebrete Rontgenstr., *14:*79, 1909.

Werzl, J. E., Burke, E. C., and Bianco, A. J., Jr.: Epiphyseal destruction from frostbite in hands. Am. J. Dis. Child., *114:*668, 1967.

Section 3

IRRADIATION INJURIES

Chapter 77

EFFECTS OF RADIATION
ON THE HANDS

Maurice Tubiana

Before considering the clinical features and management of radiodermatitis of the hands, it may be useful to review some basic concepts concerning radiation injuries in general.

PHYSICAL PROPERTIES OF IONIZING RADIATION USED IN MEDICINE

GENERAL FEATURES

An x-ray beam is composed of photons and can be defined in terms of the energy of these photons (on which the penetration of the beam depends) and their number (intensity).

The maximal energy of the photons emitted by an x-ray generator is equal (when expressed in electron-volts) to the accelerating potential (expressed in volts). However, the energy of all the photons is not the same, and their mean energy is between one third and one half of their maximal energy.

The higher the energy of an x-ray beam, the less abrupt its attenuation in the tissues, or, in other words, the greater its penetration. Low-energy x-rays are absorbed in the superficial layers and can be eliminated by filtering the beam through a metallic screen, which stops the soft x-rays. The filters used are usually made of aluminum or copper; the

thicker the filter, the greater the proportion of low-energy rays eliminated and therefore the greater the penetration of the beam. The penetrative power of a beam therefore depends on two factors: its maximal energy and the thickness of the filter. Thus, an unfiltered 120 kV. beam, a 100 kV. beam filtered through 0.5 mm. of aluminum, and a 60 kV. beam filtered through 1 mm. of aluminum show the same degree of penetration (Dutreix et al., 1969). Often therefore a beam is defined in terms of the thickness of the metal screen required to reduce its intensity by half (half-value layer).

An x-ray beam must also be defined in terms of its intensity, i.e., the number of photons or the energy flux. With an x-ray generator, this depends on the intensity of the current running through the tube (usually expressed in milliamperes).

The dose unit used in radiobiology is the Gray (Gy) or the rad (1 Gy = 100 rads, 1 Gy = 1 joule per kg.). It expresses the quantity of energy absorbed per unit of mass of irradiated tissue. The biological effects are proportional to the dose administered, and the dose in depth varies with the degree of penetration of the beam. The absorption of x-rays in the tissues is exponential, which means that if the dose is reduced to one-half at a depth of 1 cm., it will be one-quarter at

843

2 cm., one-eighth at 3 cm., one-sixteenth at 4 cm., and so on.

Beams Used in Radiodiagnosis

To obtain a clear image, the penetration of the beam, i.e., the voltage, must be chosen according to the thickness of the body segment studied. Only those rays that reach the screen or the emulsion of the radiological film contribute to the image. Therefore, in order to reduce exposure to a minimum while retaining the possibility of a clear image, it is safer to vary the intensity, i.e., the current (milliamperes) and the filter (Dutriex et al., 1969). In many countries a filter of 0.5 mm. of aluminum is mandatory in all diagnostic x-ray generators, but thicker filters of 1 to 2 mm. are sometimes optimal. To obtain sharp contrast, however, it is important that the variations of attenuation caused (e.g., by a bone) should be marked. This requires controlled energy in the beam (Dutriex et al., 1969). For each type of radiological examination, there is an optimal energy level that both protects the patient and preserves the quality of the image.

Another factor that influences the exposure of the patient, in both radioscopic and radiographic examinations, is the width of the beam, which should always be kept to a minimum.

In fluoroscopy, the dose can be considerably reduced if the examiner is fully adjusted to the dark from the very start, as the intensity required to produce a readable picture decreases progressively in the course of the 5 minutes needed for the eyes to adjust. If the examination is started prior to dark adaptation, the exposure of both the examiner and the patient is increased unnecessarily.

In normal fluoroscopic conditions (with a source-to-skin distance of about 60 cm.), the dose at the point of entry on the skin varies between 5 and 20 rads per minute, depending on the voltage and the intensity of the beam. Brilliance amplifiers make it possible to work with a beam of lower intensity, and the dose at skin level can be reduced to 0.1 to 1 rad per minute if the examination is carried out in dim light. However, the advantages offered by amplifiers and television tend to tempt one to increase the number and duration of examinations, which in turn neutralizes these same advantages.

In radiodiagnostic practice, accidents to patients are invariably due to professional error, e.g., prolonged fluoroscopy, inadequate filtrations. The fluoroscopic examinations that result in the highest exposure are cardiac catheterizations (140 rads on average), pacemaker insertion (100 rads), and reduction of fractures under visual control. Accidents to physicians are due to carelessness, e.g., ungloved hands exposed to the beam, failure to carry dosimeters, neglect of the rules of radioprotection.

The aim of radiotherapy is to deliver a high dose to the tumor without delivering too high a dose to the surrounding normal tissues. For this reason, penetration is adjusted according to the depth of the lesion. Modern equipment generates beams with a wide range of energy, from deep penetrating x-rays emitted by linear accelerators (maximal energy 20 to 30 million electron-volts) to superficial rays used in contact therapy (50 kV.), which penetrate only a few millimeters. Electron beams are also used. They deliver a fairly constant dose down to a given depth, beyond which the dose falls rapidly. This depth varies with the energy of the electron beam; when measured in centimeters, it is equal to about one-third the energy expressed in Mev.

Radiodermatitis following cancer therapy results from the high doses required to destroy the tumor. In the treatment of benign lesions, it is usually due to a faulty source-to-skin distance or to an inadequate filter. Such accidents have been reported after the treatment of warts.

In interstitial therapy and brachytherapy, many such accidents have been reported in workers who handle radioactive elements such as radium (Tubiana et al., 1963; Vennart and Cryer, 1972). The predominant factor so far as dose distribution is concerned is distance. The incidence of radiodermatitis has decreased markedly since it has become common practice to manipulate radioactive isotopes with long forceps or pincers and to reduce manipulation time to a minimum. With the introduction of artificial radioisotopes, it has become possible to develop after-loading techniques, i.e., the use of non-radioactive sheaths or casings within which the radioactive sources can be safely guided to the desired site. These techniques have improved the accuracy of the dosimetry and reduced the risks of exposure of radiotherapists and technicians.

RADIOBIOLOGY OF THE SKIN

X-rays exert their effect primarily at the level of the genetic material within the cell, i.e., the DNA molecules and the chromosomes. This may lead to mutations, to failure of cell mitosis, or to the death of the daughter cells. In contrast, cells that do not divide may appear unaffected and live their normal life span. The greater the dose received by a tissue, the greater the proportion of damaged cells. Thus, a dose of 100 rads will result in about half the cells being unable to proliferate; as the dose-effect curve is approximately exponential, 200 rads will leave only 25 per cent of the cells viable, 300 rads one-eighth of the cells, and 1000 rads one-thousandth of the cells.

The consequences in a given tissue will vary according to the rate of multiplication of its component cells. In tissues with a high proliferation rate the lesions soon become evident; by contrast, tissues with a slow rate of cell proliferation may appear normal for a long time and late effects may appear months or years after irradiation. Moreover, the shape of the initial part of the dose survival curve is different in rapidly and slowly proliferating tissues. In the latter, the cell survival is higher after small doses (less than 100 rads) and lower after high doses. Therefore, during fractionated irradiation the relative effects on slowly proliferating tissues (dermis) and rapidly proliferating tissues (epidermis) will depend upon the dose per fraction.

It is thus important to distinguish between dermis and epidermis. The epidermis consists of a few nucleated cell layers (three or four) with several superficial layers (10 to 15) composed of enucleated and thin, heavily keratinized cells. In adults, its thickness varies from 0.04 to 1.5 mm. All proliferative activity is restricted to the lowermost layer, the basal layer, which in addition to keratinoblasts contains melanocytes and Langerhans' cells. It is currently believed that there are about 20,000 small cells called keratinoblasts per square millimeter in the basal layer, about 2,000 of them being stem cells. The stem cells are self-reproductive; they are responsible for the maintenance of their own numbers and for all cell replacement, in particular after an insult. Their progeny mature into transitory proliferating keratinoblasts that are able to divide two or three times within the basal layer before migrating to the more superficial

layer where they differentiate into keratocytes (Potten, 1985). The thickness and degree of undulation of the basal epidermis depend on the body site from which the epidermis was taken. On the dorsal skin of the hand the basal layer lies at about 70 μ in depth in men and 40 μ in women. In the palm, however, the basal layer is covered by a layer up to 700 μ thick (Vennart and Cryer, 1972; White, 1975; Wray, 1964). Depending on the thickness of the epidermis, it takes a basal cell between 13 and 20 days to migrate from the basal layer to the surface, where it is desquamated. Underneath lies the dermis, which is about 1 mm. thick and is a slowly proliferating tissue. The dermis exerts considerable influence on the epidermis; after a skin graft, the characteristics of the grafted epidermis will depend on the underlying dermal bed (Vennart and Cryer, 1972).

A dose of a few hundred rads produces two types of effects: (1) erythema, resulting from early capillary dilatation and later from arteriolar changes, and (2) inhibited proliferation of cells of the basal layer. Due to this arrest of cell proliferation in the basal layer, the basal layer and the dermis are laid bare approximately 20 days after a high dose of radiation. Depending on the dose received, the lesion may be a simple dry desquamation (from a single 500-rad dose) or an exudative dermatitis that is essentially a superficial ulceration (Rubin and Casarett, 1968; Vennart and Cryer, 1972; Potten, 1985). The few surviving stem cells give rise to small islets that later become confluent at a rate that varies with the number of survivors and therefore with the dose. Cellular proliferation is rapid, the number of cells being doubled every 20 to 30 hours. The stem cells at the edges (i.e., in the nonirradiated area) also proliferate and contribute to cicatrization, as they can migrate over several millimeters (Potten et al., 1983).

The severity of the lesions is related to the surface of the irradiated area, to the dose, and to individual radiosensitivity. Exudative radiodermatitis is present in 5 per cent of cases after a dose of 1200 rads and in 50 per cent after 2000 rads. After higher doses (greater than 2500 rads in a single dose), the dermis is damaged, ulceration goes deeper, and healing is slower.

If the dose is administered in several sessions, cellular repair and proliferation that occur between sessions reduce the overall effect. Thus, 600 rads administered in a single dose has an effect equivalent to five sessions of 200 rads at 24-hour intervals. However, a very high overall dose of radiation delivered in multiple sessions (chronic irradiation) may seem to be well tolerated by the epidermis and yet produce late effects in the dermis. This is because there is more tissue repair in the epidermis, as well as compensatory cell proliferation, between sessions of irradiation. During fractionated irradiation, high doses per fraction are less well tolerated by the dermis than by the epidermis (see above).

Irradiation also causes loss of body hair (temporary from 400 rads and permanent from 1200 rads in a single dose), as well as inflicting damage to the sweat glands and sebaceous glands. While acute irradiation induces few short-term changes in the dermis and connective tissue, which are both slowly proliferating tissues, the late effects are observed in both these tissues and in the capillaries (Vennart and Cryer, 1972; Potten, 1985); hence, the recent interest in microcirculatory studies (thermal and isotopic) in preoperative assessment and the use of locally applied vasodilators (Kalleone or Padutin) in the treatment of acute lesions (Massart and Henry, 1961).

In the dermis, irradiation leads to atrophy, fibrosis (which can fix the skin to the underlying tissues), arteriolar and capillary closure with telangiectasia, and ischemia (Lagrot, 1974; Rubin and Casarett, 1968; Tubiana et al., 1963; Vennart and Cryer, 1972). These lesions occur late, often months or years after irradiation. There is little correlation between the early changes, which are primarily epidermal, and the late complications, which involve the connective tissue. Small repeated doses produce neither erythema nor desquamation but only a slow, progressive alteration in the texture of the skin, which becomes dry, atrophic and fragile and loses all its sweat and sebaceous glands. There is a concomitant thrombosing vasculitis. At that stage the slightest trauma results in a slowly healing ulceration. Cracking around the nails, hyperkeratosis, or even irregular pigmentation can also occur in the fingers with doses of 2000 or 3000 rads or more (Vennart and Cryer, 1972). Doses of only a few hundred rads produce no significant change. Some specialists have suggested the regular monitoring of fingerprints, as their erasure could be one of the earliest signs of overexposure.

The incidence of malignant change in radiodermatitis of the hand is high—20 to 50 per cent in different series. On average, this occurs 15 years after irradiation, but it has been reported as early as a few months or as late as 50 years after exposure (Vennart and Cryer, 1972). The risk of malignant change is correlated with the dose (U.N.S.C.E.A.R., 1977; Boice and Fraumeni, 1985) and increases with exposure to sunlight as a result of the co-carcinogenic effect of ultraviolet irradiation (Boice and Fraumeni, 1985). The patient often presents with an indolent ulcer in an area of dystrophic skin. While malignant lesions usually develop in diseased skin (hyperkeratosis, ulceration, radiodermal scarring), they have also been reported in apparently normal skin (Vennart and Cryer, 1972; Albert and Shore, 1986). Spindle cell tumors are the most common, but basal cell carcinoma can occur in skin showing little change. Fibrosarcomas of dermal origin have been reported but are rare.

Numerous experimental studies have been carried out on animals to assess the role of the dose, dose fractionation, and the quality of irradiation in the development of malignant lesions (U.N.S.C.E.A.R., 1977). Fractionated irradiation reduces the severity of lesions after acute irradiation or low-dose irradiation, but does not lower the incidence of malignancy and may even increase the risk (Vennart and Cryer, 1972). In humans, retrospective evaluation of the radiation received prior to the development of malignancy is often difficult, but it appears that this usually exceeds 3000 rads (Vennart and Cryer, 1972). Several series have been published on the incidence of skin cancer after radiotherapy. Rowel (in Vennart and Cryer, 1972) reported 5 cases in 100 patients who had received between 1500 and 3200 rads on the hands or face as treatment for benign dermatosis; no malignant disease was found after doses of less than 2000 rads. Delarue et al. (1975) reported only one case of skin cancer in 308 patients who had received about 1500 rads in the course of repeated radiological screening for a therapeutic pneumothorax. Among 3600 children treated by x-irradiation for ringworm of the scalp (average dose, 450 rads), basal cell carcinomas were observed in 41 cases (Albert and Shore, 1986).

It is important not to forget the effects of co-carcinogenic factors (such as chronic irritation) or repeated trauma (such as preoperative scrubbing of the surgeon's hands). Pathogenesis is essentially the same as for other forms of radiation-induced cancer; radiation produces changes within the genome of the cells and perturbs the kinetics of cell proliferation in the tissues, so that it may act as an inducer as well as a promoter (U.N.S.C.E.A.R., 1977; Boice and Fraumeni, 1985).

PROTECTION REGULATIONS FOR PHYSICIANS AND RADIOGRAPHERS

National and international recommendations have chosen 5 rads per year as the maximal permissible dose to which a professional worker can be exposed (I.C.R.P., 1959). This is equivalent to 0.1 rad per week. This permissible dose, however, is calculated in terms of the risks to the body as a whole and especially of the risk of leukemia. If only a small proportion of the body is exposed, higher doses are acceptable. In cases of irradiation restricted to the skin, international recommendations have fixed the permissible dose at 30 rads per year (I.C.R.P., 1959). When only the hands and wrists are exposed, the maximal permissible dose is 75 rads per year (or 1.5 rads per week), but in some countries, e.g., France, regulations are more strict, as they restrict the permissible dose to 60 rads per year. The safety margin is small, as malignant skin disease has been reported after doses of 2500 to 3000 rads, which would be roughly equivalent to the dose received by the skin if a professional were exposed to the maximal permissible dose for 30 years. For this reason some authors recommend a maximal permissible dose of 30 rads per year (Vennart and Cryer, 1972). It is also worth keeping in mind that the dose received by skin directly exposed to the beam for a simple x-ray film is about 1 rad, and during radiological fluoroscopy the dose is 2 to 20 rads per minute.

Hence, the need for strict measures of radioprotection. All equipment should be adequately protected and used under the conditions for which it was designed.

Exposure of the operator depends on the conditions in which he works. With a modern, well-collimated apparatus, exposure is virtually nil during film-taking or fluoroscopy if the operator is protected by a lead screen behind which radiation can arrive only after being scattered at least twice. In other cases, one should regard as a risk zone any area exposed to radiation scattered by the patient, i.e., in practice any spot from which one can see that part of the patient's body that is hit directly by the incident beam. The amount of radiation scattered is proportional to the size of the beam and its energy and is inversely proportional to the distance between patient and operator. A 0.25-mm. lead filter (or its equivalent) should be placed near the patient to prevent x-ray scatter from the latter to the operator.

In addition, the operator should wear a lead-lined rubber apron or jacket (1 mm. of lead-lined rubber is equivalent to 0.1 to 0.4 mm. of lead). One must not forget that during fluoroscopy severe exposure of the hands can occur if these are held close to the source. As the dose is inversely proportional to the square of the distance, at 35 cm. it will be double that at 50 cm. Manipulation should be as brief as possible, and the wearing of lead-lined rubber gloves (equivalent to 0.25 mm. of lead) should be encouraged, as gloves provide excellent protection. Unfortunately, few orthopedic surgeons will wear them despite the introduction of more flexible designs.

Physicians and operators are required by law to wear dosimeters (I.C.R.P., 1959). These are now available in the form of finger rings. It is also possible to roll a meter-film around a finger or to place one against the skin of the palm or the wrist.

REFERENCES

Albert, R. E., and Shore, R. E.: Carcinogenic effect of radiation on the human skin. *In* Upton, T., et al. (eds.): Radiation Carcinogenesis. New York, Elsevier, 1986, pp. 337–346.

Boice, J. D., and Fraumeni, J. F.: Radiation Carcinogenesis. New York, Raven Press, 1985.

Delarue, N. C., Gale, G., and Ronald, A.: Multiple fluoroscopy of the chest: carcinogenicity for the female breast and implications for breast screening program. Can. Med. Assoc. J., *112:*1405–1413, 1975.

Dutreix, J., Bismuth, V., and Laval Jeantet, M.: L'image Radiologique. Paris, Masson et Cie, 1969.

I.C.R.P. (International Commission on Radiological Protection): Report on Protection against X-rays up to Energies of 3 MeV. New York, Pergamon Press, 1959.

Lagrot, F.: Radiodermites des Mains. Paris, Doin, 1974.

Massart, A., and Henry, J.: A propos of a case of late radionecrosis following accidental exposure to x-rays. J. Belge Radiol., *44:*667–670, 1961.

Potten, C. S., Hendry, J. H., and Al-Barwari, S. E.: A cellular analysis of radiation injury in epidermis. *In* Potten, C. S. and Hendry, J. H. (eds.): Cytotoxic Insult to Tissue. Edinburgh, Churchill Livingstone, pp. 153–185.

Potten, C. S.: Radiation and Skin. London, Taylor & Francis, 1985.

Rubin, P., and Casarett, G. W.: Clinical Radiation Pathology. Vol. 1. Philadelphia, W. B. Saunders Co., 1968, pp. 62–119.

Tubiana, M., Dutreix, J., Dutreix, A., and Jockey, P.: Les bases Physiques de la Radiothérapie et de la Radiobiologie. Paris, Masson et Cie, 1963.

Tubiana, M., and Dutreix, J.: Radiobiologie Humaine. Paris, Hermann, 1986.

U.N.S.C.E.A.R.: Report of the United Nations Scientific Committee on the Effects of Atomic Radiations. Sources and Effects of Ionizing Radiation. 1977 Report to the General Assembly (725 pages). New York, United Nations Publication, 1977.

Vennart, J., and Cryer, M. A. (eds.): Radiobiology Forum on Radiological Protection and the Skin. Br. J. Radiol., *45:*610–620, 1972.

White, D. C.: Atlas of Radiation Histopathology. Oak Ridge, U.S. Energy Research and Development Administration, 1975.

Wray, E. T.: Radiation and skin. Proceedings of a symposium. U.K. Atomic Energy Authority. London, Harwell (H.M. Stationery Office), 1964.

Chapter 78

RADIODERMATITIS OF THE HAND

Claude Dufourmentel

and Jacques Beres

By radiodermatitis is meant the changes in the skin induced by ionizing radiation. In the majority of cases the changes are caused by x-rays, which are used more commonly for diagnostic than for therapeutic purposes. Less frequently dermatitis is produced by radium plates or needles or by other radioactive elements such as iridium and strontium, which are also used therapeutically.

ETIOLOGY

Radiodermatitis of the hands is usually an occupational disease and is commonest among members of the medical profession: physicians, surgeons, radiologists, and dentists. Physicians and surgeons were represented in about equal numbers in our survey, exposure occurring during the course of repeated screenings in tuberculosis centers, or when a gastroenterologist palpates the abdomen to guide a gastric tube or endoscope. Surgeons are exposed as a result of multiple fracture reductions performed under radiological control or foreign body explorations without adequate protection.

Radiodermatitis occurs mainly as the result of a cumulative effect, even at long intervals between doses of radiation. This important fact is true even though cell growth may occur between exposures.

It is generally accepted that the average radiation tolerance of the skin is of the order of 0.2 rad a day. For a surgeon this would correspond to one minute of exposure every 10 days, on condition that the voltage does not exceed 80 kV. and that the intensity is no greater than 3 milliamperes with an aluminum filter 1 to 2 mm. thick. The dose is then 2 rads per minute. How many surgeons are aware of these figures, and which surgeon can be certain that the time of exposure has not exceeded one minute, let alone the possibility of scattered radiation, which is far from negligible?

For over 15 years we and a number of other authors, including Pack (1939) and Lagrot (1964), have stressed the dangers of radiation during screening and have pointed out the errors of technique and faults in the equipment that can further increase these doses.

These undeniable facts are still being ignored by many. A dose of 400 to 500 rads leads to loss of hair and 600 to 1200 rads induces erythema. And how many of us remember the law that states that the radiation output varies inversely as the square of the distance between the source and the skin (and not between the source and the operative field)? Thus, if that distance is reduced from 50 to 10 cm., the skin receives as much radiation (i.e., 50 rads) in one minute as it would in 25 minutes of the "correct" exposure. In other words, the skin is exposed in one minute to a dose that would be acceptable if received in 250 days.

Let us quote Watson-Jones:

A number of surgeons have wrecked their careers as a result of reducing fractures under radiological control . . . . This is not an imaginary danger: it has actually happened to 91 surgeons. These figures refer only to cases reported in a single town and do not include non-orthopedic causes or minor cases . . . . I would like to forbid the use of radiological control in orthopedic surgery. The risks are enormous and the advantages minimal. Ninety-one surgeons are known to have paid the price—try not to be the ninety-second.

It is difficult to make the point more clearly.

There is no valid reason for a physician or a surgeon to place his hands in a radioactive field. X-ray films of fractures should be taken by a qualified radiographer and can be developed within minutes. Preoperative screening is not essential when looking for foreign bodies provided there is a bloodless field and localizing views have been taken preoperatively. A single film taken during an operation will deliver 100 times less radiation than even a brief screening. The duration of the operation is not significantly increased and unjustifiable risks are avoided.

The dangers of radiation are obviously greater if the operator is not familiar with the equipment. Searching for a foreign body can be a lengthy procedure and delays can occur if the incision is too small, if localization has been inaccurate, if a pneumatic cuff is not used or simply if the surgeon is not sufficiently prepared.

Fluoroscopes, which are now in widespread use, have not reduced the risks significantly and cannot be regarded as a substitute for the usual precautions. Although in theory the brightness of the image can be considerably amplified (up to 1000 times with the more sophisticated devices) so as to reduce the irradiation required, in practice, amplification greater than 10 times is rare. Not uncommonly the amplification achieved is a bare twofold to threefold, which in itself is not negligible, although the benefit may be counterbalanced by an impression of false security and a tendency therefore to increase the time of exposure.

Radiologists, because of their familiarity with and constant awareness of the radiation danger, hardly feature in our series. Most cases reported in this speciality date from an earlier era.

Similarly dentists have also gradually dropped the old habit of holding the film behind the teeth, a task they now entrust to their patients.

Finally in the occupational group one should mention the rare cases of technicians who although fully conscious of the dangers involved, may fall victims to the diversification of sources and continuous modifications to the equipment. The legal precautions (as defined in the Recommendations of the International Commission) are usually taken and accidents usually result from a faulty safety device. Accidental radiodermatitis in technicians is now about the only form of occupational radiodermatitis seen at an acute stage soon after exposure. One should always wait and follow the course of the disease. In certain acute forms (e.g., following irradiation by an electron beam) the condition may resolve spontaneously.

Nonoccupational radiodermatitis is much less common. However, because the same causes produce the same effects and because the radiosensitivity of the patient's tissues does not differ from that of the surgeon, the use of radiological screening in orthopedics and in explorations for foreign bodies can just as well result in radiodermatitis in the patient himself. We have seen a case in which acute radiodermatitis followed an exploration for a foreign body. Ulceration succeeded the acute phase, and malignant change to a basal cell carcinoma ended with an amputation after conservative surgery had failed.

Radiotherapy used against warts can have equally disastrous results. We saw the case of a woman who suffered ulcerating radionecrosis after radiotherapy for a wart on the dorsal aspect of the first interdigital space of the right hand. Malignant change led to amputation of the thumb and index finger, and after a recurrence the hand was amputated at the wrist.

Admittedly such catastrophes are encountered in only a minimal proportion of cases of warts treated with radiotherapy, but although amputation is rare, we have had to deal with more than a few patients in whom the complications of radiotherapy were undoubtedly far worse than the initial condition.

We do not intend to sit in judgment over the advisability of treating warts by radiotherapy, but we can confirm that this form of treatment is potentially more dangerous than it may seem and that it requires as much skill, and entails the same responsibility, as a surgical intervention.

Every surgical error is immediately obvious and can therefore be corrected, but an error in a radioactive dose may not be detected for years, by which time the diagnosis and treatment may be difficult.

Finally, a patient delighted with the result of a first course of treatment may request another course of the same therapy to treat a new crop of warts. If the areas treated overlap, the risks of radiodermatitis are considerable even after an interval of years. We can only deplore the use of such powerful therapy against such a benign lesion. The same applies to all benign lesions of the hand, such as eczema and hyperhidrosis, for which radiotherapy is still advocated by some.

CLINICAL STUDY

It is sometimes, but by no means always, possible to diagnose radiodermatitis at an early stage. In an acute form of the disease, occurring within days or weeks after exposure, the signs are spectacular and easily recognizable: pruritus, bouts of erythema, and depilation are characteristic of dry radiodermatitis (Fig. 78–1). The exudative epidermal form (sometimes called "second degree" because of its similarity to burns) presents with blisters and painful ulcerations. Painful deep ulcers with well demarcated edges result from involvement of the dermis and dermal capillaries and are characteristic products of high doses of irradiation received during reduction of fractures or exploration for foreign bodies.

The date of onset is more difficult to determine when the only signs are those of a mild radiodystrophy developing gradually, sometimes years after exposure. Similarly an early diagnosis is uncommon in occupational forms when exposure is continuous and spread over many months.

In surgeons a frequent misdiagnosis is that of allergy to gloves, talcum powder, antiseptics, or alcohol. A benign useless treatment is prescribed, surgery is delayed, and exposure to x-rays is continued; in some cases a diagnosis of eczema is made and radiotherapy

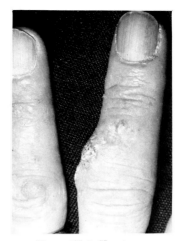

Figure 78–2. Keratoses.

is prescribed. A faulty diagnosis therefore can have the most catastrophic consequences.

A single ulcer of recent onset and wrongly believed to be traumatic in origin may be the first sign of the disease. A search for the less obvious stigmata of irradiation and a detailed history should indicate the real etiology. In any form of radiodermatitis the latent period between exposure and the manifestation of its complications may be very long indeed; in one of our patients it was 38 years.

It is important therefore to know the early signs of radiodermatitis and to question the patient about past exposure. The disease may take the form of a mild dystrophy with or without the following: atrophy of the epidermis (a dry thin skin), sclerosis of the dermis (best demonstrated by palpation), discoloration of the skin (alternating areas of hyperpigmentation and depigmentation), keratosis (Fig. 78–2), telangiectasia and the less constant carbon spots (black patches caused by interstitial hemorrhages), and changes in the skin appendages (scanty or absent hairs; friable nails with characteristic longitudinal grooves (Fig. 78–3).

Excluding the cases of acute radiodermatitis and those which present with necrosis following an apparently quiescent dystrophy (Figs. 78–4, 78–5), the commonest presentation of the disease is a skin dystrophy to which may be added any of the following features—scabs, cracks, ulcerations, dyskeratosis, erosions, exudation, bleeding, desquamation, recurrent pruritus, and lesions due to the scratching of an already fragile epidermis (Fig. 78–6).

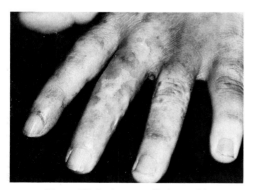

Figure 78–1. Acute radiodermatitis.

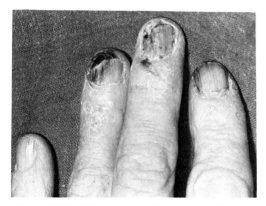

Figure 78–3. Nail lesions and tissue destruction on the middle finger. Pigmented deposits and cracks occur on several digits.

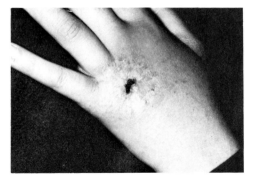

Figure 78–5. Radiodermatitis of the dorsum after foreign body extraction.

The diagnosis of radiodermatitis is simple if malignant change is obvious (Fig. 78–7). It should be suspected if ulceration is present; at an earlier stage it can be made only by histological examination.

The site of the lesions depends on the source and direction of the irradiation. In our series the disease was three times more common on the dorsal than on the palmar side.

The extent of the dermatitis is extremely variable. Of 70 cases of radiodermatitis of the hands in our study, 22 were bilateral (of which 19 were occupational); the lesions were often more marked on one side (usually the left). In 21 cases four fingers were involved and in 14 cases, three fingers only. Involvement of the thumb alone was seen in six patients, of whom two were radiologists and two were physicians.

CLINICAL COURSE

The course of the disease is somewhat unpredictable. Ulceration may start in a dystrophic, quiescent looking area; it may heal by scarring as a result of, or in spite of, topical therapy and reappear indefinitely or at least until surgery is performed. One should not be deceived by these periods of remission. This is a progressive condition: the underlying thrombosing angiitis is irreversible and can only extend. But necrosis with concomitant severe pain and risk of infection, is not the only complication.

The major long term risk in any form of radiodermatitis is malignant change, which many authors regard as inevitable (Fig. 78–7). Of our 70 patients with radiodermatitis of the hands, 14 (20 per cent) sustained malignant change—a figure comparable to those

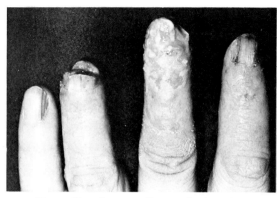

Figure 78–4. Severe radionecrotic ulceration.

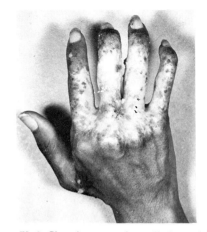

Figure 78–6. Chronic progressive radiodermatitis after irradiation of warts.

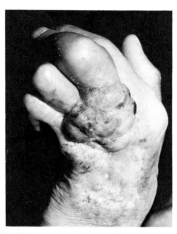

Figure 78–7. Large squamous cell carcinoma following irradiation during foreign body removal.

of Pack (1939), Rintala (21 per cent), and Mouly and Bureau (1970; 15 per cent).

Several histological forms of malignant disease occur, the commonest being squamous cell carcinoma (nine of 14 in our series, four of which progressed to invasion of regional lymph nodes). Basal cell carcinoma is rare (one case only). Bowen's carcinoma in situ (three cases) is probably an early form. Adenoacanthomas are also rare (one case) and are not malignant.

Invasion of lymph nodes seems commoner in squamous cell carcinomas occurring in the hand (one in seven according to Mouly and Bureau, 1970). This does alter the prognosis, but the incidence is probably less than was once believed: Of our four patients with axillary node involvement, only one died from the tumor.

The etiology of malignant tumors secondary to radiodermatitis of the hand in our series is worth mentioning. Twelve were occupational: nine physicians, two radiologists, and one radiographer. One followed an exploration for a foreign body. One followed radiotherapy for warts.

These findings confirm the carcinogenic action of repeated small doses, although it may be misleading to regard such doses as small. Lagrot (1964) mentions the case of a technician who reassessed the doses to which he had been exposed and reached the unlikely figure of 35,775 rads.

Carcinomas secondary to radiodermatitis of the hands have a notorious tendency to recur, even after wide excision. There may be three reasons for this: The tumors are often multifocal, the cause of the tumor (previous irradiation) is still present and further malignant change is always possible, and the tumor elicits little or no stromal reaction.

TREATMENT

The only form of curative treatment is surgery. It was not long after the discovery of x-rays by Röntgen in 1896 that Charles Allen Porter first operated in a case of digital radiodermatitis. In some cases of dystrophy that appear to remain quiescent, surgery can be postponed indefinitely as long as the lesion is kept under close watch and further exposure to x-rays is strictly forbidden. However, radical surgical treatment is almost always justifiable for radiodermatitis of the hands. The lesion should be excised like a tumor and replaced by a free graft.

The earlier the diagnosis is made and surgery performed, the better the results. The proportion of postoperative complications, failures, and reoperations in relation to the age and stage of the lesions is significant.

In young patients the indication for surgery is even stronger in view of the greater risks involved. For small lesions, electrocoagulation may sometimes be tried, and superficial lesions occasionally can be treated by dermabrasion (although the involvement of deeper layers is often not evident). In the majority of cases, however, excision and grafting remain the treatment of choice.

The operation is performed under general or local anesthesia combined with hypnoanalgesics (Fig. 78–8). A pneumatic cuff on the arm or an elastic cuff at the root of the finger is often used. Recently we have preferred to avoid the use of a tourniquet and to reduce the bleeding by subcutaneous infiltration with a local anesthetic (procaine or lidocaine) combined with epinephrine (1 in 10,000).

The excision is particularly delicate over the distal interphalangeal joint where the insertion of the extensor tendon lies close to the matrical zone. If the nail is dystrophic, it should be removed together with the matrix and nail bed. If the nail appears to be viable, one may be tempted to be conservative while remaining aware of the fact that the pathological process may continue.

The viability of the tendon is usually more difficult to assess. If the chances of survival

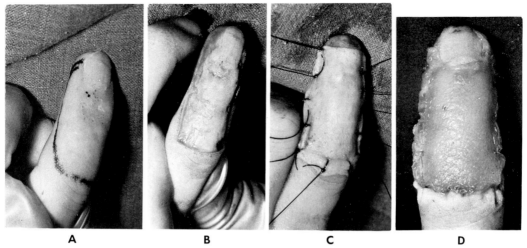

Figure 78–8. *A*, Extent of excision. *B*, The damaged tissues have been removed and the nail preserved. *C*, An overlapping full-thickness graft sutured in place with nonabsorbable material. *D*, The graft on the thirteenth day.

are poor, the area may be covered with a flap from a distance (or rarely a heterodigital flap) with a view to undertaking a tendon repair at a later stage. A skin graft will not prevent the tendon from rupturing usually at its insertion, either spontaneously or following a minor injury.

THE REPAIR

The pathological area is excised and grafted over at once. The palm receives a full thickness graft, but surgeons vary in their preferences for the dorsum. Some advocate a full thickness graft in spite of the lower chances of its taking, whereas others prefer a thinner one, which they believe will provide a more supple skin covering.

The graft should be carefully sutured in place either with nonabsorbable material or with catgut, the latter carrying the advantage that suture removal will not be required in this sensitive area. It is then held in place with a tulle gras and stockinette dressing. The dressing is changed on the second day in order to evacuate early any collections of serum or blood, which may separate the graft from its bed. If these are left longer, the graft may never become established.

Incomplete taking of the graft is a not uncommon postoperative complication. It may occur even in the absence of a hematoma and is then probably due to inadequate vascularization of the graft bed. Cicatrization

may still occur in areas where the graft has failed to take, as though the trophicity of the bed has somehow improved under the loose graft. If this is delayed, however, a complementary graft is advisable.

In the majority of cases treated at the stage of simple radiodystrophy, the graft will settle and provide a mobile digital tegument (Fig. 78–9). In some cases of deep necrosis an autoplasty may be required.

A local flap can seldom be used because adjacent tissues have also been irradiated (though to a lesser degree) and do not readily tolerate migration. Cross finger flaps are possible only for small lesions and if the adjacent finger is healthy. Brachial and thoracic flaps are used as a last resort if preservation of the digit is functionally indispensable.

Depending on the lesions, a nail, one or two phalanges of one or more fingers, a whole digital column, or the whole hand may have to be amputated. One should strive to be as conservative as possible and think in terms of function as well as of cosmetic appearance (e.g., amputation of the metacarpal when the corresponding digit has been sacrificed [except if a broad hand is desirable for professional reasons] to produce an acceptable hand with three fingers and a thumb. The extent of the amputation depends partly on the histological findings and partly on the functional possibilities of the digit to be spared.

A histological examination of the whole specimen should be requested in all cases. Once excised, the specimen should be re-

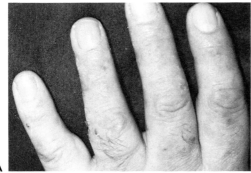

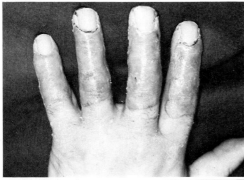

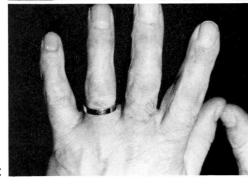

Figure 78–9. *A,* Radiodystrophy of the four fingers. *B,* The hand on the fifteenth postoperative day. *C,* The same hand five years later.

oriented digit by digit and the suspicious areas marked to ascertain that the line of excision has not crossed a potentially malignant zone.

TREATMENT OF MALIGNANT CHANGE IN RADIODERMATITIS

Two types of cases must be considered in cases of malignant change:

1. When malignant disease has been missed clinically and discovered only during histological examination, usually the excision will have been wide enough and it will suffice to keep a close watch. However, if histological examination has revealed the excision to be inadequate, it should be extended as early as possible.

2. When the malignant nature of the lesion has been diagnosed clinically, the mere presence of malignant change does not necessarily imply an amputation. However, there are cases in which the extent and depth of the lesion, joint stiffness, and major trophic changes condemn the digit or the whole hand. Radical surgery should be avoided, however, because a number of malignant lesions following radiodermatitis of the hands can be treated safely by excision and grafting alone.

Amputation becomes a necessity if such a malignant lesion recurs, together with a block dissection of the regional lymph nodes if lymphatic spread has occurred.

On the subject of treatment, we would like to make two observations:

1. In occupational radiodermatitis the diffuse nature of the lesions and their multifocal origins mean that reoperation is frequently required.

2. Each digit should be treated according to the nature and stage of its lesion, as, for example, in the case of a hand in which three adjacent fingers were involved to different degrees; the middle finger was amputated, the index finger was covered with a flap from a distance, and the ring finger was treated by excision and grafting.

We can conclude this section by again stressing the importance of prophylaxis in this relentlessly progressive condition. We would like to see discontinuation of the use of radiological screening, a practice fraught with danger for doctors and patients alike. Patients undergoing radiotherapy (and the public in general) should be better informed about the importance of previous irradiation. Finally more judicious use of x-rays should be the rule, although their undeniable diagnostic and therapeutic value is somewhat counterbalanced by the advertisement of radiotherapy as a universal and painless panacea, which is wrongfully prescribed, even in young patients, to treat benign lesions.

In this field in which complications may develop long after the initial injury, everyone should learn from the experience of others. Otherwise there is a real danger that radiodermatitis may remain a topical subject for years to come.

REFERENCES

Burdick, K. G., and Miraldif, F.: Radiodermites professionnelles. J.A.M.A., *188*(6):607–608, 1964.

Cole, H. N.: Acute and chronic radiodermatitis as seen in physicist, physician, and dentist. Postgrad. Med., *13*:133, 1953.

Conway, H., and Hugo, N. E.: Radiation dermatitis and malignancy. Plast. Reconstr. Surg., *73*:255, 1966.

Degos, A., and Touraine, R.: Deux cas de radiodermite aiguë professionnelle. Bull. Soc. Fr. Derm., *68*(2):125–127, 1958.

Diethelm, L.: Opération exécutées sous écran et protection contre les irradiations. Congrès Soc. All. Radio., 5–8 septembre 1954, Wiesbaden. Fortschr. Geb. Roentgenstrahl., *81*:32–33, 1955.

Dufourmentel, C., and Terquem, J.: Traitement chirurgical des radiodermites. Presse Méd., *61*:1239–1241, 1953.

Dufourmentel, C.: A propos des radiodermites des chirurgiens et de leurs opérés. Méd. Acad. Chir., *83*:271–284, 1957.

Gandin, J.: L'envahissement ganglionnaire dans les radiodermites professionnelles dégénérées des doigts. Ann. Chir. (Suppl. Sem. Hôp.), *13–14*:797–800, 1958.

Hartwell, S. W., Jr., Huger, W., Jr., and Pickrell, K.: Radiation dermatitis and radiogenic neoplasms of the hands. Ann. Surg., *160*:828, 1964.

Iselin, M.: Radiodermites de la main. Concours Méd., *76*(11):1068–1072, 1954.

Lagrot, F.: Les radiodermites professionnelles des doigts. Traitement technique. Ann. Chir., *18*:1511–1518, 1964.

Mohs, F. E.: Roentgen ray cancer of hands in a dentist. J. Am. Dent. Ass., *45*:160, 1952.

Mouly, R., and Bureau, H.: Les radiodermites chirurgicales. Rapport 16e Congrès Société Française de Chirurgie Plastique et Reconstructive. Paris, Octobre 1970.

Pack, G. T.: Tumors of the hand and feet. St. Louis, C. V. Mosby, 1939.

Pariente, R., Minervini, F., and Mosca, A.: Les radiodermites professionnelles de la main (traitement chirurgical). Minerva Chir., *16*(23):1494–1497, 1961.

Porter, C. A.: The surgical treatment of x-ray carcinoma and other severe x-ray lesions (based on analysis of 47 cases). J. Med. Res., *21*:357, 1909.

Chapter 79

SURGICAL TREATMENT OF POSTACTINIC LESIONS OF THE BRACHIAL PLEXUS

GIORGIO BRUNELLI

The use of radiotherapy after mastectomy for mammary carcinoma or Hodgkin's disease probably lengthens life expectancy and in some cases saves the life of the patient, but in many cases produces serious lesions involving the skin and subcutaneous layers, blood vessels and lymphatic vessels, the brachial plexus, and the ribs.

The cellular reaction to radiation is ionization. Water molecules, the principal component of cells, are broken up into hydrogen ions and oxygen ions. Normal cellular oxidation processes stop, essential enzymes are inactived, and the genetic apparatus in the nucleus is damaged, with resulting coagulation of chromatin, nuclear disintegration, vacuolization, and necrosis.

The sensitivity of the cells of different tissues differs. Most sensitive are endothelial and epithelial cells. The neural and muscular tissues are less sensitive. Fibrocytes show signs of de-formation and gigantism and produce a dense hyaline collagen without elastic fibers.

In women who have undergone a mastectomy, most frequently the area that has undergone irradiation is the axilla and often also the region above the clavicle, and sometimes even the presternum. After variable periods following exposure to radiation, the skin of these areas shows evidence of varying stages of radiodermatitis.

The blood vessels present signs of obliterative vasculitis, and hyalin changes occur in the arteries, veins, and lymphatic vessels.

Tissues become sclerotic and hard, with areas of white necrosis. Even if nerve tissue is not very sensitive to ionizing radiation, such radiation damages parts of the brachial plexus indirectly by mechanical constriction, sclerosis of the surrounding tissue and the epineurium, and ischemia due to radiovasculitis.

The clinical syndrome appears at varying times depending on the type of tissue involved, individual reactivity, the total dosage of ionizing radiation, the levels of single doses and their frequency, the type of irradiation (roentgen, telecobalt, betatrone), and the time elapsed. We have known the syndrome to appear 18 years after the last irradiation. The syndrome consists of a reduction in motor power and sensation that develops at varying rates into a stable paralysis, which is often complete, as well as paresthesia and pain in at least half the cases; the pain is often so intense as to induce the patient to commit suicide.

Our purpose in this chapter is to discuss the surgical repair of these lesions, the techniques of neurolysis of the plexus with microvascular transplantation of greater omentum in order to protect and revascularize the decompressed plexus, and the refinements in technique developed through experience.

HISTORICAL CONSIDERATIONS

Until a few years ago it was not possible to find descriptions of surgical techniques applicable to lesions caused by radiation of the brachial plexus. There are descriptions of plastic surgical techniques for reconstruction of the skin and thoracic wall but little or nothing in regard to neural lesions, even in such important recent texts on plastic surgery as those by Barsky, Kahn, and Simon (1964), Dufourmentel and Mouly (1959), Grabb and Smith (1973), and Aston and Pickrell (1977).

In 1963 Kirikuta proposed a plastic operation involving the use of greater omentum in order to reconstruct the thoracic wall and obtain good lymphatic drainage. He also mentioned the usefulness of the omentum in preventing scars constricting the plexus. He freed a segment of greater omentum, with a vascular pedicle on the right gastroepiploic artery, passing the omentum subcutaneously to the area of skin loss. A dermal-epidermal graft protected the omentum flap.

Later Dupont and Menard (1972) devised a similar technique using either a left or a right vascular pedicle for cutaneous reconstruction.

In 1974 Clodius et al. presented six cases in which microvascular transplant of the greater omentum was used in the hope that the omentum, being rich in lymphatic vessels, would decrease the lymphatic edema so commonly found in the arm. In 1978 Uhlschmid and Clodius published a seventh case in which this operation was used, but they stated that there had been no decrease in the lymphatic edema in their patient and little or no improvement in the paralysis. However, in all seven cases there was complete disappearance of pain.

Operations intended to repair actinic lesions of the plexus have been performed since the early 1970's. These at first consisted of neurolysis, but later in the 1970's rotational skin flaps were used to provide a softer covering with better vascularization. The utilization of free microvascular omentum grafts is a very recent technique.

AVAILABLE OPERATIVE TECHNIQUES: A CRITICAL ASSESSMENT

Neurolysis is the essential part of the operation, but if it is performed in isolation, it does not prevent cicatricial contractures, which are the cause of stenosis. Thus after temporary relief of painful symptoms (and even the neural deficiency), there is either a relapse or a worsening of the preoperative symptoms.

The addition of rotational skin flaps to provide a loose and vascularized subcutaneous layer has great limitations:

1. The area to be repaired is often vast and requires very large flaps, which are difficult to find in the area and leave large skin defects in the donor area, which recovers slowly (unless it is possible to use a large contralateral breast with the Sanvenero technique).

2. Usually skin that can be rotated is also suffering from the effects of radiodermatitis and so is not well suited to pad the plexus.

3. Often large rotational flaps from the shoulder or back are esthetically unattractive.

4. Rotational flaps also limit movement of the shoulder.

5. The freed plexus, however, is very deep, and the skin, even if it has a good subcutaneous layer, cannot prevent development of an enveloping scar, which causes stenosis.

Myocutaneous or pedicled muscle flaps (latissimus dorsi) have been suggested, but as far as I know have not been used. Even if the muscle is vascularized and can be adequately mobilized, it is far less suitable than the omentum for wrapping around the plexus and prevents cicatrization following neurolysis. In addition a myocutaneous flap if rotated could cover only part of the plexus.

A free microvascular myocutaneous flap would be more suitable but would have limited value in preventing the development of a scar.

The pedicled greater omentum flap thus would seem to be the best method because it is living and its transfer around the plexus allows it to survive through its own vessels. In practice this is not so. First, the pedicled flap cannot cover all of the plexus after the latter has undergone neurolysis. In fact the lesions nearly always are not only axillary but also retroclavicular and even supraclavicular and laterocervical. Second, its subcutaneous passage must not twist the pedicle or compress it; it must not even constrict it in a scar that may follow. (One must bear in mind the poor quality of the skin above it.) Third, the placing of omentum around the plexus is rendered difficult because of the connection to the stomach by the gastroepiploic artery.

Initially I used only neurolysis in three cases. In two neurolysis was combined with rotational cutaneous skin flaps. Since 1977 I have performed an ample neurolysis in all areas involved by sclerosis (axillary, retroclavicular, and supraclavicular), afterward covering the exposed plexus by means of a

Table 79–1. ACTINIC BRACHIAL PLEXUS LESIONS

No need for operation	10
Too late for useful operation	18
Neurolysis	3
Neurolysis plus skin flaps	2
Neurolysis plus free microvascular omentum transfer	34
Total	67

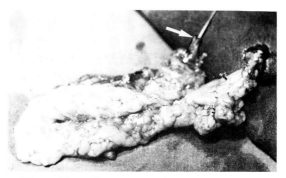

Figure 79–1. The omentum has been removed and perfused.

free omental graft whose size depends on the particular case, enveloping the plexus as completely as possible in order to pad, protect, and vascularize it without stretching (34 cases out of 43 operated on) (Table 79–1, Fig. 79–1). This omental graft is revascularized by microvascular anastomosis—a completely safe technique for anyone practicing microsurgery (since we are dealing with vessels with diameters greater than 1 mm.). If necessary, necrotic parts of trunks or terminal branches are removed and substituted with sural nerve grafts. During a certain lapse of time I have removed the calvicle with the aim of providing more space for the omentum and to ensure greater freedom of movement for the shoulder (five cases). In fact, it was not a wise idea. The scar contracture limited the range of movement of the shoulder. Therefore, I have abandoned the removal of the clavicle and I even try to preserve the bone in continuity as far as possible, passing the omentum under it, maintaining the space between the sternum and the scapula.

OPERATIVE TECHNIQUE

An S-shaped incision is made following the sternocleidomastoid muscle up to 2 cm. from the clavicle. Here the incision deviates obliquely, crossing the clavicle and coursing under the coracoid. It is continued to the middle of the anterior axillary arch and into the axillary cavity. Here the incision continues at right angles toward the arm and again at right angles in a distal direction.

The length of the cutaneous incision depends on the extent of the lesion. Once the skin is retracted, the subcutaneous layer is seen to be sclerotic and insufficiently vascularized, but there is bleeding because of the rigidity of the small blood vessels (Tables 79–2, 79–3). The pectoralis major has often been surgically removed and the pectoralis minor has often been transformed into a very hard fibrous whitish tissue; the remains of these muscles are sectioned and removed.

The middle part of the subclavius muscle is resected and then removed. In the most recent technique the clavicle is not divided except rarely to allow a better neurolysis. In these cases it is carefully reconstructed with a six-hole plate.

At this stage one proceeds to identify the terminal branches of the plexus distal to the cicatricial area. Then one follows the nerves in a proximal direction, performing a precise external neurolysis and a careful dissection of the axillary artery up to the subclavian artery. Next the subclavian vein is dissected

Table 79–2. ACTINIC LESIONS OF THE BRACHIAL PLEXUS: FREE MICROVASCULAR OMENTUM (34)—PREOPERATIVE STATE

Skin		Motor-Palsy		Sensation		Pain	
Severe radiodermatitis	9	Total		Anesthesia		Very severe	12
Moderate radiodermatitis	12	Recent	8	Recent	4	Severe	10
		Old	9	Old	4	Slight	9
Slight radiodermatitis	4	Severe in progress	7	Hypoasthesia		No pain	3
Very mild radiodermatitis	4	Severe stabilized	2	Severe in progress	15		
		Fair, recent	8	Severe stabilized	2		
				Mild	9		

Table 79–3. ACTINIC LESIONS OF THE BRACHIAL PLEXUS: FREE MICROVASCULAR OMENTUM GRAFT—OPERATIVE FINDINGS

Very severe scar (no local recipient vessels) (with partial nerve necrosis in three cases)	17
Severe scar (damaged local vessels)	13
Mild scarring	4
Total	34

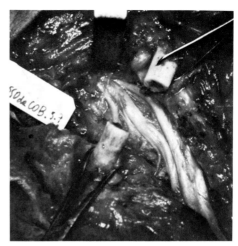

Figure 79–3. Another plexus after removal of fibrous tissue.

out; it is often attached to the scar and is easily ruptured, requiring suturing of the laceration, which is generally longitudinal.

It is difficult to clamp the blood vessels hidden in extremely hard scar tissue. In order to save time, suturing is performed while an assistant presses with two fingers above and below the point of the suture without trying to clamp the blood vessel. Prudent external neurolysis is usually enough to free the nerves or trunks, which except in the worst cases expand as soon as they are freed and have a normal appearance (Fig. 79–2). During dissection one must pay great attention to the collateral branches.

When external neurolysis of all the neural areas is completed, there may be some constricted areas of the nerve trunks. These require internal neurolysis, usually limited in both extent and depth. Severe sclerosis necessitates extensive freeing (external neurolysis) of the terminal nerves of the plexus, which are more severely affected by the condition than the divisions and cords (Fig. 79–3). When the supraclavicular fossa has also been exposed to radiation, neurolysis should be performed even on the trunks.

In only two cases have I had to perform an external neurolysis of the roots. In 12 cases it was necessary to perform internal neurolysis over a short distance in one or more trunks. In three cases the lesions were so severe that the nerve trunks were yellowish and fibrous. These had to be removed and were replaced with nerve grafts, which were then covered by the omentum (Fig. 79–4).

In the latter cases I have always operated with two teams. This is necessary so as not to lengthen inordinately the duration of the operation. The second team removes the omentum and begins one and one-half hours after the first team has started. In this way, about two and one-half or three hours after the beginning of the whole operation, the first team has finished the neurolysis (which has been facilitated by sectioning the pectoralis major if still present) while the second team can furnish the omentum for grafting. The omentum is removed by means of a median xiphoumbilical laparotomy, tying the vessels that course from the gastroepiploic arch to the greater curvature of the stomach (Fig. 79–5).

The size of the segment of the omentum extracted depends on the extent of the lesion and the thickness of the omentum. It is possible to find thick and thin segments of omentum—some rich in solid fat, others extremely loose, and still others extremely thin and transparent.

After splitting the omental layers and deciding on the size of the graft, the blood

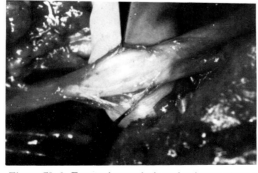

Figure 79–2. External neurolysis and epineurotomy of the lateral cord.

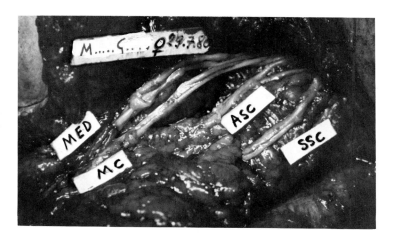

Figure 79–4. In this case because of serious necrosis a part of the nerve tissue has been removed and replaced by a sural nerve graft.

vessels are tied as are the gastroepiploic artery and vein. The right gastroepiploic vessels are then ligated and divided and will be sutured to the recipient vessels. The orifices of the small blood vessels are marked immediately with methylene blue applied by means of a sterile toothpick (Fig. 79–6). Otherwise these vessels retract into the fatty tissue and are extremely difficult to find (especially the vein).

In the first cases treated I removed a large section of omentum with four or five vascular axes branching from the arch connecting the left and right gastroepiploic arteries and veins. I tied the right gastroepiploic vein and the left gastroepiploic artery using as donors the right gastroepiploic artery (usually larger than the left) and the left gastroepiploic vein, with the intention of permitting full passage of blood in the omentum. However, I found

myself in difficulty at times owing to an omentum that was too large. Reducing its size after it had been detached was difficult and posed the danger of vascular damage causing both hemorrhage and omental ischemia.

Today the standard technique is to remove a long thin segment of omentum with two or three radial vascular axes. As stated before, the normal technique uses the right gastroepiploic vessels, but depending on whether the receiving vessels (artery and vein) are near or far from each other, the donor vessels are either the right gastroepiploic artery and vein or the right artery and left vein.

If during the operation nerve grafts are to be used, a third team by this time will have removed one or two sural nerves from the patient's legs by means of long undulating incisions to permit the atraumatic removal of the nerve for the graft without causing internal lesions, which may occur in stripping.

The second team now sutures the abdo-

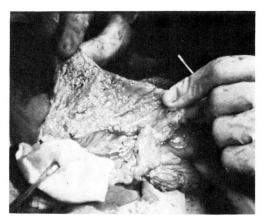

Figure 79–5. Removal of the anterior part of the omentum with its vessels (right and left gastroepiploic arteries and veins).

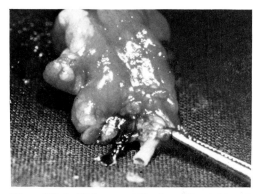

Figure 79–6. Higher magnification. The right gastroepiploic artery and vein are stained with methylene blue.

Table 79–4. ACTINIC LESIONS OF THE
BRACHIAL PLEXUS: FREE
MICROVASCULAR OMENTUM
GRAFTS—RECIPIENT VESSELS

Arteries		Veins	
Facial	17	Facial	17
Transverse cervical	6	Transverse cervical	6
Transverse scapular	2	Transverse scapular	2
Anterior circumflex	5	Tributary of superfi-	
Collateral humeral	3	cial jugular	5
Subclavian	1	Superficial jugular	3
		Subclavian	1

men. The first team must find the recipient vessels—an artery about 1 to 2 mm. in diameter for anastomosis to the gastroepiploic artery and a vein with a diameter of about 2 mm. (Table 79–4) for anastomosis to the vein.

Usually the local blood vessels in the damaged area are reduced in number and are small and hard. They may also display severe sclerosis and separation of the intima so that they are not reliable enough to ensure patency of the anastomosis. This means that recipient blood vessels must be found far from the involved area.

If there has been no irradiation of the supraclavicular fossa, the transverse blood vessels of the neck and scapula and the subclavicular vessels are suitable. Otherwise it is more convenient to search for the facial artery under the mandible and a vein leading into the external jugular vein or to perform an end to side anastomosis of the gastroepiploic vein with the jugular vein (Table 79–4).

The usefulness (or harmful effect) of perfusion of the omentum flap is a controversial subject (Fig. 79–7). In the first cases I have always performed this with a cold solution injected at low pressure with a small plastic cathether introduced into the vessel atraumatically for a few millimeters. The solution used contained an anesthetic (Marcaine), which produces paralysis of the muscular walls of the vessels and also vascular dilation, thus providing greater facility in microsurgical operation. Following experimental studies made in our laboratory which demonstrated intimal damage after the perfusion, I no longer perfuse but drop some Marcaine on the stumps of the vessels if dilation is required. Microsurgical suturing is not always easy to perform and often has to be executed deep in the tissues so that usually one cannot use approximator clamps. Suturing is easier when one uses the facial blood vessels. The suturing is performed first on the vein and then on the artery; then revascularization is permitted. First the clamps on the vein are removed and then the clamp below the arterial suture and finally that above it. The omentum immediately reinflates, reddens, and begins to pulsate (Fig. 79–8). The omentum is now laid out on the front of the freed plexus, placed lateral to the plexus, and is made to run under it. The omentum is then anchored to fibrous tissue underneath with a few stitches whose placement has to scrupulously respect the omental vessels. Great care must be taken not to damage these vessels, especially where the circumflex nerve separates from the plexus and where the radial nerve is directed posteriorly. Despite these difficulties, it is possible to envelop the omentum around the base of these branches of the

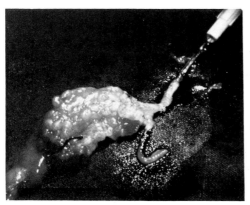

Figure 79–7. Perfusion of the omentum.

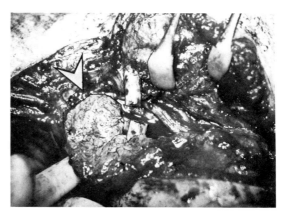

Figure 79–8. After the clamps are removed, the blood passes through the transplanted greater omentum, which is going to be placed on the freed plexus.

plexus. Sclerotic skin is sutured by means of everting stitches. Only in two cases in one series was it necessary to resort to additional grafts because of necrosis of a cutaneous flap.

INDICATIONS

In the light of surgical experience and results, we have established the following as indications—pain (the postoperative improvement of motor palsy is irrelevant), paralysis still in progression, paralysis that recently has became stabilized (four to six months), and radiodermatitis.

CONTRAINDICATIONS

The contraindications include slight paralysis without pain, total paralysis without pain that has been established for more than six months, and slow progressive paralysis that has lasted more than five years without pain.

PREOPERATIVE AND POSTOPERATIVE TREATMENT

Preoperative treatment does not differ from that with any other operation lasting five to six hours.

During the operation, before removal of the omentum, an anticoagulant and an inhibitor of platelet aggregation are administered (Calciparine subcutaneously and acetylsalicylic acid intravenously).

Postoperative treatment consists of a 12 day course of Calciparine, 330 mg. of aspirin (orally) every three days, an inhibitor of platelet aggregation, and Rheomacrodex for the first five days. Immobilization of the arm and forearm by means of a plaster cast in moderate abduction on a large cotton wool pack is recommended.

In the light of our surgical experience we can consider as mistakes a neurolysis that is too limited, the use of too large segment of omentum, and the creation of an anastomosis where the recipient blood vessels have been damaged by radiation.

COMPLICATIONS

I have seen complications in our patients only three times (± 10 per cent) because of dehiscence of the skin due to radiodermatitis. In these cases a rotational cutaneous flap resolved the problem of closing the lesion but obviously created an esthetic problem also, lengthening recovery time and reducing the mobility of the shoulder.

RESULTS

The results of surgery depend on several factors—the severity of the lesion, the time of onset of paralysis, the patient's response to radiation and to treatment, and the extent of the operation (Tables 79–5, 79–6). Table 79–5 shows the results up to the present and Figures 79–9 to 79–11 illustrate specific cases.

Pain, the most important indication for this operation, disappeared completely in almost all the cases from the day of the operation and has as yet never reappeared. Thus the results in this respect have been excellent. A more detailed analysis of the 34 patients who

Table 79–5. ACTNIC LESIONS OF THE BRACHIAL PLEXUS: RESULTS IN 67 CASES*

		Pain		Palsy		Sensation		Range of Motion		Radiodermatitis	
Neurolysis	3	Improved	1	Unchanged	3	Unchanged	2	Worsensed	3	Unchanged	2
		Worsened	2			Worsened	1			Worsened	1
Neurolysis + skin flap	2	Unchanged	2	Unchanged	1	Unchanged	1	Worsened	2	Improved	2
				Worsened	1	Worsened	1				
Neurolysis + greater omentum free microvascular transfer	34	Disappeared	28	Improved temporarily	1	Improved	2	Improved	11	Improved	21
		Improved	6	Improved	3	Temporarily improved	4	Unchanged	19	Unchanged	11
				Unchanged	20	Unchanged	19	Worsened (with clavicle resection)	4	Worsened	2
				Slightly worsened	10	Slightly worsened	9				
Metastasis	4										

*43 operations and 34 free omental grafts.

Table 79–6. POSTACTINIC LESIONS OF THE BRACHIAL PLEXUS: FREE OMENTUM
MICROVASCULAR GRAFTS (34)—ANALYSIS OF RESULTS
ACCORDING TO OPERATING COMPONENTS

	Pain		Motor Palsy		Sensation		Range of Motion	
Free omentum graft plus external neurolysis 21	Disappeared	19	Improved	1	Improved	2	Improved	11
	Improved	2	Temporarily improved	3	Temporarily improved	4	Unchanged	10
			Unchanged	17	Unchanged	15		
Free omentum graft plus internal neurolysis 6	Disappeared	4	Unchanged	3	Unchanged	4	Unchanged	6
	Improved	2	Slightly worsened	3				
Free omentum graft plus neurolysis plus nerve grafts 2	Disappeared	1	Slightly worsened	2	Slightly worsened	2	Unchanged	2
	Improved	1						
Free omentum graft plus external neurolysis and clavicle removal 3	Disappeared	3	Slightly worsened	3	Slightly worsened	3	Worsened	2
							Unchanged	1
Free omentum graft plus external and internal neurolysis plus clavicle removal 2	Disappeared	1	Slightly worsened	2	Slightly worsened	2	Worsened	2
	Improved	1						

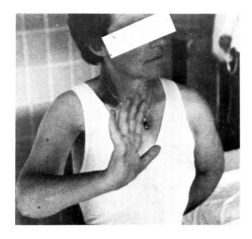

Figure 79–9. Example of a result after two years. Motion has been slightly improved. Pain is relieved, and the patient is pleased.

Figure 79–10. Another example after two and a half years. Mobility has improved, pain has disappeared, and the patient is satisfied.

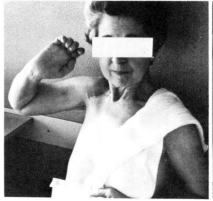
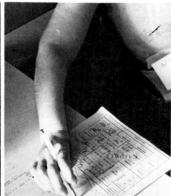

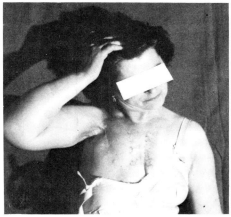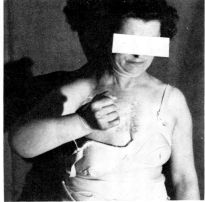

Figure 79–11. Another case after two and a half years. Mobility is improved and pain has gone.

underwent microvascular grafting of omentum is shown in Table 79–6. One can see that in all cases pain disappeared and that the improvement in the motor syndrome was not relevant. Even with severely damaged nerves that required nerve grafting there was improvement. Tactile sensitivity also improved. Passive movement worsened when a rotational flap was used; there was an improvement in passive movement in one third of cases.

REFERENCES

Abbatucci, J. S.: Les radiolesions après irradiation poru cancer du sein. J. Radiol. Electrol., 56:798, 1975.

Aston, S. J., and Pickrell, K. L.: Chest wall reconstruction. In Converse, J. M. (Editor): Reconstructive Plastic Surgery. 2. Philadelphia, W. B. Saunders Company, 1977.

Barsky, I. A., Kahn, S., and Simon, E. B.: Principles and Practice of Plastic Surgery. 2. New York, McGraw-Hill Book Company, 1964.

Basso Ricci, S., Ventafridda, V., Zanolla, R., Cassani, L., and Spreafico, R.: Presentazione di 25 casi di lesioni post-irradiatorie del plesso brachiale e loro trattamento. Tumori, 62:365, 1976.

Brown, J. B., Fryer, M. P., and McDowell, F.: Permanent pedicled-blood carry flaps for repairing defects in avascular areas. Ann. Surg., 486:1934, 1951.

Brunelli, G.: Actinic plexus treatment (neurolysis, grafts, omentum). Presentation at First Congress, International Federation of Societies for Surgery of the Hand, Rotterdam June 17–21, 1980.

Calle, R., Schlienger, P., and Viloq, J. R.: Séquelles et complications secondaires à l'irradiation exclusive des epithéliomas mammaires. J. Radiol. Electrol., 56:813, 1975.

Castaigne, P., Loplan, D., Augustin, P., Degos, J. D., and Ammouni, J. A.: A propos des paralysies du plexus brachial après cancer du sein. Presse Med., 77:49, 1969.

Dupont, C., and Menard, Y.: Transposition of the greater omentum for reconstruction of the chest wall. Plast. Reconstr. Surg., 49:263, 1972.

Fallet, G. H., Moody, J. F., and Boussina, I.: Lesions du plexus brachial survenant radiothérapie pour cancer du sein. Rhumatologie, 19:199, 1969.

Goldsmith: Long term evaluation of omental trasposition for chronic lymphoedema. Ann. Surg., 180:847–849, 1974.

Greeley, P. W.: Reconstruction of injuries following excessive radiation therapy. Am. J. Surg., 3:342, 1952.

Kirikuta, I.: L'emploi du grand epiploon dans la chirurgie du sein cancéreux. Presse Méd., 71:1, 1963.

Kogelnik, H. D.: Einfluss der Dosis-Zeit-Relation auf die Pathogeneses der paripheren Neuropathie. Strahlentherapie, 153:467, 1977.

Macomber, W. B., Wang, M. K. H., Trabue, J. C., and Kanzler, R.: Irradiation injuries, acute and chronic and sequelae. Plast. Reconstr. Surg., 19:9, 1957.

Malaspina, A., Invernizzi, A., Maffei, S., and Pisani, P.: Lesioni post-irradiatorie del plesso brachiale. Min. Med., 71:111, 1980.

Maruyama, Y., Myirea, M. M., and Logethis, J.: Neuropathy following irradiation. Am. J. Roentgenol., 60:216, 1967.

McDermot, R. S.: Cobalt-60 beam therapy—postradiation effects in breast cancer patients. J. Can. Assn., 22:195, 1971.

Millesi, H., Meissi, G., and Katzer, H.: Zur Behandiung der Verletzungen des Plexus brachialis. Vorschiag einer integrierten Therapie. Bruns' Beitr. Klin. Chir., 220:429, 1973.

Mumenthaler, M.: Armplexus im Anschluss und Roentgenbestrahlung. Schweiz. Med. Wschr., 94:1069, 1964.

Narakas, A.: Personal communication, 1980.

Notter, G., Halberg, O. K., and Vikterlof, K. J.: Strahlenschaden am Plexus brachialis bei Patienten mit Mammakarzinom. Strahlentherapie, *139:*538, 1970.

Petit, J. Y., Lasser, P., and Fontaine, F.: Indications de l'épiplooplastie au cours de l'évolution du cancer du sein traitè. Bull. Cancer, *64:*659, 1977.

Sarrazin, D., Fontaine, F., and Mouriesse, H.: Les complications de la radiothérapie des cancers du sein. J. Radiol. Electrol., *56:*805, 1975.

Steiner, C., Fallet, G. H., Moody, J. F., Roth, G., Boussina, I., Maurice, P., Alberto, P., and Pauniez, J. P.: Lesions du plexus brachial survenant après radiothèrapie pour cancer du sein. Schweiz Med. Wschr., *101:*1846, 1971.

Svensson, H., Westing, P., and Larsson, L. G.: Radiation-induced lesions of the brachial plexus correlated to the dose-time fraction schedule. Acta Radiol., *14:*228, 1975.

Uhlschmid, G., and Clodius, L.: Eine nene anwendung des frei transplantieren omentums. Chirurg., *49:*714, 1978.

INJECTION INJURIES

Chapter 80

INJECTION INJURIES
OF THE HAND

Lee W. Milford, Jr.
and Richard T. D'Alonzo

Injection wounds of the hand initially produce disarmingly little pain. The usual serious morbidity is not often realized immediately because of the lack of severe pain and the appearance of only a small wound of entrance which may be exuding the injected fluid. An immediate incision adequate to release the ischemia producing pressure and to remove the toxic fluid is essential to salvage a digit subjected to an injection wound from later disability or even amputation. Fluids accidentally injected into the body by either a high pressure grease gun or an airless paint gun have included lubricating grease, diesel fuel, brake fluid, paint, turpentine, plastics, and other materials that are now frequently used in industry (Figs. 80–1, 80–2). Pen sized tear gas guns are another source of injection injuries. Cementation pumps and molten plastic injection machines account for the usual injection injuries (Baker, 1955; Hutchinson, 1967).

In this chapter we attempt to describe the mechanism of injection injury, the pathogenesis of the lesion, and the proper method of treatment, as well as the prognosis associated with the various types of injection injuries.

In 1937 Rees reported the first case in the English language literature of an injection wound to the hand caused by an accident with a power compression tool. In this case, the lesion was caused by a high pressure fuel oil injector for a diesel engine. The estimated pressure was 4000 pounds per square inch (p.s.i.) or 281.3 kg. per sq. cm. Mason and Queen (1941) noted that Hesse had reported 183 cases in which oils had been self-injected into various parts of the bodies by persons trying to avoid Russian military service. Of these cases, 14 involved the hand. These were not high pressure injection injuries, but the oils used were similar chemically to those used recently in high pressure injections and produced similar pathological tissue changes.

Since 1937, with advances in industrial technology, the incidence of this type of injury has increased. High pressure grease guns have been responsible for more than 50 reported cases of injection injuries. Airless paint guns have been responsible for more than 25 such injuries. These two types of tools constitute a major source of injection injuries. The seriousness of this type of injury is still frequently not appreciated by physicians and only rarely appreciated by the injured worker. As late as 1964 Smith, in a

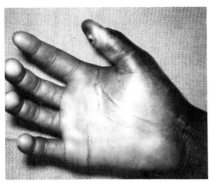

Figure 80–1. The hand of a 14-year-old black boy 48 hours after injection of brake fluid into the pulp of the right thumb. The thumb tip was already necrotic. Fluctuation was present subcutaneously over the thenar eminence and dorsum of the hand.

survey of 35 industrial shops in Glasgow employing workers who used grease guns, found that the employees in 16 of these shops were unaware of the potential hazards involved.

GREASE GUN INJURIES

The type of high pressure injection injury most frequently seen is caused by the grease gun. This industrial tool utilizes compressed air, usually at 150 p.s.i. (10.5 kg. per sq. cm.), to drive a pump, which then increases the pressure as much as 70 times in order to obtain a nozzle pressure of 5000 to 10,000

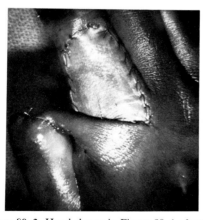

Figure 80–2. Hand shown in Figure 80–1 after necessary amputation of the thumb tip and application of a dorsal flap. Functional return was good except for the shortened thumb. On the dorsum can be seen a healed incision made to drain the fluid, which had caused surprisingly little local irritation here, as on the palmar side.

p.s.i. (351.5 to 703 kg per sq. cm.; Smith, 1964). The fluid contained in this tool may be diesel fuel, brake fluid, plastic, wax, grease, or any of a vast number of liquid lubricants and detergents. The injury commonly occurs when the worker attempts to clear the accumulated liquid from the nozzle with his fingertips and inadvertently triggers the gun, releasing the fluid, at the same time.

Initially the wound is painless and appears to be negligible, with only a pinpoint opening at the site of the injury. This opening usually exudes a small amount of the injected material. Within a few hours, however, the digit becomes tense and swollen, numb, and frequently devoid of circulation. The lesion then becomes painful.

Kaufman (1968a) has shown that the site of entry is important in predicting the extent of the injury. The index pulp is the most common site of entrance. If the entry is volar over the interphalangeal crease, the flexor tendon sheath may be penetrated with as little pressure as 750 p.s.i. (52.7 kg. per sq. cm). If the thumb or little finger is penetrated, the radial and ulnar bursae are likely to be involved. If the injury is volarly over the phalanges, the fatty subcutaneous tissue protects the sheath, and the spread of the liquid is superficial and lateral over the dorsum of the digit and hand, unless the pressure involved is much greater (5000 to 10,000 p.s.i. or 351.5 to 703 kg. per sq. cm.).

Kaufman, who also experimentally injected cadaver palms using nozzle pressures of 750 p.s.i., found generally that there were two levels of spread—superficial to the palmar fascia and deep to the palmar fascia. He had no difficulty in contaminating the mid-palmar and thenar spaces in this fashion with palmar injections. He found no cross contamination of these spaces utilizing these pressures and believed that it was not necessary to open both spaces merely because one was involved.

Mason and Queen in 1941 described three pathological stages. The early stage is illustrated by the innocuous appearing, painless digit with a pinpoint opening. This soon becomes tense, ischemic, and painful and, if not decompressed, undergoes gangrenous change within 36 to 72 hours secondary to the ischemia. Local chemical inflammatory changes occur as a result of the noxious liquid itself. This then may lead to a secondary infection resulting either from the devitalized ischemic tissue or from the potentially contaminated liquid. Immediate initial decompression is necessary to prevent gangrene of the digit.

In the intermediate stage there is subacute and chronic inflammation secondary to the formation of chemical oleogranulomas (Fig. 80–3). Hard palpable tumors become apparent. These may remain indolent for many years but more frequently are associated with fibrosis, which leads to considerable functional loss and disability of the digit.

The late stage is characterized by a breakdown of the skin overlying the oleogranulomas. Concomitantly numerous fistulous tracts with sinuses and ulcers form. Mason and Queen (1941) reported that Vinogradov had found one case of squamous cell carcinoma that arose from these ulcers.

Stark et al. in 1961 reviewed experience with their five cases and 18 additional cases in the literature. They believed that immediate wide incision with debridement and removal of the noxious liquid would decompress the ischemia as well as remove the contaminated liquid. It has been shown repeatedly that small local incisions are totally inadequate. Local digital nerve blocks are not advised, since these increase the swelling in an already compromised digit. Wide decompression through a midlateral incision along the full length of the digit is recommended. Mechanical debridement using a blunt curette is usually necessary, because most of the involved liquids are insoluble in water and most of oil solvents are toxic to tissue. There should be no hesitation about

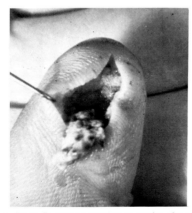

Figure 80–3. It was necessary to excise the oleogranulomas from this fingertip. This tender, firm nodule of reactive fibrous tissue resulted from injection of grease.

incising and debriding involved fibrous tendon sheaths and leaving only a small portion of the proximal and middle pulleys. Separate palmar incisions are often necessary in order to decompress the superficial spread and enable deep space drainage to occur.

Among the 18 additional cases Stark found only four patients who were treated adequately with early wide incision. In all ultimately a reasonable degree of function returned. In the remaining 14 cases, amputation of the digit was necessary. Similarly, Smith (1964) found that only seven of 22 patients whose cases were reviewed were treated initially with early wide incision. In the remaining 15 cases, amputation was ultimately necessary. In patients whose digits were not amputated, second and third reconstructive procedures were frequently necessary.

The morbidity from this injury is very high. Kaufman (1970) found that the absence from work in patients whose initial treatment was nonsurgical or only local excision ranged from one month to two years, the average being six months. In contrast, patients whose primary treatment was amputation returned to full activity in one and one-half to two months. Kaufman therefore advocated initial amputation of the digit except when either the thumb or palm was involved. Stark seems to agree with this in the neglected case, but for cases in which the patient is seen early, he believes in adequate wide excision and debridement.

Kaufman (1968b) reviewed 51 cases of patients who sustained high pressure injection injuries. He found that the digits or palm were involved in 49 patients. Of these 49 patients, with initial treatment unknown, 21 (42.8 per cent) ultimately were treated by amputation. It should be noted, however, that when automobile grease was injected, the amputation rate was eight of 28 cases (28.6 per cent), whereas when diesel fuel oil was the injected material, it was five of seven cases (71.4 per cent).

The left hand is involved twice as often as the right hand. The terminal segment of the digit is the site of injury five times as often as the middle segment and four times as often as the proximal segment. The index finger is the digit most frequently involved, as reported by Kaufman (1968b).

In the acute stage the initial treatment should consist of early liberal incision over and into the area, allowing escape of the irritant and offering a means of decompressing the ischemic digit. Coverage with a broad spectrum antibiotic is indicated. Anti-inflammatory drugs such as phenylbutazone and corticosteroids are of questionable value at best. The incision should be closed loosely to permit adequate drainage, or left entirely open. Postoperatively the hand should be elevated for 48 hours or more. Active early motion should be initiated when pain permits.

When the injury is in the intermediate state when first seen, local excision of the oleogranuloma appears to be the procedure of choice, unless fibrosis has already made the digit functionless. When it is first seen in the later state, ablation of the digit may offer the most rapid return to gainful activity.

AIRLESS PAINT GUN INJURIES

More recently another type of high pressure injection injury to the hand has been recognized. This involves the high pressure "airless paint gun." Utilization of compressed air at 125 p.s.i. (18.8 kg. per sq. cm.) forced into a hydraulic pump enables nozzle pressures of 3250 to 5000 p.s.i. (228.51 to 351.5 kg. per sq. cm.) to be obtained. Commercial painters utilize this tool to spray paint at the rate of 5 quarts (5000 ml.) per minute with sufficient force to project the paint 20 feet (6.1 m.) upward onto a surface such as a steel girder (Fig. 80–4). Other liquids used in such a gun include turpentines, toluene, lac-

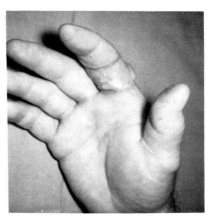

Figure 80–5. The base of the index finger had sustained a high-pressure airless paint gun injection injury 24 hours previously. It was painful, swollen, and had impaired vascularity.

quers, varnishes, shellacs, and thinners. Inadvertent injection of the paint while cleaning the nozzle also causes severe trauma. This type of injury is similar to that caused by the grease gun, in that it initially is painless and appears innocuous, but soon thereafter it becomes tense, swollen, ischemic, numb, and excruciatingly painful (Figs. 80–5, 80–6, 80–7). Unlike the injuries caused by grease guns, however, many paints are radiopaque and may be visualized radiographically, permitting an estimation of the extent of dissection and involvement.

In addition, paint is much more of an irritant to the tissues. Stark et al. in 1967 reviewed 14 cases of paint gun induced injuries and showed that the majority of the patients had systemic symptoms and signs—fever, lymphangitis, and leukocytosis. Seven of these patients required two or more operative procedures before wound healing oc-

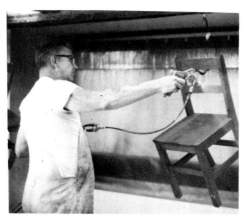

Figure 80–4. A commercial painter using an airless paint gun. Note the absence of the index ray, which was amputated secondary to an injection injury of paint from the same gun.

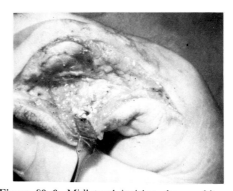

Figure 80–6. Midlateral incision shows white paint along the neurovascular bundle, which had resulted in complete thrombosis of both digital arteries.

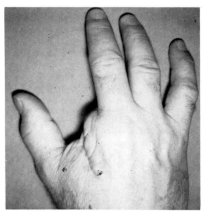

Figure 80–7. Amputation of the index ray was necessary because of the loss of blood supply to the finger. Early wide incisions might have salvaged the digit.

curred. Six of the patients ultimately needed amputation.

Stark found that one of the most important factors in successful treatment was the interval between the time of the injury itself and the time that definitive treatment was undertaken. All but one of his patients within 10 hours after injury regained useful function. In this patient a digital block was performed prior to examination. Patients treated by limited local incision with digital block obtained the poorest results. Digital block in this situation is to be condemned as a further insult to an already ischemic digit.

At the time of definitive decompression, a midlateral incision is recommended for the digit. Separate palmar incisions may be necessary because the tendon sheath, radial and ulnar bursae, and palmar spaces are all at risk and may need separate decompression and mechanical debridement. The skin may be loosely closed. Occasionally skin grafts may be necessary later. In contrast to grease gun induced injuries, Stark found that the spray gun produced no chronic fibrosis or restriction of motion.

Cyanosis may be an indication of insufficient drainage, necessitating a dorsal incision to release venous obstruction, as advised by Weeks (1967). His patient, in a case involving the injection of kerosene thinner, improved after this was done as a secondary procedure. In addition, he found it necessary to release the carpal tunnel and superficial arterial arch.

The potential for morbidity injection injuries is evident from a review of the statistics on reported cases. Eighteen amputations and 42 operative procedures were needed in treating 30 hands so injured with the airless paint gun. The time lost from gainful employment ranged from six weeks to six and one-half months.

TEAR GAS GUN INJURIES

The third group of injuries is the most recent to be described. These involve blasting injuries from the so-called "tear gas gun." The most common type is a fountain pen shaped weapon with a tear gas cartridge screwed into a penlike cylinder. The charge is activated by releasing a spring loaded mechanism. The cartridge itself is designed to discharge the gas with a force equivalent to that of a 0.38 caliber (9 mm.) bullet. It is possible to obtain a magnum cartridge that is the equivalent to the load in a 410 shotgun cartridge (Schwartzbach, 1969). This is powerful enough to gas a 9 by 12 foot (2.74 by 3.66 m.) room. It is believed that the injury caused by a tear gas gun is a result of the initial blast force from the primer, a local superficial burn of the exposed tissues, a reaction to a foreign body, and a chemical reaction to the neurotoxic and myotoxic chloracetophenone (Adams et al., 1966). The particles are mixed, so that 90 per cent of the particles are 1 to 10 μm. in diameter and 10 per cent of the particles are 10 to 30 μm. in diameter. The most common mechanism of injury is accidental discharge while holding the penlike carrier. Immediately following injury there is severe local burning pain. The entry wound is small and may appear to be benign (Fig. 80–8).

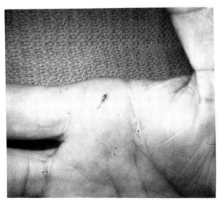

Figure 80–8. The wound of entry from a pocket tear gas gun is seated at the base of the index finger. Fortunately, the finger was salvaged.

The wound should be explored, irrigated, and mechanically debrided. Frequently healing is complicated by the persistent expulsion of retained foreign bodies. The cartridge itself has an epoxy cap, which is frequently retained in the wound if wide local debridement has not been carried out. Chloracetophenone is insoluble in water, and therefore simple irrigation is inadequate.

There is controversy in regard to primary wound closure versus leaving the wound open to granulate. Regardless of the initial method of wound closure, this type of injury has the propensity for delayed wound healing. Among eight reported cases, six patients had late sensory disturbances (bothersome paresthesias or hypesthesias; Adams, 1966; Schwartzbach, 1969; Symonds, 1967). Two of the three patients whose wounds were not closed primarily were reported to have ultimately had normal sensation.

Common to all types of injection wounds is the need for the initial emergency room physician to realize the seriousness of what appears to be an innocuous injury. There is also the necessity for immediate and complete decompression and decontamination of all tissues involved by use of appropriate generous incisions.

REFERENCES

Adams, J. P., Fee, N., and Kenmore, P. I.: Tear-gas injuries: a clinical study of hand injuries and an experimental study of its effects on peripheral nerves and skeletal muscles in rabbits. J. Bone Joint Surg., 48A:436, 1966.

Baker, J. M.: Molten plastic injuries of the hand. Plast. Reconstr. Surg., 15:233, 1955.

Hutchinson, C. H.: Hand injuries due to injection of cement under pressure. Proc. Minn. Med. Assoc., 46:83, 1967.

Kaufman, H. D.: The anatomy of experimentally produced high pressure injection injuries of the hand. Br. J. Surg., 55:340, 1968a.

Kaufman, H. D.: The clinico-pathological correlation of high pressure injection injuries. Br. J. Surg., 55:214, 1968b.

Kaufman, H. D.: High pressure injection injuries: the problems, pathogenesis and management. Hand, 2:63, 1970.

Mason, M. L., and Queen, F. B.: Grease gun injuries to the hand. Quart. Bull. Northwest. Med. School, 15:122, 1941.

Rees, C. E.: Penetration of tissue by fuel oil under high pressure from diesel engine. J.A.M.A., 109:866, 1937.

Schwartzbach, G., and Russin, M. D.: Tear gas injuries. Am. J. Orthop. Surg., 11:141, 1969.

Smith, M. G.: Grease gun injury. Br. Med. J., 2:918, 1964.

Stark, H. H., Ashworth, C. R., and Boyes, J. H.: Paint-gun injuries of the hand. J. Bone Joint Surg., 49:637, 1967.

Stark, H. H., Wilson, J. N., and Boyes, J. H.: Grease-gun injuries of the hand. J. Bone Joint Surg., 43:485, 1961.

Symonds, F. C., and Garnes, M. D.: Tear gas injury of the hand. Plast. Reconstr. Surg., 39:175, 1967.

Weeks, P. W.: Airless paint gun injuries of the hand. J. Ky. Med. Assoc., 65:1086, 1967.

ADDITIONAL BIBLIOGRAPHY NOT CITED IN TEXT

Grease Gun Injuries

Bell, R. C.: Grease gun injuries. Br. J. Plast. Surg., 5:138, 1952.

Blue, A. I., and Dirstine, M. J.: Grease gun damage. Northwest. Med., 64:342, 1965.

Bottoms, R. W.: Case of high pressure hydraulic tool injury to the hand: its treatment aided by dexamethasone and a plea for further trial of this substance. Med. J. Aust., 2:951, 1962.

Boyes, J. H.: Bunnell's Surgery of the Hand. Ed. 5. Philadelphia, J. B. Lippincott Company, 1970, pp. 559–561.

Grant, B., Wakefield, A., and Hueston, J.: Surgery of Repair as Applied to Hand Injuries. Baltimore, The Williams & Wilkins Company, 1968, pp. 178–179.

Harrison, R.: Grease gun injury. Br. J. Surg., 46:514, 1959.

Kaufman, H. D., and Williams, H. O.: Systemic absorption from high pressure spray gun injuries. Br. J. Surg., 53:57, 1966.

Rains, A. J.: Grease gun injury to the hand. Br. Med. J., 1:625, 1958.

Tanzer, R. C.: Grease gun type injuries of the hand. Surg. Clin. N. Am., 43:1277, 1963.

Paint or Spray Gun Injuries

Morley, R.: Injuries due to accidental injection of paint from high pressure paint guns. Br. J. Surg., 1:25, 1967.

Nahigian, S. H.: Airless spray gun. J.A.M.A., 195:688, 1966.

Walton, S.: Injection gun injury of the hand with anti-corrosive paint and paint solvent. Clin. Orthop., 74:141, 1971.

Waters, W. R., Penn, I., and Ross, H.: Airless paint gun injuries of the hand: a clinical and experimental study. Plast. Reconstr. Surg., 39:613, 1967.

Workman, C. A.: Power paint spray injury to the hand. Miss. Med., 60:856, 1963.

Chapter 81

BITES AND STINGS
OF THE HAND

CLIFFORD C. SNYDER
AND LARRY G. LEONARD

From the earliest times and through the ages, mankind has experienced a natural fear of venomous animals and venomous insects (Majno, 1975). Even the mention of the word venom causes a sinister apprehension in most people. An envenomation of any sort, whether the bite of a mad dog or a snake or the sting of a scorpion or a man-of-war, is immediately associated by the victim with death. Although the word venomous may refer to animals that eject a toxin through fangs or along spines, and poisonous may refer to living subjects that possess a toxin in their tissues and when eaten produce intoxication, these terms will be used synonymously. Envenomers walked, swam, and flew about this earth millions of years ago in the form of hard spiny armor covered animals and polybarbed ovipositors. When mankind first appeared about one million years ago, without protective apparel, the venomous animals and insects found the human a vulnerable prey. Although primitive man did not acknowledge his inflictions with manuscripts or prose, we need little imagination to conceive the frustrations he encountered in inhibiting these venomous attacks, the morbidity he endured, and the mortality for which he had no defense. It is fascinating to visualize fossilized pathogenic bacteria under the microscope that have been predated 300 million years, yet discouraging to realize that there were no antibiotics to combat them (Fig. 81–1).

In the early treatises of medicine, such as the papyri Ebers, Edwin Smith, Hearst, and others, there are prescriptions and treatments for inflictions by spiders, scorpions, snakes, crocodiles, hippopotamuses, lions, and even human bites. About 4000 years ago the Indian surgeon Susruta treated snake bites by opening the wounded hand widely to permit evil spirits to escape. Such therapy (escharotomy, dermatotomy, fasciotomy) has remained in use through the ages and is accepted currently by many physicians for extremity envenomations. As early as the sixth century B.C. in India, the relation of mosquito bites to malaria and of rodents to the plague was recognized (Margotta, 1968). The early Greek and Roman medical practitioners correctly identified poisonous annoyances: Hippocrates taught the therapy of spider bites, and Dioscorides wrote a five volume materia medica relating pharmacology to animal and plant poisons as well as to other medical problems. Pedanius Dioscorides, one of Nero's finest army surgeons, actually joined the Roman Legions in order to visit other countries to study the pharmacological properties of foreign plant and animal venoms. His *Materia Medica (Herbal of Dioscorides),* written in the first century, cited over 300 various bites and stings and their sequelae (Garrison, 1929). Aulus Cornelius Celsus, who lived at the beginning of the Christian era, was one of the most famous Roman medical writers (although it is doubtful that he actually was a physician), wrote the great encyclopedic work, *De Artibus.* Only the section "De re medica" survived destruction, in which Celsus remarked that the best therapy for an envenomous infliction was to open the arm and place a piece of chicken (fat) into the bite site (Wellman, 1926).

Claudius Galen (131–201 A.D.) of Pergamon, who wrote over 400 treatises and de-

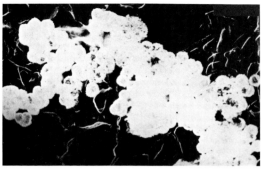

Figure 81–1. Microorganisms were on this earth at least 1.5 billion years before the earliest primate, as is represented by these fossilized germs found in rock quartz (chalcedony).

scribed many injuries by vipers, stingrays, spiders, scorpions, and marine animals, recommended wound suction, cautery, and astringents (Galen, 1975). But when the envenomation was serious, Galen actually excised the bitten area on the hand. Excision of the bite site is currently used with excellent results (Fig. 81–2). Paul of Aegina (625–690) also wrote extensively and described his prac-

tice for bites from mad dogs, lizards, snakes, scorpions, bees, spiders, crocodiles, and man, which in general consisted of sucking the wound of its poison by mouth, followed by cupping, and subsequent applications of wine or hot vinegar, onions, and theriacs (a potpourri of various ingredients) (Adams, 1846). The Greek word for wild and dangerous beasts was "theria." To cope with the hand bites by rabid dogs, attacking animals, aggressive snakes, and angry humans, physicians introduced a new and special kind of therapy, which they named "theriacs." This concoction differed from all other kinds of drugs and was used mainly for bite wounds, which were always thought to be poisonous. Theriacs became very popular and by 50 A.D. was used by all travelers, as we today depend upon vaccinations.

The Persian King Mithridates (132–63 B.C.) was a savage tyrant who always feared being poisoned (Margotta, 1968). He used his prisoners as guinea pigs by inflicting venomous bites of beasts and insects into their arms and then tested antidotes on them. He eventually compounded the best antidotes into a single

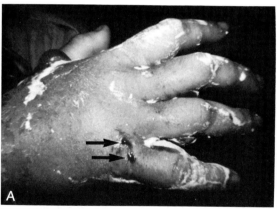

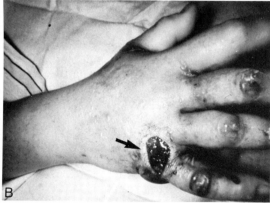

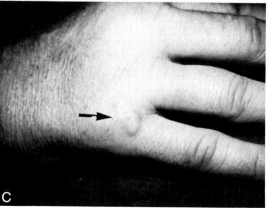

Figure 81–2. Claudius Galen in the first century utilized the excision of snakebite wounds, and this has continued as a popular method of the twentieth century. The arrows in *A* point to two bleeding fang marks; *B* shows excision of fang penetrations; *C* shows the healed wound without suturing.

preventive or theriacs for himself. He became immune to domestic poisons and reigned for 57 treacherous years. He was finally defeated by Pompey, who unsuccessfully tried to poison his captive but had to be content with seeking his death with the sword. To this day we use the term mithridatic antidotes. Two constant components of all theriacs are chunks of viper flesh and opium. Although many are sceptical about these early therapeutic measures for envenomous inflictions, one should not be too critical, because today a panacea remains wanting.

Ambrose Paré (1510–1590), a humble barber surgeon who was destined to become the idol of the French army, a councilor of state, and the surgeon to four kings of France, offered a beautiful description of bites by mad dogs, vipers, stingrays, and other "venomous beasts," including illustrations, in Thomas Johnson's *The Workes of That Famous Chirurgion Ambrose Paré* (Paré, 1634). In 1664 Francesco Redi published the first methodical work on snake poisons in which he demonstrated that venoms, in order to produce characteristics of poisoning, must be deposited (injected) under the skin; when rubbed on the skin or taken by mouth, they have no envenomating effects (Redi, 1664). It may be related that the father of modern scientific research on poisons was Felice Fontana (1720–1805), an Italian biologist who performed over 6000 experiments using over 4000 animals and 3000 snakes. The therapies he used included suction, incision, excision, herbs, oils, alkalies, acids, and hand amputations (Fontana, 1767). It was in 1860 that Silas Weir Mitchell, a Philadelphia neurologist, published his carefully devised and significant rattlesnake venom studies, which proved that venoms are proteins and noted the effects of venoms on nerves and the blood (Mitchell, 1860). The ancient fear of rabid canines and the dreaded disease of rabies was dramatically allayed by the Frenchman Louis Pasteur (1822–1895), who prepared a protective antibody and a vaccine in 1885, without ever identifying the virus (Pasteur, 1885). Using the pigeon as a subject, Henry Sewall in 1887 obtained immunity against rattlesnake venom, and his studies separately stimulated L.C.A. Calmette (1907) and Sir Thomas Frazer (1895) to immunize animals against specific venoms.

The history of human inflictions by beasts and bugs is still being written (10,000 publications each year), and our knowledge of venoms and their sequelae is increasing, yet much scientific work remains to be achieved. This is appreciated when one realizes that over 100,000 human victims continue to die from envenomation each year.

HUMAN INFLICTIONS

Although seldom in the field of medicine are two problem cases identical, human bite inflictions deliver such a unique chain of events that we are able to recognize them by a typical clinical picture—*the metacarpophalangeal syndrome.*

The human mouth is a storehouse of contaminants, which remain as a flora of organisms while in the oral cavity, but when injected into the soft tissues of the hand become a disparate cache of symbiotic microbes. Among the variety of microorganisms inhabiting the mouth are the staphylococci, streptococci, Vincent's fusiforms, *B. coli*, Proteus, spirochetes, gonococci, and pneumococci, and one must not discount the hepatitis and rabies viruses (Flynn, 1966; MacQuarrie et al., 1974; Murphy et al., 1963). The manner in which these human bite victims are injured and the usual time interval between the bite and the physician's examination are of canonical sequence. The human bite is a product of person-to-person contact ranging from alley conflicts to amorous affairs, always inflicted during a period of excitement and followed by a state of depression and confusion (Figs. 81–3, 81–4) (Boyce, 1942). The injured person fails to recognize the impending infection and delays the visit to a physician (Snyder, 1979). By the time the infuriated or inebriated victim senses the seriousness of his wound, the evidence of spreading infection is obvious (Chuinard and D'Ambrosia, 1977).

The train of incidents is typical, and we have named this sequence of signs and symptoms *the metacarpophalangeal syndrome.* For the first 24 hours after injury, the hand is noticeably swollen, with the seat of pain and tenderness established around the torn skin on the dorsum of the hand in the area of the involved metacarpophalangeal joint. After 48 to 72 hours the edema becomes pittingly prominent, the cellulitis spreads to produce more crimson tissues, the lymphangitis searches for a pathway to the epitrochlear

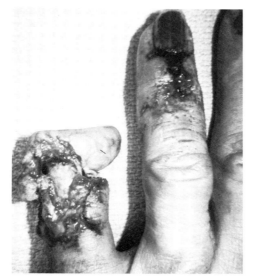

Figure 81–3. Partial amputation and dislocation of the left fifth digit due to a gnashing human bite during a hostile alley fracas.

node, the purulent exudate from the jagged wound expresses the severity of the infection, the spiking temperature curve mimics a picket fence, and the leukocytes are marching in force toward the rebellious microbes. It is only when the pain becomes unyielding that the miserable victim seeks the graces of the

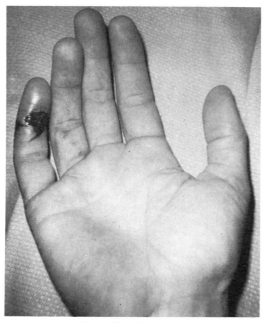

Figure 81–4. Bite inflicted by the person to herself during an exciting amorous affair, with resultant contusion-abrasion of the right little finger.

physician. Most patients strongly deny and frequently falsify the true cause of their traumatic malady (Kanaval, 1933). Regardless of the patient's hesitancy in disclosing that his present condition is the result of a fist-tooth injury, the sequence in which the pathological findings appear is the diagnostic sentinel of *the metacarpophalangeal syndrome.*

Even with the advent of antibiotics, human bite infliction, if encountered late, commonly leads to tendon, joint, and bone involvement and extensive impairment of function. The principles of treatment are based upon the complex anatomy of the tissues of the dorsum of the hand, which actually augments the spread of infection rather than limiting it (Kaplan, 1955); the mixture of organisms, in which some are symbiotic with others, leading to increased virulence; and the low resistance of the involved fibrous connective tissues. Treatment includes the immediate obtaining of a smear and culture of the wound, copious cleansing and judicious débridement of the wound, continuous irrigation of the wound, a delay in closure of the wound; the intravenous administration of antibiotics, immobilization of the hand, and hospitalization.

The hand surgeon is familiar with the complex anatomy of the metacarpophalangeal joint and the possibility of spread of the infection laterally into the superficial subcutaneous tissues of the dorsum of the hand, beneath the fascia of the proximal phalanx, beneath the extensor tendon, along the lumbrical canal or beneath the volar interosseous fascia into the middle palmar and thenar spaces, and by direct erosion of the fibrous flexor tendon sheath into the synovial membranes (Fig. 81–5). The wound and hand are gently but thoroughly washed with Betadine solution, followed by hydrogen peroxide, activated zinc peroxide, or Dakin's solution (Meleney, 1935). This converts an anaerobic medium into an aerobic state. Careful débridement of the devitalized tissue of the wound entrance should be instituted and the wound left open, without gauze packing, to encourage drainage (Jones and Shires, 1974).

Following thorough washing and flushing, the wound is catheter irrigated with a continuous drip of an organism-specific antibiotic and inspected for impending sequelae at least twice daily. If infection has already extended beyond the periphery of the wound entrance,

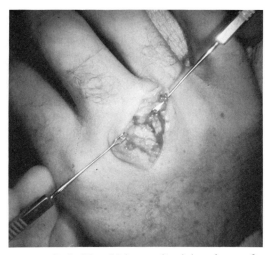

Figure 81–5. View 24 hours after injury from a fist-tooth infliction showing the lateral and deep spread of infection beneath the extensor tendon involving the metacarpophalangeal joint capsule.

x-ray examination is indicated in a search for a fracture or foreign body, and incision for wound drainage must be considered. These incisions must conform to vital anatomical structures, and attention to such contraindicates through-and-through drainage of the hand. Early curettement of joint spaces and rongeuring of bones are unnecessary if the infection of fascial planes and spaces is adequately drained. Torn tendons are not primarily repaired. An additional caution is to never incise an area of active hyperemia or cellulitis in the absence of purulence, because this will only spread with inflammatory response. Thermal and chemical cautery have no place in human bite inflictions (Mason and Koch, 1950).

Because there is always the possibility of clostridia in the wound, tetanus immune globulin or toxoid is indicated (Committee of Trauma, 1972). Prophylactic intravenous antibiotic therapy is initiated immediately and continuously, but may be changed to organism-specific antibiotics following receipt of the bacteriological report of the wound specimen. Early extremity bites are loosely dressed and immobilized with the metacarpophalangeal joints in flexion and the interphalangeal joints in extension. Once the infection has been controlled, motion exercises are encouraged. Hospitalization of the patient with an acute injury may or may not be necessary, depending upon the condition of

the wound, the patient, and the home environment.

Anesthesia for wound cleansing, débridement, drainage, and the application of dressings may be a problem. For children or hysterical and apprehensive adults, light general anesthesia is appropriate. If a full stomach is encountered, other routes should be entertained. The usual approach in adult inflictions is axillary or regional nerve block. If local infiltration anesthesia is the choice, the needle should never penetrate the wound because the infection may be dispersed.

ANIMAL BITES

Millions of people experience bites from a variety of animals each year. In the United States alone approximately three million humans were bitten by animals in one recent year. Because the upper extremity is the site of most animal inflictions, the hand surgeon must become knowledgeable about the environmental factors associated with these daily emergencies. There has been an enormous increase in the number of wild and exotic animals caught, bought, and kept as household pets, many of which are untameable and without hesitancy bite the hands that feed them. It also is common knowledge that the domestic animal population is multiplying faster than the owners to care for them. It is a perennial problem that parents continue purchasing mice, rats, rabbits, hamsters, monkeys, and other defensive biters merely to appease their children. If the parent would only spend the time to teach the child to respect and love the living creature, happiness would exceed the hazard incurred by bites.

Relative to the economic problems of animal bites, it is estimated that domestic losses due to these inflictions amount to at least 10 million dollars annually, and that medical expenses alone reach over 50 million dollars yearly. Therefore, the economic value of controlling these unnecessary human bites by animals is a problem involving everyone.

Dog Bites

Ninety of every 100 people bitten by an animal are bitten by a dog, whether it is a vicious attack or a defensive snap, or rendered in a playful mood (Robinson, 1974). The breeds responsible for the incidents are mostly German shephards, terriers, collies, and spaniels (Carithers, 1958). So be it; dogs are accountable for almost all the bites in humans (Douglas, 1975; Goldwyn, 1976). Cats account for 5 per cent of the mammalian attacks, while monkeys, rabbits, rats, bats, foxes, skunks, hamsters, raccoons, horses, camels, and bears factor in the remaining 5 per cent. Because parents are negligent and children are provocative, the majority of dog bites are observed in patients between the ages of two and 15 years. It is the child and not the dog who is usually at fault, because children have a tendency to prompt the attack by teasing and exciting the animal. The victim may be petting an unknown animal, taking food from an eating dog, avoiding a jumping canine, or picking a puppy from a mother dog. It is not uncommon for a veterinarian, an animal caretaker, or a research scientist to be bitten on the hand by a dog as a protective response.

As established by medical custom, dog bites are never closed by suturing, but instead are kept open to inhibit possible pathogenic contamination (Parks et al., 1974). This mode of therapy is certainly acceptable, especially when the wound is deep with skin and fat avulsed from the host, or when the postbite period is of a lengthy duration. In these instances the injury is treated similarly to a human bite of identical nature, that is, with copius irrigation and daily preparation for future elective coverage. The adage, "as clean as a hound's tooth," should be heeded with caution, because the dog's oral flora is as abundant with microorganisms as is that of the human mouth. *Pasteurella multocida* is the bacterium most frequently associated with dog bites (Halloway et al., 1969). There are many recorded cases in which dog bites involving the hand resulted in rabies, chronic lymphedema, fracture deformities, digital losses, and osteomyelitis (Lavine et al., 1975).

However, many dog bites are amenable to immediate attention by thorough cleansing, débridement, and loose closure with temporary wound drains (Fig. 81–6). The dog bite wounds of the hand that profit from this mode of therapy include simple, superficial, noncontaminated lacerations or those closely related to joints, tendons, nerves, and blood vessels that will lead to loss of these vital

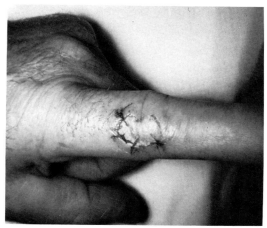

Figure 81–6. Superficial dog bites or thin avulsions may be thoroughly cleansed, debrided, and loosely closed but must be closely observed for the next 24 to 72 hours.

structures if not readily covered. The closure is achieved without buried sutures, without tension at the wound margins, and with temporary wound drains. The administration of antibiotics and tetanus toxoid or serum is instituted when indicated. Injuries by dogs can be decreased in frequency by the following:

1. Avoid strange, prowling, or ailing dogs.
2. Ignore dogs engaged in fighting.
3. Use leashes and muzzles on pet dogs in public.
4. Restrain watchdogs in the community.
5. Select family pets wisely.
6. Properly educate children in pet care.
7. Do not pet pups that are nursing.
8. Do not abruptly awaken a dog.
9. Do not interrupt a dog while he is eating.

RABIES

Epidemiology. It is hard to understand why with all the current legal statutes existent the increase in rabid animals continues unabated. Rabies remains a world-wide threat but the rabies virus and its pathogenesis continue to be poorly understood (Robinson, 1976). About one-half million people in the world are suspected of being infected by rabid animals annually and are recipients of numerous and sometimes dangerous antirabies treatments.

Of the confirmed rabies infected animals, skunks head the list of offenders; foxes rank second and bats, third. Although the infection is propagated by a multiplicity of animal carriers, 95 per cent of the human cases of rabies are inflicted by dogs.

The responsible organism is an ultramicroscopic, filterable, neurotropic virus transmitted to man by bites, skin contact, and inhalation. The incubation period varies from 10 days to one year, but the severity of the disease may lessen this prodromal period remarkably. Physicians must understand that a tear or puncture in the skin is not the only portal for entrance of the rabies virus. It may be surprising to learn that rabies infections also are introduced by eating, drinking, breathing, and handling infested materials (Constantine, 1962). It has been proven that contaminated milk has caused rabies by entering ulcerations in the intestine. Protected caged experimental animals have been placed in caves crowded with rabid bats and after 10 hours of exposure, without bites or scratches, have died of airborne rabies. There is no question that bat urine and guano harbor the rabies virus and that humans handling these excreta will contract the infection.

Symptoms. An early symptom of which the uneasy victim complains is distressing pain at the bite site, which insidiously becomes excruciating with associated exquisite tenderness. These localized complaints are soon followed by generalized skin hyperesthesia, at which time the person does not appreciate palpation. During this sequence of events there is a noticeable squinting of the eyelids and excitability in response to loud sounds, and the apprehensible patient requests darkness and quiet. There is a strong objection to light (photophobia) and noise. The patient begins to perspire profusely (sudoresis), lacrimates excessively (epiphora), and salivates incessantly (hydrophobia). As the patient's status worsens, muscle spasms and convulsions ensue, swallowing becomes difficult (dysphagia), Cheyne-Stokes respiration develops, the body temperature increases impressively, and death is unavoidable.

Diagnosis. Rabies is confirmed by the following:

1. Direct microscopic examination of the dog's brain tissue reveals Negri bodies in the motor neurons in affected animals.

2. A smear of the dog's brain tissue on a glass slide, flooded with rabies antibody and stained with fluorescein dye, is fluorescent under a special light when the virus tags onto the antibody.

3. The injection of suspected material into the brains of three week old mice will kill the mice in three weeks if the material is rabid.

4. The suspected rabid animal should be kept under surveillance for 10 days. If it lives without exhibiting suspicious symptoms, it is not rabid; but if it dies, it is suspect and must be studied.

Treatment. The incidence of rabies is high enough to warrant great concern, and the disease should always be considered. Because there is no chemotherapeutic agent or antibiotic that will control this neurotropic virus, in a diagnosed case immediate local therapy and active immunization with duck embryo vaccine supplemented with human rabies immune globulin may mean the difference between life and death. It is important to locally excise the bite area even hours after infliction and to scrub the open wound briskly with Betadine, Septisol, or Hibiclens. The wound should not be closed. Those who doubt the effectiveness of this initial treatment will find that only 5 per cent of infected research animals whose wounds were scrubbed with soap and water developed the disease; in comparison, 90 per cent of the controls whose wounds were not initially cleansed died of rabies (Snyder et al., 1979).

The most important decision for an attending physician treating an animal bite is when to treat or not treat with duck embryo vaccine and human rabies immune globulin. The physician who is unfamiliar with rabies will profit from consulting public health doctors, who are always cheerful to offer guidance. Although reactions to duck embryo vaccine are not common, these do occur and may be serious (Jones and Shires, 1974). When a reaction happens, the patient first complains of pain, pruritus, and tenderness at the inoculation site. This local reaction is followed by urticaria, chills and fever, anaphylaxis, intestinal hemorrhages, peripheral neuritis, encephalitis, paralysis, and even death. Epinephrine, if used early, will abate most anaphylactic reactions, and is administered by a slow intravenous drip as well as topically on the nasal mucosa. One should not give cortisone: although it decreases the victim's immune reaction, it paradoxically releases the potent rabies virus.

A guide to the treatment for rabies is presented in Table 81–1, but the physician must not use the therapeutic table without knowing the sequence of events involved in

Table 81–1. GUIDE TO RABIES THERAPY*

Wound Type	Healthy Family Dog or Cat†	Nonvaccinated Unidentified Domestic Animal	Rabid Domestic Animal	Wild Skunk, Fox, Bat
No lesion	No DEV, no HRIG	Observation	DEV, HRIG	Observation
Scratches	No DEV, no HRIG	HRIG	DEV, HRIG	DEV, HRIG
Superficial bite	No DEV, no HRIG	HRIG	DEV, HRIG	DEV, HRIG
Severe attack	HRIG	DEV, HRIG	DEV, HRIG	DEV, HRIG

*This guide will help the physician treat bites, but consultation with the state department of health will alleviate many worries and problems.
†DEV, duck embryo vaccine. HRIG, human rabies immune globulin.

a suspected case of rabies and the therapeutic directives.

Let us consider the questions arising in a patient involved with a possible rabid animal:

1. Was the victim viciously attacked by an unknown, possibly rabid animal or a playful family pet, and was the type of exposure a deep tissue gash, a superficial skin scratch, or a tongue licking? If the answer is a mild bite or scratch by a family pet, only treat the wound. If the wound is serious or was inflicted by a vagabond animal, proceed to question 2.

2. Is rabies endemic in the vicinity, or has there been a rabid animal in the locality recently? If the answer is no, do not treat for rabies. If the answer is yes—

3. Is the animal available? If the answer is no—

4. Is the animal a dog or cat? If the answer is no, administer duck embryo vaccine and human rabies immune globulin. If the answer is yes—

5. Was the person bitten? If the answer is no, give only duck embryo vaccine. If the answer is yes, give both duck embryo vaccine and human rabies immune globulin. If the answer to question 3 (is the animal available?) is yes—

6. Is the animal's behavior normal and is it a vaccinated dog or cat? If the answer is yes—

7. Did the animal become ill during the next 10 days? If the answer is no, no rabies treatment is indicated. If the answer is yes—

8. Does the laboratory examination of the brain confirm rabies? If the answer is no, forget the treatment. If the answer is yes, administer duck embryo vaccine and human rabies immune globulin. Remember: débride and cleanse the wound thoroughly—this is important.

Human rabies immune globulin, which is passive immunization, combined with duck embryo vaccine, which is active immunization, constitutes the best treatment available today. Human rabies immune globulin is administered in *one* intramuscular dose as early as possible following exposure. The dose is 40 I.U. per kg. of body weight, but in extensive (multiple bites and scratches) attacks or bites about the face and neck, 50 to 100 I.U.

per kg. is given. Therapy with duck embryo vaccine is instituted 24 hours after the single dose of human rabies immune globulin, and it is injected subcutaneously in various areas of the abdominal wall, back, and thighs. The dose of duck embryo vaccine is 40 I.U. per kg. of body weight. Active immunity is achieved with 14 to 21 daily injections of 1 ml. of a 10 per cent solution, depending upon the severity of the infection. The vaccine may be given in a double daily dose if the disease is critical, finishing the series in seven days. Booster injections are given 10 to 20 days after vaccination. Duck embryo vaccine is discontinued if the animal is proven nonrabid or if neurological symptoms appear.

HOUSEHOLD PET BITES

Domestic cat bites account for only 5 per cent of all bites inflicted in humans, but the severity and the complications must be reckoned with. Because cats' teeth are short and sharp, the wounds produced in hands are punctures. Infective organisms in the oral cavity of the cat and those present on the victim's skin are injected into the depths of the dermis and are difficult to clean with a cloth, sponge, or brush. Puncture wounds tend to collapse and obliterate the entrance and then become a nidus for anaerobic bacteria to multiply.

The approach to a puncture wound is to completely excise it. After débridement, most lancelike wounds should be left open, but if one is dealing with a simple wound, it may be débrided and closed. Cat and kitten bites resulting from playing without malice or assault intentions need only cleansing without further ado. Many times scratches by sharp claws are associated with the cat bite, and these may create worse problems than the bite per se. Scratch wounds usually have shallow trenches with a loss of skin. Because they need little attention, they become infected and result in multiple parallel lengthy scars. Bites by pet rabbits, guinea pigs, hamsters, rats, and monkeys are similar to wounds inflicted by cats and are treated in the same manner.

WILD ANIMAL BITES

A bite by any wild creature that flees capture and may be a rabies carrier necessitates careful attention and treatment. The incidence of rabies in wild life is high enough to warrent concern and close observation. Wild animal bites are approached therapeutically in a manner identical to that with bites inflicted by domestic species, but with much more rigor and aggressiveness. Wild animals are more susceptible to diseases and infections, and also are not available for examination and observation. Therefore early, quick, and expedient decisions must be rendered to achieve satisfactory results.

Bear Maulings

People around the world have displayed greater interest recently in hiking and camping in remote areas and wildernesses. Federal laws prohibit the carrying of guns into the national parks and forests, and therefore lovers of the out-of-doors enter the wild animal domains without protection. Inquisitive and hungry wild creatures are attracted by human voices and cooking food, and nothing will stand in their way in satisfying their instincts. In the national parks of Canada and the United States (Banff, Glacier, Yellowstone, Kootenay, Yoho), bear maulings are frequent occurrences with devastating consequences (Randall).

Grizzly bears are known for their nasty temperaments and fierce attacks. These animals average 200 to 400 kilograms in weight, stand 3 to 4 meters high, and cruise through wooded areas at 90 kilometers per hour. They have large sharp teeth and claws whose function is to pierce and tear through thick dense objects such as tree bark, the resistant scales of fish, and the hard shells of animals (Fig. 81–7). The massive neck muscles and powerful jaws are ideal for avulsing volumes of tissue from the victim. Bruins attack with teeth and claws, penetrating the soft tissues

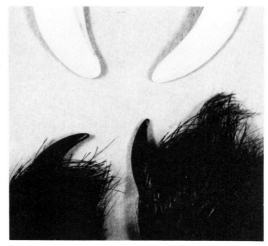

Figure 81–7. The claws of a bear are very sharp, and they can grasp and tear through tree bark and the hard shells of animals. The teeth and jaws are strong enough to avulse a human arm from its host.

deeply and avulsing large portions of muscle, tendons, and bones (Fig. 81–8). It is not uncommon for a grizzly to tear an arm from the body, rip multiple ribs along with the chest wall, bite an entire soft buttock and bony ilium from the pelvis, and avulse half a human head (Fig. 81–9).

The treatment for bear bites is instituted immediately. Wound irrigation and débridement must be thorough, and many of the wounds may be closed initially by margin approximation, skin grafts, local flaps, myocutaneous flaps, or free flaps. When there

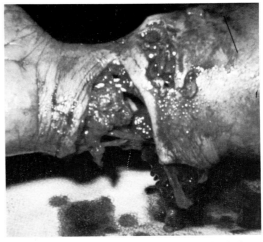

Figure 81–8. A hungry bruin looking for food ripped the skin, fat, muscles, tendons, blood vessels, and nerves of this camper's forearm with a single bite.

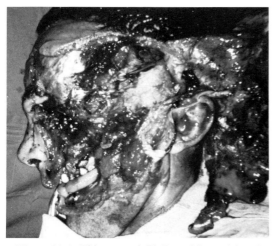

Figure 81–9. This research Ph.D., while studying the bear population in Yellowstone National Park, was surprised by an enraged grizzly, which avulsed the side of his head, eyeball, lips, and part of the mandible.

is a great loss of tissue (digits and hands), reparative surgery is staged.

Zoo Bites

Regardless of warning signs and posters noting "Do Not Feed the Animals," visitors to the zoo unmindfully reach over the metal guards and through the wire cages to feed the "begging" animal or attract a snoozing reptile. The caged creature in its excitement to retrieve the food bites the hand presented through the metal cage. Not only are the visitors victims of zoo animal attacks, but also the zoo attendants who clean the cages and work around the grounds. They often become the target of overzealous camels, zebras, burros, crocodiles, and snakes. The larger creatures, as elephants and water buffalos, inflict bruising and crushing injuries to hands associated with multiple fractures. We also have treated sharp lacerations caused by the tigers and lions that have resulted in amputations. Most zoo animal bites become infected immediately if care is delayed or lacking (Fig. 81–10). Because of the early infection and pain, all zoo bites are cleansed vigorously, débrided judiciously, and repaired as soon as reasonable. This therapeutic approach is also the regimen for the bite wounds inflicted by smaller zoo animals, such as bobcats, raccoons, weasels, minks, wolverines, badgers, and biturongs (Fig. 81–11).

REPTILE BITES

Alligator, Crocodile, and Caiman Inflictions

These reptiles have crania composed of solid membranous bone and powerful mus-

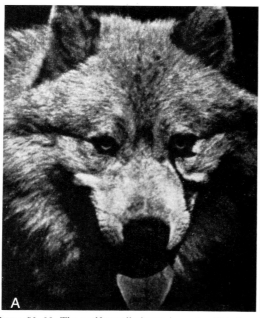

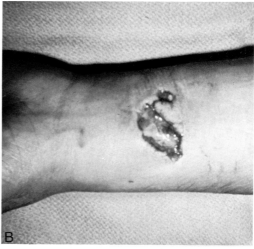

Figure 81–10. The wolf usually hunts in packs. This forearm bite shown in *B* is the typical type of wound that most canines inflict. If left unattended, it will become infected and necessitate prolonged therapy.

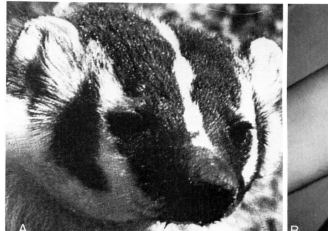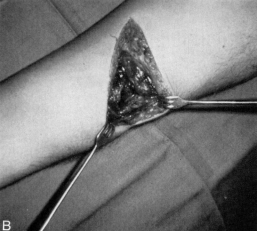

Figure 81–11. The badger has razor-sharp teeth, which incise soft tissues like a scalpel blade. Immediate débridement, repair of structures, and loose closure of the skin constitute the treatment of choice.

cles of mastication that open and close massive jaw bones. They are endowed with rows of sharp conical teeth, which are renewed as rapidly as they are lost. These reptiles are carnivorous and have a highly efficient manner of dismembering their prey. The author remembers one episode when an adult bathing in a swampy pool was attacked by a crocodile. The victim's right arm was caught between the vicelike jaws of the reptile, which with its strong tail revolved its body in the water, twisting the incarcerated arm in an attempt to tear it loose from the victim's torso. When the saurian opened its mouth to attack again, the man escaped. The humerus was fractured, and muscles, nerves, and blood vessels were avulsed (Fig. 81–12). Although a reptile's jaws can be held closed with one human hand, the same single hand is unable to pry the jaws open. The bite wounds resulting from these reptiles' attacks are devastating, including arm and hand amputations.

Two recent deaths were caused by reptiles, both in Florida. The first was in a child who fell into a reptile pit in a serpentarium, exciting the crocodile, which raced to the youngster and grasped him with steel-strong jaws through the abdomen. A bystander jumped into the pit and tried desperately to pry the reptile's jaws open, but in vain. The crocodile raised its body, walked to the pool of water, and slid with the victim beneath the surface. The boy's death was due to both the crush of the jaws and the drowning. In a second

episode a man, swimming in a central Florida river, was attacked and killed by an alligator; his remains were identified in a mangled condition.

In the treatment of crocodilian wounds the first step is to stop the bleeding, which is always present. The wounds are avulsive and necessitate thorough débridement of all devitalized muscle masses, adipose tissue, and skin. The wound is irrigated into its depths with Betadine solution and rinsed with normal saline. Depending upon the vital structures involved, the hand wound may be closed loosely or left open. Reparative surgery is delayed for a more opportune time when tendons and nerves are to be repaired.

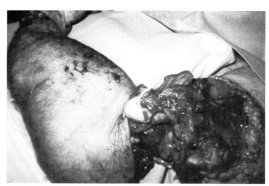

Figure 81–12. Alligator jaws are so powerful that the bite crushes and avulses both soft and bone tissues. This is a near-amputation of the upper arm and a partial severance of the wrist.

Lizards

The only known envenomous lizards are the Arizona Gila monster and the Mexican Gila monster (Mexican beaded lizard). These interesting and bizarre saurians belong to a family that roamed Asia, Europe, and other countries 50 million years ago (Bogert and del Campo, 1956). They are ecdytic (shed skin) and eremic (live in sandy areas), hibernate, are oviparous, are very envenomous, and live 25 to 30 years. There is bilateral tumidity of the lower jaw, which encases the poison (venom) gland in a position comparable to that of the parotid and submaxillary salivary glands in the human. The lobular structure of the glands encompasses numerous duct tributaries, which empty as funnels onto the gingiva of the mandible and the outer base of the anterior teeth. The teeth are grooved, enhancing the flow of the venom to the biting surfaces, and the venom inundates the entire oral cavity, in preparation for victim envenomation (Bellairs, 1970). The inferior labial venom glands of the lizard contrast with those located in the maxilla in venomous snakes.

Once the Gila monster is enraged, its attack is rapid and the jaws are vicelike in seizing a finger or hand. There are various estimates but no authentic statistics as to what the lethal dose of venom is in humans. As one may surmise, most helodermatid bites involve the hand and fingers, and the jaws may sustain the crushing tenaceous possession relentlessly "until the cows come home." (The quotation is from a young man bitten by a Gila monster.) Regardless of the minutes during which the reptile chooses to vigorously retain contact with the victim's hand, it may unfortunately be necessary to release the jaws by crude mechanical means (a bar, tree limb, pliers, wrench), or even forcefully jerk the saurian's ornamental tail (Johnson et al., 1966). All these methods of release must be undertaken with caution, because teeth may be left in the wound, and deep tears and avulsions are known complications.

The clinical findings with Gila monster bites are related to the volume of venom received, the extent of spread of the venom, the victim's resistance or allergic reaction, and his threshold to pain (Schufeldt, 1882). Pain is felt at the onset, and it may be localized or referred. The wound discomfort is soon associated with edema, as observed in all hand inflictions. The fear accompanying the biting attack is responsible for the mild shock with associated weakness, syncope, sweating, hypotension, and a rapid feeble pulse. The bitten digit or hand exhibits puncture wounds with surrounding ecchymosis due to both the sharp teeth and the powerful jaw muscles (Fig. 81–13).

The treatment in the field following retrieval of the hand from the jaws depends upon the environment. If no first aid materials are available at the scene, it is important to find the nearest medical facility. Regardless, as soon as it is feasible, one administers an analgesic (aspirin, Tylenol with codeine, morphine, Demerol) and a tranquilizer. The hand is washed enthusiastically with soap and water, then bathed in half-strength hydrogen peroxide for 10 minutes and rinsed in clinical alcohol, followed by application of a loose sterile dressing and immobilization. In the field a cheap bargain is to cleanse the wound with whiskey (a male's first aid) or mouth wash (a female's first aid). The goal is to remove as much saurian saliva from the puncture wounds and the skin of the hand as possible. Any deep inflictions, superficial lacerations, or redundant skin tags are judiciously débrided to afford smooth integumental margins in preventing anaerobic conditions and favoring eventual closure. Cooling the injured hand (not freezing) relieves pain and inhibits necrosis by decreasing metabolic activity at the site of trauma. The upper extremity is kept at the level of the heart—standing, sitting, or recumbent—and

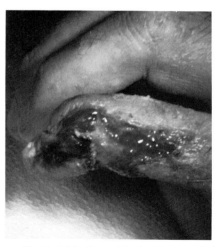

Figure 81–13. Little finger bite by the powerful jaws and sharp teeth of the Gila monster, crushing the distal interphalangeal joint and avulsing the skin from the dorsolateral surface.

not elevated high or redundantly low. Post-bite care includes observing the wound twice or more daily, with cleansing, bathing, and redressing. Although there are "antivenin kits," these are of questionable value (Russell, 1980).

Snakebites

The Committee on Emergency Medical Services of the National Research Council, seeking information relative to the first aid treatment of snakebites, invited participation at a meeting in Washington, D.C., on April 22, 1977. Five of us moderators met with federal authorities and representatives from the American National Red Cross, all with multifarious conceptions but a mutual goal—to provide advice and instructions to those (e.g., Boy Scouts, paramedics, personnel in the Department of the Interior and Bureau of Mines) who administer initial care to victims of snake envenomation. Some of the recommendations were published in the *Advanced First Aid and Emergency Care,* a manual published under the auspices of the American National Red Cross.

Another source of information is a nearly two year study conducted by the Committee on Trauma of the American College of Surgeons (1972). With the cooperation of experienced physicians with knowledge of serpentine envenomations. Our ultimate result was published in February 1981 in the form of a large poster entitled "Emergency Department Management of Poisonous Snake Bites" (Fig. 81–14). (This poster may be ordered from the American College of Surgeons' office in Chicago, Illinois.)

The reaction of a victim of a snakebite varies from extreme terror to hysteria, nervous exhaustion, syncope, and shock. This variety of reactions and the diversity of symptoms confuse the physician who is inexperienced with snakebites and may motivate him to administer unnecessary therapy to the victim (Snyder, 1972). Of 588 snakebites we have treated, 182 were inflicted in the upper extremity and 89 of these involved the hand (Table 81–2).

The environment and circumstances under which these occurred are interesting (Table 81–3). A golfer located his golfball in the rough and reached to identify it as his (and maybe better its position), when a surprised *Crotalus atrox* plunged a fang into his thumb.

Table 81–2. SITES OF SNAKE BITES ON THE HUMAN BODY*

Foot	89
Leg	279
Thigh	13
Trunk	21
Arm	5
Forearm	88
Hand	89
Head	4
Total	588†

*Snake bite envenomations involve various parts of the human body but are mainly inflictions of the extremities.
†Two deaths.

To cite another instance, one does not discount the exotic dancer whose pet indigo snake engaged its teeth into her left areola-papilla complex. Upon disengaging the amorous serpent, a second infliction occurred to the intruding hand. In a third case a female snake bounty hunter kept her pets in the house. When she opened a boudoir drawer, the awakened *Crotalus adamanteus* inserted two fangs into its mistress' hand. Children under age 14 are the recipients of most serpentine attacks, and this is the result of neglected teaching, inquisitive minds, and careless wanderings without protection (Snyder and Temple, 1979).

Incidence. Reliable statistics relating to snakebites are wanting, but they happen with greater frequency than is generally realized (Parrish, 1966). Perusal of the literature, uncertain as it is, reveals that at least 75,000 human fatalities worldwide annually are caused by snakebites. Venomous snakebites in most countries seldom terminate fatally, because of the excellent medical care, the educational information made public, and high standards of living. The morbidity is of greater concern than the mortality, which involves regional tissue sloughing and loss of skin, muscles, tendons, nerves, and bones (Fig. 81–15). Permanent anesthesia in the bitten hand area is common, as well as cau-

Table 81–3. THE ENVIRONMENT IN WHICH SNAKE BITES OCCUR

Theater stage	Hunting reserve
Serpentarium	Home yard
Research laboratory	Forest
Golf course	Swamp
Auto camper	Desert
Fraternity house	Garage
Living room	Bedroom

Emergency Department
Management of Poisonous Snake Bites

Clinical Evaluation of the Victim

1. **Assess respiratory status.**
2. **Assess circulatory status.**
3. **Determine the extent of systemic reaction from the presence of hypotension; nausea; vomiting; sweating; weakness; or neurotoxic symptoms such as dizziness, perioral paresthesia, ptosis, paralysis, or muscle fasciculations.**
4. **Inspect the area of the bite, noting one or more fang marks** (although a coral snake may leave none), **swelling, pain, or ecchymoses.**
5. **Identify the snake if possible. Most bites are from nonpoisonous snakes.** (The appearance of a snake, especially the rattlesnake, may vary considerably from these illustrations.)

Laboratory Evaluation

1. **Routine tests:**
   a. Complete blood count
   b. Type and crossmatch
   c. Prothrombin time
   d. Partial thromboplastin time
   e. Platelet count
   f. Urinalysis
   g. Blood sugar, blood urea nitrogen (BUN); electrolytes
2. **Additional tests, depending on the severity of the bite:**
   a. Fibrinogen
   b. Red cell fragility
   c. Clotting time
   d. Clot retraction time

Grade of Envenomation*

The grade of envenomation will vary with time after the bite. If the victim is seen early, severe envenomation may be underassessed. Observe at least six hours after the bite.

1. **Indications of minimal envenomation:**
   a. Local symptoms and signs (See Clinical Evaluation, 4)
   b. Few systemic symptoms and signs (See Clinical Evaluation, 3)
   c. Minimal laboratory abnormalities (See Laboratory Evaluation)
2. **Indications of moderate envenomation:**
   a. Swelling that progresses beyond the area of the bite
   b. Some systemic symptoms and signs
   c. Abnormal laboratory findings—ie, abnormal clotting factors; a fall in hematocrit or platelets
3. **Indications of severe envenomation:**
   a. Marked local symptoms and signs
   b. Severe systemic symptoms and signs
   c. Significant abnormalities in laboratory findings

*This section should be used as a rough guide to determining the amount of venom the victim received. Experts across the country are not in uniform agreement on the indications for the use of antivenin and the amount of antivenin required.

Treatment

1. **Start intravenous infusion of balanced salt solution if any evidence of envenomation exists.**
2. **Oxygen and appropriate vasopressors should be available.**
3. **Keep the bitten part level with the heart.**
4. **Release compression band** (if one has been applied) **only if:**
   • the patient is not in shock
   • an intravenous line has been established
   • antivenin is available
5. **Local care of the area of the bite**
   a. If the victim is treated within 30 minutes of the bite, **incise at least full-thickness skin to the depth of the bite. Apply suction for 20 minutes.**
   b. Some consultants with extensive experience and good results recommend early exploration of the snake bite area under local or general anesthesia as primary therapy, to diagnose the status of envenomation and to determine the depth and amount of tissue destruction.
   c. Cryotherapy is not indicated in the emergency department.
6. **Update tetanus immunization.**
7. **Antivenin** (See Grade of Envenomation)
   a. Withhold antivenin from patients without symptoms or signs of envenomation.
   b. Withhold antivenin from patients exhibiting local but not systemic symptoms or signs. **Many patients will not require antivenin.** (Copperhead venom is not usually very toxic, and rarely necessitates antivenin.)
   c. Admit all patients who receive antivenin.
   d. Administer antivenin intravenously in a continuous saline drip on the basis of grade of envenomation:
      • **Minimal:** 0-4 vials
      • **Moderate:** 5-9 vials, especially in children and the elderly
      • **Severe:** 10-15 or more vials
      Administer antivenin **only after a skin test.** Read product information carefully.
   e. Epinephrine 1/1000 in a syringe should be available before antivenin is given.
   f. Judge the amount of antivenin by improvement in symptoms and signs, not by the patient's weight. Children may need more antivenin than adults.
   g. If systemic manifestations are severe, antivenin should be given rapidly, by intravenous drip, in large doses.
8. **Watch for vascular insufficiency or compartment syndrome.** Fasciotomy may be required if distal vascularity is impaired by swelling.

Additional Antivenin Considerations
   • Polyvalent antivenin (Wyeth Laboratories) is the current antivenin of choice for all North American rattlesnake, water moccasin (cottonmouth), and copperhead bites.
   • North American coral snake antivenin (Wyeth Laboratories) should be used for eastern coral snake bites **only—not** for western or Arizona coral snake bites.

American College of Surgeons
Committee on Trauma
February, 1981

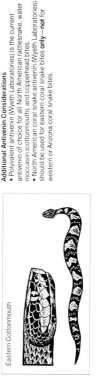

Timber Rattlesnake

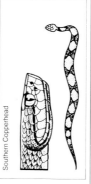

Coral Snake

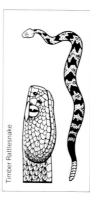

Eastern Cottonmouth

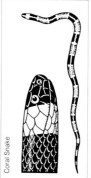

Southern Copperhead

The Committee on Trauma of the American College of Surgeons recognizes that many acceptable methods for treating poisonous snake bites are in use. The principles outlined here are a synthesis of repeated consultations with a number of physicians experienced in the treatment of snake bites.
The Committee on Trauma will furnish a list of these consultants on request. Inclusion on this list does not imply approval of this poster by an individual consultant.
Each physician should determine the accepted emergency department practice in his or her area for controversial issues such as indications for antivenin; exploration of the area of the bite; excision of the bite; fasciotomy; antibiotics, antihistamines, sedatives, and corticosteroids.

Figure 81–14. This poster developed by a group of physicians involved in treating snake bites is available from the office of the American College of Surgeons, Chicago, Illinois.

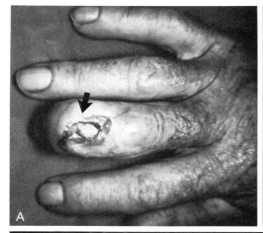
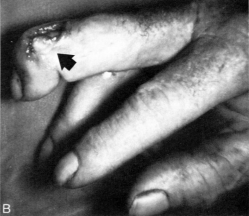
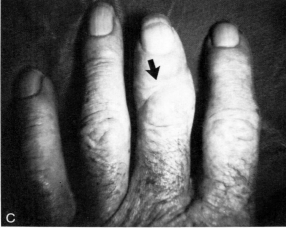

Figure 81–15. *A* and *B* exemplify a *Crotalid atrox* infliction of the middle finger with resultant loss of skin and extensor tendon and exposure of the distal interphalangeal joint. *C*, The treatment included shortening the bone, débridement of the soft tissues, and closure.

salgia, muscle atrophy, digital stiffness, and even hand loss. In many cases of snakebite, the offender remains unidentified because of the victim's fright, the speed of the serpent's escape, and the surrounding dense foliage.

Envenomers. Poisonous snakes of Mexico, United States, and Canada stem from the family Crotalidae (pit vipers) and the family Elapidae (represented by the coral snake). The pit vipers are of three genera, the Crotalus (true rattlesnakes), the Agkistrodon (moccasins and copperheads), and the Sistrurus (ground rattlers). Pit vipers are so named because of the holes that lie between and below the level of the eye and nostril, the site of a sense organ aiding in detecting the proximity of prey or enemies (Minton, 1971). The poisonous viper is differentiated from nonpoisonous snakes by its fangs, elliptical pupils, broad head with a narrow neck, and a single row of scale plates distal to the anus. Nonpoisonous snakes do not have fangs, have round pupils, and have a double row of plates

below the anal orifice. Unfortunately the coral snake, which is venomous, has no pit and has a round pupil, similar to the harmless snakes (Gans, 1978).

The venom gland of the snake is analogous to vertebrate salivary glands, and the venom is forced or propelled through the fangs for ejection (Fig. 81–16). At rest, the fangs are

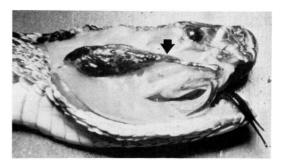

Figure 81–16. The salivary gland of the snake contains venom-producing cells proximal to the main duct *(arrow)* as it empties into the canalized fangs.

folded against the palate; when the snake strikes, they are thrust forward for penetration and ejection of venom. The instant the fangs of a striking snake touch the intended goal, the mouth closes and the venom is released. Therefore, when loose clothing is worn, the fangs touch it, the snake's mouth closes, and the venom is ejected without piercing the skin of the intended victim. Hence the depth of bite penetration depends upon covering garments, tissue thickness, fang length, and the angle of penetration. These important factors determine whether the venom is deposited above the muscle fascia or below it, a decisive element in the clinical management (Lockhart, 1965). Rattlesnakes can actually control the amount of venom they inoculate, as proven in isotope tagged venom studies in mice, rabbits, and dogs. This is important because many human victims exhibit no symptoms of envenomation (25 per cent of the bites by poisonous snakes do not result in envenomation; Wingert and Wainschel, 1975), and those treated by bizarre methods such as tobacco juice, mystic stones, cackleburr stupes, and turkey dung claim cures that are erroneous (Masterton, 1938).

The Venom. The venom of a poisonous snake is a complex of several proteins, lipids, enzymes, and other less significant constituents (Phisãlix, 1922). Several specific toxic enzymatic ingredients have been identified, including proteases, esterases, dipeptidases, hyaluronidase, and phospholipase A, each exerting destructive actions on the tissues affected. These enzymes and the toxic proteins are the reason snake envenomation yields a dramatic diversity of symptoms. When a specific snake venom is injected into a laboratory animal, it may cause an embolic phenomenon such as pulmonary embolism; the identical snake venom injected into another similar research animal may cause a hemorrhagic phenomenon such as intestinal hemorrhage. These divergent effects perplex the attending physician and confuse the method of therapy. Such should be known to the doctor so that correct therapeusis can be administered. All venoms are composed of so-called "neurotoxic" and "hematoxic" components, which are found in different ratios in various species of envenomers. The neurotoxic elements promote little action at the site of envenomation but exert their effect on distant tissues. The hemotoxic compo-

nents are responsible for tissue destruction at the site of infusion. These actions are exemplified by the following: Elapid (coral snakes, cobras, Russell vipers) venoms may cause little local pain, swelling, or tissue sloughing but may result in early respiratory and cardiac distress. In comparison, Crotalid (cotton mouth moccasin, rattlesnake) venoms produce immediate local pain, progressive swelling, ecchymosis, and eventually sloughing of tissues.

It is extremely important to differentiate between a poisonous snakebite and a nonpoisonous one, because if the former is not treated, death may ensue, and if the latter is treated with horse serum antivenin, the victim may be allergic to it, and irreversible complications, even death, may occur. Today these are liability problems, and legal developments create havoc.

Signs and Symptoms of Envenomation. The cardinal findings are the following:

1. Fang puncture wounds. There may be one to six wounds as a result of more than one attack, or because the snake may have one to six fangs, or because only one fang pierced the skin (Snyder et al., 1979; Figs. 81–17 to 81–19).

2. Swelling. There may be only mild edema and discoloration initially, or the edema may be immediate and progress suf-

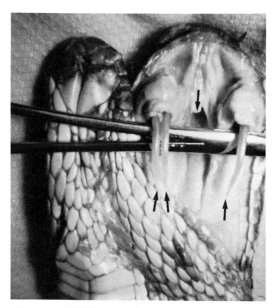

Figure 81–17. There may be one or more mature fangs present; this snake has three mature fangs. Note the cleft palate, which is normal in snakes.

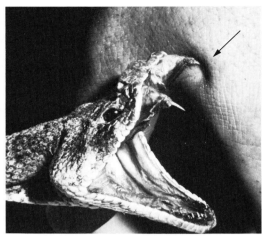

Figure 81–18. The strike of this bite will only show one fang puncture hole because both fangs did not penetrate the skin.

ficiently to obliterate superficial venous return (Fig. 81–20).

3. Pain. The victim may experience little pain at first, but later the pain may become excruciating, or the pain may be unbearable immediately and lead to syncope and shock.

Ancillary Findings. Ancillary findings include the following:

1. Erythema or ecchymosis. This is usually immediate and progressive.

2. Bullae. Bullae may be in the form of a clear serum transudate or large hemorrhagic blebs.

3. Petechiae. Venom affects the intima of blood vessels and is also responsible for capillary fragility, resulting in minute subcutaneous hemorrhages.

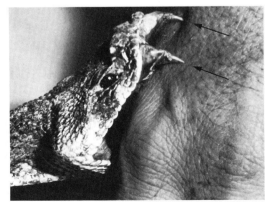

Figure 81–19. This strike registers a two-fang infliction, and therefore the skin will represent the bite with two puncture wounds.

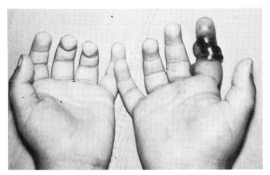

Figure 81–20. The snake-bitten right hand is very edematous (a cardinal sign), and the inflicted index finger demonstrates a large hemorrhagic bleb (ancillary finding).

4. Hyperesthesia to anesthesia. Venom affects the sensory nerve endings and produces immediate pain and then early numbness of the bite area, later changing to pain again.

5. Paresthesia. Paresthesia is a later symptom and takes the form of peculiar skin sensations, such as formication and tingling; it may terminate with causalgia.

6. Advancing pitting edema. This is due to compression of lymphatic and blood vessels and progresses proximally up a limb.

7. Cyanosis, necrosis, and tissue sloughing. These symptoms are sequential and are a result of compromise of the blood supply.

8. Anxiety, nausea, and vomiting. The central nervous system as well as the gastrointestinal mucosa is affected, and this may be accompanied by muscle twitching, convulsions, and paralysis.

9. Dyspnea, rapid feeble pulse, vertigo, dimmed vision, pinpoint pupils, and general weakness. These are all prodromal symptoms of shock.

10. Coma and death.

Laboratory Findings. Moderate to severe envenomation produces evidence of hypothrombinemia, thrombocytopenia, hypofibrinogenemia, and anemia (Huang et al., 1974). An x-ray view of the chest may reveal pulmonary edema and embolus formation. The factors that may influence the severity of symptoms are the age and size of the victim (children are affected more seriously [Snyder et al., 1968]); the time elapsed after the snakebite; the location, depth, and number of bites; the species and size of the envenomer; the amount of venom injected; the victim's sensitivity to the venom; and the efficacy of the initial first aid treatment.

Treatment. The management of persons who have been bitten by poisonous snakes varies widely because the effects vary in seriousness. Of the more than 600 patients sustaining snakebites who have come under our care over the past 33 years, about half needed only first aid therapy, and one-fourth did not even exhibit any signs of envenomation. It is necessary to clarify the differences of opinion regarding snakebites for persons whose occupations place them in snake-infested areas, including those in the armed forces, Scout leaders, personnel of the Department of the Interior and the Bureau of Mines, and game wardens and for paramedics, family practice physicians, and the general public who enjoy camping, hiking, hunting, fishing, and other recreations. Therefore, snakebite poisonings need to be classified. One understandable and applicable classification is the following:

1. Mild: fang scratch marks, no pain, minimal swelling.

2. Moderate: fang puncture(s), pain, erythema, local swelling, no systemic symptoms.

3. Severe: fang puncture(s), immediate or delayed excruciating wound pain (vipers), progressive swelling, ecchymosis, petechiae, bullae, and systemic symptoms of anxiety, hysteria, tingling, nausea, vomiting, fibrillations, vertigo, dyspnea, and syncope.

For the mild type of bite that is over one hour old, with only fang scratch marks, slight local swelling, and no pain, the wound is cleansed with soap and water or alcohol, the patient is not given antivenin, and incisions are not indicated. For the moderate snakebite, that is, for the envenomated patient who presents local findings but has no systemic effects, the fang marks are incised with one linear incision through the punctures, the wound is suctioned, but antivenin is withheld. The severe snakebite with all the cardinal and some of the ancillary findings is treated aggressively, using a tourniquet, excising the puncture wound area, administering antivenin, and hospitalizing the victim for observation and further therapy. Because some envenomers are more or less poisonous than others, all snakebites should not be attended by an "absolute standard" of therapy; instead the treatment should be individualized according to the toxic effects observed. We therefore have divided the modes of therapy into preventive therapy, emergency field therapy, and hospital emergency room therapy.

Preventive Therapy

1. Refrain from hiking or camping in known snake-infested areas, occult foliage, caves, and mines.

2. Be on the alert for snakes sunning on warm days.

3. While walking through forests and deserts, wear protective gear such as snake leggings, boots, long trousers, sleeved shirts, and gloves.

4. Do not reach into ground holes or onto poorly visible mountain ledges.

5. Avoid being alone in the woods; a companion may be a lifesaver.

6. Keep your vehicle near, whether it be two- or four-wheeled or four-legged.

7. Carry a snakebite kit on rural trips, and know how to use it (Fig. 81–21).

8. Do not keep poisonous snakes as pets; do not surprise sleeping snakes; do not molest snakes.

9. Inquire in advance about medical aid when traveling in primitive areas.

Emergency Field Therapy

1. Remember: there are no absolute rules, only practicable ones.

2. Avoid excitement, exertion, and beverages that may accelerate the circulation and rapidly propel the venom throughout the body.

3. Stay and retrieve the offender for identification, but do not exert or endanger yourself.

4. Immediately apply a flat tourniquet (belt, bandana, sock, neckerchief) proximal to the extremity bite and only snug enough to permit the introduction of one finger beneath it easily. Loosen the tourniquet a little

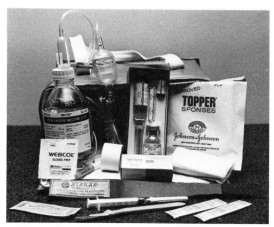

Figure 81–21. The authors' snake bite kit contains antivenin, elastic tourniquet, corticosteroids, normal saline, and other necessities.

as the swelling increases. If swelling is already present, do not apply a tourniquet. Never apply, remove, reapply, and remove a tourniquet intermittently, for this propels the venom into the general system. Release the band completely when antivenin is given intramuscularly or intravenously.

5. Cleanse the bite area, if possible, and cut from one fang mark through the other down to the subcutaneous fat. Do not use cruciate (crosshatch) incisions because they are harmful, especially on the face and hands.

6. Suction or digitally express fluid (blood and venom) gently from the incised wound without macerating it, but doing this for more than five minutes is damaging and useless.

7. Immobilize or rest the bitten limb horizontally at heart level; it should not be above or below the heart level because either position will enhance edema and necrosis. Muscular exercise should be inhibited at first because it increases circulation and venom spread.

8. Venom neutralization must be achieved. Wyeth's polyvalent antivenin is the only available therapy to date in the United States, and it has been proven to be lifesaving. The sooner it is administered, the more beneficial it is; yet it has been given 24 hours after a bite with good results. Because it is a horse serum product, the precautions as listed on the package flyer must be heeded.

Emergency Room Treatment

1. Identify the venomous injury (fang mark[s], swelling, pain) and the snake if available. Record any history of allergies (drugs, horse serum, Novocain, foods), and note whether patient has or has had hay fever, asthma, or urticarias.

2. If the victim has sustained a severe envenomation, prepare one vial of Wyeth's polyvalent antivenin (Crotalidae), and dilute this 10 ml. into 100 ml. of sterile normal saline solution and 125 mg. of Upjohn's Solu-Medrol (or methylprednisolone equivalent). During this interval, inject into the victim 0.02 ml. of a 1:100 dilution in saline of the normal horse serum (included in Wyeth's kit) to raise a small wheal intracutaneously to test for allergy. A control test of normal saline near the horse serum test facilitates interpretation of the findings. A negative reaction shows no local skin changes; a positive response occurs within five to 15 minutes, revealing a white wheal with increasing peripheral erythema, edema, and itching. If the patient has any history of allergies, the anti-

venin must be tempered to the severity of the snake bite; a safe starting dose is 0.5 ml. of 1:100 dilution. A reaction to this trial dosage is adequate warning not to use the horse serum antivenin. If the person has no allergies and the test response is negative, administer the prepared antivenin intravenously, with epinephrine, corticosteroid, and antihistamine, awaiting any untoward reactions. Children and adults are treated alike. It is hoped that our laboratory will have a human antiserum available in the future.

The local treatment of the snakebitten site is as follows:

1. If the envenomation is classed as a mild one, do not incise.

2. If the envenomation is of the moderate type, a linear incision through the fang punctures to the fascia followed by suction is the course.

3. If the envenomation is severe, the fang marks are elliptically excised with an equidistant margin of 1 cm. through the fat to the fascia. Bleeding is controlled by an occlusive dressing.

4. Escharotomy is necessary when extreme edema appears to be compromising the blood supply. Fasciotomy is indicated in subfascial envenomation and, when used judiciously can save an extremity (Glass, 1975).

5. Local remedies such as cautery, acids, alkalies, cruciate incisions, and mystical applications, some of which destroy more tissue than does the venom, are not used.

6. Cryotherapy is advocated by excellent medical serpentologists, but such treatment needs definition. We do not freeze the snakebitten area, but we do cool it. Local hypothermia reduces pain, inhibits venom release, limits edema, and decreases metabolic needs. If not governed carefully however, low temperature applications will cause bleb formation, necrosis, and gangrene. When used on digits, cold therapy is disastrous in such disease states as diabetes, arteriosclerosis, cryoproteinemia, scleroderma, Berger's disease, Raynaud's disease, and others. Once the therapeutics of cryotherapy, hypothermia, freezing, and cooling are carefully defined in relation to snakebite, an understanding will lead to better management.

7. Pressure or tight dressings are detrimental.

Tetanus immunization, antibiotics, analgesics, oxygen, calcium, transfusion, tracheotomy, and hemodialysis are all to be utilized when indicated. Hospitalization should be advised for all envenomated snakebite victims because many findings are not distinguishable early. The kin or responsible party should be advised of latent sequelae.

ARTHROPOD BITES

Arthropods are the most highly developed, specialized, and versatile of the invertebrates. There are approximately 80,000 species of arthropods, and these animals are implicated in far more poisonings to human beings than all the other phyla combined. Almost all spiders, approximately 20,000 species, are venonous. There are some 500 species of scorpions, some of which must be considered lethal. In the order Hymenoptera (bees, wasps, yellow jackets, and ants) there are numerous genera and species of potential danger to man. Among the ticks, caterpillars, assassin bugs, moths, butterflies, grasshoppers, and other arthropods there are a number of poisonous species. Arthropodal venoms represent some of the most complex and most diversified substances known. Bee venom, a good example of the complexity of an arthropod toxin, contains lipids, peptides, apamines, melittin, apic acid, sugars, free bases, amino acids, other proteins and enzymes, and a number of unidentified components. There is still considerable question as to which components of bee venom cause sensitivity, and these may not necessarily be the more toxic ones. Scorpion venoms contain 10 to 15 proteins and at least five nonproteins.

The venom of spiders needs more detailed study. Because of the small yield obtained from each spider, it takes milkings from 1000 spiders to accumulate 1 mg. of venom from the smaller species. The massive hairy tarantula is nothing but a "show-off" and is relatively harmless to man (Fig. 81–22). Ant venoms provide an example of remarkable chemical diversification because of the abundancy of species; some ants sting, some bite, and some spray their venom. More than three times as many people in the United States die from arthropod bites and stings than from rattlesnake bites. However, the majority of the arthropod inflicted deaths can be attributed to anaphylactic responses rather than to the direct effects of the venoms (Snyder et al., 1972). Yet deaths from black widow spider bites, brown recluse spider bites, and

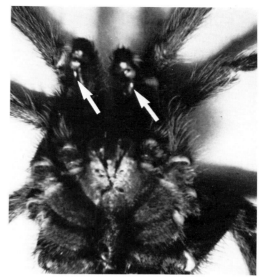

Figure 81–22. The massive hairy tarantula is a "shoo-in" for the greatest "show-off" in the phylum of arthropods, but it is relatively harmless to man. The arrows point to the two fangs.

scorpion stings as well as from multiple bee and fire ant stings do occur (Douglas, 1975).

Black Widow Spider Bites (Latrodectism)

This creature of arachnology has the justified reputation of being the most dangerous of American arthropods and is nature's archetype of the devouring female. Once mating is completed, the male is of utterly no use to future generations; therefore is it so preposterous that the female often eats her mate after she is through with him? We have observed isolated black widow couples in our laboratory that appear to have adjusted to one another, and then one morning the male is found entwined with webbing and later gone—eaten alive. Not all males are killed by their mates; some just die. The longevity of the latrodecti is 13 to 17 months.

Habitat and Features. There are four venomous genera and 20 to 25 poisonous species of Latrodectus (secret biters) spiders, and they are found on every continent in the world. Over 1000 *Latrodectus mactans* were found in a single cache in the emergency room of a Salt Lake City metropolitan hospital. It is distinguished by a glossy black body, a red-orange-yellow hourglass-shaped figure on its abdomen, and often a red tail light (Fig. 81–23). She has two small fangs

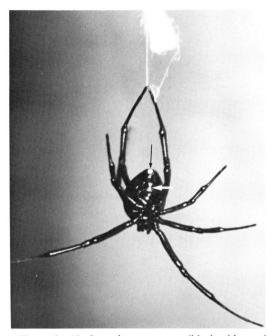

Figure 81–23. *Latrodectus mactans* (black widow spider) is a glossy black lady with a red-orange-yellow hourglass-shaped figure on her abdomen (white arrow) and often a red tail light (black arrow).

(chelicerae) through which the venom is injected into the victim. The male Latrodectus is considerably smaller, has white stripes and no hourglass, and does not envenomate. Most bites in the Mediterranean countries take place in the fields on the left hand and forearm while the farmer is collecting the corn and wheat during harvesting season (Yugoslavia, Italy, Ukraine, Syria, Lebanon, Turkey, Israel, and Northern Africa).

Toxic Manifestations. A definite history of spider bite is usually wanting, and it is only after the physician has completed examining the patient and is unable to make a diagnosis that the idea of a possible spider bite is formulated. A careful search then elicits two minute red fang marks (so close they look like one) in the skin (Fig. 81–24). The patient may then recall a sharp pinprick incident that was unperturbing and forgotten. When a black widow spider bites, there is a moment of sharp pain followed by a dull, numbing ache. Misdiagnoses of black widow spider envenomation include acute appendicitis, cholecystitis, ruptured peptic ulcer, and ureteral lithiasis. Bites on the upper extremity cause referred pain to the shoulders, back, and chest and sometimes are accompanied by dyspnea, simulating coronary thrombosis or

pneumonia. Immediately following the bite a minute punctate red mark appears with a surrounding area of erythema, and mild edema develops. This may disappear and no further signs may develop. If the venom spreads through the peripheral nerves to the central nervous system, other signs and symptoms of varying gradients evolve, such as headache, vertigo, nausea, sweating, salivation, irritability, restlessness, convulsion, paralysis, eyelid edema with ptosis, shock, and coma. Laboratory findings include leukocytosis, albuminuria, and hematuria, and though the spinal fluid pressure may be elevated, examination of the fluid yields no positive findings. Many of these patients are admitted to the hospital medical service with a pending diagnosis. It is apparent that a number of spider venoms have chemical and pharmacological properties similar to those of other venoms, and therefore it is important to encourage the public to bring the offending spider to the appropriate person for identification.

Management. The mortality from black widow spider envenomation is about 4 per cent. Most of the bites, even in children and the aged, are self-limiting and need only immediate therapy for pain and discomfort. The following is a résumé of the treatment for latrodectism:

1. Cold compresses or cooling the bite area to reduce local pain.

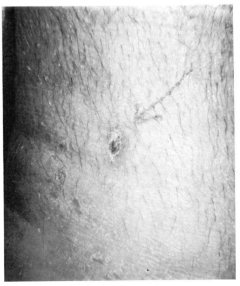

Figure 81–24. Black widow spider bite 24 hours after infliction. The minute red fang marks have been replaced by a small blue bleb.

2. Calcium gluconate, 10 ml. of 10 per cent solution intravenously, repeated at four hour intervals as necessary, for muscle spasms.

3. Diazepam, 10 mg. given slowly intravenously or by mouth if the patient is not nauseated.

4. Methocarbamol, 10 ml. given slowly intravenously, as a muscle relaxant.

5. Add analgesic cautiously; narcotics are generally required.

6. Antihistamines and corticosteroids may be used judiciously.

7. Antivenin is the only specific therapy. It is used only in severe cases of envenomation or in highly susceptible persons. The name of the product is Lyovac, and it is manufactured by Merck Sharpe & Dohme. The usual dose is 2.5 ml. intramuscularly (not intravenously) and the dose may be repeated. It is a horse serum product, and testing for sensitivity must be conducted as the package flyer indicates. Other antisera are manufactured in Mexico, Argentina, Australia, Africa, Israel, and Russia.

8. Prompt excision of the bite relieves pain and sequelae, but this is not effective if the postbite time is prolonged.

Brown Recluse Spider Bites (Loxoscelism)

This envenomer is a member of the genus Loxosceles, and it is a long time native of South and Central America, but only a recent native of the United States. Documented cases occurring in the United States have been published only since the 1950's (Fardon et al., 1967). This is the result of truck, train, ship, and air freight shipments. Soon it should make its appearance in other countries.

Habitat and Features. The average *Loxosceles reclusa* is light tan to deep brown. On its back is a dark brown, violin-shaped figure, hence its nickname, the fiddler spider (Fig. 81–25). It prefers the indoors, but lives also in outhouses, in woodpiles, and under leaves. Recently a housewife in Utah was preparing her flower garden for winter bulb planting, raking the leaves away, and a recluse spider, which she killed and retrieved, bit her hand. There was no initial pain, and she finished her planting. The next day a bleb was present, but because there was no pain, she did not seek attention for two weeks, by which time an ulcer had developed (Fig. 81–26). A

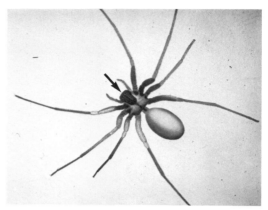

Figure 81–25. *Loxosceles reclusa* (brown recluse spider) is tan with a dark brown fiddle on its back (arrow); hence its name, the fiddler.

tentative diagnosis of basal cell cancer was made, but upon further questioning and then seeing the spider, the correct diagnosis was confirmed. The wound was excised and closed, and it healed uneventfully.

Toxic Manifestations. Although no symptoms may be apparent initially, in a few hours a small hemorrhagic blister with a white ischemic periphery surrounded by an erythematous halo appears at the site of envenomation. If seen early, this red, white, and blue configuration is nearly pathognomonic of Loxosceles poisoning. If not treated early, the lesion will become necrotic and produce systemic manifestations, including headache, fever, chills, nausea, vomiting, skin rash, and

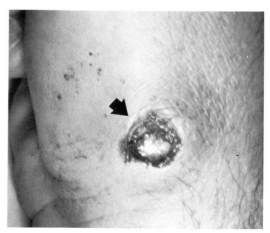

Figure 81–26. A nonhealing ulcer with the red, white, and blue phenomenon (erythema, ischemia, and cyanosis) is pathognomonic of a brown recluse spider bite, but a conclusive diagnosis would be to see the spider personally.

joint pains. Thrombocytopenia, hemolytic anemia, and pulmonary embolism have been responsible for deaths following loxoscelism. Laboratory findings may include leukocytosis, hemoglobinemia, hemoglobinuria, and renal failure.

Management

1. Corticosteroids are effective in early treatment, but must be given in adequate doses, starting with 125 mg. of Solu-Medrol intravenously immediately and repeated in 12, 24, 36, and 48 hours. This should decrease the local necrosis and eliminate the systemic sequelae. Local infiltration of the corticosteroid is as useless as shoes on a mosquito.

2. In our experience as well as that of others, excision of the lesion has been proven clinically to be effective (Fardon et al., 1967). The earlier this is done, the better the result. We excise them all and either close them per primam or with a skin graft or flap.

3. Antibiotics are used to avoid secondary infection.

4. Analgesics are given for pain.

5. Tetanus prophylaxis is given if needed.

6. Antivenin is available in South America, but is not commercially purchasable in the United States.

7. Peritoneal dialysis or hemodialysis may be indicated in severe arachnidism and renal failure.

In addition to the genera Lactrodectus and Loxosceles, at least 50 other species of spiders in the United States have been implicated in biting humans. Bites by most of these species produce localized pain, swelling, pruritus, and local tissue reaction. These too must be treated according to the degree of envenomation that persists.

Scorpion Stings

It is difficult to realize that such a fragile and delicate creature as the scorpion can be so dangerous to a human. The scorpion has been a resident of this earth nearly 400 million years, and during this time this arachnid has observed animals as large as dinosaurs and mastodons arrive and disappear, yet it has undergone little change in habits and life forms itself. There have been nearly 700 species of scorpions identified in the world, and the dangerous ones are distributed in all the Americas, Africa, Asia, and Europe. About 40 of these reside in the United States, 20 living in Arizona alone. The most danger-

ous scorpion of the United States and the one responsible for more envenomations than any other is found in the Southwest—*Centruroides sculpturatus* (Stahnke, 1972).

Habitat and Features. All scorpions are poisonous. Scorpions have a long thin body and a tail that is segmented and terminates in a conspicuous sharpness. The tail moves in all directions except down. There is a bulbous portion, the ampulla, near the tail tip, which contains two poison glands that excrete the venom (Fig. 81–27). When the scorpion "stings," the tail tip makes a small wound and the venom is deposited in the wound. As the sharp pointed tail is withdrawn, the wound also closes to prevent the escape of venom. Scorpions are nocturnal and search for water and food, such as insects, other arachnids, and small rodents. They vary in size from 1.5 to 20 cm. in length (Fig. 81–28). The subject's limbs are most frequently stung.

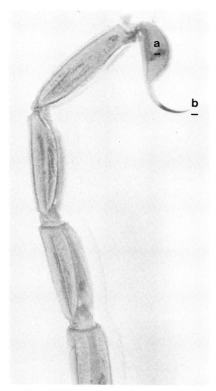

Figure 81–27. When the scorpion "stings," the poison glands in the ampulla (a) excrete the venom along the needle-sharp tail tip, which pierces the skin for deposit of the fluid; upon withdrawal of the tail tip (b), the wound closes, preventing the escape of venom.

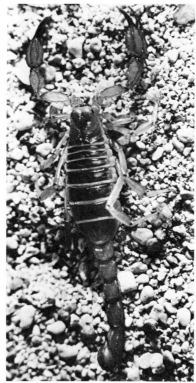

Figure 81–28. The scorpion has been a resident of this earth for 400 million years; as petite-looking as it is, the creature is very dangerous.

The Venom. There are two types of scorpion venom: One produces local effects and is relatively harmless; the other contains a neurotoxin, which is responsible for fatal reactions and has the following effects:

Signs and Symptoms

1. There is minimal local edema and little discoloration of the injected area.

2. Sharp pain is initially produced by the venom injection, followed by painful numbness.

3. Itching of the nose and mouth develop.

4. The tongue becomes sluggish and there is speech impairment.

5. The patient is unable to open his mouth and is difficult to feed; frothing may develop.

6. Restlessness, twitchings, muscular spasms develop.

7. Nausea and vomiting occur.

8. Incontinence develops.

9. Convulsions and opisthotonos develop.

10. Death results from circulatory or respiratory failure.

Management

1. Relieve pain. Apply household ammonia and papain to the sting area immediately,

or apply Valisone ointment, 0.1 per cent, or Disprosone ointment, 0.5 per cent (Schering) to the infliction. Inject 2 ml. of 2 per cent Xylocaine (Astra) with epinephrine, 1:100,000, into the affected area.

2. Inhibit nervousness, hypertension, hypersalivation, muscular fasciculations, convulsions, and shock. Give calcium gluconate, 10 ml. of a 10 per cent solution, intravenously and repeat when necessary. Give atropine sulfate, 0.6 mg. intramuscularly and Nembutal (Abbott), 100 mg. intravenously.

Hymenoptera Stings

This order of Arthropoda includes the bees, wasps, hornets, ants, and other membranous-winged insects whose venomers are females. Fortunately their attacks are more of an aggravation than a disaster, yet some are very envenomous and others kill sensitized persons. About 25 per cent of the world's population is sensitive to Hymenoptera venoms (Lockhart, 1965). At least 25 humans die of insect inflictions yearly in the United States (Jones and Shires, 1974). When a fatality occurs, the average post-sting death time is 10 minutes!

Habitat and Description. There is much variation among the species, but all members of the order have two pairs of wings, a head, thorax, abdomen, and one pair of antennae, and the females have a tubular ovipositor, which has a dual purpose of injecting poison and depositing eggs. Some hymenopteran ovipositors are barbed, and these hook into the victim and tear loose from the insect's body, causing its death; other ovipositors are smooth, and the insect is able to sting repeatedly and fly away for another day.

The *solitary bees* live alone, survive for only one season, and include many species, such as the small and large carpenter bees, miner bees, mason bees, and cuckoo bees. The *social bees* consist of the bumblebees, which are large, noisy, nonaggressive, and the most primitive of the bees, and the honeybees, which are disciplined workers. The honeybee has a hollow stinging apparatus, which is needle-sharp and extrudes when the bee is ready to strike (Fig. 81–29). When injected, this stinging apparatus is avulsed from the bee's body and left in the victim, and the honeybee flies off to die.

The *solitary wasps* have a large thorax and abdomen but a very small waist (Fig. 81–30). They are most useful to man because they

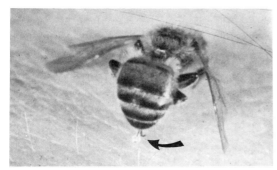

Figure 81–29. Honeybees have a hollow stinger (arrow), which is avulsed and remains in the victim as a foreign body. This should be retrieved immediately.

destroy large numbers of harmful beetles, caterpillars, spiders, and flies. Because the stinger is pointed and without barbs, they can inject multiple victims as many times as they desire.

The *social wasps* number more than 800 different species, and the common ones are the yellow jackets and hornets. They construct nests from wood fragments and leaves and, with their saliva, form these particles into a paper. It is said that the Chinese learned papermaking from these insects. Yellow jackets are very aggressive and have quick tempers. The hornet, unlike the yellow jacket that paralyzes its prey, butchers the captive alive into small portions to help transport it easily. The stinger or lancet of a wasp is not barbed, so it can be reinserted again and again, and the insect can escape without dying.

The Venom. Venoms of the bee, wasp, and hornet contain histamine and phospholipase

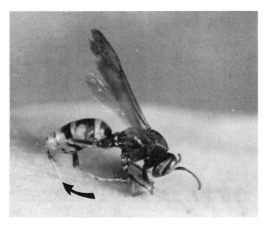

Figure 81–30. Although the wasp is called a "Southern belle" because of its thin waistline, it is most aggressive, has a nasty temper, and is able to inject its unbarbed stinger (arrow) many times into many people.

A and phospholipase B. Bee venom also consists of serotonin, acetylcholine, melittin, apamin, and a mastocytolytic peptide. Wasp venom contains serotonin, hyaluronidase, and kinin. Hornet venom is also made up of serotonin and acetylcholine and produces hypotension and increased vascular permeability. Most of the components cause pain. The kinins cause vasodilation, increased capillary permeability, diapedesis of cells, and pain.

Signs and Symptoms. These vary depending upon the amount of venom received, the degree of patient sensitivity, and the site of the sting. A single sting may pass unnoticed, yet it may cause sudden death in a sensitive victim. The effects may be sudden or delayed, and they may last for only one hour or persist for weeks. Reactions are more severe in people over 30 years and are rare in children.

1. Local reactions. Sharp pain at sting site, followed by tenderness, itching, swelling, and redness. Usually all symptoms subside and disappear; however, the reaction may become generalized.

2. Generalized reactions. Urticaria, anxiety, wheezing, abdominal discomfort, vomiting, and vertigo. These findings may abate or continue.

3. Critical reactions. Dyspnea, dysphagia, confusion, collapse, cyanosis, coma, and death.

4. Delayed phenomena. After hours or days, redness appears at the sting site, followed by urticaria, hemorrhagic bullae, skin necrosis, and anaphylaxis.

5. Eye stings. Hazardous with possible penetration of the globe, lens abscess, iris atrophy, and glaucoma. A stinger left in the eyelid may irritate the cornea or sclera for months, causing ulcers, scars, and blindness.

Treatment. Hymenoptera kill more people than any venomer in the United States. Therefore, one must consider a bee sting an acute medical problem deserving emergency attention.

1. If the ovipositor is deposited in the skin, it will appear as a black spot and possibly will be covered with a drop of blood. Retrieve it with a number 11 scalpel blade, without squeezing or pressing it because the venom sac is attached and venom may be spread farther into the wound. Do not use tweezers! Once the ovipositor has been removed, the local sting area is treated the same as an envenomation produced by an unbarbed stinger.

2. Local rubor, dolor, and calor are re-

lieved by the use of Valisone ointment, 0.1 per cent. One can inject 1 ml. of 1 per cent Xylocaine with epinephrine, 1:100,000, into affected area. Use an ice pack—no heat! Apply calamine lotion as necessary.

3. Treatment of common toxic effects from the venom per se—urticaria, joint pains, nausea, and vomiting. Inject calcium gluconate, 10 ml. of a 10 per cent solution intravenously. Benadryl, 4 mg. per kg. of body weight can be given intravenously. Xylocaine, 10 ml. of a 1 per cent solution without epinephrine in 1000 ml. of normal saline solution can be given slowly in an intravenous drip. Corticosteroids can be used. Tub bath containing a boxful of Arm & Hammer baking soda. Intravenous fluids can be given for severe anorexia.

4. Acute generalized allergic reactions need immediate attention. First start an intravenous drip of normal saline with an indwelling catheter. Give artificial resuscitation and oxygen. Inject 0.5 ml. of epinephrine hydrochloride, 1:000 subcutaneously, and repeat in five minutes if necessary. Give aminophylline, 0.25 gm. in 10 ml. intravenously, for bronchospasms. Methamphetamine hydrochloride, 30 mg. in 1.5 ml., can be given for shock and hypotension.

5. Prophylaxis: Commercial polyvalent hymenopteran antigens (Center Laboratories, Port Washington, New York) is available. Avoid exposure to areas infested by stinging insects. Avoid preparations with floral or perfume scents when hiking or camping. Wear white clothing and gloves, and do not go barefoot.

MARINE BITES AND STINGS

There are over 1000 species of marine animals and plants that are capable of inflicting injuries to fishermen, divers, swimmers, bathers, and persons involved in using the waters of the world. The injury mechanisms and their treatment may be divided into groups for simplicity (Strauss and Orris, 1974).

Marine Animals That Inflict Trauma

There are a number of marine animals that are potentially dangerous because of their size and ability to inflict injuries. Most notorious are the shark, barracuda, moray eel, giant sea bass, giant grouper, sea lion, killer whale, and octopus.

Sharks and Barracudas. Sharks and barracudas are dangerous because their behavior is unpredictable. Although shark repellent is advertised, there is no shark repellent proven consistently effective. Observations of shark behavior indicate that they are attracted to sounds resulting from water turbulence and bright objects. Swimmers with red, orange, and yellow bathing suits are like fishing lures to sharks and barracudas. Bathers should be warned not to use plastic floats and surfboards painted with bright colors. Most other marine animals that inflict injury by biting are dangerous only when molested. They may be provoked into attacking when defending their territories, teased by thoughtless divers, or protecting their young.

The most effective measures taken in Natal to reduce shark injuries are preventative (White, 1975). Twenty of 21 cases in a recently reported series occurred in areas without protection by elaborate nets along beachfronts. If damage to the protective net is suspected, swimming is banned completely. Bathing in warm water with high optical density in the late afternoon appears to be a contributory factor. Swimming should be curtailed as soon as dirty water invades the protected area. Injuries from sharks cause massive tissue loss and bleeding; therefore emergency medical care to stop the bleeding and treat shock must be instituted immediately (Fig. 81–31).

Tourniquet application may be the only feasible method of controlling bleeding from a severed or badly lacerated extremity while or after the victim is being removed from the water. In the operating room the wound will be found to be contaminated with beach sand and other debris and will require copious irrigation and estimation of damage. In the common injuries following shark attack by *Carcharodon leucas* (white shark) and related species, excision should be limited to obviously devitalized tissues, as these bites are a combination of incising and avulsing injuries and a minimum of crushing. Careful hemostasis is required, and vascular injuries require primary repair or ligation. Covering by soft tissue should be provided for major nerve and tendon injuries, for which later secondary suture repair is advised. After cleansing and débridement, loose primary skin closure is recommended with Penrose

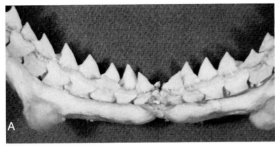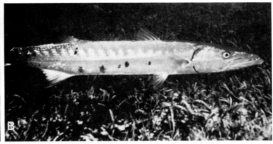

Figure 81–31. The shark (*A*) and barracuda (*B*) are devastating because of their large mouths, numerous rows of razor sharp teeth, and strong jaws. The result of injury is a massive loss of tissue, critical bleeding, and usually amputation of the extremity.

tissue drainage. If there is a large tissue defect with massive soft tissue destruction, open wound care is advised, followed by delayed wound closure or wound coverage (skin grafting). Immediate amputation of an irreparably damaged limb may be required if vascular reanastomosis is not feasible.

Animals That Sting

There is a group of aquatic animals that inflict their injuries by virtue of a stinging apparatus. Jellyfish, the Portuguese man-of-war, sea anemones, hydra, and corals are representatives of this class (Fig. 81–32). Toxins are injected by a nematoid apparatus, which functions as a microscopic trigger mechanism (Reid, 1975). Hundreds of thousands of nematocysts reside in the dangling tentacles of jellyfish, and these become imbedded on and in the skin of the victim. Professional divers, recreational swimmers, and lifeguards on beaches come in contact with these tentacles when they are swimming in waters infested by jellyfish. The poison that is discharged onto the skin produces an instantaneous painful burning, which is constant and is immediately followed by erythematous streaks wherever the tentacles touch the skin. The victim becomes very apprehensive, and if the lesions are rubbed or scratched, symptoms progress to more pain, itching, and urticaria, which becomes unbearable. If the patient is not treated, nervousness, headaches, and mental symptoms appear. In some cases collapse and paralysis have occurred within minutes.

The only treatment is emergency:

1. Inactivate the nematocysts by rinsing the hands and involved skin areas of the patient with a liquid that has a high alcohol content. If none is available—

2. Pour household ammonia onto the area of skin irritation, but keep it away from the eyes. The vegetable-proteolytic enzyme from the *Carica papaya* is an excellent analgesic. It can be purchased from the grocer as a meat tenderizer.

3. Remove the residual tentacles by coalescing them with a drying agent such as flour or baking soda; any mild alkalizing agent will neutralize the acid toxins of the nematocysts.

4. Corticosteroid solutions (fluocinolone acetonide, betamethasone) or ointments applied to the affected areas will also achieve relief.

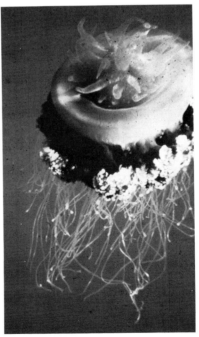

Figure 81–32. The Portuguese man-of-war injects a toxin by a nematoid apparatus in the dangling tentacles. There are thousands of nematocysts in the floating tentacles, which become imbedded in the skin and discharge the venom.

Animals with Spines

A number of marine creatures have body spines, and some of the spines have a venom apparatus. These animals are "double trouble," because the venom introduces a toxin and the spine produces a traumatic puncture wound that is prone to infection as slime and debris are introduced into the wound. A wide variety of marine animals, including segmental worms, cone shells (five recent human fatalities), sea urchins, stingrays, catfish, and spiny fish, represent this class. Injuries from this group of sea life commonly occur to the hands of commercial fishermen while releasing netted fish. The handling of sea urchins and stingrays is the cause of everyday casualties in seaboard cities and fishing villages (Fig. 81–33). Stingrays are not aggressive toward humans; rather they are very docile and avoid encounters with people (Fig. 81–34). When handled, the sharp spine in the tail becomes rigid and is the weapon to avoid.

Stingrays. Stingrays continue to be a menace along coastal waters, being responsible for thousands of stings annually. About 60 species of stingrays are known to be poisonous. This sea animal and its malicious pranks were described circa 100 B.C. by Dioscorides (Gudger, 1943). Stingrays have a furrowed spine on the tail, and it is in this groove where the venom cells and sacs are covered with epithelium. The venom is released upon penetration of the stinger. Envenomation is evidenced by intense pain, muscle spasms, vomiting, and diarrhea, which may be followed by dyspnea, convulsions, and death.

Many treatments have been proposed for stingray envenomation (Halstead and Bunker, 1953). Therapy for this infliction

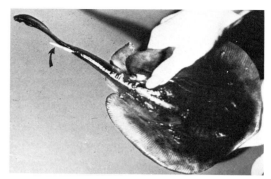

Figure 81–34. Stingrays have a spine on the tail, which is utilized to penetrate the victim; the released venom fills the furrow of the spine and is deposited within the victim's tissues.

begins with retrieving the imbedded spine, followed by soaks in less than hot Betadine solution as soon as possible, and continuing with fomentations of the same solution. Other symptomatic therapy such as antibiotics, tetanus prophylaxis, antihistamines, and steroids is instituted as necessary.

Catfish. The catfish is probably the most prevalent poisonous fish in the waters. There are about 1000 species of catfish, and some of these are endowed with rather rare characteristics: There is a male catfish that incubates its eggs in his mouth for two months; the Amazon catfish that harbors itself in the human urethra; the electrical catfish that repels attackers with its electrical plates; and the *Plotosus pincatus*, which is one of the most envenomous fish known and can cause death to a human. The catfish has dorsal and pectoral fins that erect when the fish desires, and the spines on these fins are dagger-sharp. Some spines harbor venom glands, while others have mucous cells along the epithelium covering the spine, which are toxic to vascular and neural tissues.

The typical hand injury occurs when the inexperienced tourist is removing a fish hook from a caught, wriggling, slippery channel catfish and the sharp dorsal fin or spine pierces the hand. The infliction of a salt water catfish into a hand causes an immediate painful and throbbing sensation, which may resolve in a few hours, but can become infected and even be responsible for paralysis (Fig. 81–35).

The treatment for deep spine penetrations is to incise the puncture wound and cleanse or débride it thoroughly or, if the puncture is shallow, cleanse to the depths with an

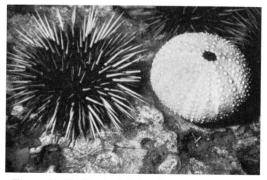

Figure 81–33. On the left is a live sea urchin with its sharp spines, and on the right is the fragile shell of the dead urchin. When it is handled, the spines stick into the victim and break off from its host.

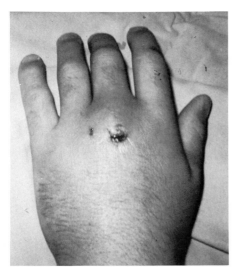

Figure 81–35. The penetration of a catfish fin or spine into this hand caused cellulitis, tenosynovitis, and infection of the metacarpophalangeal joint, terminating in paralysis of the long finger.

applicator soaked with Betadine solution and keep open. Administration of a broad spectrum antibiotic is started, and tetanus prevention is instituted. Analgesics usually suffice for the discomfort. The patient must be instructed to return to the emergency room or office the next day or sooner for a recheck.

REFERENCES

Adams, F.: The Seven Books of Paulus Aegineta. London, Sydenham Society, 1846.

Bellairs, A.: The Life of Reptiles. New York, Universe Books, 1970.

Bogert, C. M., and del Campo, R. M.: The Gila monster and its allies. The relationship, habits, and behavior of the lizards of the family Helodermatidae. Bull. Am. Mus. Nat. Hist., *109:*1, 1956.

Boyce, F. F.: Human bites: analysis of ninety cases. South. Med. J., *35:*651, 1942.

Calmette, L. C. A.: Les Venins, Les Animaux Venimeux et la Serotherapie Antivenimeux. Paris, Masson et Cie, 1907.

Carithers, H. A.: Mammalian bites of children. Am. J. Dis. Child. *95:*150, 1958.

Chuinard, R. G., and D'Ambrosia, R. D.: Human bite infections of the Hand. J. Bone Joint Surg., *59A:*416, 1977.

Committee of Trauma, American College of Surgeons: A guide to prophylaxis against tetanus in wound management. Bull. Am. Coll. Surg., *57:*32, 1972.

Constantine, D. G.: Rabies transmission by nonbite route. Pub. Health Rep., *77:*287, 1962.

Curtin, J. W., and Greely, P. W.: Human bites of the face. Plast. Reconstr. Surg., *28:*394, 1961.

Douglas, L. G.: Bite wounds. Am. Fam. Physician, *11:*93, 1975.

Fardon, D. W., Wingo, C. W., Robinson, D. W., and Masters, F. W.: Treatment of brown recluse spider bite. Plast. Reconstr. Surg. *40:*482, 1967.

Flynn, M. E.: Hand Surgery. Baltimore, The Williams & Wilkins Company 1966, p. 813.

Fontana, F.: Richerche Fichiche Sopera il Veleno Della Vipera. Lucca, J. Jiusti, 1767.

Fraser, T. R.: Immunization against cobra venom. Br. Med. J., *1:*1309, 1895.

Galen, C.: On Medical Experience. (Translated by R. Walzer.) Cambridge, Oxford University Press, 1975.

Gans, C.: Poisonous snakes. Part III. Clin. Med., *85:*13, 1978.

Garrison, F. H.: An Introduction to the History of Medicine. Ed. 4. Philadelphia, W. B. Saunders Company, 1929, p. 109.

Glass, T. G.: Snakebite. Hosp. Med., *7:*31, 1975.

Goldwyn, R. M.: Man's best friend. Arch. Surg., *111:*221, 1976.

Gudger, E. W.: Is the stingray sting poisonous? A historical résumé showing the development of our knowledge that it is poisonous. Bull. Hist. Med., *14:*467, 1943.

Halloway, W. J., Scott, E. G., and Adams, Y. B.: Pasteurella multocida infection in man. Report of 21 cases. Am. J. Clin. Pathol., *51:*705, 1969.

Halstead, B. W., and Bunker, V. C.: Stingray attacks and their treatment. Am. J. Trop. Med., *2:*115, 1953.

Huang, T. T., Lynch, J. B., Larson, D. L., and Lewis, S. R.: The use of excisional therapy in the management of snake bite. Ann. Surg., *179:*598, 1974.

Johnson, B. D., Tullar, J. G., and Stahnke, J. L.: A quantitative protozoan bioassay method for determining venom potencies. Toxicon, *3:*297, 1966.

Jones, R. C., and Shires, G. T.: Bites and stings of animals and insects. *In* Schwartz's Principles of Surgery. New York, McGraw-Hill Book Company, 1974, Ch. 6, p. 207.

Kanaval, A. B.: Infections of the Hand. Philadelphia, Lea & Febiger, 1933, p. 106.

Kaplan, E. B.: Functions and Surgical Anatomy of the Hand. Philadelphia, J. B. Lippincott Company, 1955, p. 82.

Lavine, L. S., Isenberg, H. D., Rubins, W., and Berkman, J. I.: Unusual osteomyelitis following superficial dog bite. Clin. Orthop., *98:*251, 1975.

Lockhart, W. E.: Treatment of snakebite. J.A.M.A., *193:*36, 1965.

MacQuarrie, M. B., Forghani, B., and Wolochow, D. A.: Hepatitis B transmitted by a human bite. J.A.M.A., *230:*723, 1974.

Majno, G.: The Healing Hand. Cambridge, Harvard University Press, 1975, p. 86.

Margotta, R.: The Story of Medicine. New York, Golden Press, 1968, p. 84.

Mason, M. L., and Koch, S. L.: Human bite infections of the Hand. Surg. Gynecol. Obstet., *51:*591, 1950.

Masterson, J. R.: Colonial rattlesnake lore. Zoologica, *23:*213, 1938.

Meleney, F. L.: Zinc peroxide in the treatment of microaerophibic and anaerobic infections. Ann. Surg., *101:*997, 1935.

Minton, S. A.: Venom Diseases. Springfield, Illinois, Charles C Thomas, 1971.

Mitchell, S. W.: Researches upon the venom of the rattlesnake. Smithsonian Contributions to Knowledge, *12:*145, 1860.

Murphy, R. S., Katz, and Massaro, D.: Fusobacterium septicemia following a human bite. Arch. Int. Med., *111:*51, 1963.

Paré, A.: The Workes of that Famous Chirurgion Ambrose Paré. (Translated by Thomas Johnson.) London, Thomas Cotes, 1634.

Parks, B. J., Hawkins, K. G., and Horner, R. L.: Bites of the hand. Rocky Mt. Med. J., 71:85, 1974.

Parrish, H. M.: Public Health Rept. (U.S.), 81:269, 1966.

Pasteur, L.: A review of hydrophobia. Compt. Rend., 101:765, 1885.

Phisalix, M.: Les Animaux Venimeux et Venins. Paris, Masson et Cie, 1922.

Randall, P.: Personal communication.

Redi, F.: Osservazioni Interno Alle Vipere. Florence, Stella, 1664.

Reid, H. A.: Bites and stings in travellers. Postgrad. Med., 51:830, 1975.

Robinson, D.: Canis familiaris. N. Engl. J. Med., 290:1378, 1974.

Robinson, D. A.: Dog bites and rabies: an assessment of risk. Br. Med. J., 1:1066, 1976.

Russell, F. E.: Snake Venom Poisoning. Philadelphia, J. B. Lippincott Company, 1980, p. 414.

Sewall, H.: Experiments on the preventive inoculation of rattlesnake venom. J. Physiol., 8:203, 1887.

Schufeldt, R. W.: The bite of the Gila monster (Heloderma suspectum). Am. Nat., 16:907, 1882.

Snyder, C. C.: Bites and stings, In American College of Surgeons: Early Care of the Injured Patient. Phila-delphia, W. B. Saunders Company, 1972, Ch. 7, p. 73.

Snyder, C. C., Hunter, G. R., and Browne, E. Z., Jr.: Malevolent inflictions: bites and stings. In Shires' Care of the Trauma Patient. New York, McGraw-Hill Book Company, 1979, Ch. 10, p. 176.

Snyder, C. C., Pickens, J. E., Knowles, R. P., Emerson, J. L., and Hines, W. A.: A definitive study of snakebite. J. Fla. Med. Assoc., 55:330, 1968.

Snyder, C. C., Straight, R., and Glenn, J.: The snakebitten hand. Plast. Reconstr. Surg., 49:275, 1972.

Snyder, C. C., and Temple, A. R.: Arthropod bites and stings In Gallis, S. S., and Kagan, B. M. (Editors): Current Pediatric Therapy. Philadelphia, W. B. Saunders Company, 1979.

Stahnke, H. L.: Arizona's lethal scorpion. Ariz. Med., 24:490, 1972.

Strauss, M. D., and Orris, W. L.: Injuries to divers by marine animals: a simplified approach to recognition and management. Mil. Med., 139:129, 1974.

Wellman, M.: A Cornelius Celsus. Ann. Med. Hist., 8:203, 1926.

White, J. A. M.: Shark attack in Natal. Injury, 6:187, 1975.

Wingert, W. A., and Wainschel, J.: Diagnosis and management of envenomation by poisonous snakes. South. Med. J., 68:1015, 1975.

Section 5

WAR INJURIES

Chapter 82

WAR INJURIES OF THE HAND

GEORGE E. OMER, JR.

Traumatic wounds are as old as man. Many principles in the management of extremity injuries have foundations in the warfare of prerecorded history. Gunshot wounds first occurred in Europe during the Hundred Years' War and focused attention on the treatment of firearm induced injuries. One of the first detailed accounts of gunshot wound therapy was published by Hieronymus Brunschwig in 1497 (Garrison, 1921). He was an Alsatian army surgeon and considered gunshot wounds to be poisonous. This was not an individual idiosyncrasy, as evidenced by a book published in 1693 entitled *Fifty Strange and Wonderful Cures of Gunshot Wounds*. It was written by Mattaeus Purmann, who based his writing on his experience as a Brandenburg Army surgeon during the Thirty Years' War. The most popular treatment recorded consisted of ignoring the patient's wound and utilizing a generous application of magic salve to the gun that had fired the missile (Omer, 1956). If the patient died, obviously the wrong gun had been treated.

The outstanding surgeon of the Renaissance was Ambroise Paré. His treatise on gunshot wounds, first published in 1545, was based on personal clinical experience. Under his influence, military medicine was recognized; an official directive in 1550 assigned one surgeon to each company of French infantry (Bick, 1948).

The modern soldier sustains hand injuries that range from poisoned stick puncture wounds to high velocity missile wounds. His occupation has produced an endocrine imbalance and a chronic stress reaction long before he is injured. His environment enhances the probability of infection. Treatment of the hand injury must be secondary to treatment of more lethal injuries, such as wounds of the chest or abdomen. Management of his injury is usually interrupted by successive evacuations to return him home from the battlefield, but necessitating a series of secondary medical care teams that did not perform initial care and may not comprehend the full extent of injury. These many problems can be solved by conservative initial care, meticulous evaluation and documentation of each injury, adequate patient supervision during rehabilitation, and thoughtful reconstruction of the injured hand.

CLINICAL PRINCIPLES FOR INITIAL CARE

The forces that are dissipated into the hand at the instant of injury result in many complex patterns of altered anatomy. One must learn the normal anatomy in order to concentrate on the mechanism of injury and the environment of the wound.

Gunshot wounds are internal explosions and can fracture bones remote from the missile track (Hopkinson and Marshall, 1967). It is the involvement of many tissues associated with extensive damage of small blood vessels that makes the gunshot wound a terrible clinical problem. Evaluation of such hand injuries should include radiograms in two planes of the entire extremity. All injured extremities must be thoroughly examined for arterial and neural abnormalities. Absence of a pulse, a bruit, a pulsatile swelling over the course of a vessel, even a delta area of paresthesia should indicate the need for angiography and repair of demonstrable vascular lesions anywhere in the upper extremity.

After wound inspection and examination of arterial, neural, and tendon function, a large bulky dressing and splints are applied, and the hand is elevated. The patient receives tetanus toxoid, and an infusion containing an appropriate antibiotic is started. All these procedures are instituted to prevent sepsis, since surgery is often delayed by the need to operate on other patients with more urgent wounds.

The initial surgical procedure is always performed in the operating room, with a good light, trained assistants whenever possible, adequate anesthesia, a pneumatic tourniquet, and a stable hand table. When there is a question as to the viability of a major portion of the hand, the tourniquet should not be inflated; the additional ischemia could cause permanent muscle fibrosis. Battlefield wounds are filthy and require prolonged meticulous cleansing before surgery.

Débridement has two objectives: to excise contaminated or necrotic tissue, and to incise fascial sheets that are choking edematous muscle (Whelan, 1975). A major portion of the time spent in débridement should be devoted to frequent and copious irrigation with normal saline solution.

Only a minimal amount of the skin bordering the wound need be excised, but there must be adequate exposure of the underlying injured tissue, and volar longitudinal incisions should undulate from fingertip to midforearm without crossing flexion creases at right angles. An appropriate débridement includes incisions directly into the area of injury, with isolation and evaluation of the involved neurovascular structures. The inexperienced surgeon may make the incisions too short for adequate exploration. Adequate exposure with meticulous removal of foreign bodies is time consuming but is essential to prevent infection. All devitalized muscle should be excised by sharp dissection. The criteria for viability are contractility, consistency, color, and arterial bleeding. Fragments of bone retaining soft tissue attachments should not be removed. Detached pieces of bone larger than fingernail size should be thoroughly cleansed and replaced as free grafts. Disrupted nerves and tendons should not be repaired; instead, only those portions obviously damaged are excised. The remaining nerve or tendon is replaced in the best available bed of débrided soft tissue. Transected nerves shorten with joint motion, and the epineurium of the proximal and distal portions of a disrupted nerve should be sutured with very fine wire to adjacent soft tissue to prevent retraction. Then the disruption of the nerve can be identified radiologically later. All tissue should be preserved at the most distal level of viability. A finger damaged beyond functional salvage may contribute viable skin that is useful in providing delayed coverage of the hand.

Ischemic contracture of the intrinsic muscles of the hand results after crush injuries unless decompressive fascial incisions are performed in the hand and forearm compartments. The incision for fasciotomy should include the overlying skin. Crush injuries carry a poorer prognosis for pain-free function than do gunshot wounds, because adequate dorsal and volar fasciotomies are rarely performed for crush injuries. It is often necessary to incise the volar transverse ligament to prevent ischemia of the median nerve and the flexor tendons.

An injury perforating or penetrating a joint demands formal arthrotomy and débridement. An open joint does not require immediate full thickness skin coverage. A homograft or heterograft can provide temporary cover. Synovium has rapid recuperative powers and soon covers the defect, to be covered in turn with granulation tissue receptive to split thickness autogenous skin grafts.

The techniques of débridement are difficult to translate into terms that can be understood by the inexperienced surgeon. In general, each wound is saucerized, beginning at the most superficial layer, and each deeper tissue layer is done in turn until the operation is complete. The treatment of each tissue is epitomized by the following couplets by Sir James Learmonth:

> Of the edge of the skin
> take a piece very thin.
>
> The tighter the fascia
> the more you should slash'er.
>
> Of muscle much more
> till you see fresh gore,
>
> and bundles contract
> at the least impact.
>
> Leave intact the bone
> except bits quite alone.

Vascular repair of a single injured vessel at the wrist, or more distal than the wrist, should be attempted. Magnification is indicated and is provided by eyeglass loupes. Exposure of major blood vessels and major nerves is the only indication for subcutaneous tissue shifts or transposition, but this does not include the skin. The tourniquet should be released and bleeding should be controlled before dressings are applied. Meticulous hemostasis is necessary in all débridement surgery, but is particularly important when a major arterial injury has been repaired.

Primary wound closure is not indicated for hazardous wounds of the hand (Whelan, 1975). Thoroughly débrided injuries with exposed tendons and nerves may be dressed with unsutured split thickness homogenous skin grafts or porcine skin heterografts. Heterografts or homografts decrease pain, promote the formation of granulation tissue as effectively as autografts, and must be removed, thus insuring a "second look" at the wound before definitive surgery.

Dressings are an important part of good treatment. The wound is covered with fine mesh gauze, carefully avoiding packing in areas where it might occlude drainage, such as the web spaces of the fingers. Fluffs are applied longitudinally and covered with a minimal circular dressing. Compression should be produced by increasing the number of bandages, rather than the force of the circular constriction. Iatrogenic Volkmann's ischemia of the intrinsic muscles of the hand is not uncommon after circular compression and is especially likely to occur when the patient is evacuated great distances with many other seriously injured patients. The patient should be observed and tested often for the early symptoms of ischemia—disproportionate severity of pain, a decrease in the precision of sensibility, and loss of flexor muscle strength. Muscles close to the interosseous membrane, such as the flexor pollicis longus, show the earliest symptoms of ischemia.

The hand should be maintained in the position of protection. The metacarpophalangeal joints should be in 70 to 90 degrees of flexion to maintain the maximal length of the collateral ligaments. The interphalangeal joints should be in 0 to 10 degrees of flexion to decrease the stretch on the dorsal triangular ligament. The thumb is arched in abduction and rotated to face the pulp surface of the long finger. The wrist should be in 10 to 20 degrees of extension. A circular plaster cast is applied to maintain the position of protection, but the cast is then bivalved along darted midlateral lines. The longitudinal and transverse bone arches should be maintained by molding the cast. Fingertip circulation should be observed frequently. Active finger motion should be encouraged if motion can be performed without pain.

Elevation of the wounded hand should be continuous until there is no evidence of edema, and is better maintained with a stockinette stirrup or triangular bandage sling than with pillows. The venous pump mechanism is not functional immediately after injury, and is not normal until the patient can initiate muscle activity (Omer, 1956).

Kirschner wires may be used to maintain metacarpal spacing or metacarpal length, or to stabilize unstable joint reductions (Fig. 82–1). The wires should be inserted at the time of the initial operation, but it is safer to delay Kirschner wire transfixion until the time of delayed primary closure. The wires are cut off just beneath the skin and retrieved when convenient. Radiological examination should be repeated in two planes after the insertion of Kirschner wires.

A principle as important as adequate débridement is "delayed primary" wound closure (Burkhalter et al., 1968). There is no physiological indication for primary closure of the severely injured hand, and the disasters that result far outweigh any benefit in time or expediency for the physician or the patient. Delayed primary suture should be done in three to five days if the wounds are clean on inspection and can be closed without ten-

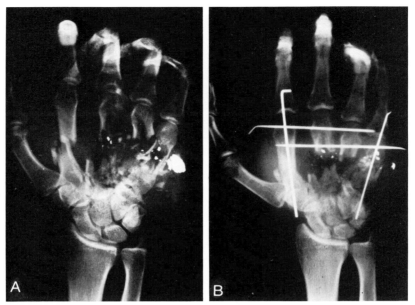

Figure 82–1. *A*, Gunshot wound involving the second through fifth metacarpals, with loss of bony substance. *B*, Kirschner wires are used to maintain metacarpal length. The transverse arches must be maintained.

sion. When the wound is necrotic, débridement should be performed again and the wound dressed with an unsutured onlay split thickness skin graft. Unsutured topical homograft or autograft skin dressings will allay infection, reduce exuberant granulation tissue formation with resultant pain and fibrosis, and help in keeping the wound clean. This cycle should be repeated until the wounds are clean and a definitive split thickness skin autograft can be applied.

Skin grafts, even on uneven surfaces, can be secured with adhesive tape instead of sutures. The undermining of skin edges for closure should be avoided. There is no place for pedicle grafts, rotation flaps, or other full thickness skin grafts until primary healing has occurred. Final healing usually results in an adequate functional surface, and is less often the cause of painful performance than is fibrotic muscle or traumatic arthritis.

Sepsis constitutes the most common complication of primary wound care and is the usual consequence of inadequate débridement and immediate wound closure. The bacterial species most often involved are *Pseudomonas aeruginosa* and *Staphylococcus aureus* (Heggers et al., 1969). Prophylactic antibiotic therapy should be directed toward eliminating the gram positive cocci by utilizing penicillin and streptomycin or penicillin and chloramphenicol.

A technique of tissue biopsy of the wound and immediate smearing for a microscope count has yielded results equivalent to those of the standard pour-plate colony counting methods (Heggers et al., 1969). A biopsy specimen of the wound granulation tissue is taken with a dermal punch, weighed and homogenized, and diluted tenfold with thioglycolate, as in the colony counting method. Exactly 0.02 ml. of the 1:10 dilution is transferred to each of two glass slides. These slides are covered and oven dried at 45° C. for 15 minutes. One slide is Gram stained, and the other is stained by the Brown-Brenn modification of Gram's stain. All fields of the two slides are observed microscopically for bacteria. The presence of a single organism on the slide is related to the presence, on culture, of more than the critical level of 10^5 bacteria per gram of tissue. The average survival of skin grafts is 92 per cent when bacterial colonization amounts to 10^5 organisms per gram of tissue or less and is less than 20 per cent when bacterial colonization amounts to 10^6 organisms per gram of tissue or more (Heggers et al., 1969). This method is fast enough to be utilized during a débridement operation and has a 97 per cent correlation with routine cultures and counts.

Loss of length of any finger or combination of fingers due to shortened metacarpals causes an imbalance of the action mechanism of the hand (Fig. 82–2). It is important to preserve the length of the injured digital ray even during primary healing. A Kirschner wire can be utilized for fixation or bent into a U to serve as a spacer until secondary bone grafting can be performed (Fig. 82–3). Metacarpal bones must remain in balanced length for the functional activity of the muscle-tendon units.

Even an isolated metacarpal injury is a problem, unless the injury involves only the metacarpal shaft and not the metacarpophalangeal joint, there is minimal angulation of the injured metacarpal shaft, the major soft tissue involvement is on the dorsal aspect of the shaft injury, and the metacarpal head is proximally displaced less than the length of the adjacent metacarpal heads. However, the extensor tendon may adhere and enhance extension of the involved finger. Then the check-reined dorsal tendon will limit flexion at the metacarpophalangeal joint and will result in the loss of power and tightness of grasp (Fig. 82–4). Eventually the uneven tendon tension may produce imbalance of the distal joints and deformity of the involved finger.

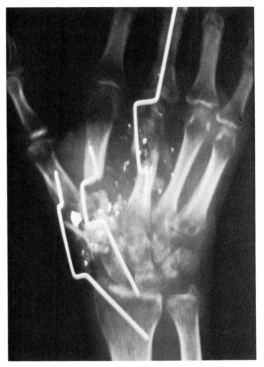

Figure 82–3. Kirschner wires bent into a "U" shape to serve as spacers until a secondary bone graft can be performed. It is important to preserve the length of the injured digital ray. The index through little rays must remain in balanced length for the functional activity of muscle-tendon units. The metacarpophalangeal joint of the middle ray received an implant arthroplasty.

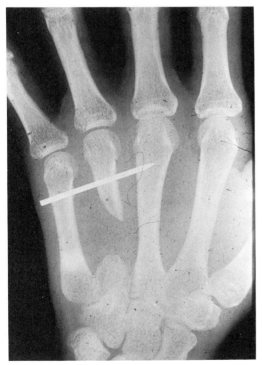

Figure 82–2. A shortened fourth metacarpal maintained by a transverse Kirschner wire. Shortening a single metacarpal will cause an imbalance in the muscle-tendon mechanism.

There is a considerable functional difference between an injury involving multiple metacarpal shafts with equal shortening of bone and muscle-tendon units, and an injury involving multiple metacarpal heads. Multiple metacarpophalangeal joint wounds involve volar and dorsal coordinated sliding tissues as well as articular surfaces. Multiple metacarpophalangeal joint wounds carry a poor prognosis for function.

In order to begin early active motion, skeletal length, angulation, rotation, and integrated arches should be restructured architecturally as precisely as possible. If the normal architecture is not retained, secondary attempts to re-establish length are rarely free of complications.

If possible, a full description of the wound and special injuries, such as disrupted nerves or tendons, should be written by the physician performing the original débridement. Operating surgeons should note normal findings regarding nerves, tendons, and vessels, as well as pathological changes. Such medical

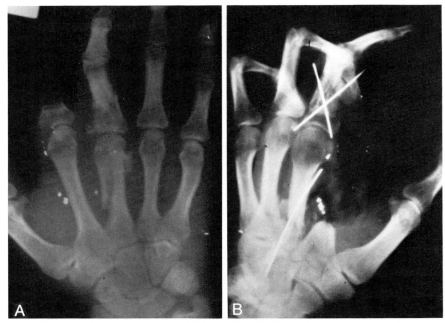

Figure 82–4. *A*, Residual of a gunshot wound with loss of the distal index finger and destroyed metacarpophalangeal joint of the middle finger. *B*, Replacement of the distal third metacarpal and proximal phalanx with the second metacarpal, metacarpophalangeal joint, and proximal phalanx.

information is of immense value to those who subsequently treat the patient. Photographs are tremendously useful for documentation.

The hand wound is not life-endangering, even when complicated by sepsis, yet all surgeons recognize the impairment resulting from a significant injury. The initial care of a war injured hand is a demanding experience, requiring meticulous attention to every detail of patient care under adverse conditions.

EVACUATION AND INTERMEDIATE CARE

For the military patient far from home, evacuation from the combat zone to the hospital providing definitive care may take days to weeks. Aeromedical evacuation is the most common method of transportation, but is usually performed with aircraft designed to haul cargo or freight. Hence the aircraft are normally noisy, dimly lit, and without humidity control or pressurization. Fatigue is a significant problem in aeromedical evacuation; prolonged exposure to thermal extremes (both hot and cold), dehydration, and the severity of the injury are significant contributing factors. Patients who have hand wounds

should be evacuated as litter patients to insure proper extremity elevation and avoid fatigue.

In patients who are evacuated with hands in simple plaster splint immobilization or in bulky dressings, the hands frequently are tied up for elevation. Often the dressings shift and constrict the extremity; the functional position is lost. Therefore, elevation during evacuation is facilitated by applying a long arm circular plaster cast with 90 degrees of flexion at the elbow, the wrist in extension, the cast extending to the midpalmar crease. All circular plaster casts should be bivalved to allow for the expansion of soft tissue at decreased barometric pressures, as well as rapid access to the underlying wound.

The plaster cast should be bivalved into anterior and posterior portions. The longitudinal plaster saw cuts should include two or three V's or darts, which prevent sliding between the two halves of the cast. The bivalved plaster cast is held with wide adhesive tape strips for transportation of the patient. Dynamic traction, such as rubber bands attached to Kirschner wires, is contraindicated during evacuation because pressure problems will not be obvious. A window should be cut in the plaster cast over an area of vascular repair. Plaster casts should be marked with pertinent medical information for the use of the receiving medical team.

Rehabilitation begins as soon as a physician assumes responsibility for the patient. Thus physical therapy instructions for active and static shoulder exercises and hand movements should be given to the patient prior to evacuation.

PAIN

CAUSALGIA

The American Civil War was the first major conflict in which high velocity missiles were used to any great extent. The dreadful pain associated with penetrating injuries of nerves was best described by S. Weir Mitchell, George R. Morehouse, and William W. Keen in their monograph in 1864, although the condition of causalgia had also been described in 1813 by A. Denmark, another military surgeon, whose patient had been wounded in the arm at the storming of Badajoz (Sunderland, 1972).

No precise definition of causalgia exists, but the characteristics of this pain have been outlined by the British Medical Research Council (Seddon, 1975):

1. The pain is spontaneous.
2. It is hot and burning, intense, diffuse, and persistent but subject to exacerbations.
3. It can be elicited by stimuli that do not necessarily have a physical effect on the limb and is aggravated by disturbing the patient's emotional or physical environment.
4. It tends to lead to profound changes in the patient's mental state.

In addition, the pain usually localizes in the hands or feet (Sunderland, 1972); it dominates the patient's life and prohibits effective rehabilitation. Causalgia develops in approximately 3 per cent of all upper extremity war wounds and usually involves the median nerve (Omer and Thomas, 1974). In one series of patients from Vietnam treated from January 1966 through July 1970, 74 per cent of the cases involved the median nerve or sciatic and tibial nerves (Omer and Thomas, 1972). There was a high incidence of multiple nerve injuries in these cases, and only 21 per cent were due to wounds distal to the elbow or knee (Table 82–1). The onset of pain had occurred within the first 24 hours after injury in 49 per cent of the cases and within the first

Table 82–1. NERVES INVOLVED IN CAUSALGIA, 1966 TO 1977

| Nerve | Number of Cases | Level of Injury | |
		ABOVE ELBOW/ ABOVE KNEE	BELOW ELBOW/ BELOW KNEE
Upper limb			
Brachial plexus	8	8	
Median	25	15	10
Ulnar	2	1	1
Radial	1		1
Lower limb			
Sacral plexus	7	7	
Sciatic	24	24	
Tibial	8	4	4
Peroneal	1	1	
Femoral	1		
TOTAL	77	61	16

week in 70 per cent of the cases (Table 82–2). The pathogenesis of causalgia is unknown. A high velocity missile injury is the most likely wound to provoke causalgia, but crush and traction injuries also produce the syndrome (Table 82–3).

Treatment should be instituted as soon as the syndrome is suspected, and chemical central sympathetic block is performed promptly to serve as a diagnostic test as well as a therapeutic procedure. The anterior approach is preferred for a stellate block, using the technique described by Kleinert et al. (1973) and paravertebral injection of the lumbar sympathetic chain, as described by Moore (White and Sweet, 1969). While the patient is free of pain, an accurate physical examination of the extremity can be performed. Subsequent central blocks may utilize an anesthetic drug with a longer duration of action, such as prilocaine or bupivacaine. Four or five blocks should be given in a series on consecutive days; one placebo of normal saline solution should be given during the series to confirm the diagnosis. The therapeutic potential for the series of blocks to give

Table 82–2. TIMES OF ONSET OF SYMPTOMS OF CAUSALGIA, 1966 TO 1970

Time	Upper Extremity	Lower Extremity	Total
Day of injury	18	20	38
First week	9	7	16
First to third weeks	5	9	14
Third to sixth weeks	3	2	5
After sixth week	1	3	4
TOTAL	36	41	77

Table 82–3. CAUSATIVE AGENTS IN
CAUSALGIA, 1966 TO 1970

Agent	Upper Extremity	Lower Extremity	Total
Gunshot wound			
High velocity wound	18	23	41
Fragment wound	12	14	26
Crush wound	3	2	5
Aircraft accident	1	2	3
Stab wound–injection injury	2		2
	—	—	—
TOTAL	36	41	77

permanent relief of pain is uncertain, but some generalizations have been made:

1. One block may give total relief.

2. One block may reduce residual pain to a tolerable level.

3. The effective duration of the first block may exceed that expected of the drug used, and subsequent blocks may give progressively longer pain-free periods.

4. The effective duration of the first block may exceed that expected of the drug used, but subsequent blocks may give progressively shorter pain-free periods.

5. The block gives relief only for the duration expected from the anesthetic drug used (Baker and Winegarner, 1969).

If the series of blocks produces effects 1 through 3, the prognosis for permanent improvement is excellent. If the blocks produce effect 4 or 5, permanent improvement should not be expected.

The technique for performing a chemical peripheral sympathectomy was developed at Brooke Army Medical Center during the Vietnam War (Omer and Thomas, 1971, 1972, 1974). When the causalgic patient is examined, the involved extremity is tapped very gently from distal to proximal to demonstrate any "trigger points" of extreme irritation (Fig. 82–5). If a "trigger point" is found, the area is surgically prepared and marked with a sterile pen. After local cutaneous anesthesia, a 16 gauge needle is inserted into the area of irritation (Fig. 82–6A). The needle is aspirated to avoid blood vessel penetration, and a flexible 18 gauge polyethylene intravenous catheter is inserted through the 16 gauge needle (Fig. 82–6B). When the technique is performed in this manner, the intravenous catheter should not penetrate a nerve or blood vessel. The large

bore 16 gauge needle is then removed, leaving the catheter in place (Fig. 82–6C). Lidocaine (0.5 ml. of a 0.5 per cent solution) is then injected into the intravenous catheter for anesthetic effect (Fig. 82–6D). If the "trigger point" pain is relieved, the catheter is capped and taped in place (Fig. 82–6E). The anesthetic block usually is insufficient for complete motor or sensory paralysis, and the pain-free patient is asked to exercise the extremity, to walk, and to perform assigned physical therapy. If the anesthetic block is not effective, an additional milliliter of lidocaine is injected, and if this also is not effective, the intravenous catheter is withdrawn.

When the anesthetic block is effective, additional periodic injections of lidocaine solution are based on the duration of pain-free activity. The patient decides the frequency of injection, dependent upon pain relief. The usual regimen has been 0.5 ml. of a 2 per cent lidocaine solution with 1:100,000 epinephrine every four hours. The volumes for individual injections range from 0.5 to 1 ml., and the periods between injections have been one to 10 hours. The average time between injections was 2.2 hours during the acute stage, lengthening to 3.4 hours as the effect of the peripheral sympathectomy decreased pain and muscle strength improved. The pe-

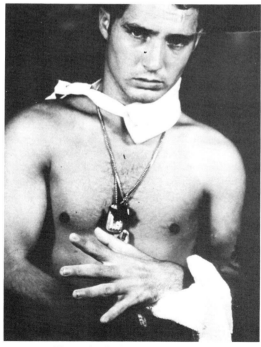

Figure 82–5. A causalgia patient.

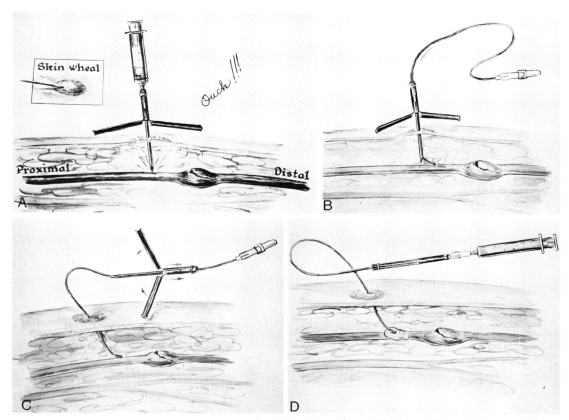

Figure 82–6. The periodic peripheral infusion sympathectomy. *A*, The "trigger-point" is injected with a 16-gauge needle after local cutaneous anesthesia. *B*, A flexible 18-gauge polyethylene intravenous catheter is inserted through a 16-gauge needle. *C*, The 16-gauge needle is then removed, leaving the flexible intravenous polyethylene catheter in place. *D*, Lidocaine, 0.5 ml. of 0.5 per cent solution, is then injected into the intravenous catheter for perineural analgesia. *E*, If the pain is relieved, the flexible polyethylene intravenous catheter is capped and taped in place. Additional periodic injections of lidocaine solution through the flex-

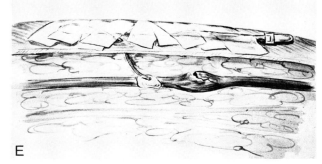

ible polyethylene catheter are based on the duration of pain-free activity. (From Omer, G. E., Jr.: Complications of treatment of peripheral nerve injuries. *In* Epps, C. H., Jr. (ed.): Complications of Orthopaedic Surgery. Philadelphia, J. B. Lippincott Co., 1978, by permission of the publisher.)

Table 82–4. RESULTS OF SURGICAL SYMPATHECTOMY FOR CAUSALGIA IN WORLD WAR II

	Excellent	Good	Poor
Upper extremity			
United States	131	22	5
United Kingdom	21	5	3
Lower extremity			
United States	65	32	2
United Kingdom	20	0	1
TOTAL	237 (77%)	59 (19%)	11 (4%)

riodic infusions are injected through the intravenous catheter without need for further skin puncture and have been continued for two weeks in a few cases. When there is more than one area of irritation, a separate intravenous catheter should be used for each "trigger point."

In contrast to a central chemical stellate block, peripheral sympathectomy is a ward procedure that can be performed simultaneously with other modes of treatment. It should block the formation of neurokinin more effectively than does the central chemical block. Peripheral sympathectomy relieves painful symptoms for variable periods of time but usually does not produce permanent relief of pain. It is much less effective when the pain has been untreated and unrelieved for three months or more after injury.

In the majority of reported cases of causalgia, the patients have needed central surgical sympathectomy, first utilized by Spurling (1930) in treating a gunshot wound of the brachial plexus. The effectiveness of central surgical sympathectomy is related not to the interruption of a sensory pathway from the periphery but to the elimination of the sympathetic efferent discharge to the peripheral arteries and sweat glands. Sympathectomy relieves only burning pain; associated painful neuromas or sympathetic dystrophy usually are not altered. During World War II surgical sympathectomy proved to be effective even years after injury (Richards, 1967; Table 82–4).

Surgical series during the Vietnam War showed 59 patients to be improved in 65 cases (91 per cent) following surgical sympathectomy (Baker and Winegarner, 1969; Omer and Thomas, 1971). The transaxillary approach is preferred to the posterior transcostal approach, with removal of the sympathetic chain from the T4 level to include the lower half of the stellate ganglion. Horner's syndrome often is not present after use of the transaxillary approach, which permits removal of only the lower half of the stellate ganglion, but it is often present following use of the supraclavicular approach and can be most annoying to the patient. When causalgia affects the lower extremity, a retroperitoneal approach through a lateral flank incision, as described by White and Sweet (1969), allows removal of the sympathetic ganglia from the second to the L5 level. For an improved result, precise postoperative sudomotor function tests should demonstrate complete sympathetic denervation of the involved extremity (Omer and Thomas, 1972) (Table 82–5).

Interviews with surviving patients whose pain was not alleviated by chemical blocks or surgical sympathectomy indicated a gradual development of tolerance to the pain after three years or more. The pain still was considered severe, but no longer dominated the patient's life, and most activities of daily living could be performed.

Table 82–5. RESULTS OF TREATMENT OF CAUSALGIA IN VIETNAM, 1966 TO 1970

	Number of Cases	Improved		Failure	
		UPPER EXTREMITY	LOWER EXTREMITY	UPPER EXTREMITY	LOWER EXTREMITY
Method					
Chemical sympathectomy					
Central block	43	7	11	11	14
Epidural (spinal cord)	4		4		
Peripheral infusion	30	5	9	2	14
	77	36 (47%)		41 (53%)	
Surgery					
Central sympathectomy	37	20	14	1	2
Destruction of nerve	2			2	
Neurolysis	1			1	
Removal of foreign body	1		1		
	41	35 (85%)		6 (15%)	

POST-TRAUMATIC DYSTROPHY

A distorted quality of sensibility, paresthesias with tingling or crawling sensations, is a transient experience in almost all patients with nerve injuries and may be related to the preponderance of unmyelinated fibers during the period of regeneration. Hyperesthesia is an exaggerated disagreeable response to tactile or painful stimuli and can be a prominent feature of the post-traumatic experience. Posttraumatic dystrophy occurs in susceptible individuals and may be related to circulatory disturbances or to neuroma formation. The established syndrome has these characteristics:

1. A high threshold to light touch with an increased distance for two point discrimination.

2. A long latent period between stimulus and response.

3. The explosive appearance of a peculiarly unpleasant pain, which is poorly localized, radiates to a wide area, and outlasts the stimulus.

4. Vigorous protective movements in response to the pain (White and Sweet, 1969).

During World War II approximately one-third of the patients who had peripheral nerve injuries had post-traumatic dystrophy (Woodhall and Beebe, 1956). There was a significantly greater risk of post-traumatic dystrophy when there was an associated arterial injury (Table 82–6).

There are only two principles in the treatment of an established pain syndrome involving an extremity—relieve the pain, and institute active use of the involved extremity.

Relief of the Pain

A neuroma can become the "trigger point" for prolonged spontaneous pain, with the possibility of subsequent narcotic addiction and emotional deterioration of a susceptible individual. Local injections have been used to relieve pain. Percutaneous injection of triamcinolone acetonide about the neuroma after a cutaneous anesthetic block with 2 per cent lidocaine was reported to relieve the pain symptoms in 50 per cent of the patients after one injection and in 80 per cent of the patients after two or more injections (Smith and Gomez, 1970). It was surmised that softening of the fibrous tissue about the neuroma was the basis for the relief of pain.

Percussion or massage of painful neuromas has been a clinical procedure in the management of military amputees since World War I. Controlled clinical studies have indicated that the technique is very useful in selected cases (Grant, 1951). Rubber mallets, mechanical vibrators, and ultrasonic treatments can be utilized to provide the repetitious percussion. Local anesthesia may be necessary over the area of "trigger pain" at the beginning of the treatment program; later the percussion or massage can be done without local anesthesia.

Transcutaneous electrical stimulation is used as a peripheral method for the production of local analgesia. The technique attempts to selectively stimulate large myelinated sensory axons and control pain by activating the inhibitory mechanisms. The direct current stimulator delivers a modified square wave pulse with controllable frequency, pulse width, and voltage. The intensity should be varied by the patient, because stimuli that are too intense overcome the inhibition mechanism and produce additional pain. Loeser et al. (1975) reported results obtained in 198 patients; 68 per cent obtained partial or short term relief, and 12.5 per cent used the stimulator for long term pain control. The best results have been obtained when the treatment is given within three months after the onset of pain.

The best surgical approach for the treatment of a painful neuroma is transfer of the entire neuroma and the proximal nerve stump to a new tissue bed where compression is unlikely and traction is minimal. The neuroma should be in an area of good circulation with a thick subcutaneous layer that is free of scar tissue. Successful results have been obtained in 82 per cent of a series of patients treated with this technique (Herndon et al., 1976). A single repeat excisional neurectomy is indicated in cases in which the patients continue to have pain (White and Sweet, 1969).

Table 82–6. POST-TRAUMATIC DYSTROPHY AND ARTERIAL INJURIES

| | Arterial Injury | | No Arterial Injury | |
Nerve	NUMBER OF LESIONS	PERCENTAGE PARES- THESIAS	NUMBER OF LESIONS	PERCENTAGE PARES- THESIAS
Median	128	54.7	237	35.4
Radial	30	43.3	250	32.4
Ulnar	136	47.1	448	38.8

The most significant types of post-traumatic dystrophy in the military population have been amputation stump (neuroma) pain and phantom limb pain. A review of the records of more than 7000 amputees from World War II and the Korean War treated at the Navy amputation center in Oakland showed that major phantom limb pain was experienced by approximately 2 per cent of amputees (Canty and Bleck, 1958). Early evacuation to CONUS hospitals for peer consultation and group therapy and the successful program of total contact hard dressings and early ambulation contributed to a reduction in the number of cases of severe phantom limb pain seen during the Vietnam War.

Active Use of the Extremity

The second principle in the treatment program is use of the involved extremity. Physical modalities may be divided into passive and active assistors. Passive activities improve circulation, decrease edema, and prepare the patient for active voluntary participation in the active exercise program. Passive modalities include elevation, traction, plaster casts, static splints (Orthoplast), faradic muscle stimulation, ice packs, hot paraffin packs, combined contrast baths, massage, and inflatable splints with positive-negative pressure. These passive modalities may need to be preceded by very delicate passive techniques when the patient is apprehensive. The skin can be lightly stroked with a feather, followed by very gentle massage, and progressing to hot paraffin baths, after which inflatable splints and similar passive modalities may be tolerated. Some passive modalities occasionally may be contraindicated; e.g., the whirlpool bath is dependent heat and may increase edema and the inflammatory reaction.

The more important phase is active exercise, which can be assisted with dynamic splints, supportive exercising slings, and special handles for tools. Special care has to be directed to key circulation areas, such as the rotator cuff muscles in the shoulder-arm-hand syndrome. General body conditioning is important, and the patient should be ambulatory, if at all possible, to meet the demands of his environment. Function can be developed with diversional games, assigned work, and activities of daily living. It is most important that physicians, physical therapists, occupational therapists, and other attendants be compassionate and yet encourage maximal effort by the patient. The best functional activity is return to active military duty. Ultimately the patient "cures" himself.

When pain has subsided, elective surgical procedures such as tenolysis and joint release may be undertaken in order to restore motion when an extensive physical medicine program has been faithfully performed by the patient. Elective surgery performed without these safeguards is ill advised.

EVALUATION FOR RECONSTRUCTION

Prior to World War II no special consideration was given to the treatment of war injured hands. In November 1944 Sterling Bunnell was appointed consultant in hand surgery to the Surgeon General of the United States Army. In May 1945 nine hand centers were established in general hospitals in the United States and reconstructive surgery of the hand became a recognized specialty. During World War II, patients who had major neural injuries of the upper extremity, without direct hand trauma, were sent to neurosurgical centers. No military hand centers were established during the Korean War; but in May 1966, during the Vietnam conflict, five hand centers were designated at Army general hospitals.

An Army Hand Center was established at Brooke General Hospital, which also served as a Veterans Administration hospital and was responsible for the medical care of soldiers and their families at Fort Sam Houston. At the Brooke Hand Center, peripheral nerve lesions of the upper extremity were considered hand surgery problems, and patients who had such lesions were not sent to neurosurgeons. Twenty-two per cent of the patients with upper extremity injuries admitted to Brooke General Hospital from Vietnam had major peripheral nerve lesions. Thirty-seven per cent of the fractures involving the upper extremity were fractures of the wrist and hand. Partial hand amputations represented 69 per cent of the total upper extremity amputations.

A clean wound, structural alignment, and prevention of deformity are important goals of initial care. Recovery of muscle-tendon activity and restoration of sensibility are necessary for a functional hand and must be evaluated prior to reconstruction. A matrix of tests should be performed in all patients to study sensibility and motor performance and to evaluate total extremity function. A basic battery for periodic quantitative examination should include Weber light touch two-point discrimination, voluntary muscle contraction on the Highet/Lovett scale with measured arc of motion, gross hand grip, tip and key finger pinch, and the Moberg timed pick-up test. Several other tests could be utilized for total extremity evaluation: peripheral nerve block anesthesia to demonstrate residual motor function, arteriography, Doppler studies, and a water displacement test of extremity volume. These quantitative tests should be repeated at regular eight to 12 week intervals to measure the changing status of the injured extremity (Omer, 1971a; Werner and Omer, 1970).

PERIPHERAL NERVE INJURIES

Additional tests can be utilized in peripheral nerve injuries to evaluate neural recovery: von Frey localization of light touch to deep pressure, Tinel's sign, precise iodine sweat test, electromyography, nerve conduction time, and sensibility to joint position and vibration. These tests are correlated with the basic tests of extremity function and routine evaluations such as radiography. The timing of operative intervention for neural surgery or reconstruction procedures depends upon the total response of the extremity and the regeneration of the injured nerve (Omer, 1968). At the Brooke Hand Center 653 patients with 917 neural injuries were evaluated with 26,900 individual tests from 1965 through 1970 (Omer, 1974a).

In managing the occult peripheral nerve injury sustained on the battlefield, extremity testing should be continued until the onset of spontaneous recovery can be expected. A prospective study was performed in 648 nerve injuries in patients who either had sustained closed injuries or in whom nerves were found not to be severed when the extremity was débrided. The clinical classification of these injuries included 331 low velocity gunshot wounds (182 lesions of single nerves and 149 neural lesions associated with multiple nerve trauma in an extremity), 264 high velocity gunshot wounds (89 lesions of single nerves

and 175 neural lesions associated with multiple nerve trauma in an extremity), 46 fracture-dislocations or crush injuries, and seven neural lesions secondary to stretch injuries. Lacerations with functional loss were diagnosed clinically as severed nerve lesions (neurotmesis) until proven otherwise at operation and were not included in the prospective study. During the period of the study patients with 454 neural lesions (70 per cent) spontaneously recovered (Table 82–7).

For those 454 nerves that underwent spontaneous recovery, the times for return of function were charted in months. After review, two time intervals after injury were recorded: The first interval was until that point at which half the nerves had recovered; the second and longer interval was that point after which only 10 per cent of nerves spontaneously recovered. The result was a scale of time from the time expected for recovery to the time when recovery should no longer be expected (Table 82–8).

EPINEURIAL SUTURING

Florens (1828) and Baudens (1836) are credited with the earliest uses of the epineurial technique for the suturing of peripheral nerves.* The procedure involves closure of the divided nerve at the epineurial layer to contain circumferentially the regenerating fasciculi. The technique was standardized during World War II.

---

*Baudens, a French army surgeon serving in Algiers, sutured the median and ulnar nerves in the axilla. He sutured adjoining tissues and thus avoided contact of the nerve with the suture material (Flynn, 1966).

Table 82–7. SPONTANEOUS RECOVERIES IN 648 UNTREATED NERVE INJURIES

Etiology	Number of Cases	Spontaneous Recoveries	
		NUMBER	PER CENT
Fractures-contusions	46	38	83
Stretch injuries	7	6	86
Low velocity gunshot wounds	331	227	68.5
High velocity gunshot wounds	264	183	69
TOTAL	648	454	70

Table 82–8. MONTHS TO SPONTANEOUS RECOVERY OF 454 NERVES

Etiology	Number of Cases	Isolated Neural Lesions		Multiple Neural Lesions	
		ABOVE ELBOW	BELOW ELBOW	ABOVE ELBOW	BELOW ELBOW
Fractures-contusions	38	2–4	1–4	1–4	1–4
Stretch injuries	6			3–6	
Low velocity gunshot wounds	227	4–7	3–6	5–8	3–7
High velocity gunshot wounds	183	3–6	3–6	5–9	5–8

The nerve is exposed through an appropriate longitudinal incision. A "guide suture" is placed in the epineurium proximal to the injury, and a second "guide suture" is placed distal to the injury in precise longitudinal alignment. These sutures are alignment markers after the nerve has been freed from scar and the neuroma and glioma (schwannoma) have been resected.

Without extensive dissection the nerve should be mobilized until there is a generous overlap of proximal and distal stumps in order to decrease longitudinal tension at the suture line. The neuroma is resected by wrapping the proximal stump with a strip of sterile glove paper and cutting across the nerve with a superior grade safety razor blade. An alternate instrument is a neurectotome, which resembles a miter box and produces a plane surface. An identical method is used with a glioma, which is more difficult to evaluate because there may be collagenization within the distal funiculi; one should err on the generous side in resecting a glioma.

There should be no surface incongruity when the two cut surfaces are matched, and this is the most demanding technical step in the epineurial repair. The tourniquet is released and all bleeding is arrested, particularly from the cut ends of the nerve. If the extremity incision is extensive, it should be closed except in the area of nerve suture. This decreases post–nerve repair handling of the extremity with potential disruption of the suture site. The nerve is carefully inspected to obtain precise longitudinal alignment. The "guide sutures," any longitudinal blood vessels within the epineurium, and the funicular patterns on the cut surfaces are all matched as accurately as possible while the first two sutures are placed 180 degrees around the circumference (9 o'clock and 3 o'clock) of the epineurium. The ends of the first two sutures are left long. The suture, of fine nylon material (10-0), is placed only in the epineurial layer. The aligned anterior arc of epineurium is repaired with interrupted sutures. It is important to match the calibers of the proximal and distal ends to maintain the surface congruity at the suture line. The nerve is then rotated 180 degrees by passing one of the initial coaptation sutures posteriorly and rotating the unrepaired posterior epineurium into view. If this maneuver distorts the nerve, it should be mobilized until there is no resistance.

The interrupted sutures in the posterior epineurium must be as neat as those in the anterior portion. A running suture is not used because a tight knot at the end of the suture line would constrict the circumference of the nerve. The "guide sutures" are removed and the wound is closed. The limb is immobilized for three weeks in a plaster bandage and then gradually allowed full active motion.

PROGNOSTIC FACTORS

World War II studies of 3418 nerve sutures established that a delay in suturing involves variable losses that average about 1 per cent of maximal performance for every six days of delay (Woodhall and Beebe, 1956). High velocity missile induced injuries involve numerous structures, and a regenerated nerve is of little value to an avulsed muscle-tendon unit. Thus a clean wound, skin closure, fracture stability, and homeostasis of the circulation seem critical to an appropriate nerve suture. During World War II, in cases in which suturing had been done earliest, within 19 days after injury, results were as good at follow-up as were those in other cases in which suturing was done early, but only after resuturing in half of the former cases. No good results were found in cases in which suturing was performed after one year; in particular, late secondary sutures always resulted in failure. At Fitzsimons Army Medical Center, Brown (1970) explored the nerves of all palsied extremities of Vietnam War casualties as soon as the wounds were healed, unless it was known from observation or from a clear operative note from the referring surgeon that a good neurorrhaphy had been done.

An associated problem in terms of prognosis is the nerve gap. World War II studies indicate that there is an average loss of about 6 per cent per centimeter from optimal motor recovery following suturing on the shortest gaps, until the critical limit is reached when suturing becomes impossible (Woodhall and Beebe, 1956).

New techniques to close nerve gaps were developed during the Vietnam War. At Letterman Army Medical Center, Mutz (1970) recorded that 3 to 5 cm. of radial nerve could be made available to close a gap by anterior transposition of the nerve following dissection of the proximal segment to the level of the posterior cord of the brachial plexus. Extensive mobilization of a nerve for approximation, such as mobilization of 14 to 20 cm., may result in the nerve's acting as a free graft (Smith, 1966).

Historically epineurial repair has been performed without magnification and with heavy reactive suture material. Circumferential tension, with a decrease in the cross sectional area, causes deflection of the fascicular alignment, with many regenerating axons ending blindly against the perineurium (Sunderland, 1953). Longitudinal tension may result in subepineurial and intrafascicular hemorrhage with fibrosis (Highet and Sanders, 1943). Histological examination of epineurial repairs done without magnification with fine suture material demonstrates fascicular malalignment with gaps, overriding, buckling, and straddling (Edshage, 1964). During the Vietnam War the use of magnification, delicate instruments, and finer, less reactive suture material improved the technique of nerve suturing. The establishment of five hand surgery centers improved the management of peripheral nerve injuries of the upper extremity.

All nerve suturing techniques involve only two principles: longitudinal alignment or functional matching of the fascicles within the perineurium, and minimal tension at the suture line, both longitudinal and circumferential.

RESULTS OF NEURORRHAPHY

The appropriate treatment for a severed nerve is neurorrhaphy, but there are many factors that prevent ideal treatment of a battlefield injury. The condition of the extremity, the level and extent of the injury, and the time until definitive care is provided influence the result of operation. Following neurorrhaphy the patient may leave the military community before the results of suturing are known. These problems limit study of the results of neurorrhaphy to relatively short follow-up periods.

A major problem in evaluating nerve repair is the definition of a successful clinical result.*

The largest clinical series prior to the routine use of magnification comprised the military injuries of World War II. An extensive review of 3415 operative procedures was recorded by Woodhall and Beebe (1956). This study has been compared with similar case studies in the British review of World War II (Table 82-9).

Later studies of delayed suturing have involved military injuries sustained during the Vietnam War, during which the use of magnification, delicate instruments, and finer, less reactive suture material improved the technique of nerve suturing. In addition, there was a decrease in battle area evacuation time, and in the majority of cases suturing was performed within the first three months after injury. An effort was made to perform suturing as early as possible; 70 per cent of the successful anastomoses were performed within six weeks after injury (Omer, 1974a). Omer reported the results in 143 cases in which epineurial suturing of upper extremity nerves was done and the patients followed for at least 12 months (Omer, 1974a); Brown (1970) recorded the results in 135 such cases, in which the patients were followed for six to 24 months (Tables 82-10, 82-11). In neither study was there adequate follow-up, and the results were not fully graded. Brown noted "some return." Omer had two criteria for "clinical return"—for an above elbow lesion, progressive motor return with independent movement and point localization of 3.84 von Frey filament without over-response (M3-S2); for a below elbow lesion, progressive motor return with independent movement and two point discrimination less than 20 mm. (M3-S3). In addition, Omer found that none of his patients with above elbow neurorrhaphy showed recovery of function of the

_____
*See Chapter 51.

Table 82–9. PERCENTAGE RECOVERIES FOLLOWING COMPLETE SUTURE
(FIVE YEAR RESULTS)

Code		Median Nerve		Ulnar Nerve		Radial Nerve	
U.S.	U.K.	U.S.	U.K.	U.S.	U.K.	U.S.	U.K.
M0–1	M0–1	10.7	3.8	8.8	0.0	12.7	10.5
	S0–1	23.0	0.0	28.5	0.0		
M2–3	M(1+)–2	38.2	63.5	43.7	80.8	41.6	28.0
	S2–(2+)	45.4	61.9	40.1	69.2		
M4	M3	29.6	14.1	34.6	14.3	24.4	24.6
	S3	13.9	29.5	18.9	28.2		
M5–6	M4–5	21.5	18.6	12.9	4.9	21.3	36.9
	S(3+)–4	17.6	8.6	12.5	2.6		
TOTAL NERVES							
–M		233	290	433	384	197	114
–S		244	278	441	390		

Table 82–10. RESULTS OF SECONDARY SUTURING OF SPECIFIC NERVES IN
NEURORRHAPHY IN VIETNAM*

Nerve	Number Repaired	No Return		Some Return	
		NUMBER	PER CENT	NUMBER	PER CENT
Ulnar	68	44	65	24	35
Median	38	19	50	19	50
Radial	5	3	60	2	40
Digital	24	10	40	14	60
TOTAL	135	76	56	59	44

*Adapted from Brown, 1970.

Table 82–11. NEURORRHAPHY IN VIETNAM RELATED TO ETIOLOGY AND
LEVEL OF INJURY*

Etiology	Number	Adequate Follow-up	Clinical Return	
			NUMBER	PER CENT
Lacerations				
Above elbow	9	8	3	37
Below elbow	90	67	30	45
High velocity gunshot wounds				
Above elbow	24	21	6	28
Below elbow	24	14	6	43
Low velocity gunshot wounds				
Above elbow	19	18	9	50
Below elbow	16	14	6	43
Fractures-dislocations				
Above elbow	1	1	0	0
Below elbow	1	0	0	0
TOTAL	183	143	60	42

*Omer, 1974a.

intrinsic muscles of the hand during the period of study. The results of the two Vietnam series were very similar and indicated that in only 40 to 45 per cent of the cases did suturing of nerves result in progressive functional return. Final recovery was not complete and therefore was not evaluated.

RESULTS OF NEUROLYSIS

Neurolysis has often been recommended as the appropriate treatment when an intact nerve is found on exploration of a nonfunctioning nerve. During World War II external neurolysis was done in 70 per cent of the cases, with saline injection in 25 per cent, and with fascicular dissection in 5 per cent of the cases. Woodhall and Beebe (1956) found no evidence that internal and external neurolyses differed in their effects on recovery. During the Vietnam War neurolysis was primarily an external technique. Brown (1970) utilized magnification to perform intraneural fascicular dissection at the Fitzsimons Army Medical Center (Table 82–12).

Omer (1974a) performed external and internal neurolysis in 59 cases in which the injured nerve was found in continuity but was bound in scar tissue. Nine nerves were those of patients not followed for at least three months, but neurolysis was successful in 60 per cent of the remaining nerves. The procedure was more successful in above the elbow lesions, in which 18 of 29 nerves showed a return of function after neurolysis, as compared with 12 of 21 nerves in below the elbow lesions.

When function of the extremity returns during the time scale for spontaneous recovery after injury, there is doubt concerning the role of a neurolysis procedure in its restoration: the intact nerve in such a case might have recovered without surgery. Of 59

Table 82–12. RESULTS OF LYSIS OF NEURAL LESIONS*

Nerve	World War II		Vietnam	
	NUMBER	FUNCTIONAL PER CENT	NUMBER	FUNCTIONAL PER CENT
Median	60	72	24	85
Ulnar	64	64	32	50
Radial	31	68	6	67
Peroneal	25	72		
Tibial	19	79		

*Brown, 1950; Woodhall and Beebe, 1956.

patients who underwent neurolysis, 12 recovered function during the time frame for spontaneous recovery (Table 82–13). Two who had sustained fractures recovered function within one month after injury; seven with low velocity and three with high velocity gunshot wounds recovered function within six months after injury. Therefore, Omer considered the net result to be that neurolysis had been demonstrably successful in restoring function in only 18 (36 per cent) of 50 neural lesions.

RESULTS OF NERVE GRAFTING

The first documented nerve grafting was performed by Philipeaux and Vulpian, in 1870 (McFarlane and Mayer, 1976). A nerve graft provides a scaffold that assists the regenerating axons in finding their way into the distal nerve stump and restoring the original pattern of innervation. Nerve grafts are often utilized under less than optimal clinical conditions, such as inadequate circulation, potential or previous infection, and a long lapse of time after the initial neural injury. The selected nerve graft must be acceptable to the host tissues without producing an inflammatory response or constrictive fibrosis; it should be small enough in diameter to vas-

Table 82–13. RESULTS OBTAINED IN VIETNAM*

Etiology	Number of Cases	Follow-up 3 Months or More	Clinical Return of Function	Return of Function in Time Range for Spontaneous Recovery	Net Result
High velocity gunshot wounds	25	24	9	3	6
Low velocity gunshot wounds	24	21	16	7	9
Fractures	5	4	4	2	2
Lacerations	5	1	1	0	1
TOTAL	59	50	30	12	18

*Omer, 1974a.

cularize readily; and it should have a fascicular pattern similar to patterns of selected
fascicles in the proximal and distal suture
lines.

The early attempts at nerve grafting during
World War II involved the use of eight fresh
homografts from patients who had undergone
amputation. None of the patients who received these grafts showed clinical regeneration, and on histological study it was found
that the best regeneration had not proceeded
more than 20 mm. into the proximal end of
the graft (Spurling and Woodhall, 1959).

The consistent failure of fresh homogenous
nerve grafts led to a trial of frozen dried
homografts. Forty-six frozen dried homografts were used in grafting at the Walter
Reed General Hospital and Cushing General
Hospital in 1944 and 1945. Clinical recovery
occurred in only two of these cases: in one,
a distal 3 cm. defect of a median nerve was
repaired, and in the other case a facial nerve
cable graft was approximated, by use of a
plasma glue technique (Spurling and Woodhall, 1959).

At the Oxford Center during World War
II, Seddon (1975) reported 58 cases in which
autogenous nerve grafting was done, with
some recovery in 35 cases; his total experience is recorded in Table 82–14. The nerve
pedicle graft was introduced during World
War II in an attempt to maintain adequate
circulation in a full thickness graft. The first
procedure involved the median and ulnar
nerves in the forearm, with the ulnar nerve
filling a gap in the median nerve (Strange,
1947).

Table 82–14. RESULTS OF NERVE GRAFTING
IN SEDDON'S COMPLETE SERIES (N = 113)

	Result		
Donor Nerves	Poor	Fair	Good
Cutaneous nerves			
Digital			
In palm	2	5	1
In digits	6	2	10
Other single strands	3	1	3
Cable	9	4	9
Inlay	1	4	6
Main nerve trunks			
Upper limb			
Free	6	2	17
Pedicle	0	5	8
Lower limb, free (all com-			
mon peroneal to tibial)	4	5	0
Total	31	28	54

Table 82–15. RESULTS OF AUTOGENOUS
GRAFTING OF MAJOR NERVES IN
VIETNAM* (N = 34)

	Function	
	No	Clinical
Type of Graft	Return	Return
Upper limb		
Cable	20	2
Pedicle	3	0
Lower limb		
Cable	7	0
Pedicle	0	2
Total	30	4

*Omer, 1974a.

Only a limited number of nerve grafts were
performed during the Vietnam War (Table
82–15). Almost all were free cable or pedicle
grafts without consideration for precise longitudinal alignment of the groups of fascicles.
No information is retrievable concerning the
nerve gap that was closed or the longitudinal
tension on the nerve graft. All were delayed
procedures (more than three months after
injury). Only four of 34 grafts (12 per cent)
demonstrated return of functional activity.

EXTREMITY RECONSTRUCTION

MOTOR FUNCTION

There are many clinical observations suggesting that restoration of precise sensibility
depends upon homeostasis and activity of the
total extremity (Omer, 1974b). Sensibility re-
education programs emphasize movement as
an important factor in appropriate stimulation of sensory organs (Omer et al., 1970a,
1970b; Omer, 1971c). In turn, the patient
alters motor patterns to obtain the best available sensory function. For example, the patient who has lost index finger volar pulp
sensibility secondary to median nerve palsy
adapts by "divorcing" the index finger and
extending it out of the pinch pattern, which
is then altered to a chuck between the thumb
and ring or middle finger. The Moberg pick-
up test is a good check of functional motor
patterns if one of the objects is a short length
of soft chalk. The chalk rubs against the
fingers and leaves a visible trail of functional
surfaces (Omer, 1971a). The abnormal motor
function that usually accompanies nerve loss
enhances the distorted sensibility patterns

and contributes to hyperesthesia. These problems are the basis for an aggressive motor re-education program, which includes visual monitoring of activity patterns and tendon transfers for improved motor function.

During the Vietnam War several surgical techniques were developed for selected early tendon transfers to serve as internal splints and enhance function while awaiting neural regeneration in the upper extremity (Brown, 1969; Burkhalter, 1974; Omer, 1968). The objectives of early tendon transfers are to stimulate sensibility re-education and to improve the coordination of residual muscle-tendon units. The muscle-tendon units used for early internal support should be synergistic with the unit to be replaced, such as a wrist flexor in substitute for a finger extensor. A synergistic tendon can utilize spinal reflex arcs and other automatic feedback mechanisms to enhance re-education. Two principles are followed: One should use as few muscle-tendon transfers as possible, since any active muscle-tendon unit used to restore a useful extremity position weakens the strength of the residual active function, and the muscle-tendon transfer must not cause deformity when neural function is recovered.

Burkhalter and associates (1973) utilized a direct transfer of the extensor indicis proprius subcutaneously around the ulnar border of the wrist into the extensor pollicis longus to restore thumb opposition in median nerve palsy. This extensor muscle-tendon transfer has the advantage of introducing new strength into the weakened power train for flexion, whereas conventional flexor muscle-tendon transfers for thumb opposition, such as the ring flexor digitorum superficialis, represent a rearrangement of volar muscle strength already committed to flexion activity.

Omer (1974c) stabilized the clawed ring and little fingers and improved thumb–index finger pinch power in low ulnar nerve palsy with a single flexor digitorum superficialis. The flexor digitorum superficialis cannot be used if the ulnar nerve innervated portion of the flexor digitorum profundus is paralyzed. The flexor digitorum superficialis is first split longitudinally, and the ulnar half is again split into two slips. The two slips of the ulnar half of the tendon are directed volar to the intermetacarpal ligament into the central slip of the extensor mechanism insertion of the middle phalanx in the ring and little fingers

for correction of metacarpophalangeal hyperextension and to improve interphalangeal function. The radial half of the superficialis tendon is directed across the adductor pollicis, distal to the volar carpal ligament and dorsal to the flexor tendons, into the insertion of the abductor pollicis brevis, for improved pinch strength and to reinforce thumb pronation.

If a power grip is a major consideration, Burkhalter extends the extensor carpi radialis longus or the brachioradialis with a multiple tailed free tendon graft through the lumbrical space, volar to the intermetacarpal ligament, to an insertion on the radial aspect of the proximal phalanx of the clawed digits (Burkhalter and Strait, 1973). This transfer introduces new power from extensor muscles into the flexion action.

These innovative muscle-tendon transfers were designed to promote active use of the upper extremity as soon as possible after injury and neurorrhaphy. In a great many other patients, more traditional muscle-tendon transfers were performed. Over a four year period at Brooke Army Medical Center, 155 patients underwent multiple tendon transfers for isolated or combined neural lesions of the upper extremity (Omer, 1974c).

SENSORY FUNCTION

Major contributions in the evaluation of sensibility, sensibility re-education, and the reconstruction of sensory capabilities were made during the Vietnam War. Omer and associates developed a battery of tests for sensibility at the Brooke Army Medical Center, based on the work of von Frey, Weber, Minor, Seddon, Tinel, Moberg, Wynn Parry, and others (Omer, 1968, 1971b; Von Prince and Butler, 1967).

Curtis and associates have developed programs for re-education of sensibility in the hands (Dellon et al., 1971, 1974). The pattern of sensory recovery is mapped at regular intervals, using the following tests: Tinel's sign, recognition of constant and moving touch, perception of vibration by tuning fork at 30 and 256 Hz, and two point discrimination distance. Several objects are used for retraining: the fingertip of the normal hand; a pencil eraser or another soft object, for early phase re-education; various sizes of square, hexagonal, and round objects such as nuts and washers; and keys, coins, safety pins, and similar objects used in daily living, for late phase re-education.

Early phase re-education is begun over the areas in which no two point discrimination has returned. The retraining object can be a pencil eraser or a fingertip of the normal hand. The patient attempts to perceive the constant touch aspect of the object. A retraining session lasts 10 to 15 minutes and is done three to five times a day. The patient observes the object, thinks how it feels, turns his head, closes his eyes, and verbalizes the sensibility. Once the constant touch is perceived, the late phase re-education is begun. The patient moves an object back and forth between the thumb and fingers in the normal hand, shifts the object to the injured hand, attempts to identify the object with his eyes opened and closed. The improvements in two point discrimination achieved by use of this program have remained intact over several years (Reid, 1977).

Surgical procedures to restore sensibility following irreparable nerve damage have concentrated on replacing precise prehension. The neurovascular island flap is utilized to transfer full thickness skin and subcutaneous tissue with an intact nerve supply. The operation should be done after indicated tendon transfers have been accomplished and the patient has supple tissues with an established range of motion for the involved extremity.

Omer and associates (1970a, 1970b) reported 15 patients with high median nerve palsy treated with neurovascular cutaneous island pedicle flaps. They emphasized that sensibility will diminish unless there is normal motor activity for precise prehension. Omer described a double cutaneous island from the ring and little finger on a common digital artery–nerve pedicle that provided precise sensibility to the volar aspect of the thumb and the thumb–index finger web (Omer et al., 1970a, 1970b; Omer, 1974b).

Patients with high median nerve palsy and high ulnar nerve palsy have lost all capacity for precise prehension. In such cases Omer has amputated the index ray through the proximal phalanx (Omer et al., 1970a, 1970b; Omer, 1974a). The insensitive skin distal to the level of the proximal phalanx of the index finger is discarded. The insensitive palmar skin proximal to the index and long fingers is excised. The fillet index finger dorsal flap is then fitted into the palmar defect to provide sensation through the superficial radial nerve.

WHITE PHOSPHORUS MUNITION WOUNDS

When an inorganic white phosphorus munition explodes, it spreads flaming droplets of inorganic phosphorus, which become embedded in the skin upon contact and spread rapidly beneath the dermis, because phosphorus is lipid soluble. Tissue necrosis results from the heat of combustion, the corrosive action of phosphoric acid, and the hydroscopic action of phosphorus pentoxide. When the munition is driven into the tissue, as from an explosive grenade, there is a wound associated with the burn. In the deep tissue wound, phosphorus is hepatotoxic and nephrotoxic; it is also a hemopoietic suppressant. Unless débridement is radical and is repeated within four to six hours, the phosphorus will continue to burn, with resulting tissue necrosis and sepsis.

Approximately a century ago 5 per cent copper sulfate was introduced for the treatment of phosphorus burns. Cupric sulfate reacts with the most superficial phosphorus to yield cupric phosphate, which coats the phosphorus particle, eliminates its contact with oxygen, and stops the burning. The black color of cupric phosphate also facilitates detection and mechanical removal. Copper sulfate is also toxic and when improperly applied in overconcentration or in continuous soaks, causes hemolysis and is nephrotoxic. We have treated renal failure in a patient who had been treated with an excessive amount of copper sulfate for a phosphorus burn of the hand and forearm that amounted to only 7 per cent body surface area (Omer and Summerlin, 1967). There were five deaths among a small series of seven patients so treated (Whelan et al., 1968).

Such a wound should be dressed in a moist occlusive dressing prior to operation to prevent ignition of the phosphorus exposed to air. At the time of débridement the involved area can be rinsed with a dilute 1 per cent solution of copper sulfate to identify the phosphorus particles (Pruitt, 1970). The copper sulfate should be promptly rinsed off with normal saline, followed by use of a dilute 3 per cent solution of sodium bicarbonate to neutralize the phosphoric acid resulting from phosphorus oxidation. The débrided phosphorus particles should be placed in water. The wound should be kept moist postoperatively and débridement should be repeated in four to six hours, and again as indicated

(Omer and Summerlin, 1967). The wound should be treated by a delayed homograft cover and secondary closure. Fractures with overlying wounds are left open and the burn wounds are treated by the topical application of mafenide daily (Dowling et al., 1968). A brisk urinary output should be maintained by administration of mannitol. These wounds heal with excessive fibrosis and keloid formation. Elective surgery performed many months after clinical healing will ignite an infection, and antibiotics should be used prophylactically.

AMPUTATIONS

Amputation may become necessary for irreversible damage or nearly complete traumatic amputation. Conservatism is the keynote, and the level of amputation should be as far distal as there is viable tissue (Heaton et al., 1966). The stump should be left open and skin placed in traction to prevent its retraction during evacuation prior to definitive surgery. Any level in the upper extremity can be fitted with modern prosthetic devices.

REFERENCES AND SELECTED BIBLIOGRAPHY

Bagg, R. J., Jr., Committee on History of Surgery in USAMEDD in Vietnam and SEA: Personal communication, 1977.

Baker, A. G., and Winegarner, F. G.: Causalgia, a review of twenty-eight treated cases. Am. J. Surg., *117*:690–694, 1969.

Bick, E. M.: Source Book of Orthopaedics. Ed. 2. Baltimore, The Williams & Wilkins Company, 1948.

Bjorkesten, G.: Suture of war injuries to peripheral nerves. Clinical studies of results. Acta Chir. Scand., *95*, Suppl. 119, 1947.

British Medical Research Council: The diagnosis and treatment of peripheral nerve injuries. Special report. *54*:1–59, 1920.

Brown, P. W.: The time factor in surgery of upper extremity peripheral nerve injury. Clin. Orthop., *68*:14–21, 1970.

Brown, P. W.: Ulnar intrinsic palsy of the hand. J. Bone Joint Surg., *51A*:800, 1969.

Bunnell, S. (Editor): Hand Surgery in World War II. The Medical Department of the United States Army. Washington, D.C., U.S. Government Printing Office, 1955.

Burkhalter, W. E.: Early tendon transfer in upper extremity peripheral nerve injury. Clin. Orthop., *104*:68–79, 1974.

Burkhalter, W. E.: Personal communication, May 30, 1975.

Burkhalter, W. E., Butler, B., Metz, W., and Omer, G.: Experiences with delayed primary closure of war wounds of the hand in Viet Nam. J. Bone Joint Surg., *50A*:945–954, 1968.

Burkhalter, W., Christensen, R. C., and Brown, P.: Extensor indicis proprius opponensplasty. J. Bone Joint Surg., *55A*:725–732, 1973.

Burkhalter, W. E., and Strait, J. L.: Metacarpophalangeal flexor replacement for intrinsic-muscle paralysis. J. Bone Joint Surg., *55A*:1667–1676, 1973.

Campbell, E. H., Jr.: Mediterranean (formerly North African) theater of operation. *In* Spurling, R. G., and Woodhall, B. (Editors): Surgery in World War II. Washington, D.C., Department of the Army, 1959, Vol. II, pp. 231–238.

Canty, T. J., and Bleck, E. E.: Amputation stump pain. U.S. Armed Forces Med. J., *9*:635–647, 1958.

Clawson, D. K.: The results of repair of the sciatic nerve. J. Bone Joint Surg., *42B*:205–212, 1960.

Clawson, D. K., and Seddon, H. J.: The late consequences of sciatic nerve injury. J. Bone Joint Surg., *42B*:213–225, 1960.

Cowan, J. S. (Editor): Second Conference on War Surgery, CINCPAC. Philippines, John Hay Air Base, March 25–28, 1968.

Dellon, A. L., Curtis, R. M., and Edgerton, M. T.: Re-education of sensation in the hand following nerve injury. J. Bone Joint Surg., *53A*:813, 1971.

Dellon, A. L., Curtis, R. M., and Edgerton, M. T.: Re-education of sensation in the hand after nerve injury and repair. Plast. Reconstr. Surg., *53*:297–305, 1974.

Dowling, J. A., Omer, G. E., Jr., and Moncrief, J. A.: Treatment of fractures in burn patients. J. Trauma, *8*:465–474, 1968.

Edshage, S.: Peripheral nerve suture, a technique for improved intraneural topography. Evaluation of some suture materials. Acta Chir. Scand., Suppl. 331, 1964.

Final Dispositions; Patients Admitted to Hospital, Active Duty Army, CY 1964–1970. Office of the Surgeon General, Patient Administration Division, J. F. Constable, May 23, 1978.

Flynn, W. F. (Editor): Hand Surgery. Baltimore, The Williams & Wilkins Company, 1966, pp. 415–454.

Garrison, F. H.: An Introduction to the History of Medicine. Ed. 3. Philadelphia, W. B. Saunders Company, 1921, pp. 193–194.

Grant, G. H.: Methods of treatment of neuromata of the hand. J. Bone Joint Surg., *33A*:841–848, 1951.

Hakstian, R. W.: Microsurgery, its role in surgery of the hand. Clin. Orthop., *104*:149–157, 1974.

Hampton, O. P., Jr.: Wounds of the Extremities in Military Surgery. St. Louis, The C. V. Mosby Co., 1971, p. 133.

Heaton, L. D., et al.: Military surgical practices of the United States Army in Viet Nam. Curr. Probl. Surg., 1–59, 1966.

Heggers, J. P., et al.: Microbial flora of orthopaedic war wounds. Milit. Med., *134*:602–603, 1969.

Heggers, J. P., Robson, M. C., and Ristrop, J. P.: A rapid method of performing quantitative wound cultures. Milit. Med. *134*:666–667, 1969.

Herndon, J. H., Eaton, R. G., and Littler, J. W.: Management of painful neuromas in the hand. J. Bone Joint Surg., *58A*:369–373, 1976.

Hessman, J., and Stockstill, L.: The casualty list. J. Armed Forces, March 30, 1968.

Highet, W. B., and Sanders, F. K.: The effects of stretching nerves after suture. Br. J. Surg., *30*:355–369, 1943.

Hopkinson, D. A. W., and Marshall, T. K.: Firearm injuries. Br. J. Surg., *54*:344–353, 1967.

Kleinert, H. E., et al.: Post-traumatic sympathetic dystrophy. Orthop. Clin. N. Am., *4*:917–927, 1973.

Kline, D. G., and Hackett, E. R.: Reappraisal of timing

for exploration of civilian peripheral nerve injuries. Surgery, 78:54–65, 1975.

Loeser, J. D., Black, R. G., and Christman, A.: Relief of pain by transcutaneous stimulation. J. Neurosurg., 42:308–314, 1975.

McFarlane, R. M., and Mayer, J. R.: Digital nerve grafts with the lateral antebrachial cutaneous nerve. J. Hand Surg., 1:169–173, 1976.

Mutz, S.: Personal communication, 1970.

Nicholson, O. R., and Seddon, H. J.: Nerve repair in civil practice. Results of treatment of median and ulnar nerve lesions. Br. Med. J., 2:1065–1071, 1957.

Omer, G. E., Jr.: The early management of gunshot wounds of the extremities. S.D. J. Med. Pharm., 9:340–346, 1956.

Omer, G. E., Jr.: Evaluation and reconstruction of the forearm and hand after acute traumatic peripheral nerve injuries. J. Bone Joint Surg., 50A:1454–1478, 1968.

Omer, G. E., Jr.: A year of trauma at the Brooke Army Medical Center—1968. U.S. Medicine, November 1, 1969, p. 9.

Omer, G. E., Jr.: Assessment of peripheral nerve injuries. In Cramer, L. M., and Chase, R. A. (Editors): Symposium on the Hand. St. Louis, The C. V. Mosby Co., 1971a, Vol. 3, pp. 1–13.

Omer, G. E., Jr.: The prognosis for functional recovery of peripheral nerves of the upper extremity following acute traumatic injury. Am. Orthop. Assoc. Thesis, 1971b.

Omer, G. E., Jr.: Restoring power grip in ulnar palsy. J. Bone Joint Surg., 53A:814, 1971c.

Omer, G. E., Jr.: Injuries to nerves of the upper extremity. J. Bone Joint Surg., 56A:1615–1624, 1974a.

Omer, G. E., Jr.: Sensation and sensibility in the upper extremity. Clin. Orthop., 104:30–36, 1974b.

Omer, G. E., Jr.: Tendon transfers in combined nerve lesions. Orthop. Clin. N. Am., 5:377–387, 1974c.

Omer, G. E., Jr., et al.: Neurovascular cutaneous island pedicles for deficient medial-nerve sensibility. J. Bone Joint Surg., 52A:1181–1192, 1970a.

Omer, G. E., Jr., and Elton, R. C.: Tendon transfers for the nerve injured upper limb. Orthop. Rev., 1:25–28, 1972.

Omer, G. E., Jr., Ratliff, H., and Lambert, P.: The neurovascular cutaneous island pedicle for deficient median nerve sensibility. J. Bone Joint Surg., 52A:1067, 1970b.

Omer, G. E., Jr., and Spinner, M.: Peripheral nerve testing and suture techniques. In Instructional Course Lectures. American Academy of Orthopedic Surgery. St. Louis, The C. V. Mosby Co., 1975, Vol. 24, pp. 122–143.

Omer, G. E., Jr., and Summerlin, W. T.: Phosphorus burns of the hand. In Symposium on Current Surgical Practices. Washington, D.C., Walter Reed Army Medical Center, 1967.

Omer, G., and Thomas, S.: Treatment of causalgia. Review of cases at Brooke General Hospital. Tex. Med., 67:93–96, 1971.

Omer, G. E., Jr., and Thomas, S. R.: Peripheral periodic infusion sympathectomy for the treatment of causalgia. J. Bone Joint Surg., 54A:898–899, 1972.

Omer, G. E., Jr., and Thomas, S. R.: The management of chronic pain syndromes in the upper extremity. Clin. Orthop., 104:37–45, 1974.

Platt, H.: On the results of bridging gaps in injured nerve trunks by autogenous fascial tubulization and autogenous nerve grafts. Br. J. Surg., 7:384–389, 1920.

Pruitt, B. A., Jr.: Management of burns in the multiple injury patient. Surg. Clin. N. Am., 50:1283–1300, 1970.

Rakolta, G. G., and Omer, G. E., Jr.: Combat-sustained femoral nerve injuries. Surg. Gynecol. Obstet., 128:813–817, 1969.

Reid, R. L.: Preliminary results of sensibility re-education following repair of the median nerve. Am. Soc. Surg. Hand Newsletter 15, 1977.

Richards, R. L.: Causalgia, a centennial review. Arch. Neurol., 16:339–350, 1967.

Sakellarides, H.: A follow-up study of 172 peripheral nerve injuries in the upper extremity in civilians. J. Bone Joint Surg., 44A:140–148, 1962.

Seddon, H. J.: Surgical Disorders of the Peripheral Nerves. Ed. 2. Edinburgh, Churchill Livingstone, 1975.

Seddon, H. J.: Three types of nerve injury. Brain, 66:237–288, 1943.

Smith, J. R., and Gomez, N. H.: Local injection therapy of neuromata of the hand with triamcinolone acetonide. A preliminary study of twenty-two patients. J. Bone Joint Surg., 52A:71–83, 1970.

Smith, J. W.: Factors influencing nerve repair. Arch. Surg., 93:335–341, 433–437, 1966.

Spurling, R. G.: Causalgia of the upper extremity: treatment by dorsal sympathetic ganglionectomy. Arch. Neurol., 23:784–788, 1930.

Spurling, R. G., and Woodhall, B. (Editors): Surgery in World War II. Washington, D.C., Department of the Army, 1959, Vol. II, pp. 234–237.

Strange, F. G. St. C.: An operation for nerve pedicle grafting. Br. J. Surg., 34:423–425, 1947.

Sunderland, S.: Funicular suture and funicular excision in the repair of severed nerves. Br. J. Surg., 40:580–587, 1953.

Sunderland, S.: Nerves and Nerve Injuries. Edinburgh, Churchill Livingstone, 1972, pp. 785, 837, 923, 1075.

Tinel, J.: Nerve Wounds: Symptomatology of Peripheral Nerve Lesions Caused by War Wounds. [Trans. by F. Rothwell.] New York, William Wood and Company, 1917.

VanderArk, G. D., et al.: Peripheral nerve injuries studied by evoked potential recordings. Milit. Med., 135:90–94, 1970.

VonPrince, K., and Butler, B., Jr.: Measuring sensory function of the hand in peripheral nerve injuries. Am. J. Occup. Ther., 21:385–395, 1967.

War Surgery, Pacific Command Conferences: 2nd Conference, 1968; 3rd Conference, 1969; 5th Conference, 1971.

Werner, J. L., and Omer, G. E., Jr.: Procedures evaluating cutaneous pressure sensation in the hand. Am. J. Occup. Ther., 24:347–356, 1970.

Whelan, T. J., Jr.: Emergency War Surgery. Washington, D.C., U.S. Government Printing Office, 1975.

Whelan, T. J., Jr., Burkhalter, W. E., and Gomez, A.: Management of war wounds. Adv. Surg., 3:227–350, 1968.

White, J. C., and Sweet, W. H.: Pain and the Neurosurgeon: A Forty-Year Experience. Springfield, Illinois, Charles C Thomas, 1969.

Woodhall, B.: Peripheral nerve–vascular injuries. In Spurling, R. G., and Woodhall, B. (Editors): Surgery in World War II. Washington, D. C., 1959, Department of the Army, Vol. II, p. 439.

Woodhall, B., and Beebe, G. W. (Editors): Peripheral Nerve Regeneration. VA Medical Monograph. Washington, D.C., U. S. Government Printing Office, 1956, p. 5.

Section 6

SPORTS-RELATED INJURIES

Chapter 83

THE SPORTSMAN'S HAND

Yves Allieu

STATISTICS AND GENERAL CONSIDERATIONS

Whether for the elite or for the ordinary performer, sports have become a feature of most societies. The increase in the number taking part, combined with the lack of preparation of some and the violent physical contacts often involved, has given rise to a new, specific, and increasingly common group of disorders. Lesions of the hand and wrist occupy an important place in this group, for they account for 8 to 20 per cent of all injuries, depending on the sport.

Accurate statistics are difficult to come by for a variety of reasons. First aid is often available on the spot, many sportsmen do not seek specialist advice, and the medical records tend to be insufficient and widely scattered. A few documents are available, however, that may help in formulating a statistical approach.

The most important survey so far is that by Polacco et al. (1967) on sports injuries in Italy between 1955 and 1959. Injuries involving the hand and wrist in that survey make up 10.25 per cent of the total. This figure is

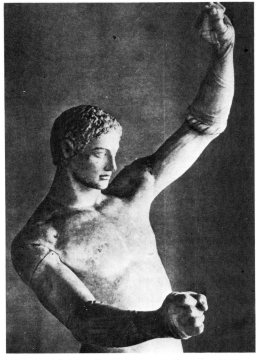

The wrestler "Pollux." Statue attributed to Pythagoras, first half of fifth century B.C. (Borghese collection).

an underestimate, however, since it includes only osteoarticular lesions. The sports most commonly concerned are boxing (48 per cent), water polo (27 per cent), volleyball (25 per cent), and gymnastics (22 per cent). Nearer the bottom of the league are football (1.96 per cent), skiing (2.47 per cent), motorcycling (4.66 per cent), and rugby football (4.6 per cent).

In France, Thiebault (1980) carried out a survey but only in amateurs. In his study, the hand was involved in 12 per cent of the injuries in all sporting specialties. The main culprits here were basketball and especially handball (over 30 per cent), in which the commonest injuries were digital osteoarticular lesions. Gymnastics, by contrast, accounted for the highest proportion of wrist injuries. This survey was based on 43,093 records involving 57 different sports, but the diagnosis of the lesions was often approximate (Fig. 83–1).

The relative importance of sports injuries in the context of traumatology of the hand is also difficult to determine in view of the selective recruitment of accident services, which does not reflect all the sporting activities in a given region. Edwards (1975) presented a figure of 8 per cent at a symposium in 1979.

Allieu et al. (1980) produced the following figures: Between 1966 and 1978 the main traumatology centers in Austria treated 2,391,227 injuries, of which 278,070 (or 11.62 per cent) were sustained in football and 3.92 per cent in other sports. It is of course significant that football and skiing have become by far the most popular sports in Austria. The proportion of hand injuries in this survey was relatively low—5.34 per cent— i.e., only 0.62 per cent of all injuries. Also, hand injuries sustained in sporting accidents represented a mere 3.76 per cent of all hand injuries.

Another approach is to try to determine the incidence of hand injuries treated in a unit that specializes in sports injuries. Thus, between 1973 and 1978, 14,521 patients were seen in a specialized center for the assessment of sports injuries in Montpellier (Allieu et al., 1980). Of those, 455 presented with a lesion of the hand or wrist. Injuries to the fingers were commonest in handball, volleyball, and the various forms of wrestling; while osteoarticular lesions of the wrist occurred most commonly in gymnastics and athletics. In fact, most of these injuries were only seen secondarily at a specialized consultation.

It is in skiing, however, that the most comprehensive statistics are available. Our figures are based on information received from practitioners in skiing resorts who are equipped to deal with traumatic emergencies on the spot. Thus, in a total of 10,923 accidents, the hand or wrist was involved in 1699 cases (hand, 1118; wrist, 581). The commonest lesion in this group (457 cases) was a sprain of the metacarpophalangeal joint of the thumb. Bezes and Julliard (1976), working in a traumatology unit treating skiing injuries in an Alpine region, reported 286 hand or wrist lesions in 5200 patients. Here again, fractures of the first metacarpal and lesions of the first metacarpophalangeal joint were high on the list.

Because of the close relationship between boxers and their managers and also because of the essentially professional nature of the sport, boxing injuries have also been studied with statistical accuracy (McCown, 1959).

These two sporting specialties highlight the importance of the recording of injuries at emergency treatment as by far the best source of information for statistical studies. In most other sports in which competitors are not subjected to medical follow-up, an accurate assessment of the incidence and nature of accidental injuries is virtually unattainable. Only with a system—at the national or international level—of on the spot recording of injuries can we hope to obtain information that can assist in the prevention of sports injuries.

The treatment of hand injuries sustained in the course of sporting activities does not differ from that of other hand injuries, but the specific psychological aspects must be emphasized. The professional sportsman is invariably anxious to resume his activities, often for financial reasons, sometimes through fear of being dropped from the team. Because of the element of haste, the practitioner directly involved with on the spot treatment is tempted to settle for a less than ideal result if this means an earlier return to normal—hence, the high incidence of late osteoarticular sequelae in retired sportsmen.

Specialized knowledge of sports is required, however, to establish some form of prophylaxis, and this involves improving the

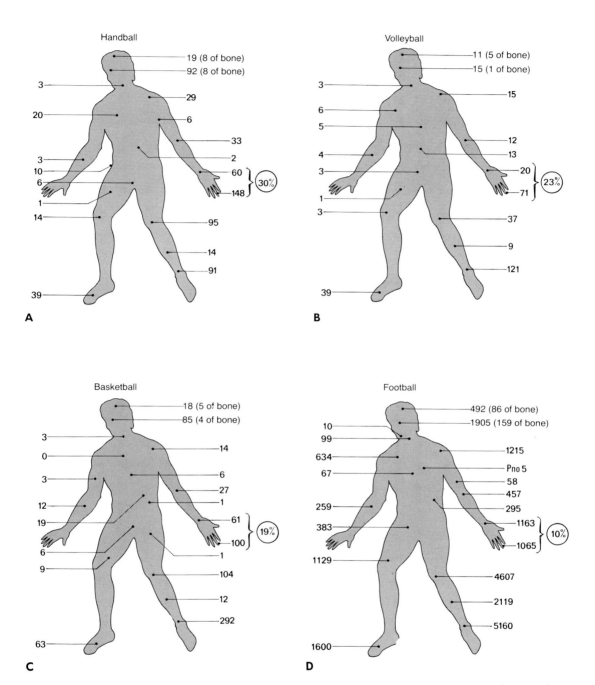

Figure 83–1. Frequency of sports injuries to the hand. Study of the Mutuelle Nationale des Sports (Thiebault).

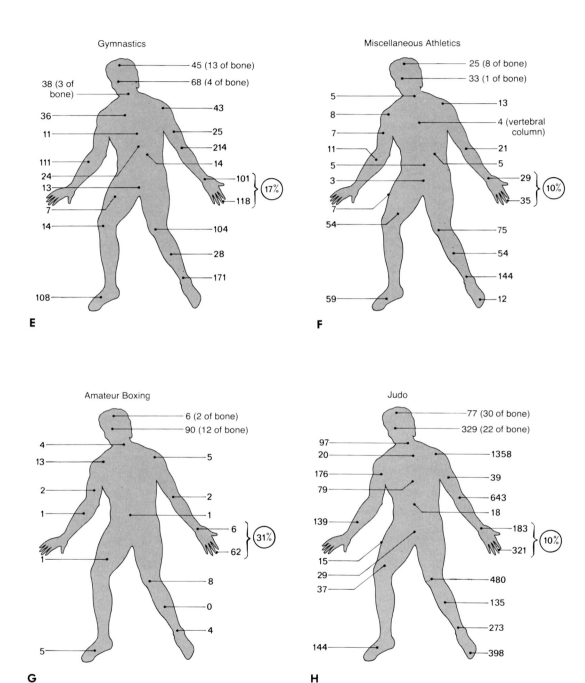

Figure 83–1 *Continued*

equipment, modifications in the practical movements, and protective measures for the hand.

NONSPECIFIC SPORTS INJURIES

The pathological group of nonspecific sports injuries includes lesions that can be seen in any instance of trauma, but there is a higher incidence in some sports and under certain conditions. We will consider, in turn, open wounds, fractures, articular lesions, tendon injuries, and neurovascular lesions.

OPEN WOUNDS

Open wounds are in no way specific, and their treatment follows the accepted rules of hand surgery. It is important, therefore, that systematic exploration be taught to on the spot practitioners. We will not consider stings and bites that occur in riding, hunting, and sea diving but will only briefly mention the granuloma resulting from a sea urchin sting, which may conceal underlying osteitis of the phalanges (Bazex et al., 1975). This type of granuloma is difficult to treat and may even require surgical exploration.

Nearer to our interest here are amputations, as may be seen when an ice skate slices off one or more fingers of the ungloved hand of a fallen skater (Bienner and Muller, 1973). Another is the avulsion of the thumb that occurs in water skiers when the nylon rope becomes tightly looped round the thumb (Iselin, 1973; Verdan et al., 1968). Digital avulsion occurs when a finger ring is caught on the hooks joining a net to a metal loop, as in basketball, or to goal posts, as in football. Six such accidents have been treated in the SOS Reimplantation Center of Montpellier-Nimes—all occurring to goal keepers. The indications and techniques of reimplantation are of course the same, but in a professional football player the duration of incapacity must be taken into account. Prophylaxis here is the obvious solution.

We are not concerned here with frostbite, the traumatic hallmark of mountaineers. Of the 276 cases reported by Foray and Lanoye (1979), 52 per cent showed involvement of at least one hand; this type of lesion is considered in Chapter 70.

OSTEOARTICULAR INJURIES OF THE WRIST

Osteoarticular injuries of the wrist usually result from a fall. They have no specific features and can occur in any sport. There is a higher incidence in gymnastics and athletics, and they are less common in boxing, rugby, football, and weight lifting.

Fractures of the Carpal Bones

Fracture of the Scaphoid. Undoubtedly one of the commonest is the fracture of the scaphoid, which is often missed in sportsmen and tends to present late at the stage of pseudarthrosis (Allieu et al., 1980; Andrivet and Benassy, 1955). In the context of sports injuries, perhaps more than anywhere, Watson Jones' aphorism applies: "Every sprained wrist is a fractured scaphoid until radiologically proven otherwise." The classic rules also apply, i.e., special scaphoid views and repeated radiological examination after two weeks (Watson Jones, 1976). Here there is the added dilemma that the professional may well refuse the prolonged immobilization; at the same time a pseudarthrosis is not always incompatible with normal sporting activities. The patient should always be warned, however, of the long term risk of osteoarthritis. Despite the need for an early return to normal, we still prefer orthopedic treatment to surgery. The treatment of painful pseudarthrosis is difficult and may well signal the end of top class professional sporting activities.

Fracture of the Triquetrum. Fracture of the triquetrum is the most common after fracture of the scaphoid. It invariably results from an avulsion of the ligament and presents as a severe "sprain" of the wrist with perilunate instability (Mayfield et al., 1980). Avulsion of the posterior horn is particularly common. Closed orthopedic treatment is the rule, followed by immobilization for one month. Pain may persist well after immobilization has ceased. The fracture usually follows a forced movement or a fall on the hand while grasping an object, such as a tennis racket or a skiing stick (Genety and Brunet-Guedj, 1976c).

Fracture of the Hamate. The incidence of fracture of the hook of the hamate is unusually high in sports, especially those requiring the forceful gripping of a handle. The injury follows a fall on the heel of the hand. The symptoms are often minimal, and there may be concomitant ulnar or median nerve signs. Radiological detection requires special carpal tunnel views. The injury has been described in injuries sustained while playing tennis, golf, or baseball or while skiing (Fig. 83–2) (Carter and Eaton, 1977; Manske, 1978; Posner, 1977; Stark et al., 1977; Takehiko, 1972).

Fracture of the Trapezium. The mechanism here is one of shearing at the level of the first web space. Such fractures are seen in cycling, motor racing, and skiing in which the handlebars, the driving wheel, or the ski stick is grasped deep in the first commissure, and in gymnastics in exercises that involve landing with the commissure opened (Desse, 1960; Neidhardt et al., 1968; Pointu et al., 1978).

Fracture of the Lunate. Fracture of the lunate is not characteristic of any sports injury. Its connection with Kienböck's disease (which is common in sportsmen) is unproven (Gentaz et al., 1972; Michon and Allieu, 1976).

Fractures of the Capitate and Trapezoid. Fractures of the capitate and trapezoid have been described following a fall, but there is no direct link with any particular sport. Frac-

ture of the pisiform has been described in tennis injuries (Helal, 1978; Quattrini, 1967).

Sprains and Dislocations

Sprains of the wrist are extremely common, yet they are often ill understood despite the excellent description by Dobyns et al. (1978). Better knowledge of the ligamentous lesions involved and of carpal instability and the systematic use of a "functional" radiological examination under local or regional anesthesia are essential if we wish to improve our treatment of this condition. Scapholunate diastasis must be specifically looked for. The anteroposterior view of the hand in supination shows the scapholunate gap and horizontalization of the scaphoid, while the strict lateral view reveals the deformity of the carpal chain.

Perilunate dislocation has been the subject of recent reviews. A relatively rare occurrence, it is seen primarily in gymnastic injuries. As described by Mayfield et al. (1980), it results from injuries involving torsion of the wrist. It is often misdiagnosed, and one of every three cases we have seen was detected only secondarily. Despite the relatively severe clinical symptoms, it is often diag-

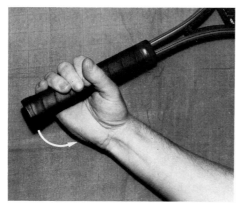

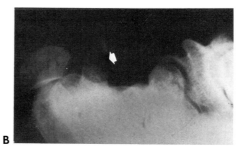

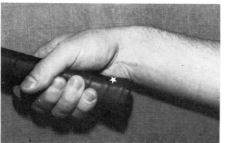

Figure 83–2. Fracture of the hook of the hamate. *A,* Mechanism. *B,* Carpal tunnel view showing the fracture.

nosed as a sprain. In two of our cases the patient had resumed his sporting activities despite an anterior dislocation of the lunate. One patient complained of difficulty with exercises on the parallel bars as a result of symptoms due to median nerve involvement. The diagnosis should not be missed if anteroposterior and lateral views are requested at the time of injury and interpreted correctly.

OSTEOARTICULAR INJURIES OF THE HAND AND FINGERS

Fractures of the Metacarpals and Phalanges

Fractures of the first metacarpal are one of the hallmarks of sports injuries. Fractures of the base are usually extra-articular, sometimes comminuted. Less common is the fracture-dislocation of Bennett, which was long regarded as characteristic of boxing injuries. Among modern sports, skiing and boxing are the commonest causes of fractures of the first metacarpal. Lesions of that bone are part and parcel of the "boxer's hand," to be considered in more detail later. However, the commonest hand fracture seen in a sporting context is that of the neck of the fifth metacarpal. It is seen not only in boxing but also in karate and results from a blow inflicted with an incompletely "locked" hand. The fracture is on the whole remarkably well tolerated even with a palmar angulation of up to 30 degrees. Untreated, the fracture may result in some degree of malunion, but it does not incapacitate.

Fractures of the metacarpal bases are commonly missed because they are less than obvious on standard radiological films. They may give rise to residual pain in the carpometacarpal joints and to deformities of the wrist (the "hunchback" wrist). Again, they are seen in injuries sustained in boxing, karate, and judo. The fracture-dislocation of the base of the fifth metacarpal deserves special mention because it may require surgical treatment.

Fractures of the metacarpal shafts are usually the result of direct rather than indirect trauma. One type of trauma characteristic of skiing (30) is the multiple fracture resulting from rotation of the metacarpal "fan." The fracture line runs obliquely across the four metacarpals toward the bases. This fracture by torsion occurs when the skier falls on a hand trapped in the loop of cord attached to the pole. The fracture is often unstable and may require surgical fixation (Fig. 83–3).

Fractures of the phalanges are in no way specific to sports injuries, in which the commonest is the crush fracture of the distal phalanx. However, the one with the worst prognosis remains the fracture of the base of the middle phalanx, which, in addition to its instability or because of it, can lead to subluxation of the proximal interphalangeal joint. Phalangeal fractures are surprisingly rare in boxing, karate, and wrestling and are more characteristic of ballgames such as basketball, volleyball, handball, water polo, and rugby.

Sprains and Dislocations of the Carpometacarpal, Metacarpophalangeal, and Interphalangeal Joints

Dislocations of the first carpometacarpal joint should always be regarded with suspicion because they may conceal a bone avulsion (e.g., Bennett's fracture with a small fragment), the management of which is invariably surgical.

Carpometacarpal dislocations are in fact fracture-dislocations, and we have already stressed the dangers of misdiagnosis. They must be reduced and, if unstable, must be treated by surgical fixation.

Sprains and dislocations of the metacarpophalangeal joint of the thumb have been studied at length in the context of skiing injuries (Bamert et al., 1976; Bezes and Julliard, 1976; Dobyns et al., 1978; Gutman et al., 1974; Hursh, 1967; Sakellarides, 1978; Stener, 1971). Instability of the severe sprain at the medial collateral ligament should be specifically looked for in functional films. They are the result of a fall on the hand with the first web space wide open around the ski pole. Recent alterations in the equipment, such as a detachable cord loop, have failed to reduce the incidence of these injuries. The best prophylactic measure is to let go of the pole prior to the fall. Interposition of the adductor aponeurosis explains the frequent failure of manipulative reduction; hence, the need for open reduction in many cases.

With the advent of acrobatic skiing, we have seen an increased incidence of sprains at the medial collateral ligament occurring as

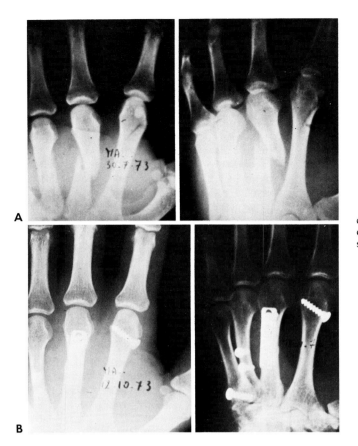

Figure 83–3. Spiral fracture of the metacarpal following a skiing accident. *A*, Preoperative state. *B*, Internal fixation by screwing and screw plate.

the skier leans on the loop of the implanted stick prior to a jump. This injury is a hallmark of the traumatology of the ski slopes, but it is also seen in judo when the thumb is trapped in the kimono, or in the course of a fall on the abducted thumb.

Dislocation of the other metacarpophalangeal joints is as rare in sports as it is in traumatology as a whole. It occasionally occurs in ballgames and in horseback riding, the little finger being the commonest victim (Coste and Desproges-Gotteron, 1960).

By contrast, sprains and dislocations of the interphalangeal joints of the fingers are extremely common in ballgames (handball, basketball, volleyball, rugby, water polo), the main culprit by far being handball (Broussin, 1977; Comtet, 1975; Curtin et al., 1976; Hromec et al., 1977; Huguet, 1977; Kruhl and Stimmine, 1964). The risks appear to be greater in the presence of minor congenital anomalies of the hand, such as congenital clinodactyly (minimal) and hyperlaxity. For

this reason on occasion we have advised against participation in handball.

The diagnosis can be difficult and requires dynamic x-ray views in "forced" positions. The treatment remains a subject of controversy. Severe sprains can be managed by orthopedic treatment, using an adjacent finger as a splint, and early mobilization, or by surgical means involving repair of the ligament (McCue, 1970). We still favor closed treatment and early mobilization.

In addition to ballgames, sources of these injuries include judo and karate (Moreau, 1957; Tibayrenc, 1975).

Repeated osteoarticular trauma in the long term can give rise to degenerative changes in the joints of the hand (Adams, 1979; Genety et al., 1979). Examination of retired sportsmen over 40 years of age shows multiple periarticular degenerative lesions. The presence of periarticular osteophytes, however, is not necessarily synonymous with osteoarthritis. It could be more accurately described as "sportogenic periarthropathy" because the articular spaces are frequently unchanged. However, genuine osteoarthritic changes can also be seen as consequences of old trauma (fractures, chronic instability), especially in retired boxers and karatekas.

TENDON INJURIES

The pathology of the tendons can be considered under two headings—tendonitis and tenosynovitis, and traumatic tendon ruptures.

Tendonitis and Tenosynovitis

Tendonitis and tenosynovitis are in no way pathognomonic of sports injuries except for the somewhat higher incidence in sportsmen. Such a disorder can take the form of an insertion tendonitis of the extensor carpi radialis brevis or longus, of the flexor or extensor carpi ulnaris, or of the brachioradialis. Or there can be tenosynovitis of the digital flexors or extensors. Most common is tenosynovitis of the radial extensors of the wrist and of those of the thumb, also known as Quervain's syndrome. Tenosynovitis of the flexor carpi radialis within the carpal tunnel is also common but less often recognized. It is seen mostly in tennis players (Genety and Brunet-Guedj, 1976b). If resistant to medical treatment, it may necessitate exploration of the tendon on the palmar aspect of the trapezium, because there may be local irritation from bone spicules. Finally there is the "trigger finger," which is usually secondary to a lesion of the digital flexors at the level of the metacarpophalangeal joints and is known to occur in fencers in the middle and ring fingers.

Traumatic Tendon Ruptures

Rupture of the Extensors. The commonest site of rupture is at the distal insertion of the tendon, resulting in the classic mallet finger. Frequently seen in ballgames, especially in baseball, it has come to be known in the United States as "baseball finger."

This lesion occurs in one of three forms— as a simple tendon rupture, as a tendon disinsertion with avulsion of a small bone fragment, and as an articular fracture of the base of the distal phalanx. It is important that the last mentioned be recognized be-

cause it is a true fracture. It occurs as a result of a "blow" to the extended finger, usually as the hand catches the ball. Simple avulsion of the tendon, by contrast, follows a violent impact on a finger with the distal interphalangeal joint in slight flexion. Avulsion, with or without a bone fragment, is treated conservatively, whereas a fracture involving the joint requires surgical repair (Fig. 83–4) (Hamas et al., 1978).

The boutonnière deformity follows rupture of the middle extensor strip on the base of the middle phalanx. Its management is far from easy: early diagnosis and bracing still carry the best chances of success. Persistent pain and swelling at the proximal interphalangeal joint can delay the return to normal sports activity.

Rupture of the extensor pollicis longus tendon is rare, but it can occur in certain sports injuries.

Rupture of the Flexor Tendons. Disinsertion of the flexor pollicis tendon has been described, mostly in the context of American football and rugby football (Blazina and Lane, 1966; Thomas, 1977; Wenger, 1973). It occurs when a player's hand, with the distal interphalangeal joint in hyperextension, grabs hold of another's shirt and the flexor profundus contracts suddenly. It is seen primarily in the ring finger, which is incapable of passive extension when the other fingers are forcefully flexed. Concomitant avulsion of a bone fragment facilitates reinsertion. In most cases, however, the blood vessels are

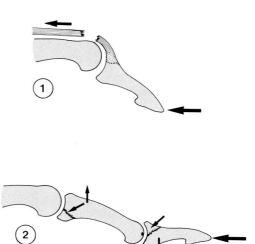

Figure 83–4. The two types of mallet finger and their mechanism.

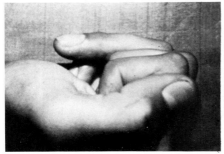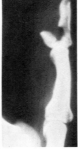

Figure 83–5. Avulsion of the flexor profundus of the ring finger with bone fragment following a rugby accident.

pulled off: tendon devascularization and the risk of adhesions then make reinsertion impossible. For the sportsman in particular, arthrodesis of the distal interphalangeal joint remains the best solution (Fig. 83–5).

NEUROVASCULAR INJURIES

Damage to Blood Vessels

The repeated microtraumas that the hand sustains in certain sports can give rise in time to an "arteriopathy," ranging from simple vasomotor problems to severe trophic disorders. The most damaging sport in this respect is probably pelota (handball), which we shall consider later, but similar disorders have been described in baseball, primarily in the ulnar collateral artery of the left index finger of professional catchers (Lowrey et al., 1976). Better padding of the glove should protect the hand but apparently interferes with catching the ball. The signs of hypovascularization (pain, cold finger) can be confirmed objectively by Allen's test, by Doppler scanning, and by scintigraphy. Vascular changes have also been described in handball players.

Damage to Nerves

Damage to the nerves usually takes the form of compression syndromes due to repeated microtrauma or prolonged pressure.

The carpal tunnel syndrome is associated primarily with fencing and motor racing. In fencers, irritation results from pressure against the handle: this can be avoided by the use of an orthopedic handle (Kreude, 1965). We have seen two racing drivers who suffered from paresthesias after prolonged driving.

Compression of the ulnar nerve at the wrist and of the vascular arches is characteristic of cycling and motorcycling (Boeda, 1972; Desse, 1960), although it also occurs in fencing (Azemar, 1969). It has been studied mostly in cyclists, in whom it apparently results from leaning on a flat handlebar (Boeda, 1972; Desse, 1960; Maurice, 1979); this leads to dorsal hyperextension and compression of the nerve at the hypothenar arch. More recently it has been known to occur in motorcyclists. We have seen three such cases, all in motorcyclists after a long ride and all using a flat handlebar. In two of the cases the palsy did not regress, and we had to intervene surgically. The ulnar nerve was markedly compressed under the hypothenar eminence, and after release of the compression, normal function returned.

Neuroma of the palmar collateral nerve of the thumb (now known as "bowler's thumb") is a recognized complication of bowling (Dobyns et al., 1972; Howell et al., 1970; Kisner, 1976; Maurice, 1979; Minkow et al., 1972). As a result of microtrauma the nerve becomes trapped within proliferating fibrous tissue; the pathogenesis is not unlike that of Morton's disease. The patient complains of paresthesia or even hyperesthesia on the medial aspect of the thumb where a firm mobile mass can be felt, which is tender to percussion. Of the 17 patients reported by Dobyns et al. (1972), seven were improved by neurolysis. In many cases, however, rest and the wearing of finger stalls may be sufficient. We have seen only one case, the incidence in the American context being appreciably greater in view of the higher proportion of professional players.

SPECIFIC LESIONS

A lesion is regarded as specific if its incidence is high in, and its localization is characteristic of, a given type of sport, or if its features are predictable.

THE STRIKING HAND

Boxing

Numerous publications have been devoted to the pathology of the hand in boxing (Burton and Eaton, 1973; Genety and Brunet-Guedj, 1976a; Illouz, 1967a,b; Eselin and Ducroquet, 1949; McCown, 1959; Polacco, 1952). We must first compare the figures of LaCava with those of McCown. In the first series, which dealt exclusively with amateurs, the incidence of fractures was 1.63 per cent as opposed to only 0.15 per cent in the second, the huge (tenfold) difference apparently being due to the inferior technique of the amateur.

The condition known as boxer's hand has been well described by Illouz (1967) and Iselin and Ducroquet (1949). Its main features are the morphological changes in the thumb, which is bent and carries a dorsal hump on the metacarpal, which appears subluxed, with reduced carpometacarpal mobility, and is shortened and broader than normal. This strange deformity with osteoarthritis of the trapeziometacarpal joint is the result of repeated injuries, malunited fractures, and untreated sprains of the joint. It has been suggested that these pathological changes are due to the configuration of the boxing glove, which prevents tight closure of the fist with the thumb locked against the other digits. The metacarpal hump is caused by hyperostosis of the base of the second and third metacarpals secondary to repeated untreated injuries (LaCava). The incidence is inversely proportional to the quality of the boxer's technique.

We must not forget the relative frequency of scaphoid fractures, which is said to have conditioned Carpentier's career (Fig. 83–6). According to Iselin, "At the age of 18, Carpentier sustained a fracture of the left wrist. He was thus forced to develop a right punch to which he later owed his fame." Lastly there is in boxers a high incidence of fractures of the neck of the fifth metacarpal, probably the commonest hand fracture in boxing.

Karate

In judo, the role of the hand consists of grabbing the opponent's kimono so as to unbalance, lift, and topple him. In karate, by contrast, the hand is the essential natural weapon, both offensive and defensive. Traditional karate is the modern sporting form of an ancient martial art, combining techniques from Okinawa and China. The earliest records are some 3000 years old. It is by definition a bare-handed fight (*kara,* empty; *te,* hand). The sport involves striking an opponent with more or less controlled blows. Training consists of hitting with extreme force such things as sandbags, wooden planks covered with straw (makiwara), or even bricks (schiwari). The fingertips are toughened by striking containers filled with sawdust, rice, or sand.

In the Western World there is now the tendency to wear some form of protection over the hands and feet. Since 1974 protective gear has become compulsory in competitions. In full contact karate, recently imported from the United States and comparable to the ancient sport pancratium, and to French boxing, the hands are protected by classic boxing gloves.

We have personally examined 43 karatekas, all black belts who had taken part in top class national and international competitions. The mechanism of the lesions varies with the quality of the technique. Excessive precipitation in the beginner is a common cause of sprains, dislocations, and fractures. Modern protective devices, however, prevent immediate injury and have transformed the classic "karate hand."

It is not easy to describe the subtleties of

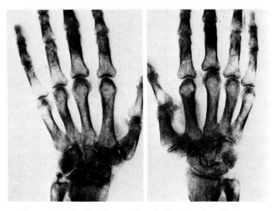

Figure 83–6. Radiograph of the hands of Georges Carpentier (1973), showing the "hunchback" appearance of the metacarpals and pseudarthrosis of the left scaphoid with osteoarthrosis of the wrist. Carpentier used the right fist "only once in every fight."

hand blows in a few words. Striking with a really devastating force requires perfect technique and intensive training. The hand, the natural weapon by excellence, can be used in a variety of ways.

The fist (seiken) is used for direct blows (tsuki) in a movement similar to the one that plunges a knife into an opponent's body. The surfaces used are those of the metacarpophalangeal joints of the index and middle fingers (kentos), which must lie directly in the line of the forearm. This locked position is highly accurate and generates immense force (Fig. 83–7).

The saber hand (shuto) strikes with the medial edge of the hand between the little finger and the wrist, i.e., the hypothenar border. Fahrer (1984) has shown the remarkable resistance of the ulnar aspect of the palm because of the organization of the fibrous tissue that is optimally adapted to sustain pressure. The spear hand (nukite) strikes with the fingertips. As for the palm (teisko), the fighter utilizes mostly the palmar aspect of the carpus, which is protected by the fleshy padding of the thenar and hypothenar eminences; great force can be generated with this blow. The reverse fist (uraken) uses the dorsal aspect of the metacarpus.

The traumatic process may involve all the tissues of the hand: skin, soft tissues, joints, capsules and ligaments, tendons, and bones. The lesions vary in time depending on the type of karate practiced—traditional (bare handed), modern (compulsory protection since 1974), or contact (with use of boxing gloves). Rubbing of the hand against a rough kimono, intensive practice of makiwara (now rare), and training with a bag can give rise to rupture and bleeding of the skin overlying the metacarpophalangeal joints of the kentos (second and third metacarpals).

Intensive training can produce hyperkeratosis of the kentos (the metacarpal joints of the second and third metacarpals), but three of our karate patients who presented this lesion had otherwise normal hands. The lesion is the hallmark of the karate hand. However, cutaneous erosions or "burns," nail scratches, and other lesions already mentioned have become extremely rare since the introduction of hand protection. Hematomas may appear in the soft tissues as a result of violent or repeated contusions of the thenar and hypothenar eminences (teisho) and dorsum of the hand as they come into contact with the hard surfaces of the elbow, knee, maxilla, or head. In demonstrations of smash-

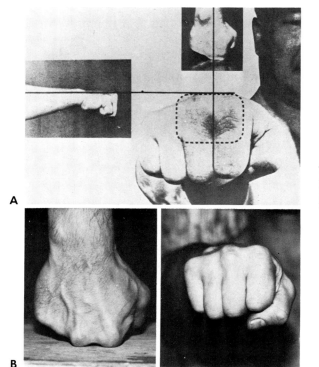

Figure 83–7. The hand of a karate expert. *A*, The karate punch (*tsuki*) exposes the metacarpophalangeal joints of the index and long fingers (*kentos*), which form the exact prolongation of the forearm. *B*, Note the hypertrophy of these joints.

ing (shiwari) with the saber hand (shuro), we have seen extensive hematomas and witnessed one case of complete anesthesia of the lateral digital nerve of the little finger, which lasted 18 months.

Osteoarticular Lesions. The pattern of osteoarticular lesions has altered somewhat since the introduction of protective devices. Prior to their use the joints most commonly affected were the metacarpophalangeal joints of the thumb and index and middle fingers, owing to inadequate locking of the hand on the lateral side. The protective devices used are such that locking is incomplete at all five metacarpophalangeal joints; hence, the rising incidence of lesions in the two medial digits. Dislocations are as common as fractures: The neck of the fifth metacarpal is now the most affected; prior to the protective era, fractures of the third and second metacarpals were just as common. This is a flagrant example of the part played by faulty equipment in sports traumatology (Fig. 83–8).

Changes in the Overall Appearance of the Hand. In the modern Western karateka, these are minimal, the most frequently encountered being hypertrophy of the kentos with an underdeveloped fibrous pad. Old phalangeal and metacarpal fractures present with asymptomatic thickening of the bone.

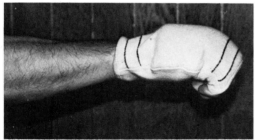
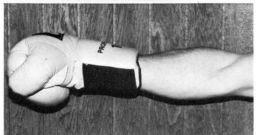

Figure 83–8. Protection of the "hitting hand" is associated with specific trauma. *A*, Protection of the hand of the karate expert prevents complete flexion of the fingers and causes a new type of injury at this site. *B*, The boxing glove exposes the thumb, which, since it cannot flex completely, is often injured.

The changes are more marked in Oriental karatekas and are due mostly to makiwara and to smashing exercises. In the West, the hand of the experienced karateka shows few major changes. Contusions, fractures, sprains, and dislocations usually involve the metacarpophalangeal joints, and deformities of the second and third joints (kentos) are typical of karate injuries (Allieu et al., 1980; Guillot and Tesson, 1977; Tibayrenc, 1975).

We do not believe that the protective devices introduced after 1974 have brought about any significant reduction in the number of accidents. By preventing the adequate locking of the fourth and fifth digital rays, they have displaced the injuries toward the medial digits. The use of boxing gloves in contact karate is likely to result in trauma similar to that seen in boxing, i.e., involving primarily the column of the thumb. It is important, therefore, that new gloves be designed to integrate the thumb more closely to the rest of the hand.

Pelota

Pelota, a regional sport played almost exclusively in the southwest of France, has a traumatic pathology of its own (Laporte, 1974; Laporte and Dunat, 1975). In addition to injuries due to accidental contact between the fingers and the wall or the ground, the hand of the pelota player is exposed to repeated microtrauma from the impact of the 100 gm. pelota, which is struck with great force with the metacarpophalangeal joints and distal phalanges. The shock is repeated several hundred times in the course of a single game; the main sufferers are the soft tissues and blood vessels in the short term, but osteoarthritis is a common late stigma.

Lesions of the Soft Tissues. The vascular congestion resulting from repeated shocks in a hand that is kept dependent between shots can transform the hand into a "washerwoman's beetle." The player has increasing difficulty in controlling his shots and tries by all means to reduce this swelling. Laporte mentions the common and spectacular practice of a player's asking a partner to stand on his hand, which he holds flat on the floor!

Hyperkeratosis is most marked at the points of impact of the pelota, i.e., the metacarpophalangeal joints. Cracks may appear in the course of a game (more so in cold weather) and usually on the dorsal aspect of the interdigital spaces.

The most severe lesion in pelota remains arteriopathy, which can present as a "white finger." The digits most frequently affected are the index and middle fingers. Acute ischemia with scabbing of the pulps is probably the result of microtraumatic arteriopathy involving the digital arteries. Digital hypovascularization can be demonstrated by arteriography (Laporte).

The accident most dreaded by players is the "nail" (in Basque, *itzia*), which presents clinically as acute pain on the palmar aspect of the metacarpophalangeal joints of the middle fingers or at an interdigital space. The only clinical sign may be a small, rounded, deep seated, palpable mass, which is tender to pressure. This clinical picture can conceal different pathological syndromes that have in common compression of the interdigital nerve. Of two patients who came to surgery (Baudet quoted by Laporte), one had an epidermoid cyst compressing the digital nerves; in the other the nerve was hypertrophied and trapped within a fibroadipose mass. Here again, the findings were reminiscent of those in Morton's disease.

Traumatic hemoglobinuria, although spectacular, is of no great clinical significance. It is due simply to release of pigment from the erythrocytes spilled as a result of the repeated shocks of the hand striking the pelota.

THE GRASPING HAND

The continuous friction and repeated skin trauma from a sporting implement grasped in a precise manner do give rise to specific forms of hyperkeratosis. A cutaneous callus may be further complicated by phlyctens, cracks, and suppuration.

A typical example of this is the hand of the gymnast, which is literally covered with calluses. Complications are common and treatment can be difficult. The same is true of rowing, whether in boats, canoes, or kayaks (Genety and Brunet-Guedj, 1976a; Genety et al., 1979; Maurice, 1979). Both gymnastics and rowing have been mistakenly held responsible in cases of Dupuytren's contracture; the contracture tends to appear late in life, long after the patient has retired from the sport, and there is probably no direct link. Severe hyperkeratosis of the palms may appear, similar to a contracture of the superficial fascia, but the deeper changes are in fact totally different.

In some sports localized hyperkeratosis corresponds to a precise grip. Thus, in golfers, bands of calluses have been described in the palm, especially in the left hand where it is said to indicate a correct grip (Chaouat and Chaouat, 1977; Chaouat et al., 1977). The calluses are usually found at the base of the third, fourth, and fifth metacarpophalangeal joints and at the base of the hypothenar eminence. Calluses elsewhere testify to a faulty grip of the club. They are asymptomatic, and the localized induration may indeed be an advantage.

In bowling the hyperkeratosis appears on the mediodorsal aspect of the proximal interphalangeal joint and the dorsolateral surface of the middle and ring fingers. Repeated pressure on the medial aspect of the thumb also can cause compression of the medial digital nerve (Fig. 83–9).

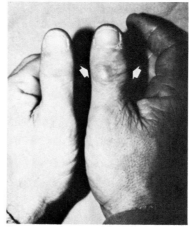

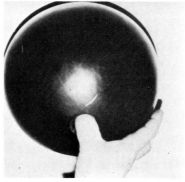

Figure 83–9. Bowler's thumb. Note the areas of medial and lateral hyperkeratosis corresponding to holding the ball. Microtrauma of the medial side may cause fibrosis that compresses the collateral nerve.

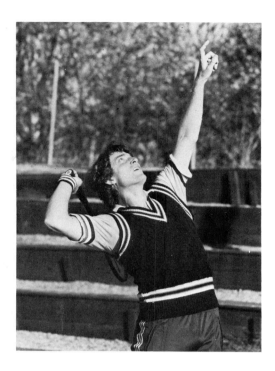

In archery the hyperkeratosis develops on the pulps of the fingers holding the string of the bow, i.e., the middle and ring fingers, despite the use of a fine protective palette (Maurice, 1979).

In tennis players calluses may be found on the medial aspect of the proximal phalanx of the thumb and palmar surface of the first web (Ferret, 1977).

Finally, in judokas, the calluses appear on the dorsum of the fingers at the level of the interphalangeal joints, which come into contact with the rough kimono.

Hand lesions in sport are multiple and varied, the most severe being those involving the tendons and the joints. The actual lesion is in no way specific, even though the treatment may pose special problems to the professional sportsman. There is clearly a place for the specialist in sports medicine and surgery, and sports injuries must not be left to amateur bone setters. Some lesions, especially of the skin, should be more widely known. Prophylaxis is often the best form of therapy, and only a better knowledge of the sport will enable the practitioner to advise on the subject of equipment and even on changes in grips and movements. The ultimate solution lies, therefore, in consultation with trainers and sportsmen themselves.

REFERENCES

Adams, I. D.: Arthrosis and sport. Roy Soc. Med., 72:185–187, 1979.

Allemandou, A.: Traumatologie chez les apprentis jockeys. Cinésiomèd., 5:31–42, 1977.

Allemandou, A., Andrivet, J., Martin, J., and Plas, F.: Pathologie du Rugby. Concours Méd., 3:317–323, 1972.

Allieu, Y., Benezis, C., Chaouat, Y., Comtet, J., Genety, A., Haim, U., Illouz, G., Laporte, G., Mansat, M., Narakas, A., Perrier, H., and Trojan, E.: Table ronde: La pathologie sportive de la main. Chir., 34:760–761, 1980.

Allieu, Y., and Michon, J.: Entorses et luxations du poignet. E.M.C. App. Loc. Mot., 14086 B10, 1976.

Andrivet, J., and Benassy, J.: Fractures et pseudarthroses du scaphoide carpien. Méd. Sport, 3:121, 1955.

Auffray, Y.: Les fractures du pyramidal. Acta Orthop. Belg., 36:313–345, 1970.

Azemar, G.: Aspect pathologique de l'escrime. Cinésiologie, 8:99–104, 1969.

Badgley, C. E., and Hayes, J. T.: Les traumatismes athlétiques du coude, de l'avant bras, du poignet et de la main. Am. J. Surg., 98:432–446, 1959.

Baird, D. B.: Delayed ulnar nerve palsy following a fracture of the hamate. J. Bone Joint Surg., 50A:570–572, 1968.

Bamert, P., et al.: Sport injuries of the thumb ray. Ther. Umsch., 33:402–406, 1976.

Bazex, A., Bazex, J., and Albarel, C.: Granulome à piqûre d'oursins avec lésions osseuses sous Jacentes. Bull. Soc. Fr. Dermatol., 82:153, 1975.

Benassy, J.: Traumatologie Sportive. Paris Masson Edit., 1976.

Bezes, H., and Julliard, R.: Les accidents du ski. A propos d'une statistique de 5200 observations. Ann. Chir., 30:583–605, 1976.

Bienner, K., and Muller, P.: Les accidents du hockey sur glace. Cah. Méd., 14:959–962, 1973.

Blazina, M. E., and Lane, C.: Rupture of the insertion of the flexor digitorum profundus tendon in student athletes. J. Am. Coll. Health Assn., 14:248–249, 1966.

Boeda, A.: A propos d'une paralysie cubitale chez une cycliste (occasionnelle). Méd. Sport, 46:34334, 1972.

Broussin, J.: Handball. Méd. Sport, 51:22–23, 1977.

Brown, E. Z., et al.: Ski pole thumb injury. Plast. Reconstr. Surg., 68:19–23, 1976.

Brown, H. C.: Common injuries of the athlete's hand. Canad. Med. Assoc. J., 117:621–625, 1977.

Burton, R., and Eaton, R.: Common and injuries in the athlete. Orthop. Clin. N. Am., 4:809–838, 1973.

Campbell, C. S.: Gamekeeper's thumb. J. Bone Joint Surg., 37B:148–149, 1955.

Campbell Reid, D. A.: Lésion isolée du fléchisseur profond. Hand, 1:115–117, 1969.

Carter, P. R., and Eaton, R. G.: Ununited fracture of the hook of the hamate. J. Bone Joint Surg. (Am.), 59:583–588, 1977.

Chaouat, Y., Simon, L., and Villiaumey, J.: Sports et rhumatismes. C. M., 99:5163–5169, 1977.

Chaouat, Y., and Chaouat, D.: Pathologie du golf. C.M., 101:2961–2966, 1979.

Commandre, F., and Viani, J. L.: The football keeper's thumb. J. Sports Med., 16:121–122, 1976.

Commandre, F., Viani, J. L., and Boeda, A. G.: Le pouce du gardien de but de football. Lyon Médit. Méd., 12:2127–2130, 1976.

Comtet, J. J.: Le doigt en maillet. Lyon Méd., *234:*767–768, 1975.

Coste, F., and Desproges-Gotteron, R.: Rhumatisme et équitation. Rev. Rhum., 27:254–258, 1960.

Coventry, M. B., and Bianco, A. J.: Ski fracture of the metacarpals. Minnesota Med., 1055–1058, 1964.

Curtin, J., et al.: Hand injuries due to soccer. Hand, *8:*93–95, 1976.

Desse, G.: Cyclisme et rhumatisme. Rev. Rhum., *27:*248–253, 1960.

Dobyns, J. H., et al.: Bowler's thumb: diagnosis and treatment. A review of seventeen cases. J. Bone Joint Surg., *54:*751–755, 1972.

Dobyns, J. H., Sim, F. H., and Linscheid, R. H.: Sports stress syndromes of the hand and wrist. Am. J. Sports Med., *6:*236–253, 1978.

Duivon, J. P.: La maladie des insertions tendineuses chez le sportif. G.M. France, *79:*3673–3680, 1972.

Dunham, W., et al.: Bowler's thumb (ulnovolar neuroma of the thumb). Clin. Orthop., *83:*99–101, 1972.

Edwards, D. M.: The spectrum of hand injuries. Hand, *7:*46–50, 1975.

Fahrer, M.: Anatomy of the karate chop. Bull. Hosp. Joint Dis. Orthop. Inst., *44*(2):189–198, 1984.

Ferret, J. M.: Les lésions chroniques du sport. Thesis in Medicine, University of Lyon, 1977.

Flatt, A. E.: Athletic injuries of the hand. J. Louisiana Med. Soc., *119:*425–431, 1967.

Foray, J., and Lanoye, P.: Gelures. E.M.C. App. Loc. Mot., *14:*33(F10), 1979.

Genety, J., and Brunet-Guedj, E.: Traumatologie du Sport en Pratique Médicale Courante. Paris, Vigot Frères Edit., 1976a.

Genety, J., and Brunet-Guedj, E.: La maladie des insertions tendineuses (enthésite, tendinite d'insertion, ténoperiostite). *In* Traumatologie du Sport en Pratique Médicale Courante. Paris, Vigot Frères Edit., 1976b, p. 71.

Genety, J., and Brunet-Guedj, E.: Arrachement de la corne postérieure du pyramidal. *In* Traumatologie du Sport en Pratique Médicale Courante. Paris, Vigot Frères Edit., 1976c, pp. 138–139.

Genety, J., Ferret, J. M., and Brunet-Guedj, E.: Lésions chroniques du sport. E.M.C. App. Loc. Mot., *15:*902(A10), 1979.

Gentaz, R., Lespargot, J., Levane, J. H., and Poli, J. P.: La maladie Kiembock. Approche tomographique. Analyse de 5 cas. Presse Méd., *18:*1270–1210, 1972.

Guillot, R., and Tesson, M.: Le karaté. Collection "Sport et Santé." Paris, Editions Médicales et Universitaires, 1977.

Gutman, J., Weisbuch, J., and Wolf, M.: Ski injuries in 1972–1973. A repeat analysis of a major health problem. J.A.M.A., *230:*1423–1425, 1974.

Hamas, R. S., Horrell, E. D., and Pierret, G. P.: Treatment of mallet finger due to intra-articular fracture of distal phalanx. J. Hand Surg., *3:*361–363, 1978.

Helal, B.: Racquet player's pisiform. Hand, *10:*87–90, 1978.

Howell, A. E., et al.: Bowler's thumb. Perineural fibrosis of the digital nerve. J. Bone Joint Surg., *52:*379–381, 1970.

Hromec, I., et al.: Hand and wrist trauma in hand-ball players. Acta Chir. Orthop. Traumatol. Cech., *44:*50–52, 1977.

Huguet, L. M.: Le basket. Collection Sport et Santé. Paris, Edit. Méd. et Universitaires, 1977.

Hursh, L. M.: Numbers and types of sports injuries. J.A.M.A., *199:*167, 1967.

Illouz, G.: Pathologie de la main chez les sportifs (boxe, ballon, ski, escrime, gymnastique, pelote basque). Vie Méd. (Enquête), *48:*227–238, 1967a.

Illouz, G.: Pathologie de la main du boxeur. Méd. Educ. Phys. Sport, *41:*43–47, 1967b.

Iselin, F.: Traumatologie de la main chez les sportif. Gaz. Méd. Fr., *80:*529–532, 1973.

Iselin, M., and Ducroquet, J.: Traumatismes de la Main chez les Boxeurs. Presse Méd., *57:*554–555, 1949.

Kalenak, A., et al.: Athletic injuries of the hand. Am. Fam. Physician *14:*136–142, 1976.

Kemm, I.: Skateboard injuries. Br. Med. J., *1:*894, 1978.

Kisner, W. H.: Thumb neuroma: a hazard of the ten pin bowling. Br. J. Plast. Surg., *29:*225–226, 1976.

Kreude, A. D.: Atteinte due au sport chez les escrimeurs. Beitr. Orthop. Trauma, *12:*719–721, 1965.

Kruhl, E., and Stimmine, W.: Typical finger injuries in playing ball. Mschr. Unfallheilk., *67:*478–482, 1964.

Laporte, G.: Hémoglobinurie des pelotaris à main nue. Bordeau Méd., *7:*647–653, 1974.

Laporte, G., and Dunat, L.: La main des pelotaris. Un modèle de pathologie traumatique. Ann. Chir., *29:*499–507, 1975.

Lemaire, V.: Une nouvelle pathologie traumatique: la pathologie des planches à roulettes. C.M., *101:*3001, 1979.

Linscheid, R. L., et al.: Traumatic instability of the wrist. Diagnosis, classification, pathomechanics. J. Bone Joint Surg., *54A:*1612–1639, 1972.

Lowrey, C. W., et al.: Digital vessel trauma from repetitive impact in baseball catchers. J. Hand. Surg., *1:*236–238, 1976.

Mäder, G., et al.: Injuries to the finger joints in athletes. Ther. Umsch., *33:*407–411, 1976.

Mahnes, F.: Les accidents propres à la pratique de l'escrime. Vie Méd. Enq., *48:*241–244, 1967.

Manske, P. R.: Fractures of the hook of the hamate presenting as carpal tunnel syndrome. Hand, *10:*181–183, 1978.

Maurice, G.: La pathologie de la main chez le sportif. Thesis, Faculty of Medicine, University of Lyon, 1979.

Mayfield, J. K., Johnson, R. P., and Kiloyne, R. K.: Carpal dislocations: pathomechanics and progressive perilunar instability. J. Hand Surg., *5:*226–241, 1980.

McCown, I. A.: Boxing injuries. Am. J. Surg., *98:*501–516, 1959.

McCue, F. C.: Athletic injuries of the proximal interphalangeal joint requiring surgical treatment. J. Bone Joint Surg., *52A:*937–955, 1970.

Michon, J., and Allieu, Y.: Fractures des os du carpe. E.M.C. App. Loc. Mot., 14046, B10, 1976a.

Michon, J., and Allieu, Y.: Séquelles des traumatismes du carpe. E.M.C. App. Loc. Mot., 14046, F10, 1976b.

Minkow, F. V., et al.: Bowler's thumb Clin. Orthop., *83:*115–117, 1972.

Moreau, F.: Les accidents du judo et leur mécanisme. Thesis in Medicine, Paris, 1957.

Neidhardt, J. H., et al.: Les fractures du trapèze (considérations sur une série de 7 cas personnels et d'une analyse de la littérature). Lyon Méd., *99:*1049–1064, 1968.

Pointu, J., et al.: Fractures du trapèze et traumatologie du sport Méd. Sport, *52:*43–48, 1978.

Polacco, A.: La déformazione professionale del carpo nei pugili (carpe bossu). Stud. Méd. Chir. Sport, *1:*3–15, 1952.

Polacco, A., et al.: Traumatologie de la main dans les sports. Friuli Méd., *22:*933–960, 1967.

Posner, M. A.: Injuries to the hand and wrist in athletes. Orthop. Clin. N. Am., *8:*593–618, 1977.

Quattrini, M.: Un caso di lussazione isolata del pisiforme nel tennis. Méd. Sport., *3:*366–370, 1967.

Rives, D.: Les lésions négligées ou méconnues de la main chez le sportif. Ouest Méd., *29:*441–445, 1976.

Rodriguez, A. L.: Injuries to the collateral ligaments of the proximal interphalangeal joints. Hand, *5:*55–57, 1973.

Roulet, J.: Maladie de Dupuytren. E.M.C. App. Loc. Mot., 15490, B10, 1974.

Sakellarides, H. T.: Treatment of recent and old injuries of the ulnar collateral ligament of the M.P. joint of the thumb. Am. J. Sports Med., *6:*255–261, 1978.

Shultz, R. J., et al.: Gamekeeper's thumb; result of skiing injuries. N. Y. J. Med., *73:*2329–2331, 1973.

Spunsll, K. H.: Athletic injuries of the hand and wrist. J. Sport Med., *3:*37–40, 1963.

Stack, H. G.: Mallet finger. Hand, *1:*83–89, 1969.

Stark, H. H., et al.: Fracture of the hook of the hamate in athletes. J. Bone Joint Surg. (Am.), *59:*575–582, 1977.

Stein-Brirck, H.: Sport actuellement: ski acrobatique. Münch. Méd. Wschr., *120:*363–366, 1978.

Stener, B.: Entorses recentes de l'articulation métacar-pophalangien ne du pouce. *In* Traumatismes Osteoarticulaires de la Main. Paris, L'Expansion Scientifique Française, 1971, pp. 59–66.

Streeton, J. A.: Traumatic haemoglobinuria by karate exercises. Lancet, *2:*191–192, 1967.

Takehiko, T.: Fracture of the hook of the hamate by a golfswing. Clin. Orthop., *83:*91–94, 1972.

Thiebault, J.: Le risque sportif: Etude de 43093 dossiers concernant 57 disciplines (sport amateur). Rev. Franç. Dom. Corp., *6:*319–352, 1980.

Thomas, C. R.: Avulsion of the flexor digitorum profondus, an athletic injury. Am. J. Sports Med., *5:*281–284, 1977.

Tibayrenc, N.: Karaté et médecine. Thesis, Paris-Broussais, 1975.

Tubiana, R.: Plaies des tendons de la main.

Tubiana, R.: Le traitement chirurgical des fractures récentes des métacarpiens et des phalanges. *In* Les Traumatismes Ostéoarticulaires de la Main. Paris, L'Expansion, Scientifique Française, 1971.

Verdan, C., et al.: Lésions graves du pouce par ski nautique. Z. Unfallmed. Berufskr., *61:*37–41, 1968.

Watson Jones, D.: Fractures and Joint Injuries. Edinburgh, Churchill Livingstone, 1976.

Wenger, D. R.: Arrachement de l'insertion d'un tendon digital profond chez des joueurs de football. Arch. Surg., *106:*145–149, 1973.

Part Five

TRAUMATIC
AMPUTATIONS
IN THE HAND

PREHENSION IN THE MUTILATED HAND

INTRODUCTION

Raoul Tubiana

Amputations in the hand are common and varied. They may be congenital, traumatic, or secondary to neurological or vascular disorders.

We shall consider here only amputations of traumatic origin. Amputations secondary to other disorders present specific problems related to the particular disease. Although the restoration of prehension remains the aim of treatment in all cases, the natural history of the disease and the often severe associated trophic changes must be taken into account in nontraumatic amputations.

Traumatic amputations differ from congenital ones, not only because of the abundance of scar tissue but because in the former the patient has not adapted to his amputation. Indeed, the older the patient, the more difficult will be the adaptation.

Traumatic amputations may be the immediate result of an accident, or they may occur secondary to necrosis. The latter type is seen mostly after crush injuries but may also follow thermal or electric burns.

Injuries of the hand have increased significantly with the use of machinery. Machinery is used not only in factories and workshops but also in every walk of life in "civilized" societies, including transport, agriculture, and the domestic environment. Accidents happen more commonly when such appliances are used by untrained personnel, for example, agricultural workers, "do it yourself" enthusiasts, Sunday gardeners, and housewives. Injuries to the hand, particularly amputations, are no longer confined to men and manual workers; they affect all ages and all strata of society.

The many varieties of injuries and amputations—recent amputations as well as secondary repair procedures—will be dealt with in the following chapters in order of increasing severity. Discussions will cover recent amputations, in which the possibilities of *replantation* must be evaluated, as well as *secondary reconstruction*.

Microsurgical techniques now have an important place in the emergency as well as definitive treatment of such amputations; however a technique should not be used because it is technically feasible but because it is best suited to the patient's needs. The use of microsurgery should not exclude utilization of standard techniques of reconstructive surgery. In well selected cases it offers new possibilities, allowing for more rapid or more beneficial reconstruction in a single stage. Only specialists with a knowledge of both standard methods and microsurgery techniques are capable of evaluating the in-

dications for replantation and for toe transfer, the chances for immediate success, and
the final functional result.

The essential point to be remembered is
that the major aim of treatment in amputations of the hand is not to restore normal
anatomical features but rather to re-establish
useful function adapted to the individual
case. Therapy must be guided by this principle.

The techniques for elective amputation in
the hand and upper limb are described in the
section on amputations in Volume IV.

Chapter 84

PREHENSION IN THE MUTILATED HAND

Raoul Tubiana

Traumatic amputations in the hand comprise a diverse group of lesions with disturbance or loss of prehension as the common denominator.

Prehension in the normal hand is covered at length in the first volume of this book (see Chapters 4 and 46). Here we should like first to stress some essential points that will help to explain the difference between prehension in the normal hand and in the mutilated hand.

Grasping of a common object under normal conditions is performed almost automatically with a great economy of gestures. After mutilation, long established nerve pathways between the central nervous system and the hand are severely disturbed and may be very difficult to restore. From the early days of life, a model of our own body image gradually develops in the parietal area of the brain that will become the permanent cortical representation of the self. This image is so deeply ingrained that it remains unchanged in the amputee.

Because of his mutilation, the patient has to adapt to his new functional possibilities. He remembers how to utilize his hand, but his previous varied range of grips is restricted or lost; sensory information is reduced, the degree depending on the extent of the injury.

The result is that the mutilated hand is "demoted" according to the severity of the lesions. Although the normal hand is a source of information and an agent of action, with multiple possibilities for dynamic adaptation well beyond those of an instrument, however perfected, the mutilated hand falls to the level of a primitive tool. The physician's role is to try to restore the more common forms of grip. Depending on the severity of the mutilation, one may hope at best to restore

a precision grip or a power grip, or simply the more rudimentary action of a vise, a pincer, a hook, a pusher, or a paperweight.

The minimum required for a precision grip is a thumb or neothumb with as nearly normal a length, mobility, and sensation as possible and a finger against which it can actively oppose.

The presence of a third digit greatly increases the control and precision of the grip.

Active flexion of the distal interphalangeal joints, with conservation of the nails, also improves the precision of the grip (Fig. 84–1), but it is important to remember that terminal grips (thumb-finger with the distal phalanges flexed) are used far less commonly than subterminal pulp grips with the distal interphalangeal joints in almost complete extension. Actually, there is a greatly reduced surface area in tip to tip pinch, and in order to compensate for this limitation, the pinch must be stronger to retain an object (Fig. 84–2). Pulp pinch involves a much larger and more malleable surface area. It is the pulp to pulp pinch that must be restored when the distal interphalangeal joints are stiff.

In a power grip the hand is wrapped around the object, and this implies mobility of the finger joints (Fig. 84–3). Under normal circumstances the metacarpophalangeal joints act as hinges: they close after the proximal interphalangeal joints in flexion movements and open before them in extension. Their action can be compensated by the proximal interphalangeal joints. The power of this full-handed type of grip depends on the width of the palm and on the survival of at least part of the peripheral digits, the fingers on the radial side being more useful for precision

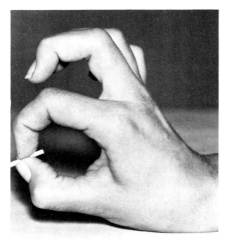

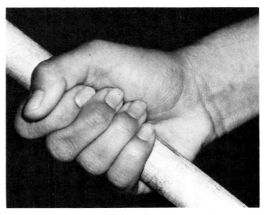

Figure 84–3. Digitopalmar power grip.

Figure 84–1. Distal pinch. The distal phalanges are flexed. Terminal grips are "precise" only if the interphalangeal joints are mobile in order to exactly adapt the grip to the size of a small object.

handling and those on the ulnar side for power grip.

The thumb is essential for a precision grip as well as for a power grip. Its function is greatly reduced if it is short and stiff, possibly limiting it to lateral pinch with the radial border of the index finger.

If the thumb is missing, the only possible grips are the digital hook, the broad digitopalmar grip, and the narrow interdigital pincer, none of which can be called precise (Fig. 84–4).

The necessity for conserving a mutilated digit, with as much length as possible, is widely appreciated. If length is conserved for control of grip, especially in the thumb and peripheral digits in mutilations, it must not be done at the expense of skin coverage of the stump. Sensibility, absence of pain, or

trophic changes and stability of the stump are more important than length. Lengthening, reconstruction, or replantation of a digit is only valuable if the functional integrity of the digit is maintained.

A mutilated thumb, even if almost completely amputated with only the base of the first phalanx remaining, may provide useful function as long as the first metacarpal is mobile, the first web space is free, and the skin cover of the stump is of good quality.

Thus the functional value of the mutilated hand depends not only on the degree of the injury, but also on other essential factors: the conservation of mobility of the remaining elements and the quality of skin cover.

When the mutilation is extensive and when the surviving fingers are stiff, the last resort is to restore pinch grip. This requires two opposable parts, at least one of which should be mobile and one, if possible, sensitive.

Reconstruction of a pincer does not guarantee that the pincer will be utilized. It is essential that the patient know how to use it. Indeed one of the basic problems in hand mutilations is adaptation to new modes of prehension. This depends on the age and intelligence of the patient, the quality of the reconstructed grip, the presence or absence of pain, the patient's occupation, his need to use his mutilated hand (patients with bilateral mutilations readapt relatively better than those with unilateral injuries), and, finally, above all, the presence of *sensibility*. Prehension is not a purely motor act: it depends on the messages of tactile and proprioceptive sensibility and their utilization by the central nervous system. Prehension cannot be reestablished by surgery, but favorable condi-

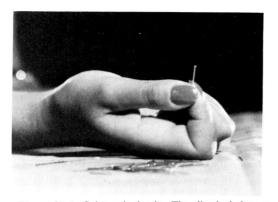

Figure 84–2. Subterminal grip. The distal phalanges are in almost complete extension.

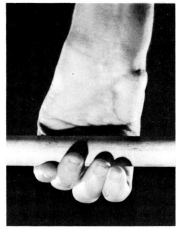
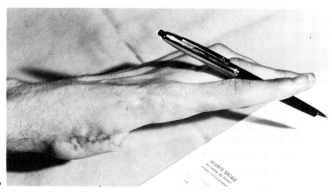

Figure 84–4. In the absence of the thumb, certain grips remain possible: *A*, Distal hook. *B*, Interdigital grip. They cannot be "precise."

tions that facilitate its re-establishment can be restored by reconstructing a pincer, excising a painful neuroma, or providing skin sensibility.

Painful fingers and fingers deprived of sensation are seldom utilized. Hence the importance of providing the gripping areas with as good a sensory skin covering as possible.

One can evaluate the existence of afferent impulses that provide protopathic sensibility for protection of the skin, but these are insufficient for stereognosis, which is necessary for the recognition of objects by touch and for gripping without the aid of vision. (See Chapter 4 in Volume I.)

Moberg (1968, 1976) stresses that Weber's test allows the simultaneous assessment of both exteroceptive and proprioceptive functions. Discrimination between two points is normally 3 to 5 mm. in the finger pulp. If this falls to 11 to 12 mm., it becomes impossible by touch alone to recognize objects or to grip without the aid of vision. Thus, the hands can be controlled only with the help of vision; this can be a particularly difficult problem in bilateral mutilations.

In the absence of sensation there is no true prehension and a *prosthesis* will not restore prehension. With the assistance of a prosthesis, the mutilated patient can perform movements resembling those of the articulated hand, but such appliances, although they allow some form of grip, remain insensitive. There is no prosthesis that recognizes touch. A sensitive grip that is capable of recognizing objects and adjusting the force of grip is certainly superior to a prosthetic pincer, which must always be controlled by

vision. Complicated prostheses are rarely used by mutilated manual workers, but a prosthesis that can be used as a simple tool and that is easy to adapt and is designed for a precise function can give great service. Surgery and prosthetics are not in competition, but are complementary methods of treatment.

Finally, there is one aspect of the mutilated hand that is too often neglected—the *psychological repercussions*. The importance of these repercussions depends on a number of factors—the level of the amputation, the age, sex, amount of anxiety of the subject, and the correct surroundings. This environment plays a role that can be predicted—centers for re-education where the injured are surrounded by similar patients or by patients who are more seriously ill and can witness functional recovery. Some patients are more concerned by the aesthetic handicap than by their functional incapacity. These patients can be provided with aesthetically acceptable prostheses for their social well-being, as proposed by Pillet. (See the chapter on aesthetic prostheses in Volume IV.)

The treatment of the mutilated hand therefore can be said to have two main objectives:

1. To re-establish methods of pinch with the help of the remaining elements. This objective is developed in the chapters that follow.

2. To facilitate the social rehabilitation of the mutilated patient, not only by insuring functional recovery but also by trying to assist in his aesthetic problems in an environment in which he can be encouraged in his attempt at readaptation.

REPLANTATION

Chapter 85

THE ROLE OF MICROSURGICAL TECHNIQUES OF TREATMENT OF UPPER LIMB AMPUTATION

Viktor E. Meyer

The development of microsurgical techniques has resulted in a considerable number of new methods of treatment, which have vastly increased the possibilities of acute and reconstructive surgery of the upper extremity. History has shown that rapid developments often lead to an overestimation of their real potential and thereby to a loss of proportion and perspective. This fact applies as well to the history of medicine and in particular to the application of microsurgical procedures in the upper extremity. It is not my intention to underestimate the tremendous value and importance of the achievements of microsurgical techniques. However, these new techniques should not unduly devalue the well established, more traditional methods of treatment. Many recent reports in the literature dealing with microsurgical methods unfortunately give the impression that the indication for a microsurgical procedure may in fact be based on personal interest of the surgeon rather than on the needs of the patient. Without doubt microsurgical techniques today offer many effective possibilities for conditions unsolvable by traditional surgery. However, there are many situations, particularly in the area of tissue replacement, in which traditional surgery still offers worthy alternatives and in many cases superior methods of treatment.

At this time it would be erroneous to omit all pedicle flap procedures from surgical training in favor of exclusive microsurgical tissue transplantation. One must understand that the neurosurgical solution must in fact be the best solution for the patient when it is employed. This is a basic tenet of any medical educational program.

Today it is generally accepted that microsurgical technique has greatly improved the results in peripheral nerve repair and even in tendon repair, especially in the repair of flexor tendons within the critical area of the osteofibrous tunnels in the digits. Also there is no doubt that in early surgery for correction of congenital deformities in young children microsurgical techniques are of great importance (Buck-Gramcko, 1981). In the following section some basic considerations relating

951

to the possibilities of replantation and revascularization as well as microsurgical tissue transplantation will be discussed.

REPLANTATION

Often there is confusion over terminology with regard to replantation. Under the heading of replantation, only cases of complete severance (amputation) should be considered. There are cases in which incomplete severance has to be transformed into a complete severance by débridement of the remaining tissue bridges. Such terms as "partial amputation" and "subtotal amputation" contradict the definition of amputation and should be discarded in favor of "incomplete severance." In fact there are cases in which small vital tissue bridges are unlikely to be of major importance in the final outcome, and the problems therefore are basically the same as in amputation cases. However, inclusion of such cases in a review of replantation confuses the evaluation with the issue of what is an "insignificant" tissue bridge (Chen et al., 1981b).

Therefore, cases of incomplete severance should rather be presented under the heading of "revascularization for survival" if there is no chance of survival without surgical restoration of the disrupted main vascular system, or "revascularization for improvement" if the part would probably survive without vascular repair. However, additional vascular repair is performed with the intention of improving the final functional result (Meyer, 1982). Often suggestions are made to divide replantation cases into macro- and microreplantations with reference to the level of the wrist joint. In fact, in the adult the diameters of vessels to be repaired proximal to the wrist joint are relatively large, making their repair easy and rapid and obviating the need for optical magnification. However, in young children the same anatomical structures may be small and difficult to repair, even using an operating microscope. Moreover, experience clearly shows that the use of magnification has improved the reliability of larger vessel anastomoses; nerve repair undoubtedly should be performed with microsurgical technique at any level in all cases. Therefore one should discourage any trend toward fragmentation, which in this well defined area of upper extremity surgery can only compromise patient care as a whole (Chen et al., 1981b).

Considering functional results, one must evaluate many factors. One must be mindful of the limited value of any percentage estimate of tissue survival because it is the result of patient selection and may or may not correlate with resulting function. However, in developing any system one must recognize that function cannot be expressed only by measurements of prehensile capability of the reattached part; success ultimately has to be measured in terms of the contribution of the replantation to subsequent overall performance of the patient.

The present guidelines for indications and contraindications for replantation are based on reports of long term functional results and possible complications. They must be considered to be dynamic rather than static in nature, because they may change in the future with improvement of surgical technique and overall treatment (Brown, 1981; Chen et al., 1981b). The following parameters, treated in detail in other chapters, are of critical importance:

The General Condition of the Patient. The general condition of the patient must be such that the risk of a long and complex surgical procedure is within reasonable proportion to the functional outcome that can be anticipated. Concomitant injuries, existing systemic or local disease, or sequelae from previous injuries may eventually preclude replantation.

The Patient's Age. The age of the patient is judged on a biological rather than a chronological basis because reattachment in healthy older individuals may be rewarding (Fig. 85–1). In general, however, the results in patients beyond 50 years of age are progressively less favorable. Replantation after the age of 60 should be performed only exceptionally. Owing to their amazing potentials for nerve regeneration, rapid bone healing, and sensory (self) re-education, children are prime candidates for replantation. Moreover, there is little tendency toward problems such as joint stiffness, tendon adhesions, and cold intolerance. The growth rate of reattached parts is nearly normal, provided there has been no damage to the epiphysis (Fig. 85–2; Jaeger et al., 1981; O'Brien, 1977). In the cases of epiphyseal damage, the esthetic and functional consequences must be anticipated and taken into consideration.

The Type of Injury. The type of injury may vary between the two extremes of a clean-cut guillotine injury and an avulsion ampu-

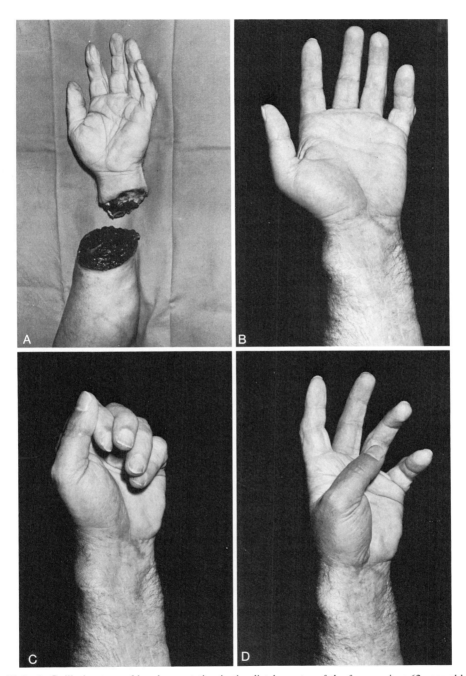

Figure 85–1. *A,* Guillotine type of hand amputation in the distal quarter of the forearm in a 62-year-old joiner. *B* to *D,* Result at two years after total primary repair. No secondary surgery was performed. This case shows that replantation may be rewarding even in older individuals if the type and level of injury are favorable. (*A,* from Meyer, V. E., Chen, Z. W., and Beasley, R. W.: Orthop. Clin. North Am., *12*:871, 1981. *C* and *D,* from Meyer, V. E.: *In* Evarts, C. M. (Ed.): Surgery of the Musculoskeletal System, Vol. 1. New York, Churchill Livingstone, New York, 1983.)

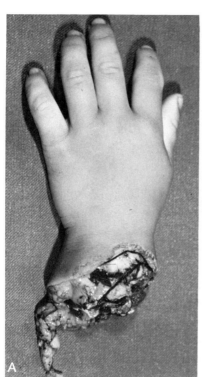

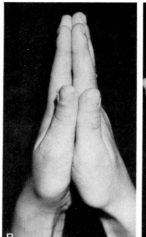

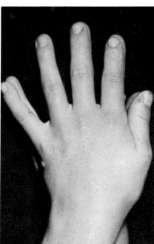

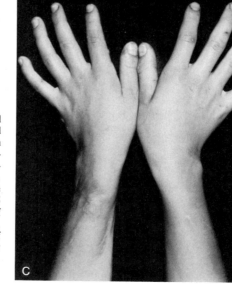

Figure 85–2. *A*, Hand of a three and one-half year old girl that was amputated by a lawn mower. *B* and *C*, Condition seven years after replantation, utilizing total primary repair. Growth of the reattached hand was within the normal range. It is interesting that the forearm with the reattached hand was at that time only 1.5 cm. shorter than normal despite 3 cm. of initial skeletal shortening. (*A*, from Meyer, V. E.: *In* Evarts, C. M. (Ed.): Surgery of the Musculoskeletal System, Vol. 1. New York, Churchill Livingstone, 1983.)

tation. It is the avulsion amputation that carries the worst prognosis for survival and functional recovery (Fig. 85–3). In avulsion amputations the severance of different anatomical structures typically occurs at multiple levels. Therefore the level of amputation in these cases should refer to the level of disruption of the nerves and muscle-tendon units rather than to the level of skeletal severance. Often a compression amputation may be transformed into a guillotine type of amputation by radical débridement and skeletal shortening. In limb replantation the necessary amount of bone shortening is often underestimated, leading to complicated soft tissue healing and delayed bone union or more frequently nonunion.

Tissue Anoxia. Tolerance to tissue anoxia can be effectively increased by cooling. At the present time this is the only practical procedure that effectively extends the anoxic period before irreversible tissue damage occurs. This is of special importance if the amputated part includes musculature, which in contrast to other tissues is susceptible to anoxia.

The Level of Amputation. The level of amputation is one key in the projection of guidelines for replantation. Proximal amputations may be associated with life-threatening problems. Although the repair of severed structures is easy because of their size, the potential for functional recovery is relatively poor because of the long distance for nerve regeneration and the often severe damage of large muscle masses (Table 85–1). However, even in apparently unfavorable cases, rewarding results may be achieved (Fig. 85–4).

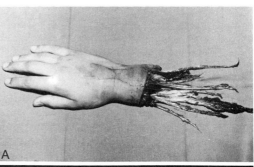
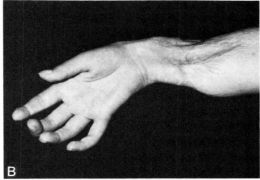
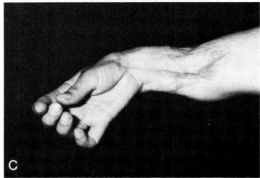

Figure 85–3. *A*, Avulsion-amputation in an 11-year-old boy demonstrates that severance of different anatomical structures typically occurs at multiple levels. This type of amputation injury has the poorest prognosis. *B* and *C*, Condition eight years after reattachment with total primary repair. After replantation, multiple split thickness skin graft procedures were necessary, as were cancellous bone grafts (because of nonunion). Skeletal growth of the reattached hand was normal. Sensibility was sufficiently protective, but two-point discrimination was more than 10 mm. However, there was some very limited prehensile capacity. (*A* to *C*, from Meyer, V. E.: Upper Extremity Replantation: Basic Principles, Surgical Technique and Strategy. New York, Churchill Livingstone, 1985.)

Table 85–1. RESULTS OF UPPER LIMB REPLANTATIONS*†‡

Level of Amputation	Number of Cases	Grades I and II (%)	Grade III (%)	Grade IV (%)
Shoulder	3	—	33.3	66.6
Arm	26	35	65	—
Proximal forearm	20	40	35	25
Distal forearm	48	79	21	—
Wrist (carpus)	30	83	17	—
Total	127	48	34	18

*Shanghai, Louisville, and Zurich.

†Minimal follow-up period: two years.

‡This review was taken from a cooperative study of three replantation centers on three different continents (Asia, North America, Europe). All three centers analyzed their patients using the evaluation system proposed by Chen (grades I to IV). A detailed description of this system is given in the article by Chen et al., 1981b.

Chen's four grades of functional recovery can be simply summarized as follows: Replantations that produced grade I and II results are classified as excellent and good, clearly worthwhile. Grade III is only fair, but worthwhile to most patients. Grade IV results are so poor that they are not worthwhile.

The review included a total of 127 cases of complete severance. Cases of incomplete severance were not included, regardless of how small the intact tissue bridge was. The follow-up was two years or more. This review, together with the basic considerations for indications previously presented, projects some guidelines for indications and contraindications for upper limb replantation. In this series, not one case of shoulder reattachment resulted in a grade I or II recovery. In the arm and proximal forearm replantations, grade I and II results were less than 50 per cent. All three centers found a striking difference between amputations through the proximal forearm and those of the distal forearm and wrist. The distal forearm and wrist were bound to be the most favorable levels for upper limb reattachment. Innervation to the forearm muscle remains intact, and the repair is of tendon rather than muscle and is in a biologically favorable area. Also the distance over which nerves must regenerate is shorter. Thus the results are often more rewarding. (From Chen Z. W., et al.: Present indications and contraindications for replantation as reflected by long-term functional results. Orthop. Clin. N. Am., *12*:849, 1981.)

In upper limb replantation, amputations proximal to but close to the wrist joint are the most favorable (Fig. 85–5; Table 85–1). In contrast, distal amputations pose little risk to the patient and in general carry a relatively good prognosis, especially in terms of nerve regeneration. However, these distal amputations require extraordinary time, effort, and skills for successful repair of the progressively smaller structures.

It is generally accepted that in all cases replantation of an amputated thumb proximal to the interphalangeal joint should be attempted even if the nerve damage is irreparable. In this situation sensibility may be restored in a second procedure by one of the various types of sensory island flap transfer (Littler, 1956).

In finger amputation the level of severance is of special importance. If amputation has occurred distal to the insertion of the flexor digitorum superficialis, function of the proximal interphalangeal and metacarpophalangeal joints can be expected to be nearly normal after replantation. In these cases the flexion arc will not be significantly impaired even if there is no motion at the distal interphalangeal joint (Fig. 85–6). Therefore these patients will have excellent functional results (Foucher et al., 1981). One must consider all socioeconomic factors prior to performing replantation, being mindful that in many professions the loss of such a finger segment does not seriously impair the overall performance of the patient.

In amputations of a single finger proximal to the insertion of the flexor digitorum superficialis, a significant impairment of the crucially important flexion arc will result and thus eventually will even impair the total hand function to a greater extent than without replantation. Therefore replantation in these cases should in general not be considered In these patients later ray amputation or transposition may be indicated, especially if the esthetic appearance of the hand is of predominant importance (Fig. 85–7). In multidigital amputations the best-preserved segments should be reattached in the most functional positions (heterotopic or transpositional replantation; Figs. 85–8, 85–9).

As previously mentioned, there are cases of incomplete severance in which microvascular reconstruction may be indicated and that should be reviewed under the heading of revascularization (Meyer, 1982). One example is the ring avulsion injury of a finger, which of course may lead to complete severance as well. However, in most instances these injuries represent various degrees of disruption of the neurovascular system (Fig. 85–10). Microvascular reconstruction has

Text continues on page 963

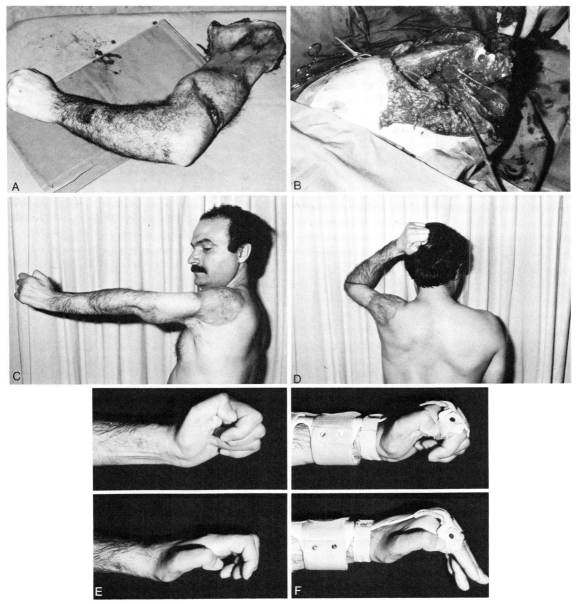

Figure 85–4. *A* and *B*, A 41-year-old laborer with avulsion-amputation in the middle third of the humerus caused by a conveyor belt. *C* to *F*, Condition two and one-half years after replantation, utilizing total primary repair. After replantation, two split thickness skin graft procedures and a Z-plasty were performed. The highly motivated patient achieved near normal shoulder and elbow motion. The prehensile capacity of the hand was seriously impaired; however, it can be improved to some degree by preventing full extension of the metacarpophalangeal joints. At the time this photograph was taken, the patient was a candidate for a tendon transfer in order to improve abduction and opposition of the thumb and tenodesis of the metacarpophalangeal joints of the fingers. Sensibility was of protective quality only. The case illustrates that even in proximal replantations following an unfavorable type of injury, sometimes unexpectedly rewarding results may be achieved. (*A* to *F*, from Meyer, V. E.: Upper Extremity Replantation: Basic Principles, Surgical Technique and Strategy. New York, Churchill Livingstone, 1985.)

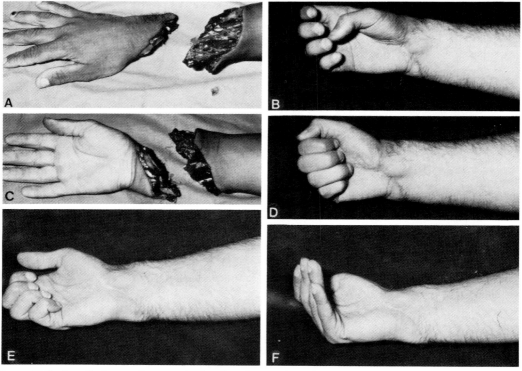

Figure 85–5. *A* to *F*, Amputations proximal to but close to the wrist joint are prime candidates for replantation, as illustrated by this case of a 20-year-old man. The photographs of the functional result after total primary repair were taken one and one-half years after the accident. This young man does not have any disability in performing his original job as a manual worker. (*A* to *F*, from Meyer, V. E.: Upper Extremity Replantation: Basic Principles, Surgical Technique and Strategy. New York, Churchill Livingstone, 1985.)

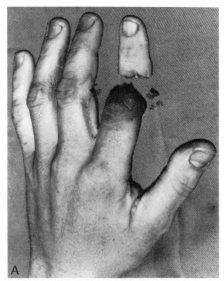

Figure 85–6. *A*, Guillotine type of amputation of the index finger distal to the flexor digitorum superficialis in a 19-year-old man. *B* and *C*, Results one and one-half years after total primary repair. Even with moderate or no distal interphalangeal joint motion, the impairment of the flexion arc of that finger was insignificant because there was a normal range of motion at the proximal interphalangeal and metacarpophalangeal joint levels. (*A* to *C*, from Meyer, V. E.: *In* Evarts, C. M. (Ed.): Surgery of the Musculoskeletal System, Vol. 1. New York, Churchill Livingstone, 1983.)

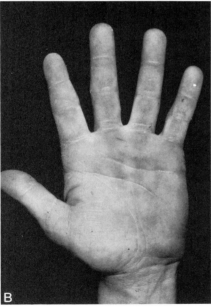

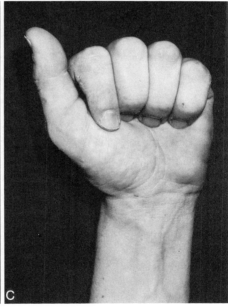

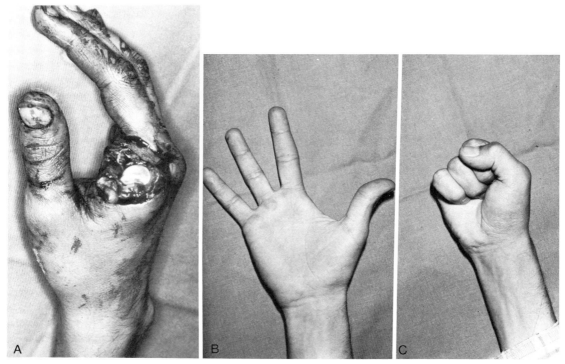

Figure 85–7. *A* to *C*, Since we started routine replantations at our clinic in 1974, we have never attempted reattachment of a single finger amputated proximal to the flexor digitorum superficialis insertion. If esthetic considerations are predominant in the individual case, we perform a ray amputation if the index finger is involved, as illustrated. In case of proximal loss of the middle or ring finger, comparable esthetic results can be achieved by ray transposition.

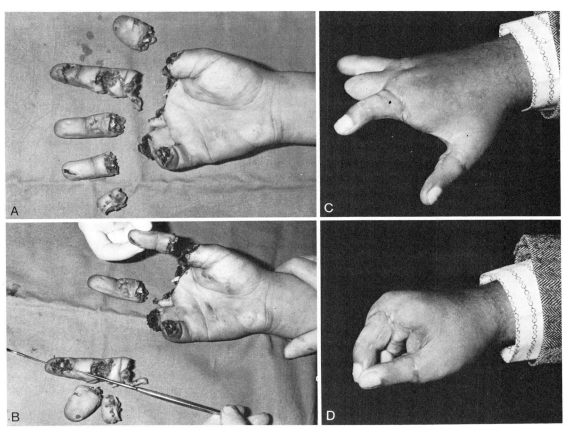

Figure 85–8. *A* and *B*, Amputation of all five digits by a circular saw in a 24-year-old carpenter. The two best-preserved segments were selected for reattachment. The long finger segment was put back into its original position and the thumb was replaced by the amputated ring finger (transpositional or heterotopic replantation). *C* and *D*, Result at ten months, with a powerful pinch of 7 kg. (*A* to *D*, from Meyer, V. E., Chen, Z. W., and Beasley, R. W.: Surg. Orthop. Clin. North Am., *12*:871, 1981.)

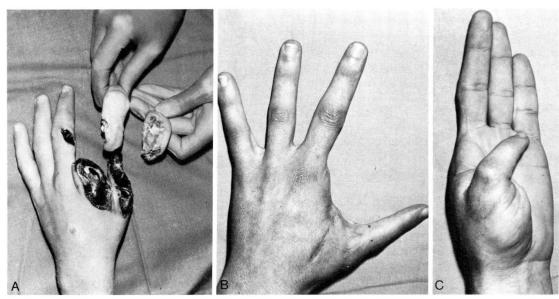

Figure 85–9. *A*, Amputation of the thumb and index finger in an 18-year-old man. The thumb segment was destroyed and not reattachable. *B* and *C*, Thumb replacement was performed by using the well-preserved index finger segment. Wound closure was easily achieved after ray amputation of the second metacarpal. The functional result is shown at eight months. The proximal interphalangeal joint of the index finger now acts as the metacarpophalangeal joint of the thumb (transpositional or heterotopic replantation). (*A* to *C*, from Meyer V. E., Chen, Z. W., and Beasley, R. W.: Surg. Orthop. Clin. North Am., *12*:871, 1981.)

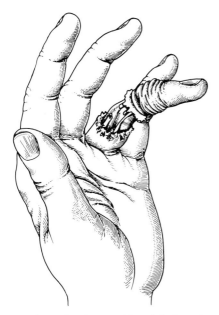

Figure 85–10. In ring avulsion injuries, the main vascular system may be either completely or partially disrupted. These injuries are typical examples of the need for microsurgical revascularization for survival or for improvement (see text).

greatly improved the prognosis in these injuries when surgery is appropriate (Fig. 85–11).

Socioeconomic Factors. With regard to the present problem of the staggering cost of health care, socioeconomic factors require due consideration. The feasibility of replantation or any other complex microsurgical procedure must not be the sole criterion for performing the operation. As already mentioned, in distal amputations of digits at the level of the interphalangeal or distal interphalangeal joint, replantation may be technically possible, but in many professions the physical impairment is of a relatively minor degree. If a replantation center could reattach all these distal parts, the public would rapidly consider replantation in all these situations as the only adequate treatment, and consequently it would be concluded that every patient has a right to have an amputated fingertip reattached. There is no doubt that this would create a sad situation for both patient and surgeon.

FREE MICROSURGICAL TISSUE TRANSPLANTATION

At this time there is no other area of reconstructive microsurgery in which development has been more rapid. A great variety of these procedures must be considered as established methods of treatment; others, however, need further clinical experience and critical evaluation. This whole area is still the subject of rapid development and change. There is no doubt that its contributions to reconstructive surgery have definitely improved the possibilities of treatment for many patients.

The main advantages of free microsurgical tissue transplantation are obvious:

1. Many complex reconstructions can be achieved in a one stage procedure that otherwise would necessitate multiple stage operations (Blair, 1982).

2. Troublesome positioning and fixation is avoided.

3. The period of immobilization of the patient and of the extremity, as well as the duration of hospitalization, may often be drastically shortened.

4. Free flap transfers offer more freedom and possibility in terms of the required tissue match of the recipient area (e.g., skin color, thickness, texture, hair growth, and amount of subcutaneous fat tissue).

5. The choice of the donor site is not restricted by the recipient area.

6. There is the possibility of restoring sensibility by the use of neurovascular flaps, which especially in the hand is of utmost importance (Gilbert et al., 1975).

7. Tissue transfers are now possible that could not be achieved with traditional methods, such as transplantations of musculature that will become functional at the recipient area (Ikuta et al., 1976; Manktelow et al., 1984).

The basic disadvantages are the relatively long operating time, the availability of appropriate recipient vessels, the possibility of early vascular thrombosis threatening the survival of the whole transplanted tissue block, the difficult and tedious postoperative surveillance needed for early detection of vascular thrombosis, and the possible morbidity or disfigurement at the donor site.

It is particularly this last point that needs

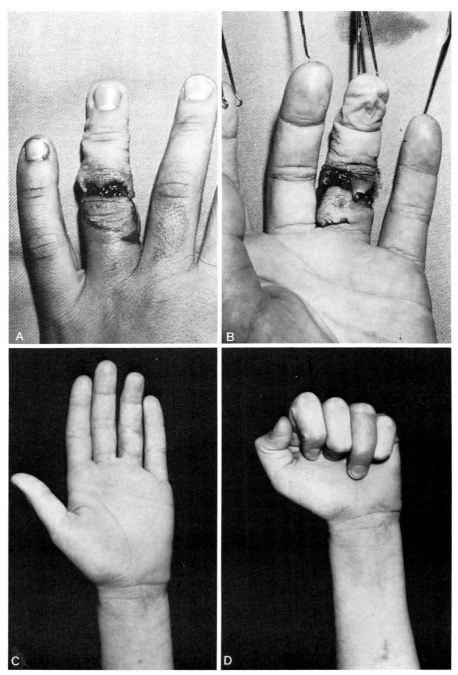

Figure 85–11. Typical ring avulsion injury in a 12-year-old boy with an oblique fracture of the middle phalanx and severance of both palmar arteries and all dorsal veins. *A* and *B*, The literally bloodless ring finger with sunken and wrinkled pulp. *C* and *D*, Functional result four months after revascularization and nerve repair. Some lack of extension and flexion of the distal interphalangeal joint remained.

careful consideration and balance against traditional methods of treatment, especially
when the donor site is in an exposed area,
when it cannot be closed directly and will
necessitate free skin grafting, or when it will
lead to obvious permanent disfigurement, as
in the great toe to hand transfer.

It is not the purpose in this presentation to
discuss the pros and cons of all of today's
available procedures. The following few examples, however, should illustrate the author's main concern.

TOE TO HAND TRANSFER

As early as the beginning of this century,
the successful use of toe to hand transfer for
replacement of a thumb and even an index
finger was reported (Eiselberg, 1900; Nicoladoni, 1900). It was not until 1969 that the
first report of a successful clinical free microsurgical total hand transfer was published
(Cobbet, 1969). Initially the transfer of the
hallux was preferred for thumb replacement.
At the present time there is a trend in favor
of the use of the second toe because of less
disfigurement and morbidity of the donor
foot (Figs. 85–12, 85–13; Chen et al., 1981a).

In a series of 12 possible candidates for
thumb replacement by a second toe to hand
transfer, eight refused to accept this operation after having seen in photographs the
esthetic result expected. This reflects the serious concern about esthetics with regard to
the hand in our patients. Through preoperative photography a realistic idea of the appearance to be anticipated can be given to
the patient in order to facilitate his participation in the evaluation of the best possible
treatment (Fig. 85–12).

Of course, toe to hand transfer also may
be considered if all four fingers have been
lost (Fig. 85–13).

Without doubt, the possibility of restoring
sensibility is a great advantage in toe transplantation (Yang and Gu, 1979).

There are rare cases in which multiple toe
transfers may be considered, e.g., the second
toe from each foot in case of complete loss
of all five digits. "En bloc" transplantation
of two toes from one foot, in cases of loss of
all four fingers, however, should not be performed, because two toes "en bloc" do not
improve prehension enough to justify the
major mutilation of the donor foot (Chen et
al., 1981a). Toe transfer in unilateral congenital deformities requires extremely careful

evaluation, because in unilateral congenital
hand or ray deficiencies it is the psychological
impact of the deformity on the patient and
his family that often is the prime problem,
not the physical handicap. Any plan of treatment for these individuals must be based on
a clear recognition of this reality.

In the bilateral amputee or in cases of
bilateral congenital absence of prehension,
however, the physical impairment is so severe
that it outweighs the esthetic considerations
(Beasley, 1969; Loosli-Guignard and Verdan,
1983; Tubiana, 1981).

As an alternative to toe to hand transfer,
transplantation of digits from the contralateral hand is possible. In general, great reserve
is indicated in the use of an uninjured hand
as donor site for such transfers. However, it
may well be considered in case of bilateral
injuries, e.g., transfer of a stiff finger from
one hand to replace a thumb on the other
hand (Büchler, 1981).

In reconstructing a thumb, excellent results
can be achieved by the use of a traditional
bone graft in combination with a so-called
microsurgical wrap-around flap from the big
toe, including the nail, which leaves the major part of the hallux intact (Morrison et al.,
1979).

Today soft tissue replacement and restoration of sensibility are among the most challenging indications for free microsurgical
tissue transplantation. Because the upper extremity is a highly mobile unit, vascularized
tissue coverage can be achieved by various
approved distant pedicle flap procedures. A
free flap is used only if the advantages convincingly outweigh the disadvantages of a
traditional procedure.

Depending on the patient, a sophisticated
microsurgical procedure can be either part of
primary repair or applied secondarily during
definite reconstructive surgery.

Groin Flap

The introduction of the groin flap with its
axial pattern vascular system represents an
important contribution for soft tissue replacements in the upper extremity (McGregor,
1972). The specific axial vascular system of
this flap was the basis for the free transplantation of that flap by means of microvascular
anastomosis (Daniel and Taylor, 1973).

Regardless of whether this flap is used as
a traditional pedicle flap or as a free microsurgical flap, its donor area is probably as-

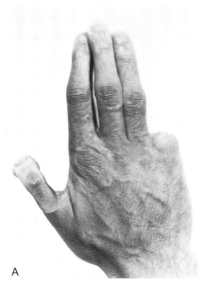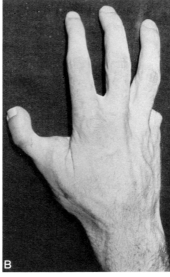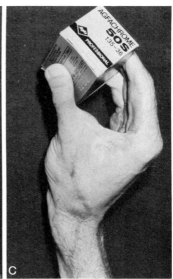

Figure 85–12. Thumb replacement by free microvascular second toe transfers. *A,* Preoperative photograph reflecting the esthetic appearance to be anticipated. *B* and *C,* Condition six months after uncomplicated second toe transfer. (*A* to *C,* from Meyer, V. E.: *In* Evarts, C. M. (Ed.): Surgery of the Musculoskeletal System, Vol. 1. New York, Churchill Livingstone, 1983.)

sociated with the least morbidity and disfigurement because the wound can be directly closed and the resulting scar lies within a hardly exposed area (Fig. 85–14). Raising the flap for free transfer requires tedious preparation and may be difficult, a fact that correlates with its small vascular pedicle and frequent anatomical vascular variations.

Other free flaps have been developed, since longer vascular pedicles with much larger vessel diameters make the procedure easier and faster (Maxwell et al., 1979). However, at this time the groin flap should still be the mainstay of coverage in hand surgery, particularly as a pedicle flap.

The anatomical relationship between the hand and foot predestines the foot to be a potential donor area for tissue replacement in the hand in even a broader sense than the aforementioned toe to hand transfer (McGraw and Furlow, 1975; Morrison et al., 1979; O'Brien and Shanmugan, 1973; Taylor and Townsend, 1979).

Dorsalis Pedis Flap

The tissue match of a dorsalis pedis flap for soft tissue replacement of the dorsum of the hand is optimal in most individuals. However, if the flap is large, the disfigurement and even the potential morbidity of the donor site are sizeable (Fig. 85–15). Conspicuous scarring and even recurrent ulcerations result, especially in the area of the extensor hallucis longus and prominent bones (Fig. 85–16). In smaller dorsalis pedis flaps, which preferably are centered over the distal third of the metatarsals, the aforementioned problems are usually not encountered.

Other Considerations

Although effective traditional methods for restoration of sensibility in the hand are well established (Littler, 1956), free transfer of neurovascular island flaps opens new perspectives. By use of a free microvascular island flap from the pulp of the big toe, sensibility in the area of pinch of the digit can be substantially improved with little morbidity and disfigurement at the donor site (Fig. 85–17; Buncke and Rose, 1979). In acute cases one must bear in mind that eventually neurovascular island flaps may be harvested from nonreplantable parts. Well selected patients may also be candidates for the use of free vascularized bone grafts to bridge extensive skeletal gaps or free muscle transplantation to restore motor function in the upper extremity (Ikuta et al., 1976; Manktelow et al., 1984; Pho, 1979; Taylor et al., 1975). Microsurgical tissue transplantation is still subject to intensive investigation, rapid

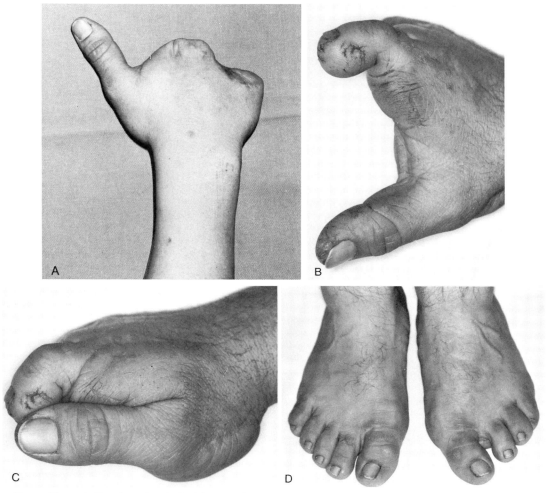

Figure 85–13. *A*, Dominant hand of a 26-year-old carpenter showing transmetacarpal loss of all four fingers. *B* and *C*, Improved prehensile capacity by second toe transfer to the second metacarpal; condition after eight years. *D*, Donor foot after eight years, with only minimal disfigurement. The patient does not have any disability of the donor foot.

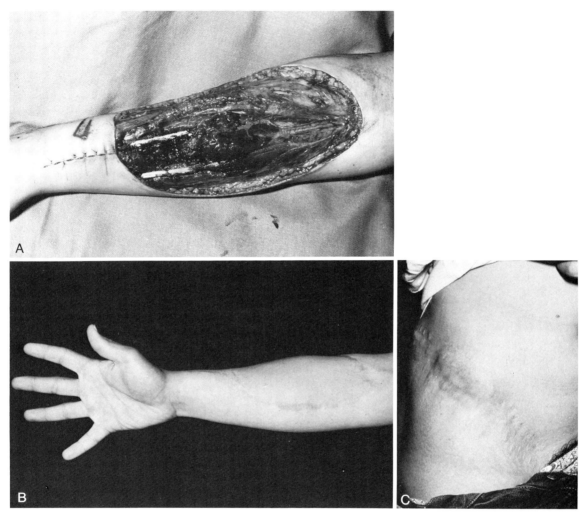

Figure 85–14. *A*, Major soft tissue and bone defect of the radius in a 12-year-old boy after an accident involving a circular saw. The photograph shows the condition after reconstruction of the radius by a bridge plate and cancellous bone grafting over a distance of 6 cm. with restoration of the severed muscle-tendon units. The metal plate is exposed in the wound. In this situation it was decided to provide definitive soft tissue coverage by a free microvascular groin flap as part of the primary procedures. *B*, Condition after two years. No defatting procedures were necessary in this case. *C*, Direct closure of the donor site resulted in minimal disfigurement in a minimally exposed body region.

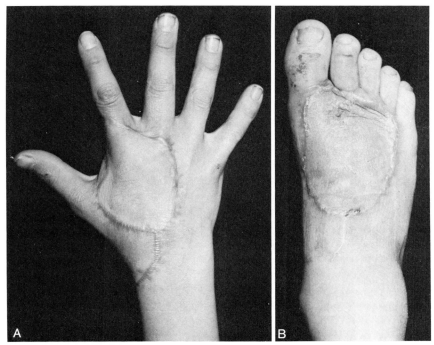

Figure 85–15. *A*, Reconstruction of the dorsum of the hand in a 13-year-old boy by a neurovascular dorsalis pedis flap. *B*, The hand had an excellent result, but a conspicuous but stable scar remained on the donor foot (condition at three years).

changes, and progress (Acland, 1981; Nassif et al., 1982; Song et al., 1982a,b).

Replantation and free microsurgical tissue transplantation are in general extremely time-consuming operations, which are beyond the realistic limit for a single surgeon. The necessity for a team of qualified surgeons is now generally accepted. However, this team approach should never favor a dilution of the responsibility with respect to the patient. To counter this potential danger, one surgeon of the team (preferably the most experienced one) should take overall responsibility regarding the patient and be the treating surgeon during the time of rehabilitation.

A replantation center requires not only a sufficient number of qualified surgeons but also a broad institutional commitment (Biemer and Duspiva, 1982; Burton et al., 1981). Microsurgical tissue transplantation can then be possible as part of the initial primary care. Basically the well accepted concept of total

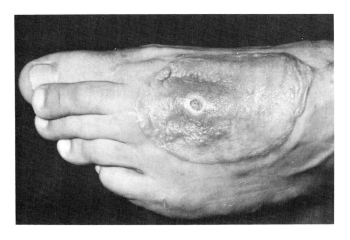

Figure 85–16. Donor foot of a 24-year-old woman after a dorsalis pedis flap transfer. Recurrent ulceration of the skin graft over the second metatarsal resulted in exposure of extensor tendons. It took three months, including six weeks of immobilization, to achieve definite healing.

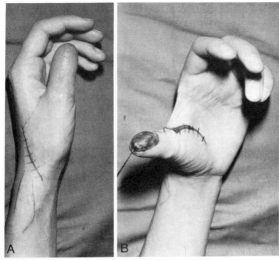

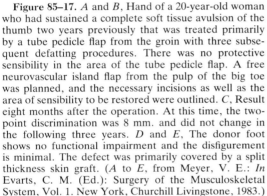

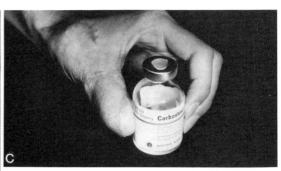

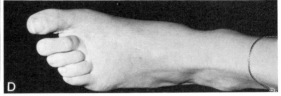

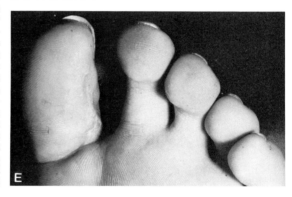

Figure 85–17. *A* and *B*, Hand of a 20-year-old woman who had sustained a complete soft tissue avulsion of the thumb two years previously that was treated primarily by a tube pedicle flap from the groin with three subsequent defatting procedures. There was no protective sensibility in the area of the tube pedicle flap. A free neurovascular island flap from the pulp of the big toe was planned, and the necessary incisions as well as the area of sensibility to be restored were outlined. *C*, Result eight months after the operation. At this time, the two-point discrimination was 8 mm. and did not change in the following three years. *D* and *E*, The donor foot shows no functional impairment and the disfigurement is minimal. The defect was primarily covered by a split thickness skin graft. (*A* to *E*, from Meyer, V. E.: *In* Evarts, C. M. (Ed.): Surgery of the Musculoskeletal System, Vol. 1. New York, Churchill Livingstone, 1983.)

primary repair in replantation surgery should be extended for primary free microsurgical tissue transplantation if indicated. Usually these transfers can be performed much more quickly in the acute case, because frequently recipient vessels are already exposed and must not be tediously dissected in scarred tissues as in many cases of reconstructive surgery (Fig. 85–14). Experience has shown that scar tissue formation often extends (especially along neurovascular structures) far beyond the site of the original injury. This is possibly the result of persistent edema, which spreads along the pathway of the loose areolar tissue embedding these structures. Consequently preparation of recipient vessels in reconstructive surgery is often difficult, time consuming, and sometimes even hazardous. These difficulties can be avoided if definitive soft tissue coverage is achieved at the earliest time possible (Fig. 85–14).

Toe to hand transfer, however, requires such careful evaluation preoperatively that in general it should not be carried out as a part of the primary procedure.

Among traditional methods of treatment for restoration of prehension, there still exists an indication for Krukenberg's operation in well selected cases, as in the bilateral amputee, especially if the patient is blind at the same time, a situation that may occur after an explosion accident. With this operation the patient may recover a considerable degree of independence (Loosli-Guignard and Verdan, 1983; Tubiana, 1981).

In most medical educational programs little or no attention is given to the present possibilities of prosthetic devices for upper extremity amputees. The existence of high quality esthetic hand prostheses is still widely ignored. In the interest of comprehensive patient care, these alternatives deserve consideration (Baumgartner, 1981; Law, 1981; Pillet, 1981).

REFERENCES

Acland, R. D., et al.: The saphenous neurovascular free flap. Plast. Reconstr. Surg., 67:763, 1981.

Baumgartner, R.: Active and carrier-tool prostheses for upper limb amputations. Orthop. Clin. N. Am., 12:953, 1981.

Beasley, R. W.: Reconstructive surgery in the management of congenital anomalies of the upper extremity. In Swinyard, C. A. (Editor): Limb Development and Deformity: Problems of Evaluation and Rehabilitation. Springfield, Illinois, Charles C Thomas, 1969, p. 476.

Biemer, E., and Duspiva, W.: Reconstructive Microvascular Surgery. Berlin, Springer Verlag, 1982.

Blair, O. R.: One-stage reconstructions. Clin. Plast. Surg., 9, 1982.

Brown, P. W.: The rational selection of treatment for upper extremity amputations. Orthop. Clin. N. Am., 12:843, 1981.

Buck-Gramcko, D.: Angeborene Fehlbildungen der hand. In Nigst, H., Buck-Gramcko, D., and Millesi, H. (Editors): Handchirurgie. Stuttgart, Georg Thieme Verlag, 1981, Vol. I.

Büchler, U., and Tschopp, H. M.: Freie kontralaterale Zeigefinger-Pollizisation. Handchirurgie, 13:10, 1981.

Buncke, H. J., and Rose, E. H.: Free toe-to-fingertip neurovascular flap. Plast. Reconstr. Surg., 63:607, 1979.

Burton, R., Beasley, R. W., Omer, G., and Meyer, V. E.: Organization for upper limb reattachment surgery. Orthop. Clin. N. Am., 12:915, 1981.

Chen, Z. W., Meyer, V. E., and Beasley, R. W.: The versatile second toe microvascular transfer. Orthop. Clin. N. Am., 12:827, 1981a.

Chen, Z. W., Meyer, V. E., Kleinert, H. E., and Beasley, R. W.: Present indications and contra-indications for replantation as reflected by long-term functional results. Orthop. Clin. N. Am., 12:849, 1981b.

Cobbet, J. R.: Free digital transfer. Report of a case of transfer of a great toe to replace an amputated thumb. J. Bone Joint Surg., 51:677, 1969.

Daniel, R. W., and Taylor, G. I.: Distant transfer of an island flap by microvascular anastomoses. Plast. Reconstr. Surg., 52:111, 1973.

Eiselsberg, V.: Ersatz des Zeigefingers durch die zweite Zehe. Arch. Klin. Chir., 61:2, 1900.

Foucher, G., et al.: Distal digital replantation: one of the best indications for microsurgery. Int. J. Microsurg., 3:263, 1981.

Gilbert, A., Morrison, W. A., and Tubiana, R.: Transfert sur la main d'un lambeau libre sensible. Chirurgie, 101:691, 1975.

Ikuta, Y., et al.: Free flap transfer by end-to-side arterial anastomosis. Br. J. Plast. Surg., 28:1, 1975.

Ikuta, Y., Tsuge, K., and Kubo, T.: Free muscle transfers by neurovascular anastomosis using microsurgical techniques—a clinical case. Plast. Reconstr. Surg., 58:407, 1976.

Jaeger, S. H., Tsai, T. M., and Kleinert, H. E.: Upper extremity replantation in children. Orthop. Clin. N. Am., 12:897, 1981.

Law, H. T.: Engineering of upper limb prostheses. Orthop. Clin. N. Am., 12:929, 1981.

Littler, J. W.: Neurovascular pedicle transfer of tissue in reconstructive surgery of the hand. J. Bone Joint Surg., 38A:917, 1956.

Loosli-Guignard, R. M., and Verdan, C.: Krukenberg's operation; indications and limitations. Ann. Chir. Main, 2:154, 1983.

Manktelow, R. T., Zuker, R. M., and McKee, N. H.: Functioning free muscle transplantation. J. Hand Surg., 9, 1984.

Maxwell, G. P., Mansons, P. N., and Hoopes, J. E.: Experience with thirteen latissimus dorsi myocutaneous free flaps. Plast. Reconstr. Surg., 64:1, 1979.

McCraw, M. J. B., and Furlow, L. T.: The dorsalis pedis arterialized flap. Plast. Reconstr. Surg., 55:177, 1975.

McGregor, I. A., and Jackson, I. T.: The groin flap. Br. J. Plast. Surg., 25:3, 1972.

Meyer, V. E.: Beitrag zur Indikation und Technik der mikrochirurgischen Revaskularisation im Vorderarm-Handbereich. Z. Unfallmed. Berufskr., 75:29, 1982.

Morrison, W. A., O'Brien, B. M., and MacLeod, A. M.: The foot as a donor site in reconstructive microsurgery. World J. Surg., 3:43, 1979.

Nassif, T. M., et al.: The parascapular flap: a new cutaneous microvascular free flap. Plast. Reconstr. Surg., 69:591, 1982.

Nicoladoni, C.: Daumenplastik und organischer Ersatz der Fingerspitze. Arch. Klin. Chir., 61:606, 1900.

O'Brien, B. M., and Shanmugan, M.: Experimental transfer of composite free flaps with microvascular anastomoses. Aust. N. Z. J. Surg., 43:285, 1973.

O'Brien, B. M.: Microvascular Reconstructive Surgery. New York, Churchill Livingstone, 1977.

Pho, R. W. H.: Free vascularized fibular transplant for replacement of the lower radius. J. Bone Joint Surg., 61B:362, 1979.

Pillet, J.: The aesthetic hand prosthesis. Orthop. Clin. N. Am., 12:961, 1981.

Song, R., et al.: The forearm flap. Clin. Plast. Surg., 9:21, 1982a.

Song, R., Song, Y., Yu, Y., and Sang, Y.: The upper arm free flap. Clin. Plast. Surg., 9:27, 1982b.

Taylor, G. I., Miller, G. D. H., and Harn, F. J.: The free vascularized bone graft. Plast. Reconstr. Surg., 55:533, 1975.

Taylor, G. I., and Townsend, P.: Composite free flap and tendon transfer: an anatomical study and clinical technique. Br. J. Plast. Surg., 32:170, 1979.

Tubiana, R.: Krukenberg's operation. Orthop. Clin. N. Am., 12:819, 1981.

Yang, D., and Gu, Y.: Thumb reconstruction utilizing second toe transplantation by microvascular anastomosis. Chinese Med. J., 92:295, 1979.

Chapter 86

TECHNIQUE AND RESULTS OF DIGITAL AND UPPER LIMB REPLANTATION

ALFRED BERGER
AND HANNO MILLESI

ORGANIZATION AND PREPARATION

During recent years a large number of replantations have been performed by different centers and have become nearly routine. A successful replantation depends on the coexistence of several factors. The patient has suffered an amputation with a degree of damage such that a replantation will still be possible. During emergency treatment someone must think of the possibility of replantation and secure the amputated part. The tissue should not suffer autolysis. The patient has to be transported to a center where replantation is possible, and equipment and trained personnel must be available, including sufficient operative capacity to allow the use of an operating room for many hours. Organization and sufficient information are necessary to create these circumstances. Guidelines, as outlined in Table 86–1, should be distributed to everybody involved in the care of trauma cases (Millesi, 1976).

In the spring of 1974 a replantation service was organized in Vienna. Two plastic surgical units (I and II, Chirurgische Universitätsklinik) with seven microsurgeons took part in this organization (Berger et al., 1979). Each of the units was on duty for 24 hours. The following discussion refers to the patients treated in the Plastic Surgical Unit of Chirurgische Universitätsklinik I.

Linking the replantation service to a plastic and reconstructive surgery unit proved to be successful because personnel and equipment were used economically. With such a unit, surgical operations can be performed routinely in cases of reconstruction and not only for replantation. This insures constant training of surgeons in microsurgical procedures. Replantation requires intensive postoperative care, energetic rehabilitation, and often several reconstructive operations. It is of great value if the same surgeon performs the replantation and supervises the rehabilitation; it can then be assumed that he will become more fully engaged to achieve a good result with "his" case. For this reason we do not like to use different surgeons for the microvascular procedures and for dealing with the other tissues, as has been suggested (O'Brien et al., 1973).

The information about the possibility of replantation has to reach all the people involved with first aid, for example, the Red Cross, accident hospitals, countryside hospitals, and general practitioners—in short, everyone who might be involved in providing first aid in a case of an accident. (As an example, Table 86–1 shows a reproduction of our information leaflet, which has been distributed by our service since 1974.) The amputated part should be secured and cooled to reduce the period of warm ischemia.

Preservation by cooling is simple to achieve. Two plastic bags and ice cubes are required. One bag is filled with ice cubes. The amputated part is put into the second plastic bag and this bag is put on top of the bag with the ice cubes with a towel in between. Cooling should be maintained at about 4° C. (Fig. 86–1). Cooling at a lower temperature causes freezing and irreversible

972

Table 86–1. GUIDELINES FOR TOTAL OR SUBTOTAL AMPUTATION

A. Total amputation
  1. Hemostasis
     a. Distal to the wrist: pressure dressing
     b. Proximal to the wrist: ligature and, if necessary, shock treatment
  2. Cooling of the amputated part not to exceed 4° C. in both directions (no freezing); necessary items:
     a. Two polythene (plastic) bags
     b. Ice cubes (deep freezing equipment is not allowed)
        1. One polythene (plastic) bag contains the amputated part and is closed in a way that no ice water or other fluids can enter that bag; the amputated part remains completely out of direct contact
        2. The second polythene (plastic) bag contains ice cubes; the first polythene (plastic) bag is placed into the second one
  3. Transportation and information for the replantation center
B. Subtotal amputation
  1. No local surgical treatment
  2. No cooling
  3. Dry sterile dressing
  4. Splint the joints in midposition; twisting of the injured part must be avoided
C. Contact the Viennese Replantation Team
  On odd days: Department of Plastic and Reconstructive Surgery, 1st Surgical Clinic
  Phone 4800, extension 2269 or 2255
  On even days: Department of Plastic and Reconstructive Surgery, 2nd Surgical Clinic
  Phone 4800, extension 2176 or 2171

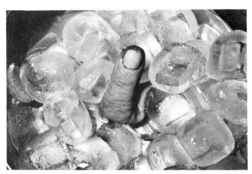

Figure 86–2. Incorrect preparation. The amputated part is in direct contact with the ice cubes, which will cause freezing of the tissues.

required, the ice cubes need to be replaced from time to time.

With the exception of cooling, nothing should be done with the amputated part. Perfusions, as performed in the early days, damage the capillary bed. A pressure dressing is applied to the amputated stump to effect hemostasis.

INDICATIONS AND CONTRAINDICATIONS

The Patient. The age and general state of the patient influence the decision. Age itself is not a contraindication, provided marked arteriosclerosis can be excluded. Professional skill and the motivation of the patient are important factors.

Involved Part. If a thumb is amputated, replantation should be attempted whenever possible. A single finger should be replanted only under certain conditions: (1) Any digit that is amputated in a child should be replanted. (2) The index finger in an adult or other single digits are replanted if the profession and motivation of the patient strongly indicate. However, if two or more fingers are involved, replantation is strongly justified. The same is true if the amputation is across the palm or more proximal.

Amount of Damage. The amount of damage depends on the nature of the trauma. Clean amputations by a knife or a rotating saw cause only local tissue damage and offer the best chances for survival. If the amputation is associated with severe crushing, the prognosis is much poorer. The same is true for avulsions (Fig. 86–3). In these cases the intima of the vessels can be damaged far proximally, and for this reason the anasto-

damage to the tissue. This will also happen if there is direct contact with the ice cubes or if, after the ice cubes have melted, the amputated part floats in the ice water (Fig. 86–2). If transportation over long distance is

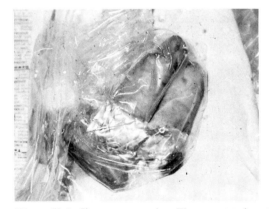

Figure 86–1. Correct preparation. The amputated part is placed in a separate plastic bag, and this plastic bag is placed in another bag that is filled with ice cubes. The tissues will be cooled to about 4° C.

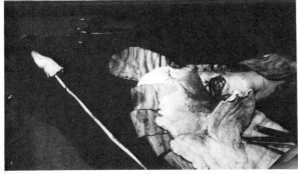
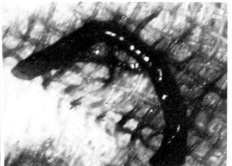
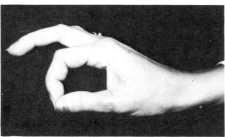

Figure 86–3. *A*, A 27-year-old woman with an avulsion injury with complete amputation of the right thumb. Replantation was performed using vein grafts. *B*, Results at eight months. Two-point discrimination was 6 mm. Movement was within the normal range and there was no sensitivity. *C*, A vein graft was taken from the volar aspect of the wrist. The graft measured 25 mm. long and 2 mm. in diameter.

mosis has to be performed at the level of completely normal vessels. Often the use of long vein grafts is necessary.

Condition of the Amputated Part. If the duration of warm ischemia is not too long, and preservation by cooling has been performed in the proper way, the conditions exist for a successful replantation. A very long period of warm ischemia, insufficient cooling, and freezing are contraindications (Berger and Millesi, 1977; Biemer and Duspiva, 1977; Owen, 1975).

REPLANTATION

After arrival, the patient is prepared for a long operation. General anesthesia is given by an experienced anesthetist, or block anesthesia is used. (Replantations proximal to the wrist level may require two teams.)

Step 1. Preparation of stumps. Under tourniquet control the structures of the proximal cross sections are identified—the type of fracture, the palmar arteries, the dorsal veins, the digital nerves, and the flexor tendons and the extensor tendons. Crushed tissue is excised. The vessel stumps are flushed with a heparin solution. They are carefully inspected to identify intimal damage. The use of a vein graft is considered.

Step 2. Preparation of the amputated part.

At the last possible moment, cooling is interrupted or continued by the use of ice cubes packed in sterile plastic bags and placed on the operation table. The cross section of the amputated part is treated in the same way as the proximal stump.

Step 3. Osteosynthesis. There are several methods of performing the osteosynthesis.

Kirschner Wire. One Kirschner wire is introduced in longitudinal direction to achieve longitudinal stability. If any shortening is required, some bone is removed and the two bone fragments are approximated. A second Kirschner wire provides rotational stability.

Plates and Screws. The use of plates and screws is indicated in amputations at the proximal level. In digital amputations this procedure would require rather extensive exposure of the bone fragments.

Compression Wires. Daniel and Terzis (1977) recommend the use of compression wires, which are introduced by the use of small drill holes.

Special Techniques. Recently special techniques for replantation have been developed to achieve intramedullary fixation (Ikuta, 1975). Zwank (1978) combines the use of Kirschner wires with screws.

Arthrodesis. If the amputation happens to cross a digital joint, an immediate arthrodesis in the position of function is a good solution.

Step 4. The next step in digital amputation is suturing of the extensor tendon.

Step 5. Suturing of profundus and superficialis flexor tendon is carried out next.

Step 6. Anastomosis of the digital arteries. The artery clamps are removed and circulation is re-established.

Step 7. Dorsal veins. Two or three dorsal veins are anastomosed either directly or by the use of vein grafts.

Step 8. Coaptation of the digital nerves either directly or by the use of nerve grafts.

Step 9. Suturing of the dorsal skin.

Step 10. Closure of the palmar skin. It is extremely important to avoid constriction. Longitudinal incisions at the peripheral skin margin produce triangular defects. These are covered with thin split thickness skin grafts, which have proved valuable.

Step 11. Immobilization using volar or dorsal splints with the avoidance of any constriction. Elevation is effected in a middle position between 45 and 60 degrees.

POSTOPERATIVE CARE

Postoperative care consists of fluid replacement, infusions of low molecular weight plasma expanders (Rheomacrodex, 2 × 250 ml. per day), acetylsalicylic acid (aspirin, 1 gram per day), dipyridamole (Persantine, three 25 mg. tablets per day), and systemically administered antibiotics. Low doses of heparin may be given (3 × 5000 units per day). The most important point is continuous observation and immediate reoperation if the circulation deteriorates. Several patients have been saved by revision of the arterial or venous anastomosis. In these cases usually a vein graft has to be used, or the anastomosis has to be redone to re-establish the circulation.

USE OF VEIN GRAFTS

Arterial and venous anastomoses have to be performed without any tension. On the other hand, sufficient resection of the ends is necessary to remove crushed tissue. This means that in many instances, because shortening should be avoided, a vein graft has to be used to establish continuity. In case of arterial or venous thrombosis, if an anastomosis has to be revised and resected, the vein graft is often the only solution. Vein grafts can be provided from the volar aspect of the forearm or from the dorsum of the foot. A segment as long as necessary is excised. The branches have to be ligated; the vein graft in arterial reconstruction is interposed in a reversed manner, its proximal end being anastomosed with the distal vessel stump and vice versa to avoid impeding the blood flow by vein valves (see Table 86–4).

The application and the results of vein grafting are presented in Table 86–2 (Piza-Katzer, 1979).

LEVEL OF AMPUTATION

Finger Tip to Nail Base. At these levels the vessels are too small to perform an anastomosis. However, the amputated part is small enough to offer a reasonably good chance of survival by simple regrafting as a "composite graft." The postoperative management is the same as for total amputation.

Nail Bed to Distal Interphalangeal Joint. At this level an arterial or venous anastomosis can be performed, although it is rather difficult because of the small diameter. Snyder et al. (1972) recommended suturing only the artery. The venous back flow is allowed to drain from the wound.

Distal Interphalangeal to Metacarpophalangeal Joint. This is the level at which amputations are most common. The description of the replantation technique refers to this segment.

Metacarpophalangeal Joint to Midpalm. Usually several digits are amputated. The arterial blood flow is restored by anastomosis of common digital arteries (1.5 to 2.5 mm. in diameter) and by venous anastomosis on the dorsum of the hand (2 mm. in diameter) (Fig. 86–4).

Proximal Half of the Palm. At this level, restoration of circulation is achieved by an anastomosis of the superficial or the deep arch.

Amputation at the Wrist Level and More Proximally. This is the true limb amputation (Fig. 86–5). The caliber of the vessels at this level is sufficiently large to allow use of conventional techniques of vascular surgery. Nerve repair should be performed using microsurgical techniques. Although the intrinsic muscles may suffer irreversible damage due to ischemia, a reasonably good result can be expected if sensibility returns because the forearm muscles are intact.

Table 86–2. AMPUTATIONS AND REPLANTATIONS*†

Primary Management with Autologous Vein Grafts

Patient No.	Age	Sex	Source of Injury	Amputation Level	Vein-Artery Graft (mm.)	Vein-Vein Graft (mm.)	Thrombosis
				Upper Extremity			
1	48	M	Circular saw	R./II/PIP		25	
2	66	M	Circular saw	L./I/MCP		30	
3	16	M	Circular saw	R./III/Ph2	18	20	24 hr.
					25	15	A + V
4	34	M	Circular saw	R./III/Ph2	20	35	
5	18	M	Circular saw	R./III/Ph1	8	10	
					18		
6	40	M	Circular saw	R./FA/3/3		30	
						40	
						40	
7	20	M	Cutting wheel	R./TT/PIP	22	18	
8	13	M	Gear shaft avulsion	R./I/Ph1	30		16 hr.
9	29	F	Avulsion	R./I/MCP		28	
10	19	M	Punching tool	R.wrist	40	30	
						50	
						60	
				L./wrist	35	40	Statim

Primary Management with Direct Repair (Vessel Suture)

11	16	M	Circular saw	L./I/IP			V/24 hr.
12	20	M	Circular saw	L./III/PIP			A/24 hr.

Severe Compound Hand Injuries or Incomplete Amputations: Primary Management with Autologous Vein Grafts

13	16	M	Meat tenderizer	R./II/Ph1	30		
14	60	F	Circular saw	L./II/Ph1	35		
15	42	M	Circular saw	L./I/MCP	20		
				L./IV/MCP	20		
16	26	M	Circular saw	L./III/Ph1	40		
17	18	M	Circular saw	R./II/PIP	5		
18	38	M	Axe	L./I/MCP	10		
				Lower Extremity			
19	8	F	Spade	L./I/MCP	8		

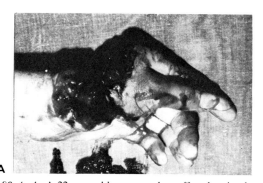
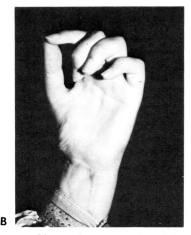

Figure 86–4. *A,* A 22-year-old woman who suffered a circular saw cut with complete amputation of the thumb and subtotal amputation of the index finger. Replantation of the thumb and of the index finger was carried out. *B,* Good functional result eight months later. Two-point discrimination was 6 mm. and good pinch and power grip were present.

Table 86–2. AMPUTATIONS AND REPLANTATIONS*† *Continued*

			Reoperation with Autologous Vein Graft					
FIRST REOPERATION, TIME AFTER PRIM. MANAGEMENT	INTERPOSITION VEIN GRAFT: ARTERY-VEIN (mm.)	INTERPOSITION VEIN GRAFT: VEIN-VEIN (mm.)	THROMBOSIS	SECOND REOPERATION	VEIN-ARTERY VEIN-VEIN		THROM-BECTOMY	REAMPUTATION
24 hr.	30	30						
16 hr.	80	35	A	7 days			X	X
Statim	70 50	60 70 80						
24 hr. 24 hr.	18	20	V	24 hr.	20	25		

*Adapted with permission from Piza, L. A.: Chir. Plast. (Berl.), 5, 1979.

†Vein grafts for bridging vessels in severe hand injuries and in amputations between 1975 and 1978. 19 patients and 21 parts—a total of 24 vein graft to artery and 22 vein graft to vein.

Primary management with vein grafts:

Seventeen patients and 19 parts—a total of 18 vein-artery and 15 vein-vein operations (16 parts survived); 3 parts had to be reoperated (a total of 4 vein-artery and 5 vein-vein; 2 parts survived; 1 part had to be reamputated (see case 8).

Two patients, after primary direct vessel anastomosis:

Secondary management with vein grafts: 2 parts (1 artery-vein and 1 vein-vein; 1 part survived). One part had to be reoperated: 1 vein-artery and 1 vein-vein (this part survived).

Of the total of 21 parts, one part had to be reamputated.

Limb Amputation at the Proximal Forearm, the Upper Arm, or the Shoulder Girdle

(Fig. 86–6). Vascular anastomosis is not the real problem in these cases. The amputated part contains a large amount of muscle, which is extremely sensitive to ischemia; the muscles suffer ischemic damage and necrosis develops. Even after good nerve regeneration, muscle function often does not return. Ischemic tissue damage may produce toxins, which are absorbed after the circulation is reestablished. The resulting toxemia endangers the patient's life. If infection occurs, septicemia may result. For this reason the decision to perform a limb replantation is more complicated. It should be performed only if the patient is in good general health. Successful replantations have been reported even up to the age of 56 years. Replantation should not be undertaken in the patient who has sustained other severe injuries.

The amputated limb must not be crushed, and it should not have been exposed to warm ischemia for more than four hours. Successful replantations have been reported after 20 or more hours if the limb was preserved by cooling. Perfusion is not necessary; a "washout" is sufficient. After careful excision of crushed tissue, a stable osteosynthesis with plates and screws is performed. The next step is arterial anastomosis to re-establish the blood flow as soon as possible. After venous

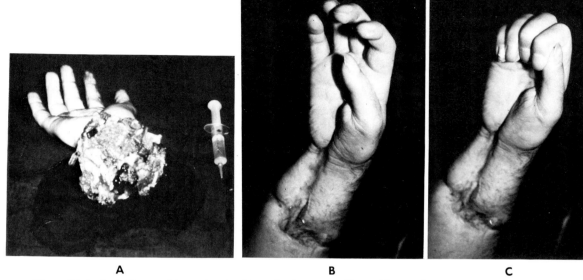

| A | B | C |

Figure 86–5. *A*, A 40-year-old man involved in a circular saw accident with complete amputation of the forearm. Replantation was done using three vein grafts 10 cm. each in length. *B*, Functional result one year later. Two-point discrimination of thumb was 8 mm.

anastomosis, muscles, tendons, and nerves are united. An extensive fasciotomy is important to avoid ischemic damage by postoperative swelling. Careful postoperative monitoring is necessary, and when the kidney function decreases to critical levels (urine outflow less than 20 ml. per hour, creatinine level over 3.0) for more than 48 hours, reamputation must be performed (Berger et al., 1979; Maurer, 1977).

RESULTS OF REPLANTATION

Evaluation of functional results after replantation surgery is extremely difficult. Several factors have to be considered. Complete amputations have to be distinguished from cases in which a connection remains with the proximal stump. If the soft tissue connection does not contain any vessels, restoration of blood flow has to be achieved if survival is to be secured. In this situation the term revascularization has become popular in spite of the fact that it involves restoration of blood flow, not of the vascular system. The prognosis, as far as survival is concerned, is not necessarily better than in complete amputations.

If the soft tissue connections are large enough to contain at least a vein, the prognosis is much better. These cases should be evaluated separately because they represent a much easier problem.

The functional result is influenced by the quality of the blood supply and the sensibility. The patient's satisfaction depends on his being able to use the replanted part. In addition to the circulation and sensibility, passive and active mobility must be evaluated. This evaluation has to be based on the severity of the injury and the extent of loss. If a single digit was replanted, it might become cumbersome if the joints are stiff and no active function is provided. By contrast, a stiff finger may be of great value to the patient if the other fingers are lost and the only successfully replanted finger is able to produce a pinch grip against the thumb. Therefore, the patient's satisfaction, which of course should be our main concern, depends on whether he is able to integrate the replanted part.

The results of our series between 1974 and 1978 are presented in Tables 86–3 to 86–6.

In whole limb replantations, the functional result will be satisfactory if muscles are available to achieve active motion. This is the case in peripheral forearm amputation but not necessarily at more proximal levels. However, even in some of these cases muscles survive and become reinnervated. Even if no

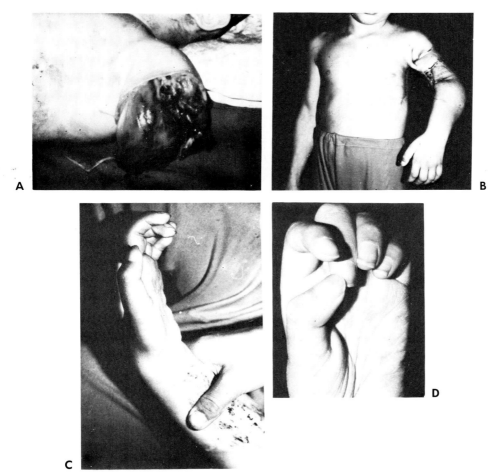

Figure 86–6. A nine-year-old boy with severe combined injury with complete amputation in the upper third of the arm. *A*, Replantation was done using local flaps. *B* and *C*, Result one and one-half years later. There was free movement of the elbow joint and protective sensibility of the median nerve. Opposition of the thumb is good. Flexion of the second and third digit is present. *D*, Replantation of the left arm, one and one-half years later. Flexion is useful and opposition is normal. Two-point discrimination of the thumb and middle finger is 10 to 12 mm.

Table 86–3. NUMBER OF CASES TREATED BY THE REPLANTATION SERVICE OF THE
I. CHIRURGISCHE UNIV -KLINIK IN VIENNA, JUNE 1974 TO THE END OF 1979

Treatment	Number of Patients	Number of Involved Parts	Number of Parts Surviving	Percentage
Total number of admitted patients	181			
No indication for replantation	60			
Complete amputations	48	57	29	51.0
Nearly complete amputation—no circulation distal to the injury	33	36	33	91.6
Restoration of original circulation	40	46	45	

Table 86–4. REPLANTATION SERVICE, I. CHIRURGISCHE UNIV.-KLINIK, VIENNA,
JUNE 1974 TO DECEMBER 1979

Type of Injury	Number of Patients	Number of Parts	Complete Amputation			Nearly Complete Amputation		
			NUMBER OF PATIENTS	NUMBER OF PARTS	SUR-VIVALS	NUMBER OF PATIENTS	NUMBER OF PARTS	SUR-VIVALS
Clean amputation	14	18	9	12	4	6	6	6
Rotating saw	45	59	28	34	20	22	25	23
Traffic accident	2	2	1	1	0	1	1	1
Degloving injury	1	1	1	1	1	—	—	—
Avulsion	9	9	6	6	4	3	3	3
Meat grinder	1	1	1	1	0	—	—	—
Crush injury	3	3	2	2	0	—	—	—
Total	75	93	48	57	29	32	35	33

Table 86–5. REPLANTATION SERVICE, I. CHIRURGISCHE UNIV.-KLINIK, VIENNA,
JUNE 1974 TO DECEMBER 1979

Level of Amputation	Complete Parts	Amputation Survivals	Nearly Complete Amputations	
			PARTS	SURVIVALS
Wrist	3	3	—	—
Metacarpus	5	4	1	1
Long fingers				
Proximal phalanx	18	7	14	12
Middle phalanx	12	6	9	9
Distal phalanx	5	0	4	3
Thumb				
Metacarpus	3	2	1	1
Proximal phalanx	8	6	6	6
Distal phalanx	3	1	1	1
Total	57	29	36	33

Table 86–6. FUNCTIONAL RESULTS IN 37 FINGERS REPLANTED OR REVASCULARIZED,
1975 TO 1977*†

			Thumb				
Case Number	Power (in Bar)	Temperature 0–2	2 PD (mm.)	Opposition	Flexion	Key Grip	Pinch Grip
25 (I)	0.01–0.38	2	6	Reduced	−	+	+ 2nd F.
72 (I)	0.21–0.25	2	4	Normal	+	+	+
49 (I)	0.5 −0.42	1	8	Normal	+ +	+	+
70 (I)	0.2 −0.32	1	10/Prot.	Normal	−	+	+
69 (I)	0.15–0.5	1–2	8	Normal	+ −	+	+
48 (I)	0.15–0.2	0–1	10	Normal	Reduced	+	+
82 (I)	0.08–0.2	2	8	Normal	Reduced	+	+
39 (M)	0.09–0.13	1–2	10	Reduced	+ −	+ −	+
66 (M)	0.17–0.28	2	−/Prot.	Very reduced	+	+ −	+
1 (M) left	0.05–0.45	0–1	6–10		Reduced	+ − (1–2)	− (1–2)
1 (M) right	0.15	2	10		−	+ − (1–3)	− (1–3)
27 (M)	0.18–0.2	2	6	Normal	Reduced	+	+

	Middle Finger					Ring Finger			
Case Number	Power (in Bar)	Temperature 0–2	2 PD (mm.)	FTPD (cm.)	Case Number	Power (in Bar)	Temperature 0–2	2 PD (mm.)	FTPD (cm.)
29 (I)	0.3–0.9	2	2–4	0	18 (I)	0.58	2	4	0
44 (M)	0.43	1	5	8	13 (I)	0.17–0.9	2	6	0
10 (M)	0.3	0	10	4	64 (I)	0.12	2	0	0
80 (M)	0.20–0.35	1	0	2.5	66 (M)	0.66	2	3	7
68 (M)	0.15	2	6	8	68 (M)	—	2	4	0
1 (M)	—	2	4	9					

	Index Finger			
Case Number	Power (in Bar)	Temperature 0–2	2 PD (mm.)	FTPD (cm.)
52 (I)	0.15–0.86	0	0	6
43 (I)	0.18–0.48	2	10	2.5
2 (I)	0.2	2	10	9
56 (I)	0.0	1	10	0
92 (I)	0.45	2	3	0
12 (I)	0.11–0.29	2	3	0.8
51 (I)	0.32	2	4–6	5
10 (M)	0.1 −0.34	1–2	10	8
44 (M)	0.43	2	6–10	5
80 (M)	0.20–0.35	1	0	3.5
68 (M)	0.15–0.2	2	6	4
39 (M)	0.09–0.26	2	10	9
1 (M)	0	2	8	5
27 (M)	0.2	1	Prot.	3.5

*Adapted with permission from Meissl, G.: Proc. Deutsch-Schweizerisch-Österreichische Unfalltagung, 1979.

†Of the fingers operated upon in our Replantation Service between 1975 and 1977, 37 have been analyzed from different points of view within a follow-up study that is still in progress.

Distribution of single (I) replantations or revascularizations:

7 thumbs, 7 index fingers, 1 middle finger, and 3 ring fingers.

Distribution of multiple (M) replantations or revascularizations:

5 thumbs, 7 index fingers, 5 middle fingers, and 2 ring fingers.

Our table shows the function of the whole finger rather than that of the replanted part only.

In the thumb the power (measured in bar) indicates the mean value at key grip and pinch grip and in the long fingers, the minimal and the maximal values.

Differentiation in temperature has been measured for cold and warm:

0 = no differentiation; 1 = 50% of differentiation; 2 = 100% of differentiation, or normal.

FTPD, distance between fingertip and palm at full flexion.

muscle recovery occurs, replantation is not
without value for particular patients. One of
our patients sustained an avulsion of the
shoulder girdle, including the scapula and
clavicle. The replanted limb survived but no
muscle function returned. Thus the case has
to be regarded as a failure. Nevertheless
preservation of the shoulder girdle was still
an advantage for the patient even if, because
of a lack of muscle function, an amputation
at the upper or forearm level has to be
performed eventually.

REFERENCES

Baudet, J., and Goumain, A. J. M.: Réimplantation
d'une main. Ann. Chir., 29:491–498, 1975.
Berger, A., Meissl, G., Millesi, H., and Piza, H.:
Komplikationen und Misserfolge durch negative Au-
swahl bei Replantation von abgetrennten Extremitä-
tenteilen. Handchirurgie, 9:59–62, 1977.
Berger, A., Millesi, H., Mandl, H., and Freilinger, G.:
Replantation and revascularisation of amputated parts
of extremities (a three year report from the Viennese
Replantation Team). Int. J. Microsurg., 1:18–21,
1979.
Berger, A., and Millesi, H.: Nerve repair after electrical
injuries. Proceedings, VII International Congress, International Confederation for Plastic and Reconstructive Surgery, Rio de Janeiro, May 20–25, 1979.
Berger, A., Meissl, G., Millesi, H., Piza, H., and
Walzer, L.: Functional results of replantation surgery
(a four year report from the Viennese Replantation
Team). Int. J. Microsurg., 1:22, 1979.
Biemer, E., and Duspiva, W. D.: Komplikationen bei
der Replantation abgetrennter Gliedmassen. Hand-
chirurgie, 9:67–70, 1977.
Daniel, R. K., and Terzis, J. K.: Reconstructive Micro-
surgery. Boston, Little, Brown and Company, 1977.
Foucher, G., Merle, M., and Michon, J.: L'ostéo-
synthèse Bilboquet. Ann. Chir., 31:1107–1108 , 1977.
Ikuta, Y.: Microvascular Surgery. Hiroshima, Lens
Press, 1975.
Krylow, V. S., Petrowsky, B. V., Stepanow, G. A., and
Akclurin, R. S.: Microsurgery in traumatic amputation
of the fingers and the hand. XV Symposium for
Surgery of the Hand, Wroclav, October 15–16, 1978.
Maurer, P. C., Oberlinner, R., Bonke, S., and Hopfner,
R.: Gefäßtraumen bei Mehrfachverletzen. In Kraft-
Kinz u. Kronberger. Kongreßbericht d. Österrei-
chischen Gesêllschaft für Chirurgie, Graz, 1977.
Meissl, G., Berger, A., Holle, J., Mandl, H., and
Millesi, H.: Funktionelle Ergebnisse in der Replanta-
tionschirurgie; Erfahrungsberichte des Wiener Re-
plantationsteams. Proc. Deutsch-Österreichisch-
Schweizerische Unfallheilkunde. Berlin, Springer Verlag, 1979.
Millesi, H.: Zufall oder Ergebnis sorgfältiger Planung—
Erfolgreiche Wiedereinpflanzung traumatisch ampu-
tierter Körperteile. Ärztl. Praxis, 28:1187–1188, 1976.
O'Brien, B. M., McLeod, A. M., Miller, G. D. H.,
Newing, R. K., Hayhurst, J. W., and Morrison, W.
A.: Clinical replantation of digits. Plast. Reconstr.
Surg., 51:490, 1973.
Owen, E. R.: Replantation of amputated extremities.
Langenbecks Arch. Chir., 339:613, 1975.
Piza-Katzer, H.: Analysis of complications in digital vein
grafts. Chir. Plast. (Berlin), 5:25–32, 1979.
Snyder, C. C., Stevenson, R. M., and Brown, E. Z.:
Successful replantation of totally severed thumb. Plast.
Reconstr. Surg., 50:533, 1972.
Zwank, L.: Abgewandelte Spickdrahtosteonsynthese bei
Fingerrreplantation durch Spickdrahtverschraubung.
Lecture, 1st Annual Meeting, German Speaking Study
Group for Microsurgery of Peripheral Nerves and
Vessels, Vienna, December 7–9, 1978.

Chapter 87

DIGITAL AND UPPER LIMB REPLANTATION

Harry J. Buncke

and Fredrick A. Valauri

The foundations of microsurgery can be traced to the early work of Murphy (1897), Carrel (1902), and Guthrie (1908), who demonstrated the feasibility of vascular anastomoses with good patency rates. Carrel and Guthrie (1906a,b) performed autotransplantation of the dog leg, kidney, and scalp, using their famous triangular vascular repair. Carrel cites Hopfner (1903) of Germany as being a pioneer in these procedures. Despite these monumental achievements of the early 1900s, there was little progress in transplantation surgery until the work of Androsov (1956) and Seidenberg et al. (1958), who experimentally and clinically anastomosed 2-mm. vessels when using vascularized bowel to reconstruct the esophagus (Seidenberg et al., 1959). Later, Jacobson and Suarez (1960) introduced the operating microscope to perform "microsurgical" repair of small vessels.

Even with the availability of suitable microscopes, the lack of small-diameter needles, suture material, and microsurgical instruments impeded success with "microminiature" (less than 1 mm.) vascular anastomoses. Buncke et al. (1965) produced 7- to 15-micron diameter nylon sutures with electroplated metallic tips (O'Brien and Hayhurst, 1973) that later led to the commercial manufacture of microsutures (Acland, 1972).

Clinical limb replantation became a reality when Malt (1964) replanted a completely severed arm. The Chinese soon followed with a series of upper and lower limb salvaging procedures (Chen et al., 1963, 1965).

Except for the fingertip replants of Douglas (1959) and Ladanyi (1970), the results of digital replants without vascular anastomoses were dismal.

In 1965, Buncke et al. (1966) microsurgically transferred the great toe to the thumb in a rhesus monkey. Later, in 1968, Cobbett (1969) performed the first great toe to thumb transfer in a human. In 1963, Kleinert (1963) repaired a digital artery to revascularize a partially amputated thumb. His case report suggested that magnification would improve the accuracy of small-vessel anastomoses. Using the operating microscope, Komatsu and Tamai (1968) performed the first replantation of a completely amputated digit.

GENERAL PRINCIPLES

Microsurgery is essential for replantation of all but the most distal amputations. Microsurgical success is multifactorial, depending upon experienced surgical teams that can perform these long procedures in an efficient and effective manner; a well-prepared emergency department staff that can stabilize and rapidly evaluate the patient by expedient physical examination, x-rays, and other laboratory tests; 24-hour availability of anesthesia, operating room, and microsurgical staffs; the availability of required microscopes, instruments, and sutures; a well-trained nursing staff for postoperative care and monitoring; occupational and physical therapists well versed in the unique needs of postreplantation rehabilitation; and social workers and psychologists to promote the patient's ability to cope with his injuries and regain an active and useful life.

The sine qua non of microsurgery is magnification. Surgical loupes, with their 4.5× to 6× magnification, are used initially for carefully assessing and identifying injured structures; the anastomoses of nerves and vessels are accomplished with the operating microscope using $6\times$ to $30\times$ magnification. The modern operating microscope usually has a foot pedal controlled with electric focusing, zoom, and X-Y control movement (voice-activated machines are now also on the market); a double-headed microscope that allows the surgeon and his assistant to utilize simultaneous binocular vision; high-intensity fiberoptic illumination; and a microscope-mounted camera and monitoring system that allow the scrub nurse to view the procedure and anticipate equipment and instrument needs. The monitors also provide the means to videotape procedures for documentation purposes (Hoerenz, 1980). The operating room hand table must be stable, with comfortable chairs that allow good posture and decrease conditions that cause fatigue.

INSTRUMENTS

Numerous instruments have been developed by many designers to fulfill several specialized needs (Bright, 1978). In general, these instruments must be fine tipped with accurately closing jaws, be of appropriate size and length to avoid hand fatigue, and have a non-glare surface to prevent eye strain. These delicate precision instruments must receive careful handling and gentle cleaning to avoid damage.

Forceps are available in several lengths with a variety of tip sizes and with toothed and non-toothed jaws. Generally, toothed forceps are used for larger structures during dissection and smooth forceps for handling vessels and tying microsutures.

Scissors are spring-loaded and are available with both sharp and blunt tips, as well as curved and straight jaws. Curved, blunt-tipped scissors are most commonly used for adventitial dissection; the straight, sharp-tipped scissors are used for trimming vessels and nerve ends.

Dilators are modified blunt forceps, used to dilate a vessel lumen mechanically prior to anastomosis. They are often used in conjunction with irrigation catheters (27 and 30 gauge) to relieve vessel spasm. Care must be taken not to damage the intima by overly vigorous dilation.

Vascular clamps, which are available in a variety of shapes and sizes, either single (Acland, 1974) or double (Zirkle and Seidenstricker, 1973), facilitate approximation of vessel ends. The clamp closing pressures of 30 gm. or less are important to prevent intimal damage (Thurston et al., 1976). Each surgeon may have preferences in the particular choice of clamps, depending on the vessel size, the topography of the wound, and the exposure of the vessels.

Needle holders, too, come in many sizes and shapes, with and without locking mechanisms, curved or straight jaws, and curved or flat jaw surfaces. Each surgeon chooses the instrument according to personal preference and the specific conditions required by the anastomosis.

Suture materials are generally monofilament nylon and are available with a variety of needle (Buncke and McLean, 1971) and suture sizes. These range from 9–0 with a 150-micron needle to 11–0 with a 50-micron needle. Suture recommendations are 9–0 for vessels proximal to the wrist, 10–0 for hand and proximal digital vessels, and 11–0 for distal digital vessels. Gentle handling is essential to avoid fracturing the suture by forceful grasping or pulling (Acland, 1975).

MICROSURGICAL TECHNIQUES

Vascular Anastomoses. Although often discussed separately, some commonality of principles applies to both venous and arterial anastomoses (Acland, 1980; Buncke et al., 1975). The proximal and distal vessel ends of the proposed anastomotic vessels must be undamaged, and there must be tension-free approximation of the vessel ends or the use of interposition vein grafts. The vessel edges and excess adventitia must be trimmed so that only clean, straight vessel ends are anastomosed with no intervening tissue. Good bleeding from the proximal artery and distal veins should be confirmed before starting the repair. This requires inspection for intraluminal thrombus, dilation, and heparinized saline irrigation beyond the vascular clamps. Anastomoses are best accomplished when the artery or vein is well exposed and easily visualized. Therefore, overhanging tissues that obscure the vessels should be retracted. Vascular clamps and gentle suction provide a dry "bloodless" field. Background materials will enhance contrast and thus facilitate suturing. A comfortable sitting position with wrists and hands well supported will reduce fatigue and improve control and manipulation of microinstruments. Moist white lap sponges and frequent wound irrigation with heparinized saline prevent microsutures from adhering to the wound area, which may cause breaking or tearing of a vessel wall if an adherent suture is drawn through the vessel.

Techniques for Suturing Anastomoses. Depending upon the vessel size, position, and the surgeon's preference, many techniques are possible (Cobbett, 1967; Hayhurst and O'Brien, 1975; Urbaniak et al., 1977). Large vessels with good exposure and adequate mobilization may be suitable for anastomoses using 0 degree, 180 degree, 90 degree, and 270 degree (or 0, 120, 240) sutures and interposing additional sutures for an 8- or 12-suture anastomosis. Furthermore, these vessels may permit turning in a double approximating clamp, thus placing the wall being sutured toward the operating microscope. Often, turning a vessel is not possible and a "back wall" technique is called for (Nathan and Rose, 1976; Harris et al., 1981). The sutures are placed in the posterior (or back) wall of the vessel and the back wall is completed first. Sutures are then placed on the front wall to complete the anastomosis. The running interrupted technique places the microsuture in a running fashion, with large loops of suture maintained between each bite (Fujino and Aoyagi, 1975; George et al., 1975). Later, the loops are cut, allowing both the operating surgeon and the assistant to tie knots simultaneously in the now interrupted sutures. Simultaneously placing and tying the sutures by the surgeon and the assistant requires a high degree of expertise and cooperation between the surgeons, but this technique is rapid and effective.

Some specific maneuvers that help in the performance of anastomoses include: (1) placing forceps within the vessel lumen and directing the needle between the blades of the forceps; this maintains the lumen, provides counterpressure, and allows the jaws of the forceps to support the vessel wall for more accurate and stable suture placement; (2) irrigating between sutures to "balloon-out" the anastomosis (Buchler et al., 1977); (3) using traction on back wall sutures to draw the back wall away from the front wall, thus minimizing the possibility of suturing the back to the front wall of the vessel; (4) having the assistant hold the adventitia to expose the inner lip of the vessel wall, which allows placing the needle while providing counterpressure to stabilize the passage of the needle through the vessel wall; and (5) using heparinized saline for irrigation and Weck* sponges to allow the vessel lumen to be seen throughout the performance of the anastomosis.

End-to-Side Anastomoses (Godina, 1979; Albertengo et al., 1981; Bas et al., 1986). Prepare the vessel end as just described. After determining a suitable point on the wall of the vessel to be used as the "side vessel," a 9–0 suture is placed in the wall and a "V" is cut full thickness on either side of this suture while traction is maintained in a centrifugal fashion. Good forward bleeding (artery) or back bleeding (vein) should be confirmed. After suitable clamps are applied following heparin irrigation, the lumen is inspected for thrombus. The more difficult side of the anastomosis should be sutured first; this may warrant a "back wall" technique (Harris et al., 1981).

When the anastomosis is completed, irrigation of the vessel surface with papaverine is often useful to relieve vascular spasm. The clamps are removed and the anastomosis is inspected for patency and seal. The fill-refill test, if done gently, will provide a reliable and innocuous test of the anastomosis (Grotz et al., 1982). If spasm is present, the adventitia should be dissected on either side of the anastomosis to look for an untied vessel branch, a frequent cause of localized spasm. Any untied branch should be ligated carefully to avoid compromising the lumen. Leaks from the anastomosis should be observed, but significant or persistent leaks should be treated by carefully placing additional sutures while the assistant irrigates the anastomosis.

Vein graft anastomoses are performed in a similar manner to venous anastomoses (Wilber et al., 1984). Whenever possible, vein graft anastomosis should be performed first at the more difficult site, as the graft will allow the anastomosis to be turned back and forth to permit fuller exposure. The easier anastomosis can then be accomplished by whichever technique is appropriate.

---

*Edward Weck & Company, Long Island City, New York.

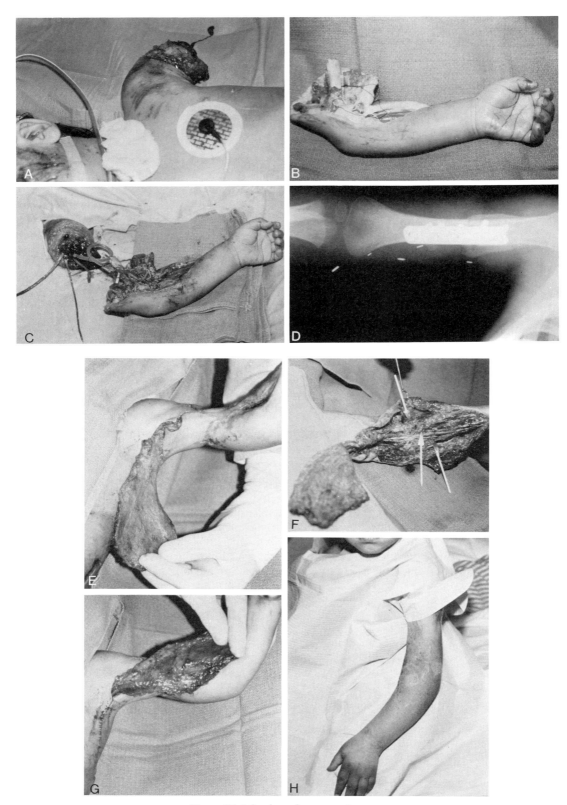

Figure 87–1 *See legend on opposite page*

REPLANTATION

Urbaniak (1982) has suggested that total replantation means the reattachment of a completely amputated part and that subtotal replantation means the restoration of viability to a partially amputated part that has suffered loss of circulation and some degree of severance of other structures, including skin, tendon, bone, or nerves. When confronted with a patient with a total amputation or a partial amputation, a surgeon must decide not only whether replantation is possible but also whether the patient is best served by replantation or by amputation. This latter point refers first to the easier decision of saving life over limb, as in the case of a multiply injured patient (Case 1; Fig. 87–1) in whom a prolonged replant procedure would jeopardize his life, and second to the more nebulous question of whether ultimate function and psychological well-being (as well as the financial burden of treatment) are best achieved by replantation or by completing the amputation.

Replantation viability does not imply replantation function. This important distinction must be made, and decisions concerning replantation versus completion of the amputation should not be based on the possibility of successful revascularization, but rather on successful restoration of function (Chen et al., 1981; Jones et al., 1982; Chase, 1970). Maximization of function in complex and multidigital and multilevel injuries can be managed by "part salvage" surgery (Chase, 1958; Alpert and Buncke, 1978; Keiter, 1980) in which "nonreplantable" amputated parts are used as heterotopic transplants to reconstruct the injured extremity (Case 2; Fig. 87–2). An example of this concept is a multiple level thumb and concomitant metacarpophalangeal level index finger amputation. The thumb is not replantable for *surgical* technical reasons, and poor function is expected from an index finger replanted at that level. However, because the amputated index finger is otherwise intact, it functions very well as a reconstructed thumb when pollicized to the first metacarpal of the stump. These decisions are usually not easy ones and must be made on a patient by patient basis and according to the experience of the treating surgeon (Hing et al., 1986; Manktelow, 1978).

Some general statements about amputations and replantations can be made: (1) sharp lacerating injuries have a better chance of successful outcome (Case 3; Fig. 87–3); (2) crush-avulsion injuries are most common; (3) distal injuries, except distal to the distal interphalangeal joint and trifurcation, have a more favorable prognosis than proximal injuries; (4) amputations of the upper extremities have a more favorable prognosis than amputations of the lower extremities; (5) short ischemic times indicate more favorable results than prolonged ischemic times; and (6) children usually fare better than adults.

Many authorities believe that certain circumstances offer good possibilities for replantation. Indications for replantations generally include nonavulsive amputation of (1) the thumb, (2) multiple digits, (3) digits distal to the superficial flexor insertion, (4) midcarpal level of the hand, (5) wrist, (6) forearm, (7) elbow or above elbow, and (8) limb and digit amputations in children.

Relative contraindications to replantations include (1) severe crush-avulsion injuries (Van Beek et al., 1978; Chen, 1973), (2) multiple level injuries, (3) multiple trauma victims, (4) patients with serious medical disease, (5) mentally unstable patients, (6) single digital amputations proximal to the superficial flexor insertion in adults, and (7) prolonged ischemic time, particularly in high amputations of the limbs in which a large

Figure 87–1. Case 1. *A* and *B*, This two-year-old boy sustained an avulsion amputation of his left arm, intra-abdominal hemorrhage from splenic lacerations, fracture of the right tibia and fibula, and facial abrasions as a result of being thrown from a car that was involved in a high-speed crash. The patient was resuscitated in the emergency room. A computed tomographic scan of his head was negative, and he underwent exploratory laparotomy for the suspected intra-abdominal injury. Concurrently, a second team of surgeons prepared the severed arm for replantation while awaiting the outcome of the laparotomy and stabilization of the patient's condition. *C*, A temporary arterial shunt was placed to perfuse the severed arm, thus restoring circulation and reducing ischemia time. *D*, Repair of the brachial artery was accomplished with an interposition vein graft after debridement and plate fixation of the humeral fragment was performed. *E* to *G*, Secondary surgery was performed, including excision of the antecubital fossa scar contracture; sural nerve grafting of the ulnar, radial, and median nerves; and coverage of this area with a pedicled latissimus dorsi muscle flap. *H*, Late result.

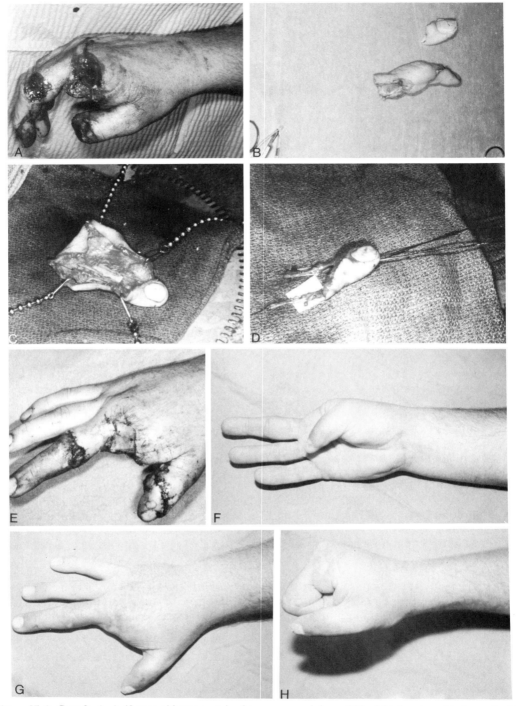

Figure 87–2. Case 2. *A,* A 40-year-old man sustained a power saw injury of his right thumb and index and middle fingers. *B,* The thumb was amputated at the distal phalanx level. The severed segment was not suitable for replantation owing to lack of suitable available vessels. *C* and *D,* The index finger had a multilevel injury, but a suitable distal fragment was used for a heterotopic (index to thumb) reconstruction of the thumb tip. *E,* The index finger stump was revised and closed, and the middle finger was revascularized. *F* to *H,* Postoperative appearance and function are excellent.

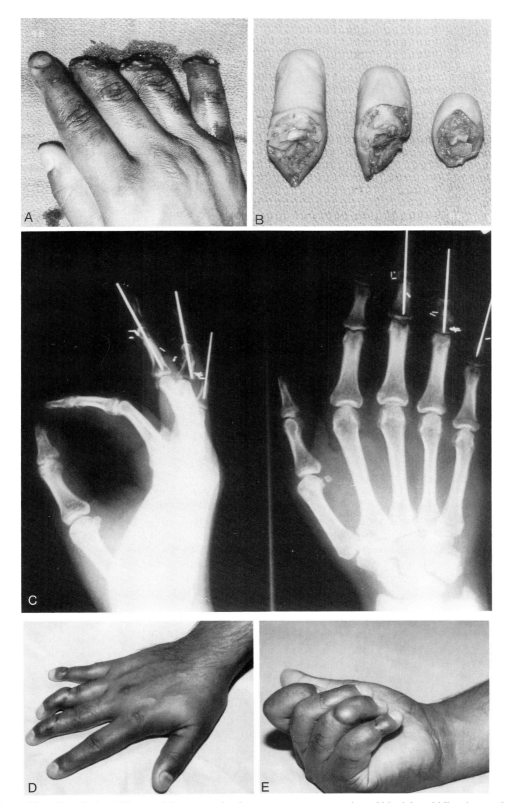

Figure 87–3. Case 3. *A*, A 28-year-old man sustained a paper cutter amputation of his right middle, ring, and small fingers. *B*, Sharp clean amputations of the middle and ring fingers at the middle phalanx level and the small finger at the distal interphalangeal joint. *C*, Kirschner wire fixation of the replanted digit. *D* and *E*, Appearance and function of the replanted digits.

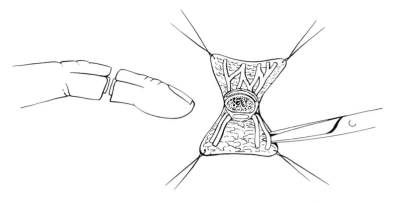

Figure 87–4. Midlateral incision for exposure of the neurovascular bundles.

muscle mass is present (Eiken et al., 1964; Usui et al., 1978; Kaufman et al., 1980).

These indications and contraindications must always be weighed for each patient. Many crush injuries can be salvaged with vein grafts (Alpert et al., 1978) to bridge the areas of injury, by immediate transference of "unreplantable" digits, or by use of emergency free flaps (Hing et al., 1985) to provide coverage of vital structures (Rose and Hendel, 1981). Such heroic measures, however, must always be tempered with sound judgment.

MANAGEMENT OF THE REPLANT PATIENT

As with any trauma patient, stabilization of vital signs and preservation of life are paramount. Once the patient is stabilized and no contraindications for replantation exist, attention should be focused on the injured part (see Case 1).

There are two techniques for preserving a severed part (Urbaniak, 1982; Van Giesen et al., 1983). One is to wrap the part in gauze moistened with saline or Ringer's solution and place it in a sealed plastic bag, which is then placed on ice. The other is to immerse the part in saline or Ringer's solution in a plastic bag, which is then placed on ice. Immersion may result in maceration, and the gauze-wrap technique may result in freezing or strangulation of the preserved part. These problems appear to be rare, however, and authors have reported success with both techniques (Urbaniak, 1982).

When the patient arrives in the emergency department, one team of microsurgeons attends to the evaluation and preparation of the patient. The other team returns to the operating room with the amputated part, where it is gently washed with pHisoHex and tap water. The part is then placed on a side table where identification and tagging of the neurovascular and tendon structures are performed under loupe magnification. Dissecting adequate lengths of neurovascular structures and proper labeling are essential time-saving activities, obviating the need for later identification of structures under the operating microscope.

Within digits, the typical approach is to make midlateral incisions (Nissenbaum, 1980) (Fig. 87–4) to identify the neurovascular structures, although some authors favor an oblique incision, which is later closed with a Z-plasty (Fig. 87–5) (Lister and Kleinert, 1979). Theoretically, the Z-plasty prevents a circumferential constricting scar, allows for flap coverage of the anastomoses, and avoids placement of the incision directly over the anastomoses. Dorsal veins are identified, dissected out from the subdermal tissue of the dorsal flap, and tagged. Occasionally, volar

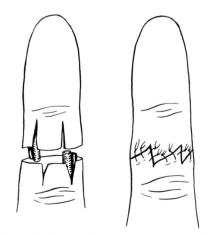

Figure 87–5. Z-plasty closure of replanted digit.

veins are evident and also should be tagged for possible use. Bone trimming, or shortening, should be performed at this time, Kirschner wires or interosseous wires should be placed in the amputated bone fragment. Each of these maneuvers provides efficient use of valuable ischemic time.

In the emergency department, the patient is resuscitated with intravenous fluids, evaluated more fully, and treated with intravenous antibiotics and tetanus toxoid. In addition, x-ray and laboratory studies are performed. Once these are completed, the patient is brought to the operating room. General anesthesia almost always is safer and less prone to complications than regional anesthetic techniques (Sanders and Anderson, 1987). Anesthesia is induced, a Foley catheter is inserted into the bladder, and a pneumatic tourniquet is placed on the proximal part of the injured extremity, as well as on the donor extremity from which nerve, vein, and skin grafts may be harvested. These areas should be scrubbed, prepped, and draped.

The amputation stump is then examined, and the structures are identified and tagged accordingly. With a multiple digital injury or a partial devascularizing injury with significant bleeding, microvascular clamps may be used to reduce blood loss when a tourniquet might further jeopardize injured and compromised tissue.

Temporary plastic shunts should be used for forearm, arm, or leg amputations so that the injured extremity may be reperfused rapidly (Case 1, Fig. 87–2C). Shunting also allows a less hurried examination and identification of the structures and bone fixation without prolonging the ischemic time. The shunts are placed first in the arteries to reperfuse the extremity, and bleeding is allowed prior re-establishing venous continuity in order to clear any toxic metabolic products resulting from limb ischemia (Melh et al., 1964). Autotransfusion of this blood can be a valuable adjunct to volume replacement (Gillott and Thomas, 1984; Tawes et al., 1986).

REPLANTATION OPERATIVE SEQUENCE

Except as noted earlier for major amputations, most amputations are treated by a relatively standard protocol as follows: (1) identification and tagging of structures, (2) débridement and lavage, (3) bone shortening and osteosynthesis, (4) repair of flexor tendons, (5) anastomoses of arteries, (6) anastomoses of nerves, (7) repair of extensor tendons, (8) anastomoses of veins, and (9) soft tissue coverage.

Once structures have been identified and labeled, débridement and removal of all foreign material and necrotic or crushed tissue are performed. Pulse lavage, with or without antibiotic solutions, is a valuable tool for wound cleansing. Occasionally, when there is severe crushing or a wide zone of injury, a "second-look" procedure the next day is essential for detecting delayed necrosis of injured tissue and may allow a replant to be salvaged before wound sepsis becomes established.

Bone shortening and osteosynthesis are an important part of the replant strategy. If properly planned, bone shortening may allow primary tension-free anastomoses of vessels and nerves without significant compromise of length and function. However, when shortening adversely affects function, vein grafting to bridge the vascular gaps is indicated. In cases in which multiple digits are involved, it is sometimes preferable to use portions of "unreplantable digits" to reconstruct other digits in a more satisfactory way.

Osteosynthesis may be accomplished in a variety of ways (Fig. 87–6) (Ikuta, 1978; Lister, 1978; Black et al., 1986; Cassel, 1984): (1) single or double parallel longitudinal wires; (2) one longitudinal and one oblique Kirschner wire; (3) crossed Kirschner wires; (4) intramedullary pins; (5) interosseous wires, by mattress, figure-of-8, or Cassel techniques; (6) plate fixation; (7) screw or bolt fixation; (8) external fixation; and (9) bone peg. We have used each of the osteosynthesis techniques based on the needs of the individual patient. Each method has its advantages.

Kirschner wires are placed with power drills, which are fast, accurate, and less traumatic than hand drills. The single Kirschner wire is simple and allows rotation, permitting some flexibility in manipulating the position of the anastomosis under the microscope. In addition, it is the least damaging to bone and requires little soft tissue dissection. It does, however, lack stability.

Double Kirschner wire techniques are more stable and often are accomplished by chevron cuts, step cuts, or ball-in-socket modifications of the bony surfaces to enhance the rigidity of the osteosynthesis. Without

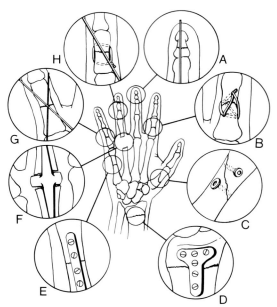

Figure 87–6. Common techniques of osteosynthesis. A = Single Kirschner wire, B = Cassel interosseous wire, C = Screw fixation, D = Plate fixation, E = Miniplate fixation, F = Implant arthroplasty, G = Double Kirschner wire, and H = Kirschner wire and interosseous wire.

careful attention to the direction of placement, however, crossed Kirschner wire and oblique Kirschner wire techniques may injure the neurovascular bundles.

We havē had limited experience with intramedullary pins. These pins are sometimes difficult to place precisely and should not be used in potentially contaminated wounds, as they may drive bacterial inoculum into the bone marrow.

Interosseous wiring may be accomplished by several techniques, as noted earlier. The Cassel wire provides excellent stability and allows early motion (Fig. 87–7). Interfragmentary wiring requires soft tissue dissection and can be somewhat cumbersome if several digits are being replanted simultaneously.

Plate fixation is more commonly indicated in the forearm, humerus, or leg than in the hand. When adequate soft tissue coverage is available, plate fixation may provide a very stable means of fixation. Screw and bolt fixations may be used (Ikuta and Tsuge, 1974) and can achieve a very stable fixation, but other techniques are often accomplished more easily.

External fixation is used at every level of amputation from the comminuted phalanx or

metacarpal fracture to fixation of the femur (Biggs and Chao, 1982; Stuchin and Kummer, 1984). The advantages of this method are that it does not require soft tissue dissection, it avoids the placing of foreign material in the wound, and, thus, it is suitable for contaminated or multiple fractures in which foreign materials or extensive dissection is contraindicated.

Bone peg technique uses a spicule of bone, usually harvested from a nonreplantable part, that is then impacted into the marrow of the proximal and distal ends of a phalanx or metacarpal fracture (Leung, 1981). Although useful in elective toe transfers, when used in trauma cases one must carefully consider the risk of placing a bone graft in a potentially contaminated wound.

When possible, ligament and capsule repair should also be performed to promote increased joint stability and function.

The use of prosthetic spacers and joint implants (Wray et al., 1984) is controversial and not commonly employed by our group. We prefer to use autogenous tissue for bridging bone gaps; however, in the contaminated wound, we use a Kirschner wire spacer, parallel Kirschner wires, or external fixation to maintain length. Later, when wound conditions are more favorable, we usually choose

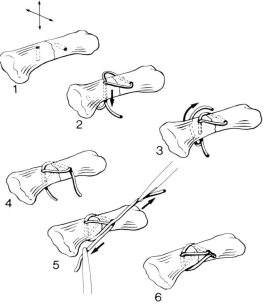

Figure 87–7. Cassel interosseous wire technique. Numbers 1 to 6 indicate order of steps during procedure.

autogenous tissue replacement. Secondary implant arthroplasties are of value but may be subject to fracture in patients performing heavy lifting or other strenuous activities.

Flexor Tendon Repair. Whenever possible, primary repair should be done, and in special circumstances, a primary tendon transfer from a nonreplantable digit may be used. We generally avoid primary placement of tendon rods if a two-stage procedure is anticipated; we prefer not to put foreign materials in potentially contaminated wounds.

In digital replants, tendons are usually recovered with tendon retrieval forceps. The assistant compresses the forearm and maintains the wrist in a flexed position to retrieve flexor tendons or in an extended position for extensor tendons. The tendons are held in place with a Bunnell needle to prevent retraction, the ends are trimmed, and half a modified Kessler suture of 3–0 prolene is placed prior to osteosynthesis. This allows any repair to be performed efficiently after osteosynthesis is accomplished. Some authors (Urbaniak, 1982) advocate placing hemi-Kessler sutures and completing the neurovascular repairs before coaptation of the flexor tendons. The argument for this is that it allows neurovascular anastomosis with the digits in extension, which permits a better view of the structures. We find, however, that seeing the structures is usually not a problem when using a Tupper handboard,* which maintains gentle retraction and extension of the digits even after flexor tendon repair. When primary repair is not possible, the end of the tendon can be tagged with a silver clip to allow x-ray identification for later second-stage repair, which might be undertaken as early as three months after primary repair.

Vascular Repair. Arterial repair is performed first, not only to re-establish circulation and reperfusion of the amputated part but also to allow assessment of viability. Anastomosis of the digital arteries can be achieved as follows: (1) at their respective proximal and distal ends primarily; (2) by interposition vein grafts with any of the combinations listed here; (3) to a crossover vessel, i.e., radial digital artery to ulnar digital artery; and (4) by vessel transposition, i.e., the use of the digital artery of the adjacent digit as the proximal vessel (Fig. 87–8).

---

*Accurate Surgical and Scientific Instrument Corporation, Westbury, New York.

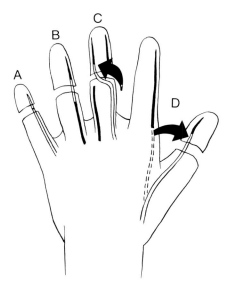

Figure 87–8. Techniques for anastomosis of digital arteries. A = End-to-end repair, B = Interposition vein graft, C = Cross-over, and D = Transposition.

Veins are usually repaired after the arteries so that good bleeding veins can be identified and specifically chosen for repair. Anastomosis of veins may be accomplished as follows: (1) by approximating their respective proximal distal ends, (2) by interposition vein grafts, (3) by mobilizing veins with selective division of branches to lengthen the vein (Fig. 87–9), and (4) by transposing cutaneous flaps containing veins.

Relatively straight grafts of varying caliber may be harvested from the greater and lesser saphenous systems. Smaller grafts for digital vessels can be found on the dorsum of the foot, in the forearm, or in the hand. Special configurations such as "Y-shaped" or multiple-branched veins can be harvested from the dorsum of the foot and are useful in repairing digital arches or common volar vessels (Fig. 87–10). Dissection should be done under loupe magnification; meticulous attention to the ligation of branch points and gentle handling of the graft are essential. Once harvested, the grafts should be labeled, documenting the direction of flow to avoid inadvertent reversal of the graft. We mark the proximal end of the graft with purple dye so that "purple is proximal" and we know that this is the direction of flow. In the event that no venous anastomosis is possible, as is sometimes the case at a replanted distal phalanx level, an artery-only replant (Serafin et al., 1973) can be sustained by removing the

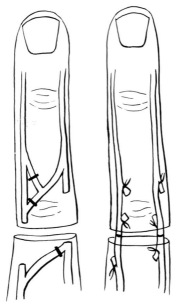

Figure 87–9. Selective division of venous branches allows end-to-end anastomosis.

nail plate (Gordon et al., 1985), by fishmouth incision of the tip of the finger (Sadahiro and Endoh, 1984), or by use of medicinal leeches (Foucher, 1980; Valauri, 1987). Alternatively, one distal digital artery can be anas-

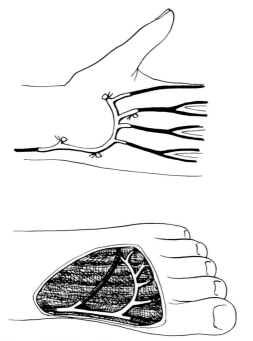

Figure 87–10. Use of the multiple-branched vein from the foot for digital arch reconstruction.

tomosed to a proximal vein (Smith et al., 1983).

Nerve Repair. Except for severe avulsive injuries, most nerves can be repaired primarily; bone shortening generally allows tension-free anastomosis. Under the microscope the ends of the nerve are examined for a "l'oeil d'escargot" sign (Villan, 1984) where the fascicles are protruding from the cut end of the nerve. Some trimming of the nerve end is usually required and may be more extensive in avulsive injuries. If primary anastomosis is not feasible because of excessive gapping, which is frequently found in severe avulsive injuries, the nerve ends are tagged with a silver clip and a secondary nerve graft is planned (Yamano et al., 1982). A primary nerve graft is indicated only rarely, as the gapping is frequently the result of crushed or torn nerve tissues at sites where the ultimate zone of nerve injury is not evident. This is particularly true in major amputations in which larger nerves may sustain injury at multiple levels. Primary repair offers no significant advantage over secondary repair (Millesi et al., 1976).

Nerve repairs are performed under the operating microscope, generally using 9–0 microsutures for digital nerves and placing only as many epineural sutures as necessary to provide a tidy coaptation without tension. Larger peripheral nerves are reapproximated by epineural repair, using 8–0 microsutures after correctly orienting the fascicular groups.

Soft Tissue Coverage. Skin should be closed loosely to prevent undue tension on damaged tissue and possible compression of underlying vascular structures. When primary closure is not possible, a meshed skin graft is sometimes suitable (Gingrass et al., 1973; McDonald and Buncke, 1981) and may be used in conjunction with local flaps. Sometimes, free flaps are performed at the initial operation, although with severe crush injuries, wet to dry dressing will suffice as a temporary cover, pending subsequent débridement and definitive coverage within the next day or two. Although pedicle flaps are also used (Elliott et al., 1979; Kleinman and Dustman, 1981), we find that the required immobilization is unsuitable for patient comfort and limb dependency and that free flaps actually are simpler to manage.

Adjunctive Procedures. Often, fasciotomies of the forearm, leg, hand, or carpal tunnel are performed in anticipation of potential or impending compartment syndromes and should be considered in any injury, particularly crush or avulsive injuries, or after prolonged ischemia (Whitesides et al., 1971; Matsen, 1975; Rowland, 1982).

DRESSINGS. Dressings should function to protect the replant, absorb wound drainage, and prevent both desiccation and maceration of the tissue (Batchelor et al., 1983). For this reason, the wound requirements govern the dressing technique.

Protection is afforded by careful splinting with either plaster splints or bulky pillow splints that function to immobilize and cushion the replanted part. The wound edges are dressed with nonconstricting Xeroform gauze initially, but if large amounts of drainage are anticipated, sterile absorbent cotton gauze is often used over a contact layer of nonadherent porous dressing such as N-terface.*

Dressing changes are limited to avoid undue manipulation of the replant, which may cause vasospasm. However, clotted blood in a gauze bandage can rapidly result in a constricting dressing if there is postoperative edema. Therefore, bloody dressings must be changed, and inspection of the dressing for potential compression and constriction should be made at frequent intervals. The replanted part is kept elevated to minimize edema and prevent venous congestion. A high room temperature (33° C.) is maintained, and a sterile towel is placed over the replanted extremity and covered with a heating pad (40° C.) for five to seven days to enhance the circulation.

MEDICATIONS. Each patient is begun on antibiotics, usually a cephalosporin (Gustilo and Anderson, 1976; Monson and Nelson, 1984), unless special sources of contamination that prompt modification of the therapy are present. Antibiotics are generally continued for one to two days unless circumstances indicate otherwise (Neu, 1984). Our routine includes aspirin (Pederson and Fitzgerald, 1984; O'Brien, 1968), 240 mg per day, begun in the emergency department usually as a rectal suppository, and dextran-40 (Bryant, 1964; Moncrief et al., 1963; Winfrey and Foster, 1964), 25 ml. per hour for five days. This is started as soon as the first arterial anastomosis is completed. Occasionally, heparin (Serafin et al., 1973; Gordon et al., 1985; Elcock, 1972) is used in lieu of dextran (Cary and Russell, 1974; Tamai, 1982) in instances

of crush injury, but caution must be exercised when there is a large zone of injury or a flap donor site that can result in significant blood loss (Ariyan and Stansel, 1976) under anticoagulation therapy. The heparin is adjusted to a dosage that maintains a partial prothrombin time of one and a half times control and is maintained for seven to ten days. Chlorpromazine (Thorazine) (Isaacs, 1977; Ketchum, 1978; Bibi et al., 1986) is used in dosages of 10 to 25 mg. orally three times per day; this may provide vasodilation as well as mild sedation. A variety of other drugs have been used occasionally on a theoretical basis (Ketchum, 1978; Chang and Petry, 1980). These include nifedipine (Procardia) for vasospasm (Nilsson et al., 1984) and isoxsuprine (Vasodilan) for vasodilation (Finseth and Adelberg, 1973; Buncke et al., 1981; Finseth and Buncke, 1984), but their efficacy remains to be demonstrated.

Because tobacco (Sarin et al., 1974; Harris et al., 1980; Yaffee et al., 1984) and caffeine-containing products may result in vasoconstriction, they are prohibited. Bupivacaine (Marcaine) blocks (Phelps et al., 1979) have been used with some success, providing pain relief and reducing vasospasm, but caution must be exercised in selecting the appropriate nerve block. For instance, a wrist block, not a digital block, should be performed for digital replants because the needle may directly injure a digital vessel, or the anesthetic solution may compress and occlude the vessel. Nerve blocks may be hazardous in heparinized patients, although the use of indwelling catheters (Neimkin et al., 1984) placed at the time of surgery can successfully circumvent this potential problem. Liberal use of analgesics in the postoperative period is essential for minimizing pain that can cause vasospasm.

POSTOPERATIVE MONITORING

Postoperative assessment may be made by clinical examination and mechanical devices. It is important to assess the turgor of the replant and the quality of capillary filling. A pale, cool digit without capillary refill implies an inflow problem; rigid, blue, rapid refill implies insufficient outflow; but a pink color with one- to two-second refill is consistent with good perfusion. If the nail bed has been removed and bleeding is absent, arterial occlusion is probably present. If dark blood is

*Winfield Laboratories, Richardson, Texas.

present, venous insufficiency should be considered. Brisk, bright red bleeding implies adequate circulation. Testing by use of pinprick can yield similar information, but if done repeatedly, this may cause undue tissue trauma and impair circulation.

Available monitoring devices include:

1. Thermistors or temperature probes that compare control area temperatures with replanted tissue temperatures (Stirrat et al., 1978; Leonard et al., 1982). Perfusion problems exist if the replant temperature falls below 30° C. or more than 3° below control area temperature.

2. Perivascular thermocouples that measure temperature proximal and distal to an anastomosis and rely on the fact that flowing blood conducts the core temperature to the periphery (May et al., 1983). Thus, when the anastomosis is occluded, flow is stopped, and the temperature distal to the anastomosis decreases. These are continuous monitors that immediately detect flow problems but are very susceptible to malposition. Possible vessel compression can occur if perivascular couplers are dislodged, and withdrawal of the coupler when monitoring is ended may injure the vessel.

3. Ultrasound Doppler devices that detect blood flow in a vascular pedicle by converting the changes in sound waves caused by moving red blood cells into an audible pulse (Buncke and Harris, 1984; Harrison et al., 1983).

4. Laser Dopplers (Fischer et al., 1983) and reflective photometers (Webster and Patterson, 1976; Smith et al., 1984) that have microprocessors that calculate the difference in light wave lengths caused by pulsative movement of erythrocytes and display readout numbers that can be followed.

5. Pulse oximeters that provide information on the presence of a pulse and oxygen saturation (Graham et al., 1986); however, their clinical reliability is yet to be proved (Duarte et al., 1987).

6. Pulse volume recording (PVR) to measure and record pulsatile blood flow displacement changes that occur when a cuff is inflated around a monitored digit or extremity (Phelps et al., 1979; Darling et al., 1972).

7. Fluorometry, which is very accurate and reproducible and is our method of choice (Graham et al., 1985). It is a washout technique performed as follows: (a) A baseline fluorescence is measured and the number is recorded. (b) One ml. of fluorescein dye is injected intravenously and a reading is taken ten minutes later. If the inflow is good, the fluorescence of the replant should rise. (c) A third reading is made one hour later and should approach the baseline if outflow is adequate. If there is no rise from the baseline, arterial obstruction is present, whereas failure to decrease toward baseline one hour after a rise implies outflow obstruction.

TREATMENT OF THE FAILING REPLANT

If a replant shows signs of failure, the diagnosis must be formulated promptly and precise corrective action taken immediately.

Vasospasm. If a digit turns pale after a dressing change, vasospasm should be suspected. Administering analgesics and performing a regional block may be effective treatment (Phelps et al., 1979).

Venous Insufficiency. A tense, blue digit indicates venous insufficiency, which may be treated by leeches (Foucher, 1980; Henderson et al., 1983; Bunker, 1981; Batchelor et al., 1984; Valauri, 1987), removal of the nail plate (Gordon et al., 1985), a fishmouth incision over the tip of the finger held open with a Penrose drain (Sadahiro and Endoh, 1984), or redoing the venous anastomosis, usually with vein grafting. Time is of the essence because prolonged venous obstruction can lead to later arterial obstruction.

Arterial Insufficiency. For suspected arterial insufficiency with vasospasm that does not resolve within several minutes after nonoperative treatment, one must explore and redo the anastomosis, usually with a vein graft. As with the venous anastomosis, look for technical errors such as kinking, twisting, or untied side branches. Thrombus in a previously unrecognized injured segment of the vessel is also seen occasionally. Vascular salvage in digits is unlikely to be successful after two to three days post-replantation (Biemer, 1981).

REHABILITATION

We work closely with physical and occupational therapists in an effort to maximize functional results (Kuder, 1986). Early passive motion is begun approximately five to seven days after surgery (Dehne and Torp,

1971; Strickland and Glogovac, 1980; Gelberman et al., 1981, 1982). Progressive active exercises followed by active resisted exercises are tailored to the needs of each patient. Additionally, modalities of ultrasound (Stevenson et al., 1986), functional electrical stimulation (FES) (Benton et al., 1981), and transcutaneous electrical nerve stimulation (TENS) (Mannheimer and Lampe, 1984), along with sensory training (Dellon et al., 1972; Dellon, 1986; Wynn Parry and Saltor, 1976) and work hardening (Mackin, 1986; Lane, 1986), are part of this comprehensive rehabilitation program.

CONCLUSION

The functional results and cost-effectiveness of replantation versus amputation have been evaluated (Jones et al., 1982). Because of the diversity of injuries, various techniques of repair, and differences in patients' motivational, vocational, and avocational needs, we can only generalize. Well-selected cases can yield excellent results when each case is considered individually with thoughtful, careful planning of the acute surgery and secondary procedures (Chen et al., 1981; Weiland et al., 1977; Morrison et al., 1978; Kleinert et al., 1980; Wilson et al., 1983). Microsurgical replantation requires the joint effort of many specialists, as well as the enthusiasm of a motivated patient (Johnson, 1986; Epps, 1986), which, together, determine the final results.

REFERENCES

Acland, R. D.: New instruments for microvascular surgery. Br. J. Surg., 59:181–184, 1972.

Acland, R. D.: Microvascular anastomosis: A device for holding stay sutures and a new vascular clamp. Surgery, 5:185–187, 1974.

Acland, R. D.: Notes on the handling of ultrafine suture material. Surgery, 787:505–511, 1975.

Acland, R. D.: Microsurgery Practice Manual. St. Louis, C. V. Mosby Co., 1980.

Albertengo, J. B., Rodriguez, A., Buncke, H. J., and Hall, E. J.: A comparative study of flap survival rates in end-to-end and end-to-side microvascular anastomoses. Plast. Reconstr. Surg., 67:194–199, 1981.

Alpert, B. S., and Buncke, H. J.: Mutilating multidigital injuries: Use of a free microvascular flap from a nonreplantable part. J. Hand Surg., 3:196–198, 1978.

Alpert, B. S., Buncke, H. J., and Brownstein, M.: Replacement of damaged arteries and veins with vein grafts when replanting crushed, amputated fingers. Plast. Reconstr. Surg., 61:17, 1978.

Androsov, P. I.: Blood supply of mobilized intestine used for an artificial esophagus. Arch. Surg., 73:917, 1956.

Ariyan, S., and Stansel, H. C.: Further hazards of heparin therapy in vascular surgery. Arch. Surg., 111:120, 1976.

Bas, L. J., May, J. W., Handren, J., and Fallon, J.: End-to-end versus end-to-side microvascular anastomosis patency in experimental venous repairs. Plast. Reconstr. Surg., 77:442–450, 1986.

Batchelor, A., Burtles, R., Sutherland, A. B., and Watson, A. C. H.: The ventilation of "boxing glove" dressings to reduce skin graft maceration. Br. J. Plast. Surg., 33:531–532, 1983.

Batchelor, A., Davison, P., and Sully, L.: The salvage of congested skin flaps by the application of leeches. Br. J. Plast. Surg., 37:358–360, 1984.

Benton, L. A., Baker, L. L., Bowman, B. R., and Waters, R. L.: Functional Electrical Stimulation—A Practical Clinical Guide, 2nd ed. Downey, Cal. Rancho Los Amigos Rehabilitation Engineering Center, 1981.

Bibi, R., Ferder, M., and Strauch, B.: Prevention of flap necrosis by chlorpromazine. Plast. Reconstr. Surg., 77:954–959, 1986.

Biemer, E.: Salvage operations for complications following replantation and free tissue transfer. Int. Surg., 66:37–38, 1981.

Biggs, B., and Chao, E.: The mechanical performance of the standard Hoffman-Vidal external fixation apparatus. J. Bone Joint Surg., 64A:566–573, 1982.

Black, D. M., Mann, R. J., Castine, R. M., and Daniels, A. U.: The stability of internal fixation in the proximal phalanx. J. Hand Surg., 11A:672–677, 1986.

Bright, D. S.: Microsurgical techniques in vessel and nerve repair. AAOS Instructional Course Lectures, Vol. 27. St. Louis, C. V. Mosby Co., 1978, pp. 1–15.

Bryant, F. M.: Study of antithrombotic properties of dextran of large molecular weight. J. Cardiovas. Surg., 5:48–52, 1964.

Buchler, U., Phelps, D., Winspur, I., and Bostwick, J.: The irrigation jet: An aid in microvascular surgery. J. Hand Surg., 2:24–28, 1977.

Buncke, H. J., and Harris, G. D.: Toe to hand transplantation in children. In Serafin, D., and Georgiade, N. G. (eds.): Pediatric Plastic Surgery. St. Louis, C. V. Mosby Co., 1984, pp. 1187–1199.

Buncke, H. J., and McLean, D. H.: The advantage of a straight needle in microsurgery. Plast. Reconstr. Surg., 47:602–603, 1971.

Buncke, H. J., Alpert, B. S., and Johnson-Geblink, R.: Digital replantation. Surg. Clin. North Am., 61:383–394, 1981.

Buncke, H. J., Buncke, G. M., and Schultz, W. P.: Experimental digital amputation and replantation. Plast. Reconstr. Surg., 36:62, 1965.

Buncke, H. J., Buncke, G. M., and Schultz, W. P.: Immediate Nicoladoni procedure in the rhesus monkey, or hallux-to-hand transplantation, utilizing microminiature vascular anastomoses. Br. J. Plast. Surg., 19:332, 1966.

Buncke, H. J., Chater, N. L., and Szabo, Z.: The Manual of Microvascular Surgery. Pearl River, N.Y., Davis & Geck, 1975.

Bunker, I. D.: The contemporary use of the medicinal leech. Injury, 12:430, 1981.

Carrel, A.: The operative technique of vascular anastomosis and transplantation of organs. Lyon Med., 98:859, 1902.

Carrel, A., and Guthrie, C.: Anastomosis of blood vessels by patching method of transplantation of the kidney. J.A.M.A., 47:1648, 1906a.

Carrel, A., and Guthrie, C.: Complete amputation of the thigh with replantation. Am. J. Med. Sci., 131:297, 1906b.

Cary, R. J., and Russell, P. S.: Replantation of severed fingers. Ann. Surg., 179:255–259, 1974.

Cassel, J.: The Cassel wire (personal communication).

Chang, W. H., and Petry, J. J.: Platelets, prostaglandins, and patency in microvascular surgery. J. Neurosurg., 2:77–85, 1980.

Chase, R. A.: The damaged index digit. A source of components to restore the crippled hand. J. Bone Joint Surg., 50:1152–1160, 1958.

Chase, R. A.: The severely injured upper limb—to amputate or to reconstruct: That is the question. Arch. Surg., 100:382, 1970.

Chen, Z. W.: Sixth People's Hospital of Shanghai: Replantation of severed fingers: Clinical experience in 162 cases involving 270 severed fingers. Chinese Med. J., 1:3, 1973.

Chen, Z. W., Chien, Y. C., and Pao, Y. S.: Salvage of the forearm following complete traumatic amputation: Case report. Chinese Med. J., 82:632, 1963.

Chen, Z. W., Meyer, V. E., and Kleinert, H. E.: Present indications and contraindications for replantation as reflected by long-term functional results. Orthop. Clin. North Am., 3:849–870, 1981.

Chen, Z. W., Chien, Y. C., Pao, Y. S., and Lin, C. T.: Further experience in restoration of amputated limbs. Chinese Med. J., 84:225, 1965.

Cobbett, J.: Small vessel anastomosis: A comparison of suture techniques. Br. J. Plast. Surg., 22:16–20, 1967.

Cobbett, J.: Free digital transfer. J. Bone Joint Surg., 51B:677, 1969.

Darling, R. C., Raines, J. K., Brener, B. J., and Austen, W. G.: Quantitative segmental pulse volume recorder: A clinical tool. Surgery 72:873–887, 1972.

Dehne, E., and Torp, R. P.: Treatment of joint injuries by immediate mobilization. Clin. Orthop., 77:218, 1971.

Dellon, A. L.: Sensory recovery in replanted digits and transplanted toes: A review. J. Microsurg., 2:123–129, 1986.

Dellon, A. L., Curtis, R. M., and Edgerton, M. T.: Re-education of sensation in the hand after nerve injury and repair. Plast. Reconstr. Surg., 53:297–305, 1972.

Douglas, B.: Successful replacement of completely avulsed portions of the finger as composite grafts. Plast. Reconstr. Surg., 23:213, 1959.

Duarte, A., Valauri, F., Buncke, G., and Buncke, H.: Pulse oximetry, experimental and clinical experience. (Submitted to Hand Surgery, June, 1987.)

Eiken, O., Nasbeth, D. C., Mayer, R. F., and Deterling, R. A.: Limb replantation. The pathophysiological effects. Arch. Surg., 88:76–87, 1964.

Elcock, H. W.: The effect of heparin on thrombosis at microvenous anastomotic sites. Arch. Otolaryngol., 95:68, 1972.

Elliott, R. A., Hoehn, J. G., and Stayman, J. W.: Management of the viable soft tissue cover in degloving injuries. Hand, 11:69–71, 1979.

Epps, C. H., Jr.: Secondary gain as a factor in results of treatment. In Epps, C. H., Jr. (ed.): Complications in Orthopaedic Surgery, 2nd Ed. Philadelphia, J. B. Lippincott Co., 1986, pp. 231–243.

Finseth, F., and Adelberg, M. G.: Prevention of skin flap necrosis by course of treatment with vasodilator drugs. Plast. Reconstr. Surg., 61:738, 1973.

Finseth, F., and Buncke, H. J.: Improvement of tissue blood flow by vasodilator therapy with isoxsuprine. In Buncke, H. J., and Furnas, D. (eds.): Symposium on Clinical Frontiers in Reconstructive Microsurgery. St. Louis, C. V. Mosby Co., 1984, pp. 438–443.

Fischer, J. C., Parker, P. M., and Shaw, W. W.: Comparison of two laser Doppler flowmeters for monitoring dermal blood flow. Microsurgery, 4:164, 1983.

Foucher, G.: Un vieux remède dans un pot neuf: la sangsue en microchirurgie. Communication à la Seizième Recontre Internationale de Microchirugie. Marseille, GAM, May 14–17, 1980.

Fujino, T., and Aoyagi, F.: A method of successive interrupted suturing in microvascular anastomosis. Plast. Reconstr. Surg., 55:240–241, 1975.

Gelberman, R. H., Amiel, D., Gonsalves, M., Woo, S. L.-Y., and Akesun, W. H.: The influence of protective passive mobilization on healing of flexor tendons. A biochemical and microangiographic study. Hand, 13:120, 1981.

Gelberman, R. H., Woo, S. L.-Y., Lothringer, K., Akesun, W. H., and Amiel, D.: Effects of early intermittent passive mobilization on healing canine flexor tendons. J. Hand Surg., 7:170, 1982.

George, P. T., Creech, B. J., and Buncke, H. J.: A rapid new technique for microvascular anastomosis (the loop technique). Plast. Reconstr. Surg., 56:99–101, 1975.

Gillott, A., and Thomas, J.: Clinical investigation involving the use of the haemonetic cell saver in elective and emergency vascular operations. Am. Surg., 50:609–612, 1984.

Gingrass, R. P., Cunningham, D. S., and Pelletta, F. X.: Skin grafting of exposed arterial vein graft: A clinical and experimental study. J. Trauma, 13:951, 1973.

Godina, M.: Preferential use of end-to-side arterial anastomoses in free flap transfers. Plast. Reconstr. Surg., 64:673, 1979.

Gordon, L., Leitner, D. W., Buncke, H. J., and Alpert, B. S.: Partial nail plate removal after digital replantation as an alternative method of venous drainage. J. Hand Surg., 10A:359–364, 1985.

Graham, B. H., Paulus, D. A., and Caffee, H. H.: Pulse oximetry for vascular monitoring in upper extremity replantation surgery. J. Hand Surg., 11A:687–692, 1986.

Graham, B. H., Gordon, L., Alpert, B. S., Walton, R., Buncke, H. J., and Leitner, D. V.: Serial quantitative skin surface fluorescence: A new method for postoperative monitoring of vascular perfusion in revascularized digits. J. Hand Surg., 10A:226–230, 1985.

Grotz, R. T., Buncke, H. J., Ochoa, E., Rand, R., and Phillips, H.: The dynamic filling test for patency in microvascular arterial anastomoses. Int. J. Microsurg., 3:293, 1982.

Gustilo, R. B., and Anderson, J. J.: Prevention of infection in the treatment of one thousand and twenty-five open fractures of long bones. J. Bone Joint Surg., 58A:453–458, 1976.

Guthrie, C.: Some physiologic aspects of blood vessel surgery. J.A.M.A., 51:1658, 1908.

Harris, G. D., Finseth, F., and Buncke, H. J.: The hazard of cigarette smoking following digital replantation. J. Microsurg., 1:403–404, 1980.

Harris, G. D., Finseth, F., and Buncke, H. J.: Posterior wall: first technique in microvascular surgery. Br. J. Plast. Surg. 34:47, 1981.

Harrison, D. H., Girling, M., Mott, G., and Eng, T.: Methods of assessing the viability of free flap transfer during the postoperative period. Clin. Plast. Surg., *10*:21–36, 1983.

Hayhurst, J. W., and O'Brien, B. M.: An experimental study of microvascular technique, patency rates, and related factors. Br. J. Plast. Surg., *28*:128, 1975.

Henderson, H. P., Matti, B., Laing, H. G., Morelli, S., and Sully, S.: Avulsion of scalp treated by microvascular repair: The use of leeches for post-operative decongestion. Br. J. Plast. Surg., *36*:235–239, 1983.

Hing, D. N., Buncke, H. J., and Alpert, B. S.: Free flap coverage of the hand. Hand Clin., *1*:741, 1985.

Hing, D. N., Buncke, H. J., and Alpert, B. S.: To replant or to transplant. *In* Habel, M. (ed.): Advances in Plastic and Reconstructive Surgery. Chicago, Year Book Medical Publishers, 1987.

Hoerenz, P.: The operating microscope. Documentation. J. Microsurg., *2*:126–139, 1980.

Hopfner, E.: Ueber Gefässnaht, Gefasstransplantionen und Replantation von amputierten Extremitaten. Arch. Klin. Chir., *70*:417, 1903.

Ikuta, Y.: Method of bone fixation in reattachment of amputations in the upper extremities. Clin. Orthop., *133*:169–178, 1978.

Ikuta, Y., and Tsuge, K.: Microbolts and microscrews for fixation of small bones in the hand. Hand, *6*:261, 1974.

Isaacs, I. J.: The vascular complications of digital replantation. Aust. N.Z. J. Surg., *47*:292–299, 1977.

Jacobson, J. H., and Suarez, E. L.: Microsurgery in anastomosis of small vessels. Surg. For., *9*:243, 1960.

Johnson, R. K.: Psychological evaluation of patients with industrial injuries. Hand Clin., *2*:567–575, 1986.

Jones, J. M., Schenck, R. R., and Chesney, R. B.: Digital replantation and amputation—comparison of function. J. Hand Surg., *7*:183–189, 1982.

Kaufman, M. H., Huchton, J. D., Patten, B. M., Vogel, R. G., and Adler, S. K.: Limb preservation for reimplantation. A review. J. Microsurg., *2*:36–41, 1980.

Keiter, J. E.: Immediate pollicization of an amputated index finger. J. Hand Surg., *5*:584–585, 1980.

Ketchum, L. D.: Pharmacological alternating in the clotting mechanism: Use in microvascular surgery. J. Hand Surg., *3*:407–415, 1978.

Kleinert, H. E., Kasdan, M. L., and Romero, J. L.: Small blood vessel anastomosis for salvage of the severely injured upper extremity. J. Bone Joint Surg., *45A*:788, 1963.

Kleinert, H. E., Jablon, M., and Tsai, T. M.: An overview of replantation and results of 347 replants in 245 patients. J. Trauma, *20*:390, 1980.

Kleinman, W. B., and Dustman, J. A.: Preservation of function following complete degloving injuries to the hand: Use of simultaneous groin flap, random abdominal flap, and partial thickness skin graft. J. Hand Surg., *6*:82–89, 1981.

Komatsu, S., and Tamai, S.: Successful replantation of a completely cut off thumb. Plast. Reconstr. Surg., *42*:374, 1968.

Kuder, P. B.: Therapists' management of the replanted hand. Hand rehabilitation. Hand Clin., *2*:179–192, 1986.

Ladanyi, I. J.: Trapianto dell falange del dito. Minerva Med., *61*:71, 1970.

Lane, C.: Therapy for the occupationally injured hand. Hand Clin., *2*:593–602, 1986.

Leonard, A. G., Brennen, M. D., and Coleville, J.: The use of continuous temperature monitoring in postoperative management of microsurgical cases. Br. J. Plast. Surg., *35*:337, 1982.

Leung, P.-C.: Use of an intramedullary bone peg in digital replantations, revascularization and toe transfers. J. Hand Surg., *6*:281–284, 1981.

Lister, G. D.: Interosseous wiring of the digital skeleton. J. Hand Surg., *3*:427–435, 1978.

Lister, G. D., and Kleinert, H. E.: Replantation. *In* Grabb, W. C., and Smith, J. W. (eds.): Plastic Surgery, 3rd Ed., Boston, Little Brown, 1979, p. 702.

Mackin, E. J. (ed.): Hand Rehabilitation. Hand Clin., *2*:1–257, 1986.

Malt, R. S.: Replantation of severed arms. J.A.M.A., *189*:114, 1964.

Manktelow, R. T.: What are the indications for digital replantation? Ann. Plast. Surg., *1*:336, 1978.

Mannheimer, J. S., and Lampe, G. N.: Clinical Transcutaneous Electrical Nerve Stimulation. Philadelphia, F. A. Davis Co., 1984.

Matsen, F. A., III: Compartmental syndrome. A united concept. Clin. Orthop., *113*:8–14, 1975.

May, J. W., Lukash, F. N., Gallico, G. G., and Stirrat, C. R.: Removable thermocouple probe microvascular patency monitor: An experimental and clinical study. Plast. Reconstr. Surg., *72*:366–379, 1983.

McDonald, H. D., and Buncke, H. J.: Split-thickness skin grafts in microvascular surgery. Plast. Reconstr. Surg., *68*:731, 1981.

Melh, R. L., Paul, H. A., Shorey, W., Schneewind, J., and Beattie, E. L., Jr.: Treatment of "toxemia" after extremity replantation. Arch. Surg., *89*:871–878, 1964.

Millesi, H., Meissl, G., and Berger, A.: Further experience with interfascicular grafting of the median, ulnar and radial nerve. J. Bone Joint Surg., *58A*:209, 1976.

Moncrief, J. A., Darin, J. C., Canizarro, P. C., and Sawyer, R. B.: Use of dextran to prevent arterial and venous thrombosis. Ann. Surg., *158*:552, 1963.

Monson, T. P., and Nelson, C. L.: Microbiology for orthopaedic surgeons. Selected aspects. Clin. Orthop. Rel. Res., *190*:14–22, 1984.

Morrison, W. A., O'Brien, B. M., and MacLeod, A. M.: Digital replantation and revascularization. A long-term review of one hundred cases. Hand, *10*:125–134, 1978.

Murphy, J. B.: Resection of arteries and veins injured in continuity—End-to-end suture: Experimental and clinical research. Med. Res., *51*:73, 1897.

Nathan, P., and Rose, M. C.: An alternative technique for microvascular suture. Plast. Reconstr. Surg., *58*:635–637, 1976.

Neimkin, R. J., May, J. W., Roberts, J., and Sunder, N.: Continuous axillary block through an indwelling Teflon catheter. J. Hand Surg., *9A*:830–833, 1984.

Neu, H. C.: Cephalosporin antibiotics as applied in surgery of bones and joints. Clin. Orthop. Rel. Res., *190*:50–63, 1984.

Nilsson, H., Jonasson, J., and Ringquist, I.: Treatment of digital vasospastic disease with the calcium-entry blocker, nifedipine. Acta Med. Scand., *215*:135–139, 1984.

Nissenbaum, M.: A surgical approach for replantation of complete digital amputations. J. Hand Surg., *5*:58–62, 1980.

O'Brien, B., and Hayhurst, J. W.: Metalized microsutures and a new micro needle holder. Plast. Reconstr. Surg., *52*:673, 1973.

O'Brien, J. R.: Effects of salicylates on human platelets. Lancet, *1*:779–783, 1968.

Pederson, A. K., and Fitzgerald, G. A.: Dose-related kinetics of aspirin. N. Engl. J. Med., *311*:1205, 1984.

Phelps, D. B., Rutherford, R. B., and Bostwick, J. A.:

Control of vasospasm following trauma and microvascular surgery. J. Hand Surg., *4*:109–117, 1979.

Rose, E. H., and Hendel, P.: Primary toe-to-thumb transfer in the acutely avulsed thumb. Plast. Reconstr. Surg., *67*:214, 1981.

Rowland, S. A.: Fasciotomy. *In* Green, D. P. (ed.): Operative Hand Surgery. New York, Churchill Livingstone, 1982, pp. 565–581.

Sadahiro, T., and Endoh, H.: Continuous blood-letting in replantation of the amputated finger. J. Hand Surg., *9*:83–88, 1984.

Sanders, N., and Anderson, K.: Anesthesia for microsurgery patients. *In* Buncke, H. J. (ed.): Clinical Atlas of Microsurgical Transplantation and Replantation. Philadelphia, Lea & Febiger, 1987.

Sarin, C. L., Austin, J. C., and Michel, W.: Effects of smoking on digital blood-flow velocity. J.A.M.A., *229*:1327, 1974.

Seidenberg, B., Hurwitt, E. S., and Cavtor, C. A.: The technique of anastomosing small arteries. Surg. Gynecol. Obstet., *106*:743, 1958.

Seidenberg, B., Rosenak, S. S., and Hurwitt, E. S.: Immediate reconstruction of a revascularized isolated jejunal loop. Ann. Surg., *149*:162, 1959.

Serafin, P., Kutz, J. E., and Kleinert, H. E.: Replantation of a completely amputated distal thumb without venous anastomosis. Case report. Plast. Reconstr. Surg., *52*:579, 1973.

Smith, A. R., Jan Sonneveld, G., and van der Meulen, J. C.: AV anastomosis as a solution for absent venous drainage in replantation surgery. Plast. Reconstr. Surg., *71*:525, 1983.

Smith, D. J., Bendick, P. J., and Madison, S. A.: Evaluation of vascular compromise in the injured extremity: A photoplethysmographic technique. J. Hand Surg., *9A*:314, 1984.

Stevenson, J. H., Pang, C. Y., Lindsay, W. K., and Zuker, R. N.: Functional, mechanical, and biochemical assessment of ultrasound therapy on tendon healing in the chicken toe. Plast. Reconstr. Surg., *77*:965–972, 1986.

Stirrat, C. R., Seaber, A. V., and Urbaniak, J. R.: Temperature monitoring in digital replantation. J. Hand Surg., *3*:342, 1978.

Strickland, J. W., and Glogovac, S. V.: Digital function following flexor tendon repair in zone 2: A comparison of immobilization and controlled passive motion techniques. J. Hand Surg., *5*:537, 1980.

Stuchin, S. A., and Kummer, F. J.: Stiffness of small bone—external fixation methods: An experimental study. J. Hand Surg., *9A*:718–724, 1984.

Tamai, S.: 20 years experience of limb replantation. J. Hand Surg., *7*:549–556, 1982.

Tawes, R. L., Scribner, R. D., Duval, T. B., Beare, J. P., Sydorak, G. R., Rosenman, J. E., Brown, W. H., and Harris, E. J.: The cell-saver and autologous transfusion: An underutilized resource in vascular surgery. Am. J. Surg., *152*:105–109, 1986.

Thurston, B., Buncke, H. J., Chater, N., and Weinstein, P. R.: A SEM study of microarterial damage and repair. Plast. Reconstr. Surg., *57*:197, 1976.

Urbaniak, J. R.: Replantation. *In* Green, D. P. (ed.): Operative Hand Surgery. New York, Churchill Livingstone, 1982, pp. 811–827.

Urbaniak, J. R., Soucacos, P. N., Adelaar, R. S., Bright, D. S., and Whitehurst, L. A.: Experimental evaluation of microsurgical techniques in small artery anastomoses. Orthop. Clin. North Am., *8*:249–263, 1977.

Usui, M., Ishii, S., Muramatsu, I., and Takahata, N.: An experimental study on "replant toxemia." J. Hand Surg., *3*:589–596, 1978.

Valauri, F. A.: Use of leeches in microsurgery. *In* Buncke, H. J. (ed.): Clinical Atlas of Microsurgical Transplantation and Replantation. Philadelphia, Lea & Febiger, 1987.

Van Beek, A. L., Kutz, J. E., and Zook, E. G.: Importance of the ribbon sign, indicating unsuitability of the vessel, in replanting a finger. Plast. Reconstr. Surg., *61*:32–35, 1978.

Van Giesen, P. J., Seaber, A. V., and Urbaniak, J. R.: Storage of amputated parts prior to replantation—an experimental study with rabbit ears. J. Hand Surg., *8*:60, 1983.

Villan, R.: Personal communication with Harry J. Buncke, 1984.

Webster, M. H. C., and Patterson, J.: The photoelectric plethysmograph as a monitor of vascular anastomoses. Br. J. Plast. Surg., *29*:182, 1976.

Weiland, A., Villareal-Rios, A., Kleinert, H. E., Kutz, J., Atasoy, E., and Lister, G.: Replantation of digits and hands and analysis of surgical technique and functional results in 71 patients with 86 replantations. J. Hand Surg., *2*:1–12, 1977.

Whitesides, T. E., Jr., Hirada, H., and Morimoto, K.: The response of skeletal muscle to temporary ischemia: An experimental study. J. Bone Joint Surg., *53A*:1027–1028, 1971.

Wilber, R. G., Shaffer, J. W., and Field, G. A.: The effect of redundancy and tension on microvascular vein grafts. J. Hand Surg., *9A*:649–652, 1984.

Wilson, C. S., Alpert, B. S., and Buncke, H. J.: Replantation of upper extremities. Clin. Plast. Surg., *10*:85–101, 1983.

Winfrey, E. W., and Foster, J. H.: Low molecular weight dextran in small artery surgery. Arch. Surg., *88*:110, 1964.

Wray, R. C., Young, V. L., and Weeks, P. M.: Flexible implant arthroplasty and finger replantation. Plast. Reconstr. Surg., *74*:97, 1984.

Wynn Parry, C. B., and Saltor, M.: Sensory re-education after median nerve lesion. Hand, *8*:250–257, 1976.

Yaffee, B., Cushing, B., and Strauch, B.: Effects of cigarette smoking on experimental anastomoses. Microsurgery, *5*:70–72, 1984.

Yamano, Y., Namba, Y., Hino, Y., Hasegawa, T., Ugawa, A., and Ise, M.: Digital nerve grafts in replanted digits. Hand, *14*:255, 1982.

Zirkle, T. J., and Seidenstricker, K. L.: An adjustable double clamp for use in microvascular surgery. Plast. Reconstr. Surg., *51*:340–341, 1973.

Chapter 88

INDICATIONS FOR REPLANTATION

DOMINIQUE LE VIET

AND VLADIMIR MITZ

Since the introduction of microscopy in hand surgery and the first replantation of a thumb, reported by Komatzu and Tamai in 1968, numerous centers have published studies of large series of replantations. After the initial excitement engendered by the new techniques had worn off, the poor quality of the functional results induced the workers in those centers to review the indications and reassess their results.

Since 1974 we have performed 150 digital replantations and 41 replantations of segments of limbs. In the light of our results we decided that the time had come to codify the indications for this type of surgical procedure. A number of relevant factors were taken into account and they will be considered in turn: the site of the lesion, associated lesions, the nature of the injury, the time lapse and mode of preservation of the limb, and the age, occupation, and motivation of the patient.

THE SITE OF THE LESION

The site of the lesion is one of the most important factors to be considered before embarking on a replantation, whether the amputation runs across a digit or a more proximal segment of the limb.

DIGITAL SECTION

The approach to the problem depends on whether one or more digits are involved.

Unidigital Amputation

Thumb. Amputation of the thumb is the prime indication for replantation surgery: it should be attempted regardless of the level. Even minimal lengthening of the first ray can bring a significant functional gain. If the line of amputation runs across the metacarpophalangeal or interphalangeal joint, the joint must be arthrodesed while the extrinsic flexor and extensor systems are reconstructed to stabilize the column of the thumb. After arthrodesis of the interphalangeal joint, a reconstructed flexor pollicis longus will increase the possibility of adduction.

The Fingers. Replantation of a single finger is seldom indicated in our view unless the amputation is distal to the distal interphalangeal joint. Stiffness of the proximal interphalangeal joint, added to the difficulty in carrying out a tendon repair in the "no man's land," means that the patient seldom derives any functional benefit from the replantation of a single digit. One should learn to resist a patient's demand by stressing the possible resulting functional disadvantages. It may be attempted, however, in female patients on cosmetic grounds and in young children. It is contraindicated, however, in a manual worker in whom a less than perfect result could interfere with the function of the hand as a whole. Besides, the mental attitude of these patients is such that they are most unlikely to request, let alone accept, secondary amputation.

Clean amputations of the distal phalanx are a different proposition. In this situation, when the distal interphalangeal joint is arthrodesed and no tendinoarticular problem arises, replantation is worth attempting even if only one finger is involved. It goes without saying that a nerve repair is essential (usually at the level of the bifurcation) in addition to restoring the arterial and the venous flow.

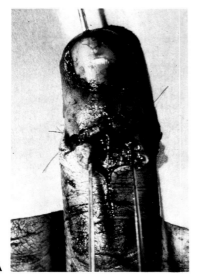
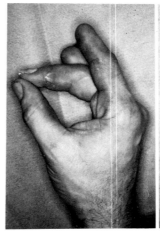
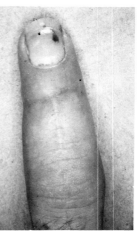

Figure 88–1. *A*, Perioperative view. A dorsal vein is sutured. *B*, Appearance at 45 days. *C*, Function at 45 days.

Even though the distal interphalangeal joint is arthrodesed, the flexor profundus should always be reinserted in order to improve the flexor power of the injured finger. These replantations often give the best functional results, at the expense of a relatively limited time off work (Fig. 88–1).

Multidigital Amputation

The functional plight of the metacarpal hand is such that replantation of one or more digital rays is imperative when several have been injured. Here again we must differentiate between injuries with and without involvement of the thumb.

Thumb and One Finger. The combined involvement of the thumb and index finger, or the thumb and index and middle fingers, represents a prime indication for replantation of the thumb. If the stump of the thumb is damaged beyond utilization, the least damaged digital stump should be pollicized. If both the index and middle fingers are damaged, priority, following pollicization, will go to replantation of the middle finger. It is important not to leave a gap between fingers, and an index stump can often make possible a useful, though elementary, pulp to pulp grip with the thumb.

Involvement of the Fingers with an Intact Thumb. Replantation is imperative if several fingers have been amputated. Since one cannot forecast the quality of the ultimate functional result, an attempt should be made to reconstruct as many digital axes as possible. If replantation of one or more fingers is unfeasible because of the severity of the lesions, the order of priority for reconstruction is: middle finger, ring finger, little finger, and the index finger last.

The concept of a bank finger is particularly important in this type of injury. It is not uncommon for one or more fingers to be unsalvageable by replantation. These digits can be used as sources of artery, vein, nerve, and tendon grafts; the primary repair, whenever possible, should be completed at the first sitting because the donors often have poor trophicity.

SECTION OF THE UPPER LIMBS

Although the indications for replantation in digital amputations tend to be relative, in total section of a limb we regard them as absolute. In view of the present state of appliances and prostheses, replantation remains the best form of treatment for amputations between the shoulder and the metacarpals.

Despite the frequency of distal mediocubital palsies and sensitivity to cold and despite the clumsiness of the fingers, the recovery of the extrinsic musculature and the psychological benefit to the patient make replantation almost always worthwhile. Obviously the result depends on the type of injury, the quality of the repair, the age of the patient, and a

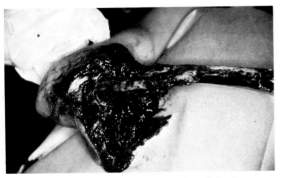

Figure 88–2. Avulsion of the muscles of the forearm. The radius and ulna are seen below the elbow.

certain element of luck that is difficult to quantify. In our own series of 41, only one patient seems possibly worse than if he had not undergone replantation. He is a 51-year-old bookbinder whose right hand was severed by a guillotine trimmer. Three years and 10 months after replantation, the hand was fixed in the position of function, exquisitely tender to touch and functionally useless. The patient refused secondary amputation (Fig. 88–2).

The contraindications to replantation of a limb segment are either local (i.e., the type of injury) or general, and one should never overlook the difficulty and the gravity of this type of procedure. Indeed, we recorded three deaths. One patient died during surgery: he had lost both arms under the wheels of a train. The other two, who had suffered multiple injuries, died postoperatively. Although in the latter cases replantation surgery cannot be blamed for the deaths, there is little doubt that prolonged anesthesia with massive transfusion hardly helped the management of these two patients. The problems of fluid and electrolyte balance and the risk of Bywaters' syndrome are such that these patients are always nursed in an intensive care unit during the early postoperative stage.

ASSOCIATED LESIONS

Associated lesions are best considered as being of two main types—staggered lesions in a severed limb and those occurring as part of a set of multiple injuries.

LESIONS LIMITED TO THE LIMB

However urgent the replantation, priority must be given to treatment of the proximal segment. In one of our cases of amputation at the forearm there was also a fracture of the humerus. Fixation of the fracture was dealt with first, because it would be illogical, not to say impossible, to carry out an osteosynthesis at the end of replantation. This patient unfortunately suffered a venous thrombosis and the distal segment had to be amputated. Mobility of the elbow was preserved, however, thanks to the initial humeral fixation.

In the haste to revascularize the replanted segment, one must not neglect the proximal lesions on whose management the ultimate result also depends.

MULTIPLE INJURIES

In addition to clean amputations resulting from industrial injuries, we have also treated amputated limbs in patients with multiple injuries following attempted suicide under trains.

Vascular shock and intra-abdominal and intrathoracic lesions, of course, are treated as priorities. Multiple fractures must also be a high priority. Even in cases in which the odds are deemed to be favorable, the decision to replant can never be taken lightly. It must be remembered that the procedure is a lengthy and hemorrhagic one that may affect the patient's chances of survival.

Among our first 20 cases we recorded six failures: four of the patients had suffered multiple injuries and two died. In our opinion the chances of failure are significantly greater in the presence of multiple injuries, when the indications for replantation should be much more strict.

NATURE OF THE INJURY

The mechanism of the injury influences not only the early prognosis but also the long term functional result. We recognize three main forms of trauma: section, avulsion, and contusion with pressure.

SECTION

This type of injury carries the best prognosis whether the instrument responsible is a knife, a trimmer, or a circular saw. At the cost of minimal shortening, it is usually possible to carry out an accurate repair, and as a rule there are no problems with skin closure. This constitutes the choice indication for replanting a segment of the upper limb. The functional results can be spectacular.

AVULSION

In both the digital amputation in which the finger is torn and the tendon is avulsed at the musculotendinous junction (Fig. 88–2) and the avulsive injury of the forearm in which skin and muscle are torn at different levels, the mechanism is violent traction in the axis of the limb.

If digital replantation is decided upon, we believe that reattachment of the tendon to the muscle body is impractical; digital mobility can be obtained only by a tenodesis effect on extension of the wrist by tethering the proximal end of the tendon to the skeleton above the radiocarpal joint. In the limb more of the muscle must be sacrificed, and this often entails considerable shortening. In this type of case the functional result in the distal part of the limb is at best mediocre.

CONTUSION WITH PRESSURE

This type of injury is the least promising because problems of vitality of skin and muscle are superimposed on those inherent in any replantation procedure. We saw such a combined crush-section injury in a limb that had been run over by the wheel of a lorry: there was extensive avulsion of skin with gross contusion of muscular tissue. After primary trimming and débridement, it is usually possible to restore arterial flow by direct suturing or bridging grafts, for the arteries lie deep and are well protected. Some form of venous drainage can often be reconstructed, again with the help of bridge grafts to the superficial veins, but it is essential that these be given a protective covering of skin. In principle, this can be achieved by the use of thin skin grafts, provided a bed of healthy muscle remains. However, in this type of injury both skin and muscles are frequently mangled.

In such cases replantation is contraindicated unless a lining of healthy skin is guaranteed. Even though arterial revascularization is possible, the absence of a good skin cover and a healthy muscular bed will lead inevitably to venous thrombosis and early failure. This in turn implies secondary amputation at a higher level because of superimposed infection (Fig. 88–3). Finally, a concomitant brachial plexus lesion (which occurred in two of our cases) represents an absolute contraindication to replantation.

DELAY AND MODE OF PRESERVATION

In the majority of our cases, circulation in the reimplanted segment was restored within seven to 10 hours after the accident. The greater the muscle mass in the amputated segment, the greater the chances of secondary fluid and electrolyte disturbances, especially if the limb has not been properly cooled. Many investigators have studied the changes in blood pH, lactate, and pyruvate levels as well as the production of muscle toxins in the course of replantation surgery.

Ideally one would wish to restore arterial flow within six hours in a limb that has been properly refrigerated, but this ideal situation is seldom attainable. Only under these conditions can one hope to prevent, or at least reduce, the irreversible ischemic destruction of the intrinsic muscles, which appear to be much more vulnerable than the extrinsic muscles.

THE PATIENT

The age, sex, occupation, dominant side, and motivation of the patient are factors that weigh heavily in the decision to replant.

The average age of our patients was 30½ years. After the age of 45 motor and sensory recovery is less likely to occur. Although the majority of our patients were men, we did carry out a few unidigital replantations in female patients on "cosmetic grounds." The patient should always be warned of the risks, the likely result, and the expected time off work.

In addition, the following facts should be made clear to the patient as early as possible after surgery: Early failure remains a possibility, a fact the patient always finds surprising. Rehabilitation may be long and slow and requires maximal cooperation on the patient's part. Improvement has been known to

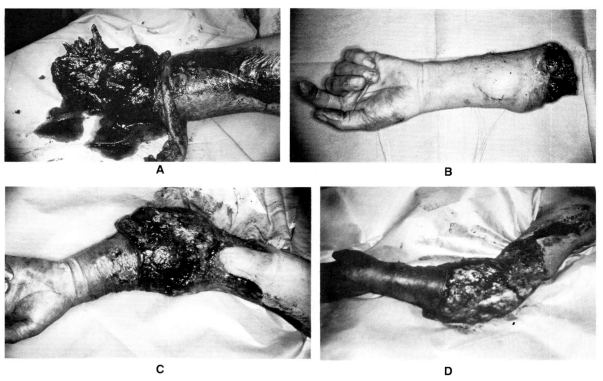

Figure 88–3. Amputation of the forearm. *A*, Appearance on arrival. A cutaneous avulsion extends above the elbow, and a contusion reaches the axilla. *B*, Healthy appearance of the amputated distal fragment. *C*, Despite major necrosis, restoration of blood supply to the hand by arterial grafting is assured. *D*, Major skin necrosis requiring amputation on the eleventh day.

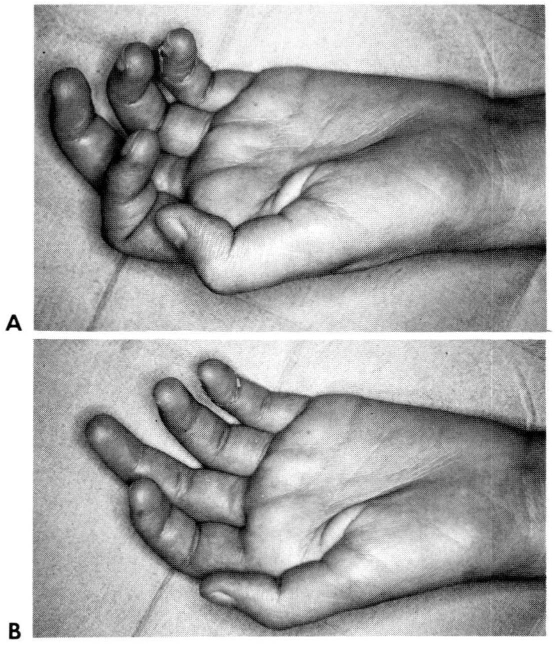

Figure 88–4. Six month result of replantation of the left forearm. *A*, Flexion. *B*, Extension.

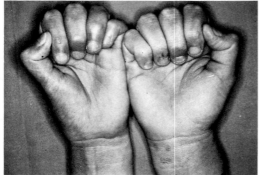

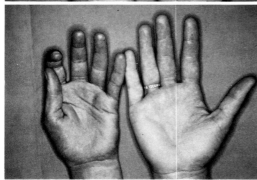

Figure 88–5. Appearance of same patient as in Figure 88–4 at two years. *A*, Flexion. *B*, Extension. Note the deficit in extension of the index finger already visible at six months.

occur up to two years after replantation (Figs. 88–4, 88–5). Sensory and motor rehabilitation must start early and be continued for months or even years. Finally, in the case of a manual worker, a change of occupation is often necessary. This should also be initiated as early as possible, preferably during rehabilitation.

CONCLUSION

We have tried to review all the factors that must be considered before deciding upon a replantation. They are many and varied, and difficult to classify. However, rather than listing the indications, perhaps one should stress the two main groups of contraindications—unidigital lesions (except for the thumb) and injuries by contusion with pressure showing extensive damage to the skin and muscles.

The object of a replantation is to effect good motor and sensory recovery. This presupposes a complete primary repair of all damaged structures (since secondary attempts are made difficult and risky by fibrosis) and a full course of rehabilitation combined with early professional readaptation. Only then can the high cost of replantation be justified.

Chapter 89

THE REPAIR OF FLEXOR TENDONS WITHIN THE DIGITAL SHEATH AT THE TIME OF REPLANTATION OR REVASCULARIZATION

JAMES B. STEICHEN
RODGER D. POWELL
AND JERRY L. ELLSTEIN

While several surgeons around the world were independently developing and learning the techniques and skills of microvascular surgery, it was not until the 1960's that these skills were polished enough to apply this technique to the attempted salvage of the completely or incompletely amputated digit. It was not until Susumu Tamai in 1965 (Komatsu and Tamai, 1968) was finally able to achieve the first successful replantation of a completely amputated thumb that a new era in traumatic and reconstructive hand surgery began. Digits that had previously been discarded because their vascular supply could not be restored were now able to be revascularized or replanted on a predictably successful basis. The primary concern of the microvascular surgeons initially was concentrated on the techniques necessary to ensure success of the vascular repairs, which were vital in guaranteeing the viability of the replanted or revascularized digit. Once the vascular repairs became more predictable and manageable, the interest in the repair and eventual function of the salvaged digit shifted more toward greater concern about the repair of the tendons, bones, and nerves (O'Brien, 1977).

Chen Chung-Wei of Shanghai, China, has contributed much to the field of microvascu-

lar surgery, and he helped us shift the emphasis from concentrating entirely on the immediate goal of vascular survival to the long-term goal of functional achievement when he stated that "survival without restoration of function is not success" (American Replantation Mission to China, 1978; Chen and Zeng, 1983).

One of the most difficult challenges for the traumatic and reconstructive hand surgeon for many decades has been the management of the severed digital flexor tendon. Many of these accomplished surgeons who have specialized in treating injuries of the hand have acknowledged that the management of an isolated digital flexor tendon severance, even without injury to other tissues in the digit (such as the digital arteries, veins, nerves, extensor tendons, and bones), is a very difficult and challenging task (Strickland, 1985a). When other structures in the digit have been injured or severed in addition to the flexor tendons, the final results of flexor tendon management and function have indeed been greatly altered and affected by the concomitant injuries of these other structures (Fig. 89–1).

The management of isolated digital flexor tendon lacerations has changed over the years, based on clinical and experimental

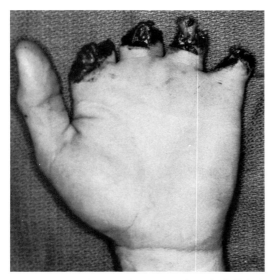

Figure 89–1. The complete amputation of all digits in Zone II is the maximum injury to a hand with trauma to all tissues, including severance of both flexor tendons, the extensor tendon, the intrinsic tendons, fracture of the bone, and complete severance of all neurovascular structures.

research related to flexor tendon healing as well as the increasing emphasis on rehabilitation after injury by trained therapists.

Decisions as to whether the best results are achieved by primary or delayed primary repair versus secondary reconstruction of the flexor tendon system have indeed changed over the last two to three decades during the parallel evolution of microvascular surgery. Decisions concerning the management of the rehabilitation phase after successful replantation and flexor tendon repair have also changed progressively as the era of microvascular surgery has continued to grow and mature.

FUNCTIONAL EVALUATION

The restoration of function following the replantation or revascularization of the completely or incompletely severed digit through Zone II of the flexor tendon system, as described by Verdan (Verdan, 1972; Kleinert et al., 1973), continues to be a challenge for the hand and microvascular surgeon.

Many different criteria have been advocated in order to evaluate the functional result obtained following successful digital replantation or revascularization. Because of

the uniqueness of the situation in which all tissues of the digit have been severed, and following the repair of all of the severed structures, the evaluation of the quality of functional return to the patient becomes more difficult.

Functional evaluations of patients with successful digital replantation or revascularization have included: (1) range of motion, (2) recovery of sensation, (3) muscle power, (4) grip strength, (5) pain, (6) cold intolerance, (7) ability to resume previous or new occupation, (8) ability to integrate the replanted parts into daily life and functional use, (9) patient satisfaction with the replanted part, and (10) cosmetic appearance. Because of the unique nature of the severity of the injury and the potential difficulties of healing these repaired structures, the evaluations have almost always included subjective as well as objective determinants. While all of the above objective and subjective criteria regarding the implanted part are indeed important to the integration into normal life by the patient, Harry Buncke has stated that of all of the factors influencing function, "experience has shown that the two most critical issues are sensibility and tendon gliding" (Buncke et al., 1981).

As a detailed analysis of flexor tendon function following digital replantation or revascularization has rarely been isolated from overall functional criteria, it seems that a review of the management decisions, techniques, and results of flexor tendon surgery in this category of patients would be important.

MANAGEMENT PROBLEMS

When the microvascular surgeon addresses the problem of tendon gliding in these injuries, two fundamental problems are presented. The first is how to restore digital motion, and the second is how to manage the severed flexor tendons.

In July of 1965, Susumu Tamai successfully performed the first replantation of a completely amputated digit. In his description of that surgery, he stated, "The flexor tendon was not sutured because it was cut in 'no man's land' and tendon graft was also postponed" (Komatsu and Tamai, 1968).

Subsequently many microvascular surgeons followed Tamai's protocol for the delayed elective repair of flexor tendons and possibly nerves because of the feeling that the initial delay in restoring blood supply to these digits that would be necessary if a delicate flexor tendon repair was performed as well as a microscopic nerve repair might jeopardize the successful revascularization of these amputated digits (Ikuta et al., 1973). Therefore, although primary repair of the severed flexor tendon in the digit was gaining acceptance throughout the world (Kleinert et al., 1973; Verdan, 1972), the microvascular surgeon at this time was more concerned about the viability of the digit, believing that if the digit survived, a secondary flexor tendon reconstruction could be performed at a later date (Urbaniak et al., 1978). The choice of the microvascular surgeon not to repair the flexor tendons initially at the time of replantation or revascularization, versus primary repair when possible, has also been evolving over the last 20 years.

SURGICAL DECISIONS AND OPTIONS

There are many choices and decisions that have to be made concerning the surgical management of the flexor tendon system.

Should Both the Flexor Digitorum Profundus and Flexor Digitorum Superficialis Be Repaired? In Zone II digital flexor tendon injuries, should both the flexor digitorum profundus and the flexor digitorum superficialis be repaired or should only the profundus be repaired and the superficialis excised (Tamai, 1978)? For many years it was recommended that a repair of the profundus only was preferred to repairing both tendons in the flexor sheath (Lendvay, 1974). The decrease in total volume of the sheath from only one tendon being repaired, versus two possibly bulbous repairs limiting the ability of the flexor tendons to glide through the intact portion of the sheath and under the annular pulleys, was believed to be an adequate reason for excision of the superficialis tendon. As our knowledge of flexor tendon anatomy and vascularity has improved and our technical skills in repairing tendons have also improved, it is currently believed that in isolated flexor tendon injuries both the profundus and the superficialis should be preserved and repaired (Lister and Kleinert, 1979). Part of the vascularity of the profundus

tendon is provided through the vincula to the superficialis tendon (Caplan et al., 1975), and, therefore, we may be destroying part of the blood supply to the profundus tendon by excising the intact superficialis tendon from the wounds.

The repair of both tendons is also thought to provide better strength and independent motion to the repaired finger as well as serving as an "insurance policy" in that if one of the flexor tendon repairs ruptures, the other repair may remain intact and provide sufficient motion, thus eliminating the need for multiple procedures to reconstruct the entire flexor tendon system. The retention and repair of the flexor digitorum superficialis also helps to provide a smooth bed for the flexor digitorum profundus tendon over the bone and possibly the joint injury. The repaired flexor digitorum superficialis may also help to prevent proximal interphalangeal joint hyperextension. It is therefore currently felt that the results in terms of flexor tendon function and digital motion are better if both the flexor digitorum profundus and the flexor digitorum superficialis are repaired.

Should the Flexor Digitorum Profundus Be Repaired If the Flexor Digitorum Superficialis Is Intact? If the flexor digitorum superficialis tendon is intact and the amputation is distal or through to the superficialis insertion, should the flexor digitorum profundus be repaired or resected from the digit? As information from more replantation centers is becoming available, the indications for replantation of an amputated digit distal to the superficialis insertion are gaining more favor and acceptance. The results of these replantations have shown that even if the flexor digitorum profundus is not repaired, or is repaired and becomes adherent, these become excellent functional digits with metacarpophalangeal and proximal interphalangeal joint motion that is satisfactory for acceptable digital function. If the profundus tendon is amenable to direct repair, however, the surgeon may wish to repair this tendon in order to preserve the possibility of profundus function and distal interphalangeal joint motion.

Is Staged Flexor Tendon Reconstruction Better? Should both the severed flexor digitorum profundus and the flexor digitorum superficialis tendon be excised from the digit and a primary passive Silastic tendon prosthesis be inserted as the first step in an elective staged flexor tendon reconstruction (Daniel and Terzis, 1977; Hunter, 1983)? In many cases of avulsion amputations of the digit, the flexor tendons may be avulsed from the digit and there is no possibility of primary repair. In these circumstances, inserting a Silastic rod primarily in order to prevent the flexor sheath from collapsing and to preserve the integrity of the annular pulleys remaining in the digit is sometimes a necessary option. If the flexor tendons may be amenable to repair, however, the surgeon must decide whether primary repair will give a better functional result than excision of the tendons and insertion of a Silastic tendon prosthesis with elective secondary tendon reconstruction after passive digital motion has been achieved. The surgeon must also be able to predict whether the wound will heal with suitable soft tissue coverage over the Silastic tendon prosthesis (Lendvay, 1977).

Should Primary Flexor Tendon Grafting Be Done? Should primary flexor tendon grafting be performed at the time of replantation or revascularization? If the flexor tendons are avulsed from the digit or are not amenable to repair, the surgeon must decide whether to insert a Silastic tendon prosthesis or to consider the possibility of a primary free tendon graft at the time of replantation (Boyes and Stark, 1971). If the surgeon feels that better results are obtained from primary tendon grafting versus repair of a damaged flexor tendon through the digit, this is another option that is available.

Should the Flexor Digitorum Profundus Plus the Flexor Digitorum Superficialis Be Shortened? Should the flexor tendons be shortened if skeletal shortening is performed at the time of replantation? Most microvascular surgeons will not hesitate to shorten the skeleton of the digit at the site of the fracture in order to facilitate the ability to resect damaged vessels, nerves, tendons, and skin back to normal healthy tissue so that primary anastomosis or end-to-end repair can be done. If indeed the bony skeleton and the digit are shortened between 5.0 and 10.0 mm., will the flexor tendons be able to adjust proximally for the slightly excess length, or is it necessary to shorten the flexor tendons as much as the skeleton is shortened in order to maintain normal length:tension ratios (May and Gallico, 1980; Meyer et al., 1981)? I feel that usually the normal debridement of the roughened flexor tendon ends is sufficient

shortening and that the muscle will absorb the slight length differential.

Should Differential Shortening of Bone and Tendon Be Done? Should there be differential shortening of the bone and tendon? If bony fixation is performed at one level, will there be less chance for a "one-wound" scar formation and adhesions of the flexor tendon to the bony repair if one end of the flexor tendon could be shortened so that the flexor tendon repair would be at a slightly different level than the bone repair? This has been recommended in an attempt to overcome the "one-wound" scar concept.

What Is the Timing of Repair? Should the timing of the repair of the flexor tendons be the same as a primary repair, a delayed primary repair, or a secondary repair or reconstruction? As there are many microvascular surgeons with differing backgrounds, training, and experience in flexor tendon repair who perform replantation and revascularization surgery, there are consequently many different approaches to the timing and repair of the severed flexor tendons. The feeling that the best chance to repair all the structures is at the time of the primary revascularization indeed seems to be the most popular concept currently, although several surgeons feel that a delay for delicate flexor tendon surgery and rehabilitation is appropriate and may indeed provide better results in terms of tendon gliding. Oddvar Eiken (1982) has recommended patch grafting the damaged or destroyed section of the flexor sheath and inserting a Silastic rod at the time of the replantation procedure. Then, after the digit has proven viability and has become passively supple, a planned staged tendon reconstruction can be performed at a later date with possibly better results than the primary repair.

SURGICAL PROTOCOL AND TECHNIQUE

Our surgical approach to the completely amputated digit (once a decision to attempt a replantation has been made and appropriate x-rays of the proximal stump as well as the amputated part have demonstrated the feasibility of the replantation attempt) involves first the dissection of the amputated part to ascertain that appropriate vessels are available for vascular repair (Fig. 89–2).

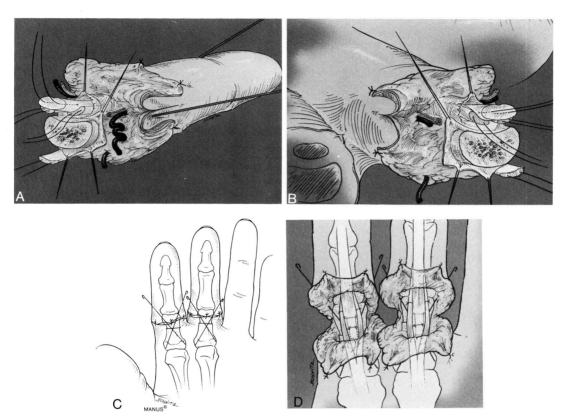

Figure 89–2. Surgical technique. *A*, The distal part is prepared by debridement of all traumatized tissue. Midlateral skin incisions are made with the dorsal and volar flaps folded distally without tension and sutured to provide retraction and visualization. The neurovascular structures are carefully and gently identified and dissected free for later anastomosis and repair. The distal flexor sheath and all annular pulleys are left intact, and the distal tendon is delivered into the wound by passive flexion of the proximal interphalangeal and distal interphalangeal joints. The flexor sheath and periosteum are dissected from the bone and reflected distally when possible, and the end of the bone is then shortened appropriately and a surface is prepared for apposition of the fracture fragments. Two 0.035 inch Kirschner wires are then drilled through the distal fragment, preserving the proximal interphalangeal joint. The core sutures are then placed in each slip of the superficialis tendon and in the profundus tendon and also placed in the extensor tendon.

B, The identical procedure is performed on the proximal stump with preparation of all structures for attachment. The core suture is pre-placed in all of the proximal tendons, including each slip of the flexor digitorum superficialis, the flexor digitorum profundus, and the extensor tendon. The intrinsic tendons are also identified at this time for repair when possible.

C, The fracture fragments are now reduced and the fingers aligned appropriately with bony resection, usually between 5.0 and 10.0 mm., which is performed as far from the nearest joint as possible.

D, The pre-placed sutures have now been tied, repairing the profundus as well as each slip of the superficialis tendon. If the flexor sheath was able to be repaired, the dorsal portion of the sheath was repaired in order to cover the fracture site prior to the sutures being tied in the flexor tendons. The sheath would be closed over the flexor tendons after they had been repaired. The extensor tendons would be sutured prior to the flexor tendons being sutured. (*A–D*, Copyright 1986, Manus.)

Mid-lateral skin incisions are made on the radial and ulnar borders, and dorsal and volar flaps are then carefully reflected distally and tagged loosely with skin sutures. Using 4.5 power loop magnification, the nerves and arteries are carefully dissected, identified, and isolated for later repair. The dorsal veins are next identified in the reflected flaps and prepared accordingly, and then the extensor and flexor tendons are dissected and visualized. All of the remaining flexor sheath and annular pulleys are left intact distally, and the distal end of the severed flexor tendons can almost always be visualized by passively flexing the distal interphalangeal or proximal interphalangeal joint, which thereby delivers the severed flexor tendons into the wound.

The exposed fracture is usually squared off with a power saw when needed. By coordinating the preparation of the proximal fracture segment as well as the fracture fragment of the amputated part and also using the x-rays to provide additional information, the fractured ends are squared off to match each other. Usually, a total of about 5.0 mm. of bone may be resected from either or both sides of the fracture, depending on which segment may be farther from the articular surface.

The extensor tendons are then shortened approximately the same amount as the bone. The flexor tendons are usually debrided of all damaged and ragged tissue, but not necessarily shortened the same amount as the bone because the flexor tendon system is believed to be able to adjust for the slight difference in length, whereas the extensor tendon system is not able to adjust at the digital level.

Once the bone has been prepared and the tendons have been debrided to healthy tissue, a 4-0 braided synthetic suture is woven in a modified Kessler-Tajima–type technique (Fig. 89–3) with locking of the suture at each point as it pierces the outside of the tendon. This places the sutures inside the tendon substance so that when the sutures are tied, the knots will lie inside rather than outside the tendon.

At this time, the exact same approach is used for the tissues of the proximal stump. The proximal ends of the severed flexor tendons can usually be gently obtained by flexion of the wrist and metacarpophalangeal joints and manually milking the tendons from proximal to distal. A small hemostat gently in-

serted in the flexor sheath can identify the distal end of the proximal flexor tendon and deliver it into the wound.

The tendon is grasped inside the tendon substance and delivered distally, and a short 25-gauge needle is then placed proximally through the flexor sheath and the flexor ten-

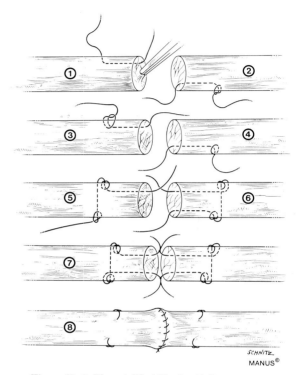

Figure 89–3. The modified Kessler-Tajima core suture is suitable for a completely amputated digit in that the sutures can be placed by one team dissecting the distal amputated part as well as by the second team that is dissecting and preparing the proximal stump. Once the tendons have been debrided, the tendon is grasped inside the core of the tendon substance with delicate grasping forceps. *Step 1:* The 4–0 braided synthetic suture is introduced through the severed end of the tendon and brought out distally between 5.0 and 10.0 mm. *Step 3:* The suture is then looped through the ipsilateral exterior edge of the tendon and locked on itself. *Step 5:* The suture is then passed transversely through the volar surface of the tendon and then looped again through the outside edge of the tendon and locked upon itself. *Step 7:* The suture is now passed back parallel to Step 1 and delivered out the opposite side of the tendon. *Steps 2, 4, and 6:* The exact same placement is carried out in the proximal end of the tendon. Step 7 shows the tendon being brought together by flexion of all the joints to take the tension off the repair site, and the core sutures are tied with multiple knots left inside the tendon substance. *Step 8:* The tendon ends are brought together with gentle tension so as not to make a bulbous repair or "accordion" the repair together, and the outer surface is then smoothed over by a continuous 6–0 nylon suture. (Copyright 1986, Manus.)

dons in order to maintain the visible presentation of the tendon in the wound (Lister and Kleinert, 1979). The 4-0 braided synthetic suture is then woven using the same modified Kessler-Tajima technique (Kessler and Nissim, 1969; Urbaniak, 1984) through the proximal flexor tendons with the ends of the suture left untied until the digits are joined. Some of the earliest cases were repaired with a modified Bunnell technique, but the modified Tajima technique has been used for the majority of the early cases and for all of the later cases.

Whenever possible, the superficialis is repaired primarily as well as the profundus, and if both slips of the flexor digitorum superficialis are separate, a separate weave is performed for each slip proximally and distally. Bony fixation is usually achieved with crossed Kirschner wires, in an attempt to preserve joint mobility so that motion may be initiated while the Kirschner wires are still providing necessary fracture fixation. Occasionally, interosseous wiring is utilized with one or two Kirschner wires added for skeletal rigidity. After the fracture has been internally fixed, the extensor tendons are repaired similarly.

Occasionally, while the fracture ends are being dissected and prepared, the dorsal portion of the flexor sheath may be able to be dissected free from the bone and preserved for later repair over the fracture site. Whenever possible, the dorsal portion of the flexor sheath is then repaired with absorbable suture in order to cover the fracture site. The preplaced sutures inside the flexor tendon substance are then tied together, in an attempt to perform as anatomical a repair as possible (Steichen and Idler, 1984).

The superficialis slips are sutured first, and then the profundus ends are tied. A 6-0 running nylon suture is then almost always used to try to smooth the surface of the profundus repair anatomically.

The flexor pulleys are preserved throughout the procedure, and whenever possible the flexor sheath is then repaired with a running 6-0 nylon following the flexor tendon repair (Lister, 1983). In many cases when the digit has been amputated in a ragged fashion, the flexor sheath is not able to be repaired at the time of replantation. It should be emphasized that the flexor tendons are repaired using 4.5 power magnification with as meticulous and atraumatic a technique as possible, employing the same delicate instrumentation used for repair of all of the severed structures (Urbaniak et al., 1985; Weiland et al., 1978).

As the measurement of tendon gliding depends upon passive mobility of the joints of the digit, attempts are made to preserve the metacarpophalangeal, proximal interphalangeal, and distal interphalangeal joints. Occasionally, when the injury has destroyed the articular surfaces or disarticulated the joints, fusion of the joint may be necessary owing to the destruction of that joint.

Occasionally, when the joint has been destroyed and the surgeon believes that adequate soft tissues can be closed over the joint, a primary Silastic arthroplasty has been performed at the time of replantation in order to preserve some joint motion. Almost always an attempt has been made to repair the damaged flexor tendons. Primary insertion of a Silastic passive tendon prosthesis in this traumatic wound has not been our normal practice.

POSTOPERATIVE MANAGEMENT DECISIONS AFTER FLEXOR TENDON REPAIR

As there are choices of management of the flexor tendon at the time of the initial surgery, there are also choices of management of the flexor tendons postoperatively. In the digit that has been severed with all structures repaired primarily, is it possible to initiate a rehabilitation program that would be normally implemented for an isolated digital flexor tendon repair? If the normal therapy program is to start early motion following flexor tendon repairs by either the Duran technique of controlled passive motion (Duran and Houser, 1975) or the Kleinert technique of "immediate controlled mobilization" (Lister et al., 1977), will this jeopardize the other repaired tendon and neurovascular structures in the digit?

Another option would be to initiate an early active motion program or perhaps a mild passive motion program with assisted active motion.

The final option would be to immobilize the replanted digit for several weeks, which would provide immobilization sufficient to heal the vessel, nerve, and extensor tendon structures and could then be followed by a progressive active and passive motion program (O'Brien and MacLeod, 1976).

PROBLEMS OF INITIATION OF EARLY MOTION

In the replanted or revascularized digit, we have felt that there are potential problems with initiation of an early flexor tendon mobilization program because of the risk of stretching the dorsal venous repairs in addition to the arterial and nerve repairs. Mobilization of the digit might increase the risk of stretching the anastomoses of the vessels, initiating vascular spasm, thrombosis, and possible vascular compromise. Disruption of the fracture or fusion fixation may also be possible (Scott, 1986).

The most important reason, however, that we have not started early motion within the first 3 weeks following replantation or revascularization has been due to possible problems with extensor tendon repair (Morrison et al., 1978). Experience has shown that whenever an extensor tendon in the digit is severed and repaired, it is necessary to immobilize that repair in a position of full extension for at least a 3 to 6 week period, depending on the location of the injury. This is important in order to prevent the extensor tendon repair from attenuating and length-

ening during its period of healing, which might make it incapable of providing full extension of the digit. A frequent finding is that whenever the extensor mechanism has been stretched or attenuated primarily, it is an extremely difficult problem to correct secondarily either by tenolysis or by attempted reconstruction. Therefore, principally based on the difficulties with management of the repaired extensor tendon in the digit, we feel that it is appropriate to immobilize the extensor tendon repair with the realization that secondary tenolysis and mobilization of the flexor tendon system may be necessary in the future.

POSTOPERATIVE THERAPY FOR REPLANTATION

Our postoperative therapy for digital replantation or revascularization has been to immobilize the digit and hand in a short-arm dressing for 3 weeks followed by the institution of active range of motion therapy for an additional 3 weeks and then dynamic splinting and passive range of motion therapy as necessary (Fig. 89–4) (Steichen et al., 1978).

Figure 89–4. *A,* A 15-year-old boy with a severe power saw injury to the right hand with complete amputation of the index finger through the metacarpophalangeal joint, the long finger through the proximal phalanx, an incomplete amputation with irreparable destruction of the ring finger, and tendon and proximal interphalangeal joint damage to the small finger.

B, Immediately postoperatively following replantation of the index and long finger with 1.0 cm. of shortening of the proximal phalanx, the flexor digitorum profundus, flexor digitorum superficialis, and extensor digitorum communis of both digits. The patient had fusion of the destroyed index metacarpophalangeal joint and primary repair of both the flexor digitorum profundus and flexor digitorum superficialis to the index and long fingers along with all other damaged structures. Ring finger amputation was completed because of the total destruction of that digit, and the small finger proximal interphalangeal joint and extensor tendon injuries were repaired.

C and *D,* Fifteen months post-replantation. The patient has limitation of full active flexion of the index, long, and small fingers, as shown here in active extension and flexion. The patient had excellent passive range of motion to the involved digits with good passive potential for improvement at this time.

E, At surgery, 15 months following replantation, the patient underwent tenolysis of the index, long, and small fingers. The profundus and superficialis tendons to the index finger were healed solidly together as a single scar unit, and after the tendons had been totally tenolyzed into the forearm area, due to the common scarring of the tendons, the proximal pull would exert its force only at the proximal interphalangeal joint, and therefore it was necessary to release the superficialis insertion in order to have both proximal muscle tendon units pull at the distal joint, which now allowed full pull-through at the proximal interphalangeal and distal interphalangeal joints. The long finger revealed a rupture of both repaired flexor tendons, which were excised, and a 5.0 mm. Silastic tendon prosthesis was inserted from the tip of the finger into the forearm. A flexor and extensor tenolysis was performed to the small finger, and owing to the quadriga effect of the adherent profundus tendon to the amputated ring finger, it was necessary to tenolyze and release the distal attachment of the profundus tendon to the ring finger in order to get full proximal excursion of the profundus tendon to the small finger. Two months following the insertion of the prosthesis to the long finger, the Silastic tendon prosthesis was removed and replaced with a free plantaris tendon graft.

F, At 5 years post-replantation, x-ray showing solid fusion of the index metacarpophalangeal joint and excellent healing of the long finger proximal phalangeal joint.

G and *H,* At 5 years post-replantation, the patient demonstrates maximal active extension and flexion. The patient has an extensor lag of the index proximal interphalangeal and the long distal interphalangeal joints, but has excellent flexion and flexor pull-through of all digits. The patient has refused a ray resection of the ring finger.

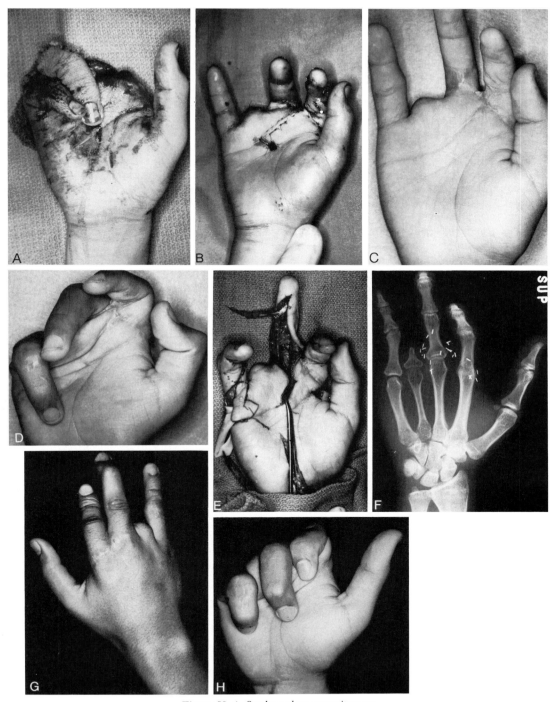

Figure 89–4. *See legend on opposite page*

RESULTS OF ZONE II DIGITAL FLEXOR TENDON REPAIRS FOLLOWING SUCCESSFUL REPLANTATION AND REVASCULARIZATION

In order to objectively evaluate the results of flexor tendon repair in digital replantation and revascularization, we evaluated the results of 26 consecutive patients with successful replantation or revascularization within Verdan's Zone II in the digital flexor sheath following severance and primary repair of their flexor tendons. This series included 44 digits, of which 31 had been replanted following complete amputation and 13 had been revascularized following incomplete amputation with total devascularization and flexor tendon severance. The 26 consecutive patients in this series were managed similarly by the same surgeon during surgery and rehabilitation. The patients were isolated from all other patients with complete and incomplete amputations that occurred either distal or proximal to Verdan's Zone II classification, and the other patients were not included in this series. A total of 63 flexor tendons were repaired, and the follow-up evaluation averaged 15.4 months with a range of from 2 to 64 months. The patients evaluated for only 2 months were those who failed to return to the office for further treatment and therapy.

Flexor tendon function was evaluated objectively by measurement of total active motion (Fess et al., 1978; Nielsen and Jensen, 1985; Schneider, 1985). The evaluations were determined in two ways. The first was to use the guidelines of the American Society for Surgery of the Hand (1978) for determining total active motion. Total active motion (TAM) is a term applied to one finger and is:

1. The sum of active metacarpophalangeal flexion + active proximal interphalangeal (PIP) flexion + active distal interphalangeal (DIP) flexion.
2. Minus the sum of incomplete active extension, if any is present.

The flexor tendon function was also evaluated based on the recommendations of Strickland and Glogovac (1980). This technique excludes the metacarpophalangeal joint from the total active motion measurements based on the concept that the metacarpophalangeal joint almost always has full range of motion postoperatively and inclusion of the metacarpophalangeal joint range of motion increases the total active motion values automatically by almost a third.

The formula of Strickland and Glogovac is:

$$\frac{\text{Active PIP + DIP flexion} - \text{extensor lag}}{175°} \times 100 =$$

% of normal active PIP & DIP motion

FLEXOR TENDON FUNCTION

The final flexor tendon function when the proximal and distal interphalangeal joints were evaluated showed that the digital replantations achieved 45 degrees of proximal and distal interphalangeal joint motion or 26 per cent of normal proximal and distal interphalangeal joint TAM, and revascularized digits achieved 57 degrees or 33 per cent of normal TAM of the proximal and distal interphalangeal joints. This meant that the entire digital group achieved final TAM of 49 degrees involving these two joints or 28 per cent of normal TAM of the proximal and distal interphalangeal joints.

When the metacarpophalangeal joint is included with the proximal and distal interphalangeal joints, the replanted digits achieved 114 degrees of final TAM or 44 per cent of normal TAM compared with the revascularized digits, which achieved 144 degrees or 55 per cent of normal TAM. The total TAM of these two groups was 123 degrees or 47 per cent.

Isolated Flexor Digitorum Profundus Versus Combined Flexor Digitorum Profundus Plus Flexor Digitorum Superficialis Repairs

There were a group of patients with Zone II digital flexor tendon injuries who for reasons determined at the time of surgery (e.g., severely injured or avulsed superficialis tendon) had only the profundus tendon repaired. It was also noted in reviewing these patients that most of the single flexor digitorum profundus repairs were performed earlier in the study, whereas most of the patients in the latter part of this study group had both flexor tendons repaired whenever surgically possible.

Twenty-five digits or 57 per cent of the

total study group had only the flexor digitorum profundus repaired. This group achieved 47 degrees or 27 per cent of normal proximal and distal interphalangeal joint TAM. When the metacarpophalangeal joint is included in the determinations, this group achieved 115 degrees or 46 per cent of normal TAM.

Nineteen digits or 43 per cent of the study group had both the flexor digitorum profundus and the flexor digitorum superficialis repaired. Evaluation of this group showed that these digits achieved 50 degrees of proximal and distal interphalangeal joint motion or 28 per cent of normal TAM of these two joints. When the metacarpophalangeal group was included, 121 degrees was achieved or 47 per cent of normal TAM.

The final results achieved in both determinations showed that the final TAM was similar whether one or both flexor tendons had been repaired.

Revascularized Digits With Fracture Versus No Fracture

The 13 revascularized digits in Zone II with flexor tendon repairs were evaluated to determine if the presence of a fracture influenced the final TAM (Strickland, 1982). Of the 13 digits in this group, seven had been fractured and six had been devascularized with the flexor tendon severed but the bony skeleton intact. The fracture group achieved 51 degrees or 29 per cent of normal proximal and interphalangeal joint TAM compared with the group without fractures, which had 61 degrees or 35 per cent of normal proximal and distal interphalangeal joint motion. When the metacarpophalangeal joint was included, the fracture group achieved 137 degrees or 53 per cent of normal TAM compared with the group without fractures, which achieved 149 degrees or 57 per cent of normal TAM.

Secondary Procedures to Increase Range of Motion

As our experience and confidence in handling replanted and revascularized digits improved over the last two decades, the number of secondary procedures to improve final function and TAM also progressively increased (Morrison et al., 1978). We now approach these digits with the same aggressive secondary reconstructive program that we would any other digit that had had the flexor tendons severed and repaired, whether or not vascular repairs had been done.

We are, however, very cautious and careful in approaching these digits for secondary reconstructive procedures and are very careful to identify the arterial blood flow to each digit preoperatively to ascertain that this is not compromised during extensive reconstructive procedures. This preoperative evaluation is done by reviewing the original operative report concerning the status of the blood flow at the end of the operative procedure as well as using Doppler flow studies to determine whether one or both digital arteries are intact. Arteriography may also be helpful occasionally in performing a careful preoperative evaluation.

The quality of the nerve return is also evaluated prior to re-entering the digit to determine whether a neurolysis may be indicated to try to improve the quality of return of sensory function to the digit.

Although in the early 1970's it was uncommon to perform many secondary procedures on these revascularized or replanted digits, we now carry out the routine procedures designed to improve the range of motion in a traumatized digit (Hayhurst, 1976). Extensor tenolysis, which may or may not include dorsal capsulotomy, is performed to increase the passive range of motion of a digit that has limited active as well as passive range of motion.

If a joint with arthrofibrosis is found to be destroyed upon exploration, we would proceed with a Silastic interpositional arthroplasty, or if stability of the digit is indicated, such as the proximal interphalangeal joint in the index finger, a fusion of the joint would be performed. Once passive motion and flexion are achieved in the digit, other reconstructive procedures consisting of a flexor tenolysis would be performed at a later date. If it is found at the time of surgery that the original flexor tendon repair had ruptured, we would proceed with staged flexor tendon reconstruction as indicated.

Secondary Procedures Affecting Digital Performance

The procedures listed in Table 89–1 were done secondarily to try to improve the final digital performance.

Table 89–1. SECONDARY PROCEDURES TO IMPROVE FINAL DIGITAL PERFORMANCE

Procedure	Number	Per Cent
Extensor tenolysis	14	25
Dorsal capsulotomy	14	25
Flexor tenolysis	14	25
Joint fusion	4	7
Joint arthroplasty	1	2
Staged tendon reconstruction:		
Hunter rods	3	6
Free tendon grafts	3	6
Tenolysis following free tendon graft	2	4
Total	55	100

Flexor Tenolysis

Thirty per cent of patients with replanted or revascularized digits underwent flexor tenolysis during their course of treatment (Cooney et al., 1985). It should be noted that other patients in this series had received recommendations for flexor tenolysis based on having a passive potential that indicated improvement could be gained by flexor tenolysis, but they failed to follow through with the recommended surgery.

Of the 13 digits that had required flexor tenolysis, it was found that six of these had repair of only the profundus, whereas seven had repair of the profundus plus the superficialis. This indicated that in this series the necessity for flexor tenolysis was not determined by whether one or both flexor tendons had been repaired.

Improvement in Motion Following Tenolysis and/or Capsulotomy

The digits that underwent either extensor tenolysis with or without dorsal capsulotomy or flexor tenolysis as required were evaluated to compare their pre-tenolysis motion versus their post-tenolysis motion.

The group prior to tenolysis had 36 degrees or 21 per cent of normal proximal and interphalangeal joint TAM compared with post-tenolysis TAM of 66 degrees, which was 38 per cent of normal proximal and distal interphalangeal joint TAM. When the same group was evaluated and the metacarpophalangeal joint was included, the group before tenolysis had a TAM of 102 degrees or 38 per cent of normal compared with post-tenolysis measurements of 128 degrees or 52 per cent of normal. This demonstrated a marked improvement in the final TAM achieved based on reconstructive procedures to mobilize the digit.

Flexor Tendon Ruptures

Ruptures of the repaired flexor tendons were diagnosed in 7 of the 63 repaired tendons, which was 11 per cent of the total tendon repairs, or 6 of the 44 digits, which was 14 per cent of the replanted or revascularized digits. Of the flexor tendon ruptures that received further treatment, three had staged flexor tendon reconstructions, and one had fusion of the proximal and distal interphalangeal joints. Further treatment was not elected by the remaining patients.

Evaluation of Flexor Tendon Function Following Primary or Secondary Fusion or Arthroplasty

Four digits required fusion of the metacarpophalangeal joint, which gave a final TAM of the proximal and distal interphalangeal joints of 114 degrees, which was 65 per cent of normal proximal and distal interphalangeal joint TAM. When the metacarpophalangeal joint was included in the determinations, the TAM was the same, but the percentage of normal was reduced to 44 per cent of normal TAM for the digit.

Nine digits required fusion of the proximal interphalangeal joint. These digits achieved only 1.1 degrees of final proximal and distal interphalangeal joint TAM, which was 0.6 per cent of normal proximal and distal interphalangeal joint TAM. When the metacarpophalangeal joint was included, the final TAM was 81 degrees or 31 per cent of normal TAM for the digit. These results showed that most of the digital motion achieved is at the proximal rather than the distal interphalangeal joint.

Five digits received proximal interphalangeal joint Silastic replacement arthroplasty, and these digits had 43 degrees of final proximal and digital interphalangeal joint TAM, which was 25 per cent of normal TAM. When the metacarpophalangeal joint was included in the final determinations, these digits achieved 130 degrees of TAM, which was 50 per cent of their normal TAM.

CLASSIFICATION SYSTEM

The classification system used to determine the results of digital replantation and revascularization based on final TAM was determined for the proximal and distal interpha-

Table 89–2. CLASSIFICATION SYSTEM FOR DETERMINING RESULTS OF DIGITAL REPLANTATION AND REVASCULARIZATION

Group	PIP + DIP Return (%)	PIP + DIP − Extensor Loss (Degrees)
Excellent	75–100	132 +
Good	50–74	88–131
Fair	25–49	44–87
Poor	0–24	0–43

langeal joint classification according to a modification of the original classification system as described by Strickland and Glogovac (1980). The 1980 classification system was based on a codification system that is essentially the one suggested by the Committee on Tendon Injuries of the International Federation of Societies for Surgery of the Hand modified to the present classification (Strickland, 1985b) (Table 89–2).

FINAL RESULTS

The final results based on the return of TAM, including the proximal and distal interphalangeal joints, is shown in Table 89–3.

If the metacarpophalangeal joint is included in the final TAM measurements (as many surgeons use in their evaluations) the final TAM achieved by the replanted digits is 114 degrees or 44 per cent of normal. The revascularized digits achieved 144 degrees or 55 per cent of normal, which means that the total group achieved 123 degrees or 47 per cent of normal TAM.

DISCUSSION

Multiple explanations have been offered for the relatively poor results of flexor tendon repairs in Zone II following successful digital replantation or revascularization based on the final TAM. Certainly it is realized that all tissue structures in the digit are involved in the trauma, repair, and scar formation process. The extent of scar tissue formation fixing many different tissues together with the single wound scar formation concept as outlined by Peacock (1984) is definitely present (Tajima 1984). This extensive scar formation, which is an attempt to heal the severe injury caused by trauma to the digit, certainly has a direct negative effect on fluid joint function as well as tendon gliding. It is also recognized that normal fluid full digital function is achieved by a combination of a well-functioning extrinsic as well as intrinsic muscle-tendon system, and the intrinsic balance in these digits is severely disrupted by the trauma that is required to amputate these digits completely.

Anatomical repair of the intrinsic system is impossible in many of these digits, and in those digits in which it is possible to identify and repair the intrinsic system, the scarring of this system usually prohibits return of its normal anatomical function.

We know that when repaired flexor tendons are not moved early, either by a controlled passive motion technique or by a technique of passive flexion and active extension, the scar that forms has a much more solid rather than elastic composition. Because we are reluctant to move these digits early, owing to our concern about attenuating the extensor tendons as well as possibly irritating the vascular repairs, which might cause vascular spasm, thrombosis, and vascular compromise, our inability to initiate routine postoperative therapy of early motion for these digits certainly contributes to the scar and resultant limited motion (Gallico and Stirrat, 1983; Creekmore et al., 1985).

Table 89–3. FINAL RESULTS OF DIGITAL REPLANTATION AND REVASCULARIZATION BASED ON TAM

	Excellent	Good	Fair	Poor	Total Digits
Replantation	0	8 (26%)	6 (19%)	17 (55%)	31
Revascularization	1 (8%)	1 (8%)	6 (46%)	5 (38%)	13
Total	1 (2%)	9 (20%)	12 (27%)	22 (50%)	44

FINAL FLEXOR TENDON FUNCTION

	Per Cent of Normal PIP and DIP	Degrees	Result
Replantation	26%	45	Fair
Revascularization	33%	57	Fair
Total	28%	49	Fair

I feel that one of the most important factors that contributes to severe scarring at the site of the flexor tendon injury, in addition to possible attentuation or rupture of the flexor tendon repairs, is the disruption of the normal blood supply to the tendon. Such disruption probably occurs as a result of the injury and the techniques necessary to achieve satisfactory revascularization.

Hunter and his associates (Caplan et al., 1975) have in the last several years beautifully described the normal vascular anatomy of the flexor tendon system. Part of this normal vascular supply is through the intact vincula connecting the superficialis and profundus tendons. Another important part of the arterial supply to the flexor tendon system is provided by the transverse or lateral vessels to this system that originate from the longitudinal radial and ulnar digital arteries to each digit (Ochiai et al., 1979).

The injury that severs or devascularizes the digit always destroys a certain length of the digital arteries. If a digit has been avulsed or severely crushed locally, it is normal and correct microvascular technique to resect all of the damaged vessel until the vessel is completely normal, as visualized clinically and through the operating microscope. It is frequently necessary to replace large lengths of damaged vessel by interpositional venous grafts or even occasionally to replace the entire proximal vessel by swinging an arterial pedicle from an adjacent digit (Fig. 89–5).

With this type of injury, plus the techniques for replacing the arterial supply to the digit, it is easy to understand how these transverse vessels to the flexor tendons system are completely destroyed. If the flexor tendons have been avulsed from the digit or if the severed superficialis is excised and thereby iatrogenically avulsed from the digit, the vincular supply to the profundus, as well as the superficialis, may also have been totally destroyed (Amadio et al., 1985). With this destruction of the normal arterial supply to the flexor tendon system must naturally come a certain amount of avascularity of the damaged and repaired flexor tendons, which may indeed contribute to the possibility of attenuation or rupture at the repair site in addition to the extensive amount of scar that may form.

Another factor that contributes to the limited TAM is stiffness or arthrofibrosis of the joints of the involved digit. The rigidity and consequent lack of active or passive mobility of these joints are due to the extent of the injury and scar formation as well as the inability to mobilize the joint early as a result of the immobilization that is thought to be necessary postoperatively. Further restrictions to flexor tendon motion and gliding are due to adhesions of the extensor mechanism, which may prevent active as well as passive motion of the digit, and these adhesions are due to the damaged and repaired extensor tendon as well as the probable combination of extensor tendon repair at the site of fracture healing. The final reason for limited flexor tendon gliding is the formation of normal adhesions within the flexor tendon sheath

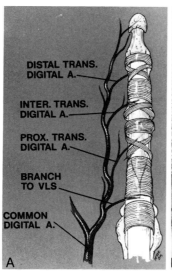
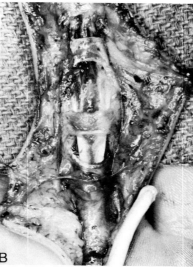

Figure 89–5. *A*, The transverse communicating branches of a single digital artery are shown entering the flexor sheath in order to contribute to the vascular perfusion of the flexor tendons.

B, With damage to a large length of the digital vessel requiring a long resection of the vessel or an interpositional vein graft, plus the avulsion of the vincula that occurs with flexor tendon retraction after severance, it is easy to see how this loss of normal blood supply to the flexor tendons may contribute to a great length of avascular tendon that may indeed lead to difficulties in healing the repaired tendon, possible attenuation of the repair site, possible rupture of the repair, and dense adhesions. (*A* and *B*, Copyright 1986, Manus.)

as a result of the injury and subsequent repair (Buncke et al., 1981).

ACHIEVEMENT OF BEST RESULTS

Based on our experience with flexor tendon repair and rehabilitation in the replanted or revascularized digit over the last 12 years, we believe that we can achieve the best results in terms of flexor tendon gliding, joint mobility, and final TAM by performing a primary repair of all structures, including the flexor tendons whenever possible. As soon as possible, an aggressive rehabilitation program needs to be started with trained hand therapists.

In spite of the surgeon's ability to perform delicate and anatomical surgery and the ability to coordinate a well-designed rehabilitation program under the direction of a trained hand therapist, if we do not have a well-motivated patient who will work to the maximum extent of his or her ability, our final results in terms of TAM will indeed be less than the surgeon expects or believes is possible to achieve.

While it is important to isolate the results of flexor tendon repairs in the evaluation of patients with digital revascularization or replantation, it is important to realize that the flexor tendons are not an isolated tissue in this severe trauma. Susumu Tamai (1978) has stated that "the criteria for flexor tendon repair are not applicable to these patients because digit replantation is not an injury only to the flexor tendon, but includes all tissues of the finger that have been repaired at the same time and at the same level." Based on his tremendous experience, Tamai (1978) has also explained that "the patient's satisfaction or gratitude may be greater than that indicated by the objective function of the replanted digit and the surgeon's evaluation."

EXPECTATIONS FOLLOWING DIGITAL REPLANTATION OR REVASCULARIZATION

Based on our experience with the successful repair and reconstruction of the completely or incompletely amputated digit, plus our review of a consecutive series of patients managed over several years by the same hand surgeon, the following conclusions are evident:

1. The final TAM achieved following successful digital replantation or revascularization in Zone II is dependent upon many variables other than only flexor tendon gliding.

2. The final TAM may be about 30 per cent of the normal proximal and distal interphalangeal joint TAM or approximately 50 per cent of the normal TAM if all three joints in the digit are included.

3. A large number of flexor tendon repairs will require secondary reconstructive procedures, including tenolysis. The secondary procedures should be performed as in procedures for other non-revascularized digits whenever the expectation of better function is present.

4. The final TAM is similar whether one or both severed flexor tendons are repaired at the time of replantation or revascularization.

5. It is important to repair the severed flexor tendons with as delicate an anatomical repair as possible and to manage their rehabilitation aggressively in order to try to provide these patients with a chance for recovery of lost function. This is important in the final overall function of the damaged hand or extremity, as emphasized by Harry Buncke (Buncke et al., 1981), who stated that "lost digits never function."

REFERENCES

Amadio, P. C., Hunter, J. M., Jaeger, S. H., Wehbe, M. A., and Schneider, L. H.: The effect of vincular injury on the results of flexor tendon surgery in zone 2. J. Hand Surg., *10A*:626–632, 1985.

American Replantation Mission to China: Replantation surgery in China. Plast. Reconstr. Surg., *52*:476–489, 1978.

Boyes, J. H., and Stark, H. H.: Flexor-tendon grafts in the fingers and thumb. A study of factors influencing results in 1000 cases. J. Bone Joint Surg. *53A*:1332–1342, 1971.

Buncke, H. J., Alpert, B. S., and Johnson-Giebink, R.: Digital replantation. Surg. Clin. North Am., *61*:383–394, 1981.

Caplan, H. S., Hunter, J. M., and Merklin, R. J.: Intrinsic vascularization of flexor tendons. *In* American Academy of Orthopaedic Surgeons Symposium on Tendon Surgery in the Hand. St. Louis, C. V. Mosby Co., 1975.

Chen, Z. W., and Zeng, B. F.: Replantation of the lower extremity. Clin. Plast. Surg., *10*:103–113, 1983.

Cooney, W. P., Weidman, K., Malo, D., and Wood, M. B.: Management of acute flexor tendon injury in the hand. Instr. Course Lect., *34*:373–381, 1985.

Creekmore, H., Bellinghausen, H., Young, V. L.,

Wray, R. C., Weeks, P. M., and Grasse, P. S.: Comparison of early passive motion and immobilization after flexor tendon repairs. Plast. Reconstr. Surg., 75:75–79, 1985.

Daniel, R. K., and Terzis, J. K.: Reconstructive Microsurgery. Boston, Little Brown and Co., 1977.

Duran, R. J., and Houser, R. G.: Controlled passive motion following flexor tendon repair in zones 2 and 3. In American Academy of Orthopaedic Surgeons Symposium on Tendon Surgery in the Hand. St. Louis, C. V. Mosby Co., 1975.

Eiken, O.: Replantation—experience and functional results. Scand. J. Plast. Reconstr. Surg., 19:65–68, 1982.

Fess, E. E., Harmon, K. S., Strickland, J. W., and Steichen, J. B.: Evaluation of the hand by objective measurement. In Hunter, J. M. et al. (eds.): Rehabilitation of the Hand. St. Louis, C. V. Mosby Co., 1978.

Gallico, G. G., and Stirrat, C. R.: Extremity replantation. Surg. Annu., 15:229–260, 1983.

Hayhurst, J. W.: Complications of digital replantation. In Daniller, A. I., and Strauch, B. (eds.): Symposium on Microsurgery, Vol. 14. St. Louis, C. V. Mosby Co., 1976.

Hunter, J. M.: Staged flexor tendon reconstruction. J. Hand Surg., 8:789–793, 1983.

Ikuta, Y., Watari, S., Kubo, T., Oyama, K., Hiramatsu, K., Nakasaki, T., Mouri, T., Yoshimura, O., Hiramatsu, H., and Tsuge, K.: The reattachment of severed fingers. Hiroshima J. Med. Sci., 22:131–154, 1973.

Kessler, I., and Nissim, F.: Primary repair without immobilization of flexor tendon division within the digital sheath. An experimental and clinical study. Acta Orthop. Scand., 40:587–601, 1969.

Kleinert, H. E., Kutz, J. E., Atasoy, E., and Stormo, A.: Primary repair of flexor tendons. Orthop. Clin. North Am., 4:865–876, 1973.

Komatsu, S., and Tamai, S.: Successful replantation of a completely cut-off thumb. Case report. Plast. Reconstr. Surg., 42:374–377, 1968.

Lendvay, P. G.: Replacement of amputated digits and extremities. In Littler, J. W., Cramer, L. M., and Smith, J. W. (eds.): Symposium on Reconstructive Hand Surgery, Vol. 9. St. Louis, C. V. Mosby Co., 1974.

Lendvay, P. G.: Pursuit of function in digital replantation. In Daniel, R. K., and Terzis, J. K. (eds.): Reconstructive Microsurgery. St. Louis, Little Brown and Co., 1977.

Lister, G. D., Kleinert, H. E., Kutz, J. E., and Atasoy, E.: Primary flexor tendon repair followed by immediate controlled mobilization. J. Hand Surg., 2:441–451, 1977.

Lister, G. D., and Kleinert, H. E.: Replantation. In Grabb, W. C., and Smith, J. W. (eds.): Plastic Surgery, 3rd Ed. Boston, Little Brown and Co., 1979.

Lister, G. D.: Incision and closure of the flexor sheath during primary tendon repair. Hand, 15:123–135, 1983.

May, J. W., and Gallico, G. G.: Upper extremity replantation. Curr. Prob. Surg., 17:634–717, 1980.

Meyer, V. E., Chen, Z. W., and Beasley, R. W.: Basic technical considerations in reattachment surgery. Orthop. Clin. North Am. 12:871–895, 1981.

Morrison, W. A., O'Brien, B. M., and MacLeod, A. M.: Digital replantation and revascularization. A long-term review of one hundred cases. Hand, 10:125–134, 1978.

Nielsen, A. B., and Jensen, P. O.: Methods of evaluation of the functional results of flexor tendon repair of the fingers. J. Hand Surg., 10B:60–61, 1985.

O'Brien, B. M., and MacLeod, A. M.: Digital replantation. In Daniller, A. I., and Strauch, B. (eds.): Symposium on Microsurgery. St. Louis, C. V. Mosby Co., 1976.

O'Brien, B. M.: Microvascular Reconstructive Surgery. New York, Churchill Livingstone, 1977.

Ochiai, N., Matsui, T., Miyaji, N., Merklin, R. J., and Hunter, J. M.: Vascular anatomy of flexor tendons. I. Vincular system and blood supply of the profundus tendon in the digital sheath. J. Hand Surg., 4:321–330, 1979.

Peacock, E. E.: Wound Repair, 3rd Ed. Philadelphia, W. B. Saunders Co., 1984.

Schneider, L. H.: Flexor Tendon Injuries. Boston, Little Brown and Co., 1985.

Scott, F. A.: Complications following replantation and revascularization. In Boswick, J. A. (ed.): Complications in Hand Surgery. Philadelphia, W. B. Saunders Co., 1986.

Steichen, J. B., Harmon, K. S., Fess, E. E., and Strickland, J. W.: Rehabilitation of the upper extremity replantation patient. In Hunter, J. M. et al. (eds.): Rehabilitation of the Hand. St. Louis, C. V. Mosby Co., 1978.

Steichen, J. B., and Idler, R. S.: Surgical aspects of replantation and revascularization. In Hunter, J. M. et al. (eds.): Rehabilitation of the Hand, 2nd Ed. St. Louis, C. V. Mosby Co., 1984.

Strickland, J. W., and Glogovac, S. V.: Digital function following flexor tendon repair in Zone II: A comparison of immobilization and controlled passive motion techniques. J. Hand Surg., 5:537–543, 1980.

Strickland, J. W., Steichen, J. B., Kleinman, W. B., and Flynn, N.: Factors influencing digital performance after phalangeal fracture. In Strickland, J. W., and Steichen, J. B. (eds.): Difficult Problems in Hand Surgery. St. Louis, C. V. Mosby Co., 1982.

Strickland, J. W.: Flexor tendon repair. Hand Clin., 1:55–66, 1985a.

Strickland, J. W.: Results of flexor tendon surgery in zone II. Hand Clin., 1:167–179, 1985b.

Tajima, T.: History, current status, and other aspects of hand surgery in Japan. Clin. Orthop., 184:41–49, 1984.

Tamai, S.: Digit replantation. Analysis of 163 replantations in an 11 year period. Clin. Plast. Surg., 5:195–209, 1978.

Urbaniak, J. R., Hayes, M. G., and Bright, D. S.: Management of bone in digital replantation: Free vascularized and composite bone grafts. Clin. Orthop., 133:184–194, 1978.

Urbaniak, J. R.: Replantation in children. In Serafin, D., and Georgiade, N. G. (eds.): Pediatric Plastic Surgery, Vol. 2. St. Louis, C. V. Mosby Co., 1984.

Urbaniak, J. R., Steichen, J. B., Weiland, A. J., Wood, M. B., and Seaber, A. V.: American Academy of Orthopaedic Surgeons Microsurgical Skills Development Laboratory Manual. Chicago, American Academy of Orthopaedic Surgeons, 1985.

Verdan, C. E.: Primary repair of flexor tendons. J. Bone Joint Surg., 42A:647–657, 1960.

Verdan, C. E.: Half a century of flexor-tendon surgery. Current status and changing philosophies. J. Bone Joint Surg., 54A:472–491, 1972.

Weiland, A. J., Villarreal-Rios, A., Kleinert, H. E., Kutz, J., Atasoy, E., and Lister, G.: Replantation of digits and hands. Analysis of surgical techniques and functional results in 71 patients with 86 replantations. Clin. Orthop., 133:195–204, 1978.

PARTIAL AND TOTAL AMPUTATIONS OF THE FINGERS

Chapter 90

DISTAL DIGITAL REPLANTATION

JACQUES BAUDET
AND L. VIDAL

We shall be concerned here with replantation of digital extremities amputated distal to the insertion of the flexor superficialis or lower than the distal third of the middle phalanx. Distal replantations pose two problems: The first is technical and can be solved only with the help of good microsurgical technique. The second problem concerns the indications for such an operation, which depend ultimately on critical analysis of the functional and cosmetic results.

HISTORICAL ASPECTS

Following the first report of replantation of a severed thumb by Kohatsus and Tamai in 1968, a number of new cases appeared in the literature (Buncke, 1965; Cobbett, 1969; Lendvay, 1968, 1970, 1973; O'Brien et al., 1973); many others have been reported since. Although some of the reports included distal

replantations, these were never considered as a separate entity.

In 1973 Seraphin et al. reported one case of successful replantation of the distal phalanx of the thumb without a venous anastomosis, and in 1976 Kubo published a similar result with the distal phalanx of the little finger in a 20 month old baby. In 1977 a similar case was described by Elsahy. It was only when larger series were published that it became possible to assess the nature and extent of the problems involved and to study the results critically (Baudet et al., 1983; Foucher, 1981; Jones et al., 1982; May, 1982; Yamano, 1985; Hagan, 1985).

CLINICAL MATERIAL

Our own experience is based on 35 patients sustaining distal amputations who were operated upon between 1972 and 1986. As shown in Table 90–1, the average age in our

Table 90–1. DETAILS OF CASES

35 Cases	26 Males	Age range:	2–72 years	
	9 Females	Mean age:	30 years	
Nature of injury	Clean section or mild contusion			16
	Severe contusion			19
			Right	**Left**
	Thumb	15	8	7
	Index	8	7	1
Digit involved	Middle	7	3	4
	Ring	4	2	2
	Little			1
	Manual workers			27
	Medical practitioner			1
Occupation	Housewife			2
	Children			5

series was 30 years (range, 2 to 72 years). The majority of our patients were male manual workers. In more than half the cases the contusion was severe. The right hand was involved more often than the left: it is more often exposed to injury, and replantation is understandably more readily attempted on the dominant side. For the same reason replantation of radial digits was more common; the thumb was involved in nearly half the cases in our series.

SURGICAL TECHNIQUE

For the convenience of both surgeon and patient and because of the availability of an anesthesia team, general anesthesia was usually preferred, but regional anesthesia is equally acceptable.

In order to reduce operating time and fatigue, two surgical teams work simultaneously. One team prepares the amputated segment, which is kept cool in swabs soaked in iced saline. They dissect the arteries, nerves, and veins and prepare the bony extremity for osteosynthesis. The other team, working with an inflatable tourniquet, treat the associated digital lesions and prepare the stump for the osteosynthesis and microanastomoses.

1. The first step in reconstruction is the repair of the bone structures. In most cases this involves an arthrodesis, which is the only solution available after the shortening required to perform the microanastomoses in a healthy zone (zone II; Fig. 90–1). An arthrodesis was carried out in 22 of our 35 patients. In only 13 cases was it possible to osteosynthesize the distal phalanx and preserve the distal interphalangeal joint (zone I and Zone III).

We prefer a form of fixation that uses Kirschner wires placed crosswise or axially in children, but fixation using a blocked nail, a corkscrew, or a cup and ball system has also been described.

2. Suturing of the tendons is unnecessary if the distal joint is arthrodesed but essential when the mobility of the joint is preserved.

3. The arterial anastomosis, the most delicate stage of the procedure, is performed next. It precedes the venous anastomoses, reduces the period of ischemia, and allows the surgeon to choose the return venous channels. It is fraught with difficulties.

The extent and severity of the contusion are difficult to evaluate accurately, and the vascular state of the distal segment can be assessed only by careful microscopy. The vessels are minute, less than 1 mm. in diameter, and their anastomosis requires 10-0 to 12-0 suture material. The restricted field makes it difficult to use double clamps: one may be forced therefore to work with single clamps and to carry out the anastomosis according to the technique of Nathan and Rose (1976), starting with the posterior plane, especially when anastomosing an intrapulpar branch of the digital artery.

In our 35 cases we were able to repair both arteries in 23 patients and only one artery in the other 12. In most cases a direct anastomosis was possible, but in two cases we had to interpose a vein graft taken from the forearm.

4. After an intravenous injection of 10 mg. of heparin, the clamp (or tourniquet) is released. While the digit recovers its "vascular" color, the nerves are reconnected by means of 8-0 or 9-0 epiperineural nylon sutures. We were able to anastomose both nerves in 28 cases, one nerve in four cases, and neither in three patients.

If revascularization is delayed, the replanted segment is surrounded with swabs

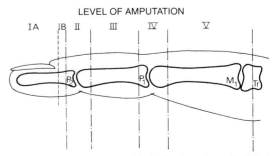

LEVEL OF AMPUTATION

Figure 90–1. Topographical classification of digital amputations according to Merle and Michon.

soaked in warm saline, and a vasodilating drug (Cinepazide or Raubasine and dihydroergocristine) is injected intravenously. The digit usually takes on a healthy color immediately (27 cases), but in eight cases it took 15 to 45 minutes.

5. Some 20 minutes after the arterial flow has been restored, the venous return is reconstructed, usually on the dorsal side. Although in theory one should try to reanastomose as many venous channels as possible, we were able to recanalize only one venous channel in 16 cases and none at all in 10 because of the severity of the contusion or the very distal site of the implantation (zone IA). As we shall see later, the surgeon must then have recourse to external venous drainage. Surprisingly, a venovenous bypass was required in only one case.

6. Finally, skin closure should be as accurate as possible except in cases of venous insufficiency when some degree of skin dehiscence may be desirable.

POSTOPERATIVE CARE

After waking up, the patient is nursed in the intensive care unit with his hand on the plane of the bed under a warming lamp. A pulse-temperature sensor is fixed to the digital extremity and another on the adjacent finger for comparison. For the first few days the replanted segment is examined night and day at half-hour intervals by trained staff.

The standard postoperative medical regimen consists of low molecular weight dextran (500 cc. per 24 hours given intravenously), a vasodilator (e.g., Cinepazide, 1200 mg. per 24 hours) given intravenously in a continuous drip, a systemic wide spectrum antibiotic, and subcutaneous doses of heparin, the dose being increased in case of thrombosis or venous congestion. The doses of these medications are decreased progressively and, when possible, they are replaced by oral medication. In every case smoking and exposure to cold are discouraged.

COMPLICATIONS

Complications can be vascular or infectious.

Arterial Thrombosis. Arterial thrombosis occurred in seven cases, i.e., 20 per cent of our series. It can occur immediately or in the early postoperative period, i.e., within a few hours after surgery (five cases). Once arterial thrombosis is confirmed, the anastomosis must be undone and the extremities retrimmed under hypothermia and reconnected, if necessary, with an interposed vein graft. Whenever possible, the proximal anastomosis is carried out end to end with the radial artery and the distal anastomosis also end to end with the collateral artery. If the latter proves impossible because of incongruence, the collateral artery is anastomosed end to side with the graft, whose distal extremity is ligated.

In only two cases was reoperation successful. Thrombosis may result from a lesion of the intima that has passed unnoticed, rarely from a technical fault (incongruence of vessels), or it may have a hemodynamic cause (turbulence along a vein graft or arterial stasis as part of a nonperfusion syndrome).

Secondary arterial thrombosis occurred twice in our series, at eight hours and 18 hours. Reoperation was successful in only one case.

Late arterial thrombosis (on the fifth postoperative day) occurred once. Survival of the replanted segment depends on its volume and the extent of the vascular connections established at the skin level when the main channel becomes obstructed. In this case the application of leeches to the exsanguinated extremity restored some of the basic dermal circulation by suction. The resulting partial necrosis was successfully treated by means of a neurovascular flap. We developed recently another salvage procedure. An automatic intermittent tourniquet is applied on the arm of the patient, who is given 4 liters per min. of oxygen through a nasal tube. Inflation produces a backflow of venous blood enhanced in oxygen through the capillary bed of the ischemic replanted part. This procedure is continued until dermal connections are definitely restored.

Venous Complications. Although early arterial thrombosis leaves no solution other than reoperation, venous complications often can be relieved by continuing use of nonsurgical ancillary methods.

In our 35 cases we encountered a venous problem in 11 cases (32 per cent). In two of these a venous anastomosis had been carried out, but in nine others it had proved impossible.

If congestion is mild, paraungual or pulpar incisions provide some relief. The patient is heparinized and a heparin solution is applied frequently to the incisions. In case of severe congestion threatening the arterial flow, the only solution is the application of leeches (*Hirudo medicinalis*): not only do they drain the extremity of venous blood, but because of the hirudin they secrete, bleeding continues more than 30 minutes after they are removed.

The leeches are used on the average for six days, although in one case application was continued for 15 days. Four to six leeches are applied daily until separation occurs (10 to 15 minutes). In some cases, especially in children, it may be necessary to restore blood volume by transfusion.

Arterial Spasm. Arterial spasm may be difficult to differentiate clinically from thrombosis. Spasm can occur at any time postoperatively, and its persistence may threaten the extremity. It may be spontaneous or may be triggered by external causes, e.g., contact with a cold liquid, interruption of warming, or antispasmodic drugs. Early treatment is imperative. The first step is to intensify the systemic treatment; it should be restarted if interrupted. If this fails, again leeches are used to try to help the extremity survive with the already established dermal channels.

Infection. Infection is fortunately rare because we use antibiotics systematically. It occurred twice in our series; in one patient the infection resolved completely without sequelae, but in the other it resulted in a pseudarthrosis.

RESULTS

In this series of 35 distal replantations, we recorded only four failures; i.e., 87 per cent yielded good functional or cosmetic results (Figs. 90–2 to 90–7).

As far as digital mobility is concerned, normal function of the proximal joints returned after two to four weeks of physiotherapy. The function of the distal interphalangeal joint depended on whether it had been arthrodesed. Insufficient flexion was a common complaint. When a functional joint was preserved, it recovered a range of mobility of 30 degrees.

Within two to four months most patients recovered proprioceptive or even some discriminative sensibility. In 10 patients the result was graded as excellent (discrimination

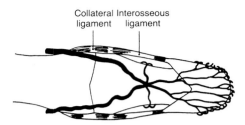

Figure 90–2. Blood supply of the pulp (after Flint).

less than 6 mm.); in 22 it was graded good (discrimination between 6 and 12 mm.). In three cases discrimination was over 12 mm.; there were trophic changes and sensitivity to cold, and sensation was graded as poor.

The cosmetic result in every case was much better than it would have been with trimming of the stump. The result was graded as excellent or very good in 80 per cent and satisfactory in the rest.

DISCUSSION

In the light of our experience, we will now consider the technical possibilities, limitations, and indications for distal replantations.

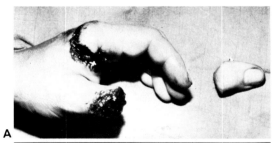

A

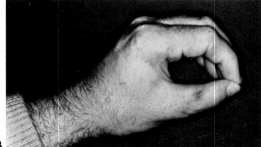

B

Figure 90–3. *A*, Amputation of the left thumb by a circular saw. Replantation was carried out with anastomosis of one artery and of two dorsal veins. *B*, Good functional and cosmetic result.

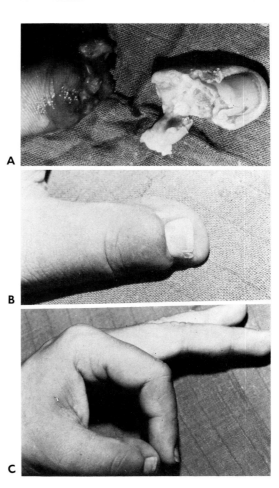

Figure 90–4. *A*, Oblique transungual amputation of the left thumb by a circular saw. Anastomosis of one artery was performed. Venous anastomosis was not feasible. Venous drainage was achieved by heparinization and bleeding. *B*, Cosmetically acceptable result with satisfactory regrowth of the nail. *C*, Excellent functional result.

TECHNICAL POSSIBILITIES

The Level of Amputation. The feasibility of a replantation depends on the level of the amputation. In most of our cases the line of amputation ran at, or close to, the distal interphalangeal joint where it is still possible to anastomose small caliber arteries. A few millimeters below the joint, the artery divides to form a pulpar anastomotic network, which

is roughly X or H shaped (Fig. 90–8). One of these preterminal divisions with a caliber of 0.5 mm. theoretically can be anastomosed and may revascularize the extremity, but the anastomosis is technically difficult and the result unreliable.

When a channeled revascularization proves impossible, two solutions are worth considering. One is simple repositioning of the severed segment. To increase the chances of

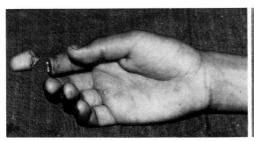

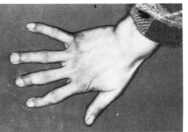

Figure 90–5. *A*, Amputation of the right index finger by a circular saw. Single arterial anastomosis was performed. Venous drainage was by application of leeches. *B*, Result: functionally excellent, cosmetically acceptable.

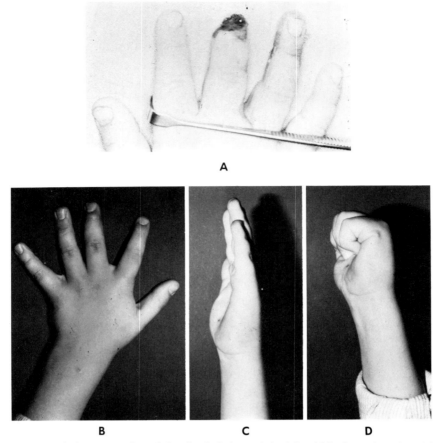

Figure 90–6. Transarticular amputation of the distal phalanx of the left middle finger by a bread-knife in a five year old child. Anastomosis of one artery was carried out and was repeated eight hours later because of thrombosis. Single venous anastomosis was performed. *B*, Good cosmetic result, excellent trophicity. *C* and *D*, Functionally satisfactory as a result of an arthrodesis in good position.

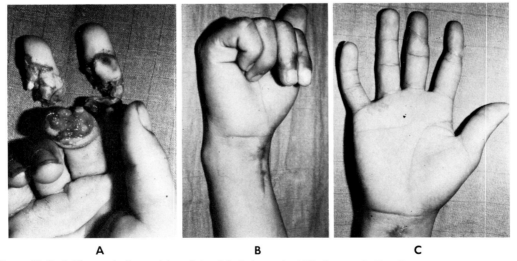

Figure 90–7. *A*, Transarticular avulsion of the right index and middle fingers. *B*, Excellent sensation and trophicity of the pulp. *C*, Inadequate prehension because of an arthrodesis in a faulty position.

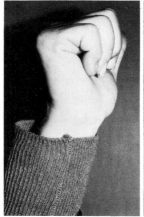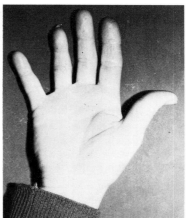

Figure 90–8. *A* and *B*, Amputation of the distal phalanx of the right ring finger by a tobacco-cutting machine in a young woman. Excellent functional result and very good cosmetic appearance and trophicity.

A　　　　**B**

revascularization, however, the extremity can be freshened and buried under a flap taken from an adjacent finger (Mantero and Bertolotti, 1975) or from a distance, e.g., thoracic skin (Brent, 1979); (Fig. 90–9).

The Nature of the Trauma. Although most of our patients sustained severe contusions, our four failures (two index fingers and two thumbs) were largely due to crushing or extensive distal vascular avulsion. It must be noted that the need to repeat the anastomosis was in itself an unfavorable factor—four failures in seven cases (57 per cent).

The Patient's Age. The patient's age was not in itself a determining factor: one successful result in a patient age 72 and one failure in one age 13.

COMPLICATIONS

An objective analysis of the complications shows that all our failures resulted from arterial thrombosis, but thanks to the conservative methods used in cases of venous congestion (heparinization, topical application of heparin, and leeches), we had no failure as a result of a purely venous complication.

This confirms previous reports of replantations without venous anastomoses when venous drainage was obtained by simple scarification (Lendvay, 1973) by repeated pulp massage or, even better, by the application of leeches (Foucher et al., 1981).

Some authors have suggested original so-

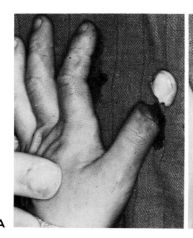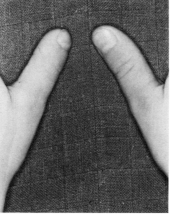

Figure 90–9. *A*, Transungual amputation of the distal phalanx of the left thumb with crushing in a four year old child. *B*, Result after simple reposition.

A　　　　**B**

lutions to this problem: One consists of dissecting a subcutaneous flap from the dorsal aspect of the replanted segment and burying it in the proximal segment (Poletti, 1981), while the other involves an arteriovenous anastomosis between a dorsal vein and the contralateral digital artery (Smith et al., 1983).

JUSTIFICATION FOR DISTAL REPLANTATIONS

This procedure is justifiable on several grounds: the high percentage of success, the good functional and cosmetic result in selected cases, and finally the socioeconomic benefit.

Our high percentage of successes (87 per cent) is the result of the work of a team well trained in microsurgery and also the competent and devoted postoperative care of our nursing staff. We believe that our efforts would be justified even with a lower proportion of successful cases.

Cosmetically, a distal replantation is clearly superior to classic trimming of the stump or even a reconstructive procedure using osteoplastic and skin flap techniques. It is fully justified in women and children no matter what digital ray is involved.

From a functional viewpoint, the digits most likely to benefit from a replantation after a unidigital amputation are the thumb, which restores the pinch, and the little finger, to lock the grip. In multidigital amputations, when the power of the whole grip is affected, replantation is indicated particularly for the radial digits. In some cases it may be preferable to replant an ulnar digit in a radial position.

When socioeconomic factors are taken into account, the advantages and disadvantages of distal replantation must be weighed against those of simple trimming of the stump.

The few series of distal replantations published so far stress the rapid motor and sensory recovery, the early return to work, and the absence of the well known complications of simple closure such as painful neuromas and hypersensitivity to pressure and cold (Foucher et al., 1981; Jones et al., 1982; Yamano et al., 1985; Hagan et al., 1985). The results we obtained would seem to confirm these observations.

REFERENCES

Baudet, J.: La surveillance post-opératoire en microchirurgie vasculaire. Rev. Chir. Orthop., 64:274, 1978.

Baudet, J., and Goumain, A. J. M.: Réimplantation d'une main. Ann. Chir., 29:491, 1975.

Baudet, J., Lemaine, J. M., Guimberteau, J. C., Girou, Y., Neretti, J., Nascimento, E., and Hourregue, F.: Les réimplantations au niveau du membre supérieur. Lettre d'information, G.E.M., N°. 6.

Baudet, J., Le Treut, A., Dilhuydy, M. H., and Goumain, A. J. M.: Valeur pronostique de la thermographie dans les interventions de réimplantation ou de sauvetage des membres. J. Radiol. Electrol., 55:239, 1974.

Berger, A., Meissl, G., and Walzer, L.: Techniques and results in replantation surgery in children. Intern. J. Microsurg., 1:9, 1981.

Bertrand, H.: Résultats fonctionnels d'une série homogène de 36 réimplantations digitales, 3 réimplantations de main et 2 réimplantations d'avant-bras. Thesis, Doctorat en Médecine N°. 354, Lyon, 1978.

Biemer, E.: Definitions and classifications in replantation surgery. Br. J. Plast. Surg., 33:164, 1980.

Braun, J. B.: Les artères de la main. Thesis, University of Nancy, December 1977.

Braun, J. B., and Borelly, J.: Etude radio-anatomique des artères de la main. Acta Anat., 99:253, 1977.

Brent, B. M.: Replantation of amputated distal phalangeal parts of fingers without anastomosis, using subcutaneous pockets. Plast. Reconstr. Surg., 63:1, 1979.

Buncke, H.: Experimental digital amputation and reimplantation. Plast. Reconstr. Surg., 36:62, 1965.

Buncke, H., Alpert, B., and Hohnson Gilbink, R.: Digital replantation. Surg. Clin. North Am., 61:383, 1981.

Casteleyn, D.: Evaluation fonctionnelle après réimplantation de membres et de doigts amputés. Acta Orthop. Belg., 47:834, 1981.

Cobbett, J.: Small vessel surgery in the hand. Hand, 1:56, 1969.

Dap, F.: Réimplantation et revascularisation du pouce. Thesis, Doctorat en Médecine, Nancy, 1982.

Elsahy, N.: Replantation of a completely amputated distal segment of a thumb. Case report. Plast. Reconstr. Surg., 59:579, 1977.

Flint, M.: Some observations on the vascular supply of the nail bed and terminal segments of the fingers. Br. J. Plast. Surg., 8:186, 1956.

Foucher, G., Hendersen, H. R., Maneau, M., Merle, M., and Braun, F.: Distal digital replantations: one of the best indications for microsurgery. Int. J. Microsurg., 3:263, 1981.

Foucher, G., Merle, M., and Michon, J.: Replantations digitales: evolution des indications. Nouv. Press. Med., 5:2392, 1976.

Hagan, H. S., Hay, E. L., and Shealy, G. J.: Distal digital replantation. JSC Med., 81:107, 1985.

Hamilton, R., O'Brien, B., Morrison, W., and MacLeod, A.: Replantation and revascularization of digits. Surg. Gynecol. Obstet., 151:508, 1980.

Harris, G., Finseth, F., and Buncke, H.: Posterior wall first microvascular anastomotic technique. Br. J. Plast. Surg., 34:47, 1981.

Hayhurst, J., O'Brien, B., and Ishida, H.: Experimental replantation after prolonged cooling. Hand, 6:134, 1974.

Ikuta, V.: Microvascular Surgery. Hiroshima, Leus Press, 1975, p. 42.

Jacobson, J., and Suarez, E.: Microsurgery in anastomosis of small vessels. Surg. Forum, *11:*243, 1960.

Jones, J. M., Schenek, R., and Buchan Chesney, R.: Digital replantation and amputation. J. Hand Surg., *7:*183, 1982.

Kenesi, C.: Essai de systématisation des artères de la main chez le foetus à terme. Presse Med., *74:*1211, 1966.

Kenesi, C., Alexandre, J. H., and Aaronc: Les artères de la main. Ann. Anat. Pathol. *15:*99, 1967.

Kleinert, H., and Kasdan, M.: Anastomosis of digital vessels. J. Ky. Med. Assoc., *63:*106, 1965.

Kleinert, H., Kasdan, M., and Romero, J.: Small blood vessel anastomosis for salvage of severely injured upper extremity. J. Bone Joint Surg., *45:*788, 1963.

Kohatsus and Tamais, S.: Successful replantation of a completely cut off thumb. Plast. Reconstr. Surg., *42:*374, 1968.

Kubo, T., Ikuta, Y., Katari, S., Okuhira, N., and Tsuge, K.: The smallest digital replant yet. Br. J. Plast. Surg., *29:*313, 1976.

Laws, J., El Sallab, R., and Scott, J.: An arteriographic and histological study of digital arteries. Br. J. Radiol., *40:*740, 1967.

Lejeune, G., Castermans, A., Carlier, A., Fissette, J., Leclercq, D., Khuc, T., Boucq, D. and Lahaye, T.: La réimplantation de 71 doigts totalement amputés. Acta Chir. Belg., *3:*181, 1982.

Lendvay, P.: Anastomosis of digital vessels. Med. J. Aust., *2:*273, 1968.

Lendvay, P.: Replacement of the amputated finger. Am. J. Med., *9:*249, 1973.

Lendvay, P., and Owen, E.: Microsurgical repair of completely severed digits. Med. J. Aust. *2:*818, 1970.

Le Quang, G.: Développements récents des techniques microchirurgicales en chirurgie réparatrice. Ann. Chir. Plast., *25:*171, 1980.

Malt, R., and Mickhann, C.: Replantation of a severed arm. J.A.M.A., *189:*716, 1964.

Mantero, R., and Bertolotti, P.: Le cross finger et réimplantation des extrémités digitales. Ann. Chir., *29:*1019, 1975.

May, J., Roth, B., and Gardner, M.: Digital replantation distal to the proximal interphalangeal joint. J. Hand. Surg., *7:*161, 1982.

Merle, M., Dap, F., Foucher, G., Bouchon, Y., and Michon, J.: Réimplantation et revascularisation du pouce. Problèmes techniques et résultats à propos de 125 cas. Mem. An. Chir., *110:*255, 1984.

Michon, J., Merle, M., and Foucher, G.: Cotation et indications des repositions digitales. Arch. Mal. Prof., *37:*870, 1975.

Nathan, P., and Rose, M.: An alternative technique for microvascular suture. Plast. Reconstr. Surg., *58:*635, 1976.

O'Brien, B., MacLeod, A., Miller G., and Newing, R.: Clinical replantations of digits. Plast. Reconstr. Surg., *52:*491, 1973.

Poletti, L.: Subcutaneous flap as an alternative to venous anastomosis in replantation surgery. Plast. Reconstr. Surg., *69:*233, 1981.

Report of the American replantation mission in China: Replantation in China. Plast. Reconstr. Surg., *52:*5, 1973.

Schoofs, M.: La réimplantation digitale. Lille Chir., *36:*75, 1981.

Seraphin, D., Kota, J., and Kleinert, H.: Replantation of a completely amputated distal thumb without venous anastomosis. Case report. Plast. Reconstr. Surg., *5:*579, 1973.

Sixth Peoples Hospital, Shanghai, China: Expansion of the study of reimplantation of severed limbs and digits. Chinese Med. J., *1:*1, 1973.

Smith, A. R., Sonnevel, D. G. J., and Van der Meulen, J. C.: AV anastomosis as a solution for absent venous drainage in replantation surgery. Plast. Reconstr. Surg., *71:*525, 1983.

Snyder, C. I., Stevenson, R., and Browne, E. Z.: Successful replantation of a totally severed thumb. Plast. Reconstr. Surg., *50:*553, 1972.

Tamai, S., Hori, Y., Fukui, A., and Shimizu, T.: Finger replantation. Int. Surg., *66:*9, 1981.

Tamai, S., Sasauchi, N., Hori, Y., Tatsumi, Y., and Okuda, H.: Microvascular surgery in orthopedics and traumatology. J. Bone Joint Surg., *59B:*1637, 1972.

Tatsumi, Y., Tamai, S., Komatsu, S., Hori, Y., Okuda, H., Kashiwagi, H., Nakamura, Y., and Mii, Y.: Functional recovery following distal replantation. *In* Proceedings, 17th Annual Meeting, Japanese Society of Surgery of the Hand, Tokyo, May 1974.

Tsai, T. M.: Experimental and clinical application of microvascular surgery. Ann. Surg., *2:*177, 1975.

Yamano, Y.: Reimplantation of the amputated distal part of the fingers. J. Hand Surg., *10A:*211, 1985.

Yoshimura, M., Nomura, S., Veno, T., Yamauchi, S., Iwai, Y., and Shimamura, K.: Evaluation of digital replantation. Acta Chir. Belg., *3:*161, 1982.

Chapter 91

TRAUMATIC AMPUTATION OF THE PHALANGES

Raoul Tubiana

Traumatic amputations of the phalanges form an extremely variable group of injuries. We will consider in turn finger tip injuries, traumatic amputations at the level of the proximal and middle phalanges (taking into account the importance of the digit), those involving several fingers, and those of the thumb (the subject of other chapters).

There are certain selective levels of amputation (described by Alnot in Volume IV), but these standard amputations are performed only rarely in emergency situations, when one usually tries to be as conservative as possible. The problem is to select the cases in which skeletal shortening can be performed in order to obtain closure without increasing the functional problems created by the injury itself. Alternatively one must judge the cases in which it is necessary to preserve the length of the stump by employing more complex plastic procedures. This evaluation is often difficult and should take into account the type of the amputation, the patient's needs, and the surgeon's ability. We will discuss these factors in detail.

First we must recall several basic considerations:

1. The general principles regarding the treatment of wounds are applicable to cases of mutilation—the avoidance of tetanus and infection by cleansing and débridement with the use of appropriate tetanus prophylaxis; limiting the destruction of tissues and repair arteries and veins to tissues one wishes to conserve; skeletal stabilization when there are associated fractures; the use of early skin cover when local conditions allow; and the prevention of stiffness and deformity.

2. The functional value of the mutilated finger depends on a number of factors, the most important of which are the length and the quality of the skin covering the stump.

3. Another important consideration from a prognostic point of view following mutilation of the fingers is the state of the rest of the hand—the other fingers and especially the thumb.

4. Whatever the stage of repair, the therapeutic indications must take into account the level of amputation; the fingers involved; the function of the other hand and the dominant hand; and the general health of the patient, his age, his occupation, and his cosmetic wishes.

5. Complex plastic procedures to cover amputation stumps with flaps (especially attempts to lengthen a digit) should be reserved for the specialist and are usually performed as secondary procedures. It is theoretically preferable to perform a one stage definitive repair at the primary operation, but this is not always possible because of the complexity of the lesions or the inexperience of the surgeon, with the risk of excessive sacrifice of tissue. In such surgery the choice of procedure is more difficult than the operative technique, and experience is therefore of great importance. The aim is not to reconstitute normal anatomical features but to restore function, and it is sometimes paradoxically necessary to sacrifice tissues at a secondary procedure that have been preserved primarily to achieve this goal. A stump conserved in an emergency may subsequently impede hand function. Its amputation, however, may be a valuable source of skin, nerve, tendon, or bone for the repair of other areas of the hand.

6. Replantation of digits has been carried out successfully in specialized microsurgical

centers. Initial enthusiasm has been modified in the light of experience now that reports of functional results are available.

The indications for replantation of digits must take into account the length of the operation and of the anesthesia and also, of course, the type and level of the amputation; they have been discussed in preceding chapters.

Chapter 92

FINGERTIP INJURIES

Raoul Tubiana

In this chapter we discuss fingertip injuries and other wounds and mutilations of the distal phalanx.

These lesions pose some intricate problems, which can be difficult to solve. Indeed the functional importance of the fingertip is such as to deserve the utmost surgical attention. Ideally treatment should aim at preserving the length of the digit, providing a thick but sensitive skin covering, and encouraging rapid healing with minimal morbidity. The type of treatment chosen should be carefully selected from the variety of surgical procedures available. Great surgical experience is essential for the application of some of the techniques, which in less than expert hands may aggravate the original loss. Yet these lesions are frequently treated in inadequately prepared centers. Erroneously regarded as a minor injury, this type of lesion may cause time to be lost from work, persistent pain, and severe loss of function in the finger. Nevertheless only occasionally are these cases referred to a specialist. To avoid such expensive complications, a precise, easy, and safe line of treatment should be defined.

We shall start therefore by outlining the emergency treatment to be followed by the hospital medical officer on duty or the isolated unspecialized surgeon. We will then discuss in greater detail the more refined procedures, which should be attempted only by the experienced hand surgeon.

Before describing the plastic procedures used for covering wounds of the digital extremities, we must first stress the important difference that exists in all the wounds of the hand between the clean laceration and the crush injury in which, in addition to the loss of the cutaneous tissue, there may be lesions of the deeper planes, especially fractures of the distal phalanx.

On the anatomicophysiological level, the essential importance of the pulp as an organ of exploration is well known. Several chapters of Volume I are dedicated to this topic. The anatomy and function of the nail have been presented in the first volume (Fig. 92–1). The rich innervation and abundant vasculature of the fingertip is provided by two palmar neurovascular pedicles. These pedicles also provide sensation and vascularization to the dorsum of the distal portion of the digit via the dorsal collateral branches of the nerves and arteries. These small dorsal arteries form a series of arcades (Flint, 1955). The rich terminal anastomotic distribution may be destroyed by wounds of the fingertip, leaving only the palmar collateral vessels, which originate at the level of the middle phalanx, for vascularization of the dorsal skin. This must be remembered when flaps are used in this region.

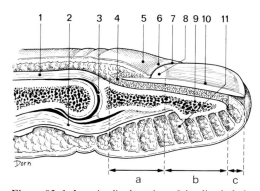

Figure 92–1. Longitudinal section of the distal phalanx showing the disproportionate thickness of the anterior and posterior covering layers. a = nail matrix, b = nail bed, c = hyponychium, 1 = extensor tendon, 2 = flexor tendon, 3 = distal interphalangeal articulation, 4 = nail fold, 5 = distal portion of nail fold, 6 and 7 = eponychium, 8 = lunula, 9 = distal phalanx, 10 = nail shelf, 11 = pulp.

1034

It is useful to remember that, as in all wounds of the hand, the therapeutic indications should include other considerations—the general condition of the patient, his age, and occupation, and the digit involved.

Fingertip injuries of the thumb merit special mention. One must re-establish a functional, sensitive, useful stump for all varieties of pinch while sacrificing as little length as possible. Conservation of the length of the thumb is considerably more important when the opposable digits are injured, shortened, or stiffened. However, even for the thumb, the quality of skin recovery of the stump is more important than the length. It is also essential to re-establish good sensation to the index finger, particularly in the zone that opposes the thumb.

BASIC TECHNIQUES

Suturing of the wound, shortening of the skeleton to allow skin suturing, the use of partial thickness grafts, and "assisted" spontaneous epithelialization have disadvantages that justify the use of more sophisticated techniques, but they have the advantage of simplicity, and the problem of the hospital medical officer on duty is to decide about the indications for each. Occasionally he may have to ask for the help of a more experienced surgeon when dealing with a particularly difficult case, such as a crush injury of the thumb or when the problem of possible replantation arises.

Antitetanus prophylaxis is necessary in all cases. An x-ray may reveal concomitant bone lesions. The wound is carefully cleaned under regional anesthetic by injection into the intermetacarpal spaces. Repeated washing with saline solution ensures removal of small foreign bodies and clots.

SIMPLE SUTURING OF THE WOUND

The line of surgical treatment is obvious if the wound presents with a skin flap that allows straightforward suturing without tension. In transverse wounds suturing can be facilitated by the excision of two small lateral triangles of skin (Fig. 92–2).

SKELETAL SHORTENING

The bone shortening procedure has the simultaneous advantage and disadvantage of being a definitive procedure. It may be necessary in crush injuries when there is a comminuted fracture of the distal phalanx. The wound is then cleaned and trimmed and the smaller bone splinters are removed sparingly to leave some bone support for the pulp and nail. An avulsed nail is best put back in place to act as a splint (Fig. 92–3).

Phalangeal shortening is more readily accepted by the older manual worker who is eager to be back at work, because it obviates the need for immobilization and avoids the risk of stiffness. It should be performed only with the prior agreement of the patient and if no more than one or two fingers are injured. It is also done if the nail is too short to be usefully conserved. However, shortening of more than 0.5 cm. to facilitate skin coverage should not be performed as an emergency procedure in the thumb, in the fingers if several fingers as well as the thumb are involved, in children, and in female patients (for cosmetic reasons). It should also be avoided, as much as possible, when a traumatic amputations reaches halfway down the nail, for further shortening will cause the nail to tilt forward.

However, when the bone is slightly pro-

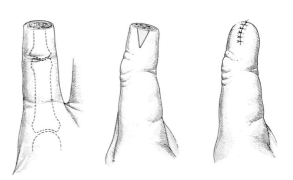

Figure 92–2. Suture of a transverse wound is facilitated by the excision of two small lateral triangular areas of skin.

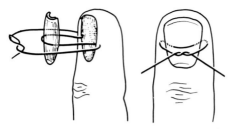

Figure 92–3. The replaced nail serves as a splint.

truding, one trims it with a rongeur and allows it to heal secondarily.

SPONTANEOUS HEALING

This technique is increasing in popularity. Previously it was used in children in whom spontaneous epithelialization with contraction occurs rapidly and a skin graft is not necessary (Das and Brown, 1978). Spontaneous healing also can be used in the adult if the injury is small and especially if it is lateral. The injury is simply covered with a gauze dressing lightly coated with petrolatum. The dressing must always allow mobilization of all the joints. It is usually changed twice a week. At each dressing the wound is washed and all joints are put through a complete range of motion.

Waiting for granulation tissue to cover a bony extremity is advisable when the use of a cutaneous flap is not indicated. In an emergency, covering the injured area with a petrolatum gauze dressing after thorough washing with saline is the least offensive treatment to be performed by the nonspecialist. Spontaneous healing in injuries larger than 1 sq. cm. takes at least five weeks in the adult. The recovery of sensation is good, and two point discrimination (Weber test) is often similar to that of the neighboring tissues when the injury is not too extensive (Allen, 1980). In spite of the simplicity of this treatment, the results are often favorable. It would be a mistake, however, to regard this as the only method of treatment. It may be contraindicated to leave a wound open at the tip of a finger with concomitant tendon, bone, or nerve lesions requiring surgical treatment. Lesions of the nail or of its bed may require special treatment, which will be dealt with later. Finally, healing time is long if the injury is extensive and exceeds 1.5 cm. in diameter, and the final result may also be painful when

the scar is in contact with underlying bone. The specialist must possess a battery of treatments that can be adapted to suit the individual case.

PARTIAL THICKNESS GRAFTS

Partial thickness grafts can be used in some emergency cases, and direct suturing of part of the wound often can be combined with skin grafting in the initial treatment. Split skin grafts may be the treatment of choice in areas where there is no bare bone. It is well known that grafts do not take readily when in contact with bone and the resulting graft may be painful. Moreover, sensation is usually very poor in such grafts. An advantage of these grafts is that they tend to contract and bring healthy adjacent tissues toward the defect.

In a large proportion of cases a second operation is required later. This may seem to be a disadvantage, but at least future repairs are not jeopardized, the lesion is not made worse, and the wound contraction will mean a reduced surface area requiring secondary repair. Split skin grafts for use in the hand may be taken from the hypothenar eminence, which provides tissue of a similar texture and type. The anterior aspect of the forearm is also a convenient donor area, but in female patients a less obvious skin area is cosmetically preferable.

All these basic techniques can yield less than perfect results, including problems of sensibility (anesthesia, pain, cold intolerance), but these problems are associated not only with these "simple" procedures but also with more sophisticated operations.

Several studies of the results of these operations have attempted to show the relative incidence of complications with these various procedures. These studies are sometimes contradictory. Bojsen et al. (1981) found that primary closure with skeletal shortening caused more complications than allowing spontaneous healing. Holm and Zachariae (1974) advocated primary suturing whenever possible. Sturman and Duran (1963) pointed out a significant number of cases of dysesthesia associated with split thickness skin grafts. Cold intolerance is a result of the wound and can develop regardless of the method of wound closure used; it is more often noted following crushing wounds.

Spontaneous healing seems to be the method causing the least number of immediate complications and sequelae. (Chow and Ho, 1982; Louis et al., 1980). It seems to us wise to advocate this last method of treatment in emergency situations except when the existence of a flap permits closure without tension.

Split thickness skin grafts are reserved for larger wounds when there is no exposed bone; the skin must be as similar as possible to that of the finger. These grafts are also indicated when the patient desires rapid healing and is unable for economic, geographic, or other reasons to undergo dressing changes two or three times a week for several weeks.

OTHER PROCEDURES AND THEIR INDICATIONS

A number of plastic procedures have been described for resurfacing the tips of the fingers. Most of them are discussed in Chapters 35 to 37 in Volume II on skin loss. We shall attempt to give precise indications for each and mention our own preference.

Skin loss in the digital extremities can be covered by full or partial thickness skin grafts, composite grafts, adjacent flaps, regional flaps taken from the hand, or distant flaps. One should aim at restoring the best possible sensation to the pulps of the thumb and index finger with at least protective sensation for the pulps and tips of the other digits. In addition, it is necessary to provide a good cushion of subcutaneous tissue at all pressure points. It must always be remembered that, as a rule, the more complex the treatment (especially if several operations are required), the longer the patient will be out of work and the more difficult the rehabilitation. These problems are exaggerated in the older patients.

According to Glicenstein (1971), time lost from regular activities is as follows: 0 to 40 days after use of a tulle gras (petroleum gauze) dressing with spontaneous closure, two months after use of an adjacent flap, and four to six months after use of distant flaps. Furthermore, rapid progress in microsurgery has opened up the possibility, in specialized centers, of replantation of increasingly small fingertip fragments, which will be described in the following chapters. It is sometimes possible to combine such replantations with the use of a neighboring skin flap.

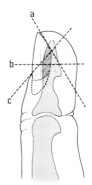

Figure 92–4. The three types of amputation of the distal extremities. a = oblique palmar amputation, b = transverse amputation, c = oblique dorsal amputation.

Let us now consider the best way of adapting these principles to the anatomy of the lesions and follow the plan of Kuhn (1967), who made a distinction between transverse amputations, oblique dorsal amputations, and oblique palmar amputations (Fig. 92–4).

TRANSVERSE AMPUTATIONS

Transverse amputations are the easiest to repair (Fig. 92–5).

1. If the lesion lies beyond the distal third of the phalanx, a simple Thiersch graft or spontaneous healing is usually sufficient when the bone is covered or only slightly exposed (Fig. 92–6).

2. If the bone is partly exposed, one can use a well cushioned protective composite pulpocutaneous graft taken from a toe. This

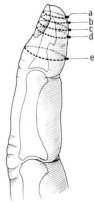

Figure 92–5. Transverse amputations. a = distal amputation, the bone is not visible, b = the bone is slightly exposed, c = amputation through middle of nail with wide exposure of bone, d = amputation through proximal third of nail, e = amputation proximal to nail.

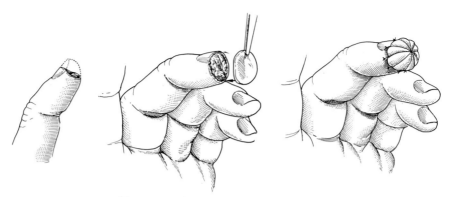

Figure 92–6. Skin graft sutured over a bolus.

technique was described by MacCash (1959) and by Ardao (1959), who used it in more than 1000 cases. It consists of cutting a domed graft from the pulp of a toe, using a broad (number 24) blade. The graft should include a few millimeters of pulp tissue in its central part. It is gently exsanguinated and sutured to the defect. The donor area usually is the fourth toe, which bears little weight and can be covered with a thin graft or simply with a tulle gras dressing to encourage contraction of its margins. The patient is allowed to walk immediately. Those who have used this technique were impressed by the rapid return of sensation (Marchac and Rousso, 1971). This is particularly indicated in the child.

3. If bone is exposed, a flap is usually preferable. Adjacent flaps have the advantage of giving sensibility. Island adjacent flaps may also be indicated here. The Kutler procedure (1947) consists of advancing two small lateral flaps (Fig. 92–7). The posterior side of the triangle should be drawn parallel to and 2 mm. from the nail to preserve as many of the sensory branches coming from the anterior part of the pulp as possible (Fig. 92–

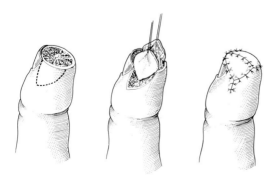

Figure 92–7. Kutler procedure.

8) (Hann, 1971). Subcutaneous fibrous adhesions, which impede the free advancement of the flap, should be divided, especially at the posterior incision.

Tranquilli-Leali (1935), Erler (1943), and more recently Atasoy et al. (1970), have shown that a larger palmar flap (Fig. 92–9), based on the V-Y principle and advanced to the defect, can provide a sensitive skin covering for the fingertip.

These two procedures, which are best carried out with the aid of magnification, are limited in their application by their small size, especially the Kutler procedure.

4. If more than half the nail bed has been lost in the injury, one has to decide whether to preserve or sacrifice the nail.

The nail requires an anterior support of at least 0.5 cm. distal to the lunula. Without support, it tilts forward over the tip of the finger, and this may be unsightly, interfere with function, and become painful. If the stump is too short, the best solution in a manual worker, is to remove the nail remnant and its matrix. If, however, it is decided to preserve the nail for cosmetic reasons in a female patient, a regional flap may be used to pad the stump. We regard this as one of the few indications for a thenar flap (Fig. 92–10) (Beasley, 1969; Smith and Albin, 1976). It is also possible, as suggested by Holevich and Paneva-Holevich (1968), to displace the nail matrix proximally (Fig. 92–11). To avoid damage to the matrix, it should be moved together with a thin layer of bone.

5. In lacerations at the level of the proximal third of the distal phalanx, there is no chance of preserving the nail. One can use the local flaps previously described. The remainder of the matrix is removed completely from the deep surface of the flap. The resection must

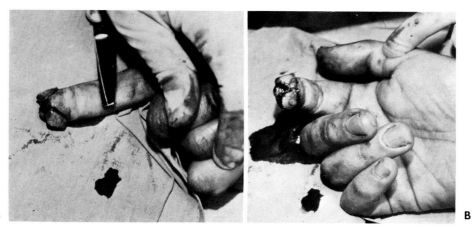

Figure 92–8. *A* and *B*, Operative technique of Kutler procedure.

be rather extensive to avoid the unsightly and often painful reappearance of nail remnants.

6. Whatever the level of the traumatic amputation, if there is an exposed bone stump to be preserved, a distant flap is preferable. The threat of necrosis makes the use of an adjacent flap dangerous. Heterodigital flaps (from another finger) are the most convenient but leave more visible scars than thenar flaps.

AMPUTATIONS OF THE TIP OF THE THUMB

All the procedures described have been used for terminal amputations of the thumb. However, we must again stress that it is important to re-establish good sensation in the thumb stump. It is better to avoid heterodigital flaps, particularly the commonly described flap taken from the lateral side of the index finger, which is a vital sensory area in the key pinch. This sensory area must be respected. Flaps taken from the dorsolateral aspect of the middle finger (Fig. 92–12) or the medial border of the index finger cause fewer local complications. When the nail is destroyed, it is preferable to use the excellent rotation flap taken from the dorsal aspect of the thumb, which can be used even in an emergency to cover a guillotine type of transverse amputation or a dorsal oblique amputation (Simonetta, 1970). The incision follows the radial border of the thumb and first

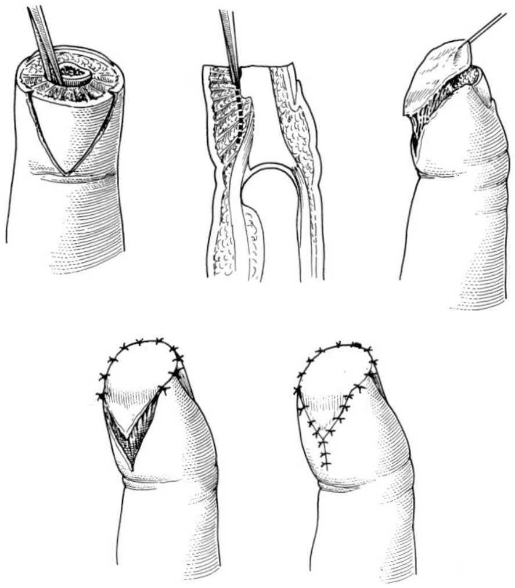

Figure 92–9. V-Y palmar island flap.

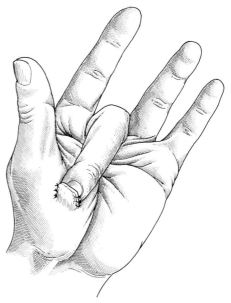

Figure 92–10. Thenar flap.

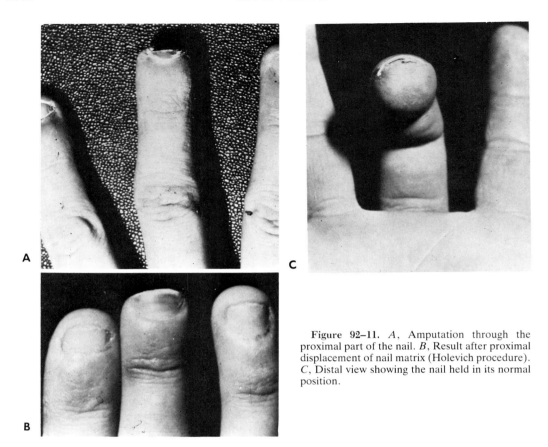

Figure 92–11. *A*, Amputation through the proximal part of the nail. *B*, Result after proximal displacement of nail matrix (Holevich procedure). *C*, Distal view showing the nail held in its normal position.

metacarpal and then runs transversely over the dorsum of the hand to the angle created between the first and second metacarpals (Fig. 92–13). The large flap, which has an ulnar base, is raised on the nerves and vessels, leaving the extensor apparatus intact. It can be rotated to produce an advancement of 1.5 cm.

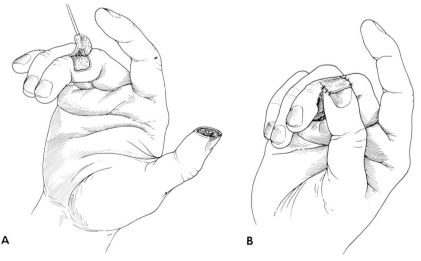

Figure 92–12. *A* and *B*, Covering of an amputation of the extremity of the thumb using a flap taken from the dorsolateral aspect of the long finger.

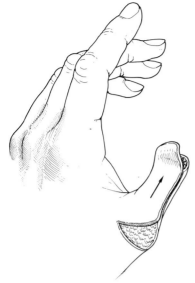

Figure 92–13. Simonetta thumb dorsal rotation flap.

OBLIQUE DORSAL AMPUTATIONS

In oblique dorsal amputations the nail is almost invariably involved (Fig. 92–14).

Partial Injury of the Nail

If the nail is only partially injured, an attempt must be made to preserve it. The nail is an important structure cosmetically and functionally and provides efficient support of the pulp in precision handling. One should always try to preserve it or at least to promote normal regeneration. This is possible only if the matrix is intact, if the nail bed is largely undamaged, if the normal adhesion between the nail and its bed is preserved, and if the phalangeal remnant is long enough (Fig. 92–15). If not, the nail will become curved and hooked.

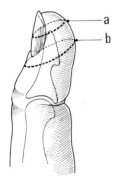

Figure 92–14. Oblique dorsal amputation. a = the nail is only partially affected, b = the nail is destroyed.

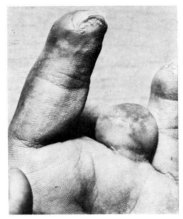

Figure 92–15. The length of the distal phalanx is insufficient. The nail curves at the extremity of the stump.

If the nail bed has been sectioned but each fragment is still adherent to the wound, these can be approximated and sutured. Instead of suturing, Matthews (1982) advises covering the nail with a layer of dental cement, which forms a protective envelope during the healing period. The cement is removed after four weeks. If the nail is detached (Fig. 92–16), the edges are trimmed and the nail is replaced in its bed and, if possible, in the matrix after perforating it to allow the release of serous fluid. It is sutured to the edges of the bed and held down as a splint with a compressive dressing.

When the nail has been damaged beyond repair, Iselin and Iselin (1967) advocate the use of a "bank nail" preserved in Cialit in order to preserve the nail bed and avoid synechiae of the matrix, which are responsible for bifid nails. If a bank nail is not available, a nail can be tailored in a Silastic sheet and inserted between the proximal nail fold and the matrix and left in place for three or four weeks in order to prevent adhesion between the eponychium and the matrix. The idea is to reconstitute an even nail bed and encourage regeneration of the nail (Fig. 92–17). As exact a reapproximation as possible

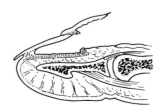

Figure 92–16. The partially avulsed nail is replaced.

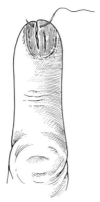

Figure 92–17. Suture of nail bed wounds using absorbable material.

of available tissue also helps. These sutures must be absorbable; otherwise their presence under the nail will be unsightly and painful. A split thickness skin graft may be used if the base of the wound is healthy, but the nail will not adhere to the graft. Lesions of the nail are notoriously difficult to treat and are dealt with in greater detail in the chapters on the nail in Volume IV.

Damage to the Matrix

If the matrix itself has been damaged beyond repair, after its complete removal, the choice lies between a graft or a flap, again depending on the quality of the bed (Fig. 92–18). However, unlike lacerations of the pulp, this lesion does not require a thick or sensitive skin cover. The aim of treatment here is to even out the nail bed, reduce the hollow caused by the absence of the nail, and, if need be, prepare the area for application of an artificial nail later.

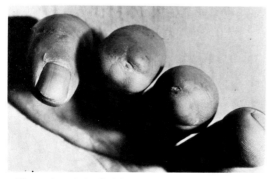

Figure 92–18. Nail debris may cause trouble because the debris may catch and is sometimes painful. Wide excision is essential since regrowth is common if the matrix is not totally removed.

If a large surface of bone is exposed, a flap is preferable; to be cosmetically satisfactory, this should be very thin. This is the situation in which heterodigital flaps come into their own if shortening is to be avoided.

Dorsolateral Flap. The dorsolateral flap taken from the adjacent finger should have a proximal or distal pedicle, according to the requirements of immobilization. If the amputation is oblique proximally toward the donor finger, a direct pedicled flap is preferred. Conversely, a distal pedicle is more easily adapted if the cut is directed to the other side of the finger.

Cross Thumb Pedicle Flap. The thumb, with its great mobility and the relative abundance of skin on the dorsal aspect of its proximal phalanx, is a donor area of choice for defects of the three middle fingertips (Tupper, 1971). By contrast, the dorsal aspects of the digits cannot always provide sufficient skin to cover extensive defects on the dorsum of the thumb. If the ulnar based Simonetta dorsal flap cannot provide the cover required for the defect, it may be necessary to raise a distant flap.

OBLIQUE PALMAR AMPUTATIONS

Oblique palmar amputations are the most serious (Fig. 92–19) because pulp sensation and digital function are directly at risk. The problems here are complex because the reconstructed pulp should be sensitive and well cushioned in order to play its role in perception, protection, and proprioception. It is at the level of the pulp that re-establishment of good quality sensation is most important. Moberg (1964) has shown that a discriminative knowledge of touch—what he calls "tactile gnosis"—is not possible if the two point discrimination is more than 5 mm. The recovery of sensibility at the level of grafts and flaps poses a number of problems.*

Logically, flaps that keep the normal relationship between the nerve ending and skin have the best chance of good quality recovery, especially when they bring their own vascular supply, avoiding ischemia. If one uses flaps with a temporary pedicle, regional flaps raised from the hand that are of similar texture gain better sensibility than distant flaps with a thick layer of fat, which acts as

*See Chapter 56 in Volume I.

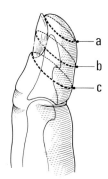

Figure 92–19. Oblique palmar amputations. a = the bone is not visible, b = amputation through the nail, the bone is exposed, c = amputation proximal to the nail.

a screen. When skin grafts are used, thick grafts that have conserved the dermal plexuses theoretically have more potential for recovery of sensibility if one admits that empty Schwann sheaths can be used as a supporting structure for new axonal growth. Cauna (1954) and Jabaley (Chapter 56, Vol. I) have shown the possibility of use of a hairless ("glabrous") skin graft without follicles that contains a high percentage of specialized mechanoreceptors.

In practice other factors also play an important role in the recovery of sensation. Most important is the condition of the receptive area. A bed of scar, granulation, or fibrous tissue is an obstacle for axonal penetration. The extent of loss of cutaneous substance also influences the result. If it is small, overlapping of the peripheral receptive fields will avoid a blind area. Finally the quality of the result depends on the absence of pain, the mobility of the digit, and the capacity for adaptation by the patient.

The multiplicity of factors explains the difference in results utilizing the same technique. The percentage of recovery of tactile discrimination as well as the percentage of painful sequelae varies from one series to another, even in successive series by the same author. Thus one must guard against a routine solution based on theoretical histological values for grafts and flaps, or on statistics that are insufficiently precise in that they fail to consider the type of skin cover and a number of other factors that influence the result. Among these are the size of the defect, the site, the condition of the bed, whether bone is exposed, the age of the lesion, the type and amount of scar tissue, associated injuries, the existence of pain, finger mobility, the age, occupation, and activity of the

patient, the length of follow-up, complications, and the length of time required for healing.

Thus it seems essential to adapt the choice of cover to the local state of the wound, keeping in mind special considerations for each case. Whatever the choice, its execution must be as technically perfect as possible, avoiding hematoma, excessive tension, hazardous dissections without magnification, and infection. Every local complication will compromise the recovery of good sensibility, for both grafts and flaps.

Some general directives may help to indicate the procedure of choice.

WHEN BONE IS NOT EXPOSED

Skin graft is possible if there is no bone showing and tissue loss is limited. The problem of recovery of sensation in skin grafts is still not clearly understood. The graft usually acquires protective sensibility, especially in the young patient. Occasionally the grafted area remains completely anesthetic and the "blind" finger is not used, whereas in other cases sensory perception may become good even though the two point discrimination test yields figures below normal. One of our own colleagues, a well known hand surgeon, had two pulp grafts in his right index and middle fingers: these are sensitive enough to allow the manipulation of microsurgical instruments without direct visual control.

Although thin partial thickness grafts have the advantage of reducing the insensitive area as they retract, total or composite grafts provide better protection (Mannerfelt, 1962; Porter, 1968). They are usually taken from areas where the skin has characteristics similar to those of the pulp—hypothenar eminence, first web space, or even the anterior aspect of the wrist, or from an amputated finger. Partial thickness grafts are useful mostly in emergency situations or for covering beveled cuts on the lateral aspects of a digit. If the graft is applied late, it is preferable to eliminate the closed screen formed by the granulation tissue progressing to fibrosis. We tend to use skin grafts for defects of the fingers not involving their tips.

WHEN BONE IS EXPOSED

If sufficient substance of the pulp has been lost to expose underlying bone, a flap is required. Only a skin transfer with its neurovascular pedicle or a contiguous homodigital flap can preserve the normal connections between the skin and its nerve supply. The quality of sensation is extremely variable in flaps moved from a distance and may even be absent if the flap is thick. It is usually sufficient for protection, and sometimes it is of very good quality and allows good function in heterodigital and palmar flaps. Palmar flaps leave less obvious scars, but the position of immobilization is less well tolerated.

These flaps may be good enough for the repair of the ulnar digits, but one should aim for a better result in the thumb, index finger, and middle finger. Three types of flaps can be used to resurface the pulp with sensation—a homodigital dorsal flap, an advanced or transposed palmar flap, or a heterodigital flap with its neurovascular pedicle. The quality of functional sensibility of these flaps is discussed in the following paragraphs.

Dorsal Homodigital Flaps

Flint and Harrison (1965) raised a flap based on the neurovascular branches of the dorsal aspect of the injured finger (Fig. 92–20), which arises from the palmar collateral bundles, at the level of the middle and distal phalanges. This obliquely cut flap provides a cover for the pulp defect. To avoid damage to the matrix, the incision should be made several millimeters proximal to it. The most distal part of this dorsal flap on the other side of the midline is likely to be the least sensitive and should be made to cover the functionally least important side of the pulp. Thus, for the index and middle fingers, the flap should be based medially so that the most distal portion of the flap covers the ulnar portion of the pulp. For the little finger, however, the base of the flap should be lateral. The thickness of this dorsal flap is less than that of palmar flaps. The quality of sensation is clearly inferior to that of those containing palmar tissue; thus the indications for these flaps are rather limited.

In the finger that is severed proximal to the base of the nail, Hilgenfeldt (1966) makes a dorsal longitudinal incision on the injured finger and slides the two dorsolateral flaps forward. Dorsal skin can be used as an island flap based on dorsal vascular and nerve branches of the palmar digital neurovascular pedicles (Joshi, 1974; Pho, 1979).

The Advanced Palmar Flap

Advancement of a triangular palmar islet using the V-Y technique, utilized for transverse amputations, may also be employed for oblique palmar amputations, although this provides only limited covering. This flap can be artificially elongated when the loss of substance is oval-shaped, suturing the two lateral angles of the triangle to the midline (Furlow, 1984), which offers an appreciable gain of as much as 1 cm. The distal extremity of the flap is curved in the shape of a cupola

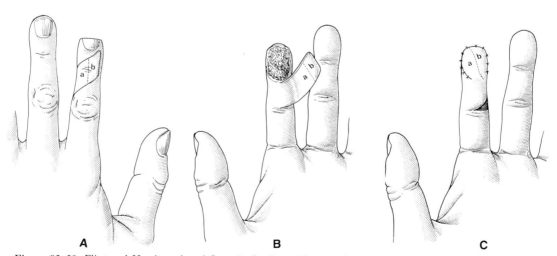

A   **B**   **C**

Figure 92–20. Flint and Harrison dorsal flap. *A*, Outline of flap on dorsal aspect of finger. For the index finger, the base of the flap is ulnar. *B*, Palmar view. a = the proximal parts of the flap where sensibility is better than in b. *C*, Placing of flap.

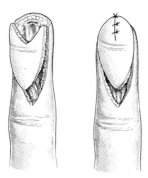

Figure 92–21. Furlow modification of the triangular island palmar flap.

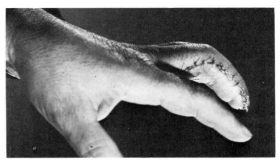

Figure 92–22. Clinical example of a Moberg-Snow advancement flap.

that fits over the end of the stump. This procedure can be used only for limited loss of palmar substance (Fig. 92–21).

Dissection of the palmar digital tissues down to the fibrous flexor sheaths allows advancement of the superficial planes of about 1 cm. The neurovascular bundles, of course, should be spared. It is possible, as suggested by Moberg (1964) and Snow (1967), to make two lateral incisions; great care must be taken to preserve the dorsal vascular branches supplying the dorsal skin of the middle phalanx, for otherwise there is a risk of necrosis (Nicoletis and Morel-Fatio, 1969). The distal obliquity of these branches makes advancement possible; we have done it on several occasions without any vascular complications (Fig. 92–22). The traction of the flap may produce a flexion deformity of the distal phalanx.

O'Brien's modification consists of raising the Moberg flap with bilateral midlateral incisions but with a proximal transverse section at the level of the second phalanx (Fig. 92–23). Thus the flap is entirely free except for its two neurovascular bundles. It is advanced to the tip and the proximal defect is grafted. This appears more risky but has the advantage of minimizing the proximal extension of the midlateral incisions, thereby reducing the risk of damage to the dorsal branches of the collateral vessels.

Hueston (1966) advocated the use of a single lateral incision, which curves in transversely at the base of the finger (Figs. 92–24, 92–25). This produces a large rotation flap based on the opposite side, which can be advanced into the pulp, the bare area at the base of the finger being covered by a full thickness free graft or a small dorsal transposition flap (Harrison, 1970). A similar technique is employed for the thumb (Fig. 92–26).

When the quality of sensitivity remains good on the side of the flap where the pedicle is preserved, recovery is often incomplete on the other side, which may lead to a real problem regarding the thumb and index. On the thumb, the longitudinal incision must always be radial and should preferably be ulnar on the index and middle fingers, at least when loss of substance is symmetrical. To compensate for this difficulty, Souquet (1985) goes behind the two neurovascular bundles and the transverse incision curves inward distally to reach the midlateral line of the opposite side in such a way as to allow for asymmetrical, albeit limited, advancement of an entirely sensitive flap.

Littler and this author have several times

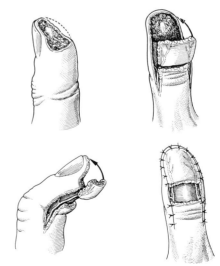

Figure 92–23. Advancement flap with transverse incision over the middle phalanx.

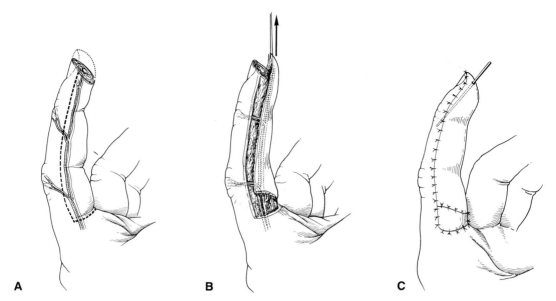

Figure 92–24. Hueston rotation flap. *A*, Drawing of flap, *B*, Advancement of flap, *C*, The loss of substance at the base of the fingers is covered by a skin graft.

used homodigital island flaps with a neurovascular pedicle to bring sensitive skin to the most used side of the pulp. However, we did not explore all the possibilities of this procedure. Dissection of the neurovascular pedicle to the base of the finger allows for pulp advancement of as much as 1.5 cm. This has been used by Venkataswani and Subramanian (1980), Mouchet and Gilbert (1982), Schund et al. (1985), and Massart et al.

(1985). The experience of these authors, in common with our own, confirms that it is this type of palmar flap that has the greatest autonomy, while retaining excellent sensitivity over its entire surface.

The flap is taken from the possible residual palmar skin of the distal phalanx as well as the middle phalanx, and from the side least useful functionally. It extends to slightly beyond the volar midline on one side and the

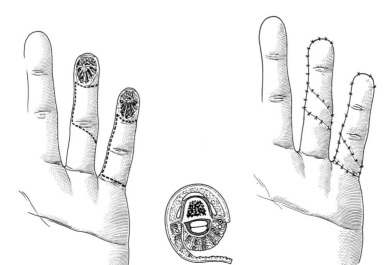

Figure 92–25. Rotation flap of palmar skin involving two fingers. The flap is separated in front of the neurovascular bundle on the side of the incision and behind the neurovascular bundle on the opposite side.

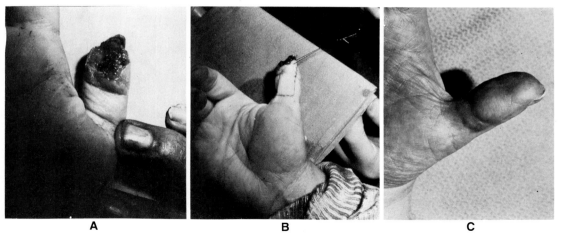

Figure 92–26. Thumb rotation flap. *A*, Loss of thumb pulp. *B*, Drawing of flap. *C*, Results.

midlateral line on the other side. It is dissected in continuity with the collateral bundle (Fig. 92–27). This is approached via a midlateral or zigzag incision to the base of the finger or to the origin of the collateral artery, if possible avoiding damage to the dorsal branch of the proximal phalanx. This flap is brought to the exposed area by slight traction to correct curving of the bundle. The radial bundle of the index finger can be "medialized," resulting in disappearance of the bend at the level of the metacarpal head (Foucher, 1986). The flap is attached to the extremity of the finger using a thin Kirschner wire. In the adult this is used at the same time to block the distal interphalangeal joint at 20 degrees of flexion to prevent excessive flexion. This thus avoids sutures distal to the

nail remnant, which would be associated with the risk of accentuating deformities. The donor zone is covered with a full thickness skin graft. Excessive traction must be avoided because of danger to the flap or the possibility of causing retraction of the interphalangeal joints. An extension orthosis is applied when the wire is removed after about 10 days. It is important not to always seek to advance the flap as far as the end of the fingers. It is not always possible to advance the flap as far as the end of the finger. Depending on the case, the distal portion of the finger may be shortened or grafted (Fig. 92–28). One can perform staged advancements at six month intervals. This possibility is interesting in multiple injuries, in which restoration of sensibility of the stump of the thumb or of an

Figure 92–27. Advancement of an island flap.

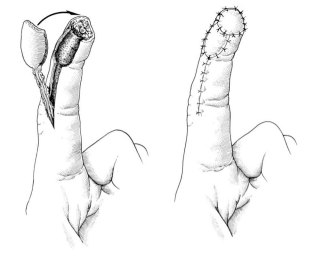

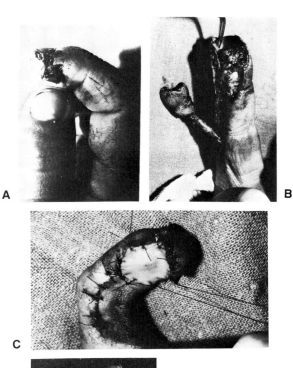

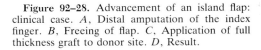

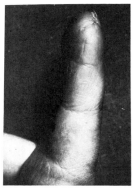

Figure 92–28. Advancement of an island flap: clinical case. *A*, Distal amputation of the index finger. *B*, Freeing of flap. *C*, Application of full thickness graft to donor site. *D*, Result.

opposable digit can be of particular importance.

The Transposition Flap

In cases of tissue loss on the lateral aspect of the pulp, the remaining pulp can be slid across to the area most useful for prehension (Littler, 1960). It may be necessary to dissect the neurovascular pedicles in the adjacent healthy zone. Thus, if the skin loss is on the radial side of the pulp of the index, a sensitive flap is carried across from the ulnar side. The donor area is covered by a graft that can be taken from the skin excised from the recipient zone. The same technique may be used to transfer sensation-intact tissue to the outer aspect of the pulp of the thumb.

Heterodigital Flaps with Neurovascular Pedicles

Extensive skin loss on the palmar aspect of the thumb may lead to such severe functional deficit that heterodigital skin island transfers are sometimes justified. These transfers are performed at the expense of a loss of sensitive skin in another digit.

The transfer is taken preferably from the anteromedial aspect of the ring or long finger (Fig. 92–29). However, it is now well known that these transfers, which carry a well pad-

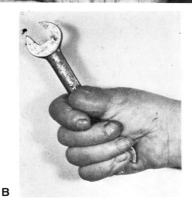

Figure 92–29. *A*, Amputation of the distal phalanx of the thumb with extensive damage to palmar skin overlying the proximal phalanx. *B*, Repair using an iliac graft and an island skin flap taken from the ring finger.

A

B

ded, well vascularized, and sensitive area of skin, are useful only if the patient can learn to reinterpret the newly displaced sensory information. Only young and active patients can be expected to adapt to this new situation; thus the indications are limited. Reconnection of the nerve pedicle of the flap to the collateral bundle of the involved finger has been done in order to facilitate reorientation (Foucher et al., 1981; Cohen and Cronin, 1983). (See the chapter on "Island Flap," Volume II, pp. 299–312.)

If the thumb has been shortened, a flap taken from the dorsum of the index finger can be used. The procedure most recently described involves a free vascularized pulp flap from the toe, which can provide a thick padded cover with good sensation to the thumb (Buncke, 1979). The technique of this flap is described later (see Chapters 113 and 114).

Author's Preference

After this lengthy enumeration of suitable procedures for loss of pulp substance, we will summarize our own indications:

If the loss of tissue is less than 1 cm. in diameter, rely on spontaneous healing. If the loss of tissue is more than 1 cm. across, the following should be considered:

1. If the bone is not exposed, a skin graft can be used for the ulnar digits, or spontaneous healing can be chosen. Advancement for the thumb and index finger can be combined, if necessary, with a skin graft on the surface that is not usually utilized in pinch. Thus, when the loss of substance is too great to allow full coverage by an advancement flap, a free graft can be used at the terminal end of the digit because its participation in pinch is small.

The flap that we use most often for the long fingers is the homodigital island flap with its neurovascular bundle, which allows the greatest advancement of the sensory flap.

2. If the bone is exposed, the size of the loss of substance will determine the technique used. If loss of substance is limited, advancement of an adjacent island flap (with blood and nerve supply preserved within the subcutaneous tissue) may be sufficient. If it involves or exceeds a hemipulp, a palmar flap with one or both bundles is necessary. For the thumb, the Hueston flap remains indicated if loss of substance is oblique and predominantly radial. Island flaps with their neurovascular bundle taken from the thumb

are a possibility, but their use is restricted by frequent variations in the arterial supply of the thumb. The dorsolateral island flap based on the dorsal branches of the digital artery and nerve of the thumb, when one can utilize it, has advantages over the heterodigital flap in that there is no disturbance in the orientation of sensibility (Pho, 1979).

3. Flaps taken from the opposite forearm are useful when skin from the same hand cannot be used or when there is a large area of loss.

When destruction of the pulp is accompanied by that of the index or other fingers, free transfer of one or more toe pulps must be envisaged. The lateral hemipulp of the great toe is preferred for the thumb, unless the possibility exists of taking a composite transfer from a damaged finger that is to be amputated.

SPECIAL INJURIES

We include under this heading multiple injuries and replantations.

MULTIPLE FINGERTIP INJURIES

When, as is often the case, several fingers are involved, every effort should be made to conserve length in each. This implies that flaps will be used more frequently, preferably palmar or dorsal homodigital flaps. The multiplicity of wounds may render the use of local or regional flaps difficult, although it is possible to combine digital with palmar flaps. One may be forced to use flaps from a distance; several small adjacent flaps can be raised on the contralateral limb, the thorax, or the groin.

REPLANTATIONS

It is tempting to replant the amputated segment. In spite of the optimistic figures obtained by Douglas (1959), it seems unreasonable in adults to attempt the replantation of a composite graft that includes a segment of phalangeal bone merely by using skin sutures. Microsurgical technique is useful for perfecting the approximation. However, early replacement of a cleanly lacerated, uncrushed fingertip, after removal of the skeletal component and exact reattachment ac-

cording to the cutaneous patterns, can result in a more or less partial take. Often the fingertip may become necrotic, but after the eschar is eliminated, the underlying tissue is found to be re-epithelialized (Fisk, 1972); comparative photographs showing distinct shortening of the digit prove this to be only a "pseudosuccess." A take is more likely if only the skin of the amputated tip is applied as a graft, after thinning the peripheral stratum corneum to make a more supple graft and avoiding dead space (Chase, 1968).

In children under five years, however, the chances of survival are much greater, and replantation by simple peripheral suturing is justifiable.

Replantation using microvascular techniques is discussed in Chapter 85.

Such distal replantations are functionally satisfactory because they are not associated with stiffness of the proximal articulations of the finger. In addition, because of distal nerve suture, sensory recovery is rapid and terminal neuromas on stumps are avoided. They are indicated in particular for the thumb. However, the small diameter of the vessels makes such operation difficult, and they should be performed only by highly trained teams (see Chapter 103).

FINGERTIP WOUNDS AND AMPUTATIONS IN CHILDREN

These injuries in children deserve special attention for several reasons. First, there is an excellent opportunity for primary healing as compared to situation in the adult. Second, one always attempts to preserve as much length as possible. For these reasons spontaneous healing is the method usually used in children; surgical indications are much rarer than in the adult patient (Bossley, 1975; Das and Brown, 1978; Illingworth, 1974). However, one can attempt replantation of distal tips.

In young children the dressing must be rigidly maintained. It is necessary to include all of the hand in the dressing and sometimes even the elbow (Sandzen, 1974).

SEQUELAE OF FINGERTIP INJURIES

The instances in which results are less than satisfactory are numerous, and the problems

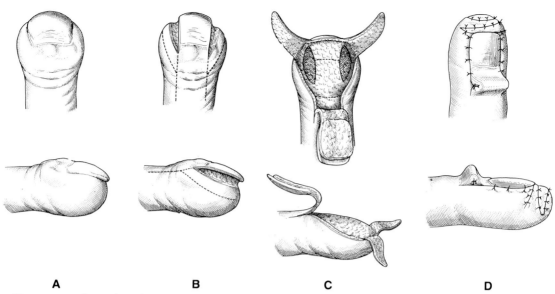

A **B** **C** **D**

Figure 92–30. Correction of a "club deformity" following digital amputation (Dufourmentel procedure). *A*, "Club" appearance of distal phalanx after transungual amputation. *B*, Freeing of the nail with its bed and matrix. *C*, The median ungual flap and the two lateral cutaneous flaps are lifted. The two ellipses represent tissue that must be resected in order to reduce the thickness of the stump. *D*, The nail is drawn back by folding of the base of the ungual flap. The two lateral skin flaps are crossed over each other distally to fill the gap caused by withdrawal of the nail. They will serve as a base when the nail regrows.

encountered are disproportionate to the size of the anatomical lesion. We shall not deal with the most disabling problems of sensibility here: the treatment of painful stumps and anesthetic pulps is described in Volume IV. We shall mention here only morphological or dystrophic sequelae.

Dystrophic Pulp. Dystrophic pulps are seen after spontaneous cicatrization or beveled palmar wounds treated with a graft. The skin is thin, adherent to the bone, and fragile, and pressure and exposure to cold are painful. An advancement flap is a remedy in these cases.

"Clubbed" Fingertip. The "clubbed" fingertip, shortened and bulbous, is very unattractive. Dufourmentel (1963) described an elegant procedure to correct this (Fig. 92–30):

1. Fashion triangular distally based flaps on both sides of the nail.

2. Free the nail with its bed and matrix; the latter should be taken close to the bone or, even better, with a small sliver of bone.

3. The volume of the fingertip is reduced.

4. The two triangular flaps are turned 90 degrees to the digital axis and are approximated to each other so as to elongate the fingertip.

5. The nail is then reapplied more proxi-

mally, creating a small fold at the base of the median flap.

Nail Problems. Sequelae involving the nail bed not only are esthetically displeasing but can also be functionally bothersome.

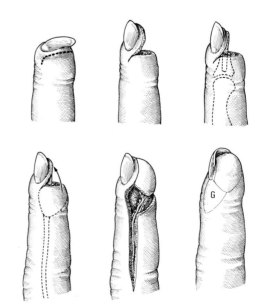

Figure 92–31. Technique for the correction of the curved nail with the aid of a bone graft and a sensory island flap.

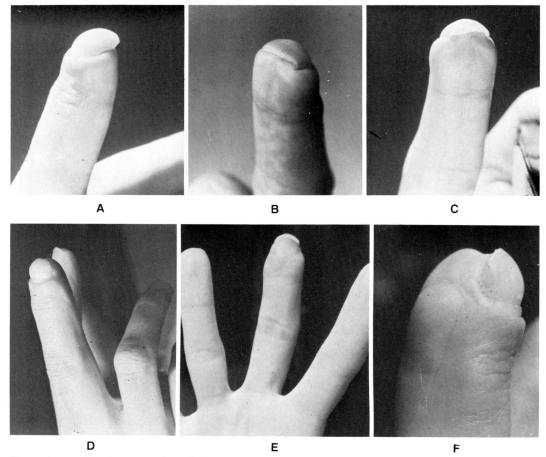

Figure 92–32. Complete correction of the curved nail. *A, B,* and *C,* Before the operation. *D, E,* and *F,* After correction with bone graft and island flap.

Nail debris is painful and must be completely removed as recurrences are common.

Curved nails are also common, unattractive, and often painful with pressure. Correction of this deformity is difficult. To avoid a recurrence, it is necessary to bring in new soft tissue, with some sensibility if possible, and also bony support (Fig. 92–31).

Proximal repositioning of the matrix is not sufficient, since the curvature may be too severe. We have used the following technique:

After elevating the nail with its bed, one osteotomizes the base of the distal phalanx parallel to the surface under the matrix. One places in this opening a thin cortical bone graft taken from the ulna to support the nail. Then one advances a pedicled island flap of palmar tissue from one side of the digit, as previously described. This sensory flap will cover the bone graft and reconstitute the distal pulp. The donor site is covered by a full thickness graft (Fig. 92–32).

REFERENCES

Aradao: Tratamiento primario de las heridas de las manos. Thesis, Montevideo, 1959.

Atasoy, E., Igakimidis, E., Kastan, M. L., Kutz, J. E., and Kleinert, H. C.: Reconstruction of the amputated fingertip with a triangular volar flap: a new surgical procedure. J. Bone Joint Surg., 52A:921, 1970.

Beasley, R. W.: Reconstruction of amputed fingertips. Plast. Reconstr. Surg., 44:349–352, 1969.

Biddulph, S. L.: The neurovascular flap in fingertip injuries. Hand, 11:59–63, 1979.

Buncke, H. J., and Rose, E. H.: Free toe to fingertip neurovascular flaps. Plast. Reconstr. Surg., 63:607, 1979.

Chase, A.: The damaged index digit. A source of components to restore the crippled hand. J. Bone Joint Surg., 50A:6, 1152, 1968.

Chow, S. P., and Ho, E.: Open treatment of fingertip injuries in adults. J. Hand Surg., 7:470–476, 1982.

Cohen, B. E., and Cronin, E. D.: An innervated cross finger flap for fingertip reconstruction. Plast. Reconstr. Surg., 72:688–695, 1983.

Das, S. K., and Brown, H. G.: Management of lost fingertips in children. Hand, 10:16–27, 1978.

Douglas, B.: Successful replacement of completely avulsed portions of fingers as composite grafts. Plast. Reconstr. Surg., 23(3):213, 1959.

Dufourmentel, C.: Correction des extrémités digitales en "massue". Ann. Chir. Plast., 2:99, 1963.

Erler, F.: Zur Versorgung von Kuppensubstanzverlusten an den Fingerendgliedern. Zbl. Chir., 70:40, 1943.

Fisk, G. R.: Conservative management of fingertips injuries. Paper read in the Spring Meeting of the British for Surgery of the Hand, May, 1972.

Flint, M. H.: Some observations on the vascular supply of the nail bed and terminal segments of the finger. Br. J. Plast. Surg., 8:186–195, 1955.

Flint, M. H., and Harrison, S. H.: A local neurovascular flap to repair loss of the digital pulp. Br. J. Plast. Surg., 18(2):156–164, 1965.

Foucher, G., Braun, F. M., Merle, M., and Michon, J.: La technique du "débranchement-rebranchement" du lambeau en îlot pédiculé. Ann. Chir., 35:301–303, 1981.

Foucher, G., Merle, M., and Michon, J.: Les amputations digitales distales. De la cicatrisation dirigée au transfert microchirurgical de pulpe d'orteil. Indications et résultats. Communication Acad. Chir., Séance 3 Déc., 1986.

Fox, J., Golden, G. et al.: Nonoperative management of finger tip pulp amputation by occlusive dressing. Am. J. Surg., 133:255–256, 1977.

Freiberg, A., and Manktelow, R.: The Kutler repair of fingertip amputation. Plast. Reconstr. Surg., 50:371–375, 1972.

Furlow, L.: V-Y "Cup" flap for volar oblique amputation of fingers. J. Hand Surg., 9-B3:253–256, 1984.

Gellis, M., and Pool, R.: Two point discrimination distances in the normal hand and forearm. Plast. Reconstr. Surg., 59:57–63, 1977.

Glicenstein, J.: Technique de réparation des amputations des extrémités distales. Ann. Chir., 25:1001–2008, 1971.

Hann, J. B.: The pattern of ramification of the volar digital nerve in the distal segment of the finger and the relationship of this pattern to the maintenance of sensibility following Kutler type revision of distal fingertip amputations. Symposium of Hand Surgery, Göteborg, 1971.

Holevich, I.: A new method for restoring sensibility to the thumb. J. Bone Joint Surg., 45B:496–502, 1963.

Holevich, I., and Paneva-Holevich, E.: Chirurgie de la main. Sofia, 1968.

Holm, A., and Zachariae, L.: Fingertip lesions. An evaluation of conservative treatment versus free skin grafting. Acta Orthop. Scand., 45:382–392, 1974.

Hueston, J. T.: Local flap repair of fingertip injuries. Plast. Reconstr. Surg., 37:349, 1966.

Iselin, M., and Gosse, L.: Le lambeau en drapeau. Son emploi systématique dans le comblement des pertes de substance limitées des doigts. Ann. Chir. Plast., 7(1):1–8, 1962.

Iselin, M., and Iselin, F.: Traité de Chirurgie de la Main. Editions Médicales Flammarion, Paris, 1967.

Joshi, B.: A local dorsolateral island flap for restoration of sensation after avulsion injury of finger tip pulp. Plast. Reconstr. Surg., 54:175–182, 1974.

Kuhn, H.: Le traitement des amputations en coup de hache des phalanges distales. Rev. Chir. Orthop. Répar. App. Moteur, 53(5):469–474, 1967.

Kutler, W.: A new method for fingertip amputation. J. Am. Med. Ass., 133:29–30, 1947.

Littler, J. W.: Neurovascular skin island transfer in reconstructive hand surgery. Trans. Int. Soc. Plast. Surg., 2:175, 1960.

McCash, C.: Toe pulp free grafts in finger tips repair. Br. J. Plast. Surg., 11:322, 1959.

Macht, S. D., and Watson, K.: The Moberg volar advancement flap for digital reconstruction. J. Hand Surg., 5:372–376, 1980.

Maqueira, N. O.: An innervated full thickness skin graft to restore sensibility to fingertips. Plast. Reconstr. Surg., 53:568, 1974.

Marchac, D., and Rousso, M.: La greffe cutanéo-pulpaire après amputation des extrèmites digitales. Ann. Chir. Plast., 16(1):51–54, 1971.

Massart, P., Saucier, T., and Bèze, H.: Restauration pulpaire par lambeau neurovasculaire homodigital. Ann. Chir. Main, 4:3, 1985.

Matthews, P.: A simple method for treatment of finger tip injuries involving the nail bed. The Hand, 14:30–32, 1982.

Moberg, E.: Aspects of sensation in reconstructive surgery of the upper extremity. J. Bone Joint Surg., 46A:817–825, 1964.

Mouchet, A., and Gilbert, A.: Couverture des amputations distales des doigts par lambeau neurovasculaire homodigital en îlot. Ann. Chir. Main, 1:180–182, 1982.

Newmeyer, W. L., and Kilgore, E. S.: Finger tip injuries. A simple effective method of treatment. J. Trauma, 14:58–64, 1974.

Nicoletis, C., and Morel-Fatio, D.: "Etranges nécrosés". Ann. Chir. Plast., 14:56, 1969.

O'Brien, B.: Neurovascular island pedicle flaps for terminal amputations and digital scars. Br. J. Plast. Surg., 21:258–261, 1968.

Pho, R. W. H.: Local composite neurovascular island flap for skin cover in pulp loss of the thumb. J. Hand Surg., 4:11–15, 1979.

Pillet, J.: A la recherche d'une main perdue. Rev. Praticien, 21(4):603–615, 1971.

Porter, R.: Functional assessment of transplanted skin in volar defects of the digits. J. Bone Joint Surg., 50A:955–963, 1968.

Russel, R. C., Van Beek, A. L., Wavak, P., and Zook, E. G.: Alternative hand plays for amputations and digital defects. J. Hand Surg., 6:399–405, 1981.

Sandzen, S. C.: Management of the acute fingertip injury in the child. The Hand, 6:190–197, 1974.

Segmuller, G.: Modifikation des Kutler-Lappens neurovaskuläre stielung. Handchir., 8:75–76, 1976.

Serafin, D., Kutz, J. E., and Fleinert, H. E.: Replantation of a completely amputated distal thumb without venous anastomosis. Plast. Reconstr. Surg., 52:579–582, 1973.

Shepard, G. M.: The use of lateral V-Y advancement flaps for finger tip reconstruction. J. Hand Surg., 8:254–259, 1983.

Snow, W.: The use of a volar flap for repair of finger tip. Amputations: a preliminary report. Plast. Reconstr. Surg., 40(2):163–168, 1967.

Souquet, R.: Le lambeau d'avancement artériel asymétrique dans les pertes de substance de la pulpe digitale (Lambeau de Hueston modifié). Ann. Chir. Main, 4:3, 1985.

Srivastava, R. K., and Kahl, J. B.: Shifting neurovascular island flap for the reconstruction of amputated digital stump. Plast. Reconstr. Surg., 66:301–302, 1980.

Tranquilli-Leali, E.: Recostruzionc dell'apice delle falangi unguali mediante autoplastica volare pedunculata per scorimento. Infort. Traum. Lavoro. 1:186–193, 1935.

Tubiana, R., and Duparc, J.: Restoration of sensibility in the hand by neurovascular skin island transfer. J. Bone Joint Surg., 43B(3):474–480, 1961.

Tubiana, R.: Traumatic amputations of phalanx and digits. In J. E. Flynn (Ed): Hand Surgery, 3rd ed., Baltimore, Williams & Wilkins, 1982, pp. 515–522.

Tuper, J.: The cross-thumb pedicle flap. A study of its functional value. Symposium of Hand Surgery, Göteborg, 1971.

Venkataswami, R., and Subramanian, N.: Oblique triangular flap: a new method of repair for oblique amputations of the finger tip and thumb. Plast. Reconstr. Surg., 66:296–300, 1980.

Vilain, R.: Les pertes de substance cutanée des doigts et de leur traitement (à propos de 100 observations). Ann. Chir., 30(4):199–212, 1954.

Vilain, R., and Michon, J.: Chirurgie Plastique Cutanée de la Main Chez l'Enfant et l'Adulte. 2nd ed. Paris, Masson, 1974.

Chapter 93

SURGICAL REPAIR AFTER TRAUMATIC AMPUTATIONS OF THE PROXIMAL AND MIDDLE PHALANGES

Raoul Tubiana

We shall be concerned here only with the mechanical consequences of traumatic amputations and mutilations. The problem of painful stumps is discussed in Volume IV.

The mechanical disorders resulting from these injuries at the level of the proximal and middle phalanges of the long fingers vary according to the length of the stump, its mobility, its sensibility, the finger involved, and the condition of the remaining fingers and other structures in the hand. We shall consider here only the problems of surgical repair after amputation of the fingers.

In some cases stumps are a definite mechanical hindrance, as, for example, when they are stiff, fixed in an unphysiological position, short, or insensitive or when they create a gap between mobile digits that makes the grasping of small objects more difficult.

If only one finger is involved, it may be preferable to remove the nonfunctional and troublesome stump.

If several fingers are involved, the indications for amputating the stumps are much less clear cut. Attempts should be made to improve their function by increasing their mobility, sensation, or length by appropriate surgery.

In other cases in which the stumps are mobile and sensitive and do not interfere with function, one has to decide whether transfer, lengthening, or amputation of the stump can in any way improve the overall function of the hand or its cosmetic appearance. Here again the problem is difficult,

depending on whether one or several digits are amputated or mutilated. In this category of patients, preservation of the thumb offers the hope of restoration of useful prehension.

INJURIES INVOLVING ONLY ONE FINGER

THE INDEX FINGER

When the index finger is amputated, its place in pinch is taken by the middle finger, but writing remains difficult if the mutilation involves the dominant hand. A long stump is useful for side to side thumb-finger and directional gripping.

When the stump is short, consideration is given to amputation of the digit at an elective level. Arguments in favor of conservative treatment include the desire to preserve the width of the hand as well as providing a potential support for a tool handle, which is particularly useful in pronation (Murray et al., 1977). These arguments are valid in manual workers, but cosmetically amputation at the base of the second metacarpal is more acceptable. Besides, it allows better opening out of the web space between the thumb and middle finger. Transferring a muscle onto the tendon of the second dorsal interosseus muscle reinforces abduction of the middle finger, which will oppose the thumb in the lateral grip. The most popular transfer involves the first dorsal interosseus muscle (Chase, 1968).

THE MIDDLE FINGER

When the amputation is through the middle phalanx, the functional deficit is usually limited. However, the more proximal the injury, the greater the handicap. As the fingers converge, a gap persists through which small objects can escape. Moreover, the lateral thumb-index grip loses much of its power in the absence of support from the middle finger. Finally, when the stump is very short, the unsupported index finger leans medially, and its tendons lose much of their efficiency as a result of the deviation of their axes. Resection of the third metacarpal would provide little help because the second metacarpal is fixed and the fourth has little mobility. The usual solution in such a case when functional loss is severe is to transpose the whole of the second ray to the position of the third.* Central ray resection without bone transposition is possible (Steichen and Idler, 1986). Closure of the defect created by the ray resection is accomplished by approximation of the adjacent metacarpals, with reconstruction of the deep transverse metacarpal ligament and dorsal dermadesis.

THE RING FINGER

The mechanical effects of amputation of the ring finger are similar to those of amputation of the middle finger but less marked, for this digit is not involved in the terminal tridactyl thumb-finger grip. The disadvantage of the empty space created by its amputation is partly compensated for by the mobility of the fifth metacarpal, which allows some degree of approximation, especially if the fourth metacarpal is excised. Translocation of the fifth ray to replace the fourth can be envisaged on cosmetic grounds, but the indications are weaker than for a second to third ray transfer.

THE LITTLE FINGER

The little finger plays an extremely important part in the digitopalmar grip. It is the key to the medial lock of the power grip and owes its action to its length and to the mobility of its joints. One should always try to preserve its length and its mobility. If the stump is short and relatively nonmobile, it gets caught easily and is best resected. The amputation should be through the shaft of the fifth metacarpal for the appearance is cosmetically superior without the protruding metacarpal head.

AMPUTATIONS AND MUTILATIONS INVOLVING SEVERAL FINGERS

The more fingers that are amputated, the greater the disturbance of prehension. Although the presence of a thumb ensures some degree of useful manual function, the range of grip-types is restricted. We shall consider in turn partial and total amputations of the fingers, amputations involving two fingers, those involving three fingers, and cases in which four fingers are lost, leaving the thumb with no opposable digit.

PARTIAL OR TOTAL AMPUTATION OF THE FINGERS

We will not dwell on the obvious distinction between partial and total amputation. When several fingers are amputated, the length of the stumps that can oppose the thumb or the palm is an important prognostic factor. The more fingers involved, the greater must be the attempt to conserve all available length. Other important factors are the suppleness and mobility of the joints of opposable digits.

AMPUTATION OF TWO FINGERS

The loss of two fingers still allows the possibility of a tridactyl grip including the thumb, a three pronged grip being usually well controlled (Fig. 93–1). If the surviving fingers and the thumb are intact, the patient will retain good manual function. Admittedly the grip will be weaker if the ulnar fingers are lost and precision will be reduced if the index and middle fingers are missing, but as a rule the patient is usually able to continue his occupation even if it involves specialized manual work. We have seen surgeons resume their profession after losing two ulnar fingers in the dominant hand. They would no doubt have been more severely handicapped by the

*See Chapter 87.

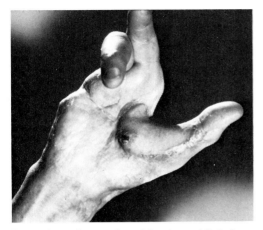

Figure 93–1. Amputation of the ring and little fingers. The contracted first commissure has been freed and lined with a flap.

loss of the radial fingers, as in their profession dexterity is more important than force.

AMPUTATION OF THREE FINGERS

The loss of a third finger worsens the prognosis considerably (Fig. 93–2). A grip between the thumb and a single digit has little stability or precision. One may be justified in trying to construct a third stabilizing opposable structure, for example, by phalangizing and lengthening the fifth metacarpal, or more simply by means of a partial prosthesis. It is essential that the remaining finger or stump be able adequately to oppose the thumb; to achieve this it may be necessary to perform a rotation osteotomy especially when

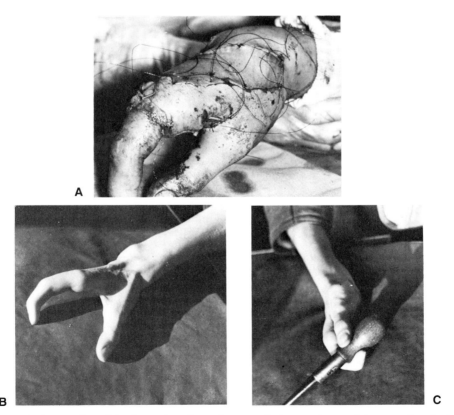

Figure 93–2. *A*, Amputation of the three ulnar fingers by an explosion causing a palmar wound at the base of the index finger with section of the flexor tendons. This wound is covered with a skin flap taken from the dorsal surface of the hand. *B* and *C*, A flexor tendon graft of the index finger restores active grip between the thumb and index finger.

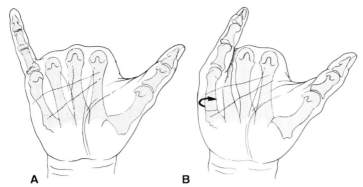

Figure 93–3. *A*, Amputation of the index, long, and ring fingers. *B*, Rotation osteotomy of the fifth metacarpal.

the opposing digit is medial and has lost some mobility and length (Figs. 93–3, 93–4). The site of the rotation osteotomy must be discussed in each case. An osteotomy performed at the base of the metacarpal is theoretically most advisable, but the rotary correction may not be realized in the digit if the metacarpophalanged joint is mobile. An osteotomy through the proximal phalanx results in more accurate correction, but there is a risk of finger stiffness.

AMPUTATION OF ALL FINGERS LEAVING AN ISOLATED THUMB

The thumb and metacarpals alone are capable of providing a strong grip between the thumb and the palm (Fig. 93–5), but control is poor (Fig. 93–6). This situation can be improved by two procedures—lengthening of the second or third metacarpal and phalangization of the fifth.

Lengthening of the Second Metacarpal. Lengthening of only the second metacarpal produces a short structure opposite the thumb, which allows a lateral grip. For this grip to be efficient, three conditions must hold:

1. The graft should be long enough, i.e., about two-thirds of the normal proximal phalanx, for the pulp of the thumb to have a broad area of contact when its interphalangeal joint is extended (Fig. 93–7). Flexion of this joint, when the stump of the index finger is too short, narrows the area of pulpal contact.

2. It is essential that the skin be sensitive at least in the zone that will come into contact with the thumb. A skin flap taken from the dorsal aspect of the thumb can be brought across to the anterolateral aspect of the proximal phalanx of the index finger.

3. The area of contact should not lie in the line of the second metacarpal but more anteriorly. For this reason the bone graft should be placed in 40 degrees of flexion.

When the web of the thumb is contracted, it may be necessary to resect the second metacarpal. The third metacarpal, not the

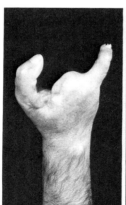
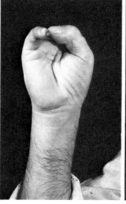
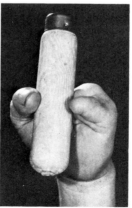

Figure 93–4. Example of osteotomy of the fifth metacarpal in a patient who lost the index, long, and ring fingers by trauma.

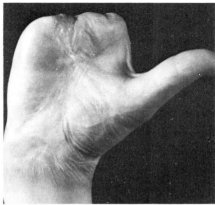

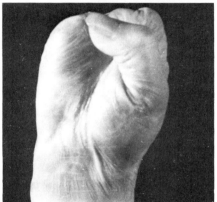

Figure 93–5. Amputation of all four fingers; the thumb is intact. Grip between thumb and palm is possible but crude.

second, is then lengthened, perhaps using a graft from the resected second metacarpal.

Phalangization of the Fifth Metacarpal. Phalangization of the fifth metacarpal combined with an osteotomy in flexion and lateral rotation of the same bone enables one to advance a mobile pillar toward the thumb (Fig. 93–8). The technical details of this procedure are discussed in Chapter 108. Lengthening of the fifth metacarpal also helps to improve the grip. This operation is particularly useful when the thumb itself has lost some of its length and mobility.

TECHNIQUES USED TO IMPROVE THE FUNCTION OF DIGITAL STUMPS

The treatment of painful stumps, from excision of neuromas to sympathectomies, is discussed elsewhere and will not be considered here.* The pain must be relieved before any reconstructive surgery is embarked upon, since a painful digital stump will not be used. The usual methods for covering the stumps with skin will not be described, except for techniques for restoring sensation. Elective reamputations are also described elsewhere (Vol. IV) and will not be discussed here. We shall describe operations to improve the mobility and sensation in the stump, to lengthen a stump, and to transplant a stump.

IMPROVING MOBILITY

Reeducation and physiotherapy alone cannot improve the mobility of the interphalangeal or metacarpophalangeal joints in the

---

*See Volume IV.

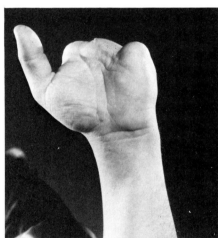

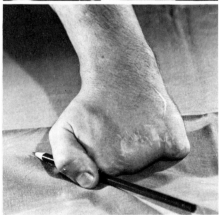

Figure 93–6. Grip between the thumb and second metacarpal lacks precision.

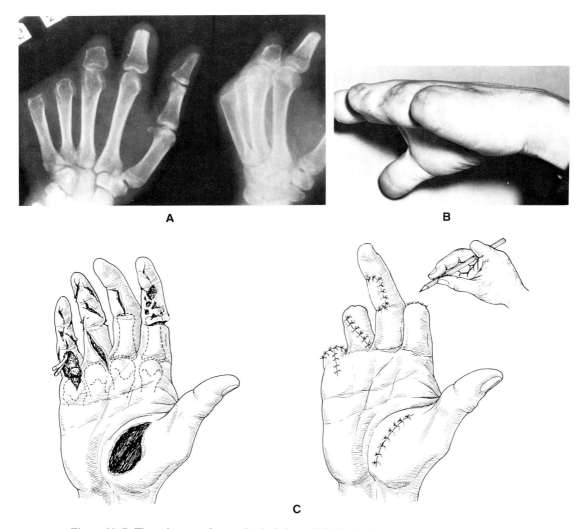

A

B

C

Figure 93–7. The existence of a proximal phalanx of the index finger improves grip precision.

presence of skin contractures and articular lesions. Instead one may have recourse to skin releases to combat contractures, to capsulectomies and even arthroplasties of the metacarpophalangeal joints, and to arthrolysis of the interphalangeal joint.

Deepening a web increases the autonomy of a short stump so that the mobility of its metacarpophalangeal joint is not restricted by contractures in adjacent fingers.

Phalangization provides increased mobility only when the metacarpals themselves are mobile, as is the case with the first and, to a lesser degree, the fifth metacarpal. As we shall see, this procedure is extensively used in severe mutilations.

An osteotomy, or an arthrodesis in a better position, helps to orientate a digital stump in a more functional position.

Finally, tendon transfers may be necessary to activate stumps whose tendons have been destroyed.

IMPROVING SENSATION

It is extremely important that the gripping area of a stump be provided with sensation. When nerve repair is impossible or has proved disappointing, the sense of touch can be improved by the transposition of sensitive skin. This sometimes can be taken from the

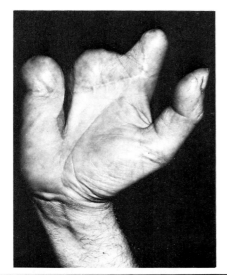

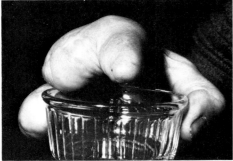

Figure 93–8. Phalangization of the fifth metacarpal, making possible its inclination in the direction of the thumb, further improves grip, which has three pressure points.

immediate vicinity, for example, by advancement from the palmar surface of the proximal part of the stump, from the dorsal aspect of the finger, or even from the palm.* Sensitive skin also can be obtained from distant sources by means of an island flap with its neurovascular bundle (Fig. 93–9). The two methods can be combined in the "creeping advancement" of an island flap (Joshi, 1974) (see Chapter 40 in Vol. II).

LENGTHENING AN AMPUTATED FINGER

It is mostly in cases of multiple amputations that the technique of digital lengthening comes into its own. The operation is rarely essential for function when the thumb is intact, but the chief indication is in the patient with a stiff or shortened thumb (Fig. 93–10).

A patient will only use a lengthened stump if the tip is painless and well padded with sensitive skin of good quality. Seldom is sufficient skin available to cover a bone graft without recourse to skin flaps. The zone of contact of the stump sometimes can be lined with a sensitive adjacent flap while less specific areas are covered with skin grafts or flaps from a distance. The extra length thus obtained is little more than 1 cm., but this can be a useful improvement.

---

*The technique is described in Volume IV in the chapter on sensory paralysis.

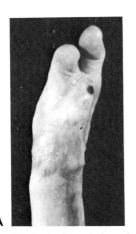
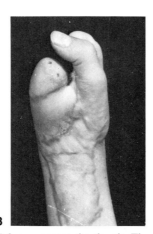
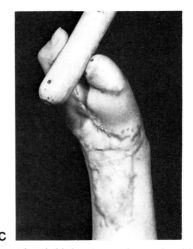

A   **B**   **C**

Figure 93–9. *A*, Amputation of all fingers except the thumb. The second and third metacarpals remain with part of their proximal phalanges. The ulnar part of the hand has been amputated. *B*, Reconstruction of ulnar support using an abdominal skin flap covering a wide iliac graft. The part of this buttress opposite the thumb is sensitized by a skin flap taken from the proximal phalanx of the long finger (indicated by two dots). *C*, Functional result: grip with three pressure points.

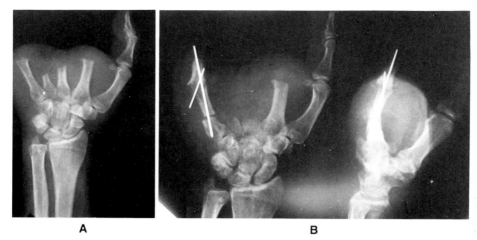

A   **B**

Figure 93–10. *A*, Mutilation of four fingers and parts of the metacarpals. The extremity of the thumb cannot reach the palm. *B*, Elongation and osteotomy of the fifth metacarpal and hollowing of the central part of the palm. The elongated fifth metacarpal is covered by the sensitive skin of the palm. A skin graft is applied to the palm. The thumb easily reaches the fifth metacarpal, the carpal joint of which is stiff.

When no adjacent sensitive skin flap is available, one solution is to borrow a narrow tube flap from a distance, perhaps from an area where the skin is thin, for example, the arm or clavicular region on the opposite side. The tube may be given sensation by means of an island flap. Lengthening by this technique produces a greater increase in length than the previous one.

The bone graft is taken from an adjacent metacarpal, the ulna, or the iliac bone. This graft must not be too long because it is essential that the skin be sutured without tension; otherwise ulceration is inevitable. Such bone grafts often resorb, and resorption is more likely if nutrition is insufficient and sensation is poor.

Lengthening by the distraction method of Matev also has a role to play in young subjects (see chapter by Matev, Volume II, pp. 535–549). Lengthening of a finger on purely cosmetic grounds is rarely indicated because the use of digital prostheses gives better results from an esthetic standpoint, particularly when a fingernail is involved.

Toe transfer may in certain cases offer an elegant solution in replacement of a distal phalanx. Rather than historic transfers by pediculated flap (the so-called "Italian method," which nevertheless sometimes gave satisfactory results; Fig. 93–11), free transfers using microsurgical techniques are now preferred (Fig. 93–12). Toe transfer techniques will be described in Chapters 103 and 104.

TRANSPLANTING THE STUMP

Digital stumps do not all have the same functional value. When several fingers are amputated, an attempt should be made to restore a tridactyl grip between the thumb, a radial finger, and an ulnar finger. It is important that the stumps be long enough to control the direction of the grip. In stumps that are not strategically placed, function can be considerably improved by transplantation in the context of a redistribution of the digital stumps.

The most commonly performed digital

Figure 93–11. Traumatic amputation of the four fingers with transfer of the second toe to the index finger by pedicle flap. (This case was kindly provided by Dr. Graner, Sao Paulo, Brazil.) *A*, Condition of hand before transfer. *B*, X-ray before transfer. *C*, Transfer of the second toe using the "Italian technique." Two skin flaps are raised, one on the toe and the other on the stump of the index finger. These two flaps are sutured together, and the hand is held on the dorsum of the foot by a plaster cast. *D*, Secondary bone graft between the phalanges of the hand and foot. *E*, Appearance of the two hands seven years after the transfer. There is good pinch function even though the "new" index finger has no active flexion at the interphalangeal joints, the patient having refused further surgery. *F*, X-ray seven years after transfer. *G*, Result 19 years after transfer.

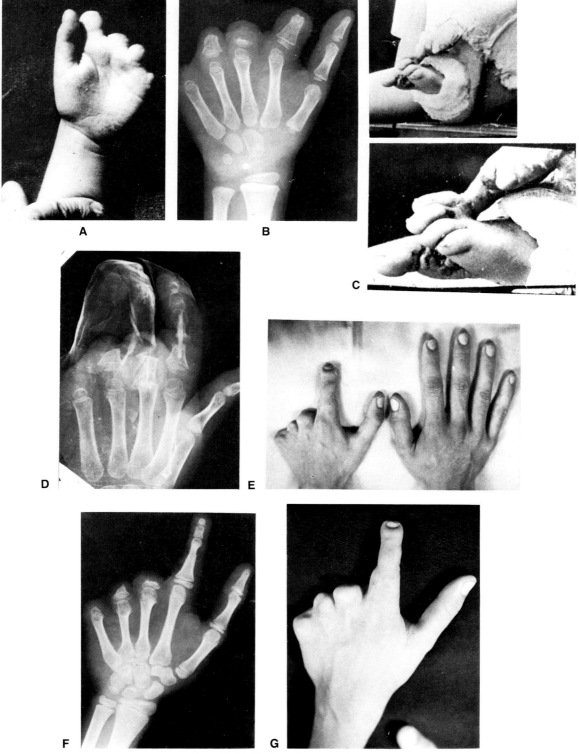

Figure 93–11 *See legend on opposite page*

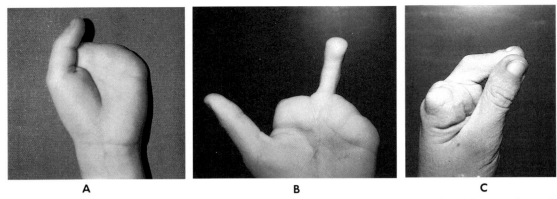

Figure 93–12. Toe transfer in opposition to a stiff thumb. *A*, Preoperative view. *B*, Transfer of the second toe. *C*, Results, with a good terminal pinch. (Courtesy of A. Gilbert.)

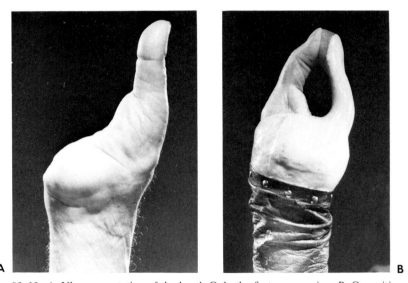

Figure 93–13. *A*, Ulnar amputation of the hand. Only the first ray remains. *B*, Opposition orthosis.

transplant is, of course, pollicization, but other types of transplant are done. They help to fill the gaps between surviving fingers and not only lengthen a stump that is too short opposite the thumb, but provide sensitive skin for it.*

We cannot close this chapter on amputations of the fingers without mentioning cosmetic digital prostheses (Fig. 93–13), which we use more and more frequently. A chapter in Volume IV is devoted to a discussion of prostheses.

---

*See Chapter 94.

REFERENCES

Chase, A.: The damaged index digit. A source of components to restore the crippled hand. J. Bone Joint Surg., *50A*:1152, 1968.

Joshi, B. B.: A local dorsolateral island flap for restoration of sensation after avulsion injury of finger tip pulp. Plast. Reconstr. Surg., *54*:175–182, 1974.

Murray, J. F., Wayne, C., and Mackensie, J. K.: Transmetacarpal amputation of the index finger: a clinical assessment of hand strength and complications. J. Hand Surg., *2*:471–481, 1977.

Souquet, R., and Mansat, M.: La main phalangienne. *In* Tubiana, R., Gosset, J., and Campbell Reid, D. (Editors): Les Mutilations de la Main. Paris, L'Expansion Scientifique Française, 1984.

Steichen, J. B., and Idler, R. S.: Results of central ray resection without bony transposition. J. Hand Surg., *11A*:466–474, 1986.

Chapter 94

TECHNIQUE OF DIGITAL TRANSPOSITION

JEAN-PIERRE RAZEMON

The aim of surgery is to improve the cosmetic appearance and function of the hand after an amputation of the middle or ring finger. In principle, the operation consists of the lateral transposition, in toto, of the index or little finger, i.e., with its own tendon apparatus and nerve and blood supply. Because the degree of displacement is limited, these structures are only slightly rerouted, and because they lie almost entirely on the palmar side of the digit, a dorsal approach is preferred as it provides better access to the skeleton.

THE INCISION

A racket shaped incision is made that surrounds the scar of the amputated finger before coursing up the dorsal aspect toward the base of the metacarpals—more precisely, to a point between the base of the metacarpal of the amputated finger and the base of the metacarpal of the finger to be transposed. This provides easy access to the two bones involved in the operation (Figs. 94–1, 94–2).

THE MUSCLES

When a finger is sacrificed, the corresponding interosseous muscles lose their functional significance, e.g., the second and third dorsal interosseous muscles when the middle finger is amputated, and the third palmar interosseous and fourth dorsal interosseous muscles when the ring finger is amputated.

Sacrifice of these muscles is essential, for transposition of a digit to the new site would otherwise result in the adding of a useless muscle mass, which is not only unsightly but may actually interfere with the function of the active interosseous muscles.

The topography of these muscles is not as complex as it may seem; by careful dissection from the periphery to the metacarpal insertion, one should be able without difficulty to separate the dorsal and palmar interosseous muscles of the same intermetacarpal space.

Transposition of the index finger following amputation of the middle finger is a simple step because the two dorsal interosseous muscles are easily accessible and can be separated readily from the corresponding palmar interosseous muscles.

When the little finger is transposed to replace an amputated ring finger, however, the interosseous stage is more delicate, for although the palmar interosseous muscle of the third interspace can be discarded, the dorsal interosseous muscle and its nerve supply must be carefully preserved. By contrast, when the fifth and third metacarpals are approximated, the fourth palmar interosseous muscle comes to lie neatly under the third dorsal interosseous muscle.

As the interosseous muscles are resected, the digital nerve is divided and the artery is tied off. It is important that the arterial ligature be placed at this stage because the vessels will be inaccessible when the metacarpal has been transposed. Therefore one should not wait until the tourniquet is released to tie off the digital artery.

Also inserted on the third metacarpal is the adductor pollicis. To preserve this attachment, one may be tempted to spare the proximal half of the metacarpal and resect the bone just distal to it. However, this

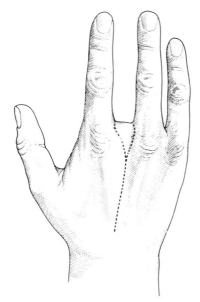

Figure 94–1. Incision line: the incision on the dorsal surface of the hand is directed toward the base between the second and third metacarpals in order to provide an easy approach to both bones.

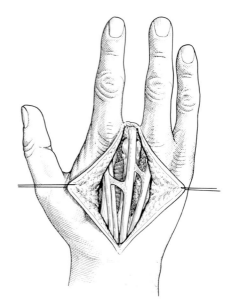

Figure 94–2. The incision exposes the extensor apparatus of the dorsum of the hand.

interferes with dissection of the muscles, as already described. It is better to disinsert the adductor completely, preserving as much periosteal and fibrous tissue as possible at the site of insertion. In fact, the adductor pollicis retains its normal power even without being reinserted on one of the remaining metacarpals (Fig. 94–3).

SECTIONING OF THE METACARPALS

The metacarpal of the amputated finger and that of the transposed finger should be resected at the same level so that muscle tension remains normal after the transposition.

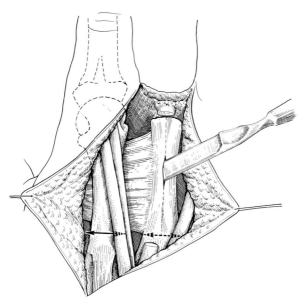

Figure 94–3. The extensor tendons of the middle fingers are resected to expose the third metacarpal and the two dorsal interossei of the second and third intermetacarpal spaces.

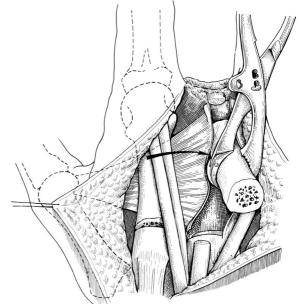

Figure 94–4. After section of the third metacarpal at its base and resection of the second and third dorsal interossei, which are inserted into it, the third metacarpal is excised. This leaves a large space in the depths of which the palmar interosseous muscles of the second and third spaces can be seen. The base of the second metacarpal is sectioned at the same level prior to transposition onto the third.

Transverse sectioning at the middle third appears to be the simplest procedure, for fixation of the two metacarpals is made easier. However, it does have some disadvantages. The first is that the interosseous muscles must be disinserted proximally, with the result that their function is impaired and their motor nerve may be stretched or ruptured. The transposed finger then loses part of its mobility and the functional gain from the operation would be minimal. The main purpose of the operation should be to allow perfect interosseous function.

There is another reason for not dividing the metacarpal at its middle third: Even though fixation at the shaft is easier, union is less readily obtained if the area of contact is reduced, and union has to occur between two different bones.

The sculpturing of a tendon and mortise joint is usually more difficult to achieve in practice than it is to plan on paper. We prefer to resect both metacarpals at the same level near their base. The Gigli saw can be used here, but great care must be taken to make sure that the adjacent muscles and their nerve and vascular supply are not injured. When the metacarpal of the amputated finger is

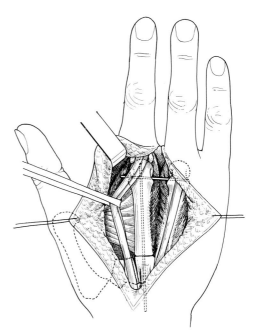

Figure 94–5. After transposition of the second ray, fixation is ensured by a longitudinal Kirschner wire on the third metacarpal and a transverse Kirschner wire fixing together the heads of the second and fourth metacarpals after confirming the perfect rotation of the distal fragment in order to avoid any overlapping of the fingers on closure of the fist.

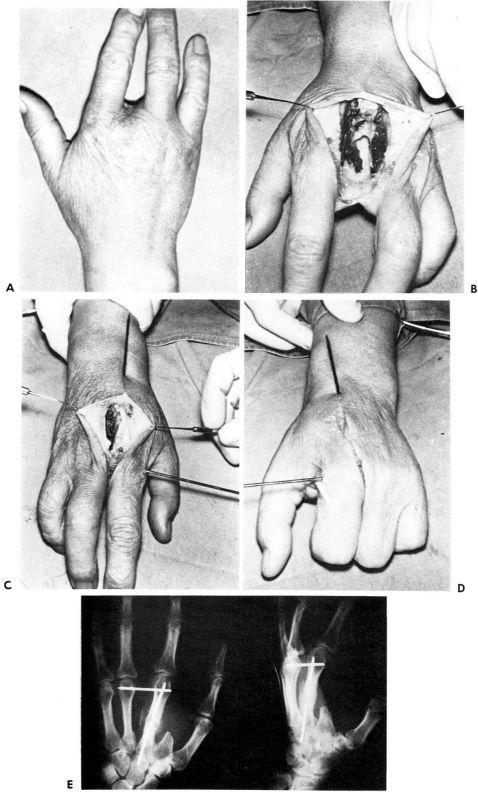

Figure 94–6. *See legend on opposite page.*

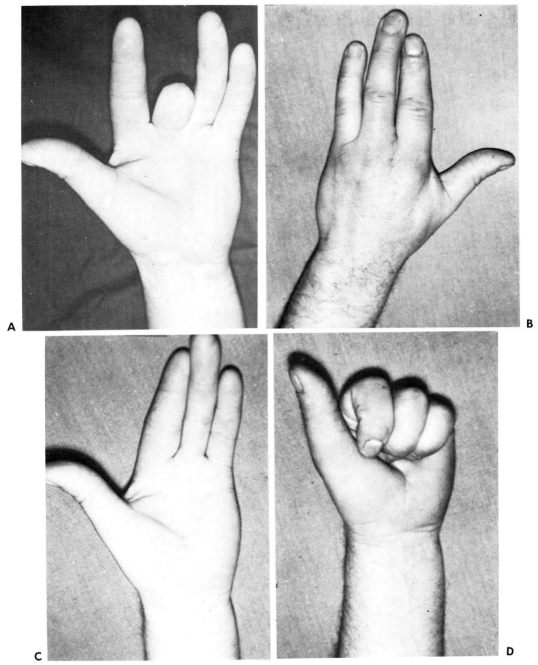

Figure 94–7. *A*, Amputation of the third ray at the middle part of the proximal phalanx. The stump is cyanosed and retracted in irreducible flexion, preventing any prehensile movement. *B*, *C*, and *D*, result of transposition of the index onto the third metacarpal. The esthetic appearance of the hand is satisfactory. The fingers are parallel, and closure of the wrist is achieved without difficulty. The difference in length between the index and ring fingers in this patient gives a particularly satisfactory result with a middle finger longer than the other four.

Figure 94–6. Perioperative photographs. *A*, Amputation of the middle finger leaves a gap between the index and ring fingers with deviation of the index. *B*, After resection of the third metacarpal, sectioned at its base, the two palmar interossei of the second and third spaces can be seen at the base of the operative site. *C*, After transposition of the index onto the third metacarpal, fixation is ensured by an intramedullary Kirschner wire. *D*, Insertion of a Kirschner wire fixing the heads of the second and third metacarpals with the fist closed. *E*, Postoperative radiographs.

resected, the extensor tendon is divided as far proximally as possible. The metacarpal is then pulled aside and the flexor tendons are also divided proximally under direct vision (Fig. 94–4).

The intermetacarpal ligament is divided on either side of the metacarpal head and the bone and its tendons removed en bloc.

TREATMENT OF NEUROMAS

The neurovascular bundles are usually readily identifiable in the base of the wound. Asymptomatic neuromas are left alone. Those that were painful and were diagnosed prior to transposition are treated by neurotomy: This is performed well proximal to the neuroma in healthy tissue after the commissural nerve has been divided into its two terminals. If a new painful neuroma develops, it occurs near the heel of the hand within the thick thenar and hypothenar muscles and not in the commissures where it is usually poorly tolerated.

TRANSPOSITION AND FIXATION

The metacarpal of the digit to be transposed is resected at the same level as that of the amputated finger. Once this has been completed, transposition is surprisingly easy.

Bone fixation can be done in one of two ways. The simplest method involves the use of two large Kirschner wires (2 to 2.5 mm.) One of the wires is allowed to protrude proximally so as not to transfix the metacarpophalangeal joint. Its length must be such

that it comes to rest in the lower part of the metacarpal. At its proximal end it is bent, to allow some extension of the wrist, and cut off under the skin (Fig. 94–5).

In order to obtain perfect fixation and prevent rotation and sliding of the bone along the wire, an extra-articular wire is placed transversely proximal to the metacarpal heads. This fixes the bone to its neighbor. It should be inserted with the fingers flexed so that rotation can be checked. Like the other Kirschner wire, it is cut off just under the skin.

The chances of malunion will be reduced if chips of cancellous bone from the head of the resected metacarpal are stuffed into any gaps and interstices at the site of the future union.

For plate fixation to be satisfactory it is necessary to lower the level of the bone cut a little so that one can obtain good fixation at the superior part. The function of the interosseous muscles can be compromised if their direction is altered. Plate fixation also poses a problem of rotation, since the posterior aspect of the metacarpal on which one places the plate is not parallel with the dorsal aspect of the second and third metacarpals. This is not a major obstacle. However, the size of the plate necessary to obtain stable fixation is such that the smooth gliding of the extensor tendons is often interfered with. Thus, in spite of the theoretical advantages of immediate mobilization, Kirschner wire fixation is more satisfactory.

The most important problem is rotation, and for the patient to properly close his fist, it is imperative that the fixation of the osteotomies be perfect. Two cases are illustrated in Figures 94–6 and 94–7.

Chapter 95

TRANSPOSITION OF THE FIFTH DIGITAL RAY BY INTRACARPAL OSTEOTOMY

DOMINIQUE LE VIET

In addition to the cosmetic problems it creates, amputation of the ring finger combines the drawbacks of amputation of a medial digit as described by Razemon (1969)—increasing convergence of the fifth finger in flexion, loss of small objects in the palm, cicatricial neuromas, and a marked reduction in squeezing power (Figs. 95–1, 95–2).

Transposition of the little finger has far fewer indications in practice than transposition of the index finger after loss of the middle finger, but it remains the solution of choice in a number of cases. In 1978 we described a technique of transposition of the fifth finger by intracarpal osteotomy. On the strength of 17 such transpositions, we de-

scribe the technique in detail here, mention its drawbacks, and analyze our results.

IMPERATIVES FOR TRANSPOSITION OF THE FIFTH FINGER

Various techniques had been suggested but always with some reticence, for the disadvantages were far from negligible. They were based, however, on two quite different principles: In the first, the fourth ray was partially or totally excised; in the second, the fifth metacarpal was transposed to the fourth. Let us consider briefly their weaknesses.

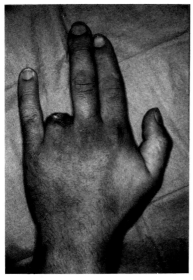

Figure 95–1. Amputation of ring finger.

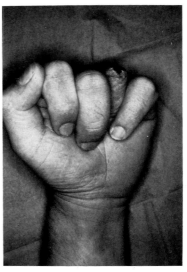

Figure 95–2. Convergence of little finger in flexion.

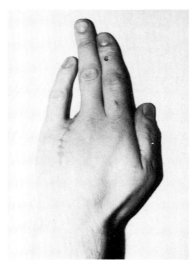

Figure 95–3. Resection of fourth metacarpal without its base. There is persistence of spread between the long and little fingers.

ABLATION OF THE FOURTH DIGITAL RAY

Ablation of the fourth digital ray is less a transposition than a forced approximation of the fifth metacarpal to the third, a procedure made easier by the laxity of the carpometacarpal joint of the little finger.

Partial amputation of the fourth metacarpal creates a space between the third and fifth fingers as the metacarpal stump prevents convergence of the fifth ray (Fig. 95–3). By contrast, after total amputation of the fourth metacarpal, the fifth ray tends to converge toward the third. The little finger thus loses some abduction and, in the course of flexion, lies under the middle finger.

TRANSPOSITION OF THE FIFTH METACARPAL ONTO THE FOURTH

The resection can be carried at the level of the shaft, with the attendant risk of pseudarthrosis, or at the base, which necessitates fixation by Kirschner wires and carries the risk of instability. Whichever technique is preferred, the procedure has three main disadvantages: It alters the supporting medial border of the hand (Fig. 95–4), it distorts the course of the hypothenar muscles, and it destroys the carpometacarpal joint of the fifth ray, a particularly mobile joint that is the main lock of the power grip.

In our opinion a transposition of the little finger should satisfy the following criteria: The ulnar border of the hand should be unaltered. The fifth metacarpal should retain its natural divergence and not converge toward the fourth. Fixation should be secure to allow early re-education. The useful carpometacarpal joint of the fifth ray should be preserved. Finally, muscle reinsertions should be avoided and the action of the interosseous muscles not tampered with.

PRINCIPLES

The technique we describe here appears to satisfy these criteria. It consists of the transfer of the whole of the fifth ray in place of the fourth and involves resection of the fourth ray, a cuneiform osteotomy of the lateral part of the hamate, and a capitohamate arthrodesis.

The fifth ray is tilted to an angle equal to the angle of divergence of the fourth metacarpal in relation to the fifth, i.e., between 7 and 10 degrees. The details of the osteotomy are described later.

SURGICAL TECHNIQUE

We shall first describe the technique and then discuss the calculation of the osteotomy angle.

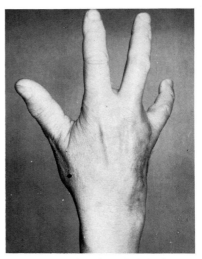

Figure 95–4. Translocation of little finger onto the fourth metacarpal. Note the depression on the ulnar border of the hand.

Incision. The skin incision runs along the fourth metacarpal, including the whole of the fourth web space and the floor of the third. This facilitates the creation of a free new third web with no traction or commissural band formation.

Dissection. The intertendinous bands connecting the third, fourth, and fifth extensor tendons are exposed and divided flush with the tendon of the ring finger and refashioned into a new intertendinous band between the middle and little fingers.

Amputation of the Fourth Ray. The stump is disarticulated, the vascular pedicles are ligated, and the flexor and extensor tendons are divided proximally. The medial and lateral interosseous nerves are divided as high as possible and buried in the interosseous muscles.

Disarticulation of the fourth metacarpal proceeds from distal to proximal. The bone is rugined subperiosteally. Disarticulation is completed by exerting traction on the metacarpal head. The only difficult step is the unhooking of the anterior aspect of the base. In order to avoid anterior rupture of the capsule, traction is combined with slight axial rotation.

The Osteotomy. With the fourth metacarpal out of the way, access is obtained to the medial aspect of the base of the third metacarpal, the lateral aspect of the fifth, and the facet of the hamate articulating with the base of the fourth.

The dorsal capsule is incised proximally, the incision running between the capitate and the hamate toward the midcarpal joint. Incision of the lower part of the extensor retinaculum provides a wider exposure of that joint.

Next the capsule is disinserted posteriorly with a knife along the medial border of the capitate, which is freshened, and in a triangular fashion with the apex proximally against the posterior aspect of the base of the hamate, which is resected. Care is taken not to incise the capsule too far medially and expose the hamometacarpal joint, because interference with that joint might destabilize the fifth ray.

The osteotomy is carried out on the posterior aspect of the hamate depending upon the results of calculations made preoperatively. These take into account the shape of the medial border of the hamate, the angle between the two lower facets of the hamate,

and the divergent angle between the fourth and fifth metacarpals. The osteotomy is started off with Pauwels' blades applied posteroanteriorly through the posterior cortex and is completed from distal to proximal using the first groove as a guideline (Fig. 95–5). The resection should be slightly more extensive anteriorly, for any alteration in the anterior concavity of the carpal condyle might result in ulnar rotation of the fifth digit. Resection of a hamate wedge in one piece is best avoided because of the risk of damage to the ulnar nerve. The anterior cortical fragment of the hamate is rugined free of the anterior joint capsule and removed with fine forceps. Finally the medial border of the capitate is roughened by the required amount.

Positioning. The bones are now brought together using Jayle's forceps levered on the upper extremity of the third metacarpal. The position of the little finger is checked in the anteroposterior axis with the hand flat and especially with the fingers flexed. At this stage the intermetacarpal ligament is provisionally sutured between the heads of the third and fifth metacarpals. Because the osteotomy is the key to accurate positioning, it may be safer in one's first cases to be overly cautious in one's resection even if corrections are required later to counteract ulnar rotation or overdivergence of the rays.

In short muscular hands it is sometimes necessary to resect the palmar interosseous muscle of the third interspace and the dorsal interosseous muscle of the fourth.

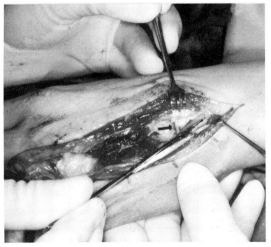

Figure 95–5. Osteotomy. Arrow shows corner of resected hamate bone.

Fixation. The osteotomy is fixed by means of a 20 to 24 mm. screw, and it may be useful to use a cancellous bone graft taken from the base of the fourth metacarpal, placed in the gap between the capitate and the hamate. The screw runs obliquely proximally and laterally; it is introduced as low as possible into the medial aspect of the hamate, medial to the extensor digiti minimi. To avoid fracturing the thin bone, the screw is directed very dorsally. In one's early cases, one is well advised to take a check x-ray view of the drill in position. This will guarantee the correct position and length of the screw, the correct degree of divergence of the little finger with the hand held flat, and the correct appearance of the midcarpal joint, which will prevent lengthening of the little finger.

Once fixation has been achieved, the medial side of the third metacarpal and lateral side of the fifth are approximated but not brought into contact, for this may cause pain on movement.

Finally the joint capsule and interosseous aponeurosis are resutured; the intermetacarpal ligament and intertendinous band are reconstructed, linking the extensor of the middle finger to that of the fifth, and the skin is closed.

Postoperative Course. The fixation should be strong enough to obviate the need for a plaster cast and to enable the patient to start re-education as soon as the pain has worn off (i.e., after three or four days). The arthrodesis between the capitate and hamate is usually united after two to three months.

TECHNICAL DETAILS

Calculating the Angle of the Osteotomy

We first envisaged a complicated calculation of the angle of osteotomy, which took into account the angle between the two facets of the lower extremity of the hamate and the angle of divergence between the fourth and fifth metacarpals. In fact, in order for the fifth metacarpal to take the place of the fourth, it is sufficient for the angle of osteotomy to be equal to the angle between the two facets of the lower extremity of the hamate.

Since the angle between the base of the fourth metacarpal and the radial border of the hamate is most often a right angle, all

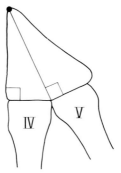

Figure 95–6. Calculation of angle of osteotomy c: $c = 1 + b$.

that is required is to draw with dye on the posterior surface of the hamate a line perpendicular to the base of the fifth metacarpal at the radial border of this base.

According to the angle between the two facets of the hamate, this line will reach either the superior pole of the hamate (Fig. 95–6) or a point at a variable distance along the radial border of the hamate (Fig. 95–7), which results in different appearances of hamate-capitate arthrodesis: perfect congruity (Fig. 95–8A), a slight superior defect (Fig. 95–8B), or a marked defect (Fig. 95–8C).

The shape of the ulnar border of the capitate must be taken into consideration when the latter is prepared. Broadly speaking there are three possibilities (Fig. 95–9): straight, requiring only minimal freshening; S shaped, when bipolar resection is required; and a broad facet for articulation with the fourth metacarpal, in which case the facet must be resected.

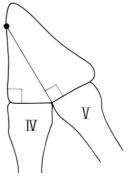

Figure 95–7. Increase of angle of osteotomy: C2 > C1.

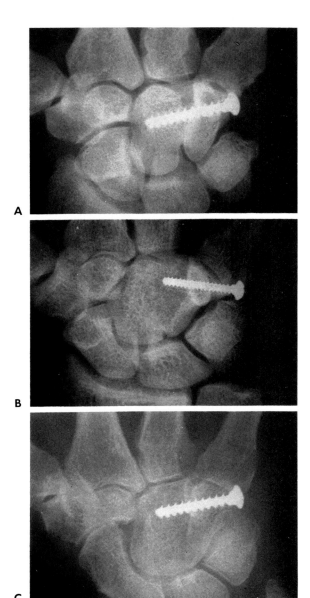

Figure 95–8. Different aspects of capitate-hamate arthrodesis. *A*, Perfect matching. *B*, Small superior gap. *C*, Large gap where a large osteotomy angle has been used.

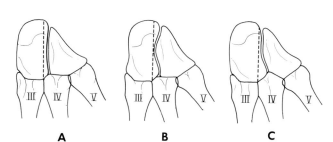

Figure 95–9. Shape of medial border of the hamate. *A*, Straight. *B*, Italic shape. *C*, Facet with IV.

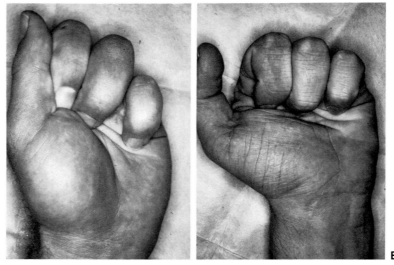

Figure 95–10. Position of little finger. *A*, Marked ulnar derotation. *B*, Satisfactory position.

These theoretical indications serve only to guide the osteotomy line and in particular to determine whether it should be extended as far as the superior pole of the hamate. With practice, when the finger seems well positioned after preoperative provisional approximation, the axes will always be satisfactory to within a few degrees.

Derotation of the Fifth Finger

Derotation of the fifth finger can be avoided by testing the position of the fifth finger in flexion. If it has occurred despite the foregoing precautions, a more extensive anterior resection is carried out, or, if this is not feasible, a small graft is taken from the base of the resected fourth metacarpal and introduced posteriorly. The intermetacarpal ligament must be resutured from the palmar side, since an approximate dorsal closure, at the expense of the capsule of the metacarpophalangeal joints, can in itself be a cause of ulnar derotation (Fig. 95–10).

CLINICAL EXPERIENCE

The series reported here includes 17 patients (3 women and 14 men) aged 18 to 53 years (average, 36.3 years). The periods of follow-up ranged from 17 to 34 months (average, 24.5 months).

ETIOLOGY

The commonest injury in our series by far (13 of 17) was a degloving of the ring finger. The left side was involved in 14 cases. In two cases the right ring finger was degloved by a ring worn on the right hand. The other four cases include three hooked fingers (resulting from sepsis) and one traumatic deformity.

INDICATIONS

Surgical transposition was indicated because of pain in seven cases and on cosmetic grounds in seven. In five cases transposition was carried out as an emergency procedure.

It is worth pointing out that during the same period we treated injuries to 70 ring fingers, of which only five were salvaged, showing that surgical transposition was not performed routinely.

COMPLICATIONS

We had no instance of sepsis in the reported series. The wrist pain, which occurs during flexion and extension and probably originates in the midcarpal joint, seldom lasts longer than about six weeks. The oldest case was in a patient followed for three years. During that time there was no osteoarthritis of the midcarpal joint in any of the wrists.

Faulty Positioning. In some of our early cases our technique resulted in faulty positioning—axial derotation (three cases) and excessive divergence between the third and fifth metacarpals (four cases). This occurred because in these earlier cases the line of osteotomy was always made to pass at the superior pole of the hamate, with the result that the angle of osteotomy was sometimes inadequate.

In our very first case we ignored a facet on the capitate that articulated with the base of the fourth metacarpal. Failure to resect this facet resulted in unsightly divergence of the little finger (Fig. 95–11).

By relying on the preoperative calculations already described, we can now avoid such errors.

Other Complications. One patient developed a pseudarthrosis in the arthrodesis between the capitate and the hamate, possibly because of excessive resection of the hamate. The patient refused the bone graft that we suggested.

One patient had some reduction of mobility of the metacarpophalangeal joint of the little finger and of the middle finger.

Finally, in one case there was gross overdivergence of the fifth finger, which resulted in palmar tilting of the head of the fifth metacarpal. The osteotomy was refashioned to correct the divergence, and the intermetacarpal ligament consolidated, with a satisfactory end result.

RESULTS

Bone Union. The intracarpal arthrodesis usually consolidates in six to 12 weeks. Good apposition is achieved with the help of the screw, which often makes interpretation of the standard x-ray films more difficult. Tomography may then be required. We have mentioned our one case of pseudarthrosis.

Carpal Tunnel Syndrome. In our series one patient developed a carpal tunnel syndrome, but this did not last long. Since this technique causes but slight narrowing of the carpal tunnel and does not interfere with the hook of the hamate (which must be preserved), we believe that the risk of carpal tunnel and Guyon's canal syndromes is minimal.

The Patient's Opinion. Fourteen of our 17 patients were satisfied with the result despite some degree of derotation or divergence. The loss of a sometimes painful stump was not regarded as a mutilation but as an improvement over their previous state (Fig. 95–12). We must stress that the short transposed

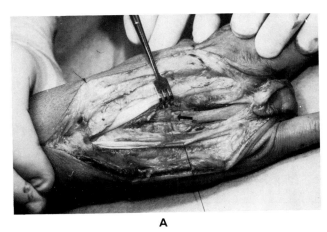

A

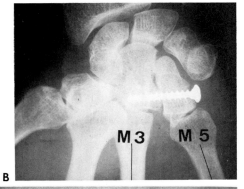

B

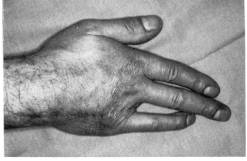

C

Figure 95–11. *Á*, The articular facet of the capitate with the fourth metacarpal is shown by an arrow. *B*, Note that this facet has been resected entirely, resulting in an excess of divergence of M5 and M3. *C*, Persistence of spread between long and little fingers.

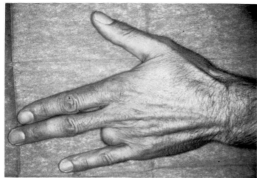

A

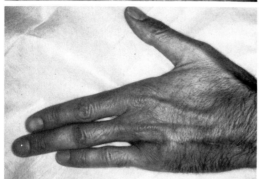

B

Figure 95–12. *A*, Preoperative view. *B*, Postoperative view.

Figure 95–13. Gripping power of both hands.

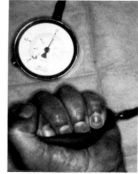
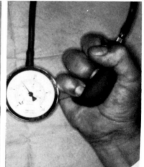

Table 95–1. RESULTS IN PATIENTS IN WHOM GRIPPING POWER WAS MEASURED

Case	Sex	Age	Preoperative Grip	% Normal Side ($\overline{m}$ = 48%)	Postoperative Grip	Difference
1	M	26	G = 0.12	12	G = 0.59	+ 391%
2	M	22	G = 0.55	58	G = 0.86	+ 56%
3	M	53	G = 0.68	56	G = 1.00	+ 47%
4	M	30	G = 0.50	50	G = 0.70	+ 40%
5	M	32	G = 0.60	46	G = 0.70	+ 16%
6	M	52	G = 0.42	42	G = 0.46	+ 9%
7	M	44	G = 0.90*	78	G = 0.76	− 16%
8	M	36	D = 0.64*	42	D = 0.42	− 34%

*The dominant side was involved.

Table 95–2. RESULTS IN PATIENTS IN WHOM GRIPPING POWER WAS NOT MEASURED

Case	Sex	Age	Postoperative Grip	Normal Side ($\overline{m}$ = 56.7%)	% Normal Side
9	M	28	G = 1.30	(D = 1.46)	89
10	M	50	D = 0.70	(G = 1.00)	70
11	M	28	D = 0.50	(G = 0.70)	71
12	F	49	G = 0.36	(D = 0.56)	64
13	M	25	G = 0.70	(D = 1.10)	63
14	M	33	G = 0.70	(D = 1.20)	58
15	F	18	D = 0.40*	(G = 0.80)	50
16	F	45	G = 0.25	(D = 0.60)	42
17	M	45	G = 0.30	(D = 0.75)	40

*The dominant side was involved.

ulnar digit gives a strange appearance to this four fingered hand. In six of seven cases, the painful neuroma disappeared.

This leaves us with three dissatisfied patients. One (case 7) was the patient left with a painful intracarpal pseudarthrosis. The other two (cases 8 and 15) complained of marked loss of power in the dominant hand that was subjected to operation.

Mobility of the Carpometacarpal Joint. Carpometacarpal joint mobility was retained in all 17 patients.

Gripping Power. We were particularly interested in this parameter. The presence of a short stump in a medial digit inevitably results in significant loss of gripping force. We believe that the narrowing of the palm that follows the digital transposition is amply compensated for by the approximation of the digits. Besides, the radialization of the medial finger produces a closer, more efficient contact during thumb-digital pinching.

Our measurements were made on a Vigorimeter graduated in k.p per sq. cm. (Fig. 95–13). The patients were divided into two groups. The first included the eight in whom gripping power was measured preoperatively (Table 95–1) and the second, the nine in whom it was not measured (Table 95–2). It is important to note that the dominant hand was involved in only four patients and that the grip was 10 to 30 per cent greater on the dominant side. The last measurements were made at least eight months postoperatively, and it is relevant that resumption of manual work resulted in an improved grip in both the operated and the nonoperated hand.

Table 95–1 shows that in six of the eight patients gripping power was improved as compared with the contralateral hand. The 391 per cent increase recorded in case 1 can

be explained by the fact that the transposition was carried out within one month after the accident on a hand that was still painful. Two patients with involvement of the dominant hand showed a decrease in grip power (cases 7 and 8). For the first we have no valid explanation; the second was due to the pseudarthrosis mentioned earlier.

In Table 95–2, because no preoperative measurements were available, we compared the gripping force on the operated side with that on the contralateral hand at the last examination. Here again, only two dominant hands were involved. In the last three cases (15, 16, 17) the result can be described only as fair. This is not surprising for patient 17 in whom both the middle and ring fingers had been amputated.

In summary, in the majority of cases the grip was retained or improved. Most of our patients were manual workers, and, with one exception, they were all able to resume their normal professional activities.

CONCLUSION

Transposition of the fifth finger by intracarpal osteotomy would seem to avoid the pitfalls usually encountered in this procedure. It is cosmetically and functionally satisfactory and aims at enhancing the value of the remaining digits. The retention of mobility at the metacarpophalangeal joints combined with the approximation of the medial digits makes up for the loss of palmar width. In our series the majority of patients were satisfied with the results and showed an overall postoperative gain in gripping power. If the technique we described is followed closely, the minor faults that characterized our early cases can be avoided. In the light of our experience, we believe that the indications for transposition of the little finger can be safely extended.

REFERENCES

Beasley, R. W.: Cosmetic consideration in surgery of the hand. Surg. Clin. N. Am., *51:*471–477, 1971.

deTaddeo, P.: Résultats de deux techniques de translocation digitale lors de la mutilation des doigts médians. A propos de 30 cas. Thesis, Paris, 1980.

Duparc, J., Alnot, J. Y., and May, P.: Amputation unidigitale des doigts. *In* Les Mutilations de la Main. Paris, GEM, 1975.

Iselin, M., and Iselin, F.: Traité de Chirurgie de la main. Paris, Flammarion Ed., 1967, p. 849.

Le Viet, D.: Translocation de l'auriculaire par ostéotomie intracarpienne. Ann. Chir., *32:*609–612, 1978.

Peacock, E. E.: Metacarpal transfer following amputation of a central digit. Plast. Reconst. Surg., *29:*345–355, 1962.

Posner, M. A.: Ray transposition for central digital loss. J. Hand Surg., *4:*242–257, 1979.

Razemon, J. P.: La médialisation digitale ou transposition du doigt chef de file dans les séquelles d'amputation des doigts médians. Ann. Chir. Plast., *14:*162–172, 1969.

Saffar, P., and Glicenstein, J.: Translocation digitale par section oblique des métacarpiens. Ann. Chir., *30:*897–907, 1976.

PARTIAL AND TOTAL AMPUTATIONS OF THE THUMB

Chapter 96

THUMB RECONSTRUCTION AFTER PARTIAL AMPUTATION OF THE THUMB

DIETER BUCK-GRAMCKO

Complete amputation of the thumb (e.g., at the level of the metacarpophalangeal joint or more proximally) and partial amputation reduce the functional ability of the hand. The loss of the tip impairs pinch and the ability to pick up small objects, as do shortening due to amputation through the proximal phalanx, deformities in nonfunctional positions, instability, fracture, nonunion with or without bone defects, sensory loss, and tender scars.

By contrast, partial amputation of the thumb results in no diminution of power grip in manual workers and causes little deficit in total hand function as long as fine touch is preserved (Pringle, 1972; Ratliff, 1972). The prerequisites for adequate use of a partially amputated thumb are a nonsensitive stump covered by healthy skin with normal sensation and minimal scar formation. Under most circumstances normal sensation is of much greater importance than the preservation of both normal length and mobility of the interphalangeal and metacarpophalangeal joints (Buck-Gramcko, 1961; Bunnell, 1944; Moberg, 1964). Nevertheless, in the primary care

of thumb injuries the surgeon should try to preserve as much length as possible, provided the bone end is covered with good viable skin and subcutaneous tissue. In the emergency room this can be achieved by some shortening of the bone, but an experienced hand surgeon may be able to use local (sensory) skin flaps with split thickness skin grafts to cover the donor sites. A direct cover of a raw bone end by skin grafts should be avoided, and abdominal skin flaps should not be used to cover partial amputations of the thumb. The complicated procedures recommended by Hilgenfeldt (1969) and Nemethi (1960) are restricted to total amputations or severe mutilations of the whole hand.

The choice of repair procedure depends on the age, occupation, hobbies, general condition, and sex of the patient, all of which influence the functional demands made on the thumb.

PRIMARY CARE

An adequate primary repair may fulfill all the requirements for later functional use of

1081

the thumb and under optimal circumstances renders further reconstructive procedures unnecessary.

DISTAL AMPUTATIONS AND AVULSION INJURIES

The provision of a good skin cover over the tip and pulp of the thumb is of special importance because of the highly specialized function of the thumb in all the activities of daily life. Painful, hypersensitive scars are more embarrassing here than in other parts of the hand, and may lead to "psychological amputation" of the thumb. Scar excision and replacement by a skin graft or a local flap may be necessary. The various procedures for effecting skin cover are applicable not only as primary procedures but also in reconstructive surgery.

Healing by Granulation Tissue. In cases of superficial skin loss in small areas healing by granulation may yield excellent results.

Free Skin Grafts. Thick split skin or full thickness skin grafts are indicated in the superficial guillotine type of amputation or in larger defects of the pulp but not when bone is exposed.

V-Y Procedures. In cases of distal amputation (not more proximal than one third of the nail) in a transverse direction (not in oblique amputations from dorsal distally to palmar proximally), the palmar triangular flap (Tranquilli-Leali, 1935) or two lateral Kutler (1947) flaps are very useful. Especially useful is the modification developed by Segmüller (1976) with microsurgical dissection of neurovascular pedicles, which insures greater mobility of the flaps, good padding, and excellent sensation. Poy (1971) used the same principle but with only one lateropalmar flap instead of two.

Advancement Flap. In cases of loss of the pulp and an intact or almost intact terminal phalanx and nail or nail bed, advancement of the complete palmar skin was recommended by Moberg in 1964. Several authors have reported good results with this technique (Buck-Gramcko, 1961; Gassmann and Segmüller, 1976; Keim and Grantham, 1969; Millender et al., 1973; Posner and Smith, 1971; Snow, 1967). The sliding of a palmar flap distally results not only in a well contoured new tip with good padding but also in immediate restoration of normal sensation,

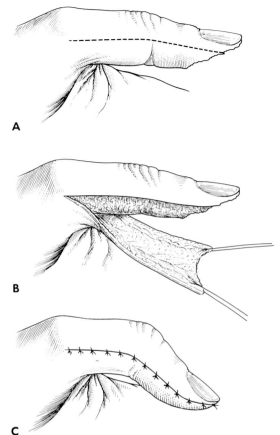

Figure 96–1. Palmar advancement flap. Avulsion injury of the pulp and incision (*A*) with careful preservation of the dorsal branches of the arteries and nerves (not shown in the drawing). The flap includes both palmar neurovascular bundles; the tendon sheath is not opened during careful dissection (*B*). Flexion of the interphalangeal and metacarpophalangeal joints provided an exact suture of the flap to the nail bed without tension (*C*).

because both the palmar neurovascular bundles are included (Fig. 96–1). This also guarantees a normal blood supply. By use of a midlateral incision on both sides as far proximally as the flexion crease of the metacarpophalangeal joint, all tissues are carefully dissected from bones and the flexor tendon sheath; the tiny branches of both arteries are coagulated to prevent hematoma formation. The interphalangeal and metacarpophalangeal joints are sufficiently flexed so that the distal end of the flap can be sutured without tension against the nail or nail bed. In closure of longitudinal incisions, it is sometimes necessary to resect small triangular areas of skin from the (longer) dorsal wound edge for better coaptation. The flexed position is maintained with a dorsal plaster splint for about two weeks. During application of the dressing and splint, the color in the distal part of the flap has to be watched carefully. If the flap blanches, more flexion is needed. Complications are rare if all details of the procedure are observed carefully. Hypersensitivity of the distal margin of the nail bed may be prevented by careful adaptation and suturing between the nail bed and the distal end of the flap. The curved deformity of the nail that occurs in cases of bone loss from the distal phalanx cannot be avoided but may be minimized by frequent trimming of the nail. The results are usually excellent, with satisfactory functional use of the thumb. In most cases full extension is gained within a few weeks and no residual extension deficit is seen.

Flexion of the joints usually allows the flap to be advanced 12 to 15 mm. If more length is necessary and is not gained by more proximal dissection, the advancement flap can be transformed into an island flap by cutting the skin transversely at the base of the flap after careful separation from the neurovascular bundles (Littler, 1964; O'Brien, 1965, 1968). Their elasticity allows the flap to be advanced a few millimeters more. The secondary defect in the proximal thumb crease is closed by a free graft (thick split or full thickness; Beasley, 1967; O'Brien, 1968) or by an additional rotation flap from the dorsoradial aspect of the region of the second metacarpophalangeal joint (Joshi, 1970). Goumain et al. (1972) have extended this procedure using an annular advancement flap created by circumferential skin division, leaving all four neurovascular bundles intact. The advancement flap can be used as an emergency or a delayed procedure.

Rotation and Transposition Flaps. Rotation and transposition flaps are not often used in emergency procedures. Most of them include sensory nerve branches and are indicated during reconstruction in cases in which restoration of sensation to the tip of the partially amputated thumb is needed. Only the laterally based dorsal or palmar flap may be used for primary repair (Argamaso, 1974; Beasley, 1967; Hueston, 1966); the defect to be covered should not be too large because the risk of impaired blood supply in the most distal parts increases with the length of these flaps. Simonetta (1978) has described a more extensive dorsal rotational flap (Fig. 96–2). Its base is generally located on the ulnar side with a broad pedicle down to the carpometacarpal joint area. The defect usually can be closed by direct suturing; a graft is seldom necessary.

Cross Finger Flaps. Cross finger flaps are indicated in cases of deeper tip or pulp loss with exposed bone, in which well padded cover is necessary. Late follow-up studies have shown that usually very satisfactory sensation is re-established (Porter, 1968; Stur-

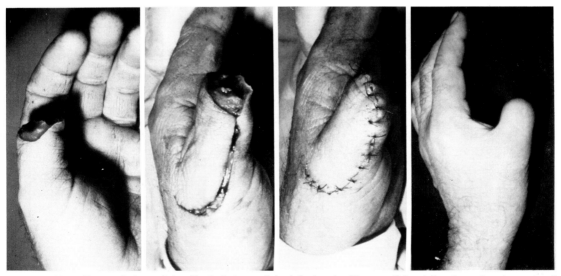

Figure 96–2. Traumatic loss of the distal phalanx of the left thumb. Closure of the defect by a dorsal rotational flap. (Courtesy of Dr. Simonetta.)

man and Duran, 1963). The best donor site is the middle finger, because a flap from the adjacent index finger adducts the thumb too tightly. Usually the flap is taken from the dorsal aspect of the middle phalanx, but Beasley (1978) has recommended the palmar surface of the middle phalanx of the middle finger as the best donor site. He emphasizes that in order to preserve a normal blood supply, the pedicle of the flap should not be dissected completely free of the radial neurovascular bundle. Later the pedicle is divided after careful identification of the neurovascular bundle using a tourniquet.

A modification is the flag flap, a dorsal flap with a small pedicle including dorsal vessels (Vilain, 1952). It is rarely applicable to the thumb.

Neurovascular Island Flap. Primary application of this special flap should be performed only by experienced hand surgeons. It was recommended by Chase (1971) and by Sullivan et al. (1973) and can give very satisfactory results. The indications for its use are in cases of soft tissue loss of the tip and pulp or more proximal avulsion injuries with denuded bone. The excellent blood supply of the island makes immediate lengthening by a bone graft possible, as Chase (1971) has reported. In general, the technique is the same as in secondary reconstructive surgery (see page 1095).

Distant Pedicle Flaps. Almost all authors agree that distant flaps are undesirable in distal thumb amputations. The reasons are poor tissue match, bulkiness, and "instability" due to the thick subcutaneous tissue, lack of sensation, and poor blood supply. If possible, local or island flaps are preferable (Bales et al., 1975; Beasley, 1967; McFarlane and Stromberg, 1962). A compromise may be the procedure recommended by Dolich et al. (1978) with a cross forearm neurocutaneous flap, a skin flap from the opposite distal forearm including the superficial branch of the radial nerve.

REPLANTATION

Tidy partial amputations of the thumb are an absolute indication for replantation using microsurgical techniques. If the surgeon in an emergency room is not familiar with these, he should refer the patient immediately to a specialized center. The functional and cosmetic results are very satisfying and justify the efforts in personnel, time, and cost. Contrary to the situation in replantation of fingers amputated at the level of the proximal phalanx or metacarpal and of whole hands, mobility is of less importance; the functional value of a thumb is not so greatly impaired if the distal joint (or even the metacarpophalangeal joint) is arthrodesed, provided the blood supply and sensation are restored. An almost normal pinch grip is possible under such circumstances (Fig. 96–3).

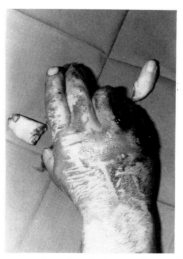 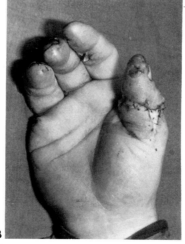 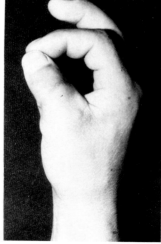

A   B   C

Figure 96–3. Replantation of a partial amputated thumb. *A,* Injury with a circular saw to all five fingers. *B,* Replantation of the thumb following primary care of nine hours' duration. *C,* Function (pinch grip) five months later.

LOSS OF AN INTERMEDIATE SEGMENT

Some special injuries (e.g., with circular saws or punch presses) can cause tissue loss from an intermediate part of the thumb. In these cases we find (usually in the proximal phalanx or metacarpal region) a more or less circumscribed loss of skin, subcutaneous tissue, tendon, nerves, vessels, and sometimes part of the bone, while the opposite side is intact. The distal part is preserved and has sufficient blood supply, so that its amputation and simple wound closure are contraindicated. Reconstruction is easier if the tissue loss is located on the dorsal aspect and the sensation of the distal part is maintained by the uninjured volar neurovascular bundles.

Palmar Aspect

Soft tissue loss on the palmar aspect of the proximal phalanx of the thumb with or without loss of the thenar eminence is usually a more severe injury than occurs on the opposite (dorsal) side because the neurovascular bundles are involved. The long flexor tendon is interrupted, with a loss of several centimeters, and the bone may be notched or totally divided; sometimes the metacarpophalangeal joint is also involved.

The most important part of the primary repair is to provide a skin cover using a pedicle flap (Fig. 96–4). The donor site is usually the lower abdomen. The defect is too small for a groin flap, and other flaps such as the cross arm flap or deltopectoral flap cause too much inconvenience by virtue of the position of the injured arm. If the continuity of the bone is interrupted, stabilization with Kirschner wires is indicated in order to maintain the length of the thumb. The bone may be restored immediately by a bone graft taken from the iliac crest. Osteosynthesis is performed with Kirschner wires or with a small plate.

The reconstruction of nerves and, in the case of intact joints, the long flexor tendon by grafts is better performed some months later when the induration of the scar and surrounding tissues has diminished and all the tissues are pliable.

Dorsal Aspect

Here the same principles of reconstruction as described for palmar intermediate injuries are applicable—skeletal stabilization by bone grafting and osteosynthesis, provision of a skin cover with an abdominal pedicle flap, and, as a secondary procedure, grafting of the extensor tendon if the joints are intact and have a good range of passive motion. Foucher and Braun (1979) described an island flap from the dorsum of the index finger for a skin cover on the dorsum of the thumb. This island is transferred on a pedicle consisting of the first dorsal metacarpal artery, one or two veins, and terminal branches of the radial nerve.

Bone reconstruction with a graft may need to be performed as a delayed procedure in cases in which a primary bone graft carries too great a risk because of contamination of the wound or when parts of the bone have been destroyed by infection. Under antibiotic cover some months later, a bone graft taken from the iliac crest is placed between the ends of the healthy bone after removal of scar tissue and sclerosed bone edges (Verdan, 1968). Usually one of the two joints is involved and must be fused by the bone graft, which is inserted following the rules of carpentry (step-like cutting of the bone ends or joining by a tenon and mortise).

RECONSTRUCTIVE PROCEDURES

In many cases of partial amputation of the thumb, reconstructive procedures are necessary because the primary treatment was only a preliminary one that was incomplete or insufficient. Cosmetic reasons alone seldom constitute an indication. Function normally has to be improved to obtain a better grip or for restoration of sensation. Occupation, age, and sex influence the decision in regard to the different procedures, as well as involvement of other fingers and whether the dominant hand is involved.

PHALANGIZATION

Phalangization of the first metacarpal involves the deepening of the first web space to provide relative lengthening of the partially amputated thumb. The gain is increased prehension for pinch and grasp. Often it can be combined with an absolute lengthening of the thumb by bone graft insertion.

The procedure is indicated in cases of loss

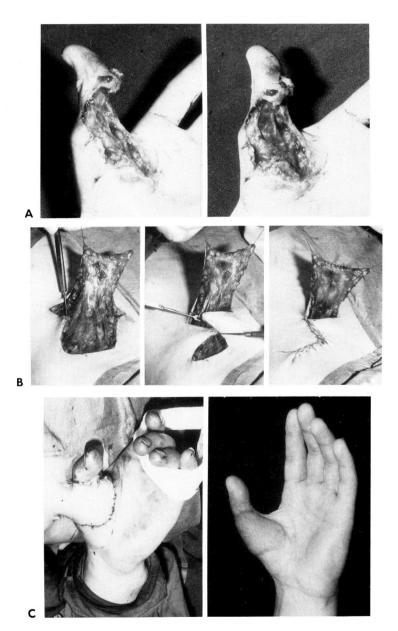

Figure 96–4. *A*, Injury by a drilling machine with loss of a palmar intermediate segment of all soft tissue. *B*, Preparation of an abdominal pedicle skin flap with closure of the donor defect by local flaps. *C*, Cover of the wound and final result.

of the thumb at the proximal half of the proximal phalanx or at the metacarpophalangeal joint, associated with partial or complete amputation of the fingers (at least the index and middle fingers). In both the dominant and the nondominant hands of heavy manual workers it is also indicated if all four fingers are intact, because thereby the grasp is improved and it is the simplest and safest method of thumb reconstruction. Prerequisites are a mobile carpometacarpal joint of the thumb, normal or almost normal sensation of the thumb stump, and, if possible, good skin in the first web space; otherwise a rotation flap from the dorsum or a distant flap becomes necessary.

In spite of the fact that Hugier (1873, 1874) performed the first phalangization as early as 1852, there have been only a few further publications on this subject (Hilgenfeldt, 1950; Kreuz, in Hilgenfeldt, 1950; Minkow and Stein, 1973; Simon, 1963; Tubiana and Roux, 1974). All authors have reported good improvement of hand function; of special value is the study of Simon (1963) on the late results in 52 patients with a follow-up time of up to 20 years.

One may use one of three possible incisions—a Z- or S-shaped incision, or an incision that creates a dorsal rectangular flap and two smaller lateral flaps on the palmar side, recommended by Peacock, 1966 (Fig. 96–5). If the skin of the first web space is scarred, a dorsal rotation flap or a distant flap may be needed. We prefer the Z-plasty as the simplest and most effective incision, as recommended by Tubiana and Roux (1974).

The muscle fascia (aponeuroses) and all fibrous structures between the metacarpals are divided. The deepening of the intermetacarpal space becomes effective only if the insertion of the adductor is divided from the sesamoid bone and reattached in about the middle of the first metacarpal to the periosteum (with a transosseous suture). Usually a small segment of the muscle belly of the transverse part of the adductor has to be resected, care being taken to preserve the muscle branches of the ulnar nerve. If the muscle shows severe fibrosis, it must be resected in order to free the passive motion of the carpometacarpal joint. Its action can be restored by a tendon transfer using the long flexor of the thumb or a flexor of an amputated finger. Usually the first dorsal interosseous muscle does not interfere with the deepening if its fascia is divided and its origin from the first metacarpal is released. In cases of severe scarring a capsulectomy of the carpometacarpal joint may be necessary. Tubiana and Roux (1974) described an arthroplasty using Silastic implants. A resection of the second metacarpal is indicated only in cases of loss of all five fingers, creating a more effective cleft hand.

We often combine phalangization with a lengthening of the thumb stump. To avoid the complication of partial resorption of the bone graft, if it was placed on top of the remaining bone, we prefer interposition lengthening as described in the next section.

We have not seen any complications in our cases. The results are difficult to grade because the conditions of the other parts have been different in all cases, but in any event there was subjectively and objectively a sig-

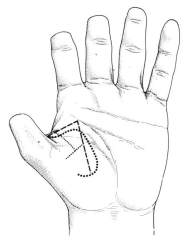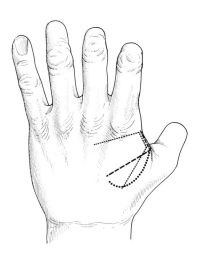

Figure 96–5. Phalangization of the first metacarpal showing the three possible incisions: straight line, Z-plasty; dashed line, dorsal rectangular flap with two lateral palmar flaps; dotted line, S-shaped incision of Kreuz.

nificant improvement in function, as reported by other authors.

LENGTHENING

The lengthening of a partially amputated thumb gives excellent functional results in cases in which pollicization is not indicated. It is applicable in cases with four intact fingers as well as in partial amputations of several or all fingers, and is often combined with phalangization (deepening of the first web space) with or without resection of the second metacarpal.

There is a great difference between the two possible ways of lengthening, the "on-top plasty" and interposition lengthening. The difference is not only in the operative technique but also in the prognosis: a bone graft placed on the tip of the remaining bone will be resorbed at least partially whereas an interposed bone graft will heal without any resorption. This is the reason I prefer interposition lengthening and have used the "on-top plasty" in only a few cases (in particular, congenital malformations with total aplasia of all the phalanges).

"ON-TOP PLASTY"

There is rarely an indication for lengthening with a bone graft and a tubed pedicle skin flap in cases of partial amputation of the thumb. The use of local skin is preferable not only for simplifying the procedure but also in respect to the blood and nerve supply.

The "cocked hat" or "thumbstall" method of Gillies fulfills these requirements, but there is disagreement about the value of this procedure. Barron (1977), Kelly (1959), and McGregor (1966) have been disappointed with the results, but Reid (1960, 1978) has reported very satisfying results. He concludes that the advantage of this procedure is that it is a single operation resulting in a strong stable thumb with good sensation and a fair appearance. The disadvantages are the limited lengthening, the occasional absorption of the graft, and the distal displacement of the web between the thumb and index finger, which, however, can be corrected readily by a subsequent Z-plasty. Hughes and Moore (1950) reported their first two cases following the suggestion of use of this method at the first clinical meeting of the British Association of Plastic Surgeons in 1946 by Gillies. They were surprised that the reconstructed thumb showed, almost at once, some degree of tactile and thermal sensibility.

Operative Technique. A dorsal semicircular incision preserves the blood and nerve supply for the "cocked hat" in its palmar pedicle. After removal of scar tissue and careful stretching of the skin, a cortical and cancellous bone graft from the iliac crest is doweled into the bone stump (Fig. 96–6). The bone graft is covered on its dorsal aspect by subcutaneous tissue, which is then skin grafted. The elongation can be up to 1.5 cm., but the longer the bone graft, the greater the

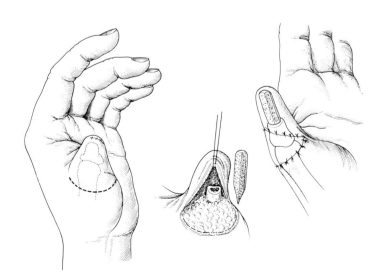

Figure 96–6. "Cocked hat" or "thumbstall" method of Gillies.

risk of later resorption and fracture of the graft.

Barron (1977) has recommended a revised cocked hat procedure, but there are no published results using this method.

Another possible way of "on-top lengthening" exists in cases of simultaneous damage of other fingers with amputation of the index finger at the metacarpophalangeal joint. It involves transposition of the distal part of the second metacarpal with its overlying soft tissues on a neurovascular pedicle. The procedure was described, as have so many details of thumb reconstruction, by Hilgenfeldt (1950) and has proved to be a successful method (Buck-Gramcko, 1964, 1970, 1971; Pitzler, 1969; Schink, 1957). The preservation of a normal blood and nerve supply to the transposed part prevents any subsequent absorption of the bone. Even if the lengthening is limited, the total hand function is much improved, because not only is the thumb ray lengthened but also a new and deep intermetacarpal space is created by the partial resection of the second metacarpal (Fig. 96–7). It is necessary to cover this new space with skin grafts or a rotation flap from the dorsum. The use of a palmar skin bridge covering the neurovascular structures, as originally described by Hilgenfeldt (1950), is not necessary; transposition on a neurovascular pedicle only gives about 2.5 cm. more lengthening. A similar procedure was described by Kelleher et al. (1968).

INTERPOSITION LENGTHENING

The interposition of a bone graft for elongation of a partially amputated thumb has to be done in the metacarpal because the remaining part of the proximal phalanx cannot be distracted sufficiently, owing to the loss of elasticity in the soft tissues, which usually show more scarring at the tip (amputation site) than in the more proximal parts. Too much scarring is a contraindication to use of this procedure and requires the replacement of scar by a skin graft or a flap. The tip of the thumb stump should have adequate sensation; otherwise a sensory flap has to be used in addition.

Elongation can be performed as a one stage procedure or by continuous distraction. The indications are the same, but with continuous distraction one can obtain more elongation (about 4 cm.), so that it is indicated in more proximal amputations (metacarpal head or metacarpophalangeal joint).

One Stage Interposition Lengthening

This procedure was mentioned by Hilgenfeldt in 1950 but not recommended. This may be one of the reasons there have only been a few publications on the subject in the last 25 years in spite of the fact that Bolton (1967) and Buck-Gramcko (1970, 1971) have published good results.

Operative Technique. Via a curved dorsal incision the first metacarpal is osteotomized transversely in its middle third. The muscle origins are carefully stripped from the proximal half of the metacarpal without damaging the radial artery. The necessary distraction of its two parts can be done by simple spreading with strong scissors or a similar instrument or by a special distraction apparatus with countercurrent threads on its two bars, as described by Stellbrink (1969). A bone graft from the iliac crest (or, in the case of resection of the second metacarpal, with deepening of the web space from this bone) is placed between the distracted parts and fixed by Kirschner wires or preferably by a plate (Fig. 96–8). Skin closure is usually possible by direct suturing; only in rare cases with much scarring or an adduction contracture is a local flap necessary (Fig. 96–9). The duration of postoperative immobilization with a plaster splint depends on the stability of the osteosynthesis. Complications such as nonunion are infrequent; resorption of the bone graft never occurs.

The gain in length is usually between 15 and 20 mm. (maximum, 25 mm.). This is sufficient for a marked improvement in hand function, not only for pinching and grasping in the presence of four intact fingers, but also in cases of complete or partial loss of other fingers. If only the small finger is intact, function can be improved by an angulatory rotational osteotomy at the base of the fifth metacarpal.

Lengthening by Continuous Distraction

This method was originally described by Matev (1970) for thumb reconstruction only in children and teenagers because of the more active and progressive ossification in this age group. More recently Matev and others have

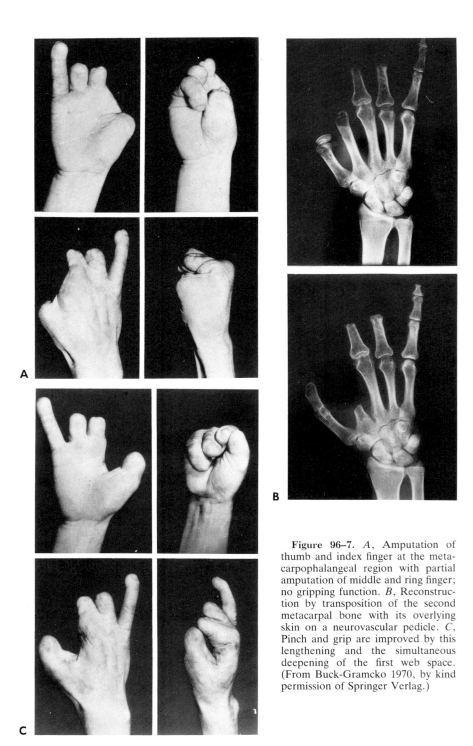

Figure 96–7. *A*, Amputation of thumb and index finger at the metacarpophalangeal region with partial amputation of middle and ring finger; no gripping function. *B*, Reconstruction by transposition of the second metacarpal bone with its overlying skin on a neurovascular pedicle. *C*, Pinch and grip are improved by this lengthening and the simultaneous deepening of the first web space. (From Buck-Gramcko 1970, by kind permission of Springer Verlag.)

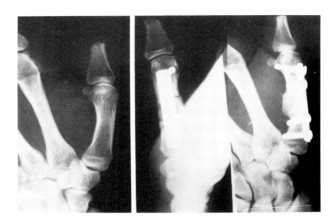

Figure 96–8. One-stage interposition lengthening of the first metacarpal bone in a case of partial loss of the thumb.

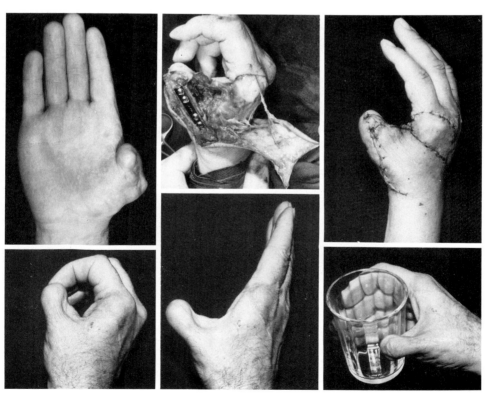

Figure 96–9. Partial amputation of the thumb. *Above middle*, Interposition lengthening was accomplished by bone graft with plate fixation. *Above right*, After scar excision, a dorsal transposition flap was necessary. *Below*, the functional result is shown three years postoperatively.

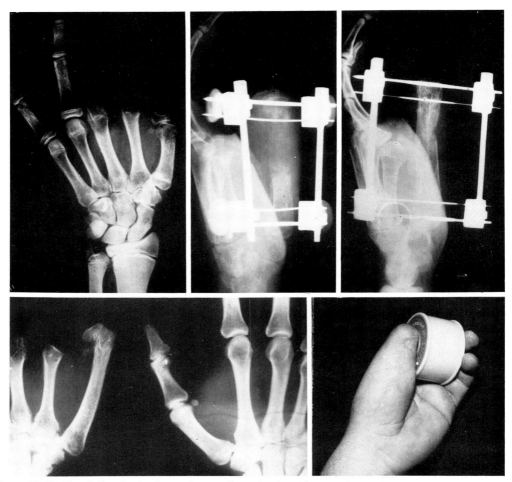

Figure 96–10. Thumb lengthening by continuous distraction in a 16 year old boy with amputation of thumb, index, and middle fingers. *Above middle*, After 30 days' distraction. *Above right*, After five months, immediately before removal of the Kirschner wires. *Below*, radiological and clinical appearance five years later; lengthening 3.5 cm. (= 75 per cent of the normal length of the metacarpal bone). (Courtesy of Dr. Ivan Matev.)

extended the use of this procedure to adults in whom the insertion of a bone graft follows the gradual distraction of the two portions of the first metacarpal (Fig. 96–10).

The operative technique and results are discussed by Matev in Chapter 58A in Volume II.

The lengthening obtained by the continuous distraction is up to 4 cm. (average, 3.5 cm.). Up to the end of 1978, Matev had treated 42 patients, the only complication being a slight infection around the Kirschner wires in one case.

SENSORY REHABILITATION

The great number of operative procedures described for restoration of sensation in a partially amputated thumb is a testament to the importance of sensation in this part of the hand. The functional value of the thumb is greatly decreased by the loss of sensation. Its restoration is an important part of reconstructive surgery of the hand.

The first step, of course, is reconstruction of the median nerve by suturing or grafting. If this is impossible or fails, or the gripping area of the remaining part of the thumb is badly scarred, sensation must be transferred to the thumb by means of skin flaps, skin islands, or even free grafted skin that includes intact nerves. This innervated skin can be taken from other areas of the hand or from other donor sites.

LOCAL SENSORY FLAPS

The two simplest ways to restore sensation to the tip of a thumb with or without partial amputation were described by Moberg (1970):

Bone Shortening. Bone shortening can be used to obtain a sensory skin cover. It is indicated in cases of irreversible median nerve palsy with intact dorsal sensation via the superficial branch of the radial nerve. Under these conditions it may be justified to resect 1 or 2 cm. of the bone or even the whole distal phalanx and to cover the new end of the thumb using a flap of dorsal skin with normal sensation (see also Buck-Gramcko, 1961).

Palmar advancement flaps have been described earlier in this chapter.

Interchange of a Sensory Island Flap. Interchange of a sensory island flap in the distal part of the thumb can improve the function if there is no sensation in the ulnar half (the main area for pinch) but there is normal sensation in the less important radial half. A skin island flap about 1.5 to 2.0 cm. long is carefully dissected out with its neurovascular pedicle and transposed to the ulnar half where a similar sized area of insensitive skin is excised as a full thickness skin graft. This can be used as a graft to cover the donor site if the skin is not too scarred. A similar procedure has been described by Joshi (1974): he uses a dorsolateral skin island raised on the palmar digital vessels and nerve. Pho (1976, 1979) has described this as a primary procedure in cases of extensive pulp loss.

Other local flaps require careful dissection in order not to destroy the fine branches of the nerves and vessels that have to be included in the flap or its pedicle. Usually these flaps are taken from areas supplied by the radial or ulnar nerve, because in most instances irreversible damage to the median nerve is the reason for the loss of sensation in the gripping area of the thumb. By blocking the different nerves with an anesthetic solution, one can determine their sensory distribution and prevent unsatisfactory results.

Radial Innervated Sensory Flaps

The radial nerve innervated skin in the hand is the source of several sensory flaps, which differ mainly in their pedicles. For the reconstruction of sensation in the distal part of the thumb with or without partial amputation, the dorsal aspect of the proximal phalanx of the index finger is the best donor area because of its proximity and minimal functional loss. Hilgenfeldt recognized this in the late 1940's and described this sensory flap in his outstanding book in 1950 and also 1964.

There are two different procedures available for transfer of sensation from the index finger to the thumb:

Transposition Flap. A transposition flap can be raised with a permanent skin pedicle including the neurovascular structures. This was the original method described by Hilgenfeldt (1950) and was used as a primary procedure by Buck-Gramcko (1961) and for secondary reconstruction by Kuhn (1961). Use of the radial nerve innervated skin area on the index finger as a transposition flap is

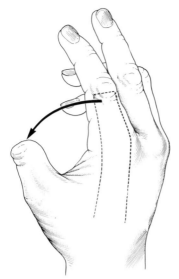

Figure 96–11. Radial-innervated sensory flap as transposition flap (Hilgenfeldt). The skin flap includes a dorsal artery, veins, and nerve branches from the superficial radial nerve.

indicated mainly in partial amputations of the thumb, in which it can cover the whole pinching area at the tip (Fig. 96–11).

Adamson et al. (1967) referred to the work of Wilson, who obtained better results by delaying this flap for six weeks. Holevitch (1963) described the use of the dorsal neu-

rovascular bundle with its surrounding loose soft tissues but without skin, which is implanted under the skin of the thumb tip for neurotization. Recently Holevitch has also used a skin island with the pedicle.

Cross Finger Flap. A cross finger flap is created so that the sensory flap also can be transferred to the pulp area of a thumb with normal length. There are several descriptions of this method, all based on the same principle (Fig. 96–12). Gaul (1969), who first carried out anatomical studies of this procedure in 1954, and Adamson et al. (1967) have dissected the branches of the superficial radial nerve as the first stage of the operation and transferred them to the thumb; Bralliar and Horner (1969) performed the dissection and transfer of the nerve pedicle during the second stage of the cross finger flap procedure, dividing the flap at its base.

Other Sources of Sensory Flaps

Beside the use of radial nerve innervated skin, there are some other ways of obtaining sensory flaps for the thumb. In most of them the nerve supplying the skin area has to be cut and carefully sutured to one of the thumb nerves so that sensation returns only after reinnervation of the skin flap.

Sensory Cross Finger Flaps. For restoration of sensation in the tip of a thumb of

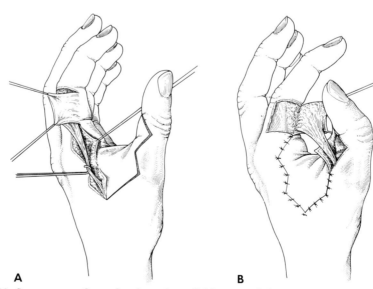

A   **B**

Figure 96–12. Sensory cross-finger flap from the radial-innervated dorsoradial aspect of the proximal phalanx of the index finger. *A*, Incision and dissection of the branch of the superficial radial nerve with its terminal arborizing fibers and surrounding areolar tissue. *B*, The nerve pedicle of the cross finger flap is transposed after mobilization to the thumb to cover its pulp.

normal length or a partially amputated one that is scarred distally or with destruction of the distal nerve, a cross finger flap can be raised on the ring finger or under special conditions on the middle finger. The flap must contain the ulnar digital nerve, which is cut as far proximally as necessary in order to reach the normal end of one of the palmar nerves of the thumb. Nerve suturing is performed without tension, and the cross finger flap is sutured to the tip of the thumb; its pedicle can be divided two or three weeks later. Hoffmann described this method in 1969, and Berger and Meissl (1975) modified it by using a dorsal cross finger flap with one or both dorsal digital nerves.

Innervated Full Thickness Skin Grafts. On the basis of the experience of McCash (1958-1959), who used skin grafts from toes to cover fingertip defects, Maquieira (1974) since 1967 has used a method of restoring sensation in the fingertips and pulps. He uses a full thickness skin graft with a nerve unit after removal of most of the subcutaneous tissue. The nerve is sutured to a nerve in the recipient area. Donor sites are the lateral pulp of the toes or fingers and the distal forearm. Maquieira has reported good results in 75 per cent of the cases. The same method was used independently by Berger and Meissl (1975).

The Neurovascular Island Flap

Transfer of sensation in the hand by means of a skin island from the ulnar side of the ring or middle finger with its neurovascular bundle as pedicle was first reported by Moberg in 1955 and has been used more extensively by Littler (1956, 1960) as well as in Europe by Tubiana et al. (1960). The donor site for the island is the ulnar aspect of the terminal phalanx of either the ring or the middle finger. The ring finger may be the functionally less important finger and has to be the donor site in all cases of damage to the main trunk of the median nerve (instead of only the branches to the thumb), but the advantage in using the middle finger is the shorter distance to the thumb, so that the skin island can be set into the distal part of the thumb without any tension and without the risk of damaging the artery or stretching the nerve, even in full radial abduction. Extended donor sites were described by Hueston (1965) with inclusion of the dorsal digital nerve branch and by Omer et al. (1970) using the adjacent surfaces of the ring and little fingers, including the intervening web.

Operative Technique. Under brachial plexus block and in a bloodless field, the skin island is outlined on the ulnar part of the distal phalanx of the donor finger. A midlateral incision is made proximal to the island and is continued in a slightly curved or zigzag fashion as far as the proximal palm. The dissection starts on the proximal border of the skin island and should free the neurovascular bundle together with the surrounded subcutaneous tissue. Without exposure of the nerve and artery, all tiny vessel branches are carefully coagulated using bipolar microforceps. The artery is dissected as far as the superficial arch. The common digital nerve is split into its two parts to the same level.

When the neurovascular bundle has been dissected without damage, the skin island is excised. Some subcutaneous tissue should be left over the bone to provide a good bed for a skin graft. In the thumb the corresponding site for the island is excised or only incised in cases in which a small island flap is used. This incision is prolonged to the proximal flexion crease where the skin is undermined to the first incision. A Penrose drain is brought through this tunnel, and the skin island is carefully pulled through to the thumb. The drain is then removed, care being taken not to twist the pedicle. The skin island is sutured to the skin of the thumb; any constriction of the pedicle should be avoided (Fig. 96–13). The tourniquet is then released and careful hemostasis is secured. The skin defect on the donor finger is covered by a full thickness or thick split thickness skin graft. Immobilization in a plaster splint with full radial abduction of the thumb is maintained for about 10 days.

Complications. In addition to damage to the neurovascular bundle during dissection and kinking of the artery, paresthesia or hyperesthesia may occur in the skin island. This is usually caused by too much tension on the pedicle if it was not dissected far enough proximally so that it is too short in radial abduction of the thumb. Another cause of pain may be a microneuroma at the margin of the island. Loss of sensation at the donor site and some reduction of sensory quality in the island skin may also be seen. Flap necrosis is a rare occurrence but has been reported by McGregor (1969).

Results. Several authors have reported results in larger series of cases of neurovascular island flap transfer (Krag and Bang Rasmussen, 1975; Murray et al., 1967; Omer et al., 1970; Reid, 1966; Tubiana, 1973, Tubiana

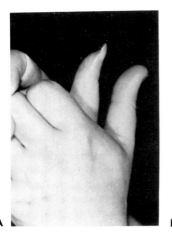
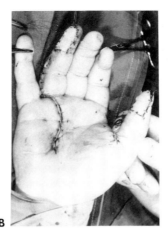

Figure 96–13. *A*, Loss of the thumb pulp with painful scar (in comparison with the contour of the normal left thumb). *B*, Replacement of the scarred pulp by neurovascular island flap.

and Duparc, 1961; Zrubecky, 1970). Generally they agree that the method is useful if the operative technique is meticulous. In the donor finger the loss of sensation has proved insignificant. Functional use of the thumb is improved considerably not only because of the improved sensation but also the increased vascular supply. The island gives an excellent durable tactile skin cover, even if the two point discrimination is less than normal. Many authors describe a progressive loss of sensibility, but a protective sensation remains. This can be explained by secondary scar compression of the pedicle and by stretching of the nerve during full radial abduction of the thumb. The hyperesthesis seen in some patients can impair the results obtained with this method.

Cortical reorientation of the localization of stimuli occurs only in a few patients and then only after a long period of time. Most stimuli are referred to the donor finger, but the function is not adversely affected by this misinterpretation. Some patients experience "double sensibility" in which stimuli are felt in the donor finger as well as in the recipient finger.

Free Neurovascular Flaps

The rapid development of microsurgery has considerably influenced reconstructive surgery of the hand. Several of the disadvantages and complications of the conventional types of neurovascular flap can be avoided by the use of a free flap with microvascular anastomoses and nerve suturing.* Even if

*A nerve cannot be repaired by "anastomosis": this Greek word means mouth, opening, estuary—and there is no opening in a nerve.

free flap transfer is a complicated procedure, its risks have been decreased as used by skilled microsurgeons. Better knowledge of the vascular and neural anatomy in the donor sites has recently advanced the clinical application of new flaps (Daniel and Terzis, 1976).

For the repair of defects in the hand the usual donor site is the foot. The similarity of the skin, the thin layer of subcutaneous fat, the large diameter of the vessels, and the minimal functional defect at the donor site make these flaps ideal. The disadvantage is the tedious, time consuming flap dissection.

In partial mutilations of the thumb, the free dorsalis pedis flap can be used as neurocutaneous cover in cases of extensive skin loss, especially on the palmar aspect. Its long neurovascular pedicle makes it possible to suture the important structures far proximally in healthy surrounding tissues (Daniel et al., 1976; Ohmori and Harii, 1976).

A free neurovascular flap from the first web space of the foot is preferable for skin cover on the thumb (and fingers) because of the similarity of the skin and the more constant nerve supply (medial plantar nerve and its digital branches instead of the very small and variable branches of the superficial peroneal nerve on the dorsum of the foot). The two point discrimination in the toe skin is better, and thus the quality of sensory reinnervation is superior to that achieved with the dorsalis pedis flap. Excellent descriptions of the anatomy have contributed considerably to the clinical use of this flap (Gilbert, 1976; May et al., 1977). The flap can include the complete web unit, can be limited to one toe, or can be extended to adjacent dorsal skin as required (Daniel et al., 1976; Strauch and Shafiroff, 1979; Strauch and Tsur, 1978).

Buncke and Rose (1979) have used a free toe pulp neurovascular flap for sensory reconstruction of an insensitive fingertip pad. The donor site is the pulp, with some part of the lateral aspect of the great toe or medial aspect of the second toe. The pedicle contains the plantar digital artery, the digital nerve, and a large vein and is sutured to the corresponding structures of the thumb (or finger). The venous reconstruction is as important as the arterial anastomosis.

REFERENCES

Adamson, J. E., Horton, C. E., and Crawford, H. H.: Sensory rehabilitation of the injured thumb. Plast. Reconstr. Surg., *40:*53–57, 1967.

Argamaso, R. V.: Rotation-transposition method for soft tissue replacement on the distal segment of the thumb. Plast. Reconstr. Surg., *54:*366–368, 1974.

Bales, C. R., Demuth, R. J., Tooze, F. M., and Graham, W. P.: Thumb length preservation following soft tissue injuries. J. Trauma, *15:*901–908, 1975.

Barron, J. N.: Cock another hat at the thumb. Hand, *9:*39-41, 1977.

Beasley, R. W.: Principles and techniques of resurfacing operations for hand surgery. Surg. Clin. N. Am., *47:*389–413, 1967.

Beasley, R. W.: Corresponding Club Newsletter, American Society for Surgery of the Hand, 1978, p. 21.

Berger, A., and Meissl, G.: Innervated skin grafts and flaps for restoration of sensation to anesthetic areas. Chir. Plast. (Berlin), *3:*33–37, 1975.

Berger, A., and Meissl, G.: Wiederherstellung der sensiblen Qualitäten der Endphalangen durch gestielte und freie sensible Transplantation. Handchirurgie, *7:*169–171, 1975b.

Bolton, H.: Elongation of the partially amputated thumb. Proceedings of the British Club for Surgery of the Hand, Lausanne, May 1967.

Bralliar, F., and Horner, R. L.: Sensory cross-finger pedicle graft. J. Bone Joint Surg. *51A:*1264–1269, 1969.

Buck-Gramcko, D.: Wiederherstellung der Sensibilität bei Teilverlust des Daumens. Langenbecks Arch. Klin. Chir., *299:*99–104, 1961.

Buck-Gramcko, D.: Daumenersatz aus dem zweiten Mittelhandknochen bei Verlust des ersten und zweiten Fingers. Langenbecks Arch. Klin. Chir., *306:*153–157, 1964.

Buck-Gramcko, D.: Verlängerung des I. Mittelhandknochens zur Funktionsverbesserung der Hand bei Verlust des Daumens und mehrerer Langfinger. Mschr. Unfallheilk., *73:*29–37, 1970.

Buck-Gramcko, D.: Lengthening of first metacarpal in cases of loss of thumb and several fingers. Transactions of the Fifth International Congress of Plastic and Reconstructive Surgery. Melbourne, Australia, Butterworths Pty. Ltd., 1971, pp. 553–558.

Buncke, H. J., and Rose, E. H.: Free toe-to-fingertip neurovascular flaps. Plast. Reconstr. Surg., *63:*607–612, 1979.

Bunnell, S.: Surgery of the Hand. Philadelphia, J. B. Lippincott, 1944.

Chase, R. A.: Early salvage in acute hand injuries with a primary island flap. Plast. Reconstr. Surg., *48:*521–527, 1971.

Daniel, R. K., and Terzis, J. K.: Neurovascular free flaps. *In* Daniller, A. J., and Strauch, B. (Editors): Symposium on Microsurgery. St. Louis, The C. V. Mosby Company, 1976, pp. 66–73.

Daniel, R. K., Terzis, J. K., and May, J. W.: Neurovascular free flaps. *In* Serafin, D., and Buncke, H. J.; Microsurgical Composite Tissue Transplantation. St. Louis, The C. V. Mosby Company, 1979, pp. 285–316.

Daniel, R. K., Terzis, J.K ., and Midgley, D.: Restoration of sensation to an anesthetic hand by a free neurovascular flap from the foot. Plast. Reconstr. Surg., *57:*275–280, 1976.

Dolich, B. H., Olshansky, K. J., and Babar, A. H.: Use of a cross-forearm neurocutaneous flap to provide sensation and coverage in hand reconstruction. Plast. Reconstr. Surg., *62:*550–558, 1978.

Foucher, G., and Braun, J. -B.: A new island flap transfer from the dorsum of the index to the thumb. Plast. Reconstr. Surg., *63:*344–349, 1979.

Gassmann, N., and Segmüller, G.: Der neurovaskulär gestielte, palmare Verschiebelappen nach Moberg. Analyse unbefriedigender Resultate. Handchirurgie, *8:*77–80, 1976.

Gaul, S.: Radial-innervated cross-finger flap from index to provide sensory pulp to injured thumb. J. Bone Joint Surg., *51A:*1257–1263, 1969.

Gilbert, A.: Composite tissue transfer from the foot: anatomic basis and surgical technique. *In* Daniller, A. J., and Strauch, B. (Editors): Symposium on Microsurgery, St. Louis, The C. V. Mosby Company, 1976, pp. 230–242.

Goumain, A. J. M., Baudet, J., and Massard, J. F.: Notre expérience des mutilations récentes du pouce. Rev. Chir. Orthop., *58:*563–574, 1972.

Hilgenfeldt, O.: Operativer Daumenersatz und Beseitigung von Greifstörungen. Stuttgart, Ferdinand Enke Verlag, 1950.

Hilgenfeldt, O.: Über einen vielfach verwendungsfähigen neurovaskulären Lappen zur Behebung von Schäden der radialen Handhälfte. Langenbecks Arch. Klin. Chir., *306:*152, 1964.

Hilgenfeldt, O.: Fingerstumpfverlängerung und Daumenbildung durch Knochenvorverpflanzung. Handchirurgie, *1:*38–45, 1969.

Hoffmann, H.: Der sensible gekreuzte Fingerlappen zur Deckung von Spitzendefekten am Daumen. Handchirurgie, *1:*82–85, 1969.

Holevich, J.: A new method of restoring sensibility to the thumb. J. Bone Joint Surg., *45B:*496–505, 1963.

Hueston, J. T.: The extended neurovascular island flap. Br. J. Plast. Surg., *18:*304–305, 1965.

Hueston, J. T.: Local flap repair of finger tip injuries. Plast. Reconstr. Surg., *37:*349–350, 1966.

Hughes, N. C., and Moore, F. T.: A preliminary report on the use of a local flap and peg bone graft for lengthening a short thumb. Br. J. Plast. Surg., *3:*34–39, 1950.

Hugier, P. -C.: Considérations anatomiques et physiologiques sur le rôle du pouce et sur la chirurgie de cet organe. Arch. Gén. Méd., *222:*404–421, 567–580, 692–706, 1873.

Hugier, P. -C.: Considérations anatomiques et physiologiques pour servir à la chirurgie du pouce. Arch. Gén. Méd., *23:*54–82, 1874.

Joshi, B. B.: One-stage repair for distal amputation of the thumb. Plast. Reconstr. Surg., *45:*613–615, 1970.

Joshi, B. B.: A local dorsolateral island flap for restoration of sensation after avulsion injury of fingertip
pulp. Plast. Reconstr. Surg., 54:175–182, 1974.

Keim, H. A., and Grantham, S. A.: Volar-flap advancement for thumb and finger-tip injuries. Clin. Orthop.,
66:109–112, 1969.

Kelleher, J. C., Sullivan, J. G., Baibak, G. J., and
Dean, R. K.: "On-top plasty" for amputated fingers.
Plast. Reconstr. Surg., 42:242–248, 1968.

Kelly, A. P.: Subtotal reconstruction of the thumb.
Arch. Surg., 78:582–585, 1959.

Krag, C., and Bang Rasmussen, K.: The neurovascular
island flap for defective sensibility of the thumb. J.
Bone Joint Surg., 57B:495–499, 1975.

Kreuz, L.: Cited by Hilgenfeldt, 1950.

Kuhn, H.: Reconstruction du pouce par "lambeau de
Hilgenfeldt." Ann. Chir. Plast., 6:259–268, 1961.

Kutler, W.: A new method for finger tip amputations.
J.A.M.A., 133:29–30, 1947.

Littler, J. W.: Neurovascular pedicle transfer of tissue
in reconstructive surgery of the hand (proceedings).
J. Bone Joint Surg., 38A:917, 1956.

Littler, J. W.: Neurovascular skin island transfer in
reconstructive hand surgery. Transactions of the International Society of Plastic Surgeons, Second Congress, London, 1959. Edinburgh, E. & S. Livingstone,
1960, pp. 175–179.

Littler, J. W.: Shifting local tissues for sensory defects.
In Converse, J. M. (Editor): Reconstructive Plastic
Surgery. Philadelphia, W. B. Saunders Company,
1964, Vol. IV, p. 1639.

Maquieira, N. O.: An innervated full-thickness skin graft
to restore sensibility to fingertips and heels. Plast.
Reconstr. Surg., 53:568–575, 1974.

Matev, I.: Thumb reconstruction after amputation at the
metacarpophalangeal joint by bone-lengthening. J.
Bone Joint Surg., 52A:957–965, 1970.

May, J. W., Chait, L. A., Cohen, B. E., and O'Brien,
B. M.: Free neurovascular flap from the first web of
the foot in hand reconstruction. J. Hand Surg., 2:387–
393, 1977.

McCash, C. R.: Toe pulp free grafts in finger-tip repair.
Br. J. Plast. Surg., 11:322–328, 1958-1959.

McFarlane, R. M., and Stromberg, W. B.: Resurfacing
of the thumb following major skin loss. J. Bone Joint
Surg., 44A:1365–1375, 1962.

McGregor, I. A.: Reconstruction of the thumb. In
Gibson, T. (Editor): Modern Trends in Plastic Surgery
2. London, Butterworth & Co. (Publishers) Ltd.,
1966.

McGregor, I. A.: Less than satisfactory experiences with
neurovascular island flaps. Hand, 1:21–22, 1969.

Millender, L. H., Albin, R. E., and Nalebuff, E. A.:
Delayed volar advancement flap for thumb tip injuries.
Plast. Reconstr. Surg., 52:635–639, 1973.

Minkow, F. V., and Stein, F.: Phalangization of the
thumb. J. Trauma, 13:648–655, 1973.

Miura, T.: Thumb reconstruction using radial-innervated
cross-finger pedicle graft. J. Bone Joint Surg.,
55A:563–569, 1973.

Moberg, E.: Discussion, In Brooks, D.: The place of
nerve-grafting in orthopaedic surgery. J. Bone Joint
Surg., 37A:299–305, 326, 1955.

Moberg, E.: Aspects of sensation in reconstructive surgery of the upper extremity. J. Bone Joint Surg.,
46A:817–825, 1964.

Moberg, E.: Useful surgical arrangement of skin with
normal sensibility to mutilated hands. In London, P.
S. (Editor): Modern Trends in Accident Surgery and

Medicine. London, Butterworth & Co. (Publishers)
Ltd., 1970, pp. 143–164.

Murray, J. F., Odd, J. V. R., and Gavelin, G. E.: The
neurovascular island pedicle flap. An assessment of
late results in sixteen cases. J. Bone Joint Surg.,
49A:1285–1297, 1967.

Nemethi, C. E.: Reconstruction of the distal part of the
thumb after traumatic amputation. J. Bone Joint
Surg., 42A:375–391, 1960.

O'Brien, B. M.: Neurovascular pedicle transfers in the
hand. Aust. N. Z. J. Surg., 35:2–11, 1965.

O'Brien, B. M.: Neurovascular island pedicle flaps for
terminal amputations and digital scars. Br. J. Plast.
Surg., 21:258–261, 1968.

Ohmori, K., and Harii, K.: Free dorsalis pedis sensory
flap to the hand, with microvascular anastomoses.
Plast. Reconstr. Surg., 58:546–554, 1976.

Omer, G. E., Day, D. J., Ratliff, H., and Lambert, P.:
Neurovascular cutaneous island pedicles for deficient
median-nerve sensibility. J. Bone Joint Surg.,
52A:1181–1192, 1970.

Peacock, E. E.: Reconstruction of the thumb. In Flynn,
J. E. (Editor): Hand Surgery. Baltimore, The Williams & Wilkins Company, 1966, pp. 561–582.

Pho, R. W. H.: Restoration of sensation using a local
neurovascular island flap as a primary procedure in
extensive pulp loss of the fingertip. Injury, 8:20–24,
1976.

Pho, R. W. H.: Local composite neurovascular island
flap for skin cover in pulp loss of the thumb. J. Hand
Surg., 4:11–15, 1979.

Pitzler, K.: Der Daumenersatz aus dem zweiten Mittelhandknochen. Bruns Beitr. Klin. Chir., 217:321–329,
1969.

Porter, R. W.: Functional assessment of transplanted
skin in volar defects of the digits. J. Bone Joint Surg.,
50A:955–963, 1968.

Posner, M. A., and Smith, R. J.: The advancement
pedicle flap for thumb injuries. J. Bone Joint Surg.,
53A:1618–1621, 1971.

Poy, N. G.: The single pedicle neurovascular island flap.
Its use in 33 cases of acute partial digital amputations.
Transactions of the Fifth International Congress of
Plastic and Reconstructive Surgery. Melbourne, Aus-
tralia, Butterworths Pty. Ltd., 1971, pp. 542–547.

Pringle, R. G.: Amputations of the thumb. A study of
techniques of repair and residual disability. Injury,
3:211–217, 1972.

Ratliff, A. H. C.: Amputations of the distal part of the
thumb. Hand, 4:190–193, 1972.

Reid, D. A. C.: Reconstruction of the thumb. J. Bone
Joint Surg., 42B:444–465, 1960.

Reid, D. A. C.: The neurovascular island flap in thumb
reconstruction. Br. J. Plast. Surg., 19:234–244, 1966.

Reid, D. A. C.: Demonstration at the Meeting of the
British Society for Surgery of the Hand, Sheffield,
May 1978.

Reid, D. A. C.: The Gillies' thumb lengthening operation. Hand, 12:123–129, 1980.

Reid, D. A. C.: Thumb lengthening by the Gillies'
method. Handchirurgie, 13:46–51, 1981.

Schink, W.: Ein Beitrag zum operativen Daumenersatz.
Chirurg, 28:371–373, 1957.

Segmüller, G.: Modifikation des Kutler-Lappens: neurovaskuläre Stielung. Handchirurgie, 8:75–76, 1976.

Simon, P.: Die Metaphalangisation. Spätergebnisse bei
der Rehabilitation Handverletzter. Z. Orthop.,
97:551–565, 1963.

Simonetta, C.: Personal communication and paper presented at the Meeting of The British Society for Surgery of the Hand, Sheffield, May 1978.

Snow, J. W.: The use of a volar flap for repair of fingertip amputations: a preliminary report. Plast. Reconstr. Surg., *40:*163–168, 1967.

Snow, J. W.: Follow-up clinic. Plast. Reconstr. Surg., *52:*299, 1973.

Stellbrink, G.: Äusseres Fixationsgerät für Fingerarthrodesen. Chirurg, *40:*422–425, 1969.

Strauch, B., and Shafiroff, B. B.: The foot. A versatile source of donor tissue. *In* Serafin, D., and Buncke, H. J. (Editors): Microsurgical Composite Tissue Transplantation. St. Louis, The C. V. Mosby Company, 1979, pp. 345–356.

Strauch, B., and Tsur, H.: Restoration of sensation to the hand by a free neurovascular flap from the first web space of the foot. Plast. Reconstr. Surg., *62:*361–367, 1978.

Sturman, M. J., and Duran, R. J.: Late results of fingertip injuries. J. Bone Joint Surg., *45A:*289–298, 1963.

Sullivan, J. G., Kelleher, J. C., Baibak, G. J., Dean, R. K., and Pinkner, L. D.: The primary application of an island pedicle flap in thumb and index finger injuries. Plast. Reconstr. Surg., *39:*488–492, 1967 (with comment, ibid., *51:*208, 1973).

Tranquilli-Leali, E.: Ricostruzione dell'apice delle falangi ungueali mediante autoplastica volare peduncolata per scorrimento. Infort. Traum. Lavoro, *1:*186–193, 1935.

Tubiana, R.: Les lambeaux cutanés palmaires en ilot. Ann. Chir., *27:*503–509, 1973.

Tubiana, R., and Duparc, J.: Restoration of sensibility in the hand by neurovascular skin island transfer. J. Bone Joint Surg., *43B:*474–480, 1961.

Tubiana, R., Duparc, J., and Moreau, C.: Restauration de la sensibilité au niveau de la main par transfert d'un transplant cutané hétéro-digital muni de son pédicule vasculo-nerveux. Rev. Chir. Orthop., *46:*163–178, 1960.

Tubiana, R., and Roux, J. -P.: Phalangization of the first and fifth metacarpals. J. Bone Joint Surg., *56A:*447–457, 1974.

Verdan, C.: The reconstruction of the thumb. Surg. Clin. N. Am., *48:*1033–1061, 1968.

Vilain, R.: Techniques elémentaires de réparation des pertes de substance cutanée des doigts. Sem. Hôp. Paris, *29:*1–7, 1952.

Vilain, R., and Dupuis, J. F.: Use of the flag flap for coverage of a small area on a finger or the palm. Plast. Reconstr. Surg., *51:*397–401, 1973.

Zrubecky, G.: Spätergebnisse nach Insellappen-Plastiken. Handchirurgie, *2:*129–131, 1970

Chapter 97

COMPLETE AMPUTATION OF THE THUMB

Raoul Tubiana

Le pouce est le maistre doigt de la main.

MONTAIGNE

Complete traumatic mutilation of the thumb does not make prehension impossible but greatly reduces the strength and precision of the grip. In spite of all the possibilities of re-education, a hand without a thumb is a hand that has lost its meaning and is only a paw (Huguier, 1874). Investigators in most countries estimate that a hand without its thumb loses 35 to 45 per cent of its function. This accounts for the interest in reconstructive procedures.

Most of the methods of reconstruction were described at the end of the last century, but techniques continue to evolve. Reconstruction of the thumb remains one of the most popular topics at hand surgery meetings. In fact, the indications are relatively infrequent.

Although surgeons like to perform this type of reconstruction, which promotes their reputation in their own eyes, patients themselves are often less satisfied with the results. The new thumb is little used or may be more of a hindrance because of its limited mobility or faulty orientation, or because it has poor sensation or is painful. In some cases manual function in general is reduced as a result of such reconstruction. This may be the result of inadequate technique or an incorrect choice of operative methods. Reconstruction of the thumb should be the prerogative of "specialists." Its indications should be carefully chosen and all precautions taken to ensure a successful functional result.

Numerous procedures have been described for reconstruction of the thumb. They can be divided into three groups according to the classification developed by Gueullette (1930):

1. Methods that use the remaining parts of the mutilated hand
   a. Phalangization of the first metacarpal
   b. Pollicization of other digits of the same hand
2. Methods of digital transplantation
   a. Using a toe
   b. Using a digit from the other hand
3. Methods of reconstruction using skin and bone grafts
   a. Skin grafting followed by bone grafting (Nicoladoni-Pierce)
   b. Simultaneous skin and bone grafting (Neuhauser-Albee)
   c. Skin grafting after transplant of a bone graft (Schepelmann-Cotte)
   d. Recent procedure using microsurgical techniques providing free sensitive skin flaps and bone grafts (Morrison, Foucher) (see Chapters 104 and 113)

Before retracing the historical aspects of these different methods, all of which have continued to improve and have their respective indications, we should like to state several principles applicable to all thumb reconstructions. A new thumb does not need to resemble morphologically a normal thumb in order to be functionally useful. However, it must fulfill the following conditions:

Length. The reconstructed thumb must not be longer than the old one. In fact it is better if it is shorter if it is going to be less mobile. Its length should be adapted to the mobility of the opposable elements.

Mobility. The new thumb should not have more articulations than a normal thumb. It can have the same number or may have fewer. The mobility of the first metacarpal is more important than that of the phalanges in re-establishing opposition with the palm and the other digits. This implies a mobile carpometacarpal joint, a supple web space, and active musculature.

Stability. A strong grip is possible only if the joints are stable. The more proximal the joint, the more important stability. Stability in the area of the grip is also important. The integuments at this level must be not only sufficiently padded but also fixed to the bone to avoid shear on the bone support.

Sensibility. It is essential that the gripping area have sensation. An insensitive thumb cannot judge the amount of force of the grip and cannot function without visual control.

Absence of Pain. A painful thumb is not used. The control of pain must always precede reconstruction.

HISTORICAL ASPECTS

The first attempt at functional restoration after mutilation of the thumb was performed by Huguier (1874), who in 1852 performed a phalangization of the first metacarpal on a man whose thumb phalanges had been ripped off by a horse bite.

"When one sees," he wrote, "that most of the advantages of the thumb are derived from its metacarpal, which in reality is its first phalanx, one may think, if it could be possible, of freeing the distal part of the bone by vertical section of the first web space to make it perform the same uses and functions as a thumb."

Phalangization of the first metacarpal remains a very useful procedure but mostly in cases of partial mutilation of the thumb. When the amputation is at the level of the metacarpal, a reconstruction has to be performed because phalangization is insufficient.

The first reconstructions seem to have been done in Lille by Guermonprez (1887): "For a long time, surgeons have been resigned to the loss of the most important digit of the hand. We think, however, that with the great advance of asepsis and anesthesia and given a sufficiently delicate surgical technique, it is no longer illogical to attempt restoration of the thumb by the use of one of the residual fingers." After a series of experiments on cadavers and macaque monkeys, Guermonprex performed three digital transfers onto the first metacarpal.

These transfers can be regarded as the precursors of pollicization. Although French surgeons had tried to reconstruct the thumb by using the remaining parts of the same hand, different methods of reconstruction were being worked out by Nicoladoni (1897), a surgeon from Gratz in Austria, methods that have developed along interesting pathways. Gueullette payed homage to Nicoladoni in these terms:

This surgeon began his works on Daumenplastik in 1895, and we are indebted to him for nearly all the procedures so far used. In 1897, he performed a graft of a finger from the other hand (the little finger); this is the procedure which was used by Joyce in 1917. In 1898, he performed a graft of the second toe. In 1899, he attempted to graft a nail for esthetic reasons onto a reconstructed thumb. In 1908, he theorized the possibility of a skin graft, together with a bone graft, a technique used by Noesske in the same year. The only missing procedure in the Nicoladoni repertoire was pollicization.

This was performed by his pupil, Lucksh (1903).

Microsurgery has put dactyloplasty back in its place in the form of free toe transplant.

A final step made possible by microsurgical techniques provides, as required, free sensitive skin flaps taken from the toes or elsewhere and bone grafts. We will describe for each of these methods the successive steps in their development.

REFERENCES

References for this chapter will be found following Chapter 101.

Chapter 98

RECONSTRUCTION OF THE THUMB BY SKIN TUBE, BONE GRAFT, AND SENSORY ISLAND FLAP TECHNIQUE

Raoul Tubiana

After complete amputation of the thumb, autoplastic procedures using adjacent skin are not sufficient to reconstruct a thumb of useful length.* Only flaps taken from a distant site can satisfy the cutaneous needs.

Nicoladoni, in 1897, was the first to describe this reconstructive technique, which sometimes bears his name. In fact, he was never able to complete his thumb reconstructions, for the three patients in whom it was planned refused to have a bone graft after the stage of skin flaps had been performed. Noesske in 1909 successfully carried out the first reconstruction of a thumb using an abdominal flap and a tibial graft.

This classic method has the advantage that no tissue is taken from the hand itself, but it does have two drawbacks that have restricted its utilization—the bone graft has a tendency to resorb, and the skin flap often shows trophic and ulcerative changes due to a poor blood supply and poor sensibility. These complications can be partially avoided if one uses a cross digit skin transplant with its neurovascular pedicle, which ensures better sensation in the pinch zone and a better blood supply (Littler, 1960; Moberg, 1955; Tubiana and Duparc, 1960).

SURGICAL TECHNIQUE

Such a procedure requires several stages (two to four), which can be combined in various ways (Fig. 98–1)—one or more for the skin flap, one for the bone graft, and one for the heterodigital skin island transplant. The stages differ according to different authors and different clinical cases. The development of techniques of free composite flaps has renewed interest in this procedure.

SKIN TUBE

The skin tube is taken from an area where the integuments are supple and relatively free of subcutaneous fatty tissue, excess of which allows too much sliding on the bone and an unstable grip. The donor area ideally should be a privileged zone, centered on a vascular pedicle, to allow a one stage application of the flap to the hand. Two such zones are the subclavicular (Fig. 98–2) and the inguinal areas. The "arterial" tube of Shaw and Payne, centered on the subcutaneous abdominal vessels, is reliable but, like all abdominal flaps, tends to be too thick. The submammary region, although not a privileged vascular zone, is sometimes chosen in female patients for cosmetic reasons.

To avoid the risk of necrosis, a single-pedicled flap, if not taken from a zone centered on a vascular pedicle, should be carefully measured so that its length is only just greater than its width. For a flap with two pedicles, the length may be twice the width. Implantation of the tube can be done in one or two stages, according to the length of the reconstructed thumb and the donor area. Because a thumb should not be too bulky, the flap will seldom be more than 6 or 7 cm.

1102

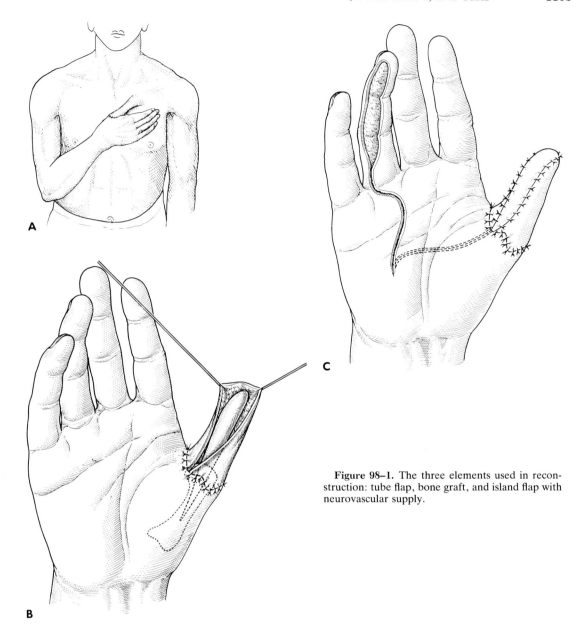

Figure 98–1. The three elements used in reconstruction: tube flap, bone graft, and island flap with neurovascular supply.

wide for an adult, the volume of the contralateral thumb being used as a model. One's calculation should include about 2 cm. for the length of the hinge of the tube. The flap can be thinned at this stage, leaving behind a thin layer of only subcutaneous flap. The "flap graft" of Colson seems unsuitable for such reconstructions, and its designer agrees with us on this point.

As an example, the inguinal flap used after an amputation of the thumb requires a tube 10 cm. long and 6 cm. wide. The pedicle is inferomedial; the axis of the flap runs obliquely, inferomedially in order to facilitate implantation on the ipsilateral aspect of the hand. The free end of the flap lies opposite the iliac crest, and this again facilitates the bone graft stage.

Use of a Subclavicular Flap. If one uses a subclavicular flap, the pedicle is superolateral and based in the contralateral acromial region. After partial thinning, the flap is tubed and its distal extremity checked for bleeding. Undermining of its edges may allow closure

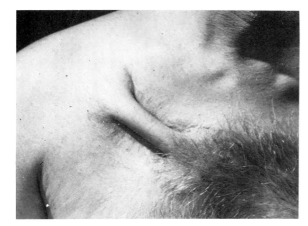

Figure 98–2. Infraclavicular skin tube flap.

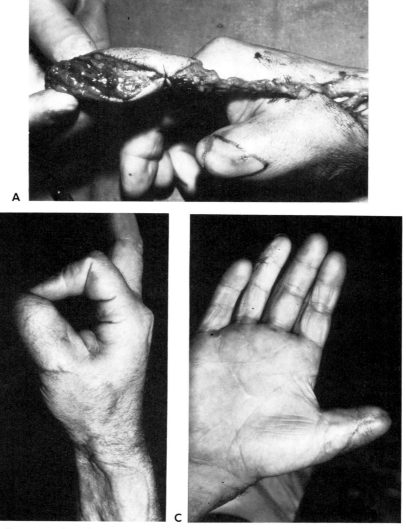

Figure 98–3. *A*, Reconstruction of the thumb in one stage with an island radial composite flap (bone and skin). *B* and *C*, Result.

of the donor area by suturing, but it is important that traction from the sutures, at the level of the pedicle of the flap, not interfere with its blood supply.

We will not discuss the technical details of skin flaps, which are dealt with in other chapters, but will only stress particular aspects relevant to thumb reconstruction. The suture line of the tubed flap on the thenar eminence should not be circumferential but elliptical or zigzag; this provides a broader base and counteracts the stenosing effects of scar contracture. The longitudinal suture of the tube should lie on the palmar side. The upper limb is immobilized in a comfortable position. The flap is left exposed as soon as possible to facilitate observation as well as mobilization of the adjacent fingers.

The use of a radial forearm ("Chinese") flap taken from the forearm in the region of the amputation considerably shortens these preparatory stages. This flap provides supple skin with poor sensitivity but a very good blood supply. It can even be used in an osteocutaneous composite flap, taking a fragment of the underlying distal extremity of the radius, offering the possibility of reconstruction of the thumb in a single stage (Foucher et al., 1984) (Fig. 98–3).

SEPARATION OF THE TUBE

Separation of the tube in our cases is carried out after four weeks. The sensory skin transplant can be performed at this stage; this has the added advantage of improving the nutrition of the tube (Littler, 1960). However, if inflammation persists, we like to postpone this maneuver until after the bone grafting; this is less traumatic to the fragile pedicle and provides extra skin covering, which is often needed. During that period a rigid dressing (we use a light plaster splint) must be applied to prevent the tube from bending.

THE BONE GRAFT AND CROSS FINGER SENSORY SKIN FLAP

Some authors insert the bone graft at the time when the flap is raised (Neuhauser, 1916; De Oliveira, 1970; Reid, 1960; Simonetta, 1975). In favorable cases only one more stage is required at which the inguinal flap is separated and the island flap applied;

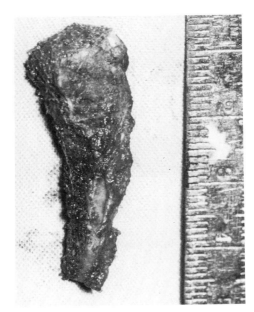

Figure 98–4. Bone graft taken from the iliac crest.

this means that the whole procedure is significantly shortened. Other authors prefer to wait for complete healing of the separated tube; it is then more supple and free of inflammation.

We like to use a solid graft from the iliac crest, 7 to 8 mm. thick. We preserve the periosteum on part of the crest so as to obtain a smoother bone surface under the future pulp. The length of the graft is adapted to each case to reconstruct a thumb 1 or 2 cm. shorter than its normal contralateral counterpart. The bone graft should be palette shaped (Fig. 98–4), present a flat gripping surface, and be about 1 cm. wide, not pointed and curved in toward the palm. It is better to aim for a subterminal pulpar pinch rather than a terminal one. The proximal end of the graft is shaped so that it can be fitted into the drilled medullary cavity of the first metacarpal (Figs. 98–5, 98–6). If the metacarpal fragment is too short and the trapeziometacarpal joint has become stiff, the graft can be embedded instead into the trapezium. Fixation can be completed by a transfixing Kirschner wire. To prevent gliding, the deep layer of the skin can be sutured to the periosteum (Chase, 1969).

The need to have a well molded bone graft mitigates against the simultaneous taking of skin and bone to preserve the vascularization of the bone graft, as had been advocated for the clavicle and the iliac crest (McGregor and

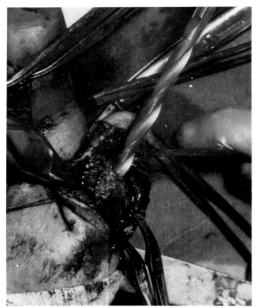

Figure 98–5. Preparation of the proximal part of the first metacarpal for insertion of the graft.

Simonetta, 1964). Similarly, the technique of placing the bone graft deep to the skin and later transplanting both bone and skin after the latter has established new vascular connections has now been largely discarded.

THE NEUROVASCULAR SKIN ISLAND TRANSPLANT

This technique, described in Volume II, provided a flap large enough to restore sensation to a broad surface on the neothumb as well as to cover its extremity. We commonly use half of the palmar surface of the two distal phalanges (Fig. 98–7). It is also possible to extend the donor area to the territory of the proximal phalanx; this was suggested by Hueston (1965), who also utilizes the territory of the dorsal branches of the collateral nerve, and thus obtains transplants 6 to 7 cm. long and more than 2 cm. wide. The donor zone must be chosen so that it produces a minimum of functional disturbance. We like to use the medial aspect of the middle finger not only because it provides the largest flap and has little gripping and pinching function, but also because, like the thumb, it is supplied by the median nerve, and that seems to facilitate the integration of the neothumb. If this area is not available, we use the medial skin of the ring finger, or any other sensory territory with the exception of the anterolateral aspects of the index and middle fingers.

The sensory flap is transferred by either the "open sky" or the tunneling technique (Fig. 98–8). The pedicle should be protected

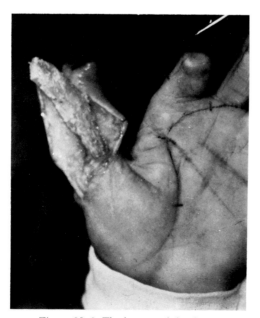

Figure 98–6. The bone graft in place.

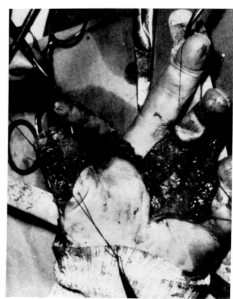

Figure 98–7. Preparation of a heterodigital skin island flap.

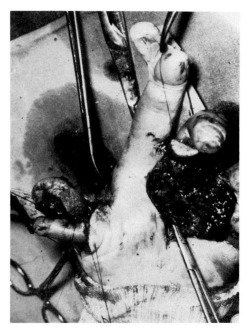

Figure 98–8. The island flap is transferred to the "new" thumb through a subcutaneous tunnel.

from tension and compression at all times. The skin transplant is laid on the palmar aspect of the neothumb, between the edges of the incised tube, on the pinch zone, i.e., the tip and anteromedial aspect of the neothumb. This extra skin also facilitates closure of the tube after the inclusion of the bone graft.

Rather than using an island of sensitive pulpar skin, some surgeons prefer to transfer the dorsal skin of the index finger.* Such flaps are certainly inferior in regard to blood supply, quality of sensation, and padding, but they sometimes can prove useful.

RESULTS

The chief handicap of the reconstructed thumb is that it possesses no joint of its own and depends for its mobility on that of the first carpometacarpal joint.

The sensation of the reconstructed thumb should be analyzed. In the territory of the island flap, sensation is not far from normal,

*See Chapter 39A in Volume II.

although two point discrimination is inferior to that of the normal thumb. At first the sensation is referred by the patient to the donor finger; progressively, after a variable length of time, comes a stage of "dual sensation" when the thumb and donor finger are perceived simultaneously. Although errors of perception do persist, experience has shown that the more the patient uses his neothumb, the more accurate his sensory interpretation becomes. Integration occurs much sooner in young active patients, but it is much delayed or never occurs if for some local (pain, instability) or psychological reason, the patient does not use his new digit. Such neurovascular skin flaps should be used only in hands that are free from pain.

Obviously the cross finger flap improves the nutrition of the neothumb. It brings with it both sensation and a blood supply; hence, the normal color of the new digit, the rapid consolidation of the bone graft, and the reduction in bone resorption (Fig. 98–9).

COMPLICATIONS

Successive technical improvements have significantly reduced the incidence of complications, and in trained hands this procedure has become extremely reliable. Risks do persist, however.

Infection. Early infection is rare, but recurrence remains a permanent danger if soft tissue or bone infection has followed the initial injury. At least six months should elapse between the last infectious episode and reconstruction.

Complications Involving the Tube Flap. Ulceration of the extremity can result because of poor vascularization of a badly designed skin flap, trauma to an anesthetic area, or pressure from too long a bone graft. Ulceration may lead to osteitis, which is difficult to treat and may result in loss of the bone graft. If the skin flap is too thick, the neothumb will be bulky and ungainly. Besides, a thick fat pad will tend to roll around the bony pivot and prevent the pinching of fine objects.

Complications Involving the Bone Graft. In addition to the faulty orientation of the graft mentioned earlier, there is the risk of instability and the possibility of resorption.

Pseudarthrosis results from inadequate fix-

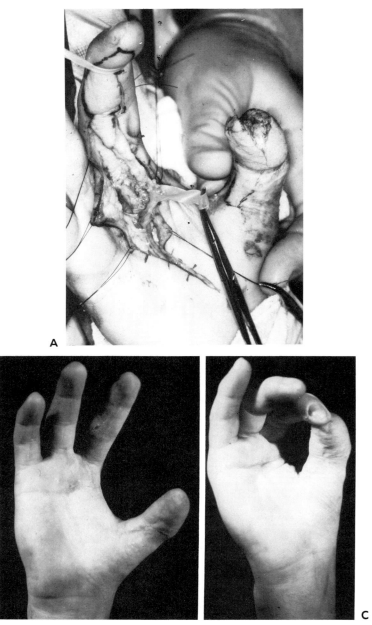

Figure 98–9. Complete amputation of the thumb and index finger, with persistence of the proximal half of the first metacarpal. *A*, Skin tube flap with iliac bone graft. A large island skin flap was taken from the long finger. The receptor zone for the neurovascularized flap is drawn on the anteromedial portion of the tube. The skin taken from the tube will be used to graft the donor area on the long finger. *B* and *C*, Early result. The neurovascularized flap is seen to cover the tip of the "new" thumb.

ation or ischemia. Introducing the graft into the metacarpal is not enough to produce a stable fixation, especially when the remaining metacarpal stump is short; fixation has to be reinforced by Kirschner wires or a screw, or by plating and adding small cancellous bone grafts.

Resorption of the bone graft depends on a variety of factors—the length and origin of the graft, the method of implantation into the skeleton, the blood supply, and possibly the quality of sensation in the overlying soft tissues, which will influence the utilization of the neothumb. Bone resorption is more frequent and more extensive when the neothumb is little used or not utilized at all.

Complications Involving the Sensory Island Flap. These are discussed in Chapter 39A in Volume II. Necrosis is rare, but painful hyperesthesia may result from tension in, or compression of, the pedicle. The quality of sensation and its integretation depend on utilization of the new thumb; it may even regress if the thumb is not utilized. Utilization is partly conditioned by the correct siting of the flap on the anteromedial aspect of the neothumb.

The majority of these complications are avoidable and should not weigh against the procedure that can provide a useful thumb without the use of another finger or toe.

As an example, here is the case of a surgeon and friend who suffered amputation of the thumb on a sailboat at the start of his brilliant career. He has been kind enough to summarize his own case:

At the end of July 1953 I was injured during a manoeuvre by a windlass. As shown in the x-ray (Fig. 98–10), the left thumb was amputated at the base of the proximal phalanx, with rupture of the flexor and extensor tendons of the thumb without any hematoma at the lower end of the forearm. I retrieved the amputated thumb, then being six hours from the coast. I reached the Giens Hospital where the surgeon, with my agreement, felt that the tendons had to be sacrificed and merely sutured the bone and the phalanx and the skin (Fig. 98–11), all in a plaster cast leaving the tip of the thumb visible. I first hoped that the bone might "take" and would then only need to be covered. Alas, three weeks later the end of my gangrenous thumb just hung limply from the suture when the plaster was removed. Paul Tessier suggested a tube flap using the skin of the medial surface of the arm, secondarily supported by an iliac graft, to provide a thumb which would not be normal in size but shorter by the length of the nail. I agreed and all went well. The repair was completed at

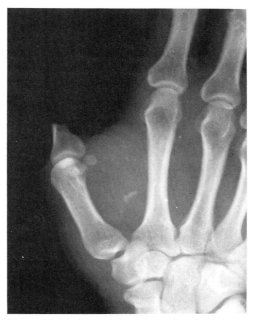

Figure 98–10. Amputation of the thumb at the base of the proximal phalanx.

the end of January 1954. Clinically, during the first six months I had the feeling of a wooden thumb, seemingly completely independent of the rest of me. Since I thought about it constantly, I felt that those near to me saw only my "new thumb." I tended to hide it from shame in my trouser pocket or jacket. However, without any

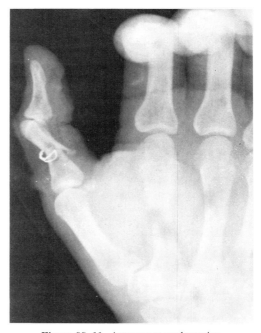

Figure 98–11. Attempt at replantation.

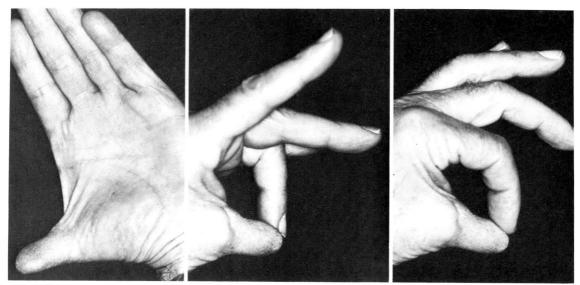

Figure 98–12. Reconstruction of the thumb by a skin tube and bone graft. The "thumb" 30 years later.

rehabilitation I was able to start operating again at the end of January 1954, only using gloves made-to-measure. Thanks to the concern of my chief, Alain Mouchet, who did not for an instant give the impression that all would not return to normal and who throughout my period of recovery had me assist him, I never really stopped working.

Tactile sensitivity came back in a year, and I can distinguish different materials without using the opposing finger. Cold sensitivity took a little longer to return and is now completely normal.

From time to time I have to shave the hairs which grow on the graft, but I have never taken any precautions when scrubbing before surgery.

As an anecdote, at the Congrès de Chirurgie in October 1954 attended by many foreign surgeons, I performed a hiatal hernia repair. My friend V. amused himself by asking the watchers if they had noticed anything unusual in the behavior of the surgeon. Nobody had noticed anything, and all were surprised to learn that the surgeon who had just operated in front of them had had no left thumb one year and a half before. I should also add that I have continued to sail (Fig. 98–12).

If a conclusion must be drawn for this case, without denying due merit to the surgeon who completely fulfilled his task, the use of an amputated hand depends essentially upon the willpower of the patient.

REFERENCES

Chase, R. A.: An alternate to pollicization in sub-total thumb reconstruction. Plast. Reconstr. Surg., 44:421, 1969.

De Oliveira, J. C.: Some aspects of thumb reconstruction. Br. J. Surg., 57:85–89, 1970.

Foucher, G., Merle, M., and Michon, J.: Le traitement de mutilations Traumatique du pouce. Aspects nouveaux et apport microchirurgical. Chirurgie, 110:56–62, 1984.

Hueston, J. T.: The extended neurovascular island flap. Br. J. Plast. Surg., 18:304, 1965.

Littler, J. W.: Neurovascular skin island transfer in reconstructive hand surgery. In Transactions of the International Society of Plastic Surgeons, Second Congress. Edinburgh, E. & S. Livingstone, 1960.

Littler, J. W.: On making a thumb: one hundred years of surgical effort. J. Hand Surg., 1:35–51, 1976.

McGregor, I. A., and Simonetta, C.: Reconstruction of thumb by composite bone. Br. J. Plast. Surg., 17:37, 1964.

Moberg, E.: Transfer of sensation. J. Bone Joint Surg., 37A:305, 1955.

Nicoladoni, C.: Daumenplastik. Wien. Klin. Wochenschr., 10:663, 1897.

Nicoladoni, C.: Daumenplastik und organischer ersatz der fingerspitze (anticheiroplastik und daktylo-plastik). Arch. Klin. Chir., 61:606, 1900.

Peacock, E. R., Jr.: Reconstruction of the thumb. In Flynn, J. E. (Editor): Hand Surgery. Baltimore, The Williams & Wilkins Company, 1966.

Reid, D. A. C.: Reconstruction of the thumb. J. Bone Joint Surg., 42B:648, 1960.

Simonetta, C.: Chirurgie réparatrice des pertes de substance et des amputations du pouce. Thesis, University of Lausanne, 1975.

Tubiana, R., and Duparc, J.: Opération palliative pour paralysie sensitive à la main. Mém. Ac. Chir., 24–25:666–670, 1959.

Tubiana, R., and Duparc, J.: Un procédé nouveau de reconstruction d'un pouce sensible. (Rapport de R. Merle d'Aubigné). Mém. Ac. Chir., 86:8–9, 1960.

Tubiana, R., and Ramadier, J. O.: Reconstruction autoplastique du pouce. Ann. Chir., 31:235, 1955.

Tubiana, R., Stack, G., and Hakstian, R. W.: Restoration of prehension after severe mutilations of the hand. J. Bone Joint Surg., 48B:455–473, 1966.

Chapter 99

POLLICIZATIONS

Raoul Tubiana

Pollicization consists of transferring a digit to replace the thumb. We shall be concerned here only with pollicizations performed after traumatic amputations; pollicizations for congenital absence of the thumb are considered in Volume IV. They raise different problems of indications and techniques for a number of reasons: The child adapts more readily to his infirmity, there is better integration at a young age, and there is none of the scar tissue that complicates traumatic amputations. Finally, most of the pollicizations carried out for traumatic amputations are only partial, whereas almost all pollicizations for congenital absence of the thumb are total and require reconstruction of a carpometacarpal joint.

HISTORICAL REVIEW

It took a number of successive steps to arrive at a reliable technique of pollicization. First there were the attempts of Guermonprez at transferring "digital remnants" to the first metacarpal. The first recorded case is interesting and is reported here:

On the 11th April, 1885, Marie de B. . ., a carder aged 45, made the mistake of removing some foreign bodies while her machine was on, at the very moment when the ribbon was running over the teasle. Her thumb got caught in the material.

The patient was taken to the Hopital de la Charité in Lille where her dangling index finger was amputated . . .

One month after the accident, her thumb was reconstructed from the remnants of the middle finger, after the procedure had been tried several times on a cadaver. . . The patient was anesthetized with chloroform, an Esmarch band applied, and the hand fixed on a small sandbag. The operation was then carried out under aseptic con-

ditions. . . . The third interdigital space was dissected to free the middle finger over a distance of 6 to 8 mm. from the lowest palmar crease, and this without damaging the blood vessels (Fig. 99–1). The newly created thumb was then carried to a position perpendicular to the metacarpal (Fig. 99–2). . . .

An unsuccessful attempt was made to suture the glenosesamoidal ligament of the thumb to the phalangeal portion of the extensor tendon of the middle finger. . . .

Four months after the accident, when all edema had disappeared, the patient was anesthetized once more. The scar was excised, the glenosesamoidal ligament and the tendon of the middle finger were exposed, and the fifth stage was completed without an Esmarch bandage and without hemorrhage. The ligament and tendon were secured to each other with three buried sutures of "Florence hair." The new thumb was straightened and its position corrected. . . . The ligament and tendon were secured to each other with three buried sutures.

This woman has now resumed her previous occupation as a carder. The new thumb, however, is not perfect (Fig. 99–3); it cannot flex, extend, or oppose, but though immobile it constitutes a strong support opposite the ring and little fingers.

Soon thereafter, Guermonprez performed two more digital transpositions, and his pupil Hanotte reported the three cases in a thesis published in Lyon in 1888.

A few years later, in 1903, Lucksh, a pupil of Nicoladoni, presented a patient whose thumb had been lost and replaced by the adjacent index finger. The transposition was performed by the pedicled flap technique. The palmar cutaneous bridge had been divided after three weeks and the transposed finger was anesthetic.

Somewhat later, Hulsmann (1919) and then Porzelt (1935) tried to preserve sensation by transferring the two distal phalanges of an adjacent finger to the first metacarpal.

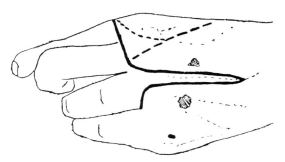

Figure 99–1. Lines of incision (Guermonprez).

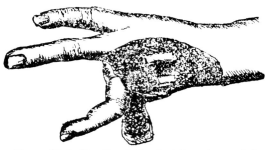

Figure 99–2. Results of the first five stages of the operation (Guermonprez).

They preserved two pedicles (palmar and dorsal) after excising the bone from the proximal phalanx. The first web space was inevitably contracted—the operation, as Hilgenfeldt later pointed out, consisting of "translation of a finger" to the neighboring metacarpal (fingerverschiebung).

In 1919 Noesske transferred an index finger along with part of its metacarpal to the thumb, and Perthes in 1921 carried the whole of the ray of the index finger to replace the first ray. He thus created a long triphalangeal thumb but was unable to make it extend because the intrinsic muscles had been resected.

In 1929 Bunnell pollicized an index finger amputated at the proximal phalanx. He transferred the second metacarpal along with the proximal phalanx onto the trapezium and thus obtained a sensitive uniphalangeal thumb equipped with a mobile joint.

The following stages led to a technique for pollicizing any of the four fingers to create a thumb that is biphalangeal, mobile, sensitive, stable, and opposable. A number of surgeons attempted such ambitious reconstructions with variable degrees of success, but the real progress followed the work of three surgeons who described their technique in detail and analyzed their results—Hilgenfeldt, Gosset, and Littler.

From 1943 onward Hilgenfeldt carried out a series of pollicizations, transferring one of the other digits, usually the middle finger.

He was kind enough to send us his case reports translated into French, and we wish to express our grateful thanks. In 1950 he summed up the immense experience he had acquired and outlined the guiding principles for every pollicization. He stressed the importance of mobility, not so much of the phalanges but mostly of the metacarpal, which implies a mobile trapeziometacarpal joint and a free commissure. Sensation, both cutaneous and "organic," is equally important.

Gosset in 1949 published his technique for pollicization of the index finger. He described an original incision pattern that produced a palm pedicled commissural flap, which has since been adopted by most surgeons (Fig. 99–4). Later he developed a preference for pollicizing the ring finger and published his technique (1964) and results (1972; thesis by Langlais).

In 1952 Littler applied the principle of neurovascular island transplantation for digital transfers. Greater room for maneuvering was obtained by recessing the cutaneous bridge. In Chapter 100 he describes his method of index finger pollicization.

PRINCIPLES OF THE METHOD

Any finger can be transferred to replace the thumb. We shall discuss the advantages of each digit in turn, but first we shall con-

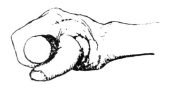
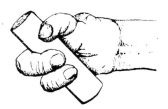

Figure 99–3. Grasping a large object (Guermonprez).

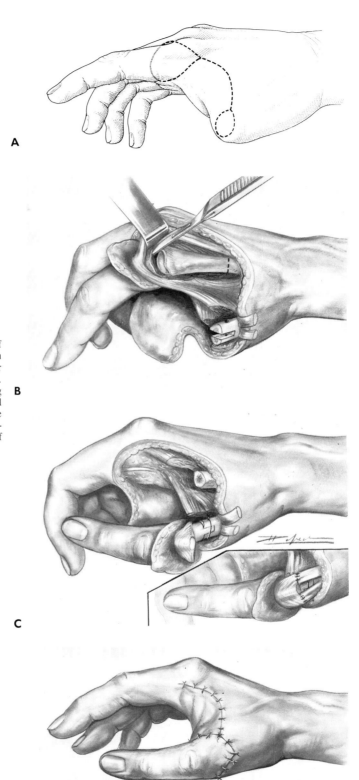

Figure 99–4. Technique of pollicization of the index finger by J. Gosset. *A*, Incision line to provide a dorsal flap with a palmar pedicle. *B*, The index finger is disarticulated. *C*, Bone and tendon arrangement; lodging of a phalangeal tendon into a metacarpal mortice. The two extensor tendons of the thumb are transferred to the extensor apparatus of the index finger. *D*, Suture of skin flaps at the end of the operation.

sider those principles that apply to all pollicizations.

THE INCISIONS

The incisions must be so designed to respect or reconstruct a good commissure for the neothumb. Hilgenfeldt (1950) advocated a narrow longitudinal palmar pedicle anterior to the vascular pedicles and flexor tendons of the pollicized finger. However, this cutaneous bridge is not really necessary according to Littler (1952), who prefers a digital "island" transfer with the neurovascular bundles. In traumatic amputations pollicization is often complicated by extensive scar formation. Extra skin is then required in the form of a graft or flap.

BLOOD SUPPLY, SENSATION, AND MOBILITY

The pollicized finger must have a good blood supply, sensation, and mobility and must be of an adequate length. All these points are very important.

Blood Supply. Dissection of the neurovascular bundles is best carried out under magnification. It is obviously preferable for the transferred finger to have intact vascular pedicles, but a finger can be pollicized even if one of its collateral arteries has been destroyed, and we ourselves have done it with success more than once. Roullet (1971) went further when he described a method of transposition of the index finger when the two palmar pedicles have been destroyed. The blood supply comes from the deep interosseous artery when the index finger is transferred *en masse* along with its dorsal and palmar interosseous muscles; Roullet describes this technique in Chapter 102. A preoperative angiogram can be of assistance prior to the transfer of an injured finger.

The venous return occurs via the small deep veins that accompany the palmar arteries. It is advisable, when possible, to try to preserve one or two dorsal veins, but this is only feasible when the index finger is transferred (Fig. 99–5). If no vein can be carried along with the transfer, there remains the possibility of a venous microanastomosis.

Sensation. The pollicized finger should be painless but it should have sensation. Any

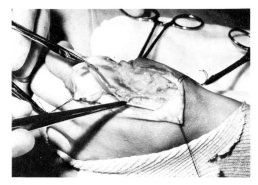

Figure 99–5. With pollicization of the index finger, it is possible to preserve the dorsal subcutaneous veins.

painful neuroma must be treated, whether in the transferable finger or stump of the thumb. One should be aware that at first the transferred finger is not perceived as a thumb but retains its individuality. As with heterodigital skin transplants, therefore, there is some difficulty in utilization that requires a period of adaptation; this depends essentially on the mobility of the new thumb and the extent to which it is used. Hilgenfeldt (1950) claims that integration of the neothumb is improved if the flexor pollicis longus is united to the flexor digitorum profundus of the pollicized finger.

Length and Mobility. The transferred finger should be approximately the same length as the contralateral thumb (the tip of the thumb normally does not quite reach the proximal interphalangeal joint of the index finger). It should not be longer or have more than two phalanges. The length of the transfer depends on the level of amputation. Our practice, as with most other surgeons, is to adjust the length of the transfer at the expense of its proximal part.

Several factors must be taken into account here, namely, the presence or absence of the first metacarpal and the state of the transferred finger, whether intact or injured. The techniques differ appreciably when pollicization is undertaken for partial as opposed to total loss of the first ray (Fig. 99–6). When part of the first metacarpal has been spared and the transferred finger is of normal length, the proximal phalanx of the latter is trimmed down to produce a thumb of normal length. Its proximal interphalangeal joint will replace the metacarpophalangeal joint, and its distal interphalangeal joint will become the inter

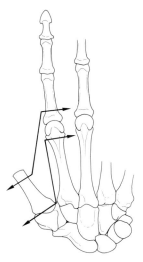

Figure 99–6. Adjustment of the length of the pollicized fingers. The length of the transferred digit depends upon the length of residual first ray skeleton. When a proximal portion of the first metacarpal persists, only the phalanges of the pollicized digit are transferred. The proximal interphalangeal joint will become the metacarpophalangeal joint of the new thumb. If the entire first metacarpal is absent, the whole finger is transferred. The metacarpophalangeal joint of the finger, particularly in the child, can be used to replace the first carpometacarpal joint.

phalangeal joint of the thumb. The néothumb thus will have a terminal phalanx onto which is inserted the flexor digitorum profundus tendon (useful for precision grip) and which carries a nail (a cosmetically important aspect). Some surgeons prefer to shorten the distal rather than the proximal phalanx to reduce laxity of the extrinsic tendons. Thus Butler (1964) excises the distal phalanx but preserves the nail and its matrix on a pedicle, which is transposed to the middle phalanx. If the pollicized finger has itself been injured and has lost its distal phalanx, its metacarpophalangeal joint is preserved and the metacarpal trimmed as required.

When the thumb and its metacarpal have been totally destroyed, the metacarpophalangeal joint of the pollicized finger may be used to reconstruct a trapeziometacarpal joint. This operation is frequently performed in young children for congenital absence of the thumb; it will be described in detail later. The hyperextension of the basal metacarpophalangeal articulation may be an embarrassing sequel (Buck-Gramcko, 1971, 1977). It can be prevented by fixing the metacarpal head in flexion between 70 and 90 degrees.

We have performed this operation in children and in young adults after traumatic mutilations that had resulted in total loss or stiffness of the trapeziometacarpal joint.

In the manual worker one may be justified in aiming for good stability rather than mobility of the basal joint in cases in which the interphalangeal joint of the transferred finger has retained its mobility. The base of the proximal phalanx of the pollicized finger is buried in the carpal mass with an anteposition of about 40 degrees and its rotation adjusted so that the pulp can oppose that of the remaining fingers. This arthrodesis undoubtedly restricts the range of movement of the neothumb, especially the movements of anteposition and retroposition. This constitutes a distinct disadvantage when the other opposable digits themselves have reduced mobility. Gosset (1974) put forward the idea of preserving, with the base of the proximal phalanx, a capsular ring, which is sutured to the fibrous tissue around the trapezium. The bones are held together with a Kirschner wire; a fibrous pseudarthrosis results, which in two of his patients provided useful mobility.

We ourselves used an articular prosthesis at the base of the thumb on two occasions. In the first case we performed a trapeziectomy in a severely damaged carpus and replaced the bone with a Swanson silicone trapezium implant. The implant became subluxed and the resulting mobility was mediocre, but there was no residual pain. It may have been better to use the Caffinière ball and socket coupled prosthesis, which was not available at the time but which has been used since (Fig. 99–7). In the second case we used a large digital Swanson implant, one of whose stems was implanted in the proximal phalanx and the other in the proximal end of the first metacarpal whose basal joint was stiff. When seen five years later, the patient had a stable and mobile thumb and had resumed his occupation as an agricultural worker.

THE BONES

When the bones are fixed at the level of the first metacarpal, the rotation must always be carefully adjusted to allow the pulps to face the neothumb in opposition. A scratch on the bone before its resection serves as a useful landmark when rotation is applied. A

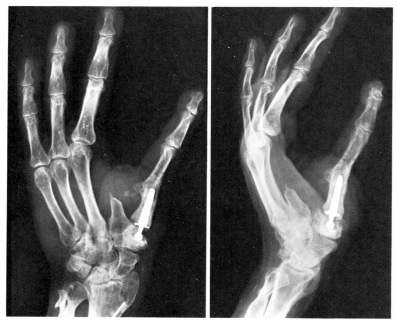

Figure 99–7. Pollicization of the index finger. A La Caffinière trapeziometacarpal prosthesis is used. (Patient of Dr. Hautier.)

90 degree rotation, which is often advocated, is definitely insufficient; a 130 degree rotation of the pollicized finger is usually required to ensure opposition with the middle and ring fingers (Fig. 99–8). Correct positioning of the pollicized finger should be feasible without tension; the bones may require further shortening if the tension is too great. This of course is done before the bones are fixed. The overall arrangement of the bones depends on whether the metacarpal has been totally or partially destroyed.

Fixation can be secured by two Kirschner wires inserted crosswise (Fig. 99–9). Littler (1953) uses an intramedullary graft, which, once rotation has been applied, is fixed to the shafts by two horizontal Kirschner wires (Fig. 99–10). The fitting of a phalangeal tenon into a metacarpal mortice, as advocated by Gosset (1949), makes positional adjustments more difficult (Fig. 99–4C). Another solution is internal fixation by means of a small metal plate.

Musculotendinous Attachments

It is essential that the neothumb be provided with a musculature; this is probably the most complex part of the operation. Dissection and bone fixation require great care, but tendon arrangement also requires imagination for the problems are different for each case.

One must restore not only the extrinsic musculature but also the intrinsic muscles, which are essential for the stability and mobility of the phalanges.

There are various ways of reactivating the musculature of the neothumb; the choice depends on the local conditions and espe-

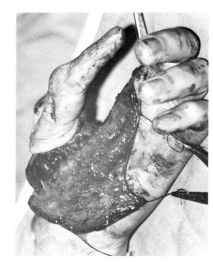

Figure 99–8. Adjustment of rotation of the pollicized digit.

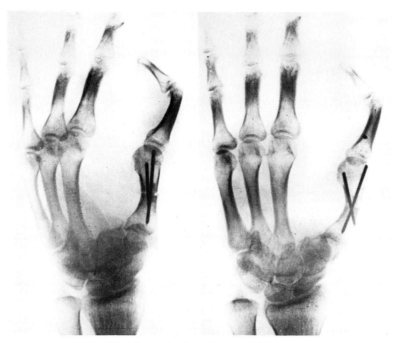

Figure 99–9. Bone fixation using two Kirschner wires.

cially on whether the thenar muscles have been destroyed.

Let us now consider how the main movements of the thumb can be restored.

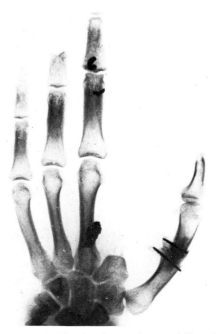

Figure 99–10. Fixation by an intramedullary bone graft fixed by two transverse parallel Kirschner wires.

Extension. The simple transfer of an extensor of the thumb to the extensor communis of the transferred finger is insufficient because it will result in an extensor lag of the distal phalanges. The intrinsic muscles must be replaced, and this can be done in several ways. If the thenar muscles have survived, the adductor pollicis is reattached to the palmar interosseus muscle and the abductor pollicis to the dorsal interosseus muscle (Fig. 99–11).

However, if the thenar musculature has been destroyed, one can use the extensors of the thumb and of the pollicized finger (Fig. 99–12). The transfer of the index finger allows its interosseous muscle to be used. One carefully frees them with a periosteal rongeur from the second metacarpal and by dividing their distal insertions on the base of the first phalanx as well as their dorsal aponeurotic expansions. When the osteosynthesis has been performed, the lateral extensor tendons of the index finger are separated from the central extensor tendon as far as the level of the old proximal interphalangeal joint (at the metacarpophalangeal joint of the new thumb) (Figs. 99–13, 99–14). These bands (the lateral extensor tendons) are threaded and adjusted, the radial band to the first dorsal interosseous muscle and the ulnar band to the first palmar interosseous muscle, which then assume the

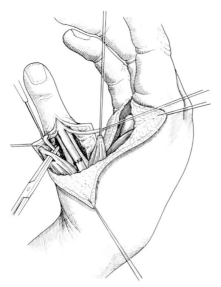

Figure 99–11. Re-establishment of the extensor apparatus. Simple suture of the extensor communis tendon of the finger to the long extensor of the thumb is not sufficient. The action of the intrinsic muscles must be restored. If the thenar muscles are still in place, as is the case here, the lateral extensor tendons are sutured on the underside to the adductor and on the radial side to abductor pollicis brevis.

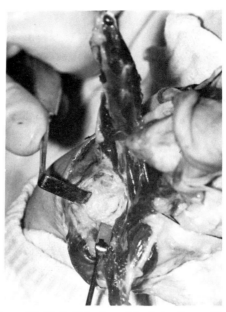

Figure 99–13. Pollicization of the index finger. *Center*, the extremity of the stump of the first metacarpal is exposed between two retractors. *Top*, the first dorsal interosseous muscle, which will be transferred to the ulnar lateral extensor tendon of the index finger to function as the first palmar interosseous. *Bottom*, the adductor muscles of the thumb, abductor pollicis brevis and flexor pollicis brevis, which will also be used to re-establish opposition and reinforce extension of the thumb.

roles of an abductor and an adductor of the thumb, respectively.

Flexion. Flexion is restored by means of the flexor tendons, which are transferred along with the finger after their fibrous sheaths have been divided at the level of the metacarpophalangeal joint. Flexion is usually satisfactory after pollicization of a partially amputated finger. The muscles will adapt progressively, and their shortening is not a

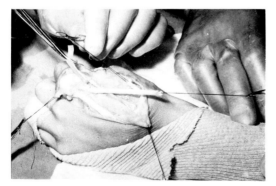

Figure 99–12. In this pollicization of the index finger, the radial neurovascular bundle (around which a rubber loop is passed) is retracted by a forceps, exposing the tendon of the first dorsal interosseous muscle. The proximal part of the muscle, pulled by a traction stitch, can be seen at the bottom of the photograph.

problem in children. In the adult, when the proximal phalanx has been used to replace the metacarpal with a resulting shortening of the transferred finger of, say, 4 to 5 cm., it may be necessary to reintervene a few months after the pollicization to readjust the length of the finger flexors in the forearm. When there is little or no scar tissue at the wrist, the flexor profundus tendon of the pollicized finger is divided in the forearm, pulled down to the palm, and rerouted proximally along the course of flexor pollicis. It is then resutured, preferably to the tendon of flexor pollicis longus at the musculotendinous junction. The flexor superficialis is independent and adapts readily; only rarely must it be shortened in the forearm.

Adduction. Adduction in the pollicized finger depends on one utilizable intrinsic muscle and the long muscles. It must be counterbalanced by means of abductors; otherwise the pollicized finger will become (as happens too often) uselessly fixed in adduction.

Restoration of Anteposition. It may be necessary to restore anteposition when the

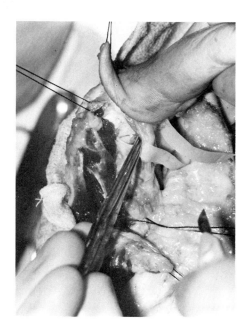

Figure 99–14. When the thenar muscles are destroyed, the best use must be made of the extrinsic muscles of the index finger and thumb and of the usable interosseous muscles. Here, the tendon of the extensor communis indicis is divided at the level of the wrist and will be sutured to the tendon of the long extensor of the thumb, which is identified by a traction stitch. The tendon of the extensor proprius indicis is divided at the level of the metacarpophalangeal joint and passed through the tendon of the first palmar interosseous (identified by a traction stitch) and through an ulnar lateral extensor tendon of the transferred index.

lateral thenar muscles have been destroyed. Buck-Gramcko (1977), in total reconstructions of the first ray, sections the extensor communis of the index finger and sutures its proximal end to the base of the proximal phalanx (which is attached to the first metacarpal). He thus reconstructs a long abductor of the thumb.

Harrison (1964) has suggested the use of the extensor tendon of the pollicized finger to restore opposition, the tendon being divided in the forearm, reflected around a pulley, and sutured to a motor muscle. Other solutions consist of transferring another tendon, or even the abductor digiti minimi muscle; the latter solution has the added advantage of restoring the contour of the thenar eminence.

CHOICE OF FINGER FOR TRANSFER

Any of the four fingers can be pollicized, and one should choose the least useful and the one whose loss will least affect the overall function of the hand. Various authors interpret these "rules" in different ways.

Index Finger. Transfer of the index finger enables the surgeon to preserve two dorsal veins; the digital pedicle is displaced without crossing or angulation. The architecture of the hand is minimally altered by displacement of a peripheral digit. Muscular reactivation is made easier by the presence of two long extensors and the possibility of using the two interosseous muscles (dorsal and palmar). All these advantages explain why the index finger is most often pollicized, especially when one wishes to reconstruct a first ray that has been totally destroyed (Fig. 99–15).

However, the commissure reconstructed by means of a dorsal flap is deeper than normal. It is undeniable that the index finger plays an important part in thumb-finger grip as well as in pulp to pulp grip and lateral grip. Although substitution by the middle finger is possible, opposition of the pollicized index finger to the middle finger requires a greater range of mobility than opposition of a neo-thumb to an intact index finger.

Middle Finger. The middle finger is Hilgenfeldt's preference for pollicization (1950), and he justifies his choice with the following arguments: Its volume is closest to that of the thumb. In power grip, the more peripheral index and little fingers are the most useful. The little finger is less powerful than the index finger and requires the adjacent ring finger to stabilize it; hence, his preference for the middle finger.

Transfer of the central digit, however, is not without repercussions on the balance of the hand. Resection of the head of the third metacarpal may lead to rotation and overriding of its neighbors; preservation of the head

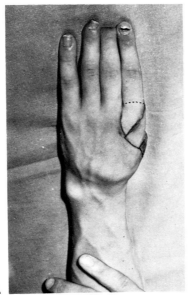 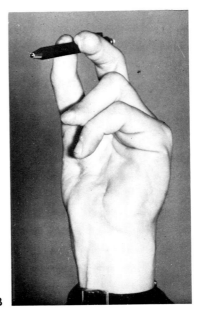

Figure 99–15. Complete amputation of the first ray and pollicization of the index finger. *A*, Incision lines. *B*, Results.

is cosmetically less acceptable. It is therefore advisable when the middle finger is pollicized to transfer the ray of the index finger onto the third metacarpal.

Ring Finger. The ring finger, whose use is advocated by Le Tac (1952), is also preferred by Gosset (1964) and an ever increasing number of surgeons. It is functionally relatively less important than its fellows and is far enough from the thumb so that its transfer can restore partial tension to the flexors. Its transfer also causes less alteration of the architecture of the hand, since the great mobility of the fifth metacarpophalangeal joint to some extent can approximate the little finger to the middle finger.

Little Finger. Finally, the little finger, although slender, can be pollicized. Contrary to widespread belief, it is a far from unimportant digit, and its transfer markedly reduces the stability of the palmar grip. Although we would not choose it for transfer in preference to the other fingers, as Kelleher and Sullivan (1958) have done, we must concede that its pollicization could be envisaged.

All these arguments in favor of pollicization of one digit or another when one is transfering a healthy digit are of value. Under these circumstances the ring and index fingers are the ones usually transferred, and the techniques for their pollicization will be described. However, sometimes a digit has been partially amputated and thus the question of its being used as a transfer arises. These problems are discussed in the following chapters.

REFERENCES

References for this chapter will be found following Chapter 101.

Chapter 100

POLLICIZATION OF THE INDEX FINGER

W. LITTLER

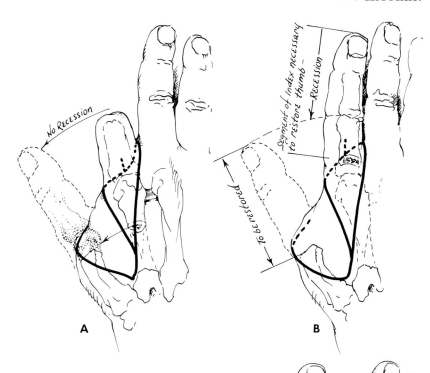

Figure 100–1. *A,* An index finger amputated at the proximal interphalangeal level requires no recession when transposed to substitute for a thumb lost proximal to the metacarpal head. Enough of the second metacarpal is preserved to restore length when joined through an intramedullary bone graft to the first metacarpal remnant (bone graft obtained from resected portion of the second metacarpal). *B,* When a normal index finger is utilized, a recession to the proximal interphalangeal level is required, approximately 4.5 cm. A length of index finger corresponding to the length of the thumb lost is transposed on its neurovascular pedicle together with the flexor and extensor tendons. The first metacarpal will in this case be joined to the proximal phalanx. Skin incisions are made encircling the digit at the metacarpophalangeal level and forming a (volar based) triangular dorsal flap for exposure and preservation of the web. *C,* Since the original description, simulating that of Gosset (1949), the larger triangular dorsal interosseous flap has been broken to form two smaller but safer flaps, one volar based and the other dorsal based.

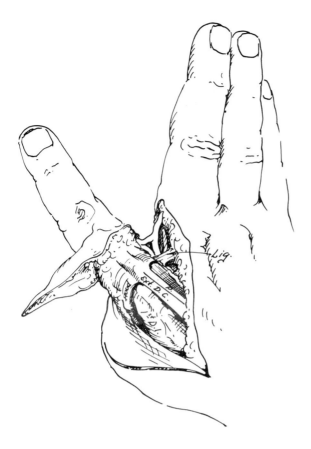

Figure 100–2. Dorsal exposure showing the extensor tendons and aponeurosis (4 T.D.C.), the intermetacarpal neck ligament (to be divided), and the common volar artery with its digital branches.

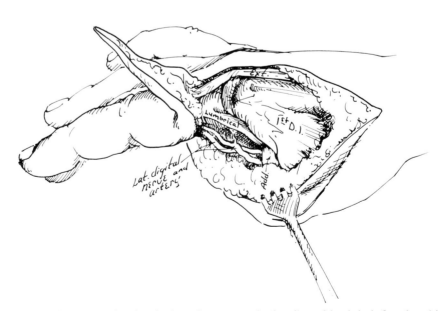

Figure 100–3. Lateral exposure showing the lateral neurovascular bundle and lumbrical, first dorsal interosseous, and adductor muscles. The lateral digital artery often originates from the princeps pollicis.

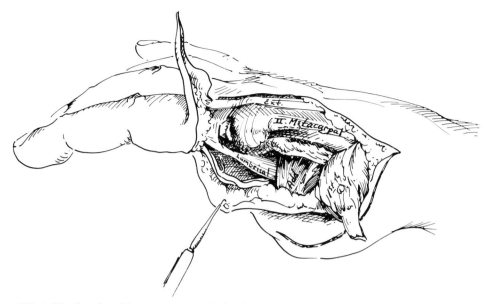

Figure 100–4. The first dorsal interosseous muscle has been detached from its second metacarpal and insertion on the proximal phalanx. The adductor pollicis and lumbrical muscles are more clearly defined.

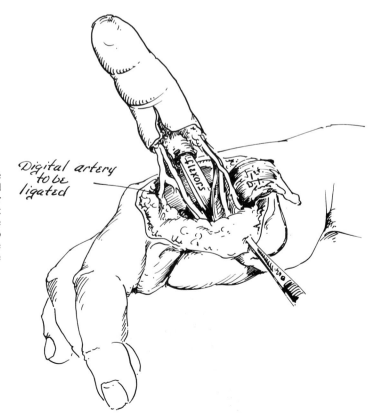

Figure 100–5. Volar aspect of the dissection demonstrating the radial and ulnar neurovascular bundles, the flexor tendons, and the lumbrical muscles. It is essential at this point to section the vertical septa of the palmar fascia to facilitate the lateral shifting of these structures. The digital artery to the middle finger is ligated.

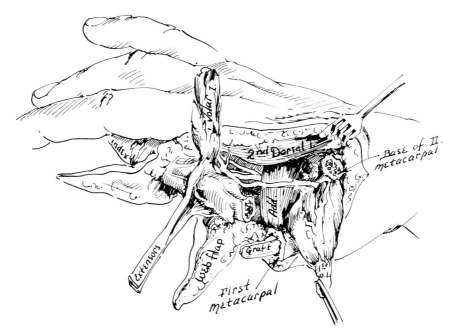

Figure 100–6. Completed dissection from the dorsum. The second metacarpal shaft has been resected and fashioned for use as an intramedullary graft to unite the transposed phalangeal unit to the first metacarpal. The adductor pollicis muscle forms the floor of this dissection and occupies an intermediate relationship between the extensor tendons and metacarpal dorsally and the flexor tendons and neurovascular bundles ventrally. For illustrative purposes, the extensors are divided. The volar interosseous muscle is generally discarded, although when the digit is recessed it can be preserved to function as an adductor by separating its lateral tendinous band from the dorsal aponeurosis and proximal phalanx. The drawing shows the distal portion of the second metacarpal; however, this is discarded and a normal finger is used.

Figure 100–7. *A* and *B*, Completed transposition. The first metacarpal is firmly joined to the proximal phalanx of the index fingers through an intramedullary bone graft and oblique Kirschner wire in approximately 10 degrees of flexion and pronation. This restores a more natural longitudinal arch and better opposition at this stage, and end-to-end suture should be made between the extensor pollicis longus and the extensor digitorum communis. The flexor pollicis longus can be sutured to the index profundus at a later date (three to four months) to provide greater strength and independence. *C*, Closure of flaps following transposition of finger.

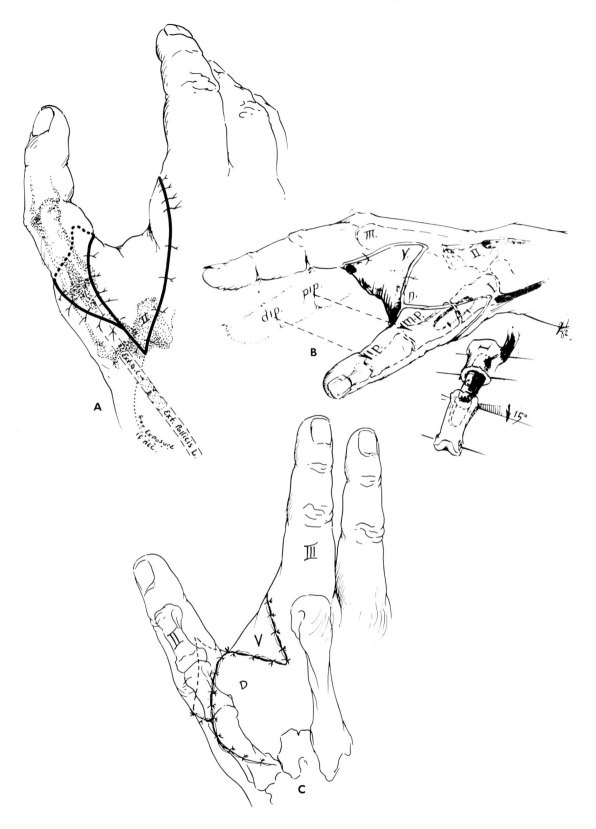

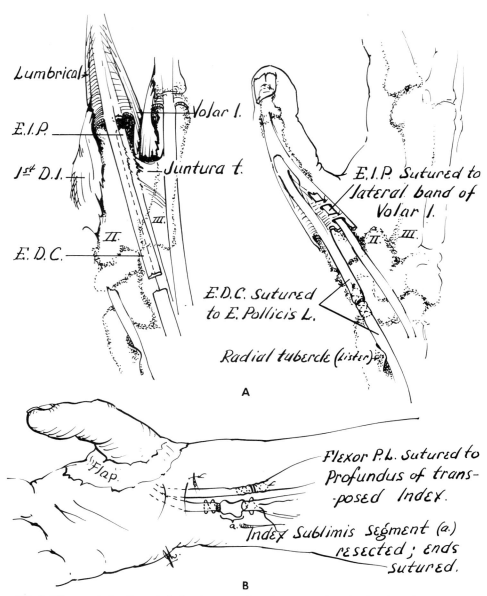

Figure 100–8. When an index finger is isolated, recessed, and transposed to the thumb position, the intrinsic and extrinsic musculature can suffer a marked loss of amplitude. In some cases a readjustment of tendon length (and insertion) is therefore important if power and a full range of extension and flexion are to be regained. *A,* The important intrinsic interphalangeal extension is retained through a suture of the extensor indicis proprius tendon to that of the volar interosseous (ulnar lateral band of index extensor aponeurosis). The extensor digitorum communis is sutured to the extensor pollicis longus. *B,* More independence and flexor power are gained at a second stage by suturing the flexor pollicis longus to the index profundus and by resecting an appropriate segment from the index sublimis tendon.

Illustration continued on opposite page

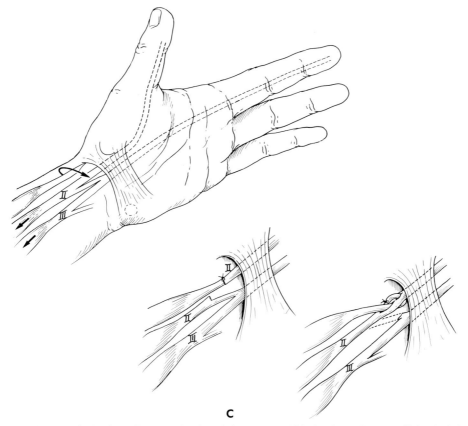

C

Figure 100–8 *Continued. C,* If the flexor profundus of the transposed index finger is not sufficiently independent of the adjacent (long, middle) finger, any flexor junctotum tendinum must be released. *D,* Index attachment must be released if following transfer of the normal (cortically controlled) long thumb flexor to the index profundus, independent terminal phalangeal flexion (of the transposed index finger) is to be gained.

Chapter 101

OTHER TECHNIQUES OF POLLICIZATION

RAOUL TUBIANA

Even if pollicization of the index finger has been the most common method used in our experience, it is important to understand techniques for pollicization of the other digits (Fig. 101–1). We shall therefore describe the procedure for the ring finger, which is the second most commonly used; the techniques for pollicization of the middle and little fingers differ only in minor detail.

POLLICIZATION OF THE RING FINGER

The technique for pollicization of the ring finger, which has been well described by Gosset (1964, 1975), follows in principle the one described by Hilgenfeldt (1950) for pollicization of the middle finger (Figs. 101–2 to 101–5).

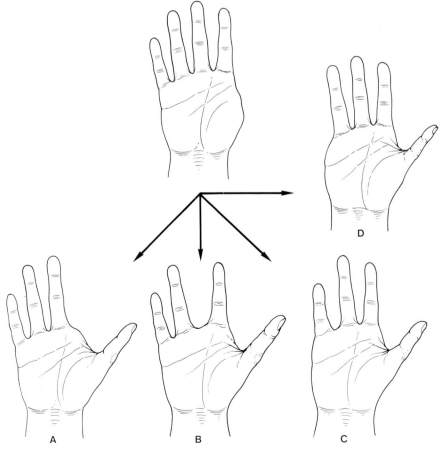

Figure 101–1. All the fingers can be pollicized.

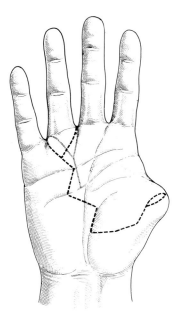

Figure 101–2. Pollicization of the ring finger. Incision lines.

Skin Incisions

The straight thenar incision runs along the medial border of the thenar eminence until it reaches the vertical axis of the third intermetacarpal space. The circular incision at the

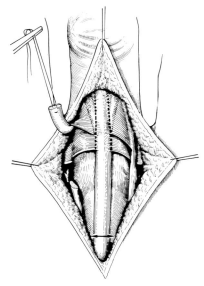

Figure 101–4. Dorsal view. The common extensor tendon is divided over the course of the metacarpophalangeal joint. The interosseous tendons are also divided and retracted before being reattached.

base of the ring finger delineates a proximally pointed V shaped dorsal flap, which overlaps the line of the metacarpophalangeal joint.

The palmar incision, made along a longi-

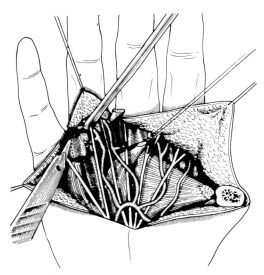

Figure 101–3. Palmar stage. The common palmar digital nerves of the third and fourth spaces have been split. The medial proper palmar artery of the long finger and the lateral proper palmar artery of the little finger have been divided. Division of the transverse intermetacarpal ligament on either side of the pollicized digit is accomplished. The lumbrical canal is opened and the lumbrical tendon is divided.

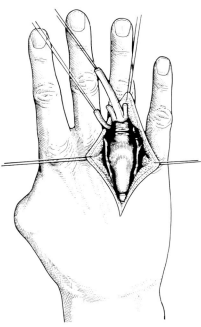

Figure 101–5. Dorsal stage. The dorsal veins of the ring finger are divided. The extensor communis tendon is divided at about 3 cm. proximal to the metacarpophalangeal joint. The proximal phalanx is sectioned at the required length, preserving the two tendons of the interosseous muscles inserted into its base.

tudinal axis, runs a curvilinear or zigzag course to avoid a perpendicular crossing of the flexion creases. It runs from the base of the ring finger to the thenar incision in the axis of the fourth metacarpal. The thenar and palmar incisions form a V whose two arms are of approximately equal lengths. We do not regard as essential the long narrow (1 cm. wide) palmar skin flap that runs from the base of the finger to the heel of the hand, which Hilgenfeldt uses in pollicization of the middle finger and Gosset in pollicization of the ring finger "in order to spare gliding elements of the cutaneotendinous pedicle."

PREPARING THE STUMP OF THE THUMB

After resection of the neuromas of the collateral nerves of the thumb in healthy tissue, the bed is prepared for the tendinous neurovascular pedicle of the ring finger. This pedicle follows the course of the resected flexor pollicis longus. The next step consists of searching for the extremities of the divided extensor tendons on the dorsum of the thumb. The extremity of the first metacarpal is prepared to receive the proximal phalanx of the transposed ring finger.

PREPARING THE DIGIT FOR POLLICIZATION

Palmar Stage. The skin of the intermetacarpal space is retracted, the superficial palmar fascia opened, and the fibrous septa resected.

Isolation of the neurovascular bundles of the third and fourth intermetacarpal spaces: The aim of the dissection is to preserve the blood supply and the innervation of the finger to be pollicized. The innervation includes the digital nerve to the ulnar side of the third space and the digital nerve to the radial side of the fourth space. From the vascular point of view, these are all the digital arteries that must be taken with the finger to be transferred. This means that the collateral branches to the ulnar side of the middle finger and the radial side of the little finger must be ligated and divided.

The deep palmar fascia is incised on either side of the metacarpal and the lumbrical canal is opened to free the flexor tendons.

Dorsal Stage. Next the dorsal veins are divided. We believe that one of them should be preserved and dissected far enough to allow an anastomosis with another vein on the dorsum of the stump of the thumb.

Freeing of the extensor apparatus requires particular care. The common extensor tendon or tendons are divided 2 to 3 cm. proximal to the metacarpophalangeal joint. The juncture tendinum are divided. One should strive to preserve the hood of the interosseous muscles on either side of extensor communis and down to the tendons of the interosseous muscles, which are themselves divided, the two segments being sutured to a tendon transfer. The metacarpophalangeal joint is now disarticulated.

TRANSFER OF THE POLLICIZED FINGER

Liberation of the finger is completed by dividing the proximal part of the fibrous flexor sheath together with any other fibrous tissue that may be holding it. Freeing of the finger is continued along the whole length of the palmar incision and into the forearm in order to give maximal freedom to the flexors of the ring finger in relation to those of the other fingers.

The proximal phalanx is shortened as required to match the length of the contralateral thumb. Next the digit is displaced like an island flap along with its tendinous and neurovascular pedicles. Bone fixation is carried out, as mentioned earlier, taking into account the degree of rotation required.

Any tendinous redeployment should make use of the extensor tendons of the thumb and eventually those of utilizable thenar muscles. If one is to achieve good extension, it is important that the expansions of the interosseous muscles be reactivated. Gosset (1975) has advised, when possible, that the short extensor of the thumb to the external expansion of the interosseous muscles and the long extensor to the internal expansions.

The tourniquet is released to allow complete hemostasis. The skin is sutured after the posterior V shaped flap of the pollicized finger is fitted into the corresponding anterolateral slit of the thenar stump.

The neothumb is immobilized in plaster with the distal phalanx free and the thumb in opposition. The plaster cast is kept on for 25

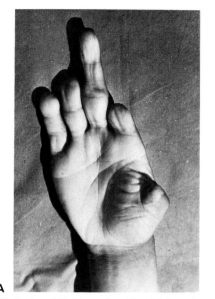 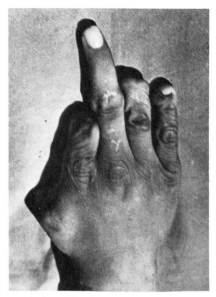

Figure 101–6. *A* and *B*, Example of hand injury due to an explosion. The thumb has been amputated at the level of the metacarpophalangeal joint, the index finger at the distal part of the proximal phalanx, and the ring finger at the distal interphalangeal joint.

days. Then, as with other pollicizations, an opposition splint is worn for several weeks between sessions of re-education.

POLLICIZATION OF A PARTIALLY AMPUTATED FINGER

Despite the good results obtained and the near perfection of present techniques, a number of surgeons hesitate to transfer a healthy digit when it is possible to use a digit that is already injured or amputated, provided of course the latter has a good blood supply and sensation. Such stiff or shortened digits, a useless embarrassment in the absence of the thumb, are literally transformed once they replace the thumb, especially when the first carpometacarpal joint has retained its mobility (Figs. 101–6 to 101–8).

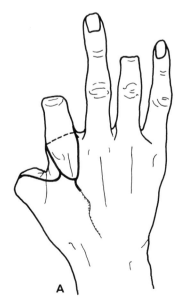 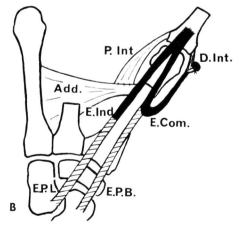

Figure 101–7. Pollicization of the mutilated index finger. *A*, Incision lines (dorsal view). *B*, Muscle and tendon arrangement.

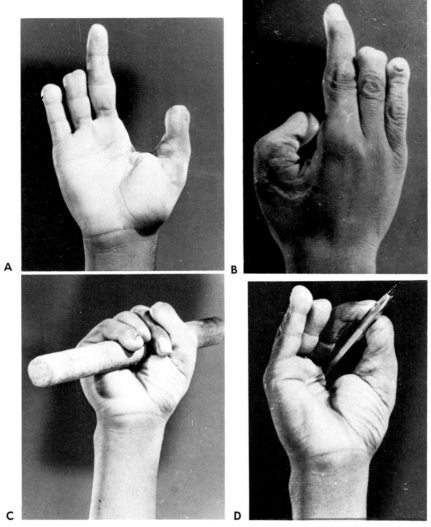

Figure 101–8. *A* to *D*, Result. The value of the short stump of the index finger is considerably increased by its pollicization.

In one case when the blood supply and sensation of an injured index finger seemed inadequate to allow its pollicization, Snell (1962) transferred a heterodigital island flap to that finger prior to pollicization. Roullet (1971) describes in Chapter 112 his technique for the block transfer on accessory pedicles of the index finger, showing how far one can go in utilizing an injured finger. One always has to concede that pollicization of mutilated fingers with an imperfect vascularization and sensibility and stiffened joints does not offer the same prospects for use or the same quality of results as transfer of a healthy digit. The indications are always difficult to decide.

POLLICIZATION WITH RECONSTRUCTION OF THE WEB SPACE

When the web space has been destroyed in an injury or contracted by scarring, it must be reconstructed along with the thumb (Fig. 101–9). The web space is freed and skin replacement must be planned. If the bed is scarred, a skin graft is unlikely to take, and multiple or extensive scars may preclude the use of a local skin flap. The only resort then is a flap from a distant site. This is best prepared in advance and carried to the finger in the form of a tube flap (Fig. 101–10). The

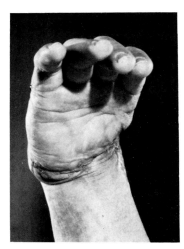

Figure 101–9. Traumatic amputation of the whole first ray. There is extensive scarring of the radial aspect of the hand and wrist.

two pedicles of the tube are fixed to the radial border of the hand, taking into account the future position of the neothumb. The actual pollicization is carried out only when the tube is mobile enough to be spread open (Fig. 101–11).

RESULTS OF POLLICIZATION

A successful pollicization provides a mobile sensitive neothumb whose function approaches that of a normal thumb. Cosmetically the new thumb may be criticized for its slimness but it has a nail and its appearance is still better than that obtained by any other reconstructive method. The results, however, are not invariably good. They depend on the surgical technique, the finger chosen for pollicization, the state of the rest of the hand, and the patient himself.

THE INFLUENCE OF TECHNIQUE

The actual technique is of prime importance. Indeed the surgeon takes on a heavy responsibility when, in a hand already deprived of its thumb, he undertakes the transposition of a healthy finger. The technical traps are numerous and may give rise to multiple complications, which more experienced surgeons, rightly proud of their results, too often tend to minimize.

Vascular Complications. Vascular complications may lead to partial or total loss of the

Figure 101–10. *A* and *B*, An abdominal tube flap has been inserted both in front of and behind the index finger to be pollicized.

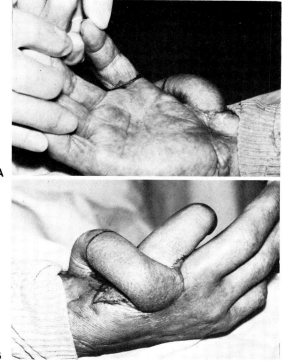

A

B

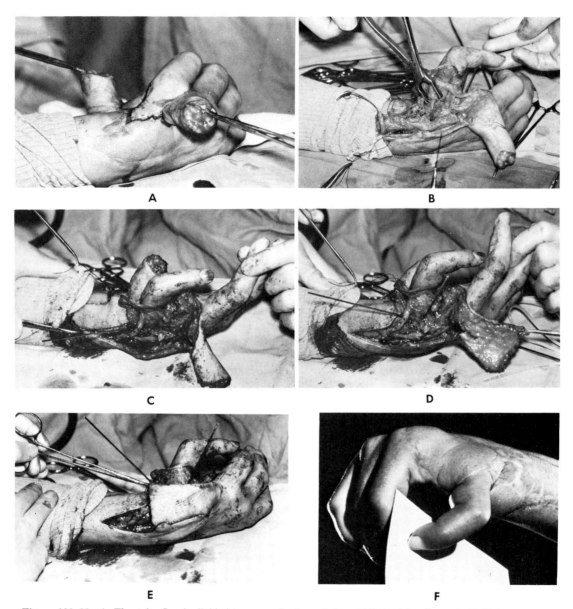

Figure 101–11. *A*, The tube flap is divided transversely through its middle incision lines. *B*, Pollicization of the index finger. The base of its proximal phalanx is fixed into the trapezium. *C*, Bone and tendon arrangement. *D*, The two halves of the tube flap are then opened longitudinally. *E*, The palmar portion of the flap covers the new web, and the dorsal part covers the radial aspect of the hand and wrist. *F*, Result.

pollicized finger. This is admittedly rare when the finger has a normal arterial supply, and it can be avoided by delicate handling of the digital pedicles and careful ligation of the small arterial branches whose avulsion might lead to thrombosis of the digital artery. The small venae comitantes should be preserved because they take over the responsibility for digital venous return when the dorsal veins are sacrificed.

If we exclude accidental injuries, vascular complications are due mostly to excessive tension in the tissues or to kinking of the pedicles. They may also result from arterial anomalies, as when the digital collateral vessel arises from the deep palmar arch or forms a ring around the digital nerve.

The risk of vascular complications is greater when an injured finger is transferred; an arteriogram is then of great assistance.

Malposition. Faulty rotation is the commonest form of malposition; it prevents the pulp of the neothumb from coming into contact with the digital pulps. However, we have observed other faulty positions, such as adduction of the metacarpal, and irreducible flexion of the interphalangeal joints, which hold the thumb down against the palm, thus rendering it useless. Hyperextension of the metacarpophalangeal joint, which replaces the trapeziometacarpal joint, is usually encountered after reconstructions in children.

Reduced Active Mobility. A reduction in active mobility is the result of insufficient "muscular control" of the neothumb. Reduced flexion is relatively less of a handicap (if the first metacarpal has retained its mobility) than poor extension, which prevents the grasping of larger objects. An extensor lag deficit of the interphalangeal joints, which is not uncommon, is due to failure to reactivate the intrinsic muscles.

Skin Contractures. Skin contracture is the result of the faulty design of incisions or follows skin necrosis. It is far from uncommon and can severely restrict the mobility of the new thumb.

Other Complications. We shall only list the other possible complications—painful neuromas, osteitis, pseudarthrosis at bone junctions, and painful scar contractures at the donor site. Their common effect is to reduce or prevent utilization of the neothumb, and they may represent a handicap greater than that present prior to the pollicization.

OTHER FACTORS INFLUENCING THE RESULTS

The result also depends on which finger is pollicized. We have already stressed the importance of the choice of the transferred finger; the condition of that finger, whether healthy or mutilated, must also be taken into account. Gosset (1964) has expressed the view that the ring finger is the finger of choice; he backs his view with his own results and with the arguments we have mentioned.

Together with Langlais (1984), Gosset expressed his results on the basis of the following point scoring system:

Mobility and power of the thumb	5 points
Tactile sensation and stereognosis	1 point
Proprioception	1 point
Professional value	2 points
Cosmetic appearance	1 point

His 16 transfers of healthy ring fingers scored 8 of 10 points, whereas pollicizations of healthy index fingers averaged only 6. All these patients had "integrated" the neothumb after two to three years, with a "return of proprioception."

Pollicizations of mutilated digits were much less successful, averaging a score of 3 of 10. For this reason Gosset made a distinction between "typical" pollicizations, in which a healthy finger is transferred, and "atypical" ones in which he used an injured finger.

The functional result also obviously depends on the state of the rest of the hand. This aspect is considered further in the next chapter when we shall discuss complex mutilations involving the thumb and fingers.

Finally, the result depends on the patient himself. His morale and desire for recuperation significantly influence the prognosis. One should perform pollicizations only in active subjects who, knowing all the facts, accept the principle of digital transfer. The procedure is best avoided in the passive, the pusillanimous, the compensation minded, those who tacitly accept their deformity, and the anxious, who dread the very idea of this type of surgery.

REFERENCES

Albee, F.: Synthetic transplantation of tissue to form a new finger with restoration of the function of the hand. Ann. Surg., 69:379, 1919.

Buck-Gramcko, D.: Pollicization of the index finger: method and results in aplasia and hypoplasia of the thumb. J. Bone Joint Surg., *53A*:1605, 1971.

Buncke, H. J., Buncke, C. M., and Schulz, W. P.: Hallux-to-hand transplantation, utilizing micro-vascular anastomoses. Br. J. Plast. Surg., *19*:332, 1966.

Buncke, H. J., et al.: Thumb replacement: great toe transplantation by micro-vascular anastomosis, Br. J. Plast. Surg., *26*:194, 1973.

Bunnell, S.: Physiological reconstruction of a thumb after total loss. Surg. Gynecol. Obstet., *52*:245, 1931.

Bunnell, S.: Digit transfer by neurovascular pedicle. J. Bone Joint Surg., *34A*:772, 1952.

Butler, M. B.: Ring finger pollicization, J. Bone Joint Surg., *46A*:1069, 1964.

de la Caffiniere, J. Y., and Malek, R.: Chirurgie Réparatrice du Pouce, Paris, Masson et cie, 1981.

Campbell Reid, D. A.: Reconstruction of the thumb. J. Bone Joint Surg., *42B*:444, 1960.

Campbell Reid, D. A.: The neurovascular island flap in thumb reconstruction. Br. J. Plast. Surg., *19*:234, 1966.

Campbell Reid, D. A.: Pollicisation—an appraisal. Hand, *1*:27, 1969.

Campbell Reid, D. A., and Gosset, J.: Mutilating Injuries of the Hand. G. E. M. Monograph 3. Edinburgh, Churchill Livingstone, 1979.

Carcassonne, F.: Contribution à l'étude des restaurations anatomiques et fonctionnelles du pouce dans les traumatismes de la main. Lyon, Bosc et Riou, 1930.

Clarkson, P. W., and Chandler, R.: On making thumbs. Plast. Reconstr. Surg., *29*:325, 1962.

Cobbett, J. R.: Free digital transfer. Report of a case of transfer of a great toe to replace an amputated thumb. J. Bone Joint Surg., *51B*:677, 1969.

Cotte: Restauration anatomique et fonctionnelle du pouce. Lyon Chir., 1919.

Gillies, H., and Millard, R.: The Principles and Art of Plastic Surgery. Boston, Little, Brown and Company, 1957.

Gosset, J.: La pollicisation de l'index, J. Chir. (Paris), *65*:403, 1949.

Gosset, J.: Les Mutilations de la Main. Paris, L'Expansion Scientifique Française, 1975.

Gosset, J., and Sels, M.: Technique, indications et résultats de la pollicisation du 4ème doigt. Ann. Chir., *18*:1005, 1964.

Graham, W. C., et al.: Transposition of fingers in severe injuries of the hand. J. Bone Joint Surg., *29*:998, 1947.

Guermonprez, F.: Essai de Cheiroplastie. Tentative de Restauration du Pouce. Paris, Dupont, 1886.

Guermonprez, F.: Notes sur Quelques Résections et Restaurations du Pouce. Paris, P. Asselin, 1887.

Guermonprez, F.: Autoplastie de la Main. Lille, Quarré, 1893.

Gueullette, R.: Etude critique des procédés de restauration du pouce. J. Chir. (Paris), *36*:1, 1930.

Hanotte: Restauration fonctionnelle du pouce. Thesis, University of Lille, 1888.

Harrison, S. H.: Restoration of muscle balance in pollicization, Plast. Reconstr. Surg., *34*:236–240, 1964.

Hilgenfeldt, O.: Operativer Daumenersatz. Stuttgart, Ferdinand Enke Verlag, 1950.

Holevich, J.: A new method of restoring sensibility to the thumb. J. Bone Joint Surg., *45B*:496–502, 1963.

Hueston, J.: The extended neurovascular island flap. Br. J. Plast. Surg., *18*:304–305, 1965.

Huguier, P. C.: Remplacement du pouce par son métacarpien, par l'agrandissement du premier espace interosseux, Arch. Gen. Med., *1*:78, 1874a.

Huguier, P. C.: Considérations anatomiques et physiologiques pour servir à la chirurgie du pouce (oeuvre posthume). Paris, Asselin Edit., 1874b.

Iselin, M., and Iselin, F.: Traité de Chirurgie de la Main. Paris, Flammarion, et Cie, 1967.

Joyce, J. L.: A new operation for the substitution of a thumb. Br. J. Surg., *5*:499, 1918.

Joyce, J. L.: The results of a new operation for substitution of a thumb. Br. J. Surg., *16*:362, 1929.

Kelleher, J. C., and Sullivan, J. G.: Thumb reconstruction by fifth digit transposition. Transactions, 3rd International Congress of Plastic Surgeons, Washington, D.C., 1963, p. 968.

Komatsu, S., and Tamai, S.: Successful replantation of a completely cut-off thumb: case report. Plast. Reconstr. Surg., *42*:374, 1968.

Kuhn, H.: Reconstruction du pouce par "lambeau de Hilgenfeld." Ann. Chir. Plast., *6*:259, 1961.

Lambert, O.: Résultat éloigné d'une transplantation du gros orteil en remplacement du pouce, Bull. Soc. Med. Paris, 689, 1920.

Langlais, F., and Gosset, J.: Results of thumb reconstruction. *In* Campbell Reid, D. A., and Gosset, J. (Editors): Mutilating Injuries of the Hand. Edinburgh, Churchill Livingstone, 1979, pp. 78–80.

Le Tac, R.: Reconstitution du pouce détruit par pollicisation de l'annulaire ou du 5ème doigt. Mem. Acad. Chir., *7278*:262, 1952.

Littler, J. W.: Subtotal reconstruction of the thumb, Plast. Reconstr. Surg., *10*:215, 1952.

Littler, J. W.: Neurovascular pedicle method of digital transposition for reconstruction of the thumb. Plast. Reconstr. Surg., *12*:303, 1953.

Littler, J. W.: Neurovascular skin island transfer in reconstructive hand surgery. *In* Transactions, International Society of Plastic Surgeons (Second Congress, London, 1959). Edinburgh, E. & S. Livingstone, 1960.

Littler, J. W.: On making a thumb: one hundred years of surgical effort. J. Hand Surg., *1*:35–51, 1976.

Luksch, L.: Uber eine nene methode zum ersatz des verlorenen daumens. Verh. Dtsch. Ges. Chir., *32*:221, 1903.

Matev, J. B.: Thumb reconstruction after amputation of the metacarpophalangeal joint by bone lengthening. J. Bone Joint Surg., *52A*:957, 1970.

McGregor, I., and Simonetta, C.: Reconstruction of thumb by composite bone skin flap. Br. J. Plast. Surg., *17*:37, 1964.

Merle d'Aubigne, R., Tubiana, R., and Ramadier, J. O.: Reconstruction du pouce. Rev. Chir. Orthop., *38*:456–475, 1952.

Moberg, E.: Discussion. *In* Brooks, D.: Nerve grafting in orthopaedic surgery. J. Bone Joint Surg., *37A*:305, 1955.

Neuhauser: Daumenplastik. Berl. Klin. Wochensch., 1287, 1916.

Nicoladoni, C.: Daumenplastik, Wein. Klin. Wochenschr., *10*:663, 1897.

Nicoladoni, C.: Daumenplastik und organischer ersatz der fingerspitze (anticheiroplastik und daktylo-plastik). Arch. Klin. Chir., *61*:606, 1900.

Nicoladoni, C.: Weitere erfahrungen über daumenplastik. Arch. Klin. Chir., *69*:697, 1903.

Noesske, K.: Uber den plastischen ersatz von ganz oder

teilweise verlorene fingern, insbesondere des daumens, und über handtellerplastik. Munch. Med. Wschr., *56:*1403, 1909.

Noesske, K.: Ueber ersatz des samt metakarpus verlorenen daumens durch operative umstellung des zeigefingers. Munch. Med. Wschr., *67:*465, 1920.

Perthes: Uber plastichen daumenersatz und besonders beim verlust der ganzen Daumenstrahlen. Arch. Orthop. Unfallchirug., *19:*199, 1921.

Pierce, G. W.: Reconstruction of thumb after total loss. Surg. Gynecol. Obstet., *45:*835, 1927.

Porzelt: Reconstitution du pouce par transplantation du gros orteil. Arch. Klin. Chir., *135:*340, 1925.

Roullet, J.: Technique de la translation "en masse" en vue de la pollicisation. Ann. Chir., *25:*1009–1014, 1971.

Snell, J. A.: A further use for the neurovascular island flap principle in hand surgery: the piggy-back flap. Br. J. Plast. Surg., 968, 1963.

Shebelmann: Plastischer ersatz bei totaldefekt des rechten daumens. Z. Orthop. Chir., *34,* 1914; *35,* 1916; *39,* 1919.

Simonetta, C.: Chirurgie réparatrice des pertes de substance et des amputations du pouce. Lausanne, Imprimerie Held S. A., 1975.

Tanzer, R. C., and Littler, J. W.: Reconstruction of the thumb by transposition of adjacent digit. Plast. Reconstr. Surg., *3:*533, 1948.

Teich-Alasia, S., and Garelli, R.: Etude du retour de la sensibilité dans les lambeaux transplantés. Ann. Chir. Plast., *35,* 1964–1965.

Tubiana, R., and Duparc, J.: Un procédé nouveau de reconstruction d'un pouce sensible (rapport de R. Merle d'Aubigné). Mem. Acad. Chir., *86:*8–9, 264, 1960.

Tubiana, R., and Duparc, J.: Restoration of sensibility in the hand by neurovascular skin island transfer. J. Bone Joint Surg., *43B:*474, 1961.

Tubiana, R., Duparc, J., and Moreau, C.: Restauration de la sensibilité au niveau de la main par transfert d'un transplant cutané hétérodigital muni de son pédicule vasculo-nerveux. Rev. Chir. Orthop., *46:*163, 1960.

Verdan, C.: The reconstruction of the thumb. Surg. Clin. N. Am., *48:*1033, 1968.

Verdan, C.: Les procédés ostéo-plastiques de reconstruction du pouce. Proceedings, Tenth Congress, S.I.C.O.T., 1966, p. 808.

Chapter 102

TRANSLATION POLLICIZATION

Jacques Roullet

Injury to the digital pedicles in severe mutilations of the hand does not, per se, preclude the possibility of pollicization. As long as part or the whole of a digital ray has survived destruction of the branches of the superficial palmar arch, this ray can be used in the repair of an amputated thumb. However, transposition is possible only if the ray to be transferred is adjacent to the recipient ray because the vascular pedicles to which the replacement digit owes its survival do not have the versatility of digital arteries. The solution therefore is pollicization *en masse* (or block) (Figs. 102–1 to 102–6).

The success of this operation depends on the condition of the deep interosseous artery. In the course of a planned amputation of the ray of the index, this vessel can be assessed in terms of its location, volume, and

branches. Arising from the deep palmar arch, it can be found coursing along the crest of the second metacarpal between the first dorsal and palmar interosseous muscles. Flanked by two relatively wide bore veins, the deep interosseous artery, which runs within a sheath of fatty tissue, constitutes the main channel of a potential vascular pedicle, which can be mobilized except for its fan of terminal branches. Indeed, as it approaches the palmar fibrocartilage, the artery divides into five branches: The middle axial branch supplies the joint while the other four run in pairs on either side of the joint, strapped down by the tendons of the interosseous muscles to anastomose with the palmar and dorsal collateral arteries. These four digital branches are slender, superficial, and vulnerable. When transposing this digit to the ray of the thumb, therefore, one should mobilize the whole mass made up by the first two dorsal and

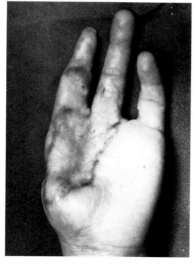

Figure 102–1. Amputation of the thumb, degloving of the radial half of the middle palmar space, and amputation of the ring finger. The defect is covered with a full thickness graft. The digital pedicles and flexors of the index and middle fingers have been destroyed. The muscular stump of the base of the thumb is functional. The little finger is intact.

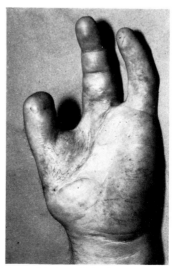

Figure 102–2. Block pollicization of the index finger, which has been secondarily shortened to a more manageable length to facilitate transfer of sensitive skin over to the palmar side.

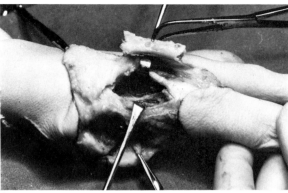

Figure 102–3. First stage of the operation: resection of the shaft of the second metacarpal. The deep interosseous pedicle can be seen deep in the wound.

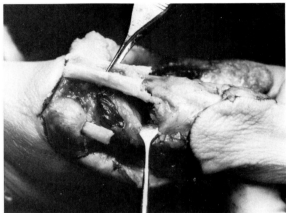

Figure 102–4. Preparation for implantation of the pollicized finger at the proximal third of the metacarpal. Osteosynthesis is achieved by means of an encased graft cut from the shaft.

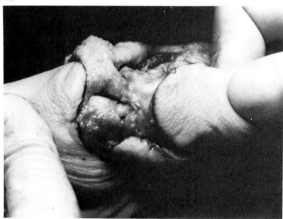

Figure 102–5. Block transfer of the index finger.

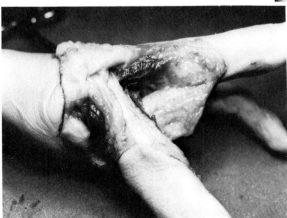

Figure 102–6. Implantation of the finger on the base of the thumb.

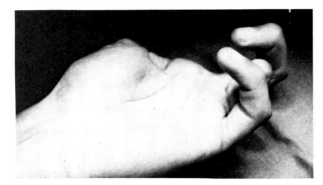

Figure 102–7. Severe mutilation of the hand with thumb muscles intact. At the base of the thumb, one notes a deep scar, indicating division of the digital arteries. Hilgenfeldt's operation is thus contraindicated.

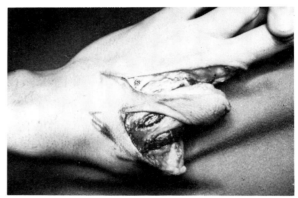

Figure 102–8. Preparation of a dorsal pedicle under a skin bridge.

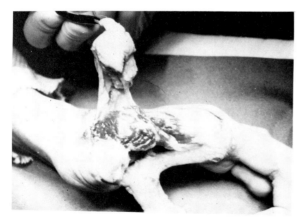

Figure 102–9. Volar aspect of the neurovascular pedicle. Soft tissue covers the proximal third of the index metacarpal before transposition.

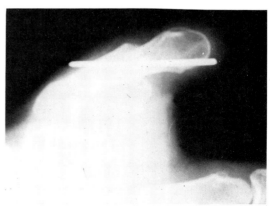

Figure 102–10. Transposition of the stump of the metacarpal to the stump of the thumb.

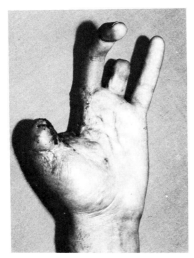

Figure 102–11. Postoperative appearance of the palm.

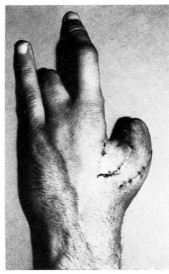

Figure 102–12. Postoperative appearance of the dorsum of the hand.

palmar interosseous muscles together with the precious pedicle within.

If the second ray has been lost as a result of trauma and it is proposed to pollicize the third, this technique is even more imperative, because the deep interosseous pedicle of the third ray is less capacious than that of the second.

SURGICAL TECHNIQUE

The choice of skin incision is dictated by the presence of unhealthy scars, by the need to repair the collateral nerves, and by the very object of the operation, which consists of resection of the second metacarpal from the dorsal side in order to free the corresponding muscular and vascular pedicles. The incision therefore comprises a dorsal and a palmar extension as well as a middle part, which will correspond to the future web space. The second metacarpal is resected subperiosteally, sparing the base into which is inserted the extensor carpi radialis longus. Depending on the requirements of each case, the metacarpophalangeal joint may be retained, or the shaft of the first phalanx can be exposed via an intra-articular and subperiosteal approach. This frees and mobilizes the digital extremity at the end of its muscular interosseous pedicle, which contains the deep interosseous vascular pedicle. Transposition is made possible by applying torsion to the interosseous muscle mass; the distal segment of the second ray is aligned with the proximal segment of the first ray, thus achieving the main object of the operation.

An alternative technique consists of pollicization on a dorsal pedicle (Figs. 102–7 to 102–12). In classic pollicization, using a distal pedicle, the dorsal vascular pedicles of the fingers make a beneficial contribution and contain wide bore veins. Experience has shown that these pedicles can provide an adequate blood supply even in severe, deep, and extensive mutilations. It seems likely that enlargement of the dorsal vessels makes up for the paucity of the superficial and deep palmar blood supply. Such a pedicle can be used in the transfer of a digital stump to a vestigial thumb ray.

The dorsal arteries, veins, and nerves are scattered in the subcutaneous fatty tissue, and separate dissection of each structure would constitute quite a challenge. It is preferable, therefore, that they be transferred intact within the ensheathing tissues, preserving the overlying bridge of skin; this is almost a Hilgenfeldt operation "in reverse."

REFERENCE

Roullet, J. A., and Landreau, Y.: Technique de la translation "en masse" de l'index en vue de sa pollicisation. Ann. Chir., 25:1009–1014, 1971.

Chapter 103

THUMB RECONSTRUCTION USING MICROVASCULAR TECHNIQUES

ALAIN GILBERT

The principle of reconstructing a mutilated thumb by use of a toe was first described by Nicoladoni in 1895 but it was not until 1898 that he operated on his first patient using the second toe. Although an attractive possibility, this technique had been little used because of practical difficulties in carrying it out.

In 1930, Gueulette found in the literature reports of 17 toe transplantations and one forefoot transplantation; he even found one case of homotransplantation of a big toe that had not been rejected at the end of three months. The overall results in these reports were not very good: Gueulette found that of the 17 transplantations, four underwent complete and four partial necrosis.

In 1965, at the Third International Congress of Plastic Surgery in Washington, Freeman reviewed reports of the operations that had been performed by members of American Association of Plastic Surgeons. He found 61 transfers among the 43 reports published. In this group of cases, the results seemed better, for there were no instances of necrosis and in more than half the cases the results were considered good or excellent.

With the advent of microsurgical vascular techniques, there has been a renewal of interest in the technique and in overcoming the long and arduous immobilization imposed upon the patient.

The first successful clinical case, reported by Cobbett in 1969 was soon followed by reports by Buncke (1973), Tsai (1975), O'Brien (1974), Ohmori and Harii (1975), and Gilbert (1976). Although the number of cases is still small, it is probable that they will increase as microsurgical techniques develop.

1142

ANATOMY

The technique of toe transplantation is based on the vascular anatomy of the forefoot, particularly the well-defined regional vascular supply of the first intermetacarpal space and first two toes. More than 70 anatomical dissections carried out have made it possible to construct a "vascular map" of the region that well illustrates the technical difficulties of the operation.

THE FIRST DORSAL INTEROSSEOUS ARTERY

The dorsal interosseous artery arises from the dorsalis pedis artery as it enters the intermetacarpal space (Fig. 103–1). It remains dorsal and courses toward the commissure. The pathway of this vessel is fundamental because it determines the operative technique used. There are three variations (Fig. 103–2).

Type I: The artery stays superficial, running above the interosseous muscle, or, more simply, is covered near its origin by a fibrous or muscular arcade formed by an insertion of the interosseous muscle on the first cuneiform. It can also penetrate to the interior of the muscle.

Type II: The artery penetrates more deeply into the commissure and courses the deep surface of the interosseous muscle. It becomes superficial again at its anterior border.

Type III: The artery still lies superficially, running along the interosseous muscle, but it is very atrophic and rarely reaches the web space. The plantar network is then dominant.

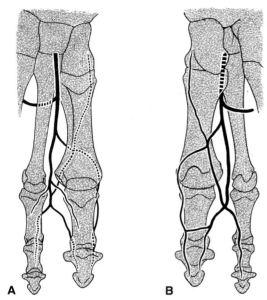

Figure 103–1. Vascular network of the first web space. *A,* Dorsal view. *B,* Plantar view.

THE VOLAR INTEROSSEOUS ARTERY

The volar interosseous artery is an anterior branch of the dorsalis pedis artery arising proximal to the plantar arch. It runs volarly toward the lateral sesamoid bone of the first toe, near which it anastomoses with the medial plantar artery. It ascends then toward the first web space; at this level there is a thick branch anastomosing the two first inter-

osseous arteries (dorsal and plantar). The digital arteries usually arise from the dorsal interosseous artery.

The dorsal arterial network is used more frequently as a pedicle to the toe transplant because it is more easily dissected, but in view of these anastomotic relations, the plantar arterial network can be used as an alternative.

THE VENOUS DRAINAGE

The venous drainage is similar to that in the fingers—dorsal, subcutaneous, and superficial. All the small veins of the dorsal region of the toe join together in two or three trunks, which rejoin the distal arch. There are two accessory venous systems that are satellites of the interosseous arteries. These veins also rejoin the venous arch at the origin of the dorsal interosseous artery. During surgery one can sacrifice the deep network, and it is possible to separate all the superficial vessels of the dorsal network, which forms an arch drained laterally by the small saphenous vein and medially by the great saphenous vein.

THE NERVES

The toe pulps are innervated by the plantar collateral nerves, which have to be looked for in the sole of the foot. One point of

Figure 103–2. Anatomical variations of the first dorsal interosseous artery in relation to the interosseous muscle and the intermetatarsal ligament.

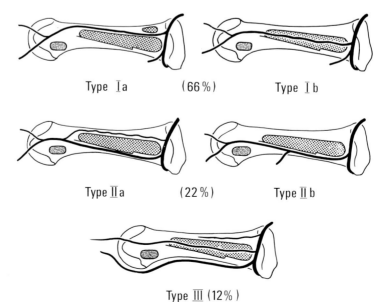

Type Ia (66%)   Type Ib

Type IIa (22%)   Type IIb

Type III (12%)

particular importance is that the medial collateral nerve of the big toe often is not found at the medial border but is almost dorsal to the metacarpophalangeal joint. The dorsal skin of the first and second toes, as well as the skin web between them, is innervated by the medial terminal branch of the deep peroneal nerve.

THE TENDONS

The extensors do not bring any problems. The tendon of the extensor digitorum brevis eventually can be used to reactivate opposition in a new thumb. The flexors are difficult to dissect because they are deeply buried in the sole.

PREPARATION FOR SURGERY

Preparation for surgery must be done, whenever possible, in close cooperation with the patient. Both first and second toes are usually available to transplant, each having its advantages and disadvantages.

The use of the second toe leaves the foot morphologically and functionally almost intact. It presents, in the child, three growth plates. Being more delicate and thinner, it is advantageous in the woman. The first toe provides a stronger thumb with a better aesthetic appearance than the second one, but the aesthetic result and the functional deficit in the foot are undoubtedly more severe (Figs. 103–3 and 103–4). The majority of the patients choose the second toe, in view of the foot deficit.

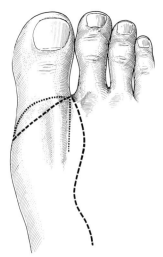

Figure 103–3. The incision for a first toe transfer.

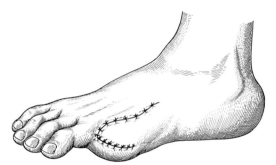

Figure 103–4. Closing the foot after first toe transfer.

Placement of the incisions depends on preoperative planning in order to foresee any cutaneous deficit. It is most important to ensure satisfactory skin coverage in the foot, and if there is to be a deficit, it is better for it to be on the hand. When a small defect is foreseen, we prefer to plan the rotation of a local flap, or even an Ollier's or Wolf graft. For more extensive raw areas, it is wise to provide skin coverage in a first stage and to perform the toe transplant in the second stage.

The arteriography is not performed routinely, but it is very useful, as it helps to determine the size of the first dorsal interosseous artery and to show the hand arterial network particularly after trauma or in congenital abnormalities.

THE OPERATION

The operation can be performed by two teams, but it is often preferable for only one surgeon to dissect both the recipient hand and the donor site on the foot.

In the case of post-traumatic reconstruction or if one is absolutely sure to find good quality and sufficiently large vessels in the hand, it is undoubtedly better to start by dissecting the foot. However, if one is dealing with congenital malformations, particularly the aplasia of the thumb, it is wise to start by dissecting the hand first, to be absolutely sure of the technical possibilities to perform the whole operation. In certain instances, one must cancel the toe transplantation or at least it must be postponed.

THE TOE DISSECTION

The toe dissection is performed on a bloodless field by means of a tourniquet applied

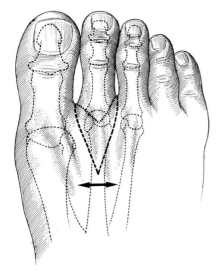

Figure 103–5. The incision for a second toe transfer.

around the thigh. We will describe, as an example, the dissection of the second toe. The dissection of the first toe is very similar, but it is rarely used.

Starting with a "racket-shaped" type of cutaneous incision, we are able to include the dorsal venous network which is dissected proximally up to the venous arch (Fig. 103–5). One of the branches of the venous arch is divided to free a single vascular pedicle, which is thick (2.0 mm.) and has a good length (4.0 to 8.0 cm.). The dissection continues to a deeper plane and the dorsal interosseous artery is freed from its origin at the dorsalis pedis artery and distally as far as the web space. Special attention is to be paid to this dissection, which must be performed very carefully to avoid spasm or vascular lesion.

It is preferable to use surgical ties or vascular metal clips instead of coagulation to overcome the risk of thrombosis. It may be necessary to divide the interosseous ligament to free the artery when it runs deeply. Near the web space one can easily see the division of the interosseous artery into its two collateral branches (digital arteries). The branch to the first toe must be ligated, as well as the anastomotic branch to the volar interosseous artery. The extensor tendons are divided at the base of the second metacarpal bone.

A smaller racket-shaped type of incision is now made on the volar side to complete the previous one. The two thin digital nerves are dissected free, from the web space proximally up to the origin of the contralateral digital

nerve and then they are divided. The flexor tendons must be divided, as proximally as possible, to ensure length. The metatarsophalangeal joint capsule is then sectioned, and the toe is then attached by the vascular pedicle only. The tourniquet is then released.

THE HAND DISSECTION AND THE TOE TRANSFER

The hand dissection is performed on a bloodless field, obtained by means of a tourniquet inflated around the arm. The recipient arteries and veins are exposed through a dorsal incision which must go as proximally as possible to allow the microanastomosis to be performed in larger vessels.

Following the vessels, the digital nerves and the tendons are exposed and dissected free from surrounding tissues for a short length (Fig. 103–6). The bone stump is then osteotomized to allow the osteosynthesis with the proximal phalanx of the toe.

As soon as all the recipient structures are dissected and ready for the transplant the vascular pedicle of the donor toe is divided, and it is transferred to the hand. The first step is to perform the osteosynthesis by means of two Kirschner wires (Fig. 103–7). Thereafter, the tendons are sutured (usually one flexor tendon and one extensor tendon only). The arterial anastomosis is performed under microscope, soon followed by the nerve anastomoses. The vascular clamps are then released and the tourniquet is deflated to allow the revascularization of the toe. The ischemia time is usually less than 40 min. (Fig. 103–8).

The venous anastomosis is then performed while the persistent arterial blood flow and the blood pressure improve any present vascular spasm. The skin is closed, and a light dressing is applied, leaving exposed the tip of the toe (Fig. 103–9).

POSTOPERATIVE TREATMENT

The hand is slightly elevated, and the tip of the toe is observed hourly for color, temperature, and circulation for the first 24 hours. A short course of antibiotics is started immediately after the operation but no other medicine is given to the patient. On the third postoperative day, he is allowed to walk under supervision. The Kirschner wires are

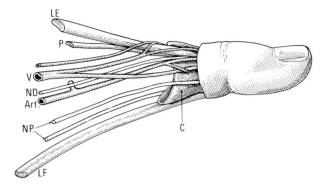

Figure 103–6. The first toe at the end of the dissection. LE = extensor hallucis proprius, P = extensor digitorum brevis, V = dorsal vein, ND = dorsal nerve (terminal branch of superficial peroneal nerve), ART = dorsalis pedis artery, NP = plantar nerves, LF = flexor hallucis longis, and C = articular capsule.

removed between the fourth and sixth postoperative weeks, and physiotherapy is then started.

RESULTS

From 1974 through to 1986, 142 toe transplants were performed in 117 patients. This includes 63 thumb reconstructions, 46 of the patients being adults and 17 being children (in the children's group eight reconstructions were performed for congenital amputations and nine for traumatic amputations). Twenty-six patients were submitted to a double transplant as a two-stage procedure. The second stage, performed after a delay of 6 to 18 months, involved the second toe of the opposite foot always (Fig. 103–10). The youngest patient operated on was 11 months old, and the oldest was 57 years old.

In our series only three cases were unsuccessful. The first was one attempt to recon-

struct the thumb immediately after a crush injury in a six-month-old child. The second unsuccessful case was an attempt to reconstruct a digit in a 25-month-old child. In this second case, the postoperative arterial thrombosis, lately diagnosed, was followed by an unsuccessful revision of the anastomosis. The third one was a similar problem in a 30-month-old child.

AESTHETIC RESULTS

The thumb usually appears too thin when the second toe is used to perform the reconstruction (Fig. 103–11). In the majority of

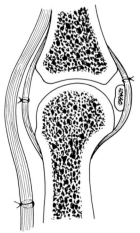

Figure 103–7. Arthroplasty between the base of the toe phalanx and the head of the first metacarpal with capsular reconstruction.

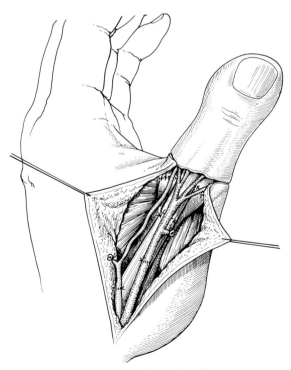

Figure 103–8. The vascular and tendinous sutures.

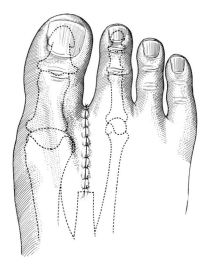

Figure 103–9. Closure of the foot after raising the second toe and post of the second metatarsal joint.

the individuals the big toe is undoubtedly more similar to the thumb than the second toe. Its nail is wider and longer than the one of the second toe.

In spite of this, when the patient is called upon to decide which toe to transplant, he usually prefers the second toe, refusing to accept the important foot amputation caused by the first toe transplant. In our series only 4 of the 117 patients chose the big toe transplant.

The resection of the second toe and metacarpal bone ends up in an aesthetically more acceptable result than the one resulting from the resection of the first toe (Fig. 103–12). The permanent flexion deformity of the distal interphalangeal joint of the second toe, which is commonly found after its transplant, can be prevented by its immobilization for six weeks with a transfixing Kirschner wire and by suturing the extensor tendon under maximum tension.

The best cosmetic result is undoubtedly obtained by a partial toe transplant, which allows one to reconstruct an almost perfect distal thumb. The two major disadvantages are by one side the absent interphalangeal joint motion and by the other side the delay in the healing frequently encountered at donor site.

FUNCTIONAL RESULTS

The sensation, as tested in teenagers and adults, always recovered with a two point

discrimination going from 3.0 to 14.0 mm. The results were similar to the ones obtained after a digital nerve microanastomosis. In our series, hyperesthesia was never a complaint.

It is very difficult to evaluate the results in children, but when the operation was performed between the ages of 15 and 30 months, the recovery seems to be very good, with the sensibility of the reconstructed thumb similar to that of the one of the opposite side. The range of motion of a toe ranged from 40 to 90 degrees, which is always less than the one of a thumb.

The motion recovery is never excellent, depending on the condition of the thenar eminence muscles and the trapezium-metacarpal joint. These structures must be examined and their condition is assessed before the surgical plan is made. On the foot side, it must be stressed that the patients having had a first toe transplant would have a running impairment, which is never found in the second toe transplant patients.

GROWTH OF THE RECONSTRUCTED THUMB

Follow-up studies in children revealed that the growth of the reconstructed thumb was similar to the growth of the equivalent nontransplanted toe. Overgrowth and undergrowth of the transplanted toe were never too important. This conclusion highly supports the use of this technique for thumb reconstruction in children.

INDICATIONS

CONGENITAL AMPUTATIONS

The majority of congenital amputations result from constricting annular bands, being most of the time normal proximal structures (nerves, vessels, tendons). These amputations are usually at metacarpophalangeal joint level, the first metacarpal bone and the thenar eminence muscles being normal. In these cases, the results are excellent.

The hypoplasia of the thumb is a good case for pollicization. This condition is usually associated with other abnormalities (nerve, vessel, muscle, and bone malformations), which make the transplantation technically difficult to perform and ending up with poor functional results.

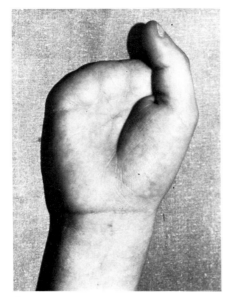

Figure 103–10. Child, 11 years old. Post-traumatic amputation of four fingers, preserving the base of the proximal phalanx. *A,* The thumb is normal. *B,* One year after transfer of a second toe. *C,* Excellent terminal pinch. *D,* Active flexion for the finger is 45 degrees at the metacarpophalangeal joint and 45 degrees at the proximal interphalangeal joint. *E,* Another second toe is transferred for cosmetic reasons.

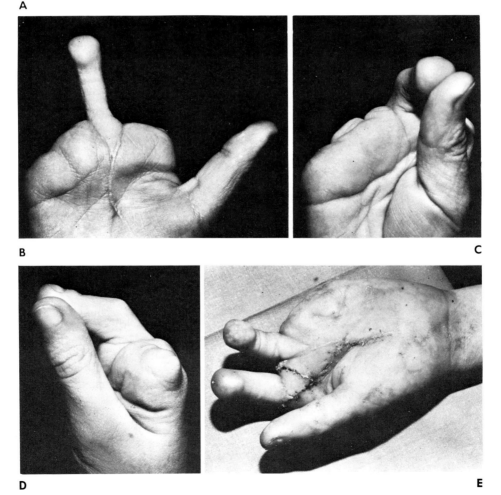

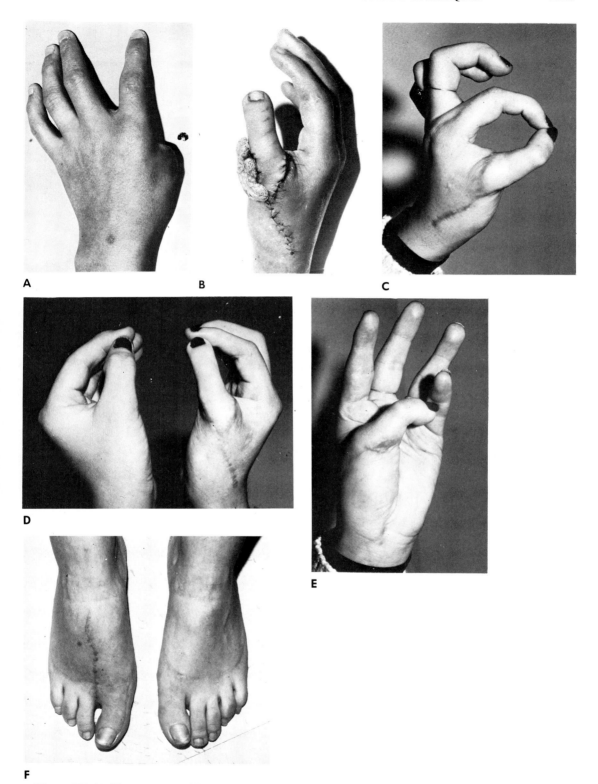

Figure 103–11. Young woman, 20 years old. Traumatic amputation of the right thumb at metacarpophalangeal level. *A,* Preoperative aspect. *B,* At the end of the transfer, a skin graft is often necessary. *C,* Ten months postoperative: the terminal pinch. *D,* Cosmetic aspect of the thumb. *E,* Opposition of the thumb. *F,* The foot after raising the second toe.

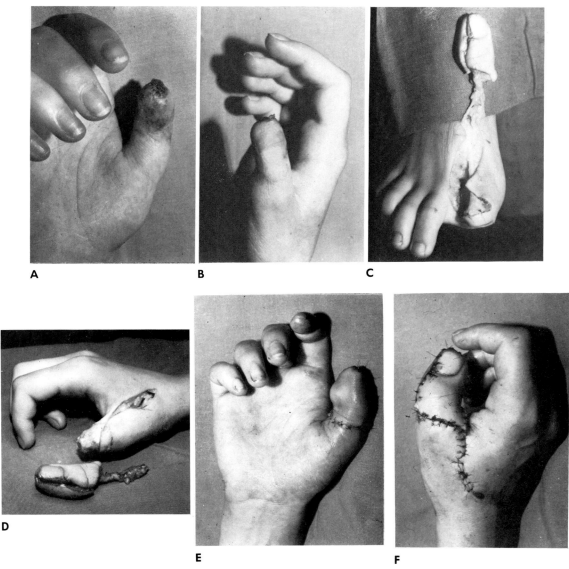

Figure 103–12. Another example of toe transfer. *A* and *B*, Preoperative views. *C*, The first toe flap is prepared and reduced in size. *D*, The flap detached and ready to be transferred on the thumb. *E* and *F*, Early result.

In the "one-finger-hand," in the "two-finger-hand," or when it is impossible to perform a pollicization, one can reconsider the possibility of performing a toe transplant to reconstruct the thumb. In these cases the newly reconstructed thumb will be a fixed post counteracting the function of the finger, which must have a full range of movements.

Traumatic Amputation

It is not always easy to make a correct surgical plan to reconstruct the thumb after a traumatic amputation, and it must be done in view of trying to offer a good grip and strength. Several factors dictate the indication: level of amputation, age of the patient, handedness, profession, and associate injuries. The level of amputation is the main factor orienting the decision:

1. Amputation distal to the half of the proximal phalanx. It is an indication to transplant a part of the toe including the nail. The aesthetic result will be excellent. As the metacarpophalangeal joint is intact, the motion of the reconstructed thumb will be functionally acceptable.

2. Amputation between the base of the proximal phalanx and the metacarpophalangeal joint level. This is the best indication for a toe transplant, as all the thenar eminence muscles are preserved. The first toe transplant will give the best aesthetic result.

3. Amputation between the metacarpophalangeal joint level and the middle third of the metacarpal bone. It is sometimes necessary to transplant the second toe with the distal half of the second metacarpal bone, to provide length, but when the thenar eminence muscles are destroyed, the functional results are poor. At instances, it is also necessary to provide skin coverage.

4. The complete amputation of the thumb including all the first ray. A toe transplant will give a poor result in this case. The result of a pollicization is by far better than that of the toe transplant, which can, however, be considered as an alternative in the case of technical impossibility to perform a pollicization.

CONCLUSION

The toe transplant is undoubtedly an improved technique to reconstruct an amputated thumb, as the classic methods are frequently time-consuming and give unsatisfactory results. It shall, however, be performed only for the above specified indications and by a team well trained in vascular microsurgery.

REFERENCES

Bencke, H.: Digital transplantation. Clin. Plast. Surg., 4:295, 1975.

Clarkson, P.: On making thumbs. Plast. Reconst. Surg., 29:525, 1962.

Cobbett, J.: Free digital transfer. J. Bone Joint Surg., 51B:577, 1969.

Freeman, B.: Reconstruction of the thumb by toe transfer. Plast. Reconst. Surg., 17:393, 1965.

Gilbert, A.: Composite tissue transfers from the foot. In Symposium on Microsurgery. St. Louis, The C. V. Mosby Company, 1976, p. 230.

Gilbert, A., and Dessapt, B.: Lambeaux libres avec microanastomosis vasculaires. Chirurgie, 102:980, 1976.

Gilbert A., Morrison, W., Tubiana R., Lisfranc, R., and Firmin, F.: Transfert sur la main d'un lambeau libre sensible. Chirurgie 101:621, 1975.

Harii, K., Ohmori, K., and Ohmori, S.: Successful clinical transfer of ten free flaps by microvascular anastomosis. Plast. Reconstr. Surg., 53:259,1974.

Harii, K., Ohmori, K., Torii, S., Murakami, F., Kasai, Y., Sekiguhi, J., and Ohmori, S.: Free groin flaps. Br. J. Plast. Surg., 28:225, 1975.

MacCraw, J., and Furlow, L.: The dorsalis pedis arterialized flap. Plast. Reconst. Surg., 55:177, 1975.

MacGregor, I., and Jackson, I.: The groin flap. Br. J. Plast. Surg., 25:3, 1972.

Millesi, H.: Personal communication.

O'Brien, B., Morrison, W., Ishida, H., MacLeod, A., and Gilbert, A.: Free flap transfers with microvascular anastomoses. Br. J. Plast. Surg., 27:220, 1974.

Ohmori, K., and Harii, K.: Transplantation of a toe to an amputated finger. Hand, 7:134, 1975.

Tsai, T.: Experimental and clinical applications of microvascular surgery. Ann. Surg., 181:169, 1975.

Chapter 104

THUMB RECONSTRUCTION BY USE OF A WRAP-AROUND FLAP FROM THE BIG TOE

WAYNE A. MORRISON

Current methods of thumb reconstruction remain imperfect because of inadequate function, significant secondary defects, or cosmetic limitations. Metacarpal lengthening, cocked hat procedures, and phalangization all fail to provide necessary length, a padded tip, and a nail. Osteoplastic reconstructions are prone to swivel and lack a nail, and the island flap poses problems of finger identification and secondary defects. Bone grafts also have a reputation for absorption. Pollicization and big toe transfers sacrifice significant tissue and retain the esthetic characteristics of their origin. Second toe transfers, although causing a minimal secondary defect, still remain second toes on the hand.

A composite neurovascular flap from the big toe containing skin, pulp, and nail can be transferred to the hand by microvascular anastomosis where it is wrapped around an iliac crest bone graft tailored to the shape and length of the missing thumb. This reproduces a thumb with a nail and a nonswiveling, well padded pulp, which esthetically appears identical to its predecessor. There is no confusion with finger identification, and a minimal secondary defect remains because the hallux is preserved by using a cross toe flap from the second toe and a split skin graft (Hamilton et al., 1979; Morrison et al., 1980a, b).

METHOD

TOE FLAP

Flap markings are shown in Figures 104–1 and 104–2. The ipsilateral hallux is chosen as

the donor so that the flap seam will be along the nondominant radial side when the flap is transferred to the thumb. Moreover the larger digital nerve to the big toe is on the lateral side so that the innervation to the ulnar pulp remains undisturbed. The circumference and length of the wrap-around flap are determined by measuring the opposite normal thumb. The difference in circumfer-

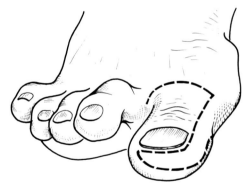

Figure 104–1

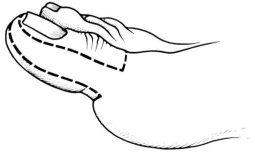

Figure 104–2

Figures 104–1 and 104–2. Toe markings showing the medial and tip skin flap which is retained on the toe.

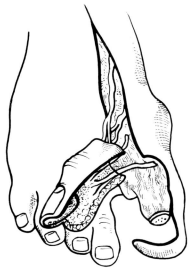

Figure 104–3. Toe flap mobilized on its dorsal vessels. The distal half of the distal phalanx is included in the flap.

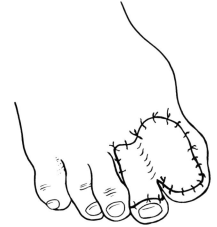

Figure 104–4. Toe defect closed dorsally with a split skin graft covering the dorsum of the big and second toes.

ence between the thumb and the hallux determines the width of the protective skin bridge that is retained along the medial border and the tip of the toe. This is innervated by a large dorsal branch of the medial digital nerve of the big toe arising proximal to the metacarpophalangeal joint. The hallux, including the nail and its matrix, is totally degloved except for the medial and tip strip, and the flap is isolated on its dorsal arterial and venous systems as far proximally as the dorsalis pedis artery and the long saphenous vein to permit anastomosis to the radial artery and cephalic vein at the anatomical snuff box region in the hand (Fig. 104–3). The deep peroneal nerve is also included with the flap for connection with terminal branches of the radial nerve. In a minority of cases the dorsal metatarsal artery is too small to support the flap and the plantar vessels must be used. In this situation they are usually of good caliber but are short. The plantar digital nerves are divided proximally and transferred with the flap. The distal half of the distal phalanx underlying the nail matrix is included with the resection to prevent breaking of the nail and to act as a vascularized bone segment distal to the free iliac crest bone graft, thereby reducing resorption of the graft.

Toe Defect

The toe defect is closed first by trimming the distal phalanx stump and folding the tip

flap laterally around the toe. The plantar area is resurfaced by a cross toe flap from the dorsal surface of the adjacent second toe (Fig. 104–4). The dorsal defects of the big and second toes are grafted with thick split skin (Fig. 104–5). The cross toe flap is divided under local anesthesia at four weeks.

Bone Graft

An iliac crest bone graft is taken and shaped to form the new skeleton of the thumb. It is interposed between the vascularized segments of bone proximally and distally

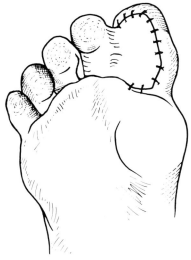

Figure 104–5. Toe defect, plantar view, closed with a cross toe flap taken from the dorsum of the second toe.

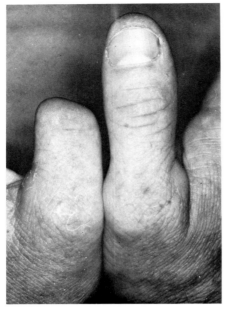

Figure 104–6. Case 1. Preoperative view. Amputation through the head of the proximal phalanx.

to minimize resorption. No angulation of the graft is attempted, and it is transfixed into position with Kirschner wires.

THUMB RECONSTRUCTION

The recipient vessels used are the large radial artery and cephalic vein at the anatom-

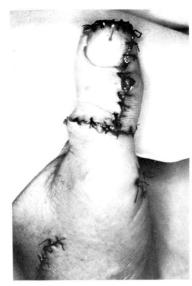

Figure 104–8. Foot flap wrapped around bone graft.

ical snuff box region, well away from the site of the previous injury. The stumps of the thumb digital nerves are located on the palmar surface and trimmed. With the bone graft in position and the recipient vessels and nerves defined, the toe flap is detached from its blood supply in the foot and transferred to the hand where it is wrapped around the bone graft. The corresponding vessels and nerves are connected.

The technique relies on the success of small vessel anastomoses and nerve repairs. The

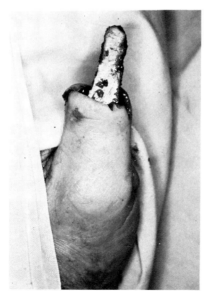

Figure 104–7. Iliac crest bone graft.

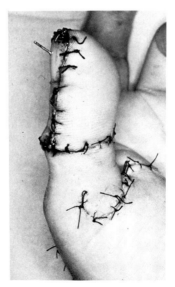

Figure 104–9. Lateral view.

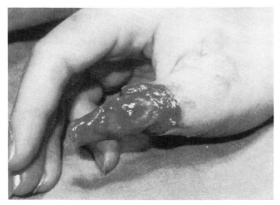

Figure 104–10. Case 2. Preoperative view. Degloving of thumb.

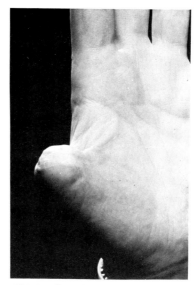

Figure 104–12. Case 3. Preoperative view. Amputation at the metacarpophalangeal joint.

vessels used are large by design. By mobilizing the toe flap on the dorsal system, the dorsalis pedis artery becomes the donor vessel, and its large diameter and long pedicle greatly increase the reliability of microvascular transfer. Similarly, large recipient vessels are chosen at the wrist.

Resulting function depends on the quality of nerve repair and the sensory capacity of toe skin. Although two point discrimination often falls short of normal in these transfers, as it does in any form of toe transfer, functionally the thumb has no substitute, and thus it is used automatically and undergoes its own form of sensory re-education. There are now many reports of toe flaps whose two point discrimination has narrowed consider-

ably after transfer to the hand (Buncke and Rose, 1979; Foucher et al., 1980; Strauch and Tsur, 1978). The brain registers thumb as thumb, and no further secondary defect is added to an already compromised hand.

The bone grafts have not become resorbed appreciably with this technique, presumably because of the excellent circumferential vas-

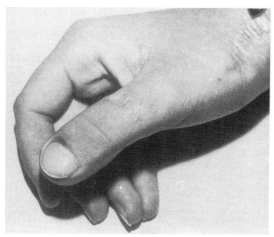

Figure 104–11. Case 2. Postoperative view. Delayed primary "wrap-around" flap to resurface defect.

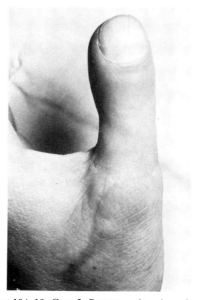

Figure 104–13. Case 3. Postoperative view after seven years.

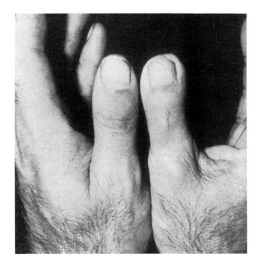

Figure 104–14. Case 4. Thumb reconstruction of proximal phalangeal level five years after surgery, comparing thumbs.

cularization afforded by the wrap-around flap (Frykman et al., 1987).

No joint is transferred so that there are relative limitations of this method as a reconstruction for amputations proximal to the metacarpophalangeal joint. The operation is contraindicated in children because it fails to provide the growth potential of pollicizations and whole toe transfers.

Esthetically the thumb can be shaped to the exact proportions of the opposite normal thumb; it is not limited by the underlying skeletal size of the index, big, or second toes. It therefore potentially creates the most aesthetic thumb short of replantation (Figs. 104–6 to 104–14).

Finally the secondary defect in the foot is minimal provided adequate care is taken to shorten the distal phalanx and inlay a generous cross toe flap from the adjacent second toe (Fig. 104–15).

REFERENCES

Buncke, H. J., and Rose, E. H.: Free toe to finger tip neurovascular flap. Plast. Reconstr. Surg., 63:607–611, 1979.

Foucher, G., Merle, M., Maneaud, M., and Michon, J.: Microsurgical free partial toe transfer in hand reconstruction. A report of 12 cases. Plast. Reconstr. Surg., 65:616–609, 1980.

Frykman, G. K., Morrison, W. A., Gumley, G. J., O'Brien, B. M., MacLeod, A. M., and Ciurleo, A.: The functional results of thumb reconstruction by microneurovascular wrap-around flaps. J. Hand Surg. (Am.), in press, 1987.

Hamilton, R. B., O'Brien, B. M., and Morrison, W. A.: The cross toe flap. Br. J. Plast. Surg., 32:213–216, 1979.

Morrison, W. A., O'Brien, B. M., and MacLeod, A. M.: The surgical repair of amputations of the thumb. Aust. New Zealand J. Surg., 50:237–243, 1980a.

Morrison, W. A., O'Brien, B. M., and MacLeod, A. M.: Thumb reconstruction using a free neurovascular wrap-around flap from the big toe. J. Hand Surg., 5:575–583, 1980b.

Strauch, B., and Tsur, H.: Restoration of sensation in the hand by a free neurovascular flap from the first web space of the foot. Plast. Reconstr. Surg., 62:361, 1978.

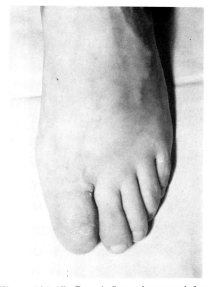

Figure 104–15. Case 4. Secondary toe defect.

Chapter 105

FUNCTIONAL COMPARISON BETWEEN POLLICIZATION AND TOE TO HAND TRANSFER FOR THUMB RECONSTRUCTION

Jacques Michon,
Michel Merle,
and Guy Foucher

METHOD

The results of 33 pollicizations and 21 toe to hand transfers for thumb reconstruction were compared to determine the comparative value of both methods and their advantages and disadvantages and to try to clarify the indications for the use of each method. The functional results of thumb reconstruction were tested in the following six categories and scored as indicated:

1. Mobility (0 to 4). Two points were given for carpometacarpal joint and 2 points for the metacarpophalangeal and interphalangeal joints.
2. Strength (0 to 4). Measured by pressure on the rubber bulb of a manometer, compared to the unaffected side.
3. Sensibility (0 to 4). None or painful = 0; protective = 2; 10 mm. = 3; normal = 4.
4. Cosmetic appearance (0 to 4)
5. Pinch accuracy (0 to 4)
6. Grasping power (0 to 4). Calculated by combining possibility of opening and closing digits and thumb (0 to 2) with strength of grasping, evaluated with the rubber bulb of a manometer and compared with the results with the unaffected hand (0 to 2).

Categories 1 to 4 directly tested qualities of the new thumb; categories 5 and 6 tested the global function of the hand, including the thumb.

The total score for a normal hand would be 24. Our classification of total test scores

for the reconstructed thumb was as follows: 20 and above, excellent; 18 to 20, good; 12 to 17, moderate; 6 to 11, fair; and 0 to 5, failure.

Final scores were calculated by three different methods: study of physiotherapist records at the end-of-treatment check-up, special meetings and discussion involving cases with imprecise records, and information questionnaires sent to patients who could not come to the clinic (six cases).

All patients were followed for more than one year after the reconstruction.

According to preoperative anatomical conditions, the cases were divided into four groups: group I—missing thumb with four normal fingers; group II—missing thumb with some amputated or disabled fingers; group III—metacarpal hand, including cases with an isolated remaining little finger; group IV—distal thumb amputations with retention of the metacarpophalangeal joint or more.

Two cases of congenital absence of the thumb were excluded from this presentation. Both involved operations done on teenagers, one by pollicization of the index finger and the other by second toe transfer. Neither reconstruction was used well by the patient, a result that can be explained by the advanced age of the patients at the time of operation. The reconstruction did not change their well established mental picture of a hand without a thumb. The treatment in congenital cases

Table 105–1. SUMMARY OF RESULTS IN GROUP I

Evaluation	No. of Cases	Total Score
Pollicization		
Excellent	2	20, 21
Good	2	18.5, 19.5
Moderate	1	17
Toe to hand transfer		
Excellent	1	20.5 (big toe)
Good	2	18 (second toe) 17.5 (big toe)
Moderate	3	13.5, 13, 12.5 (second toe)
Failure	1	0 (necrosis, second toe)

ideally should be carried out in the very early years of life.

RESULTS

GROUP I: MISSING THUMB WITH FOUR NORMAL FINGERS

We compared five cases of pollicization with seven cases of toe to hand transfer. The findings are summarized in Tables 105–1 and 105–2.

Pollicization was demonstrated to produce higher scores in thumb reconstruction when all the remaining digits were normal (Fig. 105–1). Nevertheless detailed examination of the scores showed a decrease of the power grip (which was not over 2.5 to 3.0 in five patients) in every case of pollicization. In one case, when transferring the ring finger to the thumb, a little finger was simultaneously transferred onto the fourth metacarpal. In this case the power grip was diminished to 1.5, with restricted function of the flexor tendons of the fifth and third digits. This unfavorable effect of transfer on prehension may restrict the indications for pollicization in manual workers, in favor of transfer of the big toe by a microvascular procedure.

In 50 per cent of the cases of second toe transfer, secondary flexion contracture at the proximal interphalangeal joint level developed in varying degrees (Fig. 105–2). In the toe transfer group, better results were achieved with big toe transfer, with marked superiority over second toe transfer in both mobility and power of the new thumb. In all cases of toe transfer, power grip remained normal or very slightly diminished (scores were 3 to 4).

On the basis of the findings in group I, we would recommend pollicization as the method of choice for thumb reconstruction when all other digits are intact, particularly if the patient is involved with precision hand work. For manual workers, however, transfer of the big toe may be the proper solution. This is true in spite of some restriction of sensibility and mobility at the metacarpophalangeal and interphalangeal joint levels, if conservation of strength and endurance is required.

GROUP II: MISSING THUMB WITH SOME AMPUTATED OR DISABLED FINGERS

We studied 17 cases of pollicization and five cases of toe transfer. In this group polli-

Table 105–2. RESULTS OF TESTING IN GROUP I

Case	Level	Digit Transferred	Total	Thenar Mobility	Thenar Power	Thenar Sensibility	Cosmetic Appearance	Pinch	Grasp
Pollicization (five cases)									
1	Metacarpal	Fourth	21.0	3.5	3.5	4.0	3.0	4.0	3.0
2	Metacarpal	Fourth	21.5	4.0	3.5	4.0	3.5	3.0	3.5
3	Metacarpal	Fourth	18.0	2.0	3.5	4.0	3.0	3.0	2.5
4	Metacarpal	Fourth	18.5	3.0	3.0	4.0	3.0	3.0	2.5
5	Metacarpal	Fourth	17.0	3.0	3.0	4.0	3.0	2.5	1.5
Big toe transfer (two cases)									
1	Metacarpal	T1	17.5	2.0	3.0	2.5	3.0	3.0	4.0
2	Metacarpal	T1	20.5	3.5	3.0	3.0	4.0	3.0	4.0
Second toe transfer (five cases)									
1	Metacarpal	T2	13.0	2.0	2.0	2.0	2.0	2.0	3.0
2	Metacarpal	T2	11.5	1.5	2.0	2.0	1.5	1.5	3.0
3	Metacarpal	T2	Necrosis	—	—	—	—	—	3.5
4	Metacarpal	T2	18.0	3.5	2.0	2.0	3.0	3.5	4.0
5	Metacarpal	T2	13.5	2.5	2.0	2.0	2.0	2.0	3.0

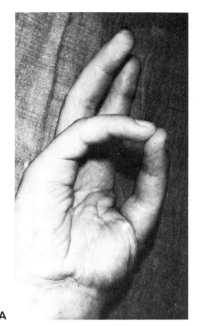
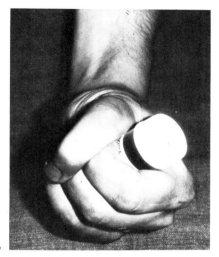

A   B

Figure 105–1. *A* and *B*, Excellent function of a pollicization of an intact ring finger.

cization made use of fingers that were more or less damaged in all cases, and for better comparison, we isolated a series of seven "on top plasties" in which the transposed index finger was amputated at the metacarpophalangeal or proximal phalangeal level (Tables 105–3 and 105–4; Figs. 105–3 to 105–5).

In group II statistical comparison becomes much more difficult and controversial, be-cause anatomical conditions may vary consid-erably from one patient to another. If the pollicizations are examined in detail, two conclusions may be reached:

1. If disability in the transferred digit is minor, results in the reconstructed thumb will be good. However, if joints or tendons have been jeopardized, the results may be disap-pointing.

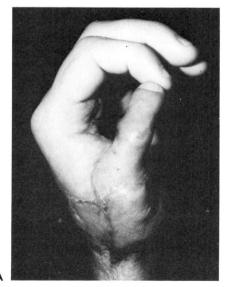
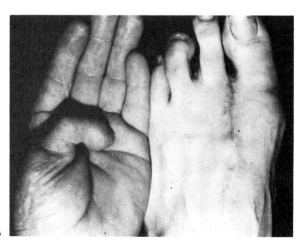

A   B

Figure 105–2. *A* and *B*. Transfer of second toe to thumb. Functional and cosmetic deficits to the foot are minimal.

Table 105–3. SUMMARY OF RESULTS IN GROUP II

Evaluation	No. of Cases	Total Score
Pollicization		
Moderate	6	17.5, 17.0, 15.0, 14.0, 14.0, 12.5
Fair	4	10.5, 9.5, 8.0, 5.0
On top plasty (Fig. 105–3)		
Moderate	4	14.5, 13.5, 12.5, 12.0
Fair	3	11.5, 11.5, 6.0
Big toe transfer (Fig. 105–4)		
Good	2	18.5, 16.0
Second toe transfer (Fig. 105–5)		
Moderate	3	14.5, 12.5, 12.0

2. The degree of utility of a pollicized digit is in inverse proportion to the severity of amputation or functional disability in the remaining digits. Displacing one already compromised element on the hand also decreases prehension capacity and strength. This explains our high proportion of fair and failure results in group II, all corresponding to poor initial conditions—polyamputated hands or multiple stiff or crippled digits. The addition of a poor hand and the transfer of a compromised digit in that hand further compromise the result.

On the contrary, toe transfer brings in a new intact element, which through precise technique can be free of scars, can have its own secure blood supply, and does not deprive the hand of any of its previous possibilities. Toe transfer thus provides a functional addition with no loss. In group II our functional scores again provide evidence of the superiority of the big toe, compared to the second toe, in retaining mobility and power.

For both reconstructive methods the functional quality of the reconstruction depends on the conservation and activity of the carpometacarpal joint and the thenar muscles. Neither arthroplasties nor tendon transfers, correlated with any type of reconstruction,

Table 105–4. RESULTS OF TESTING IN GROUP II

Case	Level	Digit Transferred	Total	Thenar Mobility	Thenar Power	Thenar Sensibility	Cosmetic Appearance	Pinch	Grasp
Pollicization (10 cases)									
1	Metacarpal	Third	15.0	2.0	2.0	3.0	3.0	2.0	3.0
2	Metacarpal	Fourth	17.5	3.0	2.5	4.0	3.0	2.0	3.0
3	Metacarpal	Fourth	15.0	2.0	2.0	3.5	3.5	2.5	1.5
4	Metacarpal	Second	12.5	2.0	2.0	2.0	2.5	2.0	2.0
5	Metacarpal	Second	17.0	2.0	3.0	4.0	3.0	3.0	3.0
6	Carpal	Third	10.5	2.0	1.5	2.0	2.0	1.5	1.5
7	Carpal	Third	9.5	1.5	1.0	3.0	1.5	1.0	1.5
8	Carpal	Second	8.0	1.0	1.0	1.5	1.5	1.5	1.5
9	Carpal	Second	5.0	0.5	0.5	2.0	1.0	0.0	1.5
10	Carpal	Second	14.0	2.0	2.0	3.0	2.0	2.5	2.5
On top plasty (seven cases)									
1	Metacarpal	Second	14.5	2.0	2.5	3.0	2.5	2.0	2.5
2	Metacarpal	Second	12.5	2.0	2.0	2.5	2.0	2.0	2.0
3	Metacarpal	Second	6.0	1.0	0.0	2.0	1.5	0.0	1.5
4	Metacarpal	Second	11.5	1.0	2.0	1.5	1.0	3.0	3.0
5	Metacarpal	Second	13.5	2.0	3.0	4.0	1.5	1.0	3.0
6	Metacarpal	Second	11.5	0.5	2.0	4.0	1.0	2.0	2.0
7	Metacarpal	Second	12.0	2.0	2.0	3.5	2.0	1.0	1.5
Big toe transfer (two cases)									
1	Metacarpal	T1	16.0	2.0	3.0	2.5	3.0	2.5	3.0
2	Metacarpal	T1	18.5	3.0	4.0	2.0	3.0	4.0	2.5
Second toe transfer (three cases)									
1	Metacarpal	T2	12.0	1.5	1.5	3.0	2.0	1.5	2.5
2	Metacarpal	T2	14.5	2.0	2.0	4.0	3.0	2.0	1.5
3	Metacarpal	T2	12.5	2.5	1.0	2.0	2.0	2.0	3.0

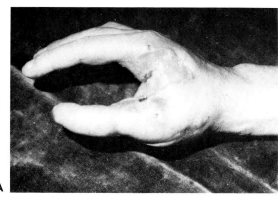

A

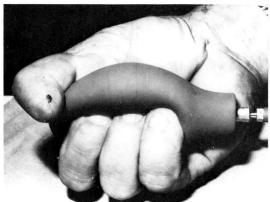

B

Figure 105–3. Result of pollicization of a distally amputated index.

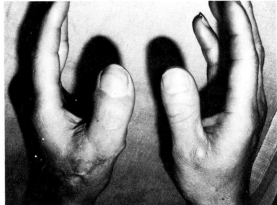

A

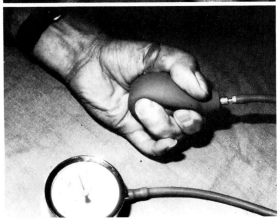

B

Figure 105–4. *A* and *B,* Despite absence of the index finger and stiffness of the little finger, transfer of the big toe has restored a powerful grip to a carpenter.

1161

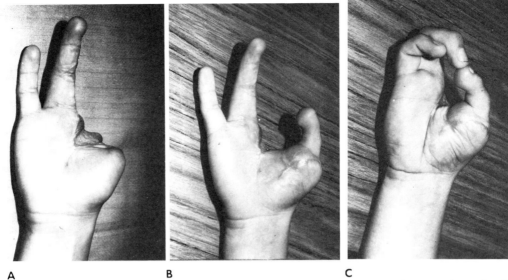

A   B   C
Figure 105–5. *A*, Amputation of thumb, index, and middle finger. *B* and *C*, Second toe transfer to thumb.

could achieve really adequate powerful motion in the new thumb in the absence of a carpometacarpal joint.

To summarize our findings for group II, the indications for toe transfers seem stronger, in proportion to the severity and extension of anatomical and functional deficits in the remaining digits, while the advantages of pollicization decrease in proportion to the deficit in the remaining fingers. Since the quality of pollicization is directly dependent on the integrity of the transferred finger, the use of a partially amputated or disabled finger must be balanced against limitations of thumb function. Transfer of the big toe is always an addition to hand function in every case, especially for manual workers and for patients with severe and multiple finger mutilations. However, the major contraindication to this procedure is the effect on foot function, which for active patients may be a real problem in their professional or leisure lives. In most cases they can walk extensively and painlessly but may have difficulty in running and in practicing sports.

GROUP III: METACARPAL HAND, INCLUDING ISOLATED REMAINING LITTLE FINGER

In the metacarpal hand, no possibility for real grasping exists, so that total scores were reduced to a maximum of 20 points. This total also applies to the metacarpal hand where the fifth finger was still present. An excellent result meant a score of 16 or above. A score of 12 or above was classified as a good result, 8 or above as moderate, 4 or above as fair, and scores under 4 as failures.

Five pollicizations were evaluated. Three toe transfers were performed, but only two could be evaluated. The scores are presented in Tables 105–5 and 105–6.

The result achieved in the total metacarpal hand by second metacarpal pollicization was only a very weak and unrefined lateral forceps pinch. The reconstruction was a little more useful if the elementary short thumb was in position to oppose a good mobile fifth digit. However, a good position was very difficult to obtain. This problem might have

Table 105–5. SUMMARY OF RESULTS IN GROUP III

Evaluation	No. of Cases	Total Score
Pollicization		
Moderate	3	10.5, 9.5,* 9.0
Fair	2	7.5*, 7.0
Toe transfer		
Good	1	12.0
Moderate	1	10.5
Unknown	1	(?)

*Scores for patients with a remaining fifth digit.

Table 105–6. GROUP III: METACARPAL HAND WITH OR WITHOUT FIFTH FINGER

	Total Score	Mobility	Thenar Power	Sensibility	Cosmetic Appearance	Prehension
On top plasty, 5 cases	8.7	1.6	1.4	3.1	1.3	1.3
Second toe, 2 cases	11.75	2.5	1.5	4.0	2.0	1.75
Best toe	13	2.5	2.0	4.0	2.0	2.5
Best pollicization	10.5	1.5	2.0	4.0	1.0	2.0

been improved by rotation osteotomy of the fifth metacarpal. We did not perform this procedure in this series of patients.

Toe transfer can very easily be oriented in the exact direction of a little finger at the time of osteosynthesis to achieve a precise and delicate pinch, even with restricted mobility. In the total metacarpal hand our choice has been to prepare for thumb reconstruction by elevating the ulnar side of the stump with an iliac bone graft and groin flap, combined with removal of the second metacarpal to deepen the first web space. Two months later the toe is transferred by microsurgical technique, oriented to face the osteoplasty (Fig. 105–6).

In our first case the elevation osteoplasty was too short and inadequately covered dorsally by a free skin graft. A strong pinch could not be obtained after toe transfer. However, such a technical failure is not an argument against the principles of this method, as demonstrated by a useful functional result in another patient (Fig. 105–7).

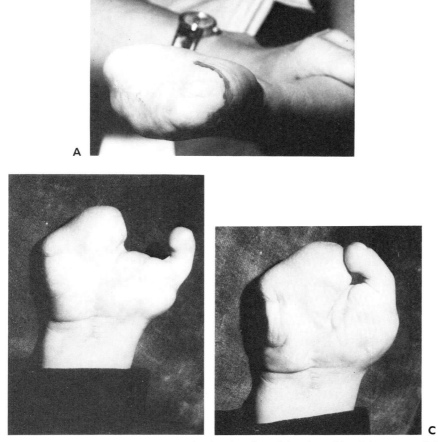

Figure 105–6. *A*, Metacarpal hand. *B*, Reconstruction by elevation of the ulnar side of the stump. *C*, Transfer of the second toe on the first metacarpal.

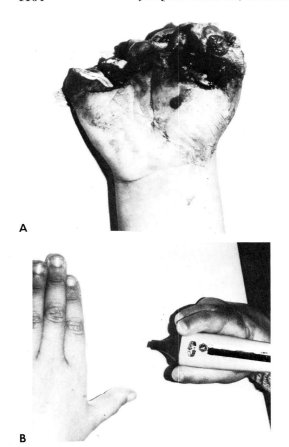

Figure 105–7. *A*, Total metacarpal hand covered primarily by a groin flap. *B*, Result after transfer of three toes in two operations.

In the future we would strongly consider the use of the big toe in similar cases, since we know from patients in the other groups that mobility and power would definitely be better. Furthermore, microsurgical techniques now allow more sophisticated reconstructions.

GROUP IV: DISTAL AMPUTATIONS OF THE THUMB

In group IV we further consider distal amputations of the thumb when the metacarpophalangeal joint was entirely preserved. In this category, 10 cases were evaluated. Two had undergone pollicizations of the two distal phalanges of a finger. Three patients were treated by on top plasty of the multilated index finger. Five similar patients were treated with partial toe transfer of the big toe or a combined second and big toe partial

transfer (Fig. 105–8). The scores in these cases are presented in Tables 105–7 and 105–8.

In cases of amputations distal to the metacarpophalangeal joint, both methods can achieve very good results. In our opinion, however, it seems unnecessary to sacrifice a useful digit for distal reconstruction. This restricts the indications for pollicization to digits with proximal injuries with good blood and sensory supplies to the distal phalanges. Partial transfer of a big toe or a combined second and big toe transfer seems to use the best solution for all other cases of distal amputations of the thumb.

DISCUSSION

To evaluate the different techniques more precisely, we studied results from the viewpoint of thumb function independent of the rest of the hand—mobility, power, and sensibility. It was immediately obvious that the level of amputation of the thumb was a very important factor. Amputation at the carpal level is a difficult condition because the carpometacarpal joint must be reconstructed, and our attempts to use Silastic implants have been more or less disappointing in this condition. In most cases the thenar muscles are also destroyed, and tendon transfers could not achieve adequate normal function in such a difficult area.

To summarize our findings, on top plasty (pollicization of a partially amputated finger) seldom achieves a satisfactory thumb. The average of results of second toe transfers is in the moderate range, although, a few cases yielded good results. The metacarpophalangeal and interphalangeal joints of the second toe have more or less limited mobility, and their power is often weak. The appearance is also somewhat disturbing. The two competitive alternatives in treatment are pollicization and transfer of the big toe. Both methods restore good mobility, real power, and a thumblike aspect. As we have already pointed out, pollicization of a normal digit gives better mobility and a more precise pinch, but also weakens the grasp power.

SUMMARY

The functional results of two methods of thumb reconstruction—pollicization and toe

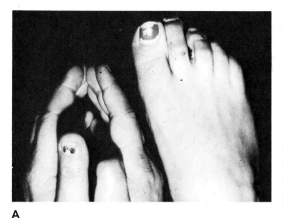

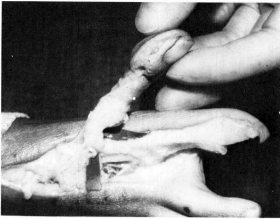

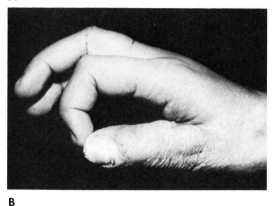

Figure 105–8. Distal amputation of the thumb in a young woman. *A*, Neither the big toe nor the second toe is of the correct caliber. *B*, Partial transfer of the big toe "to measure," seen during the dissection. *C*, Satisfactory cosmetic and functional result.

transplantation—were evaluated in four groups of patients: group I, those missing the thumb but with four other normal digits; group II, those missing the thumb with partially mutilated or amputated other digits; group III, those with a metacarpal hand; and group IV, those with a distal thumb amputation. In each group the results were compared in five categories: sensibility, mobility, power grip, precision grip, and cosmetic appearance.

In group I, pollicization provided superior

sensibility and mobility, but power grip was best achieved by transfer of the big toe. Second toe transfer and pollicization both resulted in some weakness, compared with the normal hand. Precision grip, related to the quality of sensibility, was better achieved by pollicization than by any free transfer.

In group II, although pollicization of a mutilated digit is more controversial, in some cases a very good functional level was reached, directly related to the amount of preoperative sensibility and the mobility of the proximal interphalangeal joint in the transferred digit. Reduction of strength and prehension depended on the number and quality of the remaining nontransferred digits. Toe transfer yielded better results in all five categories, because the severity of digit mutilation increased.

In group III, pollicization of the second metacarpal achieved a very rudimentary pinch, with toe transfer allowing for much greater prehension possibilities.

In group IV, distal thumb amputations were treated with distal digital pollicization as

Table 105–7. SUMMARY OF RESULTS IN GROUP IV

Evaluation	No. of Cases	Total Score
Distal pollicization		
Excellent	1	20.0
Good	2	19.5, 18.0
Moderate	2	13.0, 12.5
Partial toe transfer		
Excellent	3	21.0, 21.0, 20.5
Good	2	19.5, 17.0

Table 105–8. RESULTS OF TESTING IN GROUP IV

Case	Level	Digit Transferred	Total	Thenar Mobility	Thenar Power	Thenar Sensibility	Cosmetic Appearance	Pinch	Grasp
Pollicization (two cases)									
1	Distal to metacarpal joint	Second	13.0	2.0	2.0	4.0	2.0	2.0	1.0
2	Distal to metacarpal joint	Third	20.0	3.0	3.0	3.5	4.0	4.0	2.5
On top plasty (three cases)									
1	Distal to metacarpal joint	Second	12.5	2.0	3.0	3.0	1.5	2.5	1.5
2	Distal to metacarpal joint	Third	19.5	3.0	3.0	4.0	3.0	2.5	4.0
3	Distal to metacarpal joint	Third	18.0	3.0	3.0	4.0	2.0	3.0	3.0
Partial toe transfer (five cases)									
1	Distal to metacarpal joint	Partial toe	20.5	3.0	3.5	4.0	3.0	3.0	4.0
2	Distal to metacarpal joint	Partial toe	21.0	4.0	3.0	4.0	2.5	3.5	4.0
3	Distal to metacarpal joint	Partial toe	21.0	3.0	4.0	4.0	3.0	3.0	4.0
4	Distal to metacarpal joint	Partial toe	19.5	3.0	3.0	4.0	2.5	3.0	4.0
5	Distal to metacarpal joint	Partial toe	18.0	3.0	3.0	3.0	2.5	3.5	3.0

well as partial toe transplantation. Both methods were beneficial, but the indication for pollicization was extremely limited.

Finally, the results of big and second toe transfer for thumb reconstruction indicated that big toe transfer provided superior results in both functional and cosmetic aspects.

REFERENCES

Buck-Gramko, D.: Pollicization of the index finger: method and results in aplasia and hypoplasia of the thumb. J. Bone Joint Surg., 53(A):1605, 1971.

Buncke, H. J.: Toe digital transfer. Clin. Plast. Surg., 3:49, 1976.

Buncke, H. J., Buncke, C. H., and Schulz, W.: Immediate Nicoladoni procedure, utilizing microminiature vascular anastomoses. Br. J. Plast. Surg., 19:332, 1966.

Buncke, H. J., and Rose, E. H.: Free toe fingertip neurovascular flaps. Plast. Reconstr. Surg., 63:607, 1979.

Buncke, H. J., and Shah, K. G.: In Serafin, D., and Buncke, H. J. (Editors): Toe-Digital Transfers in Microsurgical Composite Tissue Transplantation. St. Louis, The C. V. Mosby Company, 1976, pp. 216–229.

Foucher, G., Merle, M., Maneaud, M., and Michon, J.: Microsurgical free partial toe transfer in hand reconstruction: a report of 12 cases. Plast. Reconstr. Surg., 65:616, 1980.

Gilbert, A.: Composite tissue transfers from the foot: anatomic basis and surgical technique. In Daniller, A. J., and Strauch, B. (Editors): Symposium on Microsurgery. St. Louis, The C. V. Mosby Company, 1976, pp. 230–241.

Gosset, J.: La pollicisation de l'index. J. Chirur. (Paris), 65:403, 1949.

Gosset, J.: La reconstruction de pouce amputé. Monographie, Groupe d'Etude de la Main, Expansion Scientifique, Paris, 1974.

Harkins, P., and Rappet, J.: Digital transposition in the injured hand. J. Bone Joint Surg., 57(A):1064, 1972.

Harrison, S.: Restoration of muscle balance in pollicization. Plast. Reconstr. Surg., 34:236, 1964.

Herbon, J., et al.: Traumatic amputation of the thumb and three fingers: treatment by digital pollicization. J. Bone Joint Surg., 57(A):708, 1975.

Himura, M. S., and Buncke, H. J.: Biomechanical

analysis of toe to thumb transplants: a look at both sides. J. Hand Surg., *1*:81, 1976.

Kaplan, I.: Primary pollicization of injured index finger following crush injury. Plast. Reconstr. Surg., *37*:531, 1966.

LeQuang, C.: Transferts d'orteils. Rev. Chir. Orthop., *4*:299, 1978.

Letac, R.: Reconstruction du pouce d'etruit par pollicisation de l'annulaire ou du cinquiéme doigt. Mem. Acad. Chir., *78*:262, 1952.

Littler, J. W.: Subtotal reconstruction of the thumb. Plast. Reconstr. Surg., *10*:215, 1952.

Littler, J. W.: The neurovascular pedicle method of digital transposition for reconstruction of the thumb. Plast. Reconstr. Surg., *12*:303, 1953.

Littler, J. W.: On making a thumb: one hundred years of surgical effort. J. Hand Surg., *1*:35, 1976.

Matev, J.: Reconstruction of the thumb through gradual elongation of the thumb metacarpal. J. Bone Joint Surg., *52*(A):1058, 1970.

May, J. W., and Daniel, R. K.: Great toe to hand free tissue transfer. Clin. Orthop., *133*:140, 1978.

May, J. W., Smith, R. J., and Peimer, C. A.: Toe to hand free tissue transfer of thumb construction with multiple digit aplasia. Plast. Reconstr. Surg., *53*:107, 1974.

Millesi, H.: Reconstruction of the thumb by transfer of toe tissue. Chir. Plast., *1*:347, 1973; Plast. Reconstr. Surg., *53*:107, 1974.

O'Brien B.: One stage toe to hand surgery. *In* Microvascular Reconstructive Surgery. London, Churchill Livingstone, 1977, pp. 183–204.

O'Brien, B., and MacLeod, A. H.: Microvascular free toe transfer. Clin. Plast. Surg., *5*:223, 1978.

O'Brien, B., MacLeod, A. H., Sykes, P. J., and Donahoe, S.: Hallux to hand transfer. Hand, *7*:128, 1975.

O'Brien B., MacLeod, A. M., Sykes, P. J., Threefall, Y. N., and Browning, F.: Microvascular second toe transfer for digital reconstruction. J. Hand Surg., *3*:123, 1978.

O'Brien, B., MacLeod, A. M., and Sykes, P. J.: Hallux to hand transfer. Hand 7:128, 1979.

Ohmorii, K., and Harii, K.: Transplantation of a toe to an amputated finger. Hand, *7*:134, 1975.

Ohtsuka, H., et al.: Two toe to finger transplants in one hand. Plast. Reconstr. Surg., *60*:561, 1977.

Sallis, J.: Primary pollicization of an injured middle finger. J. Bone Joint Surg., *45*(B):503, 1963.

Strauch, B., and Shakiroff, B.: The foot, a versatile source of donor tissue. *In* Serafin, D., and Buncke, H. J. (Editors): Microsurgical Composite Tissue Transplantation. St. Louis, The C. V. Mosby Company, 1979, pp. 345–356.

Tamai, S., et al.: Hallux to thumb transfer with microsurgical technique: a case report in a 45 year old man. J. Hand Surg., *2*:152, 1977.

Tubiana, R.: Hand reconstruction. Acta Orthop. Scand., *46*:446, 1975.

White, W. F.: Pollicization of the missing thumb, traumatic or congenital. Hand, *1*:23, 1969.

White, W. F.: Fundamental priorities in pollicization. J. Bone Joint Surg., *52*:438, 1970.

Yoshimura, M. D.: Toe to hand transfer. Plast. Reconstr. Surg., *1*:74, 1980.

Chapter 106

SURGICAL INDICATIONS IN MUTILATIONS OF THE THUMB

Raoul Tubiana
and Alain Gilbert

The indications for reconstruction of the thumb are difficult to codify. A number of procedures have been described and are being continuously modified. Because cases requiring reconstruction of the thumb are few, it is uncommon for one surgeon to become familiar with all the techniques described. When one has adopted a technique and improved it over the years, he usually tends to remain faithful to it and may display some dogmatism with respect to surgical indications.

The various procedures available do not exactly fit all situations and are to some extent complementary. The surgical indications depend to a large extent on two local factors—the level of amputation and the state of the rest of the hand. Other factors of a more general nature, however, must be taken into account—those relating to the patient (his age, sex, profession, hobbies, and psychological background) and those relating to the surgeon (the facilities available and his experience).

It is difficult to outline a standard therapeutic approach. Each case merits individual evaluation. This phrase, so frequently used in medical textbooks, is particularly appropriate here. At the most, broad lines of orientation can be offered, with the risk of apparent contradictions from one patient to another.

Reconstruction of the thumb should be undertaken only in specialized centers offering the possibility of choice between all reconstruction methods without restriction of a technical nature.

CRITICAL REVIEW OF TECHNIQUES USED

These techniques have been described in earlier chapters, and there follows a review only of their respective advantages and disadvantages.

Osteoplastic reconstruction by skin tube, bone graft, and sensory island flap: This has an essential advantage: it does not involve the use of a remaining finger, ensuring better patient acceptability. However, the multiplicity of operative stages is a serious disadvantage. Further problems are the absence of inherent mobility and an imperfect cosmetic result due to absence of a nail.

Progressive lengthening of the first metacarpal by distraction, as described by Matev,* is indicated mostly in young patients. It can lead to bone lengthening of up to 3 cm. without opening the skin, but treatment lasts several months.

Kessler has suggested progressive lengthening of 2.5 to 3 cm over two or three weeks followed by a bone graft, which consolidates in six weeks. The whole treatment program is thus shortened to about two months. Repeated, but much shorter, lengthening is also possible.

Pollicization has obvious advantages—a single operation, a short inpatient stay, potentially good mobility, and an acceptable cosmetic result. It has the major disadvantage of using a remaining finger.

_____

*See Chapter 58A in Volume II.

1168

Microsurgical (toe) transfer also presents several advantages—a one stage surgical procedure, a less predictable but often excellent cosmetic result, and the fact that no finger is sacrificed. These are balanced by two main drawbacks—reduced mobility, and length limited by lack of available tissue. The risk of vascular insufficiency, where the surgeon is experienced, are minimal and should not now be regarded as a contraindication.

Over the last few years a technique for partial toe transfers has been developed in which only the cutaneous envelope and nail of the toe are transferred and adapted to a classic bone-graft thumb column. This technique makes it possible to mold the new thumb, and the cosmetic results can be remarkable (Morrison, see Chapter 104). The main drawback is of course lack of mobility of the part reconstructed with the help of a bone graft. Foucher (see Chapter 113) described another technique utilizing the proximal interphalangeal joint of the second toe.

In a few, admittedly rare, cases, it is possible to transfer a finger from the contralateral hand if the finger has been mutilated or the hand paralyzed but with patent arteries. This is sometimes indicated in the reconstruction of complex mutilation involving the thumb and fingers together. The essential advantage is the better mobility of the transferred finger. The risks of this operation are on a par with the anticipated gain.

FACTORS INFLUENCING RECONSTRUCTION

Apart from the level of amputation, which is generally the essential factor governing choice and will serve as the usual guide, other factors are important and may sometimes predominate.

The patient's age is an important factor in considering reconstruction of the thumb. Reconstruction in children should make provision for growth, and only procedures, such as pollicization or whole toe transfer, that allow for growth can be used. In older patients techniques involving extensive dissection or vascular anastomoses should be used only with the utmost caution. Reconstruction does not have to be complete, and simpler procedures, such as phalangization, can prove useful alternatives.

The wishes of the patient must be taken into account. Thus in a young woman cosmetic considerations may override all others, and the sacrifice of a finger may be unacceptable. More than the length of the thumb, the depth of the first web and especially the presence of a nail are basic factors in terms of cosmetic appearance.

Social and professional requirements sometimes dictate the indications. A patient whose occupation involves heavy manual work needs a stable and sensitive thumb; a jeweller needs a long sensitive thumb; a musician needs all five fingers. Pollicization of the ring finger may be unacceptable to a woman.

The complexity and consequences of a reconstructive procedure should be carefully explained to the patient. Many patients recoil from an osteoplastic procedure that involves the taking of an iliac graft, an abdominal skin flap, or a sensory island flap. Others may refuse a toe transfer through fear of mutilation of the foot. Also the "loss" of a finger is often too much to contemplate. The advantages and disadvantages of each procedure should be explained to the patient or to the parents of a mutilated child, but the decision ultimately rests with the surgeon. When there is an obvious lack of motivation and cooperation, no surgery should be offered.

Finally, the thumb lesion must be seen in its context: i.e., the state of the other fingers and the contralateral hand. The indications of course are different if one or more fingers are mutilated. If, as is common, the index finger has also been partially amputated, pollicization becomes the obvious choice provided the stump of the index is sensitive, healthy, and painless. If several of the fingers have been amputated at the same time as the thumb, a toe transfer represents the only solution. In the rare case of a bilateral mutilation, a finger may be transferred to the contralateral hand. All these factors should be taken into account before the final surgical decision is taken.

DISTAL AMPUTATION OF THE THUMB (DISTAL TO THE HEAD OF THE PROXIMAL PHALANX)

In a number of cases, and depending on the patient's professional occupation, reconstruction may be unnecessary. However, this was the most widespread view before the availability of techniques leading to reconstruction of a near normal distal phalanx.

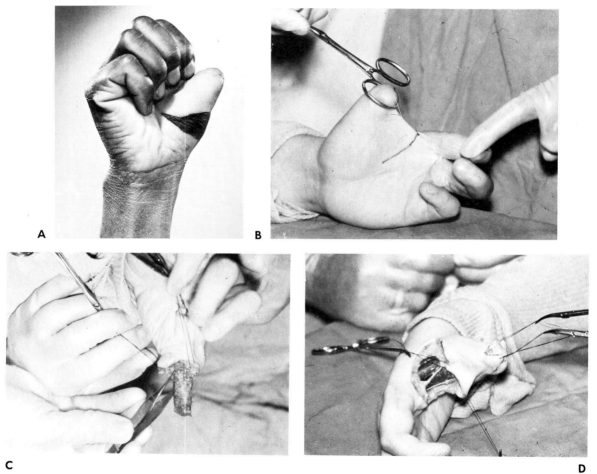

Figure 106–1. Distal amputation of the thumb. Gillies "cocked hat" and its modification. *A*, Result in a black patient clearly showing the skin graft at the radial part of the base of the thumb. *B*, "Reversed cocked hat" (Barron) flap line in a 32 year old male. *C*, Insertion of an iliac bone graft. *D*, The flap covers the bone graft. *E* and *F*, Result one year later.

Illustration continued on opposite page

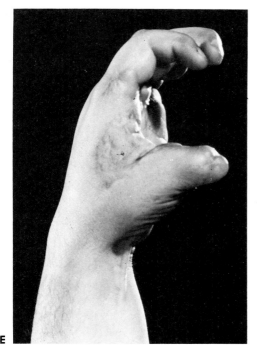

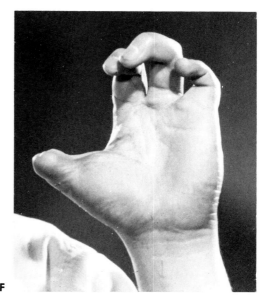

E

F

Figure 106–1 *Continued*

The aim is to provide a thumb of sufficient length to facilitate pinch grip but also a well-padded and sensitive pulp and, if possible, a nail, which considerably improves cosmetic appearance and stabilizes the pulp. Before the era of microsurgery the only possibility was limited lengthening covered by sensitive skin using techniques such as the "cocked hat" of Gillies (Fig. 106–1) and phalangization. These older reconstructive techniques still have a place but the best cosmetic results are usually achieved with a bone graft covered by a partial toe transfer including the nail. Reinnervation is usually good, and the loss of interphalangeal joint mobility is not much of a handicap if the other joints are mobile (Fig. 106–2).

AMPUTATION AT THE BASE OF THE PROXIMAL PHALANX OR AT THE METACARPOPHALANGEAL JOINT

The fundamental factor in these cases is whether the thenar eminence has survived, for this will determine the likelihood of success of any reconstructive procedure. All procedures can be considered here (Fig. 106–3). The choice again must take into account the overall state of the hand and the patient's occupation, sex, and age.

Thus amputation at the proximal third of the proximal phalanx in the thumb of the left hand in a manual worker should be treated by phalangization with or without a lengthening procedure. The same lesion in a 20 year old female patient implies a cosmetic rather than functional problem: a toe transfer offers a solution for both. If the amputation runs across the metacarpophalangeal joint, simple lengthening does not always suffice, especially if the dominant hand is involved and the patient is involved in precision work. If the other fingers are intact, it is preferable to use reconstructive methods that do not utilize the rest of the hand. Autoplastic reconstruction yields good functional results, but the cosmetic appearance may leave a great deal to be desired.

In these cases the toe transfer finds its best indication, and if the big toe is used, the ultimate appearance can come close to that of the normal thumb. This increases the strength of the hand but leaves greater sequelae in the foot. If the other fingers are

Text continued on page 1176

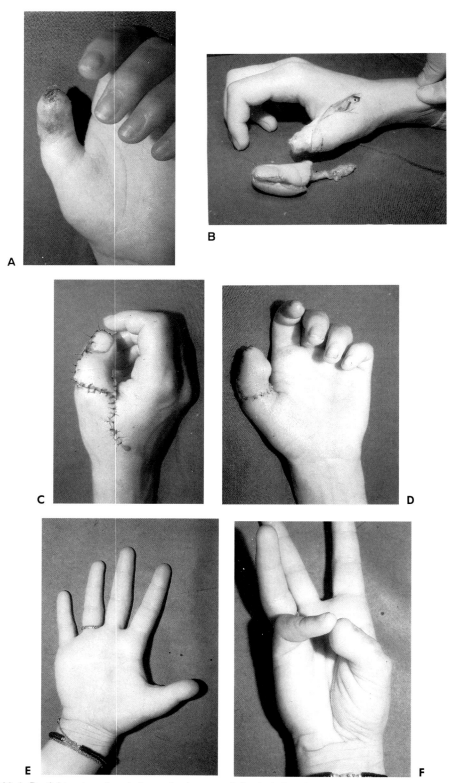

Figure 106–2. Partial toe transfer. *A*, Loss of substance of distal phalanx in a 17 year old girl. *B* to *D*, Partial graft of big toe. *E* and *F*, Postoperative result.

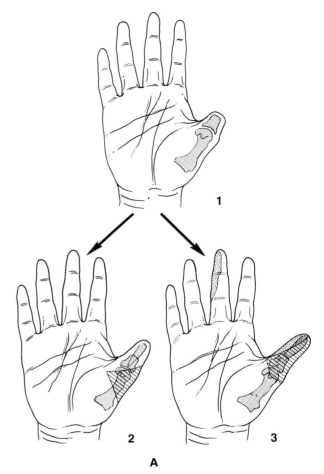

Figure 106–3. Possible reconstruction technique following amputation at the base of the proximal phalanx. *A*, Distal lengthening by short bone graft and Gillies flap: (1) lesion, (2) Gillies technique, (3) osteoplastic reconstruction with tube flap, bone graft, and sensitive island flap.

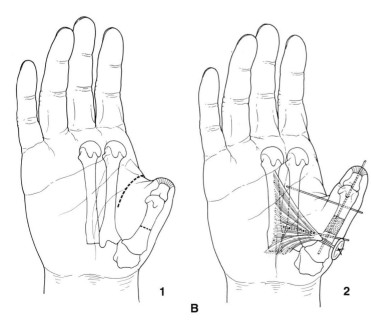

Figure 106–3 *Continued B*, I stage metacarpal lengthening with bone graft, phalangization, and transfer of adductor muscle: (1) incision line, (2) operative diagram.

Illustration continued on following page

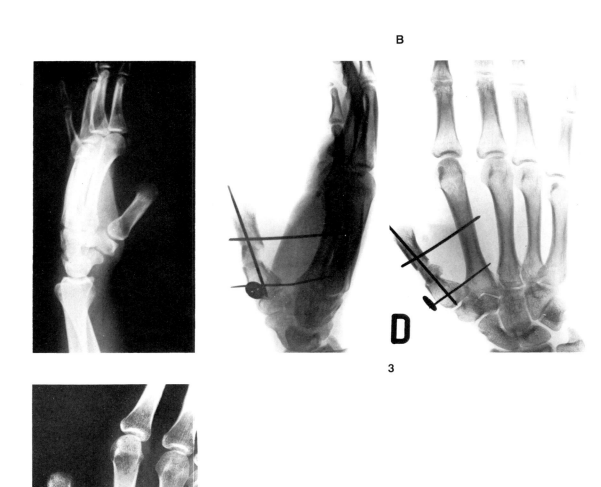

Figure 106–3 *Continued B* (3) clinical case, 30 year old male, one stage metacarpal lengthening with phalangization of first metacarpal; result.
Illustration continued on opposite page

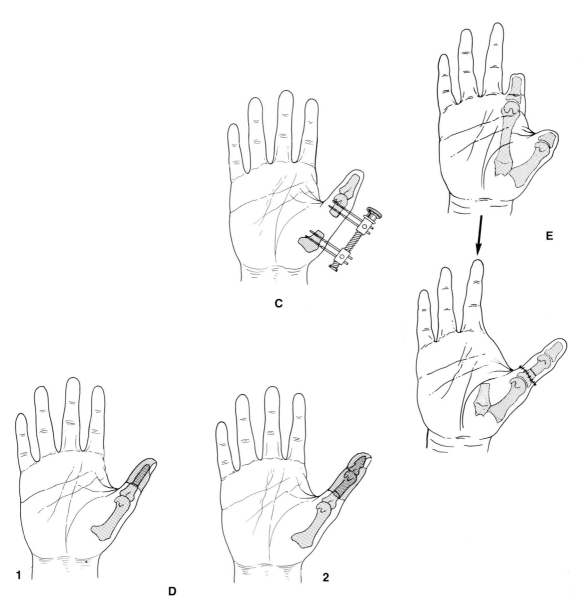

Figure 106–3 *Continued C*, Progressive lengthening. *D*, Toe transfer: (1) reconstruction "to measure" by partial toe transfer and (2) total toe transfer for distal mutilations. *E*, Pollicization of the stump of a mutilated finger.

mutilated, especially if there is an associated distal mutilation of the index finger, pollicization is worth considering (Fig. 106–4).

The results are much less spectacular, however, if the thenar eminence has been destroyed. Osteoplastic reconstruction carries much less hope of success because of the lack of mobility, and a toe transfer or a pollicization is far more promising if one is seeking articular mobility.

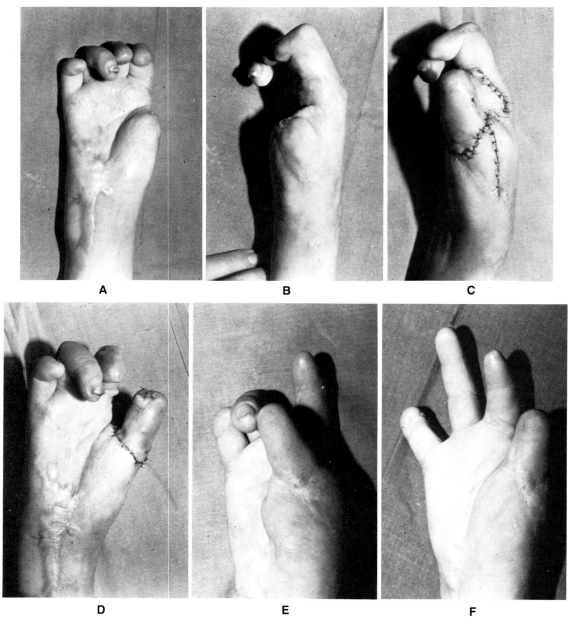

Figure 106–4. Amputation of thumb with partial amputation of index finger of an 11 year old boy. *A* and *B*, Preoperative state. *C* and *D*, Immediate postoperative state after pollicization of the mutilated index finger. *E* and *F*, Result one year later.

AMPUTATION AT THE MIDDLE OR PROXIMAL THIRD OF THE FIRST METACARPAL

In amputation at the middle or proximal third of the first metacarpal (Fig. 106–5), the thenar eminence has usually been destroyed, but if it survives, we are back to the situation just described. The primary consideration is the survival of the trapeziometacarpal joint, which with the help of tendon transfers can be reactivated. Autoplastic reconstruction

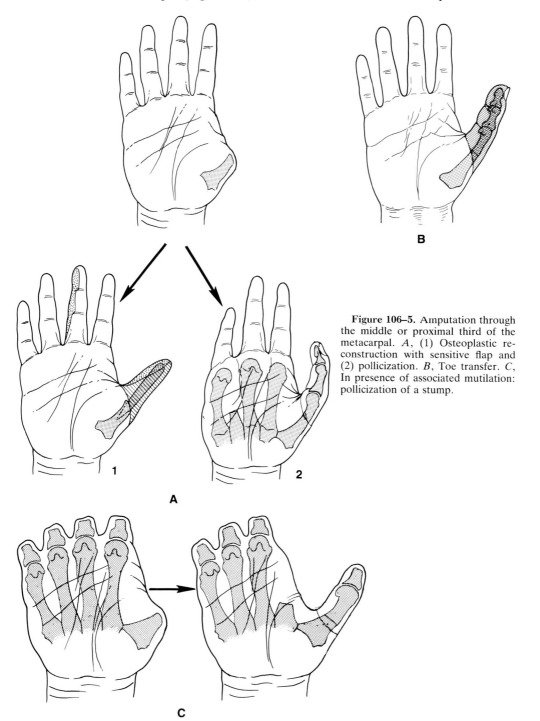

Figure 106–5. Amputation through the middle or proximal third of the metacarpal. *A*, (1) Osteoplastic reconstruction with sensitive flap and (2) pollicization. *B*, Toe transfer. *C*, In presence of associated mutilation: pollicization of a stump.

**Table 106–1. SUMMARY OF INDICATIONS FOR THUMB RECONSTRUCTION
ON THE BASIS OF VARIOUS FACTORS**

Amputation Site	Young	Old	Manual Worker	Precision Grip	Woman	Associated Digital Injuries
Base of proximal phalanx	Partial toe transfers	None	None	Partial toe transfers or big toe	Partial toe transfers	Pollicization of mutilated digit or big toe
Metacarpophalangeal or trans-metacarpal	Toe transfers	One stage lengthening	Progressive lengthening	Toe transfers	Big toe or partial toe transfers	Big toe or pollicization
Base of the first metacarpal	Pollicization	Pollicization or orthosis	Pollicization or big toe	Pollicization	Pollicization	Pollicization or big toe or osteoplastic reconstruction

can still yield good results provided it is associated with tendon transfers.

Toe transfers are always worth considering, and there remains the choice of toe. The big toe cannot be taken along with its metatarsal because this would unbalance the foot. The second toe can be raised together with its metatarsal, but this poses two problems: The metatarsophalangeal joint enjoys a significant range of dorsiflexion, hence, the need for

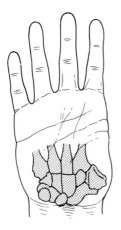
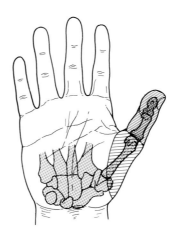
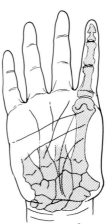
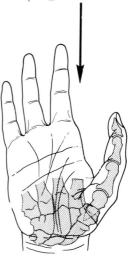

Figure 106–6. Complete amputation of the first metacarpal. *A*, Reconstruction using distant skin flap and toe transfer (with metatarsal). *B*, More often, pollicization of an adjacent finger gives much better mobility.

anterior capsuloplasty; and the extensive skin loss can be partly covered by the raising of a dorsal flap from the foot, but this often must be complemented by a local flap or a flap taken from a distant site.

In cases of toe transfer it is possible to carry out a simultaneous opposition transfer by taking the extensor digitorum brevis tendon up to the wrist. The first choice, however, is a pollicization, and the ring finger is the ideal candidate because its metacarpal is not required.

COMPLETE AMPUTATION OF THE METACARPAL

In cases of complete amputation of the metacarpal (Fig. 106–6), loss of the thenar eminence means loss of mobility. This type of injury often results from accidental explo-sions that give rise to other digital mutilations and to multiple vascular and neural lesions.

This situation represents the best indication for pollicization of the index finger when the latter is utilizable. The mobility of the new thumb in fact depends entirely on that of the transplanted segment. The skeletalized tube will at best be a fixed segment relying exclusively on the mobility of the other fingers.

When pollicization proves impossible (as in severe mutilations or persistence of a single digit), there remains the possibility of transferring the second toe along with its metatarsal (Fig. 106–7). This is carried out in two stages: First an abdominal skin tube is implanted at the site of the future thumb, and later the second toe with its metatarsal is fixed inside the tube. The mobility of the new thumb can be improved by means of tendon transfers combined with a trapeziometacarpal arthroplasty. In exceptional circumstances, free transfer of a finger taken from the opposite hand may be envisaged.

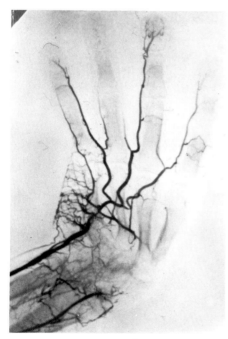
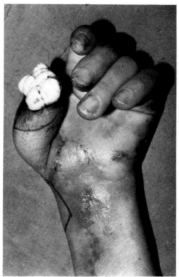
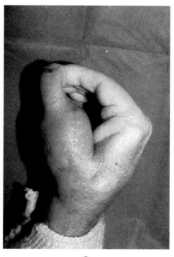

| A | B | C |

Figure 106–7. Complete amputation of first metacarpal in a 45 year old male. *A*, Preoperative arteriography contraindicates pollicization of the index finger. *B*, Classical osteoplastic reconstruction using an inguinal skin flap. *C*, Result of transfer of second toe with its metatarsal. (Case of Dr. Lignon.)

COMPLEX AMPUTATIONS

Chapter 107

MUTILATIONS INVOLVING THE THUMB AND SEVERAL FINGERS

RAOUL TUBIANA

This chapter covers a variety of clinical combinations. The treatment must be adapted to each case of mutilation and aim at restoring one or more useful types of grip.

To begin with, one assesses the reconstructive possibilities in terms of the remaining structures. Are there mobile digital stumps capable of moving toward, and away from, each other, or of reaching the palm? Is it possible to cover the gripping zones with sensitive skin of good quality?

Before examining the techniques of repair, let us first try to classify these lesions.

CLASSIFICATION OF MUTILATIONS

It is difficult to fit these extremely varied lesions into a precise framework and to codify their treatment. Pulvertaft's classification (1966) has the merit of clarity (Fig. 107–1). It recognizes radial hemiamputations, with loss of the thumb and radial fingers; ulnar hemiamputations, which carry a much better prognosis; central hemiamputations, with loss of the index, middle, and ring fingers; and distal hemiamputations, in which all the fingers are lost and only the metacarpals remain.

Multiple amputations are often less easy to classify. In a functional plan, prime importance is attached to the first ray. It is important to distinguish between partial and total amputations of the thumb and associated amputations of the first ray with amputation of an adjacent single ray or multiple other rays of the hand.

Additionally these mutilations are often associated with subsequent sequelae—stiffness and diminution of sensation, motor power, or vascularization—that considerably reduce the functional value of the remaining elements and compromise the chances of successful reconstruction. One must take these sequelae into account when establishing a program of reconstruction.

We shall follow a plan that considers mutilations of increasing severity. In view of the importance of the thumb and first metacarpal, we will consider partial amputations of the thumb associated with amputations of the adjacent ray or multiple other rays; complete amputations of the thumb associated with amputations of the adjacent ray or multiple other rays—the loss of all the digits (this eventuality corresponds to the metacarpal hand, which again can be subdivided into many types); and finally total amputations of the hand, which can be transmetacarpal or above wrist.

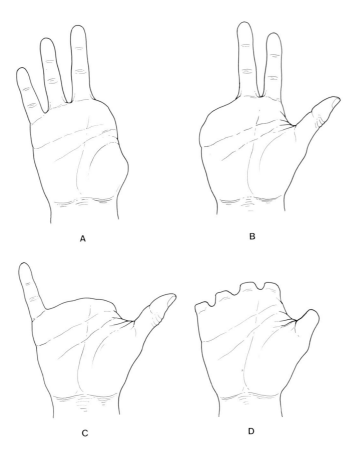

A   B

C   D

Figure 107–1. Pulvertaft's classification. *A*, Radial hemiamputation. *B*, Ulnar hemiamputation. *C*, Central hemiamputation. *D*, Distal hemiamputation.

PARTIAL AMPUTATION OF THE THUMB WITH AMPUTATION OF ONE OR SEVERAL OTHER RAYS

We must distinguish between cases in which the fingers are partially amputated—those in which they are totally amputated and those in which there is injury to the metacarpals.

Partial Amputation of the Thumb with Partial Amputation of the Fingers

This group covers a wide range of lesions (Fig. 107–2). One must appreciate the functional value of the remaining elements. Are there fingers or parts of fingers that can reach the thumb or palm? Can one discard one part or another and achieve contact with power? Is the skin cover in the area of grip sensitive and of good quality?

The functional prognosis is favorable if many mobile segments remain. Contact between these segments of different lengths must be facilitated by means of reorientating osteotomies or transpositions. The problem varies from one case to another, but the primary aim is to make the movements of the first ray as useful as possible. This can be achieved by deepening the first commissure by phalangization of the thumb, or lengthening the stump of the thumb with a transposed injured finger. Transfer of a healthy finger, if any persists, is out of the question because it must be preserved for palmar gripping. One obviously must take into account any osteoarticular, tendinous, or neural lesions of the persisting fingers or stumps.

Lengthening of any digit other than the thumb is justified only in cases of multidigital lesions. In the "phalangeal hand" only the proximal phalanges persist, and even limited lengthening of a finger to enable it to oppose the thumb can bring about significant functional improvement.

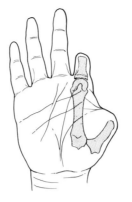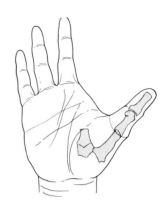

Figure 107–2. Partial amputation of the thumb associated with partial amputation of the fingers. In the case shown here the logical solution is pollicization of the mutilated index finger.

Partial Amputation of the Thumb with Amputation of All the Fingers

In these cases all the metacarpals have survived together with a fragment of phalanx of the thumb (Fig. 107–3), and one should strive to improve the strategic value of the remaining mobile structures—the first ray and the fifth metacarpal. If the stump of the thumb has no mobile joint, its metacarpophalangeal joint can be fixed in a slight flex-

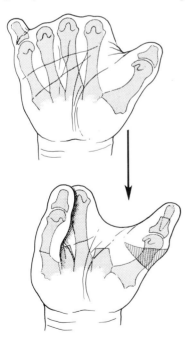

Figure 107–3. Partial amputation of the thumb associated with amputation of all the fingers. The functional value of the first ray is increased by phalangization and lengthening of the first metacarpal. This can be associated with phalangization and osteotomy of the fifth metacarpal.

ion to enable it to reach the head of the fifth metacarpal. Phalangization of the first metacarpal would considerably improve the functional value of this hand. Simultaneous phalangization of the fifth metacarpal can sometimes also be useful.*

Partial Amputation of the Thumb with Partial Amputation of the Fingers and the Metacarpals

A second "arm" must be constructed opposite the mobile first ray to create a pincer. If the remaining fragment of the fifth metacarpal is long and mobile enough, one must try to lengthen it (if necessary, by means of bone grafts taken from the other metacarpals and covered with sensitive skin). The fifth metacarpal is often too short and has lost its mobility. An opposition post can then be constructed from an iliac graft (Fig. 107–4). This is then covered on its anterolateral aspect by sensitive ulnar skin. A skin flap from a distant site is used to cover the medial side of the bone graft.

A toe transfer, performed with the help of microsurgical techniques, represents an alternative method for constructing an opposition post for the thumb.

COMPLETE MUTILATION OF THE THUMB WITH MUTILATION OF THE FINGERS OR METACARPALS

Here again we distinguish between cases in which the fingers are partially or totally

---

*The technique of these phalangizations is discussed in detail in Chapter 108.

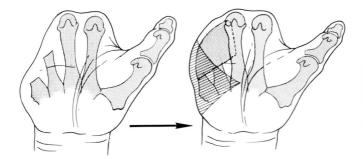

Figure 107–4. Partial amputation of the thumb associated with amputation of the fingers and ulnar metacarpals. An iliac graft is lodged between the third and the remaining part of the fourth metacarpal to form a buttress. The radial part of this graft, in front of the thumb, is covered by sensitive skin.

amputated and those in which amputation of the thumb coexists with mutilation of the metacarpals.

Complete Mutilation of the Thumb with Partial Mutilation of the Fingers

A thumb must be constructed to oppose the remaining digits or digital stumps. The choice of procedure for thumb reconstruction is determined to a great extent by the importance of associated injuries of the other rays. If a single ray is amputated, it is most commonly the index finger; then the other fingers, particularly the middle finger, may effectively oppose the reconstructed thumb, satisfying the criteria already outlined.* If multiple other rays are partially or totally destroyed, the hand is more compromised. One must distinguish those cases in which multiple parts of digits remain, when one is fit to be transposed onto the first metacarpal (Fig. 107–5). The surgeon must take into account the general architecture of the hand, the relative length of the first metacarpal, the transferable part, the opposable elements, and their mobility. If the first carpometacarpal joint is destroyed or stiff, it is better to transfer a stump with at least one mobile joint rather than create a fixed opposition post. Reorientation of the stumps opposable to the new thumb or phalangization of the fifth metacarpal will improve the grip (Fig. 107–6).

When a digital transfer appears risky, a post can be constructed opposite a mobile structure in the form of a sensitive skeletalised skin tube (Fig. 107–7), but in these cases there is an increasing tendency to perform toe transfer. In older age groups a prosthetic solution may be preferable.

Total Amputation of the Thumb with Amputation of All the Fingers

Loss of the thumb and all the fingers constitutes the "metacarpal hand." All commissures are lost, and the hand is reduced to the state of a pusher, or a hook if the wrist is mobile. However, when the first metacarpal has retained some mobility, prehensile function can be restored. The problems of reconstruction depend on the residual length of the metacarpals.

Long Metacarpals. When the metacarpals are long, there is the possibility of reconstructing a three pronged hand by phalangizing the first and fifth metacarpals, the second and fourth being resected to deepen the "interdigital" spaces. The third metacarpal is retained to preserve the insertions of the adductor pollicis and also because this middle support enhances the precision of the grip.* The first metacarpal can be profitably lengthened to facilitate the grasping of large objects, the second metacarpal supplying the graft. Hilgenfeldt (1960) and Michon (1973) have improved this technique by performing "a composite autoplasty," which lengthens the first metacarpal by translation of a palmar flap receiving its blood and nerve supply from the pedicles of the index finger and containing the distal part of the second metacarpal.

The fifth metacarpal sometimes can also be lengthened, but this requires reorientation by osteotomy to allow contact with the first (Tubiana, 1958). We have tried to improve the mobility of the mobile metacarpals by freeing them as far up as possible and performing muscle or tendon transfers (Tubiana and Roux, 1974).

The fixed structure formed by the third metacarpal stabilizes grip.

*See Chapter 97.

*For the surgical technique, see Chapter 108.

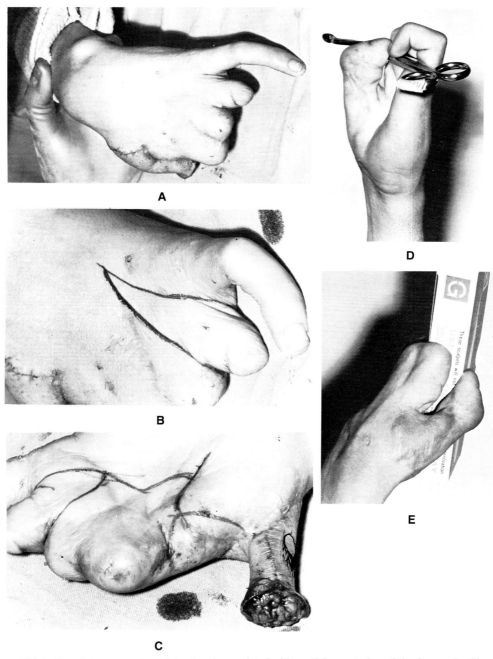

Figure 107–5. Complete amputation of the thumb associated with partial amputation of the fingers. In this old case the fifth ray and stumps of the first phalanges of the index, long, and ring fingers resisted. The thumb and distal third of the first metacarpal were absent. There was a degree of mobility of the remaining part of the first metacarpal. Transposition of the fourth metacarpal with its stump of proximal phalanx into the first metacarpal was carried out. A tube flap had previously been brought up to the radial aspect of the hand for reconstruction of the first web. In such a case, a toe transfer would be used at the present time.

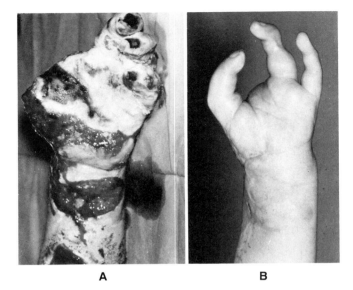

A   B

Figure 107–6. *A*, Crush injury of the hand with radial hemiamputation. *B*, Transfer of the long finger onto the first metacarpal. Pinch between stiff fingers was re-established.

Partially Amputated Metacarpals. When the metacarpals are partially amputated, the possibilities of reconstruction depend essentially on the survival of the proximal part of the first metacarpal, which will be lengthened by the procedures described earlier. Some form of opposition posts are then erected from the ulnar part of the hand stump and stabilized by an iliac graft implanted on the fourth metacarpal, and the whole covered with a skin flap. Use of a removable prosthetic opposition post constitutes another possibility.

If the first metacarpal is destroyed and useless, the possibilities of repair are much more limited. An attempt can be made at phalangizing the fifth metacarpal, if it is long enough, and creating a commissure, thus enabling the hand to grip small objects. This can be a useful procedure in young subjects. When all the metacarpals are short, the functional situation is the same as in total amputation of the hand. However, even when all mobilizing operations on the metacarpals prove hopeless, wrist movements can be put to use. In all these types of severe mutilation,

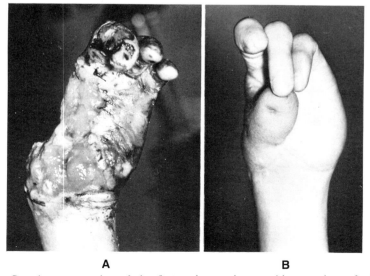

A   B

Figure 107–7. *A*, Complete amputation of the first and second rays with extensive soft tissue damage. *B*, Construction of a buttress opposite to the ulnar digits.

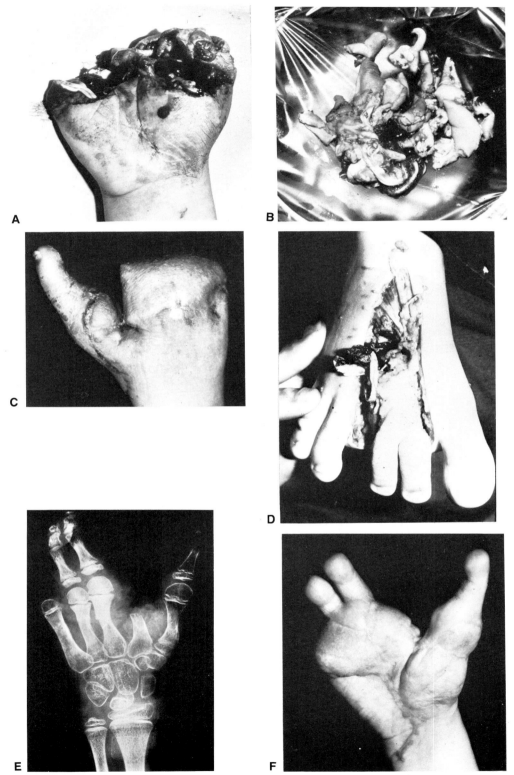

Figure 107–8. Transmetacarpal amputation in a child. (Case of Dr. G. Foucher.) *A*, At admission. *B*, The preserved finger fragments were unusable. *C*, Reconstruction of the thumb using a second toe. A skin flap was used previously to cover the extremity of the stump. *D*, Transfer from the other foot of the second and third toes. *E*, X-ray. *F*, Result.

microsurgery opens new possibilities of reconstruction.

MICROSURGICAL TECHNIQUES IN SEVERE AMPUTATIONS

Toe transfers, as we have seen, have modified some of the indications for reconstruction of the thumb. The use of microsurgical techniques will have even more important consequences in the treatment of severe amputations affecting both the thumb and fingers. These techniques offer the possibility of transfer of sensitive skin taken from the back of the foot, from the web between the first and second toes, or from the pulp of a toe, as well as partial toe transfers, the transfer of one or two toes, which may restore pollicidigital pinch grip; and transfer of a finger taken from the opposite hand, which may restore digitopalmar pinch grip.

These new techniques offer a wide range of possibilities for repairing severely amputated hands and can be modified for each case. The extent of the amputation, the condition of the other hand, sequelae at the donor site, and general factors concerning the patient (age, occupation, ability to cooperate) must all be taken into consideration.

With regard to the donor site, partial toe transfers obviously involve the least sequelae. Transfer of the second toe is much better compensated for than transfer of the great toe. Two toes may be taken, one for each foot, allowing for pinch grip in opposition or,

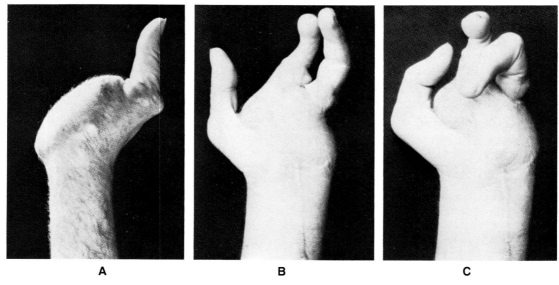

A   B   C

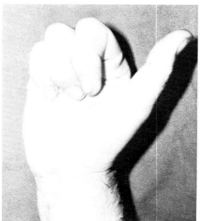

D

Figure 107–9. Heterolateral digital transplantation. (Case of Mr. W. Morrison.) *A*, Preoperative state, patient aged 45 years, old transmetacarpal amputation. *B*, Transfer of the second toe to the second metacarpal and of the ring finger taken from the opposite hand transferred medial to the toe. Photo taken 18 months after operation, fingers extended. *C*, Fingers flexed: note the difference in flexion between the finger transfer and the toe transfer. *D*, The donor hand.

more ambitiously, tripodal pinch grip if it has been possible to reconstruct the thumb by another method. The taking of two adjacent toes (the second and third), as performed by Foucher (Fig. 107–8), now seems to have become a fairly widespread technique in China.

It must be remembered that toe transfer, although it provides a sensitive digit capable of replacing a thumb or even a finger to achieve terminoterminal pinch grip, has neither the length nor adequate flexion to provide digitopalmar pinch grip or to replace the whole first ray. Movements of the toes differ from those of the fingers: flexion of the metacarpophalangeal joint is dorsal, which can be prevented by capsuloplasty, but there is no palmar flexion. The proximal phalanx is much longer than the distal phalanges, which have only limited capacity to flex and extend. The fingers are longer, more sensitive, and much more mobile.

The toe is only an imperfect substitute, and it is clear that in severe amputations there is the temptation to transplant a finger from the other hand. This involves considerable risk, which nevertheless in exceptional cases may be very useful. Büchler (see Chapter 109) reports a case of transfer of the contralateral index finger, and Morrison in four cases used the ring finger, considering this to be less functionally useful than the index finger for the donor hand (Fig. 107–9). While we can admire the technical prowess of these surgeons and the quality of their results, which could not have been obtained by other methods, it must be stressed that although transfer of a contralateral finger has been shown to be technically possible and effective, this criterion is not sufficient to justify use of the procedure frequently. Preference generally must be given to methods involving the least risk for the patient. Only specialists familiar with a wide range of procedures, including the more traditional ones, are capable of evaluating certain rare indications.

TOTAL AMPUTATION OF THE HAND

One must distinguish here between transmetacarpal amputations and more proximal amputations. When a carpal segment has survived, activated by the wrist flexors and extensors (inserted on the base of the metacarpals), the persistent mobility of the stump can be extremely useful in creating a natural and powerful hook. These movements also can be used to establish a sensitive grip against a prosthesis or to activate a prosthesis.

A patient with a unilateral amputation will seldom use a prosthesis except a cosmetic one. The problem is quite different with bilateral mutilations. It is in these cases that Krukenberg's operation can be considered; this is discussed in Chapter 111.

REFERENCES

Hilgenfeldt, O.: Operativer Daumenersatz. Ferdinand Enke Verlag, Stuttgart, 1950.

Michon, J., and Dolich, B. H.: The metacarpal hand. Hand, 6:285–290, 1974.

Michon, J.: The metacarpal hand. In Campbell Reid, D. A., and Tubiana, R. (eds.): Mutilating Injuries of the Hand. G.E.M. Monograph 3, 2nd ed. Edinburgh, Churchill Livingstone, 1984, pp. 88–92.

Pulvertaft, R. G.: Traumatic mutilation of the hand. Severe combined mutilations of the thumb and fingers. Xe Congrès SICOT, Paris, 1966, pp. 819–827.

Tubiana, R.: Phalangisation du 5ème métacarpien. Acta Orthop. Bel., 24(suppl. III):120–121, 1958.

Tubiana, R., and Roux, J. P.: Phalangization of the first and fifth metacarpals. J. Bone Joint Surg., 56A:447–457, 1974.

Chapter 108

PHALANGIZATION OF THE METACARPALS

Raoul Tubiana

Phalangization of the metacarpals consists of deepening the web spaces in order to improve the "pincer" function of the hand when the digits have been amputated. This procedure is most commonly performed on the first and fifth metacarpals, which possess the greatest potential mobility.

The second and third metacarpals articulate with the distal row of carpal bones by joints that are virtually fixed. They constitute the stable element of the metacarpal arch. The fourth metacarpal has limited mobility, about 10 degrees in the anteroposterior plane, which contributes to the cupping of the palm.

The peripheral metacarpals, the first and the fifth, possess a well developed intrinsic musculature of their own—the thenar and hypothenar muscles. The mobility of the first metacarpal is considerable, since it can oppose all others. In the fifth metacarpal, mobility is much less marked although extremely useful.

The main purpose of phalangization of the first metacarpal is to deepen the first cleft sufficiently to restore lateral mobility and, if possible, opposition. Phalangization of the fifth metacarpal, a more demanding procedure although less spectacular in its effect, is done in an attempt to develop in a structure with limited mobility a function comparable to that of the first metacarpal.

HISTORICAL ASPECTS

Phalangization of the first metacarpal was described in 1873 by Huguier, who reported in detail two patients treated in 1854. Since then this procedure has been performed on numerous occasions, and the technique has been improved by Kreuz (1944) and Hilgenfeldt (1950).

Phalangization of the fifth metacarpal dates back to the First World War (Burkhardt, 1916). In 1958 we combined an osteotomy with phalangization of the fifth metacarpal. Later we described in detail the technique of phalangization of the first and fifth metacarpals and published our results (Tubiana and Roux, 1974).

PHALANGIZATION OF THE FIRST METACARPAL

ANATOMY AND PHYSIOLOGY

The tissues of the first intermetacarpal space function as a hinge, and opposition of the thumb depends on their remarkable mobility. Opposition is a complex movement that brings into play the three segments of the thumb ray.* The first metacarpal, with which we are concerned here, performs a movement of anteposition followed by one of flexion-adduction combined with "automatic" longitudinal rotation in pronation. This is possible only if three conditions are met:

1. The skin, especially on the dorsal aspect of the web, must be supple. Scars and skin retraction are liable to limit the freedom of movement of the first metacarpal. Extra skin covering must be provided in every phalangization.

2. Two triangular muscles cross each other in the cleft between the first and second metacarpals (Fig. 108–1).

Anteriorly lies the adductor pollicis, which originates chiefly from the third metacarpal and terminates in a tendon that inserts on the medial sesamoid of the thumb and, by an expansion, on the extensor apparatus of the

---

*See Chapter 4 in Volume I.

1190

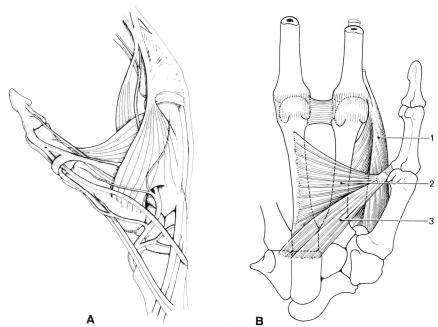

Figure 108–1. Dorsal view of the first web. *A,* The following are shown, from the dorsal surface to the palmar surface: the extensor tendons of the thumb, the radial artery in the floor of the anatomical snuffbox, the first dorsal interosseous muscle, the adductor muscle, the first lumbrical. *B,* Palmar view. 1 = first dorsal interosseous muscle, 2 = transverse adductor muscle, 3 = oblique adductor muscle.

thumb. Its transverse fibers form the tense cord of the commissure. Posteriorly lies the first dorsal interosseus muscle, which originates from both the medial border of the first metacarpal and the lateral border of the second metacarpal. It inserts on the base of the proximal phalanx of the index finger. Any significant deepening of the cleft requires partial release of the origins of these two muscles. Superficially, they are covered by a double layered aponeurosis, and part of each layer is a sheet lining the deep aspect of the two muscles. All these fibrous structures tend to contract after an injury and restrict mobility. During operative release they should be incised layer by layer.

3. The trapeziometacarpal joint must be mobile. Contracture of the capsule not uncommonly accompanies contractures of the skin and aponeuroses. The dorsal capsule of the trapeziometacarpal joint, and especially the oblique posteromedial ligament, must be incised if it is contracted.

OPERATIVE TECHNIQUE

The Skin

The incision should provide free access to the anterior and posterior commissural structures and take into account the possible need for extra skin, depending on the extent of the contracture.

When the first web shows little or no scarring and the skin is utilizable, one or more Z-plasties can be fashioned astride the commissure. The anterior limb of the Z usually runs parallel to the opposition crease of the thumb and the posterior limb, parallel to the medial border of the first metacarpal (Fig. 108–2). This limb should be placed so that it can be extended up to, or even beyond, the first carpometacarpal joint if one intends to free the posterior extrinsic tendons in their radial grooves (Fig. 108–3). Transposition of the local flaps may not be sufficient to ensure mobility of the first web, and an additional cover in the form of a full thickness graft is often necessary. This can be taken from the medial aspect of the arm and applied to the posterior aspect of the commissure (Fig. 108–4). Steps should always be taken to prevent contracture of the commissure and especially of the graft. Thus, to maintain the width of the open web, the first two metacarpals may have to be held apart by means of two transverse Kirschner wires left in place for about three weeks. Further immobilization then can be achieved by the use of an adjustable splint, which keeps the web fully open.

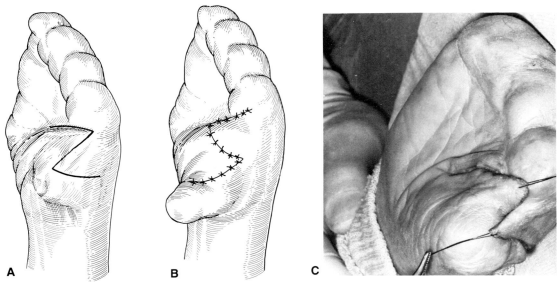

Figure 108–2. *A*, Z-plasty of web. *B*, Closure after crossover of the two flaps. *C*, Operative view of the two flaps of the Z.

If there is some contraction of the web but the skin of the dorsum of the hand has remained supple, there is the possibility of using a broad flap borrowed from the dorsum of the hand. Ideally it should be designed so that its apex lies distally on the posterior aspect of the proximal phalanx of the index finger and so that it has a broad base (Figs. 108–5, 108–6) (Delbet and Tessier, 1961). When the phalangization has been com-

pleted, the defect on the dorsum of the hand is covered with a free skin graft. We prefer a large rotation flap rather than the posterior advanced rectangular flap sometimes suggested.

A third possibility, when the dorsal skin of the hand is of poor quality or in short supply, is to cover the defect with a flap taken from the anterior aspect of the contralateral arm above the elbow crease. The first digital ray

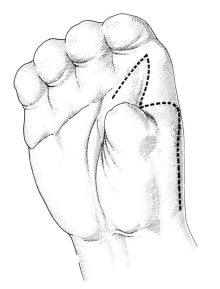

Figure 108–3. The dorsal incision may be prolonged if necessary to free the dorsal structures.

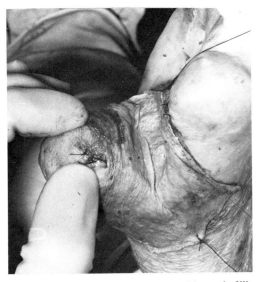

Figure 108–4. Thick split-thickness skin graft filling the web after its freeing.

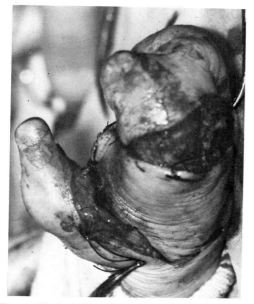 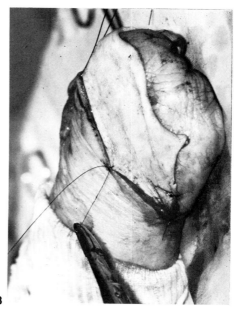

Figure 108–5. *A*, Transfer to the web of a large rotation flap taken from the dorsum of the hand. *B*, The dorsal donor region is covered by a graft.

is kept separate from the second by the complete thickness of the arm. It is now possible to use the new generation of forearm flaps or a free flap taken on the dorsum of the foot, sometimes combined with a toe transfer. Despite its advantages, the inguinal flap is often too thick. The size of the skin plasty must conform to that of the cutaneous functional units of the hand.

In all cases an attempt should also be made to preserve or restore the skin cover with good sensation over terminal pressure areas.

Fascia and Muscle

The two neurovascular bundles of the thumb and the radial collateral bundle of the index finger are isolated at the outset. Pos-

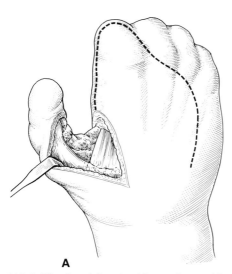 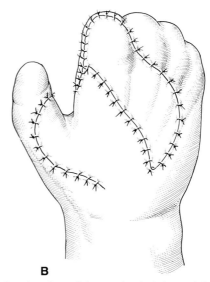

Figure 108–6. The dorsal flap should extend over skin of the dorsal surface of the proximal phalanx of the index if it is of good quality. *A*, Transfer of flap. *B*, Transfer of flap into web.

teriorly the sensory branches of the radial nerve are also dissected out and protected. The anterior and posterior aponeuroses are incised throughout their full lengths (Figs. 108–7, 108–8). All the fibrous structures that stretch between the first two metacarpals are incised (Fig. 108–9).

What is done to the muscles depends on the prevailing conditions. The origin of the first dorsal interosseous muscle on the first metacarpal is usually released (Fig. 108–10). If necessary, its action as an abductor of the index finger can be restored by transferring the extensor indicis proprius to the site of insertion of the first dorsal interosseous muscle. By contrast, the adductor pollicis muscle must be preserved as much as possible. Disinsertion of the adductor pollicis from the third metacarpal permits spreading of the first web but scarcely any deepening (Fig. 108–11). This technique is used to overcome contraction of the web. In order to deepen, it is necessary to divide the sesamoid insertion of the adductor (Figs. 108–12, 108–13). Its indispensable action must be restored after a phalangization. In cases of incomplete amputation of the thumb, partial deepening of

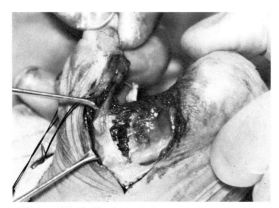

Figure 108–8. Section of the posterior aponeurosis starts spread.

the commissure is sufficient, and only the origin of the distal fibers of the adductor needs to be released from the third metacarpal. Any significant deepening of the first cleft requires division of the sesamoid tendon of the adductor, with reimplantation of the tendon halfway down the shaft of the first metacarpal by transosseous fixation (Fig. 108–14).

If the muscle is grossly fibrotic and discolored, it is preferable to release part of its insertion and to replace its action by tendon transfer using a powerful muscle (Fig. 108–15). For this purpose we have used the tendon of the flexor pollicis longus muscle or the flexor of an amputated digit. The transferred tendon is implanted into the first metacarpal through a small tunnel in the bone (Fig. 108–16). When the whole muscle is fibrosed, it may have to be excised prior to the transfer.

The movements of the first metacarpal may be restricted by adhesions of the tendons on

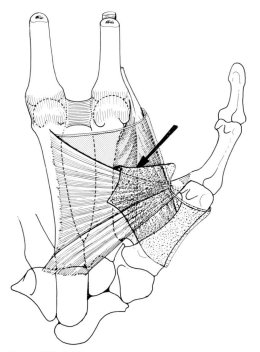

Figure 108–7. The aponeuroses of the first web. The adductor and first interosseous muscles are each covered by aponeuroses on their superficial and deep surfaces. These contracted aponeuroses must be incised or excised in order to obtain spreading of the web.

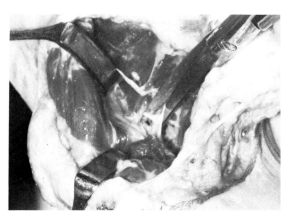

Figure 108–9. Section of the contracted deep intermuscular fibrous aponeurosis.

Figure 108–10. The insertions of the first dorsal interosseous muscle on the first metacarpal are detached with a periosteal elevator.

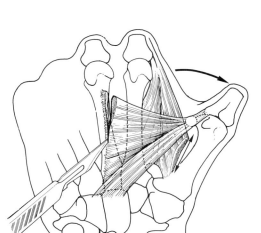

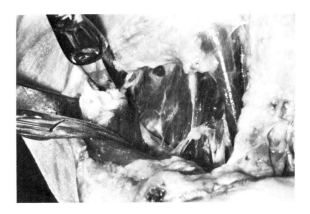

Figure 108–11. Disinsertion of the adductor pollicis from the third metacarpal.

Figure 108–12. Diagram showing reimplantation of the adductor tendon.

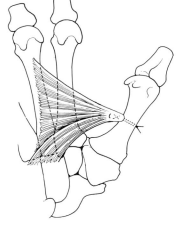

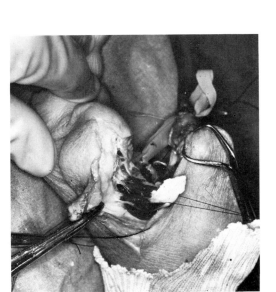

Figure 108–13. Section of a healthy adductor muscle tendon.

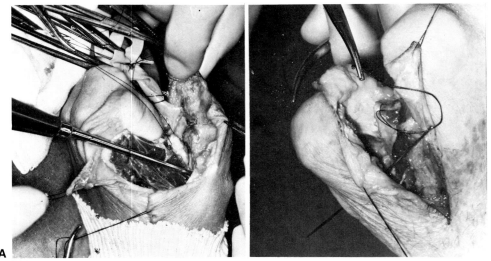

Figure 108–14. Reinsertion of the adductor tendon on the proximal part of the first metacarpal. *A*, Fashioning of a bone tunnel. *B*, Transosseous suture on a button or bolus.

the posterior aspect of the wrist (Fig. 108–17). We have encountered this complication after crushing injuries of the forearm with ischemia and sometimes after mutilation of the extremities. These adhesions must then be freed. One should make sure that the first carpometacarpal joint has sufficient mobility; if movement is still restricted after a dorsal capsulectomy, an arthroplasty may be needed (Fig. 108–18).

PHALANGIZATION OF THE FIFTH METACARPAL

This phalangization consists of deepening the fourth interdigital cleft in order to increase the mobility of the fifth metacarpal, at the same time creating an intermetacarpal pincer. The technique, which we described in 1958, has since been modified (Tubiana and Roux, 1974).

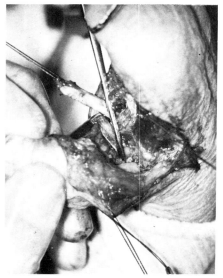

Figure 108–15. The adductor is partially fibrosed. Its action will be reinforced by transfer of the tendon of flexor pollicis longus, which is seen on a traction suture.

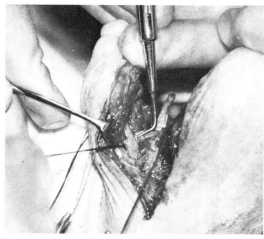

Figure 108–16. Passage of the flexor pollicis longus tendon through the bone tunnel.

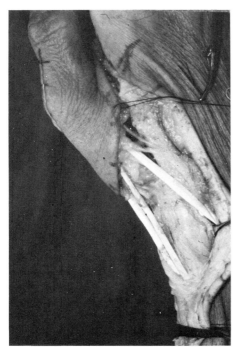

Figure 108–17. Freeing of the posterior extrinsic tendons of the thumb, which are sometimes adherent in the osteofibrous grooves of the radius.

ANATOMY AND PHYSIOLOGY

The goals of this operation are to deepen the fourth cleft and increase the mobility of the fifth metacarpal. The requirements are as follows:

1. The hypothenar muscles must be intact. Two of the hypothenar muscles, the flexor digiti minimi brevis and the abductor digiti minimi, have a flexion action in anteposition. This action is exerted indirectly through the metacarpophalangeal joint, since the two muscles have no metacarpal attachments (Fig. 108–19). Although far from negligible, this action is less important than that of the opponens digiti minimi, which is the prime mover of the metacarpohamate joint and the only muscle with attachments on both the carpus and the fifth metacarpal. Electromyographic studies in the normal hand confirm that the essential action of this muscle occurs during the final part of opposition and is associated with cupping of the palm. The fourth dorsal interosseus muscle inserted on the base of the fourth finger is sacrificed. The third palmar interosseus muscle on the other hand, because it exerts its action through the metacarpophalangeal joint, pulling the little finger toward the axis of the hand, can be used as a transfer to provide more opposition (Fig. 108–20).

2. The mobility of the metacarpohamate joint can be improved, but the problem here is a difficult one. The joint is a particularly complex one, formed by two roughly cylindrical surfaces (one convex on the metacarpal and the other concave on the hamate), which slide on each other. At the same time the articular facets on the contiguous surfaces at the base of the fourth and fifth metacarpals form a synergistic joint. The plane of the articular facet of the hamate is oblique lateromedially and posteroanteriorly, forming an angle of 25 degrees with the frontal plane. The shaft of the fifth metacarpal is not exactly

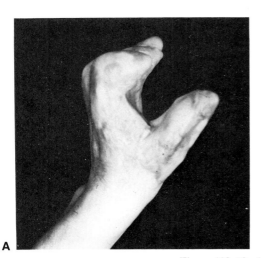

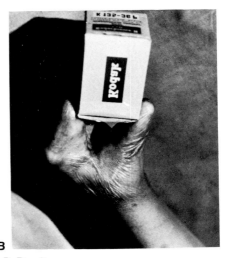

Figure 108–18. *A* and *B*, Results.

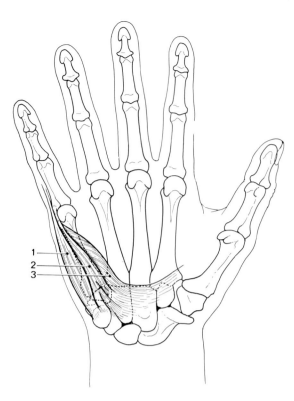

Figure 108–19. Diagram of hypothenar muscles. 1 = abductor digiti minimi, 2 = flexor digiti minimi brevis, 3 = opponens digiti minimi.

Figure 108–20. The interosseous muscles of the fourth space. 1 = the third palmar interosseous muscle, which will be retained and sometimes transferred, 2 = the fourth dorsal interosseous muscle, which will be resected, 3 = the second palmar interosseous muscle. *A*, Dorsal view. *B*, Palmar view.

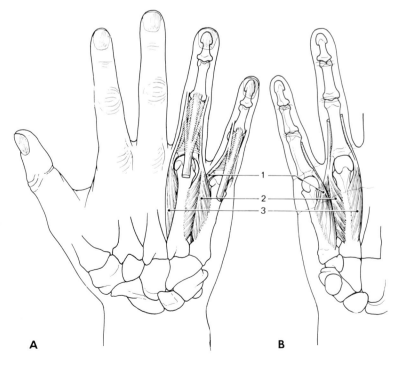

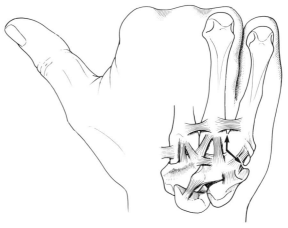

Figure 108–21. The carpometacarpal joints of the fourth and fifth metacarpals. Posterior view. The proximal intermetacarpal ligament must be left intact. By contrast, the capsule and the posteromedial oblique ligament may be incised to permit anteposition of the fifth metacarpal.

perpendicular to the articular plane, being inclined radially to form an angle of 80 to 85 degrees. This relationship explains why movements at the carpometacarpal joint of the little finger are exclusively flexion and extension or, by analogy with the first metacarpal, anteposition and retroposition, and why these motions occur in a plane that is oblique in relation to the sagittal plane. The slight degree of opposition of the little finger, which accompanies cupping of the palm, becomes more marked when the finger is flexed. Normally flexion (or anteposition) of the fifth carpometacarpal joint is limited to 15 to 20 degrees in a plane that is oblique posteroanteriorly and mediolaterally, although usually a few degrees of retroposition (extension) is possible.

The structures restricting anteposition are the intermetacarpal aponeurosis and the carpometacarpal ligaments, not the skin, neurovascular bundles, or muscles.

The Intermetacarpal Aponeurosis. The intermetacarpal aponeurosis has two leaves, which stretch between the distal parts of the fourth and fifth metacarpals. The anterior leaf lies immediately under the flexor tendons and the fourth lumbrical muscle. It forms the transverse intermetacarpal ligament, sometimes more exactly called the intervolar ligament because it connects the adjacent articular volar plates of the fourth and fifth metacarpophalangeal joints. The posterior leaf is thick and lies deep to the extensors and superficial to the plane of the bones. Both leaves are consistently present. If these two layers are divided, anteposition of the fifth metacarpal increases to 25 or 30 degrees.

The Dorsal Capsuloligamentous Structures. The dorsal capsuloligamentous structures include a thick capsule shared by the metacarpohamate and intermetacarpal (between fourth and fifth) joints; a proximal intermetacarpal ligament (Fig. 108–21), which stretches between the bases of the fourth and fifth metacarpals and ensures intermetacarpal stability; and a tough oblique posteromedial ligament. In the cadaver, division of the posteromedial ligament and posterior capsule allows 50 to 55 degrees of anteposition without reducing lateral stability, provided the proximal intermetacarpal ligament is intact.

OPERATIVE TECHNIQUE

An incision is made over the dorsal and palmar aspects of the fourth metacarpal (Figs. 108–22, 108–23). The skin incision should be sinuous or zigzag to guard against contractures, and so arranged that skin with intact sensation will cover the lateral aspect of the fifth metacarpal, or at least the end of the stump.

On the dorsal aspect, the dorsal longitudinal veins should be preserved if possible. The transverse connections of the extensor apparatus are divided. On the palmar aspect, the common palmar digital artery to the ring and little fingers is identified, and the branch to the ulnar side of the ring finger is divided and ligated, preserving the branch to the little finger (Fig. 108–24). The common palmar digital nerve from the superficial branch of the ulnar nerve to the ring and little fingers

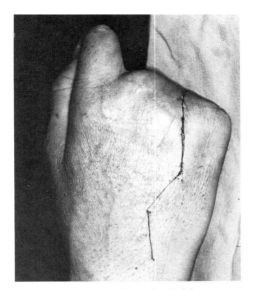

Figure 108–22. Posterior incision.

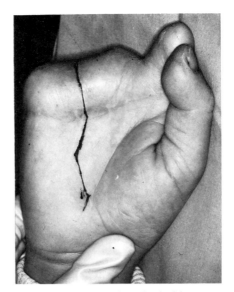

Figure 108–23. Anterior incision.

is identified and split longitudinally as far proximally as the level of the deep palmar arch of the ulnar artery (Fig. 108–25). Finally the fourth lumbrical is resected.

The second stage consists of carefully identifying and dividing the two leaves of the distal intermetacarpal aponeurosis. The fourth dorsal interosseous muscle, which is to be sacrificed, is dissected off the lateral aspect of the fifth metacarpal supraperiosteally with an elevator until the proximal intermetacarpal ligament is exposed. This lig-

ament must be preserved to ensure the lateral stability of the phalangized metacarpal.

Mobilization of the fifth metacarpal will provide a useful intermetacarpal grip either when the thumb has normal length and mobility or when the little finger has a phalangeal stump and a mobile metacarpophalangeal joint. The possibility of achieving grip by phalangization of the fifth metacarpal is considerably reduced if the whole thumb and all the phalanges of the little finger have been lost. If such is the case, additional maneuvers

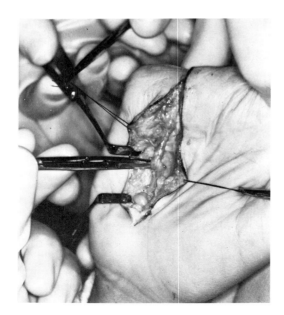

Figure 108–24. Palmar stage. Freeing of the neurovascular bundle of the fourth space.

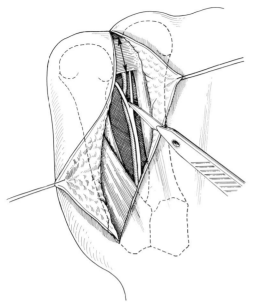

Figure 108–25. The common palmar digital nerve of the fourth space is split.

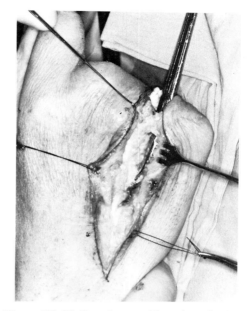

Figure 108–27. Dorsal stage. There is a distal reinforcement of the dorsal aponeurosis, forming a veritable posterior intermetacarpal ligament, which must be divided.

should be considered (Figs. 108–26, 108–27, 108–28).

1. Resection of the fourth metacarpal, leaving just its base. This procedure widens the newly constructed commissure but adds little in the way of active mobility. A part of the resected metacarpal is sometimes used as a bone graft to lengthen the fifth metacarpal.

If that is done, the end of the bone graft should be covered, if possible, by a flap of adjacent skin with intact sensation.

2. Osteotomy at the base of the fifth metacarpal. This osteotomy, which is carried out

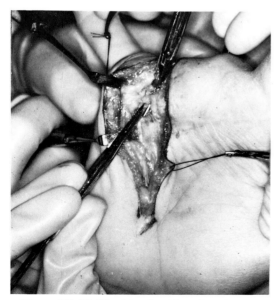

Figure 108–26. The interglenoid or deep intermetacarpal ligament is divided.

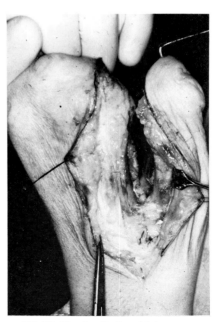

Figure 108–28. The fourth dorsal interosseous muscle has been completely removed.

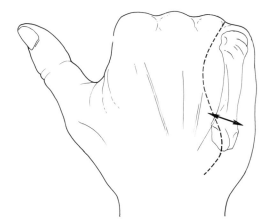

Figure 108–29. Osteotomy of the base of the fifth metacarpal.

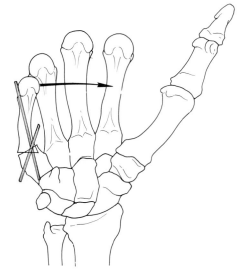

Figure 108–31. Angulation of the fifth metacarpal, forward and radially. Fixation by two Kirschner wires leaves the carpometacarpal joint free.

through a dorsal incision, is done about 15 mm. distal to the carpometacarpal joint (Figs. 108–29, 108–30). The distal part of the metacarpal is then angled forward and radially and is fixed with two Kirschner wires (Fig. 108–31). This maneuver must be performed with great care so as to preserve stability without producing stiffness of the carpometacarpal joint.

The aims of the osteotomy are to increase the range of anteposition by about 25 degrees and shift the arc of motion to a more useful sector, and to improve the opposition of the phalangized metacarpal to the thumb (or neothumb) by reorientating the bone in such

a way that an area of intact skin faces the other limb of the pincer.

3. Improving the mobility of the metacarpohamate joint. This is done either by dividing the oblique posteromedial ligament (the stabilizing proximal intermetacarpal ligament being preserved)—which increases the range

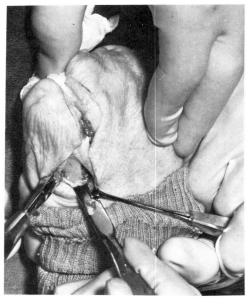

Figure 108–30. Photograph of osteotomy.

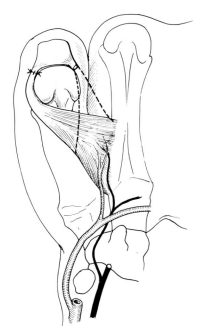

Figure 108–32. Diagram of transfer of the third palmar interosseous muscle.

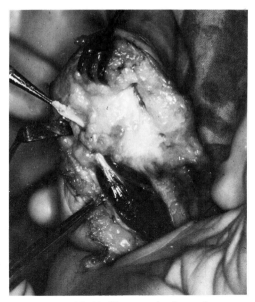

Figure 108–33. Photograph of transfer.

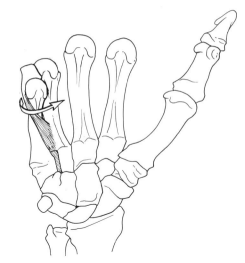

Figure 108–34. The transfer increases the "opposition" of the fifth metacarpal.

of anteposition—or by means of an arthroplasty using a coupled prosthesis.

4. Transfer of the terminal tendon of the fourth palmar interosseous muscle. This tendon, which is inserted on the lateral aspect of the base of the proximal phalanx of the little finger, is slipped under the hypothenar muscles and transferred to the medial side of the phalanx. The muscle thus acquires a pronating action, which reinforces opposition of the phalangized metacarpal (Figs. 108–32, 108–33, 108–34). It has been shown by electromyography that the interosseous muscle complements the opponens muscle, whose action fades during anteposition beyond 30 degrees (Tubiana and Roux, 1974). Other transfers are possible depending on which

structures have survived the injury. Finally the newly created cleft is covered with a skin graft and kept open with a well molded dressing (Fig. 108–35).

INDICATIONS FOR PHALANGIZATION OF THE METACARPALS

Phalangization of the metacarpals has been performed mostly on mutilated hands, but there are other indications.

PHALANGIZATION OF ONLY THE FIRST METACARPAL

Phalangization of the first metacarpal only is indicated in the following circumstances:

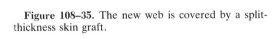

Figure 108–35. The new web is covered by a split-thickness skin graft.

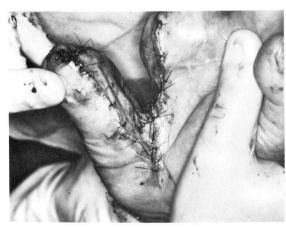

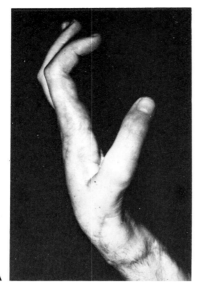 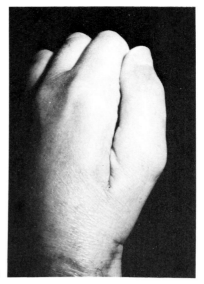

A   **B**

Figure 108–36. Ischemic contracture of the muscles of the hand with contraction of the first web. *A*, Phalangization of the first web associated with tendon transfer. *B*, Restoration of useful lateral pinch grip.

Isolated Contracture of the First Web. Isolated contracture of the first web without amputation of the thumb occurs after burns, in iatrogenic contractures following immobilization in a faulty position (adduction-retroposition) (Fig. 108–36), and in stiff paralyzed hands. Tendon transfers are sometimes necessary to restore anteposition (Fig. 108–37). A splint must be worn postoperatively to keep the deepened web open.

Partial Amputation of the Thumb. In cases of partial amputation of the thumb through the proximal phalanx, major reconstructive procedures are seldom required; deepening of the commissure alone usually permits the grasping of larger objects. If the phalangeal segment is too short, phalangization may be combined with moderate lengthening (1 cm.) of the thumb by a bone graft covered with a flap of adjacent intact skin (Fig. 108–38).

Thumb-Finger Amputation. Phalangization of the first metacarpal is particularly

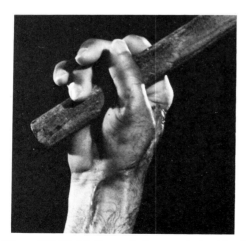

Figure 108–37. Median and ulnar paralysis with stiffness of the fingers and contraction of the first web. Partial phalangization of the first metacarpal restores passive movements of the thumb ray. There is an associated tendon transfer.

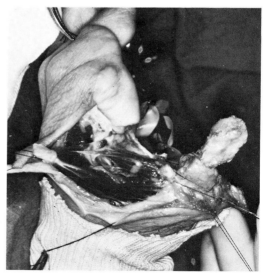

Figure 108–38. Lengthening of the first metacarpal associated with phalangization.

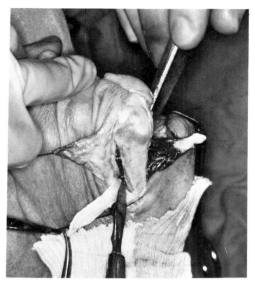

Figure 108–39. Excision of the second metacarpal in a case of contracture of the first web with amputation of the index finger.

longus is inserted) in order to create a wider and deeper commissure (Fig. 108–39).

PHALANGIZATION OF ONLY THE FIFTH METACARPAL

This operation is indicated after traumatic amputation of the four fingers in order to provide the thumb with a mobile opposition post (Fig. 108–40). The shorter or stiffer the thumb, the more useful the phalangization will be.

In more severe mutilations, however, further steps may be taken to enhance the effect of the phalangization, such as resection of the fourth metacarpal to widen the newly constructed cleft and to narrow the palm, and lengthening of the phalangized fifth metacarpal when the thumb is unduly short. However, the fixed limb of a pincer should not be made longer than the mobile limb.

Finally the function of the metacarpohamate joint can be enhanced either by altering its sector of mobility by means of an osteotomy of the fifth metacarpal, or by increasing its mobility by means of a capsulectomy or arthroplasty (Fig. 108–41).

COMBINED PHALANGIZATION OF THE FIRST AND FIFTH METACARPALS

This is performed when all five digits have been lost. Contrary to a widespread belief (Iselin, 1961), this procedure can restore useful pincer function even if the metacarpals

useful in combined amputations of the thumb and adjacent fingers because it can create a pincer between the first and second metacarpals. Lengthening of the first metacarpal by whatever procedure is of value only if the sensory supply to the skin on the tip of the stump is intact and if there are digital segments left that the neothumb can usefully oppose.

When the first web is contracted and the index finger has been lost, it is preferable to resect the second metacarpal (preserving its base on which the extensor carpi radialis

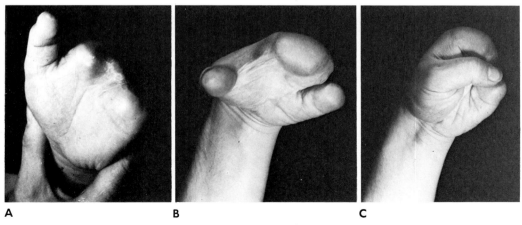

A   B   C

Figure 108–40. A, Amputation of all four fingers, thumb intact. B, Phalangization of the fifth metacarpal. C, Result.

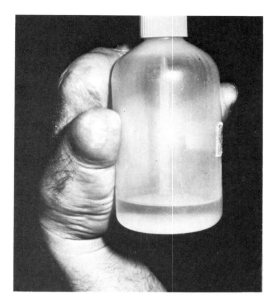

Figure 108–41. Amputation of all four fingers of the right hand, thumb stiff. Phalangization of the fifth metacarpal with capsulectomy of its proximal joint (section of the posteromedial oblique ligament) providing spread allowing a wide grip.

are not lengthened. The essential element of the pinch under these circumstances is obviously a mobile first metacarpal (Fig. 108–42). If the latter is absent or stiff, an isolated phalangization of the fifth will be of little use.

When the amputation is at the level of the metacarpal heads, resection of both the second and the fourth metacarpals produces two deep clefts (Fig. 108–43). The third metacarpal is not disturbed in order to preserve the origin of the adductor pollicis muscle. Be-

sides, the presence of this third post permits more precise grasping of large objects, while small objects such as pins and sheets of paper can be held between the phalangized first and fifth metacarpals.

Lengthening of the phalangized metacarpals is mechanically useful, but clinically it is beneficial only if the skin is of good quality and sensation is present.

Combined phalangization, sometimes performed bilaterally, has been known to restore

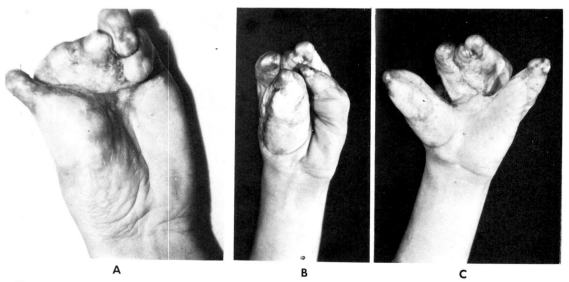

| A | B | C |

Figure 108–42. *A*, Burn with crushing of hand in a press. Only stumps of the fingers remain. *B* and *C*, Note the amplitude of movements which the two phalangizations allow.

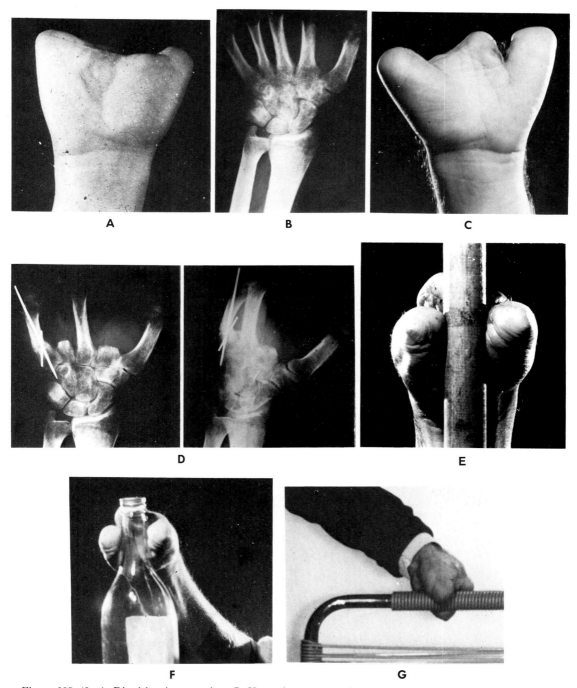

Figure 108–43. *A*, Distal hemi-amputation. *B*, X-ray shows amputation of the distal part of the metacarpals. *C*, Phalangization with slight lengthening of the first and fifth metacarpals and resection of second and fourth metacarpals. *D*, X-ray showing in particular the osteotomy of the fifth metacarpal. *E* to *I*, Functional results showing restoration of a powerful wide grip and a precise grip.

Illustration continued on following page

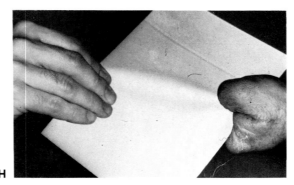

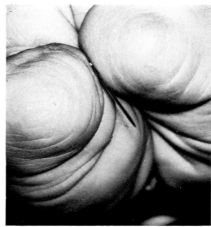

Figure 108–43 *Continued*

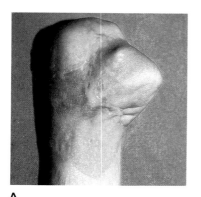

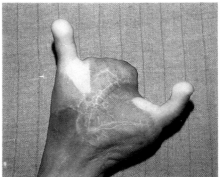

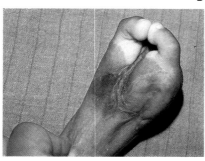

Figure 108–44. Metacarpal hand. Sequelae of burns. *A*, The entire stump covered
with skin grafts. *B*, Phalangization of the
first and fifth metacarpals combined with
the transfers of two toes (the second toe
of each foot). *C*, Result (A. Gilbert). Phalangization of the first and fifth metacarpals
considerably increased the effectiveness of
the toe transfers.

independence to helpless patients with severe bilateral mutilations.

The benefit brought by phalangizations in cases of severe mutilations of the hand underlines the importance of preserving as much length as possible in the first and fifth rays at the time of the initial treatment. Although this is usually kept in mind when one is dealing with the thumb, it is often forgotten in the context of the fifth finger, which is too readily sacrificed.

Elongation of the mobile metacarpals using free tissue transfers, now made possible by microsurgical techniques, increases pinch grip ability, but it must be pointed out that simple phalangization of the peripheral metacarpals is capable of considerably improving the function of amputated hands. Surgeons dealing with such patients must be familiar with phalangization techniques, which may still be of great value and when combined with toe transfer can further enhance their effectiveness (Fig. 108–44).

REFERENCES

Burkhard, O.: Mittelhandfinger. Feldärzrl. Beil. Munch. Med. Wschr., *63*:1409, 1916.

Delbet, R., and Tessier, P.: Personal communication.

Hilgenfeldt, O.: Operativer Daumenersatz and Beseitigung von Greifstörungen. Ferd. Enke, Stuttgart, 1950.

Huguier, P. C.: Considérations anatomiques et physiologiques sur le rôle du pouce et sur la chirurgie de cet organe. Arch. Gén. Méd., *22*:404–421, 567–580, 692–706, 1873.

Huguier, P. C.: Considérations anatomiques et physiologiques pour servir à la chirurgie du pouce. Arch. Gén. Méd., pp. 54–82, 1874.

Iselin, M.: Considérations sur l'amputation métacarpienne. Mem. Acad. Chir., *87*:534–537, 1961.

Kreuz, L.: Die Herrichtung des Unterarmstumpfs zum naturlichen Greifarm nach dem Verfahren Krukenbergs. Zbl. Chir., *71*:1170–1175, 1944.

Simon, P.: Die Metaphalangisation. Spätergebnisse bei der Rehabilitation Handverletzter. Z. Orthop., *97*:551–565, 1963.

Tubiana, R.: Phalangisation du 5ème métacarpien. Acta Orthop. Belg. (Suppl. 3), p. 120, 1958.

Tubiana, R., and Roux, J. P.: Phalangization of the first and fifth metacarpals. J. Bone Joint Surg., *56*:447–457, 1974.

Chapter 109

PROXIMAL RADIAL HEMIAMPUTATION: RECONSTRUCTION OF PREHENSION BY FREE CROSS HAND DIGITAL TRANSPLANTATION

Ueli Büchler

Although the isolated loss of the thumb in an otherwise normal hand can be regarded as a "local" problem, mutilating injuries that involve adjacent rays as well require different reconstructive considerations. Very often, amputations occur along an oblique line, which includes the proximal thumb and increasingly distal levels of the more adjacent ulnar rays. In the extreme case of proximal radial hemiamputation of the hand, we are faced with not only loss of the entire first ray (including its important mobile basilar trapeziometacarpal joint), but also the loss of index and middle rays, and to a variable extent the more distal ring and small digits. We shall deal here with this rare type of lesion, which poses difficult reconstructive problems.

PLANNING THE RECONSTRUCTION: GENERAL CONSIDERATIONS

Even when the elements of a mobile grip are preserved in the ring and little fingers, it is usually not advisable to utilize either digit to construct a neothumb. The function of the ulnar half of the hand is already diminished and must not be weakened further. It follows that there is no local tissue available for reconstruction of a thumb and that the ele-

ments of a new grip must be transferred from a distance.

Reconstruction of prehension should be planned along simple and realistic lines to restore precision pinch and power grasp. As a minimum, three goals must be met—improvement of function on the ulnar side, creation of a central commissure, and construction of a radial pincer arm.

FUNCTION ON THE ULNAR SIDE

The fourth and/or fifth rays should be sensate with power, length, and mobility that approaches or exceeds the level of the proximal interphalangeal joint.

In the simplest case in which the little finger is preserved up to the proximal interphalangeal joint, a supination osteotomy of the fifth metacarpal is the answer (Fig. 109–1b).

When functionally useful elements of both ulnar rays are preserved, their reorientation is best achieved through a combined flexion-supination osteotomy of the hamate. This repositions both rays together and provides for a wider area of ulnar hand support. Steps must also be taken to correct metacarpophalangeal joint stiffness if present.

If all active elements have been lost on the ulnar side, the transfer of one or two toes may be considered (Fig. 109–1c).

1210

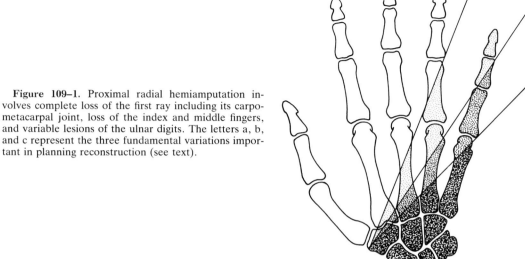

Figure 109–1. Proximal radial hemiamputation involves complete loss of the first ray including its carpometacarpal joint, loss of the index and middle fingers, and variable lesions of the ulnar digits. The letters a, b, and c represent the three fundamental variations important in planning reconstruction (see text).

THE CENTRAL COMMISSURE

The importance of a central commissure cannot be overstressed. A power grasp is possible only if the arms of the pincer can stand far enough apart; the intervening space should be cleared of inactive metacarpal remnants. Before a neothumb is constructed, one must make sure that sufficient soft tissue is available to line the future commissure.

All procedures mentioned so far will constitute the first stage and precede reconstruction of the thumb.

RESTORING A RADIAL PINCER ARM

The most difficult surgical step in proximal radial amputations is the construction of a radial pincer arm whose function approaches that of the normal thumb—a tall order if we remember that the intrinsic musculature of the thumb as well as its carpometacarpal joint has been destroyed. Only with a free tissue transfer can we hope to create a neothumb that is sufficiently long, stable, mobile, sensitive, and powerful.

Because pollicization of a finger yields the best results in cases of destruction of the first ray and in congenital aplasia of the thumb, it would seem logical in this form of hemiamputation to transfer a finger from the other hand rather than a toe.

If we compare the functional potential of a transferred finger, a transferred big toe, and a transferred toe, the pollicized contralateral finger seems to offer the most advantages (Figs. 109–2, 109–3). To begin with, the range of movement of the finger is more than five times greater than that of any toe. If, as is the rule, the absent carpometacarpal joint is replaced by the metacarpophalangeal joint of the pollicized finger, the neothumb is capable of abduction and adduction in addition to some degree of circumduction. In such cases the most proximal joint is now situated in the correct anatomical position, i.e., at the base of the neothumb. If instead a toe is used, its defined length would require a proximal lengthening bone graft to place the new metacarpophalangeal joint more distally.

A major disadvantage of using a toe metatarsophalangeal joint is that the range of movement is tilted in favor of extension. When a toe is transferred to the thumb position, the metatarsal must be osteosynthesized subcapitally to a bone graft at an angle of 65 degrees, which shifts into flexion the normal extension arc of motion.

The main and obvious drawback is that the loss of a finger imposes a considerably greater loss of function of a hand than loss of a toe on a donor foot. Depending on the finger transferred, the theoretical functional loss is between 5 and 25 per cent. If half of the

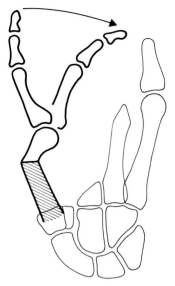

Figure 109–2. In proximal radial hemiamputation, transfer of a toe does not allow ideal reconstruction of a thumb. The transferred toe is too short and has an insufficient range of motion. Moreover, the transfer requires osteoplasty of the metacarpal head to the trapezoid.

normal value of a thumb is restored to the recipient hand (equals 20 per cent), the donor deficit is justified. This should make the operation recognized and refundable by insurance companies. Admittedly the decision to "sacrifice" a digit from an intact hand is one that cannot be taken lightly by either the patient or his surgeon, but the potential ben-

efit outweighs the functional loss in the donor hand, which is usually adequately compensated.

CROSS HAND POLLICIZATION BY FREE DIGITAL TRANSFER

One prerequisite in reconstruction of a neothumb is an adequate reserve of soft tissue in the thenar region. If this is not available, a flap from a distant site (raised as a preliminary procedure) or a Chinese flap may be necessary.

Because every finger is a possible candidate for transfer, the choice depends on which "lost" ray produces the least morbidity. For a number of reasons, we favor the ray of the index finger (Büchler and Tschopp, 1981; Littler, 1953; Murray et al., 1977).

The patency of the arteries of the donor digit and of its neighbor should be checked by Allen's test and by sonography, and an angiogram of the receiving hand is strongly advocated.

DONOR HAND

At the base of the donor finger, as much skin is raised with the transfer as is compatible with simple primary suture closure. Along with the transfer, one common digital palmar artery is taken from its origin together with one or two dorsal veins up to the wrist. The

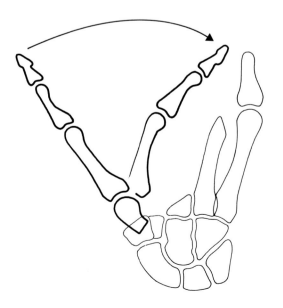

Figure 109–3. Transfer of a finger from the intact hand makes use of the known advantages of pollicization. The metacarpophalangeal joint replaces the last carpometacarpal joint, and the length of the digit allows sufficient range of motion.

two proper digital nerves are raised in full length, care being taken to avoid interfascicular dissection of the median and ulnar nerves. The extensor and flexor tendons are divided at the musculotendinous junction. The intrinsic muscles that cannot be transferred are left in situ and serve to stabilize the adjacent digital rays. The metacarpal is osteotomized at the neck, 1 cm. proximal to the capsule of the metacarpophalangeal joint. The rest of the procedure follows the usual steps of resection and transposition.

Receiving Hand and Transfer

The corresponding structures are then identified in the injured hand and prepared to receive the transplant. The neck of the metacarpal is fixed to the carpus by means of a stable osteosynthesis; the metacarpal head should be flexed at 30 degrees to the imaginary axis of the thumb, with its plane of flexion orientated toward its ulnar "opponent." When the index finger is transplanted, the extensor proprius tendon is mobilized and prolonged by a portion of the central slip out to the level of the distal third of the proximal phalanx; the aponeurosis is closed by direct suturing. The abductor pollicis longus is connected to the extensor communis, and the extensor pollicis longus to the previously mobilized extensor proprius. On the palmar side, the A_1 A_2, and A_3 pulleys are incised to enhance the adductor action of the extrinsic flexor tendon. Several flexors are available in the forearm to reactivate the transplant, e.g., the flexor pollicis longus for the flexor profundus and the flexor superficialis II for the superficial flexor of the transplant. It is preferable not to carry out the intrinsic substitution at the same session. Sensory bundles of the median nerve are then prepared for suturing but without disturbing the intraneural topography. The donor artery is anastomosed if possible end to side to the radial artery, and the vein is connected end to end to a branch of the cephalic vein. The whole procedure on average takes about six hours.

Rehabilitation

As the tendons are tethered by Pulvertaft weaves, early active mobilization is allowed. The inevitable intrinsic deficit necessitates passive extension exercises. Since the original muscles are utilized, the re-education and coordination of extrinsic functions are usually simple.

Intrinsic Transfer

For the purpose of re-education we like to reactivate intrinsic functions at a second operation when the main goal is to restore a powerful adductor of the thumb. The choice here lies between another superficial flexor, the extensor carpi radialis longus, or the extensor carpi ulnaris. Depending on the power of abduction present, the tension of this transfer (extended by a graft) is adjusted to prevent a claw deformity from developing later in the neothumb. Although circumduction is invariably limited, an additional transfer (running in the direction of a theoretical abductor) will improve extension of the proximal interphalangeal joint. It can be inserted on a previously mobilized radial band of the extensor apparatus. If the distal interphalangeal joint proves unstable, it should be arthrodesed in a position of function.

CASE PRESENTATION

A 20 year old patient suffered a proximal radial hemiamputation of the dominant hand in an explosion. The first two rays, the middle and ring fingers, as well as the two distal phalanges of the fifth finger were destroyed in the injury.

Because only the proximal phalanx of the fifth finger had survived, no reconstruction was attempted on the ulnar side, but an osteotomy of the metacarpal was carried out. To deepen the central commissure, the third metacarpal was resected at its base. At a second operation the ray of the index finger from the contralateral hand was transferred to replace the missing thumb, using the technique already described.

Two and one-half years later the patient was pleased with the overall function and appearance of this hand and experienced no pain, even from heavy work. The neothumb had excellent trophicity and useful sensation, i.e., a two point discrimination of 8 to 11 mm. The maximal span of the pincer was 8 cm. and the two arms came into close apposition whatever the position of the wrist. The gripping power was between 4 and 8 kg. (Figs. 109–4, 109–5).

Under direct visual control very small objects could be pinched with no difficulty, and larger objects could be lifted effectively with no auxiliary

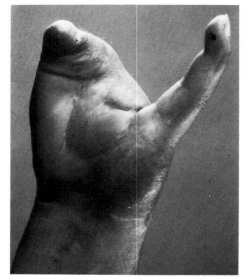

Figure 109–4

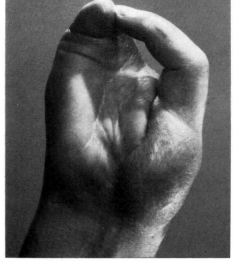

Figure 109–5

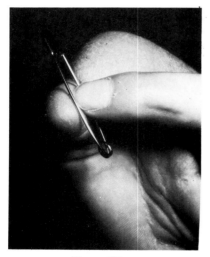

Figure 109–6

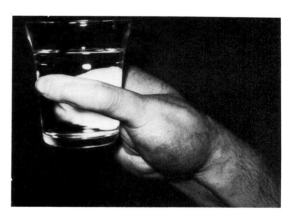

Figure 109–7

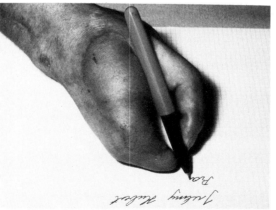

Figure 109–8

Figures 109–4 to 109–8. Result of transfer of a contralateral finger for reconstruction of the thumb in a case of proximal radial hemiamputation. Sensation and function of the reconstructed hand are described in the text.

help. However, some tools could be stabilized only by using a more or less circular grip. The injured hand remained dominant, proving that the patient had successfully learned the full possibilities of use of the reconstructed thumb (Figs. 109–6 to 109–8). The donor hand lost none of its practical value but was shown to have lost 15 per cent of its effectiveness in both precision and power gripping.

REFERENCES

Büchler, U., and Tschopp, H. M.: Freie kontralaterale Zeigefingerpollizisation. Handchirurgie, *13:*36–45, 1981.

Buck-Gramcko, D.: Pollicization of the index finger. J. Bone Joint Surg., *53A:*1605–1617, 1971.

Buncke, H. J., and Shah, K. G.: Toe-digital transfers. *In* Serafin, D., and Buncke, H. J. (Editors): Microsurgical Composite Tissue Transplantation. St. Louis, The C. V. Mosby Company, 1979, pp. 573–586.

Littler, J. W.: The neurovascular pedicle method of digital transposition for reconstruction of the thumb. Plast. Reconstr. Surg., *12:*303–320, 1953.

Murray, J. F., Carman, W., and MacKenzie, K.: Complications and hand strength following transmetacarpal amputation of the index finger. J. Hand Surg., *2:*471–481, 1977.

O'Brien, B., MacLeod, A. M., Sykes, P. J., Browning, F. S. C., and Threlfall, G. N.: Microvascular second toe transfer for digital reconstruction. J. Hand Surg., *3:*123–134, 1978.

Souquet, R., and Mansat, M.: La Chirurgie Secondaire dans les Mutilations de la Main. Paris, Libraire Maloine, 1980, p. 9ff.

Tubiana, R.: Phalangisation of the 1st and 5th metacarpals. J. Bone Joint Surg., *36A:*447–457, 1974.

Chapter 110

BILATERAL HAND MUTILATIONS

Raoul Tubiana

We shall be concerned here only with severe mutilations, i.e., those in which at least one of the elements of the thumb-finger pinch has been lost in each hand. In our series, heat and electrical burns were the commonest causes of such mutilations, followed by crush injuries at work and following traffic accidents. There were also a few cases of frostbite and explosion injuries.

The problems arising from severe bilateral mutilations differ from those of unilateral mutilation not only in the severity of the injury and its psychological effects but also in the therapeutic approach. Here one must draw on the combined possibilities of reconstructive surgery and prosthetics.

Severe mutilations of both hands constitute a major disability, which cannot, and must not, be regarded simply as two unilateral lesions. The problems may appear to be similar at first, but they are more complex and, to some extent, quite new. Whereas in the unilateral lesion surgery aims at providing the patient with a useful instrument to assist the contralateral intact hand, in cases of severe bilateral mutilation the surgeon must try to restore the lost autonomy. He does this by combining surgery and prosthetics. The therapeutic approach involves difficult decisions because it must take into account the site and extent of the lesions as well as the age, occupation, and psychological state of the patient.

The psychological repercussions are considerable, for a bilaterally mutilated patient is initially anxious and, not surprisingly, tends to lose hope. For this reason it is important to restore his confidence by explaining what treatment is available, what can be attempted for each hand, and what surgical program is

envisaged while taking into account his own wishes. It cannot be repeated too often that the restoration of a natural sensitive grip will help the patient considerably in adapting to his infirmity. Encouraged by the early results, the patient himself often requests further surgery. This trusting collaboration can go a long way toward instilling psychological and functional confidence in these unfortunate patients. In the field of reconstructive surgery few patients bring more satisfaction to their surgeon. Urged by sheer necessity, patients with bilateral mutilations often achieve remarkable functional results, comparatively much superior to those with unilateral injuries.

With these facts in mind, we have divided these mutilations into three groups according to their severity and surgical possibilities— mutilations in which one can hope to restore good bilateral manual prehension, mutilations that are severe on one side and more limited on the other, in which one can hope to restore good prehension on one side at least, and severe bilateral mutilations (Tubiana, 1969).

THE FIRST GROUP: BOTH MUTILATIONS ARE RELATIVELY LIMITED

When the lesions, which can be symmetrical, are such that one can expect to restore useful prehension on both sides, each hand can be reconstructed by one of the procedures used for unilateral injuries. However, several points must be stressed.

1. Simultaneous immobilization of both limbs should be avoided whenever possible.

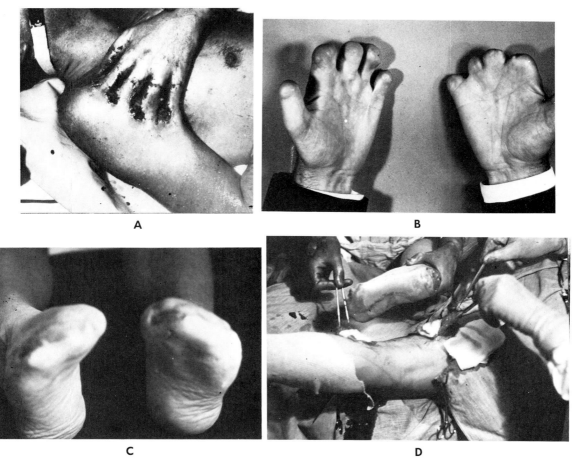

Figure 110–1. Severe frostbite in a climber in the Himalayas, resulting in the loss of fingers and toes and ulceration of the heels. Covering of the extremities by skin flaps. (R. Merle d'Aubigné and R. Tubiana.) *A*, The stumps of the four fingers and of the thumb were covered with small tubular flaps taken from the right shoulder. *B*, The left hand after the operation. The same operation was performed on the right hand. *C*, All toes were lost from both feet and both heels were ulcerated. *D*, The heel and extremities of the metatarsal were covered with skin flaps taken from both sides of the popliteal fossa. This patient was able to return to mountaineering and skiing.

2. The surgical indications can be stretched to try to achieve the best result in each hand. Thus a toe transplant is more likely to be considered and readily accepted in cases of bilateral mutilations.

3. It is important to reduce the number of operations to a minimum, by combining, for example, reconstruction on one hand with the preparation of a skin flap for the other. This requires careful advance planning. Thus, in one patient with frostbite of both hands and feet, each hand was operated on at the same time as one foot. The hand stump was covered with skin flaps taken from the contralateral shoulder, while the heel and distal extremities of the feet were covered at the same session by skin flaps from either side of the contralateral popliteal fossa (Fig. 110–1).

In another patient in whom both thumbs and index fingers were crushed, the wounds were first covered over by skin grafts (Fig. 110–2). On one side the thumb was reconstructed by means of a subclavicular tube flap and osteoplastic transplants from the middle finger along with the neurovascular bundle. On the other side, the index stump, being longer, was pollicized (Fig. 110–3).

THE SECOND GROUP: THE MUTILATION IS MUCH MORE SEVERE ON ONE SIDE

The patient must recover his autonomy as soon as possible, and thus one operates first on the better side. This was the case with a

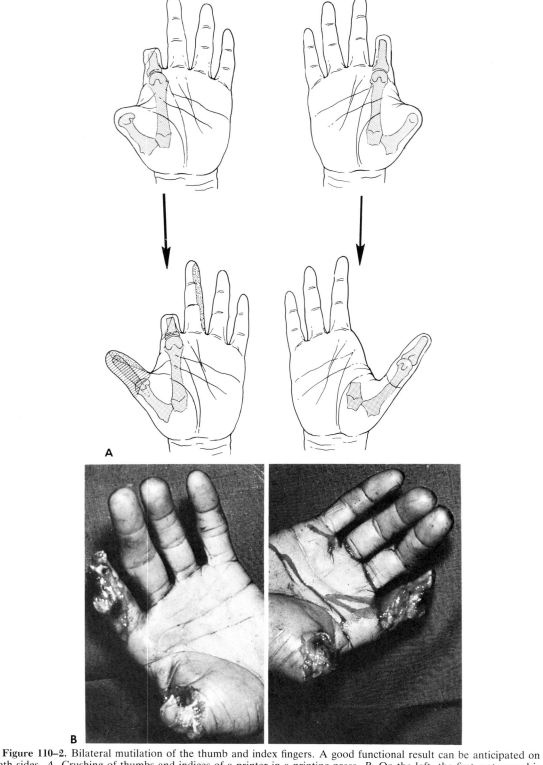

Figure 110–2. Bilateral mutilation of the thumb and index fingers. A good functional result can be anticipated on both sides. *A*, Crushing of thumbs and indices of a printer in a printing press. *B*, On the left, the first metacarpal is long; the stump of the index finger is short and covered by poor quality skin. The thumb is reconstructed using a tube flap with bone graft and a neurovascularized island flap taken from the long finger.

Illustration continued on opposite page

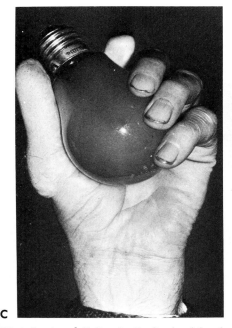
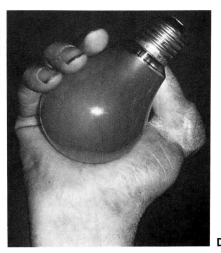

C D

Figure 110–2 *Continued C*, Result. *D*, On the right, the first metacarpal was shorter and the stump of the index finger longer. Pollicization of the mutilated index finger was done.

young girl who had both hands crushed and burned in a laundry press (Fig. 110–4). On the left side the thumb was amputated, but the first metacarpal and a phalangeal fragment were preserved. The first metacarpal was therefore promptly phalangized and the stump was covered with a skin flap. The injury on the right side was much more severe: the thumb and little finger had been amputated, the palm was crushed, and there was loss of mobility and sensation of the three remaining fingers. Healthy skin had to be grafted first before the nerves and tendons could be repaired. The same abdominal tube flap was utilized to cover the palm and to provide an opposing post in front of the

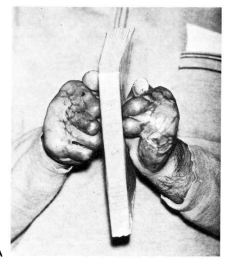
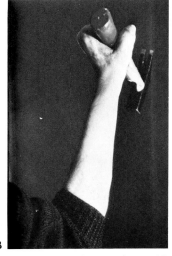

A B

Figure 110–3. Another example of Group I bilateral mutilation. *A*, Sequelae of severe burn of both hands with mutilation of the fingers and coalescence of the webs, making any grip impossible. *B*, Result after phalangization of the right first web.

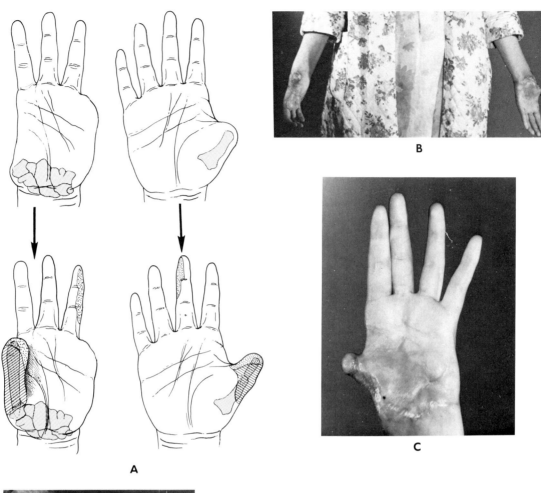

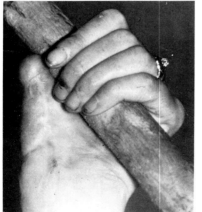

Figure 110–4. *A*, Severe mutilation on one side, limited injury on the other. *B*, Laundress whose hands were trapped in a pressing machine. *C*, On the left, amputation of the thumb. *D*, Phalangization of the first metacarpal.

Illustration continued on opposite page

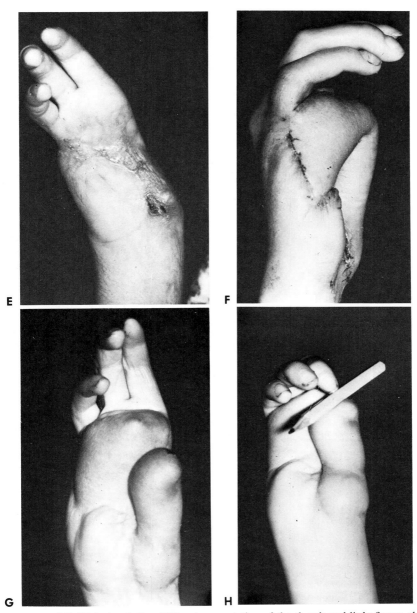

Figure 110–4 *Continued E*, Right hand. In addition to amputation of the thumb and little finger, the tendons and digital neurovascular bundles are destroyed in the palm. *F*, A large abdominal tube flap is brought to the palm. *G*, This is used to cover the palm and reconstruct a thumb. *H*, Restoration of flexion and sensitivity of the fingers by tendon and nerve grafts.

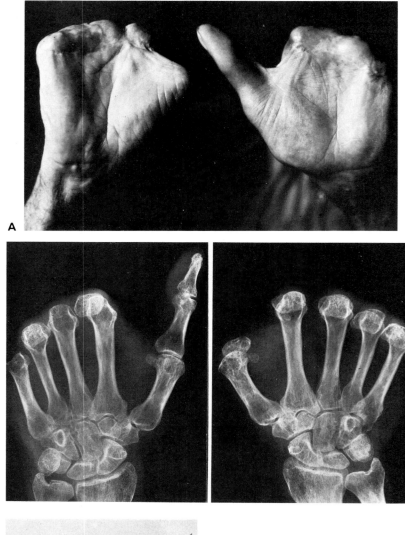

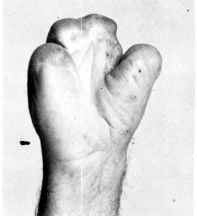

Figure 110–5. *A*, Engineer with both hands mutilated by an explosion. *B*, X-ray of both hands. *C*, Phalangization of the first and fifth metacarpals on the right.

Illustration continued on opposite page

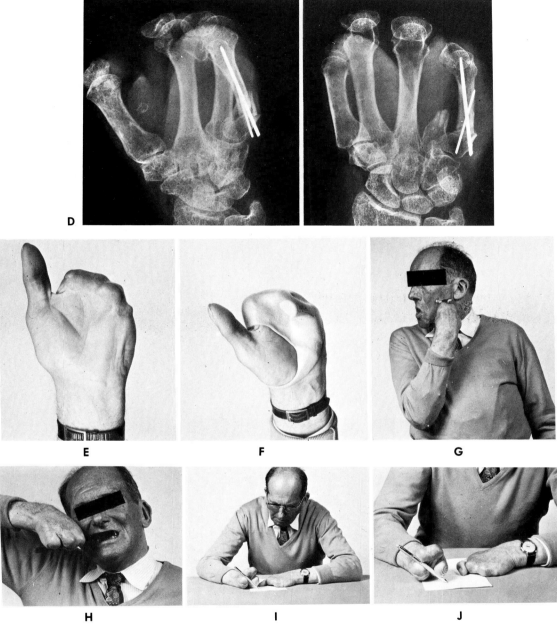

Figure 110–5 *Continued D*, X-ray of the right hand. Resection of the fourth metacarpal and osteotomy of the fifth metacarpal. *E*, On the left, amputation of all four fingers; the thumb remains. *F*, Orthosis with buttress opposing the thumb. *G* to *J*, Functional result. The patient became completely independent. The phalangized right hand remained dominant. He scarcely uses his prosthesis.

middle and the index fingers. Sensation and mobility were duly restored with nerve and tendon grafts.

A 45 year old engineer (Fig. 110–5) suffered mutilation of both hands by an explosion, with loss of all fingers and of the thumb on the right. On the left, the thumb remained, but the four fingers were lost. He was fitted with an orthosis to elongate the ulnar part of the hand opposite the thumb. Phalangization of the first and fifth metacarpals was performed on the right side, which gave a very good functional result because the right hand remained the dominant hand. The patient used his orthosis only for a transient period. He was quickly satisfied with

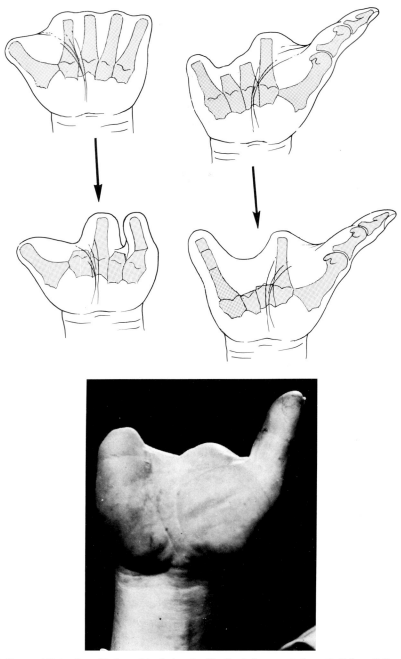

Figure 110–6. Severe bilateral mutilation of both hands. On the left, amputation of all five digits and even part of the metacarpals. The thumb remains on the right. Lengthening and phalangization of right fifth metacarpal were carried out, and strong and sensitive grip was thereby re-established. This was followed by phalangization of first and fifth metacarpals on the left.

his phalangizations alone, which restored his independence.

In another fairly similar patient, in whom the residual metacarpals were shorter, phalangization was performed at the outset with elongation of the fifth metacarpal on the side where the thumb was preserved (Fig. 110–6). In this group of patients it is sometimes possible to take from the least damaged side a mutilated or stiffened finger that has nevertheless retained a good blood supply. The finger may be transferred to the other hand using microsurgical techniques if its contribution restores pinch grip that otherwise would be impossible.

THE THIRD GROUP: BOTH HANDS ARE SEVERELY MUTILATED

Here all remnants must be utilized in an attempt to restore useful grips to both limbs. As a rule it is wise to wait for the result of the operation on the first side before embarking upon repairs on the second. Thus when faced with two metacarpal hands of which one only has a mobile first metacarpal, one can hope to create a grip on that side, but no metacarpal pinch is possible on the side where the thenar eminence has been destroyed.

The less severely mutilated hand is operated upon first. If some useful function has been restored, one can then make the most of the remnants on the other side and perhaps be content with utilizing the powerful movements of the wrist, with its sensitive skin, against a prosthetic post. If, however, only a

weak and narrow pinch has been restored on the better side, the surgeon will aim at creating a broad and powerful grip on the other side. This may entail "proximalizing" the mutilation and performing Krukenberg's operation. The main advantage of this operation is that it creates a sensitive grasp (Fig. 110–7).* The main criticism of the procedure is the unsightly forearm digitation (Fig. 110–8). However, in fact most of the patients in whom we have performed a Krukenberg operation have been extremely satisfied, and one may wonder whether the cosmetic factor, always highly subjective, should be given pride of place in such cases. Undoubtedly the best judge is the patient himself, and for him the functional aspect far outweighs the cosmetic. Evidence for this is overwhelming.

I am somewhat shocked by the reactions of those doctors, physiotherapists, and prosthetists who, having only photographic experience of this operation, cringe with horror when it is suggested. Their unfavorable reaction often causes the patient to refuse an operation that could considerably reduce his plight. This attitude seems even more unreasonable when one considers that the unsightly pincer can be cleverly disguised by an easily fitted prosthesis, which itself can be activated by the two arms of the pincer (Fig. 110–9). Moberg, who has assessed our results, not only shares our view but goes even further when he, quite justifiably, advocates this procedure for unilateral mutilations. We have performed Krukenberg's operation mostly for bilateral amputees, and it can be done on

*See Chapter 111.

Figure 110–7. Krukenberg's operation. The opposable surfaces of the branches are covered by sensitive skin.

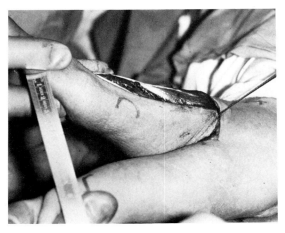

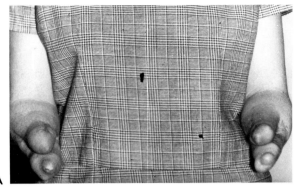

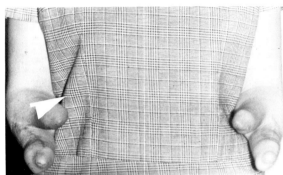

Figure 110–8. Amputation of both hands in a young girl by explosion of a grenade. Bilateral Krukenberg's operation. *A*, Branches closed. *B*, Branches open.

Figure 110–9. *A* and *B*, Movements of forearm branches activate the thumb movements in a hand prosthesis.

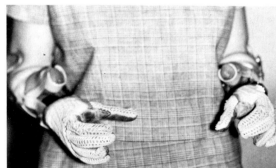

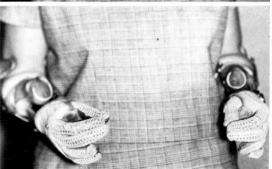

both sides, especially in patients with hand and eye injuries—a not uncommon occurrence after explosive injuries.

However, in cases not of amputation but of severe bilateral mutilations or unilateral amputation associated with amputation on the other side, Krukenberg's operation is usually indicated on one side alone in order to preserve one long limb that can reach the scapular, lumbar, and gluteal regions.

In one young male patient who suffered bilateral mutilations as a result of a mine explosion, good sensitive prehension was restored on both sides (Fig. 110–10). On the right side, where the hand had been completely amputated, Krukenberg's operation was performed. On the left, an index stump was pollicized.

Krukenberg's operation can be performed even for midforearm amputations, since most of the muscles required for activating the pincer have proximal origins. Thus to open

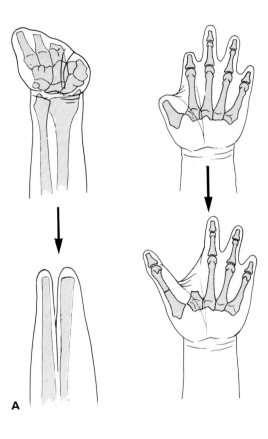

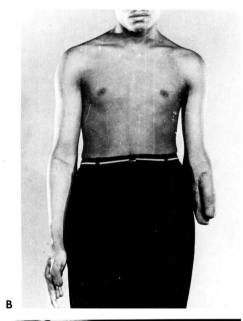

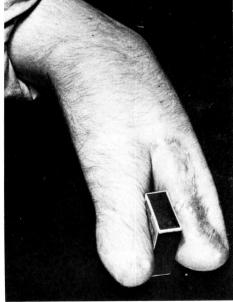

Figure 110–10. Severe bilateral mutilation of hands. *A*, On the right, complete amputation of the thumb and partial amputation of the index, ring, and little fingers. Pollicization of the mutilated index finger was done. *B*, On the left, amputation proximal to the wrist. Krukenberg's operation was carried out. *C*, results of Krukenberg's operation.

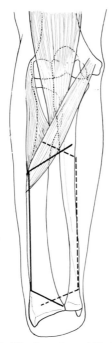

Figure 110–11. The branches of Krukenberg was essentially activated by muscles inserted into the proximal one third of the forearm: biceps, supinator, and pronator teres. Incisions for two skin flaps: anterior with ulnar pedicle (solid line); posterior with radial pedicle (dotted line).

the Krukenberg grip one needs the abductors of the radius, i.e., the biceps and brachioradialis, and to close it, the radial adductors, which are the pronator teres and supinator (Fig. 110–11). The ulna as a rule enjoys little mobility but should be stabilized by the triceps and brachialis. All these muscles have a proximal attachment. We have been forced in some cases to perform a very short Krukenberg operation with arms only 7 cm. long, but they retained their agility and sensitivity (Fig. 110–12).

This procedure is justifiable only if the ends of the pincer arms are provided with sensation, which explains its limited indications following burns. It is important that the tissues be mobile and well vascularized, and the muscles in good condition. Similarly the indications are restricted in ischemic syndromes and electrical burns.

It is essential that the patient should be fully informed preoperatively about the nature of the procedure envisaged. He may be encouraged by seeing the results obtained in other patients.

PROSTHETIC APPLIANCES

Prosthetic appliances can be of great cosmetic and functional assistance to patients with hand mutilations. It is our belief, however, that the decision to fit appliances should be made by the surgeon in conjunction with the prosthetist and the patient and not by a prosthetist alone without the advice of a surgeon experienced in the management of mutilations.

The possibilities of prosthetics must be carefully examined for each patient. Theoretically, with total hand prostheses the patient could be spared a long series of operations, but whatever the progress achieved in the field of prosthetics, these prostheses are all devoid of sensation and are conceived as an instrument and not as part of the body.

The possibility of a prosthesis should not preclude an attempt at reconstructive surgery whenever the latter offers a chance of restoring a sensitive grip. One should avoid the hurried fitting of prostheses, which might jeopardize the optimal utilization of all available stumps. A cosmetic prosthesis for social wear can do a lot to help a patient adapt to his infirmity. Similarly, carefully chosen and adapted appliances at the end of the cycle of surgical repairs can improve certain specific grips. The relative advantages and disadvantages of surgical reconstruction and prosthetic fitting must be compared. As an example, Krukenberg's operation is popular in countries where facilities for prosthetic fitting are limited.

CONCLUSION

In this chapter, mention has been deliberately limited to traditional reconstruction procedures. Obviously, the contribution of microsurgical techniques will enrich the possibilities of reconstruction without the treatment plans described here undergoing any fundamental change. Furthermore, in order to offer patients the best possible chance of recovery, these serious mutilations must be treated by teams capable of all reconstruction techniques, and appliance technicians must participate in organizing the treatment plan. We have achieved this at our Institute for Hand and Upper Limb Surgery. The following chapters indicate the contribution of microsurgery to the secondary reconstruction of these mutilations.

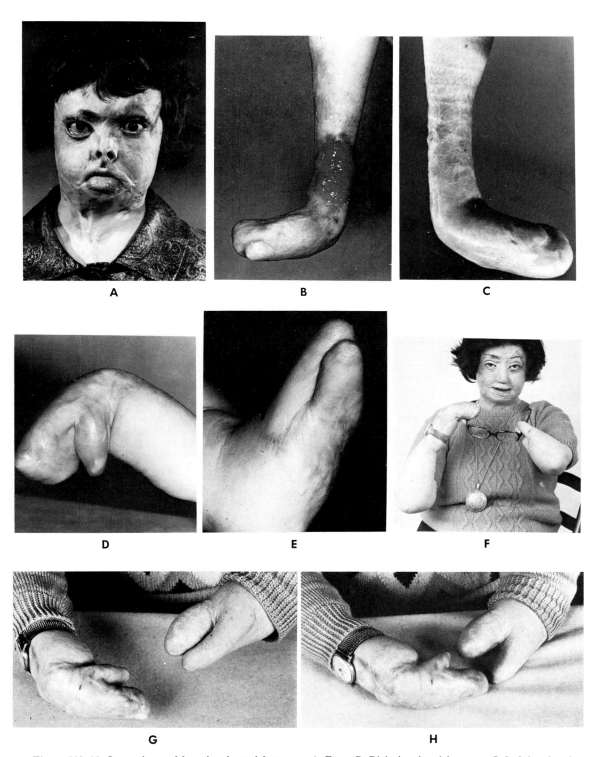

Figure 110–12. Severe burn of face, hands, and forearms. *A*, Face. *B*, Right hand and forearm. *C*, Left hand and forearm. *D*, On the right, the full length of the limb is preserved. The wrist was slightly mobile. Skin flap to forearm and phalangization of first metacarpal were done. *E*, On the left, the wrist was stiff in flexion and the hand was completely fixed. Krukenberg's operation was performed at level of healthy skin. Branches were only 7 cm. long. *F*, Overall result. *G* and *H*, The two pincers thus created are mobile. Complete restoration of independence.

Illustration continued on following page

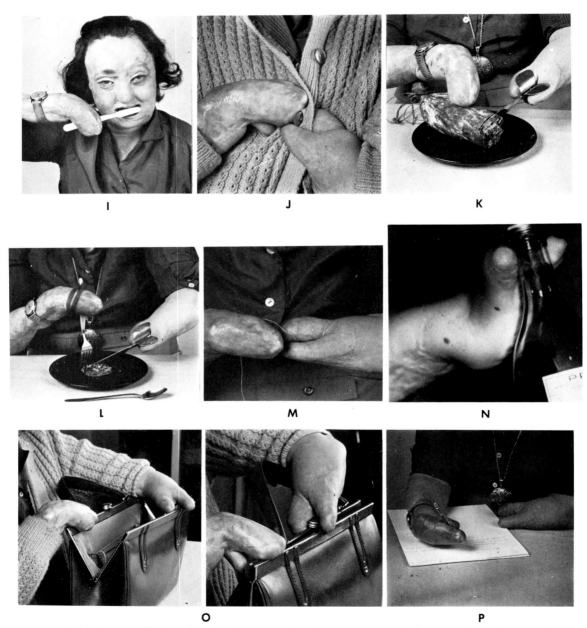

Figure 110–12 *Continued* The patient is able to wash herself (*I*), dress herself (*J*), cook (*K*), eat (*L*), sew (seen here threading a needle) (*M*), and do her housework (*N*). The Krukenberg pincer is strong. Seen here lifting a liter container. She is able to go to market (*O*), write (*P*), and write well (*Q*). *R*, She works as a secretary; she types.

Illustration continued on opposite page

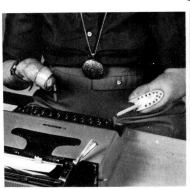

Q

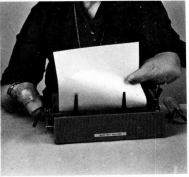

R

Figure 110–12 *Continued*

REFERENCES

Hilgenfeldt, O.: Operativer Daumenersatz und Beseitigung von Greifstörungen. Stuttgart, Ferdinand Enke, 1950.

Huguier, P. C.: Considérations anatomiques et physiologiques sur le rôle du pouce et sur la chirurgie de cet organe. Arch. Gén. Méd., 22:404–421, 567–580, 692–706, 1873.

Huguier, P. C.: Considérations anatomiques et physiologiques pour servir à la chirurgie du pouce. Arch. Gén. Méd., 54–82, 1874.

Krukenberg, H.: Ueber plastische Umwertung von Amputationstumpfen. Stuttgart, Ferdinand Enke, 1917.

Simon, P.: Die Metaphalangisation. Spätergebnisse bei der Rehabilitation Handverletzter. Z. Orthop., 97:551–565, 1963.

Tubiana, R.: Phalangisation du 5ème métacarpien. Acta Orthop. Belg. Suppl. 3:120, 1958.

Tubiana, R.: Repair of bilateral hand mutilations. Plast. Reconstr. Surg., 44:323, 1969.

Tubiana, R., and Elbaz, J. S.: Les mutilations graves bilatérales des mains. Ann. Chir. Plast., 10:116–122, 1965.

Tubiana, R., and Roux, J. P.: Phalangization of the first and fifth metacarpals. J. Bone Joint Surg., 56:447–457, 1974.

Tubiana, R., Gosset, J., and Campbell Reid, D. A.: Les Mutilations de la Main, 2nd ed., Monographies du G.E.M., Paris, Expansion Scientifique Francaise, 1984.

Chapter 111

KRUKENBERG'S OPERATION

P. MAURER

Krukenberg's operation, or digitation of the two forearm bones, is seldom performed, because in spite of the very good functional results, patients and surgeons tend to reject it on cosmetic grounds. Yet the resulting pincer has the significant advantage of sensibility, and its appearance, outside working hours, can be concealed by "social" prostheses activated by movements of the two claws.

TECHNIQUE

The technique has been well described and later modified by Kalio (1948) who advocates incisions that allow the lining of the internal prehensile part of the pincer with normal sensible skin.

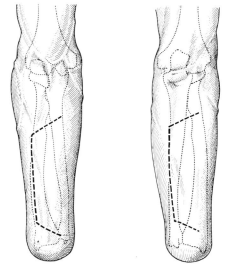

Figure 111–1. Outline of the anterior and posterior incisions.

1232

SKIN INCISIONS

The skin incisions are designed to produce an anterior and a posterior flap (Fig. 111–1). Anteriorly the incision begins three fingerbreadths below the elbow crease just inside the midline and runs obliquely laterodistally to within one fingerbreadth of the lateral border of the forearm. Thence it is continued alongside the lateral border down to the extremity of the stump, thus producing a medially based horizontal flap.

Posteriorly the incision follows a similar but reversed oblique course, starting 1 cm. from the medial border of the forearm. It then runs vertically down along the medial border, producing a laterally based horizontal flap.

DIVIDING THE FOREARM MUSCLES

The anterior skin flap is raised together with the superficial fascia to expose the superficial muscles of the forearm. After identifying the inferior border of the pronator teres, access to the deeper structures is obtained by passing between that muscle and the flexor carpi radialis, palmaris longus, and extensor carpi ulnaris on the medial side.

This maneuver exposes the superficial aspect of the flexor digitorum communis superficialis, which is split into a medial and a lateral half, between the tendons to the middle and ring fingers, up to the common flexor arch, which is then divided. The median nerve is also divided at that level as it emerges from the pronator teres, and the distal segment is resected.

More deeply the flexor communis profundus is separated from the flexor pollicis. These two muscles are disinserted from the

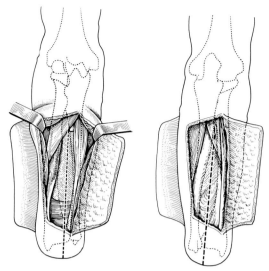

Figure 111–2. Raising the two flaps and separation of the muscles in the anterior and posterior compartments.

anterior aspect of the interosseous membrane, which is laid bare along its entire length. At the level of its upper border the interosseous neurovascular bundle is identified; the vessels are ligated and the nerve is resected (Fig. 111–2).

The muscle bellies are preserved when they are not too voluminous. In well muscled subjects, however, in whom they may interfere with closure of the pincer by bulging in the commissure, any of the following may be resected: flexor carpi ulnaris, palmaris longus, and flexor superficialis. The deep flexors are preserved.

On the extensor side the skin flap is raised together with the superficial fascia; access is obtained first by passing between the medial and lateral heads of the extensor communis. The extensor digiti minimi is then separated from the extensor indicis and the abductor pollicis longus, and the interosseous membrane is exposed (Fig. 111–3). The neurovascular bundle is identified at the proximal end of the membrane; the vessels are ligated and the nerve is resected.

SEPARATING THE TWO BONES OF THE FOREARM

The next step is to free the two surfaces of the interosseous membrane and to resect it entirely by dividing its attachments to the radius and ulna. The upper end of the membrane, including Weitbrecht's ligament, should also be completely resected, after which the two bones are pulled apart.

FASHIONING THE DISTAL END OF THE STUMP

Ideally the bones should be resected 1 to 2 cm. proximal to the upper border of the pronator quadratus. A longer stump might give rise to trophic changes. Sectioning may be done more proximally but not proximal to the insertion of the pronator teres, which is one of the muscles responsible for closing the claw.

The tendons are divided just distal to the site of bone sectioning. The radial and ulnar vessels are ligated as distally as possible.

SUTURING

The tendons are divided into two groups and sutured to the extremities of the bone stumps. The two skin flaps are sutured so as to form a commissure and line the inner faces of the pincer. The superolateral corner of the anterior flap is sutured to the inturned superolateral corner of the posterior flap, and the superomedial angles are also sutured to each other. The free proximal borders of the two flaps are then joined to form the commissure.

Thus the two flaps surround the two arms

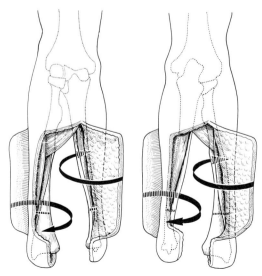

Figure 111–3. Lines of rotation of anterior and posterior flaps.

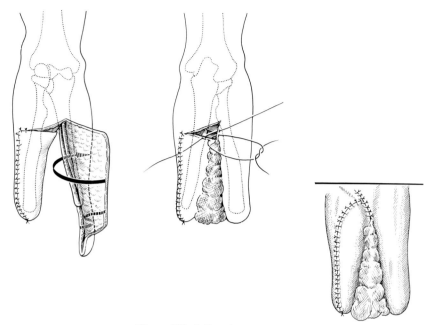

Figure 111–4. Suturing the flaps.

of the pincer—the anterior flap clothing the ulnar arm and the posterior flap, the radial arm. The free borders of each flap are sutured all along their bases. This suturing may be impossible if the flaps are too short, in which case they are approximated by sutures driven through the underlying muscles, bare areas being covered by free skin grafts.

Finally the extremities of the two arms of the pincer are covered by folding over of the flaps from within outwards (Fig. 111–4)

DRESSINGS

The skin grafts are dressed with tulle gras, which is sutured to adjacent flap edges. The two arms of the claw are wrapped in and kept wide apart by swabs and cotton wool. The dressing is changed on the third or fourth day, except over the skin grafts.

RE-EDUCATION

Re-education is started on the third or fourth day and should aim to teach the patient to open and close the pincer. The pincer is opened spontaneously by the supinator and closed by the action of pronator teres. However, these movements of supination and pronation tend to interfere with precision

handling without providing much power to the grip.

The patient must be trained, therefore, when opening the pincer to stabilize the ulna by contracting the triceps and flexing the radius by contracting the biceps. This implies simultaneous contraction of the triceps and biceps (and brachialis), which are normally antagonists; hence, the difficulty of achieving this movement.

Similarly, closure of the pincer is carried out by the simultaneous contraction of the antagonistic pronator teres and supinator.

The aim is to mobilize the radius in the sagittal plane. To achieve this, the physiotherapist immobilizes the ulnar arm of the pincer in 30 degrees of flexion and instructs the patient to move the radius. Control of this movement is learned gradually. Later, re-education is pursued without the ulna being fixed.

Control of the pincer is obtained after several weeks of practice. Mobilization does not occur in a purely sagittal plane, because there persists a tendency to utilize the movements of pronation and supination.

FUNCTIONAL RESULTS AND INDICATIONS

In strongly motivated subjects, the results can be excellent and function is superior to that obtained with a prosthesis, mostly because of sensibility. However, the holding of small objects and toilet of the anal region remain difficult with a Krukenberg pincer, and the functional results may be offset by the unsightly appearance of the limb.

For this reason the operation is not recommended in cases of unilateral mutilation as the patient retains his functional autonomy with one intact hand and will seek a cosmetically acceptable limb rather than enhanced function. If functional assistance is required, a prosthesis usually suffices.

Krukenberg's operation comes into its own in bilateral mutilations. In spite of recent advances in prosthetics, we prefer the pincer: its greatest value is in the blind because of the retention of a sensitive limb and also because the subject feels less repulsion at an unsightly stump, which he cannot see.

Finally, the following combinations can be considered after discussion with the patient: a bilateral Krukenberg operation, a Krukenberg operation on one side and a prosthesis on the other, or a prosthesis adapted to a Krukenberg arm. This provides reasonably good function as well as an acceptable cosmetic appearance in social circumstances, the patient being at liberty to discard his prosthesis in private life.

In any case no decision should be taken without showing the patient a film or, even better, a mutilated cosufferer who has successfully undergone the operation.

REFERENCE

Kallio, K. E.: Recent advance in Krukenberg's operation. Acta Chir. Scand., 97:165–188, 1948.

Chapter 112

PEDICLE TRANSFER OF THE HAND

JACQUES ROULLET

The transfer of the right hand in a right hemiplegic to the left wrist is undoubtedly unique.

We had the opportunity to treat a 47 year old right hemiplegic who had mutilated his left hand with a chain saw (Figs. 112–1, 112–2). Following his stroke but prior to this injury, the man lived relatively independently on a farm. Following the injury he became totally dependent on a care facility. The patient was not in favor of a Krukenberg operation but agreed to accept transfer of the paralyzed right hand to the left stump if it could be done without significant risk.

A free microsurgical transfer would have involved anastomoses high in the left forearm and would have compromised the possibility of a later Krukenberg operation. Moreover, the operation had to be carried out in such a fashion that if the transfer was a functional failure, a Krukenberg operation could still be done. Thus the only technique was a variety of a tubed pedicle transfer (Figs. 112–3 to 112–6). This was done in stages.

In the first operation the muscles of the lower two-thirds of the right forearm were detached from the bone and the hand was pedicled to the left wrist with a tube containing one ulnar artery, veins, and nerves. The wrist was disarticulated at one midcarpal joint, saving as much capsule as possible. The stump on the left was disarticulated at the same level. The extensor tendons were repaired at this stage, as was the superficial branch of the radial nerve.

In an operation one month later with the two arms suspended above his head, the flexor tendons and median nerve were repaired. Six months later the tube was divided and the hand remained viable. Finally several months later the ulnar nerve was repaired and the long flexor of the thumb was transferred to allow opposition.

The result was remarkable (Figs. 112–7 to

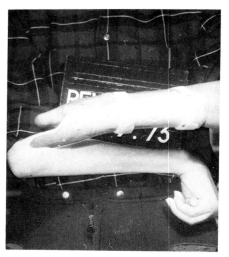

Figure 112–1. Preoperative state with one of the multiple splints tried.

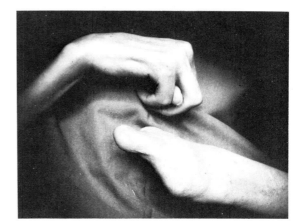

Figure 112–2. Spasticity of the right hand and mutilation of the left.

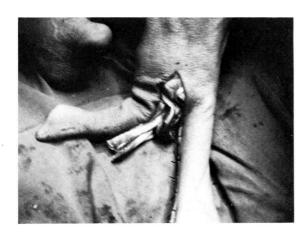

Figure 112–3. Preoperative construction of the tube containing the ulnar pedicle.

Figure 112–4. Preoperative x-ray.

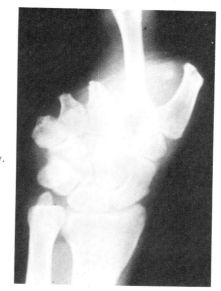

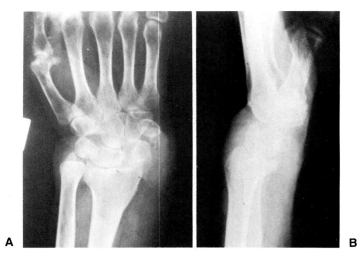

A   **B**

Figure 112–5. *A* and *B*, Postoperative x-rays.

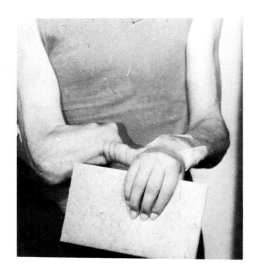

Figure 112–6. Intermediate stage. Observe the effect of the intrinsic spasticity on the metacarpophalangeal joint.

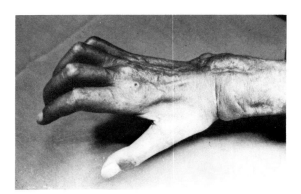

Figure 112–7. Postoperative atrophy of the intrinsic muscles.

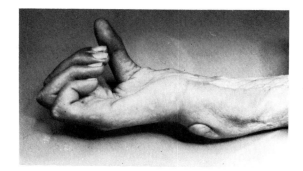

Figure 112–8. Flexion one year postoperatively.

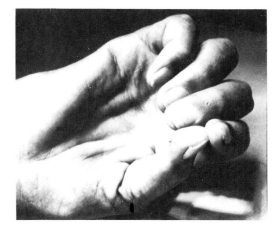

Figure 112–9. Metacarpophalangeal instability of the thumb following a ski injury. Opposition of the thumb following tendon transfer of the flexor pollicis longus.

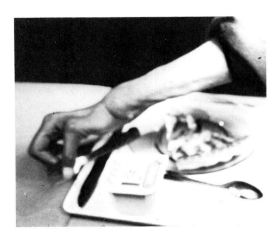

Figure 112–10. Useful grip despite metacarpophalangeal instability.

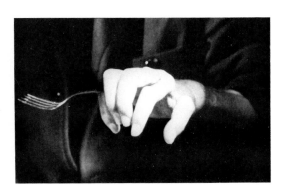

Figure 112–11. Stable platform for holding a fork.

112–11). Prosupination and flexion-extension of the wrist were good. He recovered the ability to open and close the hand in a useful and powerful fashion. The intrinsic muscles remained paralyzed. Progressive recovery of sensation was observed. The improvement of the patient's morale was enormous. The day following the removal of the dressing after the last operation he returned directly to his mountain home. Follow-up after eight years showed him to be leading a life of relative independence.

EDITOR'S NOTE

At our outpatient clinic at the American Hospital in Paris we have seen another case of translocation of the hand performed by Dr. J. W. May of Boston. This case had the added benefit of more recent microvascular techniques. The patient presented following a gun-blast injury with a previous complete right brachial plexus paralysis, a right thumb amputation, and a left transmetacarpal ulnar hemiamputation with sparing of the first ray. In 1983 Dr. May performed a free transfer of the paralyzed right hand to replace the destroyed part of the left hand. The result was excellent, the fingers having active mobility sufficient for a good grasp. The right side had been fitted with a prosthesis, making the patient independent.

Chapter 113

PARTIAL TOE TRANSFERS IN RECONSTRUCTIVE SURGERY OF THE HAND

GUY FOUCHER

AND F. M. BRAUN

The introduction of microsurgery has added a new dimension to reconstructive surgery of the hand, especially when the thumb is involved. It enables one to carry out a nearly ideal reconstruction in the form of replantation; it also increases the safety factor in a number of established procedures such as pollicization. The use of the microscope facilitates endoneurolysis of an interdigital nerve as well as arterial repair after accidental preoperative vascular trauma. Finally, anastomosis of dorsal veins, to prevent postoperative congestion, has become a relatively simple surgical step.

Microsurgery, in addition, has opened the way for new techniques of reconstruction such as toe transfers. Since the first experimental transfer reported by Buncke et al. (1967) and the initial successful transfer carried out in a human patient by Cobbet (1969), a number of procedures inspired by these pioneer transfers have been described: pulp transfer (Buncke, 1967; Cobbett, 1969), skin transfer of the first web (Gilbert, 1976; Morrison, 1980), and vascularized articular transfer (Foucher and Merle, 1976).

Recently other techniques have been introduced for composite transfers in distal digital reconstruction (Foucher et al., 1980). All are based on anatomical features and described elsewhere in this book. However, we wish to stress a few important points regarding the donor site:

It is possible to raise a toe, in part or in toto, through only one dorsal incision even when the plantar plexus or flexor tendon is to be included in the transfer.

The second metatarsal must be resected very proximally when the skeleton of the second toe is to be transferred. This facilitates skin closure on the foot without interfering with weight bearing, as was shown by our podoscopic studies of footprints. Besides, early resection when raising the toe makes it easier to dissect out the plantar artery.

The stage of ischemia at the donor site should be reduced to a minimum by adequate preparation. The nerve is sutured first, immediately after bone fixation and ideally in a bloodless field. Next the artery is anastomosed end to end or end to side, depending on which artery is used. When one of the long fingers is the site of the transfer, the interdigital artery is usually chosen as the receptor. We prefer this technique to that described by O'Brien, who invariably carries out an end to end anastomosis with the radial artery. The caliber of the digital artery is sufficient to allow an adequate flow, and congruence with the donor vessel is usually excellent. To reduce dorsal scarring further, the vein can be sutured and can be tunneled through a small horizontal incision after subcutaneous undermining. We like to allow bleeding through one of the lateral branches while the chosen vein is being clamped and anastomosed. Japanese surgeons often use the proximal part of the digital artery for transfers on one of the long fingers. We avoid this technique for two reasons: it makes use of an artery with a limited flow and provides a relatively poor blood supply to the receptor finger.

In reconstruction of the thumb, we usually carry out an end to side anastomosis with the radial artery, using a T-shaped segment of the intermetatarsal artery whenever possible.

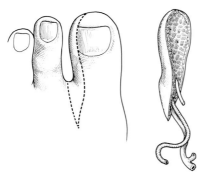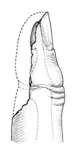

Figure 113–1. Free pulp flap (after technique of Buncke).

PARTIAL TOE TRANSFER IN DISTAL DIGITAL RECONSTRUCTION

Five techniques for this procedure deserve consideration. The choice depends on what is needed to obtain a "custom made" reconstruction.

The tissues that can be transferred are the pulp alone; the nail complex; a composite skin graft with the nail complex; a composite graft including the pulp, bone, and nail complex; or a composite transfer including the pulp, bone, and nail matrix.

THE FREE PULP FLAP

The free pulp flap is indicated in cases of extensive beveled tissue loss from the thumb and index finger when a Littler island flap is not feasible because of associated lesions or is insufficient to cover the defect (Fig. 113–1). It is also useful for restoring sensation to a post-traumatic phalangeal or metacarpal hand covered by insensitive abdominal skin.

As a rule we prefer as donor the big toe, which provides a wider flap with better discrimination than the second toe (10 to 25 mm. versus 7 to 18 mm.; May et al., 1977). Also the diameter of its collateral nerve is more like that of the receptor digit. When the second toe is chosen, the resulting scar is minimal, but the two collateral nerves must be connected in a Y fashion to the receptor to make up for the incongruence.

Depending on the digit to be reconstructed, we advise using the homolateral big toe for the thumb and the contralateral foot for the index finger, because this provides the best discrimination to the pulp.

GILBERT-MORRISON'S COMMISSURAL FLAP

We shall not dwell at length on this flap, which is described elsewhere in this work. It is an excellent choice for a transfer, and we have used it to line retracted webs. However, scarring at the donor site is not insignificant, and we believe that we can obtain a similar result with many other free flaps, such as the groin flap, Chinese flap, posterior interosseous flap, and lateral arm flap. We reserve the flap with its two sensible pulps for grossly mutilated hands requiring reconstruction of the web and sensation in a short pincer.

TRANSFER OF THE NAIL COMPLEX

Transfer of the nail complex is only rarely indicated and our experience is limited to one case, but the technique has not been described previously. Contrary to what has been written in the past (Lendway, Morrison), it is possible to take the nail and its bed, the nail matrix, and its skin lining without any bone. It is also possible to raise only one lateral groove to obtain a nail of perfect size. At the donor site the exposed bone is covered with a plantar cross-toe flap from the second toe. We carried out such a transfer in a 10 year old boy, an excellent pupil and a musician, whose problems were cosmetic and functional. Sensation was abnormal and writing difficult. Both problems were solved by the transfer. More frequently vascularized bone has to be transferred at the same stage to support the nail. This vascularized bone is not prone to late resorption and secondary nail deformity.

THE "WRAP-AROUND" DIGITAL FLAP

This is another rarely indicated procedure that can prove useful however in cases of multidigital skin avulsion when microsurgical reposition is not possible. We used it in a girl who had sustained extensive skin avulsion in the index and middle fingers together with severe bony lesions of the index finger. The latter was amputated proximally, and we covered the middle finger with skin obtained by a filleted graft taken from the second toe. This provided an excellent skin cover with a good ultimate functional and cosmetic result. The proximal interphalangeal joint of the middle finger recovered a 90 degree range of motion.

This technique is not unlike that described by Morrison for reconstruction of the thumb.

COMPOSITE TRANSFER OF PULP, BONE, AND NAIL BED

This original technique allows partial lengthening of a digit in amputations running through the proximal or middle part of the nail, leaving an intact matrix (Fig. 113–2*B*, *C*). The tissue loss in these cases results in the growth of a dystrophic hooked nail, which can be functionally disabling. These can be treated by a delayed primary, or secondary, repair involving a composite transfer from the big toe, which includes the pulp, a fragment of bone adjacent to the distal phalanx, as well as the distal part of the nail bed. The nail bed flap is tilted 90 degrees onto the raw bone surface to allow reconstruction of the distal digital fragment. In cases in which we used this technique the result was functionally and cosmetically satisfactory. The advantages of this composite flap must be weighed against those of the distal compound transfer taken from the second toe (Buncke, 1976a; Fig. 113–2*A*).

COMPOSITE TRANSFER OF PULP, BONE, NAIL BED, AND MATRIX

A combined requirement for pulp, bone, nail bed, and matrix can be dealt with in several ways:

1. Transfer of the distal part of the second toe is sometimes sufficient (Fig. 113–3). It is suitable for distal amputations running across the neck of the middle phalanx or the distal interphalangeal joint, especially when the index finger is involved. The decision is only taken after comparing the second toe with the contralateral healthy digit. The transfer may be justified on cosmetic grounds or on functional grounds in the presence of a painful neuroma.

2. When the thumb is involved, the foregoing transfer is inadequate, and the choice of reconstructive procedure lies between the "twisted two toes" flap and transfer of the big toe. The simplest technique, which is sometimes sufficient, consists of transferring from the big toe the pulp and a piece of nail matrix cut to measure, together with the subjacent bone (Fig. 113–4). If the skin available is insufficient to clothe the bony transfer, a small lateral flap is used.

3. When the thumb is a large one and loss of tissue is more proximal (e.g., running across the head of the proximal phalanx or the interphalangeal joint), a double transfer may be required—a composite transfer from the big toe including the pulp and nail, and another composite flap from the second toe including a laeral flap and skeleton and, if required, the extensor and flexor tendons (Fig. 113–5). The skeleton of the second toe is turned around 180 degrees to be wrapped in the flap from the big toe. At the donor site only one toe is reconstructed by clothing the intact skeleton of the big toe with the skin of the second toe. The result is cosmetically acceptable, and the transfer can be given mobility (through the transplanted joint and tendons). We prefer this technique to

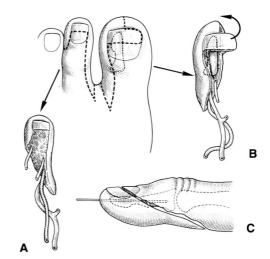

Figure 113–2. Composite transfer. *A*, Technique of Buncke. *B* and *C*, Personal technique.

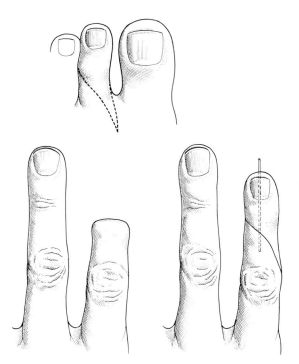

Figure 113–3. Digital elongation by partial distal transfer of the second toe.

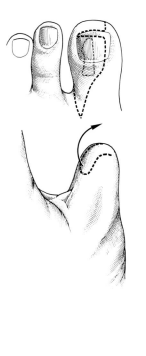
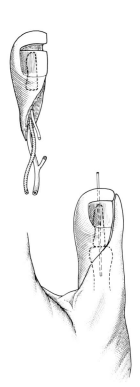

Figure 113–4. Composite transfer (skin, bone, nail) for thumb reconstruction.

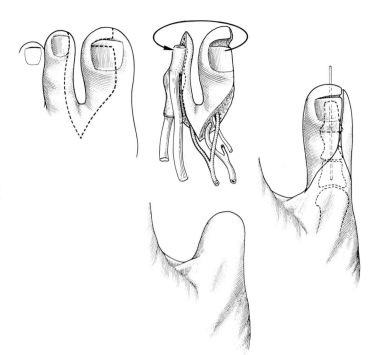

Figure 113–5. Double composite transfer (skin, nail, bone, joint, tendons) with inversion of elongation of thumb "to measure."

Morrison's "wrap around" technique in which an iliac graft is used as skeleton. Owing to a nonvascularized graft there is the risk of resorption as well as sclerosis around the nerves, poor sensation and stiffness. Finally, because of the lack of growth plates Morrison's procedure is of course not applicable in children.

RESULTS

The choice of partial-toe transfer technique among the ones now available depends on the nature, extent, and site of the injury as well as on cosmetic considerations.

In regard to the functional result, sensation is consistently good, even better than that at the donor site and that obtained with whole toe transplants, possibly because the nerve suture is made very distally and under ideal conditions. In addition these flaps are used over highly mobile osteoarticular structures, creating a context that favors sensory re-education. In 38 transplants on the thumb and index finger with a mean following of 39 months and an average of 23 years, the mean moving two point discrimination has been 9 mm. and the clinical (static) two point discrimination has been 11 mm. Also experience

has shown that when the digit is used regularly for fine gripping, the ultimate result can be improved by a specific program of sensory rehabilitation.

MICROSURGICAL JOINT TRANSFER

This type of transfer was first suggested by Buncke in 1976 following his studies in experimental animals. Most research workers had confirmed that in the absence of vascularization, experimentally transplanted joints showed histological evidence of articular cartilage destruction and early disappearance of epiphyseal cartilage. Clinically the results can be satisfactory for a time (Colson, 1984; Erdelyi, 1963). In a few cases (all very young children), some authors reported that the epiphyses remained open (Erdelyi, 1963; Graham, 1948, 1954; Peacock, 1956). However, experimental studies of vascularized transplants confirm that histological changes are minimal and that the epiphyses remain healthy (Buncke et al., 1967; Goldberg et al., 1980, 1983; Hurwitz, 1979; O'Brien, 1977; Slome, 1966).

We had the opportunity to perform the first free transplant of a vascularized joint taken from the second toe (a case we reported in 1976 [Foucher and Herle, 1976]). Since then we have carried out six additional vascularized transfers, two island transfers from a bank finger, one transfer pedicled on an intrinsic muscle (Chase's method), and five nonvascularized free transfers. The procedures are not comparable; the indications are different, and the vascularized transplant offers the advantage of transferring a composite flap capable of replacing, at one operation, bone, joint, tendon, and skin. Besides, if growth is desirable, only a vascularized transfer will do.

Initially the choice lies between the metatarsophalangeal joint and the proximal interphalangeal joint of the second toe (which we used in all our cases). The former has limited flexion but 35 to 45 degrees of hyperextension, and the fact that it needs to be rotated (to change the sector of mobility) means that some of the advantages of the composite transfer are lost, namely, in regard to the skin and tendons. Moreover, the transfer is bulky and unsuitable at the proximal interphalangeal joint.

The interphalangeal joint of the second toe, by contrast offers definite advantages. Flexion in most cases approximates 90 degrees and can usually be improved if the patient wears a specially designed orthosis at night. The skin and tendons can be raised in one piece, and the size of the transplant matches well that of the proximal interphalangeal joint of a finger. However, one frequently observes a 20 to 30 degree extension deficit.

From a technical point of view, it must be stressed that the articular transplant should be centered on a plantar vascular system. This is possible even if the dorsal intermetatarsal artery is used as the vascular source, provided the distal anastomosis described by May et al. (1977) is carefully dissected. Fixation must be stable enough to allow early mobilization. Our best results following the use of centromedullary fixation (with or without cement) appeared to be better than those obtained when Kirschner wires were used.

In such cases it is difficult to be sure whether the transplanted joint has retained its vascularization. In one case the vascularization was well demonstrated on an arteriogram. In the remaining cases, only the skin monitored the vascular patency.

As for function, we must point out that all our patients showed an extension deficit of 20 to 30 degrees, the exact cause of which we have been unable to establish. Possible factors involved are pre-existing claw deformity of the toe, difficulty in adjusting the tension in the extensor tendon, length of the interposed bone segment, bowstringing of the flexor tendon that bridges the transplanted joint anteriorly, or sliding of the lateral extensor tendons of the receptor finger.

The indications for toe transfers must be considered therefore in comparison with a Swanson implant, an arthrodesis, and a nonvascularized transplant. Regardless of the technique used, the results of the first and third of these are usually mediocre. In one of our patients we carried out a vascularized transfer at the proximal interphalangeal joint of the index finger and a nonvascularized transfer on the middle finger. The range of mobility obtained was almost identical in both digits—an extension deficit of 30 degrees and an active flexion range also of 30 degrees, but on the x-ray the vascularized joint had a minimal aspect and the nonvascularized was entirely destroyed. These two techniques therefore are best regarded as complementary, since only the vascularized transfer offers an elegant solution to the problem of extensive loss of dorsal tissue at the proximal interphalangeal joint of a badly mutilated hand in an adolescent. Only by this method can a bone, a joint, a tendon, and an area of skin be transplanted simultaneously and ensure future mobility and growth.

REFERENCES

Blauth, W., and Schneider-Sickert, F.: Congenital Deformities of the Hand. An Atlas of Their Surgical Treatment. New York, Springer Verlag, 1980, pp. 136–153.

Boyes, J. H.: Bunnell's Surgery of the Hand. 4th Ed. Philadelphia, J. B. Lippincott Co., 1964, pp. 318–320.

Buck-Gramcko, D.: Pollicization of the index finger. Method and results in aplasia and hypoplasia of the thumb. J. Bone Joint Surg., 53A:1605–1617, 1971.

Buncke, H. J., Daniller, A. I., Schulz, W. P., and Chase, R. A.: The fate of autogenous whole joints transplanted by microvascular anastomoses. Plast. Reconstr. Surg., 39:333–341, 1967.

Bunnell, S.: Surgery of the Hand. Surgical Repair of Joints. Philadelphia, J. B. Lippincott Co., 1948, pp. 300–304.

Burwell, R. G.: Skeletal allografts for synovial joint reconstruction (editorial). J. Bone Joint Surg., 52B:10–13, 1970.

Campbell, C. J., Ishida, H., Takahoashi, H., and Kelly,

F.: The transplantation of articular cartilage. An experimental study in dogs. J. Bone Joint Surg., 45A:1579–1592, 1963.

Campbell, C. J.: Homotransplantation of a half or whole joint. Clin. Orthop., 87:146–155, 1972.

Carroll, R. E., and Green, D. P.: Reconstruction of hypoplastic digits using toe phalanges (abstract). J. Bone Joint Surg., 57A:727, 1975.

Colson, P., and Hovot, R.: Chirurgie réparatrice du pouce. Greffe articulaire. Lyon Chir., 42:721–724, 1947.

Colson, P.: Osteoarticular Transplants in the Hand, Ed. II. Paris, Masson, 1984, pp. 678–684.

Comtet, J. J., Bertrand, H. G., and Moyen, B.: Free autogenous composite joint graft use in multiple finger injuries. Int. J. Microsurg., 2:121–124, 1980.

Cuthbert, J. B.: The late treatment of dorsal injuries of the hand associated with loss of skin. Br. J. Surg., 33:66–71, 1945.

Daniel, G., Entin, M. A., and Kahn, D. S.: Autogenous transplantation in the dog of a metacarpophalangeal joint with preserved neurovascular bundle. Can. J. Surg., 14:253–259, 1971.

Depalma, A. F., Sawyer, B., and Hoffman, J. D.: Fate of osteochondral grafts. Clin. Orthop., 22:217–220, 1962.

Depalma, A. F., Tsaltas, T. T., and Mauler, G. G.: Viability of osteochondral grafts as determined by uptake of S^{35}. J. Bone Joint Surg., 45A:1565–1578, 1963.

Dingman, R. O.: Follow-up clinic. Plast. Reconstr. Surg., 47:594, 1971.

Dingman, R. O., and Grabb, W. C.: Reconstruction of both mandibular condyles with metatarsal bone grafts. Plast. Reconstr. Surg., 34:441–451, 1964.

Donski, P. K., Carwell, G. R., and Sharzer, L. A.: Growth in revascularized bone grafts in young puppies. Plast. Reconstr. Surg., 64:239–243, 1979.

Donski, P. K., and O'Brien, B. M.: Free microvascular epiphyseal transplantation. An experimental study in dogs. Br. J. Plast. Surg., 33:169–178, 1980.

Ducuing, J.: Contribution expérimentale à l'étude des greffes articulaires totales. Paris, Masson Edit., 1912.

Eades, J. W., and Peacock, E. E.: Autogenous transplantation of an interphalangeal joint and proximal phalangeal epiphysis. Case report and ten year follow-up. J. Bone Joint Surg., 48A:775–778, 1966.

Entin, M. A., Alger, J. R., and Baird, R. M.: Experimental and clinical transplantation of autogenous whole joints. J. Bone Joint Surg., 44A:1518–1536, 1962.

Entin, M. A., Daniel, G., and Kahn, D.: Transplantation of autogenous half-joints. Arch. Surg., 96:359–368, 1968.

Erdelyi, R.: Experimental autotransplantation of small joints. Plast. Reconstr. Surg., 31:129–139, 1963.

Erdelyi, R.: Reconstruction of ankylosed finger joints by means of transplantation of joints from the foot. Plast. Reconstr. Surg., 31:140–150, 1963.

Edwards, E. A.: Anatomy of the small arteries of the foot and toes. Acta Anat., 41:81–96, 1960.

Ferlic, D. C., Clayton, M. L., and Holloway, M.: Complications of silicone implant surgery in the metacarpophalangeal joint. J. Bone Joint Surg., 57A:991–994, 1975.

Field, P. L., and Hueston, J. T.: Articular cartilage loss in long-standing immobilisation of interphalangeal joints. Br. J. Plast. Surg., 23:186–191, 1970.

Flatt, A. E.: Studies in finger joint replacement. A review of the present position. Arch. Surg., 107:437–443, 1973.

Foucher, G., and Merle, M.: Transfert articulaire au niveau d'un doigt en microchirurgie. Groupe d'avancement pour la microchirurgie. In lettre d'information du GAM n°7, 1976.

Foucher, G., Merle, M., Maneaud, M., and Michon, J.: Microsurgical free partial toe transfer in hand reconstruction, a report of 12 cases. Plast. Reconstr. Surg., 65:616–626, 1980.

Foucher, G., Denuit, P., Braun, F. M., Merle, M., and Michon, J.: Le transfert total ou partiel du deuxième orteil dans la reconstruction digitale. A propos de 32 cas. Acta Orthop. Belg., 47:854–866, 1981.

Foucher, G., Van Genechten, F., Merle, M., Denuit, P., Braun, F. M., Debry, R., and Sur, H.: Le transfert à partir d'orteils dans la chirurgie reconstructrice de la main. A propos de 71 cas. Ann. Chir. Main, 3:124–138, 1984.

Foucher, G., Hoang, Ph., Citron, N., Merle, M., and Dury, M.: Joint reconstruction following trauma. Comparison of microsurgical transfer and conventional methods. A report of 61 cases. J. Hand Surg., 1986 (accepted for publication).

Foucher, G., Braun, F. M., Merle, M., and Michon, J.: Le transfert du deuxième orteil dans la chirurgie reconstructrice des doigts longs. Rev. Chir. Orthop., 67:235–240, 1981.

Foucher, G., Van Genechten, F., and Morrison, W. A.: Composite tissue transfer to the hand from the foot. In Jackson, I. T., and Sommerlad B. C. (Eds.): Recent Advances in Plastic Surgery. Edinburgh, Churchill Livingstone, 1985, pp. 65–82.

Foucher, G., Schuind, F., and Hoang, Ph.: Free vascularized joint transfers. Presentation at the first meeting of the American Society for Reconstructive Microsurgery, Las Vegas, 1985.

Freeman, B. S.: Reconstruction of thumb by toe transfer. Plast. Reconstr. Surg., 17:393–398, 1956.

Freeman, B. S.: Growth studies of transplanted epiphysis. Plast. Reconstr. Surg., 23:584–588, 1959.

Freeman, B. S.: Results of epiphyseal transplants by flap and by free graft. A brief survey. Plast. Reconstr. Surg., 36:227–230, 1965 (follow-up, Clinic, 48:72, 1971).

Furnas, D. W.: Growth and development in replanted forelimbs. Plast. Reconstr. Surg., 46:445–453, 1970.

Gibson, T., Davis, W. B., and Curran, R. C.: The long-term survival of cartilage homografts in man. Br. J. Plast. Surg., 11:177–187, 1958.

Gilbert, A.: Composite tissue transfers from the foot: Anatomic basis and surgical technique. In Daniller, A. L., and Strauch B. (Eds.): Symposium on Microsurgery. St. Louis, Mosby, 1976, pp. 230–242.

Gill, A. B.: Transplantation of entire bones with their joint surfaces. Ann. Surg., 61:658–660, 1915.

Goebbel, R.: Ersatz von Fingergelenken durch Zehengelenke, München Med. Wehnschi., 60:1598–1601, 1913.

Goldberg, N. H., and Watson, H. K.: Composite toe (phalanx and epiphysis) transfers in the reconstruction of the aphalangic hand. J. Hand Surg., 7:454–459, 1982.

Goldberg, V. M., Porter, B. B., and Lance, E. M.: Transplantation of the canine knee joint on a vascular pedicle. J. Bone Joint Surg., 62:414–424, 1980.

Goldberg, V. M., and Heiple, K. G.: Experimental

hemi-joint and whole-joint transplantation. Clin. Orthop. *174*:43–53, 1983.

Graham, W. C., and Riordan, D. C.: Reconstruction of a metacarpophalangeal joint with a metatarsal transplant. J. Bone Joint Surg., *30A*:848–853, 1948.

Graham, W. C.: Transplantation of joints to replace diseased or damaged articulations in the hands. Am. J. Surg., *88*:136–141, 1954.

Gregory, C. F.: The current status of bone and joint transplants. Clin. Orthop., *87*:165–166, 1972.

Gross, A. E., McKee, N. H., Pritzker, K. P. H., and Langer, F.: Reconstruction of skeletal defects at the knee. A comprehensive osteochondral transplant program. Clin. Orthop., *174*:96–106, 1983.

Gu, Y. D., Wu, M. M., Zheng, Y. L., Yang, D. Y., and Li, H. R.: Vascular variations and their treatment in toe transplantation. J. Reconstr. Microsurg., *1*:227–232, 1985.

Haas, S. L.: Experimental transplantation of the ephiphysis with observations on the longitudinal growth of bone. J.A.M.A., *65*:1965, 1915.

Haas, S. L.: Free transplantation of bones into the phalanges. Surg. Gynec. Obst., *23*:301, 1916.

Haas, S. L.: Further observations on the transplantation of the epiphyseal cartilage plate. Surg. Gynec. Obst., *53*:958, 1931.

Harris, W. R., Martin, R., and Tile, M.: Transplantation of epiphyseal plates. An experimental study. J. Bone Joint Surg., *47A*:897–914, 1965.

Herndon, C. H., and Chase, S. W.: Experimental studies in the transplantation of whole joints. J. Bone Joint Surg., *34A*:564–578, 1952.

Hoffman, S., Siffert, R. S., and Simon, B. E.: Experimental and clinical experience in epiphyseal transplantation. Plast. Reconstr. Surg., *50*:58–65, 1972.

Huang, S. L., Hou, M. Z., and Yan, C. L.: Reconstruction of the thumb by a free pedal neurovascular flap and composite phalanx-joint-tendon homograft: A preliminary report. J. Reconstr. Microsurg., *1*(4):299–303, 1985.

Hurwitz, P. J.: Experimental transplantation of small joints by microvascular anastomoses. Plast. Reconstr. Surg., *64*:221–231, 1979.

Imamaliev, A. S.: Transplantation of hemijoint in experiment. First report. Ortop. Traum. Protez., *21*:43–46, 1960.

Imamaliev, A. S.: Hemi-articular transplantation in experimental and clinical conditions. Ortop. Traum. Protez, *23*:9–15, 1962.

Impallomeni, G.: Sul trapianto delle articolazini. Arch. Orthop., *28*:342, 1911.

Johansson, S. H., and Engkvist, O.: Small joint reconstruction by perichondrial arthroplasty. Clin. Plast. Surg., *8*:107–114, 1981.

Judet, H.: Essai sur la greffe des tissus articulaires. C. R. Acad. Sci. Paris, *146*:193–196, 600–603, 1908.

Judet, H., and Padovani, J. P.: Transplantation d'articulation complète avec rétablissement circulatoire immédiat par anastomoses artérielle et veineuse. Mem. Acad. Chir., *94*:520–526, 1968.

Judet, H., and Padovani, J. P.: Transplantation d'articulation complète avec rétablissement circulatoire immédiat par anastomoses artérielle et veineuse chez le chien. Rev. Chir. Orthop., *59*:125–128, 1973.

Kettelkamp, D. B., Alexander, H. H., and Dolan, J.: A comparison of experimental arthroplasty and metacarpal head replacement. J. Bone Joint Surg., *50A*:1564–1576, 1968.

Kettelkamp, D. B., and Ramsey, P.: Experimental and clinical autogenous distal metacarpal reconstruction. Clin. Orthop., 74:129–137, 1971.

Kettelkamp, D. B.: Experimental autologous joint transplantation. Clin. Orthop., *87*:138–145, 1972.

Kuo, E. T., Ji, Z. L., Zhao, Y. C., and Zhang, M. L.: Reconstruction of metacarpophalangeal joint by free vascularised autogenous metatarsophalangeal joint transplant. J. Reconstr. Microsurg., *1*:65–74, 1984.

Leung, P. C., and Kok, L. C.: Transplantation of the second toe. A preliminary report of sixteen cases. J. Bone Joint Surg., *62A*:990–996, 1980.

Lexer, E.: Substitution of whole or half-joints from freshly amputated extremities by free plastic operation. Surg. Gynec. Obstet., *6*:601, 1908.

Lexer, E.: Joint transplantations and arthroplasty. Surg. Gynecol. Obstet., *40*:782–809, 1925.

Lloyd, G. J., McTavish, D. R., Soriano, S., Wiley, A. M., and Young, M. H.: Fate of articular cartilage in joint transplantation. Can. J. Surg., *16*:306–320, 1973.

Lopez, A.: Articular grafts. Med. Exper., *47*:501–507, 1962.

Lugnegard, H.: Autologous transplantation of a finger phalanx with articular surface. Report of a case. Acta Chir. Scand., *126*:185–190, 1963.

McKeever, F.: In discussion. Herndon and Chase. J. Bone Joint Surg., *34A*:578–582, 1952.

Mathes, S. J., Buchannan, R., and Weeks, P. M.: Microvascular joint transplantation with epiphyseal growth. J. Hand Surg., *5*:586–589, 1980.

May, J. W., Chait, L. A., Cohen, B. E., and O'Brien, B. M.: Free neurovascular flap from the first web of the foot in hand reconstruction. J. Hand Surg., *2*:387–393, 1977.

May, H.: The regeneration of joint transplants and intracapsular fragments. Ann. Surg., *116*:297–303, 1942.

Menon, J.: Reconstruction of the metacarpophalangeal joint with autogenous metatarsal. J. Hand Surg., *8*:443–446, 1983.

Mooney, V., and Ferguson, A. B.: The influence of immobilization and motion on the formation of fibrocartilage after joint resection in the rabbit. J. Bone Joint Surg., *48A*:6–10, 1966.

Morrison, W. A., O'Brien, B. M., and Macleod, A. M.: Thumb reconstruction with a free neurovascular wraparound flap from the big toe. J. Hand Surg., *5*:575–583, 1980.

Moyen, B.: Paper at the 8th International Meeting of Microsurgery. Panel on toe transfer. May 1982 (unpublished).

O'Brien, B. M.: Microvascular Free Small Joint Transfer. Microvascular Reconstructive Surgery. Edinburgh, Churchill Livingstone, 1977, pp. 248–249.

O'Brien, B. M., Gould, J. S., Morrison, W. A., Russel, R. C., Macleod, A. M., and Pribaz, J. J.: Free vascularized small joint transfer to the hand. J. Hand Surg., *9*(5):634–641, 1984.

Pap, K., and Kronpecher, S.: Arthroplasty of the knee. Experimental and clinical experiences. J. Bone Joint Surg., *43A*:523–530, 1961.

Parrish, F. F.: Treatment of bone tumors by total excision and replacement with massive autogenous and homologous grafts. J. Bone Joint Surg., *48A*:968–972, 1966.

Peacock, E. E.: Reconstructive surgery of hands with injured metacarpophalangeal joints. J. Bone Joint Surg., *38A*:291–302, 1956.

Porter, B. B., and Lance, E. L.: Limb and joint transplantation. A review of research and clinical experience. Clin. Orthop., *104*:249–274, 1974.

Planas, J.: Free transplantation of the finger joints. Rev. Espan. Cir. Plast., *1*:21–26, 1968.

Pritzker, K. P. H., Gross, A. E., Langer, F., Luck, S. C., and Houpt, J. B.: Articular cartilage transplantation. Human Pathol., *8*:635–651, 1977.

Rank, B. K.: Long term results of epiphyseal transplants in congenital deformities of the hand. Plast. Reconstr. Surg., *61*:321–329, 1978.

Reeves, B.: Orthotopic transplantation of vascularised whole knee joints in dogs. Lancet, *1*:500–502, 1969.

Reeves, B.: Studies of vascularized homotransplants of the knee joint. J. Bone Joint Surg., *50B*:226–227, 1968.

Rinaldi, E.: Metacarpal loss treated by metatarsal substitution. Ital. J. Orthop. Trauma, *2*:335–340, 1976.

Ring, P. A.: Transplantation of epiphyseal cartilage; an experimental study. J. Bone Joint Surg., *37B*:642–647, 1955.

Roffe, J. L. Latil, F., Chamant, M., Huguet, J. F., and Bureau, H.: Intérêt chirurgical de l'étude radio-anatomique de la vascularisation artérielle de l'avant-pied. Ann Chir. Main, *1*:84–87, 1982.

Rutishauser, E., and Taillard, W.: L'ischémie articulaire en pathologie humaine et expérimentale. La notion de pannus vasculaire. Rev. Chir. Orthop., *52*:197–223, 1966.

Sarrafian, S. K., and Topouzian, L. K.: Anatomy and physiology of the extensor. Apparatus of the toes. J. Bone Joint Surg., *51A*:669–679, 1969.

Schreiber, A., Walker, N., and Nishikawa, M.: Autologe Gelenkentransplantationen mit mikrochirurgischer gefassplastik. Helv. Chir. Acta, *43*:151–155, 1976.

Schreiber, A., Walker, N., Nishikawa, M., and Yargarsil, M. G.: Transplantation d'articulation avec la technique de microchirurgie vasculaire. Acta Orthop. Belg., *45*:403–411, 1979.

Seligman, G. M., George, E., Yablon, I., Nutik, G., and Cruess, R. L.: Transplantation of whole knee joints in the dog. Clin. Orthop., *87*:332–344, 1972.

Slome, D., and Reeves, B.: Experimental homotransplantation of the knee joint. Lancet, *2*:205–206, 1966.

Smith, P. J., and Jones, B. M.: Free vascularised transfer of a metatarsophalangeal joint to the hand. A technical modification. J. Hand Surg., *10B*:109–112, 1985.

Snowdy, H. A., Omer, G. E., and Sherman, F. C.: Longitudinal growth of a free toe phalanx transplant to a finger. J. Hand Surg., *5*:71–73, 1980.

Straub, G. F.: Anatomical survival, growth and physiological function of an epiphyseal bone transplant. Surg. Gynecol. Obstet., *48*:687–690, 1929.

Swanson, A. B.: Arthroplasty in traumatic arthritis of the joints of the hand. Orthop. Clin. North Am., *1*:285–298, 1970.

Tietze, A.: Ersatz des Resezierten Unteren Radiusendes durch eine Grosszehenphalange. Chir. Kongre. Verhandl., *1*:77–81, 1902.

Tsai, T. M., Ogden, L., Jaeger, S. H., and Okubo, K.: Experimental vascularized total joint autografts. A primate study. J. Hand Surg., *7*:140–146, 1982.

Tsai, T. M., Jupiter, J. B., Kutz, J. E., and Kleinert, H. E.: Vascularized autogenous whole joint transfer in the hand. A clinical study. J. Hand Surg., *7*:335–342, 1982.

Tsai, T. M., Singer, R., Elliott, E., and Klein, H.: Immediate free vascularized joint transfer from second toe to index finger proximal interphalangeal joint. A case report. J. Hand Surg., *10B*:85–89, 1985.

Vercauteren, M. E., and Van Vynckt, C.: A free total toe phalanx transplant to a finger. A case report. J. Hand Surg., *8*:336–339, 1983.

Volkov, M.: Allotransplantation of joints. J. Bone Joint Surg., *52B*:49–53, 1970.

Watanabe, M., Katsumi, M., Yoshizu, T., and Tajima, T.: Experimental study of autogenous toe-joint transplantation; anatomic study of vascular pattern of toe joints as a base of vascularised autogenous joint transplantation. Orthop. Surg. (Tokyo), *29*:1317–1320, 1978.

Watanabe, M., Katsumi, M., Yoshizu, T., and Tajima, T.: Experimental study and clinical application of free toe-joint transplantation with vascular pedicle. Orthop. Surg. (Tokyo), *31*:1411–1416, 1980.

Whitesides, E. S.: Normal growth in a transplanted epiphysis. Case report with a 13 year follow up. J. Bone Joint Surg., *59A*:546–547, 1977.

Wilson, J. N.: Epiphyseal transplantation. A clinical study. J. Bone Joint Surg., *48A*:245–256, 1966.

Wilson, J. N., and Smith, C. F.: Transplantation of whole autogenous joints in the hand. J. Bone Joint Surg., *48A*:1651–1654, 1966.

Worsing, R. A., Engber, W. D., and Lange, T. A.: Reactive synovitis from particulate silastic. J. Bone Joint Surg., *64A*:581–585, 1982.

Wray, R. C., Mathes, S. M., Young, V. L. and Weeks, P. M.: Free vascularized whole joint transplants with ununited epiphyses. Plast. Reconstr. Surg., *67*:519–525, 1981.

Wray, R. C., and Young, V. L.: Drug treatment and flap survival. Plast. Reconstr. Surg., *73*:939–942, 1984.

Yablon, I. G., Brandt, K. D., Delellis, R., and Covall, D.: Destruction of joint homografts. An experimental study. Arthritis Rheum., *20*:1526–1537, 1977.

Yoshizu, T., Watanabe, M., and Tajima, T.: Etude expérimentale et applications cliniques des transferts libres d'articulation d'orteil avec anastomoses vasculaires. *In* Tubiana, R. (Ed.): Chirurgie de la Main. Tome II. Paris, Masson, 1984, pp. 539–551.

Zaleske, D. J., Ehrlich, M. G., Piliero, C., May, J. W., and Mankin, H. J.: Growth plate behavior in whole joint replantation in the rabbit. J. Bone Joint Surg., *64A*:249–258, 1982.

Zaleske, D. J.: Revascularized joint transplants. *In* Friedländer et al. (Eds.): Osteochondreal Allografts. Boston, Little Brown, 1983, pp. 377–385.

Zrubecky, K.: Freie Verpflanzung von zehengelenken. Handchirurgie, *2*:67–71, 1970.

Chapter 114

REVASCULARIZED AND REINNERVATED TRANSFERS IN MUTILATIONS OF THE HAND

CLAUDE LE QUANG

Thanks to microsurgical techniques that enable the surgeon to restore the circulation and nerve supply, it is now possible to transfer a variety of tissue segments across a distance. Such transplants not only survive but recover their functional potential when this depends on sound motor or sensory innervation. Not surprisingly, the hand has benefited most from such complex transfers, because, more than anywhere else, the hand poses the problems of restoring skin cover, sensation, and motor function. It is also significant that the first successful microsurgical transfer in man was effected in reconstructing the thumb using a big toe; this was carried out by Cobbett in 1969.

We shall restrict our discussion here to neurovascular transfers involving only the skin and subcutaneous tissue, or these in combination with other tissues. The first group, simple neurovascular transfers, involve sensitive skin flaps, whereas the second, the composite neurovascular transfers, are used to restore muscle function, in addition to providing a sensitive skin cover (musculocutaneous flaps with motor reinnervation), or to reconstruct part or all of a digital column (toe or finger transfer).

SENSORY NEUROVASCULAR FLAPS

The transfer of a "sensitive" skin flap along with its sensory nerve pedicle provides a skin covering that will recover its sensation within a reasonable time provided the sensory nerve or nerves of the flap are sutured to equivalent nerves at the receptor site, as was shown by Daniel et al., (1975). The juxtaposition of

the vascular and sensory territories of the pedicles in a given flap can be controlled by blocking the relevant nerve or nerves with a local anesthetic. The anesthetized zone should correspond approximately to the area of supply of the vascular pedicle.

Reinnervated free flaps are especially useful in parts of the body that require a good skin cover and subcutaneous padding as well as tactile sensation—the extremities of the limbs (e.g., the pressure points in the foot and prehensile surfaces of the hand). Potential donor sites are numerous and are to be found essentially on the chest (deltopectoral, axillary, external mammary), on the upper limb (forearm flap), and on the foot.

Because the receptor site is on the hand, the flap must have specific characteristics—thinness, a small size, occasionally complex shapes, and good sensory discrimination. By reason of its anatomical similarity, the foot is the donor site of choice, supplying, according to needs, its dorsal skin, its first commissure, and the pulp of the toes.

DORSALIS PEDIS FLAP

The dorsal foot flap, described by MacCraw and Furlow (1975), was the first sensory flap to be used clinically (Daniel et al., 1976). It can include most of the dorsal surface of the foot and carries with it the dorsalis pedis vessels, the dorsal interosseous branches of the first interspace, as well as the dorsal venous arch (Fig. 114–1). (We discuss the technique of raising the flap when we consider the uses of the first interdigital web space.) The bare area at the donor site re-

1250

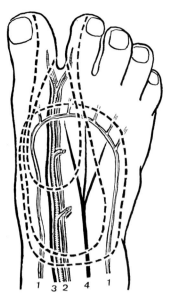

Figure 114–1. Flap from the dorsum of the foot with variants (dotted line). 1 = medial and lateral saphenous veins, 2 = dorsalis pedis artery and vein, 3 = anterior tibial nerve, 4 = musculocutaneous nerve.

quires a full thickness skin graft, which may remain fragile for a long time over the extensor tendon of the big toe. This flap is thin and carries little subcutaneous fatty tissue, but it receives a long vascular pedicle (one artery and two veins) as well as a sensory nerve supply from the musculocutaneous branch of the lateral popliteal nerve. The neurovascular pedicles can be lengthened by upward dissection along the leg. Before raising this flap, however, an angiogram should be obtained to confirm the presence of a good arterial supply to the foot and to avoid the risk of ischemia of the forefoot, especially of the big toe.

The dorsal region of the foot is of particular interest to the hand surgeon because it is a potential provider of several types of composite transfers. As we shall see, the classic dorsopedal flap can be extended toward the first two toes and the intervening web. Along with the skin, any of the following can be transferred: the extensor digitorum brevis, the extensor tendons, the second metatarsal, and the whole of the second toe.

TOE PULP FLAP

The toe pulp flap, as described by Buncke and Rose (1979), includes the lateral hemi-

pulp of the big toe or all the pulp of the second toe (Figs. 114–2, 114–3). This transfer can be taken from any toe, but for anatomical reasons the first two toes are usually preferred. Within the subcutaneous pad is included the neurosensory pulp complex along with its vascular and nervous pedicles.

The technique is simple. The bifurcation of the interosseous plantar pedicle of the first interspace is approached through the floor of the first web. The plantar interosseous artery and its collateral vessel supplying the relevant pulp are identified; the other collateral is ligated. For the second toe the whole of the pulp is taken, including the thick adipose pad, the incision running 2 to 3 mm. from the nail and, in depth, flush with the periosteum of the terminal phalanx and close to the peritenon of the flexor longus tendon. In the big toe, where part of the pressure zone must be left in situ, only the lateral half of the pulp is transferred, the incision again running 2 to 3 mm. from the lateral edge of the nail. Care must be taken, in detaching the deep surface of the pulp, not to divide the fine terminal branches of the collateral nerve. The sensory trunk is dissected up to the root of the toe and farther up, if necessary, within the digital nerve itself. The surface area of sensitive skin can be extended by including in the flap the plantar or lateral surface of the toe, which is then practically "degloved."

The overall result is a pulpar flap of chosen dimensions whose pedicles include for the second toe, the medial collateral plantar ar-

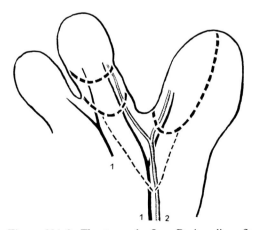

Figure 114–2. The toe pulp flap. Broken line, flap including the pulp of the big toe or second toe. Dotted line, commissural or web flap. 1 = digital nerve, 2 = first plantar interosseous artery.

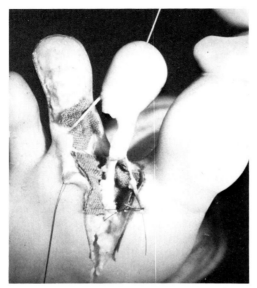

Figure 114–3. Raised pulp flap of the second toe.

tery and the two collateral plantar nerves, and for the big toe, the lateral collateral plantar artery and nerve. If a longer arterial pedicle is required, it is possible to use the dorsalis pedis artery together with its dorsal interosseous branch to the first interspace and the latter's branch to the first or second toe. This pedicle is inconstant, however, and should be demonstrated by a preoperative angiogram, as we shall see in the section on toe transfers. Conversely, because the satellite veins of the plantar arteries are sometimes too few or too small, one may use one or two superficial dorsal veins whose continuity with the pulp is preserved by means of a sheet of subcutaneous tissue isolated on the lateral aspect of the toe.

Depending on its size, the residual defect can be managed by "controlled" cicatrization assisted by approximating sutures or covered with a thin graft which will contract in time with little, if any, effect on function.

DORSOCOMMISSURAL FOOT FLAP

The dorsocommissural foot flap, derived from the dorsalis pedis flap of MacCraw and Furlow (1975), has a morphology that adapts well to the web spaces of the hand. Depending on the area involved, it can be extended upward toward the dorsum of the foot or distally to include the skin overlying the adjacent pulps. The whole area of skin should

lie within the territory of the dorsalis pedis artery and its first dorsal interosseous branch (when present); hence the need for preoperative angiography.*

The surgical technique for raising a dorsalis pedis flap differs little from that used in transfer of the second toe, at least for the stage of exposure of the vessels on the dorsum of the foot (Figs. 107–1, 107–2). The skin incision runs just medial to the internal pillar of the dorsal venous arch. The dorsalis pedis vessels are approached close to the lateral border of the extensor hallucis longus tendon. The vessels are dissected more laterally in depth and separated from the periosteal plane. In dissecting the dorsalis pedis artery and its dorsal interosseous branch (which can lie deep in the first interspace), it is important to preserve the layer of subcutaneous tissue connecting the superficial aspect of the vascular pedicle (or of the overlying interosseous vessel) to the deep layer of the skin because it transmits small nutrient cutaneous vessels. The first tendon of the extensor brevis digitorum is included in the dissection and is divided as it runs obliquely between the vessels and the skin. Two veins must be included in the dorsal flap—a satellite of the dorsalis pedis artery and a superficial vein arising from the dorsal arch, usually from the saphenous vein.

In raising the two hemipulps adjacent to the first web space, the dissection is carried out anteroposteriorly, flush with the phalanges but preserving the periungual fold. The corresponding plantar collateral nerves are dissected as far proximally as possible and the plantar collateral vessels are ligated distal to the bifurcation. With each hemipulp is included the corresponding dorsal collateral artery up to the bifurcation of the first dorsal interosseous vessel from which it arises. Separation of the first commissure should be effected at a deep level to avoid damage to the bifurcating artery. Once the dorsalis pedis artery has been ligated just distal to the origin of the dorsal interosseous and at the posterior extremity of the first space (a potentially difficult maneuver), the whole transfer can be lifted in one piece, including its two main segments. Proximally the small muscular and osteoarticular vessels are ligated, and this now allows exposure of the dorsalis pedis artery and its satellite veins

*The vascular anatomy of the commissural zone of the foot has been studied in detail by Gilbert (1976).

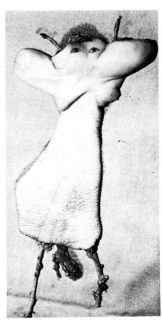

Figure 114–4. Raised Y-shaped dorsopedal flap.

farther up the foot if a longer vascular pedicle is required. The sensory nerves to be raised include the anterior tibial nerve and its medial branch, which accompany the dorsalis pedis vessels, and the terminals of the musculocutaneous branch of the lateral popliteal nerve.

A large Y-shaped flap can now be lifted, which carries the following pedicles: one long wide bore artery (the dorsalis pedis), two large veins (dorsalis pedis and saphenous), and four readily accessible nerves (musculocutaneous for the dorsum, anterior tibial for the dorsal part of the commissure, and two plantar collaterals for the pulps; (Fig. 114–4).

The bare area at the donor site is covered with a large dermoepidermal skin graft. Function is seldom affected, but there remains the risk of ulceration at points of friction.

QUALITY OF SENSATION

The quality of sensation provided by the various neurovascular flaps varies according to their sites of origin. If two point discrimination is compared, in a normal control, between the trunk and lower limbs, the results show a considerable difference. The anterolateral chest and the forearm skin have

poor discrimination (20 to 30 mm.). The figures for the dorsum of the foot (18 to 20 mm.) and the first commissure (15 mm.) show an appreciable improvement; the pulp of the toes is the highest, with a discrimination of 6 to 8 mm., which, though still inferior to digital pulp, can be improved further with practice. There is a wide range of discriminatory potential therefore, and the donor site can be chosen to approach the requirements of the receptor zone.

COMPOSITE NEUROVASCULAR TRANSFERS

We shall now consider composite transplants involving different tissues that can all be autonomized, transferred, and reimplanted as one. The microsurgical transfer of such heterogeneous blocks of tissue requires at least one common vascular pedicle (simple musculocutaneous flap, osteocutaneous flap, osteomuscular transfer) and at most a vascular pedicle associated with a nerve pedicle (neurovascular, musculocutaneous flap, toe transfer). We shall describe transfers of the latter type in the knowledge that in certain privileged sites, multiple associations are possible. We shall detail only the commonest of those (Le Quang, 1980).

NEUROVASCULAR MUSCULOCUTANEOUS TRANSFERS

Neurovascular musculocutaneous transfers include the muscle and its overlying coat of subcutaneous tissue mounted on a single feeder pedicle. Several anatomical types can be fashioned with various patterns of blood and nerve supply.

Two main systems of vascularization have been devised (Fig. 114–5):

One Piece Vascularization. The one piece (monobloc) vascular type includes all forms of "true musculocutaneous flaps" in which the nutrient artery first enters the muscle before sending off numerous perforating feeders to the skin via the fascia and subcutaneous layers. As a rule the venous circuit is modeled on the arterial system. This type of flap is the commonest because it can be reproduced for most superficial muscles that lie subjacent to the skin. The best instance is the latissimus dorsi, but a number of other

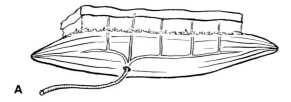

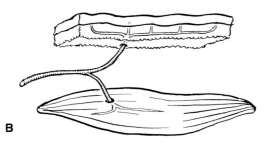

Figure 114–5. Blood supply of musculocutaneous flaps. *A*, Monobloc. *B*, Dissociated.

muscles display similar characteristics in the trunk (pectoralis major, rectus abdominis), in the neck (sternomastoid, trapezius), and in the limbs (gluteus maximus, gracilis, rectus femoris, tensor fasciae latae, gastrocnemius). It is important, in raising a flap of this type, that the continuity between the skin and subjacent muscle be preserved over the widest area possible. The variations between sites is such, however, that the minimal area of contact required is difficult to define. At best one can say that, in practice, the zone of contact does not have to coincide with the point of penetration of the artery into the muscle, and that depending on the number of perforating vessels, the zone can be relatively small compared with the overall extent of the flap.

Dissociated Vascularization. The dissociated vascular type constitutes the second system of irrigation of musculocutaneous flaps. These are, in fact, "muscular and cutaneous" flaps, the association between skin and muscle resulting from anatomical coincidence. Each component carries its own feeding artery, but because the two arteries arise from a common trunk, the flap happens to have a common pedicle. This type of flap is seldom used, and we shall describe only one clinical example in which a dorsopedal

skin flap is raised in conjunction with the extensor digitorum brevis. Here the skin and muscle can be separated without risk provided their common pedicle is safeguarded.

As far as innervation is concerned, there are three main groups of neurovascular musculocutaneous flaps:

Group 1 includes flaps whose nerve supply is limited to the sensory innervation of their cutaneous component. An example of such a sensory musculocutaneous transfer is the axillary flap when twinned with a segment of latissimus dorsi as well as the posterior fibers of the lateral perforating branches of the corresponding intercostal nerves. By reason of its thickness and its poor sensory discrimination, it is seldom used in hand surgery.

Group 2 includes transfers whose innervation depends entirely on the nerve supply to the muscle. They are the commonest. These musculocutaneous flaps with motor reinnervation are represented by most of the one piece (monobloc) vascular flaps mentioned earlier. They constitute a significant advance in microsurgery of the nerves and vessels because in addition to the safe and inert skin cover, they have a dynamic functional potential because of the mobilization of a whole muscle.

Group 3 includes even more ambitious transplants involving a reinnervated muscle under a sensitive skin flap, superficial sensation and muscular contraction being restored by means of two nerve sutures. These are the musculocutaneous flaps with sensorimotor reinnervation.

We shall not describe all the potential donor sites but only those most frequently utilized.

Latissimus Dorsi Flap

The latissimus dorsi flap is derived from the axillary flap described by De Coninck and Boeck (1975) and used clinically by Baudet et al. (1976). It is taken from the lateral chest wall, and its pedicle is centered on the inferior scapular vessels and their thoracodorsal branches (Fig. 114–6). In the majority of cases the muscular branch arising from the thoracodorsal (or sometimes from the inferior scapular) penetrates the deep surface of the latissimus dorsi, close to its anterior border, in the lower axilla, often splitting before penetrating the muscle. This vessel irrigates the muscle itself as well as the overlying skin

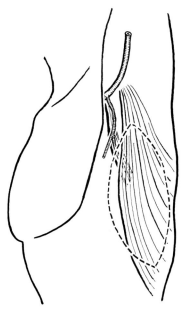

Figure 114–6. Musculocutaneous–latissimus dorsi flap with its vascular pedicle and motor nerve.

via its musculocutaneous branches. The motor nerve to the latissimus dorsi joins the pedicle to which it becomes closely related in its last few centimeters. This is the principal motor nerve; there are in addition deeper accessories that do not need to be included in the transplant. The latissimus dorsi therefore provides a readily accessible pedicle made up of one artery, one vein, and one nerve, all of a fair size and up to 10 cm. in length. In this flap, contact between skin and muscle must be preserved. Virtually the whole of the muscle can be raised along with its skin lining, but in practice the anterior part of the muscle, which bears the pedicle, is sufficient.

The sensory nerves of the skin flap penetrate the muscle close to its anterior border. These are the nerves of the sensory axillary flap; they include the posterior fibers of the lateral perforating branches of the fourth, fifth, sixth, and seventh intercostal nerves, which emerge along the anterior axillary line.

It should be obvious that the latissimus dorsi flap has multiple clinical applications. In local transposition plasties the muscle can be used by itself or included in a musculocutaneous flap pedicled on its nutrient vessels. As a microsurgical musculocutaneous transplant, the latissimus dorsi flap can be used as a simple free flap, as a sensory

neurovascular free flap (for the pressure zones of the foot), as a functional transfer with motor reinnervation, or with combined sensorimotor reinnervation. The donor zone is usually closed by approximation of the edges after extensive pectoral and dorsal undermining; if this is not feasible, a thin skin graft is applied.

Gluteus Maximus Flap

The gluteus maximus flap is derived from the lower gluteal flap, which we have described elsewhere (Le Quang, 1980b). The donor site is particularly suitable because it straddles the gluteal fold. It brings with it a large segment of the inferoposterior part of gluteus maximus, at whose free border the inferior gluteal vessels enter to supply the muscle and overlying skin. Because this is a monobloc type of flap, the muscle must not be separated from its skin cover, which can reach quite a broad area (Fig. 114–7). The vascular pedicle, comprising the inferior gluteal artery and one or two venae comitantes, can be as long as 10 cm. if it is dissected high enough.

The motor nerve of the gluteus maximus at this level arises from the perineal branch of the sciatic nerve, which follows the vascular pedicle, superficial to the sciatic nerve itself, and gives off sensory branches to the skin on either side of the gluteal groove. This musculocutaneous flap can be used either as a local island plasty (for defects in the sacral region), as a simple free flap, or as a reinnervated (motor or sensorimotor) flap. Separating the motor from the sensory contingent within the sciatic nerve, however, can be a daunting task. Despite its size, the defect left by this relatively large flap can be closed by direct suturing, the residual scar being largely concealed by the gluteal fold.

Medial Gastrocnemius Flap

The medial gastrocnemius provides an extremely reliable musculocutaneous flap now extensively used in the repair of homolateral and contralateral skin defects in the lower limb (Feldman et al., 1978). The feeding vessels in the sural artery and its satellite vein (and the motor nerve to the medial head of gastrocnemius)—enter the deep surface of the muscle as they cross its popliteal border 3 to 4 cm. below its condylar insertion. This

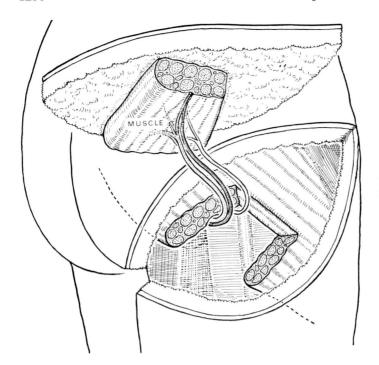

Figure 114–7. Musculocutaneous–gluteus maximus flap with its ischial vascular pedicle.

neurovascular pedicle is stout and short but can be lengthened by dissection within the muscle itself (Fig. 114–8). Raising the muscle and its pedicle is a relatively simple maneuver, but farther down, the terminal tendinous lamina of the gastrocnemius must be split off the fleshy part of the soleus some of whose fibers travel downward toward the origin of the Achilles tendon. The sensory supply to the skin of the flap is as follows: The upper third of the posterior aspect of the leg is innervated by a terminal branch of the sural nerve and the lower two-thirds is supplied by branches from the lateral saphenous nerve, which runs vertically downward between the two heads of gastrocnemius, alongside, and in the same superficial plane as, the lateral saphenous vein.

Here again contact between skin and muscle must be retained over a broad enough area. The donor zone is covered by a thin skin graft, which will result in some degree of scarring on the calf.

Extensor Brevis Flap

The extensor brevis flap differs from the preceding flaps in that it belongs to the dissociated vascular type. It combines the skin from the dorsum of the foot with the extensor digitorum brevis muscle, and the two can be raised separately. The cutaneous component, which corresponds to the MacCraw-Furlow flap mentioned earlier, is supplied by arteriolar branches from the dorsalis pedis and the first dorsal interosseous. The muscle also receives one or two identifiable branches from the dorsalis pedis (Figs. 114–9, 114–25B). The dorsalis pedis artery and its two venae comitantes therefore constitute the common vascular pedicle from which the blood supply to both skin and muscle branches off separately. To this we must add the dorsal venous arch of the foot, which drains the skin flap.

The motor nerve of the extensor brevis (which is often two separate nerves) arises from the anterior tibial nerve as its lateral bifurcation, behind or just below the extensor retinaculum, at roughly the same level as the arteries to the muscles. The motor component can be readily separated from the medial (sensory) bifurcation by careful dissection within the anterior tibial nerve. The sensory innervation of the dorsal skin of the foot is provided by branches of the musculocutaneous nerve.

The extensor brevis flap therefore is equipped with a pedicle consisting of one artery, two or three veins, a motor nerve, and a sensory nerve, all of good size and length. Its reinnervation can be either motor

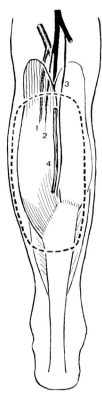

Figure 114–8. Musculocutaneous–medial gastrocnemius flap. 1 = gastrocnemius artery and vein, 2 = motor nerve (branch of the medial popliteal), 3 = sensory nerve (lateral saphenous), 4 = superficial lateral saphenous vein.

alone or motor and sensory. The donor site should be covered with a split skin graft after a few days to allow for some spontaneous burgeoning over the exposed extensor tendons.

TRANSFER OF THE SECOND TOE

Transfer of the second toe to the hand epitomizes the composite type of neurovascular transplant because it involves the displacement of innervated pulp, bone, joints, and tendons. Our preference, regardless of the finger requiring reconstruction, is for the second toe whose loss to the foot is least noticeable (Le Quang, 1978). Yet due recognition must go to Buncke et al. (1966, 1973), Cobbett (1969), and O'Brien et al. (1975), who pioneered the microsurgical transfer of the big toe to the hand, and to Ohmori and Harii (1975), who later had recourse to the second toe to lengthen a mutilated index finger.

We will describe the surgical technique for transfer of the second toe whose vascular pedicle is centered either on the dorsal arterial system (the more common occurrence) or on the plantar system. One must recall that the second toe is normally vascularized by four collateral arteries: two plantar and two dorsal. The bulk of the blood supply comes through the two medial collateral vessels of the first web space. The plantar medial collateral artery arises from the first plantar interosseous artery, which itself comes from the plantar arch (posterior tibial system). This plantar pedicle is fairly reliable, but it is short, tortuous, and deep.

The second pedicle is centered on the dorsal system: The dorsal medial collateral artery arises from the first dorsal interosseous artery, which in turn comes off the dorsalis pedis (anterior tibial system). The dorsal arterial pedicle offers the advantages of being longer, straighter, and more superficial than the plantar artery (at least the dorsalis pedis, since the first interosseous artery lies deeper), but it is less predictable; in 10 to 20 per cent of the cases it cannot be used because the dorsalis pedis or first interosseous artery is absent or inadequate and a plantar pedicle must then be raised.

Careful assessment of the arterial supply of the foot and the hand is imperative. The

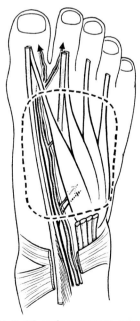

Figure 114–9. Musculocutaneous–extensor digitorum brevis flap.

clinical examination and Doppler test alone cannot provide definite confirmation of the presence of an adequate dorsal arterial axis in adipose patients nor can they reveal whether the first dorsal interosseous artery lies below.

Angiography therefore is an essential part of the preoperative examination. Carried out at least three weeks prior to surgery, it provides valuable information concerning the arterial and venous circulation in the foot. The anteroposterior view (in which excessive flexion of the ankle is avoided so as not to compress the dorsalis pedis artery) will confirm the presence of a "long" dorsalis pedis that is continued by an adequate dorsal interosseous artery and, from the latter, a branch to the second toe. Oblique views will reveal the depth of the dorsal interosseous artery in the first interspace. Finally, the angiogram shows whether the plantar network is sufficient to supply the big toe after interruption of the dorsalis pedis.

Raising of the Second Toe Transplant on the Dorsoarterial Pedicle

Raising of the second toe on the dorsal arterial pedicle (Fig. 114–10) is carried out under control by an inflatable cuff. The dorsalis pedis artery and its venae comitantes are approached directly through a straight dorsal incision, and, when required, the dissection is carried upward to the anterior retinaculum. The dorsalis pedis is ligated just distal to the origin of the first dorsal interosseous artery. The vascular dissection in the floor of the first intermetatarsal space must be performed with the utmost care in view of the risk of damaging, or even ligating by mistake, the origin of the dorsal interosseous artery. As it plunges plantarward, the dorsalis pedis often curls into a loop from the convexity of which it gives off the interosseous branch, which can be mistaken for its terminal anastomosis with the lateral plantar artery. The presence of numerous, and sometimes voluminous, satellite veins further complicates the task of the dissector working in a restricted space. It is essential to dissect out and clearly visualize the arterial trifurcation (formed by the dorsalis pedis, the first dorsal interosseous, and the lateral plantar arteries), which can lie deep between the bases of the first and second metatarsals. The extensor brevis tendon of the big toe is di-

vided on either side of the vascular pedicle: lying as it does between the vessels and the skin, it can interfere with the dissection, especially if a dorsal skin flap is required.

At this time, the osteotomy of the second metatarsal bone and the mobilization of the second toe enable and make the vascular dissection easier in the intermetatarsal space and toward the plantar area.

The dorsal interosseous artery is dissected, in continuity with the dorsalis pedis, down to the first commissure and raised along with a layer of interosseous muscle tissue. Near the base of the second toe, at the terminal bifurcation of the interosseous artery, the larger branch going to the big toe is ligated, but the smaller one destined to the second toe is carefully preserved. An arterial pedicle consisting of the dorsalis pedis and first dorsal interosseous arteries is thus created, which can reach up to 10 cm.

Next two distinct venous networks are dissected—first, a superficial subcutaneous vein arising from the dorsal venous arch, which drains into the medial saphenous vein, and second, the one or two deeper veins that accompany the dorsalis pedis artery.

Along with the second toe, one can raise a long racket shaped dorsal skin flap centered on the dorsalis pedis axis, and preserve the thin strips of tissue connecting the vessels to the subcutaneous layer.

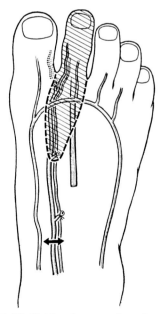

Figure 114–10. Raising the second toe by the dorsal route (diagrammatic representation).

The other structures exposed through the dorsal incision include the extensor tendon, the tendon of extensor brevis coursing to the second toe, and a sensory branch of the musculocutaneous nerve; these all should be divided as high up as possible. The anterior tibial nerve and its medial terminal branch make only a small contribution to the sensory supply of the second toe, but because a thorough dissection might result in damage to the dorsalis pedis vessel, it is usually safer to raise the whole of the neurovascular pedicle.

On the plantar side a small triangular piece of skin is lifted along with the base of the toe—but much smaller than the racket shaped flap on the dorsal side. A zigzag incision is made from the apex of the triangle toward the arch of the foot to expose the first and second interosseous plantar pedicles as well as the flexor tendons. The two plantar collateral nerves of the toe are identified at the interdigital bifurcation, dissected out proximally, and separated from the fibers coursing to the third toe.

The flexor tendons are exposed through the thick plantar fascia and, like the nerves are divided as far proximally as possible, the flexor longus tendon lying behind the muscle body of flexor brevis. The lumbrical and interosseous tendons are divided next, and the toe is detached at the level required; this can take the form of a metatarsophalangeal disarticulation, or an osteotomy of the second metatarsal if the metacarpophalangeal joint of the finger must be replaced.

The next problem is to decide the fate of the plantar arteries. The lateral plantar collateral artery is ligated as it comes off the commissural bifurcation. It seems safer, however, to preserve the continuity of the plantar collateral vessel, the first plantar interosseous artery, and the dorsalis pedis artery until the cuff has been released. The medial plantar collateral artery is only tied after it has been ascertained that the toe is adequately vascularized through the dorsal pedicle alone, the plantar pedicle having been provisionally clamped. If the dorsalis pedis proves inadequate, only the first plantar interosseous artery will be used to feed the transplant.

Raising the Second Toe on the Plantar Arterial Pedicle

This alternative becomes a necessity when the vascular anatomy of the foot is "unfavor-able"—a short dorsalis pedis artery or absence of the first dorsal interosseous artery. The toe is raised on its plantar pedicle formed by the medial plantar collateral and the first plantar interosseous artery, which is divided as high as possible after ligation of the lateral plantar collateral of the big toe. The dissection on the dorsal side poses few problems, but the skin flap must be kept small because there is no dorsalis pedis supply. By contrast, the dissection on the plantar side is much more delicate, for it is carried out through a deep adipose layer and the course of the artery is tortuous. As it crosses the medial intermuscular septum, the plantar interosseous curves medially, close to the sesamoids, under the head of the first metatarsal. It is seldom possible to follow the artery beyond this bend, and thus the whole arterial pedicle is only 3 to 4 cm. long. The plantar interosseous artery is sometimes accompanied by a vein of fair caliber, which can serve as a second drainage channel for the toe since there is no dorsalis pedis satellite vein.

Regardless of the vascular pedicle used, the surgical wound is closed by simple approximation of the first and third toes and reconstruction of the intermetatarsal ligament. Proximal sectioning of the second metatarsal is often superfluous.

Sequelae in the Donor Foot

The sequelae in the donor foot are relatively minor and constitute an additional argument in favor of use of the second rather than the big toe for digital reconstructions. In practice, sacrifice of the second toe in a normal foot entails little cosmetic or functional loss (Fig. 114–11). The patient remains capable of standing, walking, climbing, running, or indulging in most common sporting activities.

DIGITAL TRANSFER

The technique of digital transfer, using another finger, is one with which every hand surgeon should be familiar. In a few, admittedly rare, cases—as we shall see in the next section (Fig. 114–18)—it is possible to transfer a functionally "devalued" finger from one hand to another (Brownstein, 1977).

For obvious reasons, the digit chosen is usually a long, partly mutilated finger, which is stiffened, only slightly mobile, and some-

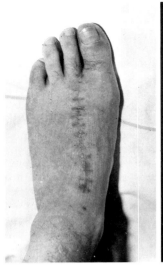 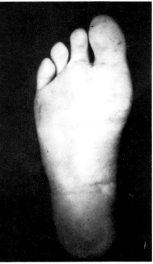

Figure 114–11. Sequelae of transfer of the second toe. *A*, Dorsal view. *B*, Plantar view.

A

B

times shortened, but has good distal sensation and overall trophicity. In other words, to be a candidate for transfer, the finger must have an intact neurovascular pedicle long enough to be sutured to the equivalent structures at the receptor site. As for reimplantations (except that here longer pedicles are available), it is necessary to raise, along with the donor finger, a collateral artery with the digital artery from which it arises, one or two dorsal veins, the two palmar collateral nerves (or at least the nerve supplying the functionally more important half of the pulp), and one or two dorsal sensory branches. The flexor and extensor tendons are divided as high as possible, and the finger is raised together with a racket shaped dorsal skin flap centered on the venous pedicle. The skeleton is divided at the level required to match the receptor hand. The dissection is relatively simple in a normal hand, but difficulties can arise with the arteries in an injured hand.

Preoperative angiography is an important adjunct, for it helps in the choice of a feeder artery to supply the donor finger down to the pulp while insuring that the transfer does not jeopardize the blood supply of the adjacent finger. Late films provide valuable information regarding the venous return.

It is essential that the deficit in the donor hand be reduced to a minimum. The transfer of the "devalued" digit is combined whenever possible with amputation of the corresponding digital ray so as to improve (or at least not reduce) the overall performance of the hand, amputation at the upper third of the second metacarpal for the index finger, or metacarpal resection for the ring and middle fingers combined with transposition of an adjacent finger.

INDICATIONS

The indications for the various forms of neurovascular transfers described are numerous and cover a multiplicity of hand mutilations and their sequelae. We can now consider their clinical applications for partial (pulpar) and total digital reconstructions and for the repair of complex mutilations.

PULP RECONSTRUCTION

Pulp reconstructions in lesions of the digital extremities must aim at restoring the curvature of the pulp as well as its capacity for sensory discrimination. Only another pulp can achieve this goal adequately, by means of a cross finger pulpar island flap with a permanent neurovascular pedicle.

Pulp transfer from a toe is a particularly suitable solution whenever a digital pulp is not available for transfer. In practice this applies to multidigital mutilations in which all surviving pulp tissue must be preserved at all cost. Since the vessels and nerves of the finger mirror those of the toe, the pedicles are anastomosed in the finger or in the hand, and if required a palmar artery or dorsal vein is rerouted from an adjacent digital ray. Here again a preoperative angiogram of the mutilated hand is essential.

It must be remembered that the conventional pulpal flap carries no recognizable vein in its purely palmar pedicle, whereas in a pulp transfer from a toe venous channels must be re-established by anastomosis. Otherwise the penalty will be necrosis.

Finally, at the cost of minimal sequelae in the foot, toe pulp can reconstitute digital pulp to perfection in regard to both the curvature and the sensory discrimination, which can be restored to 4 to 6 mm. Besides the toe pulp is not subject to the same errors of localization as cross finger pulp flaps; in the latter the nerve or nerves of the flap are reconnected to those of the receptor finger. As a rule, for repairs on the thumb, the lateral pulp of the big toe is utilized, whereas for other digital extremities, the pulp of the second toe is preferred (Fig. 114–12).

DIGITAL RECONSTRUCTION

The aim in a digital reconstruction is to reconstitute a digital column of adequate length with good mobility and sensation and as nearly normal an appearance as possible. The reconstruction may involve the thumb or one or more digits.

Reconstructing the Thumb

When the line of amputation runs through, or proximal to, the base of the proximal phalanx, the pollex-finger grip with the remaining digits can be restored only by lengthening the mutilated thumb. If the first carpometacarpal joint is intact, the reconstruction should concentrate on length, sensation, and morphology rather than on distal mobility. Two microsurgical techniques are available, which utilize either a toe or another finger.

Transfer of the Second Toe. Transfer of the second toe is now a well established technique. When the toe is raised on its dorsal arterial pedicle (dorsalis pedis), an end to side anastomosis is carried out with the radial artery as it emerges from the anatomical "snuff box." This is replaced by a side to side anastomosis, however, if the preoperative angiogram leaves any doubt as to the adequacy of the blood supply from the ulnar artery. In the rare cases in which the toe is transferred on its shorter plantar pedicle, the plantar interosseous artery is anastomosed in the palm to the princeps pollicis or to a palmar collateral artery.

If the first dorsal interosseous artery is absent, the plantar and dorsal arterial pedicles can be raised simultaneously; the plantar interosseous artery is then anastomosed (end to side or end to end) to the distal segment of the dorsalis pedis, whose proximal extremity is then connected to the radial artery on the dorsum of the hand. This technique offers the double advantage of circumventing the short pedicle without having recourse to a vein graft while ensuring a good blood supply to the dorsal skin flap (Fig. 114–13).

The next surgical steps pose no particular problems. Bone fixation comes first, using

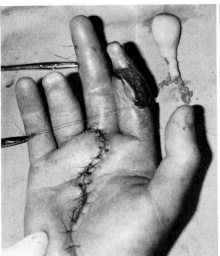 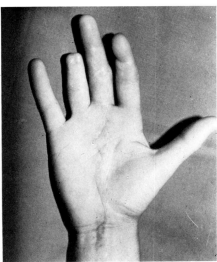

A   **B**

Figure 114–12. Multidigital mutilation. Reconstruction of the pulp of the index finger using the pulp of the second toe. *A*, At operation. *B*, Result six months later.

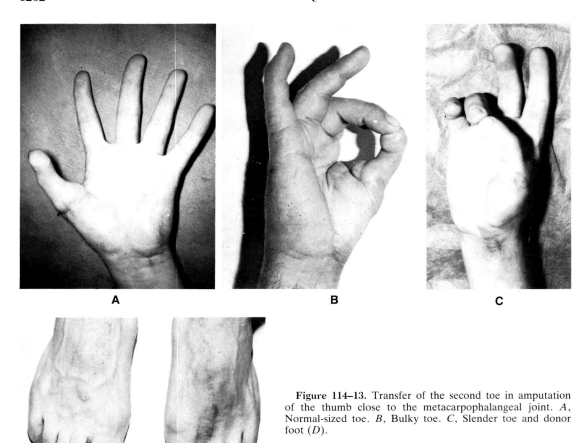

A   B   C

Figure 114–13. Transfer of the second toe in amputation of the thumb close to the metacarpophalangeal joint. *A*, Normal-sized toe. *B*, Bulky toe. *C*, Slender toe and donor foot (*D*).

D

two Kirschner wires planted crosswise so as to keep the pulps opposed. The vascular anastomoses are carried out next, starting with the arteries (vide supra), after which the two veins of the toe are connected to a vena comitans of the radial artery and to a dorsal superficial vein.

The extensor and flexor tendons of the toe are sutured at the wrist whenever possible; that of the extensor brevis is branched onto the lateral thenar muscles.

The distal interphalangeal joint of the toe is maintained in extension for four to six weeks by means of a Kirschner wire to counteract its tendency to drift into flexion. Nerve suturing is done last, and as far as possible from the vascular anastomoses.

The clinical result can be assessed after six months. One can expect a new thumb that integrates fully with the hand both functionally and cosmetically. Two point discrimination can be as good as 8 to 12 mm., and overall trophicity compares favorably with that of the adjacent digits. However, hypersensitivity to cold may persist for several years; hence, this technique is contraindicated in the patient whose occupation involves exposure to low temperatures. The overall mobility of the column of the thumb is adequate (since the carpometacarpal joint and thenar muscles have been preserved), even if the metacarpophalangeal joint has been arthrodesed and phalangeal mobility remains poor.

The chief indication for transfer of the second toe is in cases of amputation of the thumb in the zone between the base of the proximal phalanx and the middle third of the first metacarpal (Fig. 114–13). The presence of a metacarpophalangeal joint of course improves the mobility of the new thumb. In amputations running through the first metacarpal, therefore, the absent metacarpophalangeal joint is replaced by the metatarsophalangeal joint of the second toe, which is raised along with a segment of the metatarsal together with a long racket shaped dorsal skin flap. The metatarsal bone is fixed in flexion to counteract the hyperextension of the first phalanx of the second toe. This is completed with a split skin graft on the exposed anterolateral aspect of the transplanted toe (Fig. 114–14). In the thumb, segmental mobility is perhaps less important than adequate length, good sensation, and sufficient overall mobility to allow opposition. The initial morphology of the second toe is of little significance (Fig. 114–13).

Multidigital amputations involving the thumb and one or more fingers constitute a good indication for toe transfer, the choice lying between the big toe and the second toe (Fig. 114–15). Despite the good results with thumb reconstructions using the big toe, we retain our preference for the second toe, which is much less disabling as far as the foot is concerned.

In isolated amputation of the thumb, however, the advantages of toe transfer must be weighed against those of other lengthening and replacement procedures. The presence of four healthy fingers in the hand constitutes a "reserve" of pollicizable digits and obviates the need for the reconstruction of a mor-

phologically and functionally subnormal entity.

The choice of reconstructive procedure has to take into account general factors (age and occupation) as well as local ones (level of amputation and associated lesions). Thus, in relatively distal amputations (near the metacarpophalangeal joint), the toe transfer is one of several solutions. In more proximal injuries, however (i.e., those involving the thenar muscles or the first carpometacarpal joint), and in cases in which one other digit has been functionally devalued, pollicization must be preferred to a toe transfer. Finally, the toe transfer can be used in association with a conventional method (skin tube secondarily skeletalized and sensitized by a toe and its metatarsal) (Fig. 114–16) or to rescue a partial failure with another technique (Fig. 114–17).

Transfer of a Finger from the Other Hand. Transfer of a finger from the other hand can be envisaged in a few suitable cases. The principle is the same as that of the "promotive pollicization" of an injured finger of the same hand, but here microanastomoses are required. We have seen that the candidate for transfer must not be too severely damaged: it usually takes the form of a stiff or shortened finger that has retained an intact and anastomosable neurovascular pedicle. As with the metacarpal amputation of a mutilated index finger, the sacrifice does not reduce and may even enhance the function of the donor hand. The finger, which has been devalued by shortening and stiffness, can

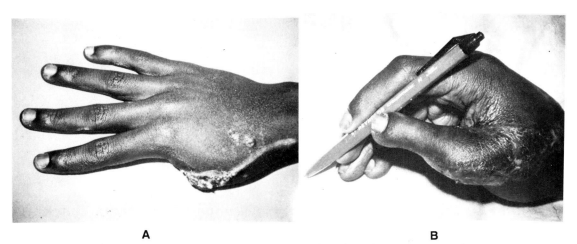

A   **B**

Figure 114–14 Transfer of the second toe in proximal amputation of the thumb. *A*, Amputation at the distal third of the first metacarpal. *B*, Postoperative result.

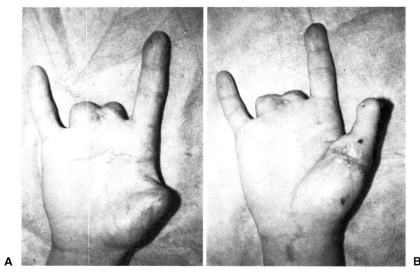

Figure 114–15. *A* and *B*, Transfer of the second toe in multidigital amputation.

supply a new thumb, which, more than length or distal mobility, requires trophicity and good sensory innervation.

Surgical integration of the digit with the hand is carried out along the same lines as for the transfer of the second toe. Depending on the length of the pedicle, the donor artery is anastomosed to the radial artery on the dorsum of the hand or to a palmar artery. If the veins of the mutilated finger have been severely damaged, a vein graft may prove necessary. The functional and cosmetic result should be quite satisfactory provided the injuries to the transferred digit have not been crippling (Fig. 114–18).

Reconstruction of a Finger

The first choice in reconstructing a finger is undoubtedly transfer of the second toe, provided microanastomoses are deemed possible. This operation is even more clearly the choice when the mutilation is more severe. The technique is the same as for the thumb, and depending on whether a dorsal or palmar pedicle is used, anastomosis is effected with the radial artery or with the digital artery or a palmar collateral vessel.

The clinical result, assessed in terms of mobility and precision and power of the restored grip, depends not only on the state of

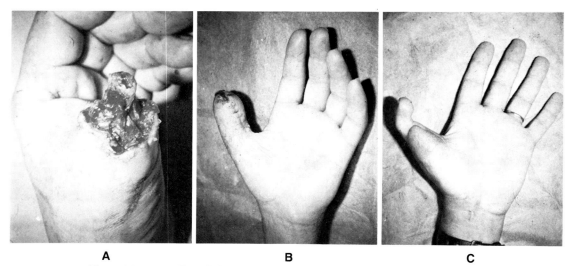

Figure 114–16. *A*, *B*, and *C*, Transfer of the second toe combined with a tube flap.

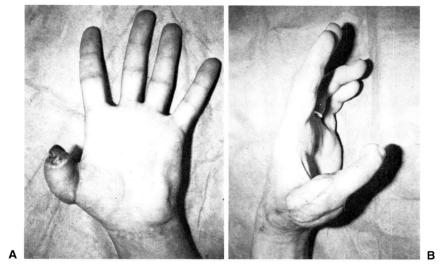

Figure 114–17. *A* and *B*, Transfer of the second toe after failure with Nicolandoni's technique.

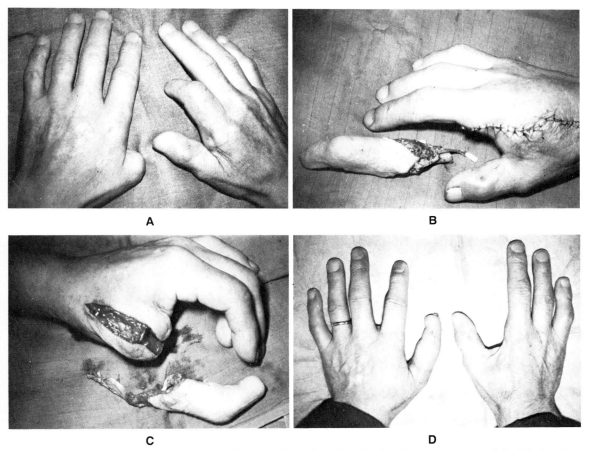

Figure 114–18. Reconstruction of the thumb using a finger from the other hand. *A*, Amputation of the left thumb; stiff shortened index finger. *B*, Raising the index finger. *C*, Transferring the index finger to the contralateral thumb. *D*, Postoperative view of both hands.

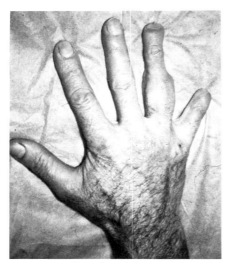

Figure 114–19. Transfer of the second toe in distal amputation (proximal interphalangeal) of a ring finger.

proximal phalanx. However, even when the toe is fixed to a metacarpal stump and the (somewhat reduced) mobility is entirely dependent on the transplanted interphalangeal joints, the reconstructed pincer can be adequate if the toe is accurately oriented toward an opposable thumb.

In distal monodigital or bidigital amputations, surgery is justifiable only on cosmetic grounds. The functional result is often mediocre because the active mobility of the finger is markedly inferior to that of its neighbors (Fig. 114–19).

By contrast, surgical reconstruction has a definite place in proximal multidigital amputations, especially when the thumb has been spared (Figs. 114–20, 114–21). Unlike the traditional techniques of lengthening by transposition of a neighboring stump, transfer of the second toe preserves all the viable structures in an already grossly mutilated hand and restores bidigital or tridigital sensation and motor grip.

In amputations involving the five digits, one must recognize those with an oblique section leaving a partially opposable thumb stump against which a transferred toe can

the thumb remnant but also on the level of sectioning of the digit being reconstructed. The most promising cases are those in which the metacarpophalangeal joint has survived, since the transferred toe will acquire more mobility once it is sited on the base of the

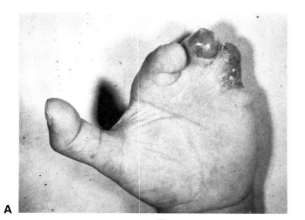

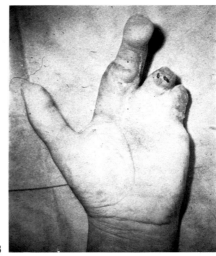

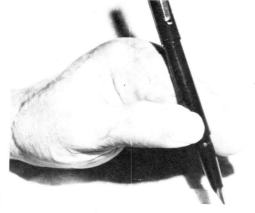

Figure 114–20. *A, B,* and *C,* Transfer of a second toe to a phalangeal hand with sparing of the thumb.

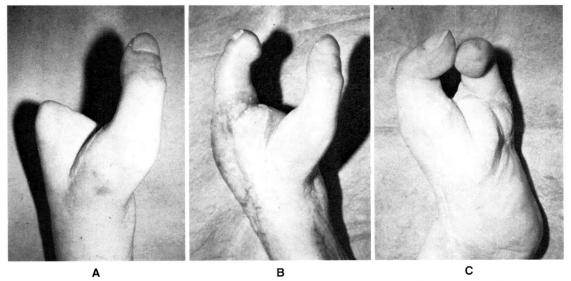

A   **B**   **C**

Figure 114–21. *A, B,* and *C,* Transfer of the second toe to a metacarpal hand with thumb sparing.

achieve a relatively powerful grip even if distal contact is not restored (Fig. 114–22). If the stump of the thumb is too short (e.g., the carpometacarpal hand), one can consider a double transfer of second toes in an attempt to reconstruct some sort of pinch grip. In such multiple proximal amputations, prior positioning of a tube flap atop one of the digital columns to be lengthened can prove extremely useful (Fig. 114–23).

RECONSTRUCTION IN COMPLEX MUTILATIONS

The reconstruction of complex mutilations can be extremely difficult to plan in the presence of multiple severe lesions. With the help of microsurgical flaps, they can be achieved in a minimal number of stages. After major tissue destruction, angiography is the best guide to the choice of receptor vessels. The great variety of flaps now available from the foot means that, using microsurgical techniques, we can now solve many of the problems posed by severe mutilations, which until recently were as good as untreatable.

Repairs Involving Sensory Flaps

Repairs involving the provision of sensory flaps are indicated particularly after injuries

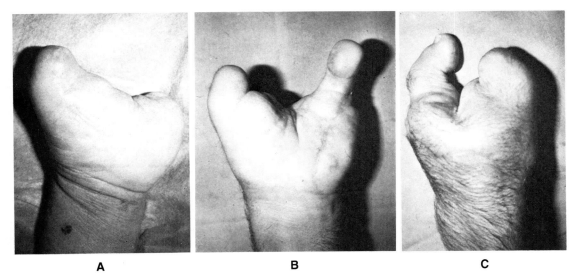

A   **B**   **C**

Figure 114–22. *A, B,* and *C,* Transfer of the second toe to a metacarpal hand with thumb stump only.

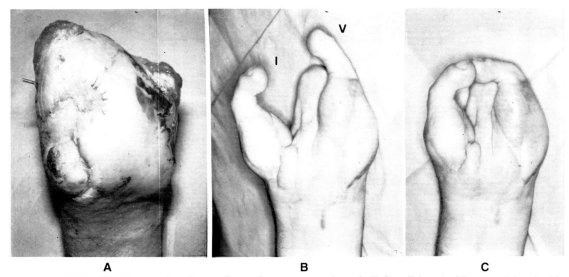

Figure 114–23. Double transfer of second toes for an amputation of all five digits. *A*, Metacarpal hand with proximal amputation of the first ray at the level of the carpal-metacarpal joint. *B* and *C*, Results after toe transfers on the first and fifth rays (the thumb has been lengthened by a groin tube flap and has mobility as a result of a musculoplasty of the abductor digiti minimi).

that cause extensive tissue loss in the zones of prehension of the hand, i.e., the palm, the webs, and the fingers. In these areas the new skin covering should be well padded but not too bulky, with the finest possible sensory discrimination, especially at and near the finger tips. The sensitivity of the innervated transplant reappears progressively between the third and sixth postoperative months, but it can be improved further over the following six months with sensory re-education. The final sensory result can be fully assessed only after one year. Tactile sensation is the first to return—appreciation of touch followed by two point discrimination. Pain and heat perception return later still.

When transplanted to the hand, the skin flap from the dorsum of the foot seldom develops more than protective sensation (i.e., two point discrimination greater than 15 mm.). By contrast, commissural and pulp skin recover real discrimination (i.e., less than 15 mm.). It is interesting that transferred toe pulp reinnervated by a digital nerve shows a tactile sensitivity superior to that in a control (nontransferred) toe with a two point discrimination of 4 to 6 mm. as compared with 6 to 8 mm. We have already considered the problem of reconstructive repair of pulp alone.

For the palm of the hand, the thin dorsopedal flap usually brings adequate sensation (Fig. 114–24). This flap can be readily extended by including skin from the first web if an interdigital commissure requires a cover. The sensory nerves chosen for suturing in the hand should be such that no important hand zone is made anesthetic. As a rule, one should be able to pick a branch whose territory coincides approximately with the defect; this offers the additional advantage of avoiding errors of localization at the cortical level.

For more extensive lesions involving most of the hand, one uses the dorsopedal flap prolonged by the first web and including one or both adjacent hemipulps. This complexly shaped sensory flap is particularly useful for one stage overall repairs after avulsion injuries with crushing or deep widespread burns resulting in multidigital amputations with extensive destruction of soft tissue.

Emergency rescue treatment (excision and partial skin grafting) usually produces a fixed retracted phalangeal hand with dystrophic anesthetic stumps. The particular Y shape of the dorsocommissural foot flap matches the tissue loss resulting from surgical relief of the contracture at the palm and commissures and provides a safe sensory cover for the digital stumps (Fig. 114–25).

In some cases it may be convenient to include in the transfer not only one hemipulp from the big toe but also the whole of the second toe whose skin can serve to clothe one phalangeal stump. The vessels of the transfer are usually anastomosed end to side to the radial artery and to its venae comitantes at the wrist; the sensory nerves are connected to their equivalents in the hand as distally as possible. This type of neurovascular transfer restores to the hand a wide range of sensitivity—gross from the dorsum of the foot and more discriminating from the toe pulp.

Musculocutaneous Repairs

Musculocutaneous repairs aiming at restoring motor function must be considered after severe mutilations in the upper limb combining skin lesions with damage to both the intrinsic and extrinsic musculature of the hand.

The treatment of these complex injuries must be preceded by exhaustive and accurate assessment of the lesions in the affected segment. The ranges of active and passive mobility must be carefully determined. A complete clinical radiological and electrophysiological examination is used to quantify the osteoarticular and neuromuscular damage. Trophicity and circulation are best evaluated by angiography. Only when a comprehensive assessment has been completed can one decide whether a microsurgical transfer is justified, whether a long or short muscle should be used as donor, and which receptor neurovascular pedicles are likely to yield the best result.

The immediate success of the transfer is judged on the basis of survival of the skin flap. Secondary or functional success is evaluated by the return of muscle contractions as confirmed by palpation and electromyography. The ultimate criteria of success, however, are active mobility of the fingers, gripping power, and overall manual function. However, despite prolonged re-education, restored motility can be thwarted by joint stiffness; the overall muscle power in the transfer depends on that of surviving synergists and antagonists.

Repair of the intrinsic muscles of the hand seldom enters the context of microsurgical transplants. Nevertheless some crush injuries can result in complex lesions of the hand and wrist with secondary necrosis of skin, tendons, intrinsic muscles, and neurovascular tracts. A one stage repair is then out of the question, but the number of operations can be reduced if one uses a musculocutaneous transfer with motor and sensory reinnervation.

If repair of the flexor tendons and of the sensory part of the median nerve is postponed until a second stage, the first surgical stage can be devoted to providing a skin covering for the palm and restoring intrinsic motor power by means of the combined transfer of a dorsopedal skin flap and the extensor digitorum brevis muscle, the latter being used to replace the interosseous muscles. The main artery of the flap is anastomosed end to side

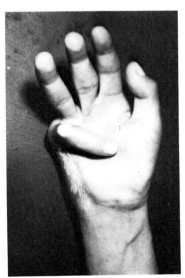 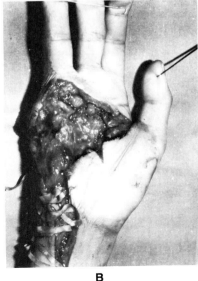 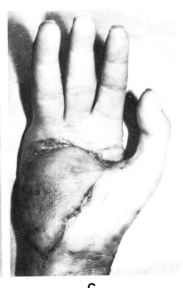

A   **B**   **C**

Figure 114–24. *A, B,* and *C,* Repair of a burnt palm using a sensory dorsopedal flap.

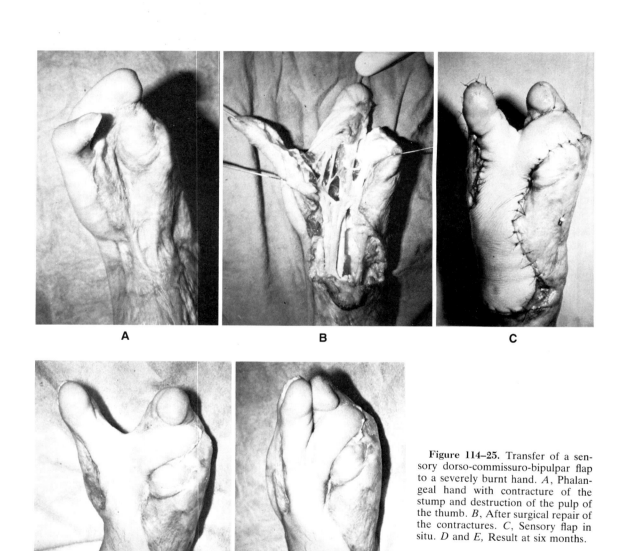

A   B   C

D   E

Figure 114–25. Transfer of a sensory dorso-commissuro-bipulpar flap to a severely burnt hand. *A*, Phalangeal hand with contracture of the stump and destruction of the pulp of the thumb. *B*, After surgical repair of the contractures. *C*, Sensory flap in situ. *D* and *E*, Result at six months.

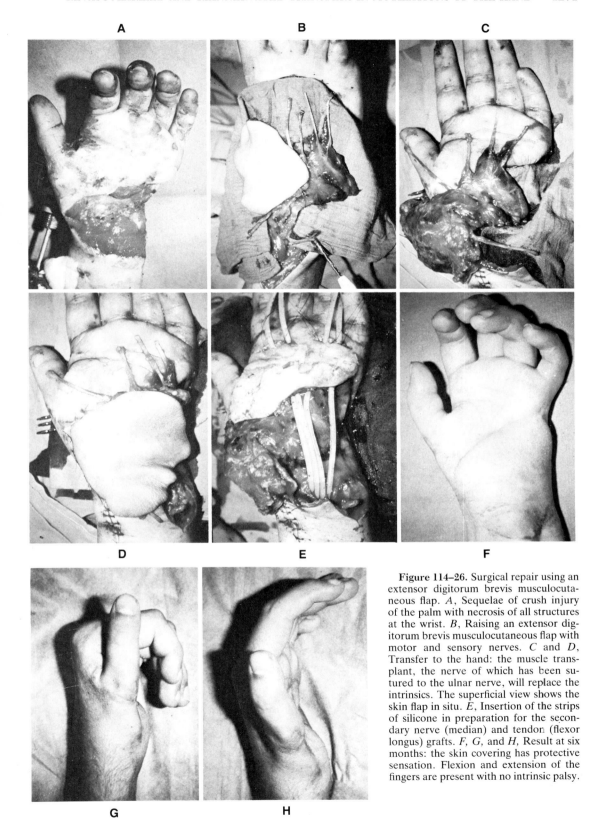

Figure 114–26. Surgical repair using an extensor digitorum brevis musculocutaneous flap. *A*, Sequelae of crush injury of the palm with necrosis of all structures at the wrist. *B*, Raising an extensor digitorum brevis musculocutaneous flap with motor and sensory nerves. *C* and *D*, Transfer to the hand: the muscle transplant, the nerve of which has been sutured to the ulnar nerve, will replace the intrinsics. The superficial view shows the skin flap in situ. *E*, Insertion of the strips of silicone in preparation for the secondary nerve (median) and tendon (flexor longus) grafts. *F*, *G*, and *H*, Result at six months: the skin covering has protective sensation. Flexion and extension of the fingers are present with no intrinsic palsy.

with the radial or ulnar artery; the dorsalis pedis vein is anastomosed to a vena comitans and the superficial dorsal vein of the foot to a superficial vein at the wrist. The sensory nerve of the transplant is sutured to the sensory component of the ulnar nerve and the motor nerve of extensor brevis to its motor component. Finally the tendons of extensor brevis are "lassooed" around the metacarpophalangeal pulley of the fingers (as described by Zancolli [1978]), and silicone bands are laid down under the transfer to facilitate grafting of the flexor tendon and median nerve, which is carried out about three months later at a separate session. Ideally one should achieve a sensitive palm with active flexion of the fingers and intrinsic muscle activity (Fig. 114–26).

Reconstruction of the extrinsic musculature is considered primarily in the management of the sequelae of a severe Volkmann contracture with quasitotal loss of the muscles of the anterior compartment of the forearm (Ikuta, 1976). A muscle transplant in this situation must satisfy a number of criteria— a long powerful muscle made up of parallel fibers with adequate contractility (i.e., an excursion of 4 to 7 cm.); a single, wide bore arteriovenous pedicle; a single, axon rich motor nerve with no admixture of sensory fibers; and the absence of major functional loss at the donor site. The candidates for transfer are many; they include the pectoralis major, latissimus dorsi, gracilis, and gastrocnemius.

The latissimus dorsi flap is perhaps the least disfiguring. The artery of the flap is anastomosed with either of the two main arteries of the forearm, but in the most severe cases only one of the two may have survived. The donor artery is anastomosed end to side with the intact forearm artery or end to end with the stump of the divided arterial tract if it is likely to provide a sufficient output.

Re-establishing the venous return is less of a problem. If no deep vena comitans is available at the site, a healthy superficial one usually can be found near the elbow crease.

The nerve of the revascularized muscle is sutured to a healthy motor branch of the median nerve of equivalent size, usually the interosseous nerve. The belly of the donor muscle is anchored in the upper third of the forearm, and its tendinous extremity is sutured separately to the deep flexor tendons and to the tendon of the flexor pollicis longus.

The latissimus dorsi must therefore be transplanted complete with its own terminal tendon. The difficulty here lies in adjustment of the tension: laxity will produce insufficient flexor power while overtautness may lead to ischemia of the muscle. The simultaneous transfer of the skin flap will also reduce the risk of ischemic necrosis of the muscle after skin closure (Fig. 114–27).

COMPLICATIONS

Every surgeon contemplating a microsurgical neurovascular transfer must keep in mind the potential vascular and neural complications.

VASCULAR COMPLICATIONS

Vascular complications represent the chief risk in this type of transplant surgery, since ischemic necrosis, if it sets in, will involve all the tissue structures supplied by the single pedicle. Meticulous handling of the transplant, careful preparation of the receptor site and anastomoses, preventive measures against vasoconstriction and platelet clumping, and judicious selection of cases are all essential, but do not constitute a definite guarantee against intravascular thrombosis, which must therefore be detected early.

Venous thrombosis usually occurs within the first 24 hours and sometimes even by the end of the operation, but its clinical manifestations may be delayed by three to six hours, depending on the expansibility of the venous bed of the transplant. Careful watch must be kept therefore for the first minor signs of venous stasis, such as exaggerated bleeding at a skin edge or an injection site (especially if the blood is darker), acceleration of the capillary pulse, early congestion in the distal segment of the flap, or superficial cooling with unusual reddening of the skin. Intervention at this early stage makes it possible to verify the competence of the venous anastomosis and if necessary to switch to another receptor vein, since inadequate flow downstream from the anastomosis is a commonly overlooked cause of stasis. Such intervention may rescue the whole transplant if the obstacle to flow occurs before a thrombus reaches the arterial network (Fig. 114–28).

Arterial thrombosis is more readily diag-

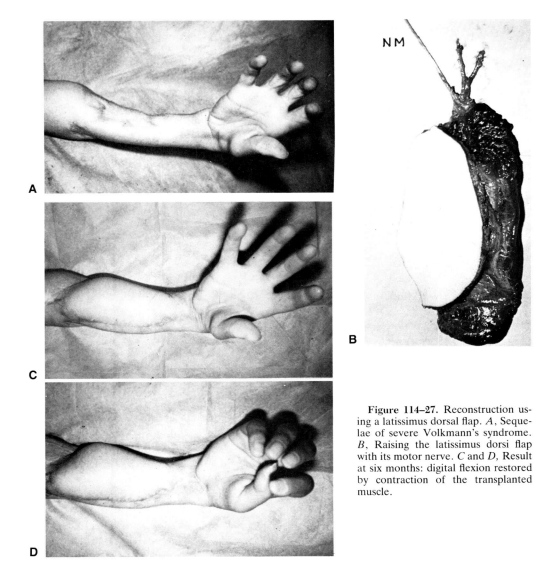

Figure 114–27. Reconstruction using a latissimus dorsal flap. *A*, Sequelae of severe Volkmann's syndrome. *B*, Raising the latissimus dorsi flap with its motor nerve. *C* and *D*, Result at six months: digital flexion restored by contraction of the transplanted muscle.

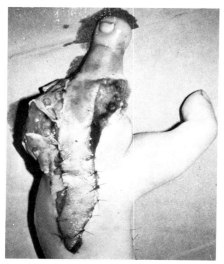

Figure 114–28. Venous thrombosis of a transferred second toe. Reoperation at 24 hours ensured survival of the whole transplant.

nosed, since it results in the immediate interruption of the blood flow. The first telltale signs are the absence of bright red bleeding from skin edges and injection sites after venous blood has been gently squeezed out of the transplant. Arterial thrombosis can occur at the end of the operation at the site of a faulty anastomosis or later, within the first three days, as a result of compression of the vascular pedicle. Such compression is often

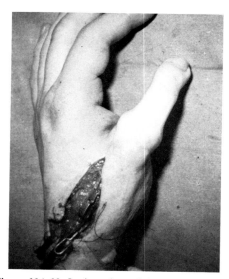

Figure 114–29. Lesion of arterial pedicles at tenolysis four months after second toe transfer. Ischemic discoloration persisted after release of the pneumatic cuff. The artery was repaired using a vein graft, with survival of the whole transplant.

the result of a hematoma (made worse by poor drainage), tight skin closure, or the systemic administration of anticoagulant medication.

Resuturing of the arterial anastomosis, even at an early stage, brings no guarantee that normal flow will be restored or that the transplant will survive: surgical manipulations to clear the thrombotic obstruction starts off the vicious circle of recurrent vascular spasm and widespread thrombosis.

There is in addition the risk of a secondary arterial lesion attendant upon reoperation close to a vascular anastomosis. Late accidental interruption (after the first month) of the feeding vessels will not give rise to acute ischemic necrosis but may well trigger off a state of chronic vascular insufficiency, especially in the case of composite transplants (e.g., second toe transfers); hence, the need for surgical review of the arterial supply, even at a relatively late stage (Fig. 114–29).

COMPLICATIONS INVOLVING THE NERVE SUPPLY

Complications involving the nerve supply do not threaten the immediate survival of the transplant but can jeopardize future function. Despite the unpredictability of peripheral nerve surgery, usually in the more favorable cases one can hope for functionally adequate sensory and motor reinnervation. The risk of denervation can be reduced by meticulous microsuturing, by the choice of a suitable receptor nerve, and by promoting trophicity through a good blood supply. We have never observed painful neuromas in our reinnervated transplants; by contrast, we have seen hyperalgia recede after reinnervation through a digital nerve from which a neuroma was resected.

Finally we must stress the frequent sensitivity to cold, which is commonest after toe transplants and may last for several years.

REFERENCES

Baudet, J., Guimberteau, J. C., and Nascimento, E.: Successful clinical transfer of two free thoraco-dorsal axillary flaps. Plast. Reconstr. Surg., *58:*680, 1976.
Brownstein, M.: Thumb reconstruction by free transplantation of a damaged index ray from the other hand. Case report. Plast. Reconstr. Surg., *60:*280, 1977.

Buncke, H., Buncke, C., and Schulz, W.: Immediate Nicoladoni procedure in the rhesus monkey or hallux-to-hand transplantation utilizing microminiature vascular anastomosis. Br. J. Plast. Surg., *19:*332, 1966.

Buncke, H., MacLean, D., Geroge, P., Creech, B., Chater, N., and Commons, G.: Thumb replacement: great toe transplantation by microvascular anastomosis. Br. J. Plast. Surg., *26:*194, 1973.

Buncke, H., and Rose, E.: Free toe-to-fingertip neurovascular flap. Plast. Reconstr. Surg., *63:*607, 1979.

Cobbet, J.: Free digital transfer: report of a case of transfer of a great toe to replace an amputated thumb. J. Bone Joint Surg., *51B:*677, 1969.

Daniel, R., Terzis, J., and Midgley, R.: Restoration of sensation to an anesthetic hand by a free neurovascular flap from the foot. Plast. Reconstr. Surg., *57:*275, 1976.

Daniel, R., Terzis, J., and Schwarz, G.: Neurovascular free flap. A preliminary report. Plast. Reconstr. Surg., *56:*13, 1975.

DeConinck, A., Boeck, W., Vanderlinden, E., and Claessen, G.: Autotransplants avec microsutures vasculaires, anatomie des zones donneuses. Ann. Chir. Plast., *20:*163, 1975.

Feldman, J., Cohen, B., and May, J.: The medial gastrocnemius myocutaneous flap. Plast. Reconstr. Surg., *61:*531, 1978.

Gilbert, A.: Composite tissue transfer from the foot: anatomical basis and surgical technique. *In* Daniller, A., and Strauch, B. (Editors): Symposium on Microsurgery. St. Louis, The C. V. Mosby Company, 1976, p. 230.

Ikuta, Y., Kubo, T., and Tsuge, K.: Free muscle transplantation by microsurgical technique to treat severe Volkmann's contracture. Plast. Reconstr. Surg., *58:*407, 1976.

LeQuang, C.: Transfert d'orteil. Rev. Chir. Orthop., *64:*299, 1978.

LeQuang, C.: Développements récents des techniques microchirurgicales en chirurgie réparatrice. Ann. Chir. Plast., *25:*171, 1980.

LeQuang, C.: Two new free flaps developed from aesthetic surgery. II. The inferior gluteal flap. Aesth. Plast. Surg., *4:*159, 1980b.

MacCraw, J., and Furlow, L.: The dorsalis pedis arterialized flap. A clinical study. Plast. Reconstr. Surg., *55:*177, 1975.

O'Brien, B., MacLeod, A., Sykes, P., and Donahoe, S.: Hallux-to-hand transfer. Hand, *7:*128, 1975.

Ohmori, K., and Harii, K.: Transplantation of a toe to an amputated finger. Hand, *7:*134, 1975.

Zancolli, E. A.: Structural and Dynamic Bases of Hand Surgery. 2nd Ed. Philadelphia, J. B. Lippincott Co., 1978, p. 168.

INDEX

Page numbers in italics indicate a figure; page numbers followed by the letter t indicate a table.

42099